Essentials of
Medical Surgical Nursing

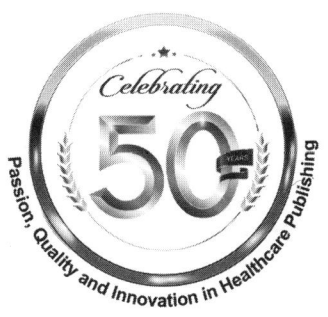

Essentials of Medical Surgical Nursing

Second Edition

BT Basavanthappa MSc (N) PhD
Professor and Principal (Retired)
Government College of Nursing, Bengaluru, Karnataka, India
PhD Guide for Research Work
Member
Faculty of Nursing, RGUHS, Karnataka, India
Academic Council, RGUHS, Karnataka, India
Examiner
UG and PG Courses on Nursing, Various Universities
Ex-Programme Incharge
IGNOU, BSc Nursing Course, Karnataka and Goa, India
Life Member
Nursing Research Society of India, New Delhi, India
Trained Nurses Association of India, New Delhi, India
President
RGUHS, Nursing Teachers Association, Karnataka, India
Winner
Bharat Excellence Award and Gold Medal
Vikas Ratan Gold Award
UWA Lifetime Achievement Award
Shree Veeranjaneya "Shrujanashri" Award
Indira Gandhi Gold Medal
Best Teacher Award (RGUHS)

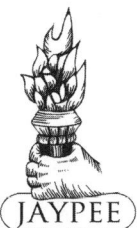

JAYPEE BROTHERS MEDICAL PUBLISHERS
The Health Sciences Publisher
New Delhi | London

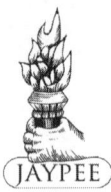 **Jaypee Brothers Medical Publishers (P) Ltd**

Headquarters
Jaypee Brothers Medical Publishers (P) Ltd
EMCA House, 23/23-B
Ansari Road, Daryaganj
New Delhi 110 002, India
Landline: +91-11-23272143, +91-11-23272703
+91-11-23282021, +91-11-23245672
Email: jaypee@jaypeebrothers.com

Corporate Office
Jaypee Brothers Medical Publishers (P) Ltd
4838/24, Ansari Road, Daryaganj
New Delhi 110 002, India
Phone: +91-11-43574357
Fax: +91-11-43574314
Email: jaypee@jaypeebrothers.com

Overseas Office
J.P. Medical Ltd
83 Victoria Street, London
SW1H 0HW (UK)
Phone: +44 20 3170 8910
Fax: +44 (0)20 3008 6180
Email: info@jpmedpub.com

Website: www.jaypeebrothers.com
Website: www.jaypeedigital.com

© 2021, Jaypee Brothers Medical Publishers

The views and opinions expressed in this book are solely those of the original contributor(s)/author(s) and do not necessarily represent those of editor(s) of the book.

All rights reserved. No part of this publication may be reproduced, stored or transmitted in any form or by any means, electronic, mechanical, photocopying, recording or otherwise, without the prior permission in writing of the publishers.

All brand names and product names used in this book are trade names, service marks, trademarks or registered trademarks of their respective owners. The publisher is not associated with any product or vendor mentioned in this book.

Medical knowledge and practice change constantly. This book is designed to provide accurate, authoritative information about the subject matter in question. However, readers are advised to check the most current information available on procedures included and check information from the manufacturer of each product to be administered, to verify the recommended dose, formula, method and duration of administration, adverse effects and contraindications. It is the responsibility of the practitioner to take all appropriate safety precautions. Neither the publisher nor the author(s)/editor(s) assume any liability for any injury and/or damage to persons or property arising from or related to use of material in this book.

This book is sold on the understanding that the publisher is not engaged in providing professional medical services. If such advice or services are required, the services of a competent medical professional should be sought.

Every effort has been made where necessary to contact holders of copyright to obtain permission to reproduce copyright material. If any have been inadvertently overlooked, the publisher will be pleased to make the necessary arrangements at the first opportunity. The **CD/DVD-ROM** (if any) provided in the sealed envelope with this book is complimentary and free of cost. **Not meant for sale**.

Inquiries for bulk sales may be solicited at: jaypee@jaypeebrothers.com

Essentials of Medical Surgical Nursing

First Edition: 2011

Second Edition: **2021**

ISBN: 978-81-947090-8-4

Printed at: Sterling Graphics Pvt. Ltd.

To
My parents
and
My nursing profession
and
My dear students

Preface

It gives me immense pleasure and satisfaction to introduce second edition of *Essentials of Medical Surgical Nursing* to nursing community. In offering this text, I remain grateful for the support given to my all titles on Nursing and who have provided constructive feedback as well as encouraging commands.

This book is intended to provide an easily comprehensible, non-intimidating and concise text on the subject matter of Medical Surgical Nursing to the nursing students. There was a felt need among nursing students and teachers to have a handy book on "Medical Surgical Nursing" which caters to the needs of Indian students. It has been written in accordance with the needs of the present existing syllabus prescribed for the nursing course at degree level. The information provided is based on established knowledge and practice and also backed by scientific principles. Every attempt has been made to maintain simplicity and lucidity of language and style.

I hope this book will continue to serve as good source not only for nursing students but also a source reference and revision to the nurses who are in service and educational settings.

I am aware that for manifold reasons, errors might have crept in. I shall feel obliged, if such errors are brought to my notice. I sincerely welcome constructive criticism from readers that would help me to enrich my knowledge.

BT Basavanthappa

Acknowledgements

I owe a great deal of thanks to many who encouraged and supported me with their time and encouragement throughout.
- Shri G Basavannappa, Former Minister of Karnataka State for having initiated and support me to take up this "Noble Nursing Profession" as my career.
- Dr (Mrs) Manjula K Vasundhra, Former Professor and HOD of Community Medicine, Bangalore Medical College, who continuously encouraged me to write texts in the field of Nursing since nursing is a major force in Medical and Health services.
- My father Shri Thukkappa, who continues to grace for the progress of my career and all-around development of my personality for the welfare of the community.
- My mother Smt Hanumanthamma who continues to be a bright spot in the lives of all who knew her and whose grace gave me strength to progress of my life.
- My wife Smt Lalitha, who gives meaning to my life in so many ways. She is the one whose encouragement keep me motivated, whose support gives me strength and whose gentleness gives me comfort.
- My lovely children BB Mahesh and BB Gaanashree, for all the joy they provided me and all the hope that they instill me and who bare with patient throughout my works of the nursing texts. They keep me young at heart.
- Finally my warmest appreciation goes to M/s Jaypee Brothers Medical Publishers (P) Ltd., New Delhi, for sharing my vision for this book and giving me the chance to turn vision into reality.

Contents

1. **Introduction to Medical Surgical Nursing** 1
   - Evolution of Medicine and Nursing in India 1
   - Hindu Writings on Diagnosis and Prognosis 2
   - Hindu Surgery 2
   - Chronological Events 2
   - Nursing in India 4
   - Auxiliary Nursing 5
   - Registration of Nurses 6
   - The Nurse's Responsibility for the Future of Nursing 7
   - Concepts of Health and Illness 8
   - Illness, Sickness and Disease 10
   - Illness Behaviour Stages 11
   - Sick Role Behaviour 12
   - Effects of Hospitalization 13
   - Effects of Illness on Family Members 14
   - Infection and Inflammation 15
   - Asepsis 16
   - Role of Nurses in Surgical Settings 18
   - Intensive Care Unit 20

2. **Management of Common Signs and Symptoms** 25
   - Management of Fluid and Electrolyte Balance 25
   - Management of Fever 27

3. **Nursing Management of Respiratory Problems** 43
   - Nursing Assessment of Respiratory System 43
   - Diagnostic Studies of Respiratory System 45
   - Acute Bronchitis 47
   - Pneumonia 48
   - Tuberculosis 51
   - Bronchiectasis 54
   - Empyema 55
   - Lung Abscess 55
   - Occupational Lung Diseases 56
   - Lung Cancer 57
   - Nursing Management in Thoracic Surgery 58
   - Chest Trauma and Thoracic Injuries 60
   - Rib Fractures 61
   - Flail Chest 61
   - Pneumothorax 62
   - Pleural Effusion 63
   - Pulmonary Embolism 64
   - Pulmonary Hypertension 67
   - Cor Pulmonale 69
   - Lung Transplantation 70
   - Pulmonary Contusion 71
   - Chronic Bronchitis 71
   - Emphysema 72
   - Asthma 74
   - Cystic Fibrosis 76

- Respiratory Failure 78
- Chronic Obstructive Pulmonary Disease 79
- Management of COPD 84

4. **Nursing Management of Digestive Disorders** 93
   - Nursing Assessment of Digestive System 93
   - Diagnostic Studies in Digestive System 96
   - Radiological Studies 97
   - Endoscopic Examination 99
   - Liver Biopsy 100
   - Problems of Mouth 100
   - Oral Infections and Inflammation 100
   - Oral Cancer 102
   - Nausea and Vomiting 104
   - Gastroesophageal Reflux Disease (GERD) 106
   - Hiatal Hernia 110
   - Achalasia 111
   - Esophageal Carcinoma 112
   - Gastritis and Dyspepsia 114
   - Acute Gastritis 114
   - Chronic Gastritis 115
   - Upper Gastrointestinal Bleeding 115
   - Peptic Ulcer Disease (PUD) 116
   - Cancer of the Stomach 120
   - Irritable Bowel Syndrome (IBS) 122
   - Diarrhea 122
   - Fecal Incontinence 124
   - Constipation 125
   - Acute Abdomen 127
   - Abdominal Trauma 128
   - Appendicitis 128
   - Peritonitis 129
   - Diverticulitis 130
   - Inflammatory Bowel Disease (IBD) 130
   - Ulcerative Colitis 131
   - Crohn's Disease 132
   - Intestinal Obstruction 133
   - Colorectal Cancer 134
   - Ostomy Surgery 136
   - Anorectal Disorders 137
   - Jaundice 138
   - Hepatitis 139
   - Cirrhosis of Liver 141
   - Cholelithiasis 143
   - Primary Sclerosing Cholangitis (PSC) 145
   - Acute Pancreatitis 146
   - Chronic Pancreatitis 147

5. **Nursing Management of Cardiovascular Disorders** 149
   - Nursing Assessment of Cardiovascular System (CVS) 149
   - Physical Examination 150
   - Diagnostic Studies of CVS 152
   - Hypertension 156

- Coronary Artery Disease (CAD) 163
- Angina Pectoris 164
- Myocardial Infarction 166
- Shock 171
- Cardiogenic Shock 178
- Heart Failure 179
- Cardiac Dysrhythmias 183
- Inflammatory Heart Disease 193
- Myocarditis 194
- Infective Endocarditis 195
- Rheumatic Heart Disease 197
- Valvular Heart Disease 197
- Cardiac Surgery 201
- Arterial Disorders 203
- Acute Arterial Occlusive Disorders 205
- Chronic Arterial Occlusive Disease 206
- Buerger's Disease 208
- Raynaud's Disease 208
- Amputation and its Management 209
- Disorders of Veins 209
- Varicose Veins 211
- Venous Stasis Ulcer 212
- Pulmonary Embolism 212

6. Nursing Management of Hematological Disorders 213
- Nurses Assessment of the Hematological System 213
- Hematological Disorders 217
- Disorders of Erythrocytes 217
- Erythrocytosis 226
- Anemia caused by Blood Loss 227
- Disorders of Hemostasis 227
- Thrombocytopenia 227
- Thrombocytosis 229
- Disorders of Coagulation 229
- Disseminated Intravascular Coagulation (DIC) 231
- Disorders of WBCs 233
- Neutrophilia 234
- Leukemias 234
- Lymphomas 237
- Blood Transfusion 240

7. Nursing Management of Genitourinary Disorders 245
- Nursing Assessment of Genitourinary System 245
- Urine Studies 246
- Inflammatory Disorders of Urinary System 249

8. Nursing Management of Disorders of Reproductive System 275
- Nursing Assessment of the Male and Female Reproductive System 275
- Diagnostic Studies of Reproductive System 278
- Reproductive Problems of Females/Women 281
- Cervicitis 282
- Bartholinitis (Bartholin's Cysts) 283
- Pelvic Inflammatory Disease (PID) 283
- Premenstrual Syndrome 284

- Dysmenorrhea ... 285
- Amenorrhea ... 286
- Dysfunctional Uterine Bleeding (DUB) ... 287
- Endometriosis ... 288
- Uterine Prolapse ... 289
- Fistulas ... 291
- Neoplasms of the Female Reproductive Tract ... 292
- Uterine Leiomyoma (Fibroids) ... 295
- Endometrial Cancer ... 295
- Ovarian Cysts ... 296
- Ovarian Cancer ... 297
- Vulvar Cancer ... 298
- Surgeries of the Female Reproductive System ... 299
- Infertility ... 300
- Problems of the Breast ... 301
- Benign Breast Problems ... 301
- Fibroadenoma of Breast ... 302
- Breast Infections ... 303
- Nursing Management of the Patient Undergoing Mastectomy ... 307
- Male Breast Problems ... 308
- Epididymitis ... 309
- Orchitis ... 310
- Testicular Torsion ... 311
- Testicular Cancer ... 312
- Problems of Prostate ... 313
- Benign Prostatic Hyperplasia (BPH) ... 314
- Cancer of the Prostate ... 316
- Problems of the Penis ... 317
- Erectile Dysfunction/Impotence ... 319
- Sexually Transmitted Diseases ... 320
- Chlamydial Infections ... 323
- HIV Infection and AIDS ... 327

9. Nursing Management of Endocrine Disorders ... 333
- Nursing Assessment of the Endocrine System ... 333
- Disorders of Pituitary Gland ... 334
- Prolactin Hypersecretion ... 336
- Growth Hormone Hypersecretion ... 337
- Hypopituitarism ... 338
- Hyperfunction of Posterior Pituitary ... 339
- Syndrome of Inappropriate Anti-Diuretic Hormone ... 339
- Diabetes Insipidus (DI) ... 341
- Disorders of the Thyroid Gland ... 342
- Hyperthyroidism ... 342
- Hypothyroidism ... 345
- Cancer of the Thyroid Gland ... 347
- Disorders of Parathyroid Gland ... 349
- Hypoparathyroidism ... 350
- Disorders of Adrenal Gland ... 352
- Cushing's Syndrome ... 352
- Iatrogenic Cushing's Syndrome ... 354
- Aldosteronism ... 355
- Adrenocortical Insufficiency ... 356

- Disorders of Pancreas 357
- Diabetes Mellitus (DM) 357
- Complications of Diabetes Mellitus 361
- Hyperglycemic Hyperosmolar Non-Ketonic Coma (HHNC) 362
- Chronic Complications of DM 362
- Hypoglycemia in DM 363
- Hypoglycemia in Non-DM 363
- The Diabetic Foot 364

10. Nursing Management of Integumentary Disorders and Burns 367
- Common Skin Problems 371
- Parasitic Infections 371
- Fungal Infections 372
- Bacterial Infections 374
- Viral Infections of the Skin 376
- Allergic Conditions of the Skin 377
- Lupus Erythematosus 381
- Papulosquamous Diseases 381
- Acne 382
- Bullous Diseases 383
- Tumors of the Skin 383
- Malignant Lesions of the Skin 385
- Nursing Management of Dermatological Surgery 386
- Pressure Ulcers 387
- Burns 388
- Classification of Severity of Burns 391

11. Nursing Management of Musculoskeletal Disorders 397
- Diagnostic Studies of the Musculoskeletal System 400
- Soft-Tissue Injuries 403
- Dislocation and Subluxation 404
- Carpal Tunnel Syndrome (CTS) 405
- Repetitive Strain Injury (RSI) 405
- Rotator Cuff Injuries 405
- Meniscus Injury 406
- Bursitis 406
- Muscle Spasms 406
- Fractures 406
- Traction 409
- Fracture Immobilization 411
- Internal Fixation 413
- Management of Complications of Fracture 413
- Inflammatory and Degenerative Disorder—Musculoskeletal System 415
- Gout/Gouty Arthritis 424
- Septic Arthritis 426
- Lyme's Disease (LD) 427
- Seronegative Arthropathies 428
- Psoriatic Arthritis 429
- Reiter's Syndrome 429
- Systemic Lupus Erythematosus 429
- Systemic Sclerosis 431
- Crest Syndrome 431
- Sjögren's Syndrome 431

- Polymyositis/Dermatomyositis 432
- Fibromyalgia Syndrome (FMS) 433
- Infectious Bone Diseases 433
- Low Back Pain 435
- Management of Spinal Surgery 438
- Scoliosis 440
- Common Hand and Foot Problems 441
- Musculoskeletal Tumors 443
- Muscle Tumors 444
- Nursing Management of Bone Tumor 444
- Metabolic Bone Diseases 444
- Osteoporosis 446

12. Nursing Management of Immunological Problems 449
- Primary Immune Aberrations and Disease 457

13. Nursing Management of Infectious Diseases 487
- The Infectious Process 489
- Standard Precautions 490
- Transmission-Based Precautions 492
- Disinfecting Skin 492
- Changing Infusion Sets, Caps and Solutions 492
- The Patient with an Infectious Disease 493

14. Perioperative Nursing 495
- Definition of Perioperative Nursing and Nurse 495
- Scope of the Perioperative Nursing 495
- Role of Nurse in Perioperative Care 496
- Preoperative Care 497
- Intraoperative Care 504
- Postoperative Care 511
- Discharge from the POCU 521

15. Nursing Management of Disorders of Eye 523
- Nursing Assessment of the Visual System 523
- Visual Impairment 527
- Eye Infections and Inflammation 530
- Eye Trauma and Injury 531
- Glaucoma 533
- Cataract 534
- Retinal Detachment 536
- Strabismus 537
- Eye Tumors 538

16. Nursing Management of Disorders of Ear, Nose and Throat 539
- Nursing Assessment of Auditory System 539
- Hearing Impairment (Hearing Loss) 540
- Disorders of External Ear 543
- Problems of Middle Ear and Mastoid 545
- Problems of Inner Ear 548
- Disorders of Nose and Sinuses 550
- Disorders of Throat 556

17. Nursing Management of Neurological Disorders 563
- Nursing Assessment of the Nervous System 563
- Pain 565

- Diagnostic Studies of the Nervous System 569
- Intracranial Problems 570
- Head Injury 577
- Infections and Inflammation of Brain 580
- Brain Abscess 582
- Intracranial Tumors 582
- Spinal Cord Tumors 583
- Intracranial Surgery 584
- Cerebrovascular Accident/Stroke 585
- Epilepsy/Seizure Disorder 591
- Headache 595
- Multiple Sclerosis 597
- Parkinson's Disease 599
- Myasthenia Gravis 603
- Alzheimer's Disease 604
- Amyotrophic Lateral Sclerosis (ALS) 605
- Guillain-Barré Syndrome 606
- Trigeminal Neuralgia (TIC Douloureux) 607
- Bell's Palsy 608
- Spinal Cord Injury 609

18. Nursing Management of Oncological Conditions 613
- Cancer 613

19. Management of Emergency and Disaster Nursing 635
- Emergency Nursing 635
- Principles of Emergency Care 638
- Disaster Nursing 638
- Hospital Emergency Preparedness Plans 639

20. Critical Care Nursing 643
- Evolution of Critical Care Nursing 643
- Critical Care Unit/ICU 645
- Critical Care Patient 645

Index 657

CHAPTER 1

Introduction to Medical Surgical Nursing

EVOLUTION OF MEDICINE AND NURSING IN INDIA

The history of medicine in India goes back through the centuries to about 3000 BC. The beginnings are shrouded in the mist of ancient myths. The experience and concern in health development date back to vedic period between 3000 BC and 1400 BC. The Indus Valley Civilization showed relics of planned cities and practice of environmental sanitation. According to Dr Wheeler on the basis of his research studies from South, Arikamedu (Pondicherry) to North Mohenjodaro and Harappa, only one culture had been followed. An ideal healthful living of the people, such as every house of Mohenjodaro and Harappa had separate good water supply. In every backguard of the houses, there was a wide royal street and by the side of the street there was an arrangement of safe drinking water. Actually, this was followed by Dravidians who lived at that time. After the invasion of Aryans, the Dravidian got relegated to South. The specialist of pictograph reader, Father Heras says that it was a fact that ancient people of Mohenjodaro were proto-Dravidians, a fact also hinted by Sir John Marshall that there was a link between all that is the Dravidian culture, including Mohenjodaro and Karnataka. The Ayurveda and other system of medicine practised during this time suggests the development of comprehensive concept of health by the ancient sages of India.

Traditional Medicine and Surgery in India

Indian medicine is ancient. Its earliest concepts are set out in the sacred writings called the Vedas, especially in the metrical passages of the Atharvaved, which may possibly dates as far back as the second millennium BC. According to a later writer, the system of medicine called Ayurveda was received by a saint Dhanvantari from Brahma, and Dhanvantari was defined as the God of medicine. In later times, his status was gradually reduced, until he was credited with having been an earthly king who died of snakebite. Legends tell of Dhanvantari's relations with snakes and illustrates the skill with which early Indian practitioners treated snakebite.

The period of Vedic medicine lasted until about 800 BC. The Vedas are rich in magical practices for the treatment of diseases and in charms for the expulsion of the demons traditionally supposed to cause diseases. The chief conditions mentioned are fever, cough, constipation, diarrhea, dropsy, abscesses, seizures, tumors and skin diseases (including leprosy). The herbs recommended for treatment are numerous.

Golden Period of Indian Medicine

The golden age of Indian medicine, from 800 BC until about 1000 AD may be termed the Brahmanistic period. It is marked especially by production of the medical treatises knwon respectively as the Charaka-Samhita and Sushruta-Samhita, attributed respectively to the physician Charaka and Susruta, traditionally a surgeon. Both these works were formerly regarded as being of great antiquity, and hence claims arose for the priority of Indian scientific medicine over its Greek counterpart.

Another school asserted that these works were written many centuries after the beginning of the Christian Era. The most recent estimates place the Charaka-Samhita its present form as dating from the Ist century AD, and there were earlier versions. The Sushruta-Samhita probably originated in the last centuries of the pre-Christian Era and became fixed in its present form in the 7th century AD at the latest. Other medical treatises of lesser importance are those attributed to Vagbhata (8th century). All later treatises were based on these works.

Because the Hindus were prohibited by their religion from cutting the dead body, their knowledge of anatomy was limited. The Sushruta-Samhita recommends that a body be placed in a basket and sunk in a river for seven days. On its removal, the parts could be easily separated without cutting. As a result of these crude methods, the emphasis in Hindu anatomy was given to the bones, and then to the muscles, ligaments and joints. The nerves, blood vessels and internal organs were very imperfectly known.

The Hindus believed that the body contained three elementary substances, microcosmic representatives of the three divine universal forces, which they called spirit (air), phlegm, and bile. These were comparable with the humours of the Greeks. Health depends on the normal balance of these three elementary substances. The spirit has its seat below the navel the phlegm about the heart, and the bile between the heart and the navel. The seven primary constituents of the body—blood, flesh, fat, bone, marrow, chyle, and semen are produced by the action of the elementary substances. Semen was supposed to be produced from all parts of the body and not from any individual part or organ. Both Charaka and Sushruta state the existence of a large number of diseases (Susruta says 1,120). Rough classifications of diseases are given. In all texts "fever" of which numerous types are described, is regarded as important, phthisis (wasting disease, especially pulmonary tuberculosis) was apparently common, and the Hindu physicians knew the symptoms of cases likely to terminate fatally. Smallpox was common, and it is probable that smallpox inoculation was practised.

HINDU WRITINGS ON DIAGNOSIS AND PROGNOSIS

In diagnosis, the Hindu physicians used all five senses. Hearing was used to distinguish the nature of the breathing, alteration in voice, and the grinding sound produced by the rubbing together of broken ends of bones. They appear to have had a good clinical sense, and their sections on prognosis contain acute references to symptoms that are of grave import. Magical beliefs still persisted, however, until late in the classical period, the prognosis could be affected by such fortuitous factors as the cleanliness of the messenger sent to fetch the physician, the nature of his conveyance, or the types of persons whom the physician met on his journey to the patient.

Indian therapeutics was largely dietetic and medicinal. Dietetic treatment was important and preceded any medicinal treatment. Fats were mostly used internally and externally. The most important methods of active treatment were referred to as the "five procedures"; the administration emetics, purgatives, water enemas, oil enemas, and sneezing powders, inhalations were frequently employed, as were leeching, cupping and bleeding.

The Indian Materia Medica was extensive and consisted mainly of vegetable drugs, all of which were from indigenous plants. Charaka knew 500 medicinal plants, and Sushruta knew 700. But animal remedies (such as the milk of various animals, bones, gallstones) and minerals (sulfur, arsenic, lead, copper sulfate, gold) were also employed. The physicians collected and prepared their own vegetable drugs. Among those that eventually appeared in western pharmacopoeias are cardamom and cinnamon.

As a result of the strict religious beliefs of the Hindus, hygienic measures were important in treatment. Two meals a day were prescribed with indications of the nature of the diet, the amount of water to be drunk before and after the meal, and the use of condiments. Bathing and care of the skin were carefully prescribed, as were cleaning of the teeth with twigs from neem trees, anointing of the body with oil, and use of eyewashes.

HINDU SURGERY

In surgery, ancient Hindu medicine reached its zenith. Detailed instructions about the choice of instruments and the different operations are given in the classical texts. It has been said that the Hindus knew all ancient operations except the arrest of hemorrhage by the ligature. Their operations were grouped broadly as follows: excision of tumors; incision of abscesses, punctures of collections of fluid in the abdomen; extraction of foreign bodies; pressing out of the contents of abscesses; probing of fistulas; and stitching of wound.

The surgical instruments used by the Hindus have received special attention in modern times. According to Sushruta, the surgeon should be equipped with 20 sharp and 101 blunt instruments. The sharp instruments included knives of various patterns, scissors, trocars (instruments for piercing tissues and draining fluid from them), saws and needles. The blunt instruments included forceps, specula (instruments for inspecting body cavities or passages), tubes, levers, hooks and probes. The Sushruta-Samhita does not mention the catheter, but it is referred to in later writings. The instruments were largely of steel. Alcohol seems to have been used as a narcotic during operations.

Especially in two types of operations the ancient Hindus were outstanding. Stone in the bladder (vesical calculus) was common in ancient India, and the surgeons frequently carried out the operation of lateral lithotomy for removal of the stones. They also introduced plastic surgery. Amputation of the nose was one of the prescribed punishments for adultery, and repair was carried out by cutting from the patient's cheek a piece of tissue of the required size and shape and applying it to the stump of the nose. The results appear to have been tolerably satisfactory, and the modern operation is certainly derived indirectly from this ancient source. The Hindu surgeons, also performed an operation for the cure of anal fistula and in this they were definitely in advance of the Greeks.

In the past there had been much speculation as to whether the Greek derived any of their medical knowledge from the Hindus. Mid-20th century opinion held that there was certainly intercommunication between Greece and India before the time of Alexander the Great.

CHRONOLOGICAL EVENTS

A brief description of chronological events related to development of health and medicine in India is given below:

3000 BC: In the Indus Valley Civilisation, one finds evidence of well developed environmental sanitation programs such as underground drains, public baths, etc. 'AROGYA' or 'Health' was given high priority in daily life and this concept of health included physical, mental, social and spiritual well-being.

2000 BC: Rigveda marks the beginning of the Indian system of medicine. Medicine was considered part of VEDAS or Scriptures. 'Ayurveda', a 'Science of life and art of living' said to be founded by Sage 'Atreya'. Good health implies an ideal balance between tridoshic factors, i.e. wind, bile, phlegm (Vata-Pitta and Kapha) according to Ayur-Veda. Health promotion and health education were also emphasized by following 'Dinacharya'.

1000 BC: Atharvaveda mentions the twin aims of medical sciences as health and longevity and curative treatment. Hygiene and dietetics are considered important in treatment. Beneficial effects of milk are described in detail.

800 BC: A codification of medical knowledge scattered through vedas by Bhela called Bhela-Samhita.

700 BC: A codification of medical knowledge by Agni-Vesa, said to be disciple of Atreya, called Agnivesa Samhita became the basis of later Charaka.

600 BC: A treatise by Kasyapa mainly dealing with paediatrics.

500 BC: 'Chivaravastu', a book written by unknown author is found. It mentions prince Jivika, the court physician of Bimbasara, King of Magadh, as a marvellous physician and surgeon. He is credited with such difficult operations as piercing the skull to operate on the brain, surgery of the eyes, etc. and medical treatment of dropsy, internal tumors and varicose veins.

272 BC-236 BC: King Asoka, a convert to Buddhism, built number of hospitals. More emphasis was laid on the preventive aspects. Doctors, nurses, and midwives were to be trustworthy and skillful. The nurses were usually men and old women. This period saw famous medical schools at Taxila and Nalanda.

237 BC-201 BC: St Buddha instituted a state medical system, appointed doctors for every 10 villages on the main roads of India. Pharmaceutical gardens were also maintained.

200 BC-100 BC: Patanjali explored the yoga system of philosophy of men and physical discipline—the starting point of yoga therapy later continued.

100 BC: Charaka-Samhita, the first classical exposition of Indian system medicine deals with an almost all the branches of medicine, anatomy, physiology, etiology, prognosis, pathology, treatment procedure, and sequence of medication and an extension Materia Medica for more than 600 drugs. This treatise formed the basis of the Atreya School of Medicine in India, in (100) AD. The qualification of attending nurse, enshrined in the Charaka-Samhita, i.e. knowledge of preparation and compounding of drugs for administration, cleverness, devotedness to patient under care and purity of both mind and body.

200-300 AD: Sushruta-Samhita appears to have been revised by Nagarjuna, laid main emphasis on surgery. This great treatise described more than 300 operations, 43 different surgical processes and 121 different types of instruments. The Materia Medica is also extensive covering more than 650 drugs of animals, plant and mineral origin. This treatise forms the basis of Dhanwantari School (300 AD).

Sushruta defines ideal relations of doctor, patient, nurses and medicine as the four feet upon which a cure must rest.

500-600 AD: Vagbhata wrote Astanga Hridaya (8 limbs and heart). The eight limbs refer to the eight traditional branches of Ayurvedic knowledge, i.e. therapeutics, surgery, ENT, mental and superstitious diseases, infantile diseases and treatment, toxicology, arresting physical and mental decay, and rejuvenation or regaining lost virility potency and procreative ability.

This book is the most concise and scientific exposition of Ayurveda. It is in verse form, making it easy to memorise. It incorporates the teachings of the sages Atreya and Dhan-Wantari and the Rasayana school of medicine. It is distinguished but its knowledge of chemical reactions and laboratory processes. This book has been translated into foreign language.

600-800 AD: Sodhala (700 AD) two treatises, Gandanighraha, a medical treatise and Sodhala, a medical Lexicon.

Vrudukunta (750 AD) writes Siddayoga, the earliest treatise on Rasa Chikitsa now existing intact. The Rasa Chikitsa system considers mercury as the king of all medicines. Siddayoga explain the various preparations of mercury and other metals, alloys, metallic compounds, salts and sulphur. This school of medicine is called SIDDHA school. All of them are made of metals, salts and sulphur. It is supposed to be a continuation of the pre-Aryan medical system in India. It is popular in Eastern and Southern India.

Siddha Nagarjuna two treatises on the Siddha systems, Rasarathanakara and Arogya Manjari. Madhavacharya (700-800 AD) wrote Madhava Nidana. This is a compilation from the earlier works of Agnivesa, Charaka, Sushruta, Vagbhata. It is specially useful as a chemical guide to preparations. It is famous all over India as the best Ayurvedic work on the diagnosis of diseases.

800-1300 AD: A number of treatises were written in India during this period. Arkaprakasha, a book on tincture extraction, Sarangadhara Samhita, Chikitsa, Sangraha and Yoga Ratnakara are the better known among them.

The period also witnessed a spirit of writing on the Rasa Chikitsa system. Rasha Hridaya by Govind Vagbhata, Rasaratnakara by Siddha Nityananda, Rasara-Tnasammukta by Vagbhata (another), Rasarnava by Sambhu, Rasendrachintamani by Ramachandra, and Rasendra Choodamani by Somadeva.

1300-1600 AD: Bhavamisra wrote Bhava Pra-Kasha. This is the most renowned Indian treatise during the period. It contains an exhaustive list of diseases and their symptoms and complete list of drugs including many not mentioned in the earlier works. It includes etiology and treatment of syphilis, a disease brought into India by Portuguese seamen.

Other works of this period are Chikitsaliye by Trisata, a manual on diagnosis; Chintamani by Ballbhendra on aetiology and diagnosis; and Vaidyamrutha by Moreswara on the treatment of diseases.

Another class of works produced during this period are Medical Lexicons by Madanapala, Nagahari, Bimapala, and Rajavallabha.

1600: East India Company established British Rule in India. Western medicine and surgery started to be practised and became popular in India.

NURSING IN INDIA

Beginning of Modern Nursing

In the past, the progress of nursing in India has been hindered by many difficulties, such as: the low status of women, the system of purdah among Muslim women, the caste system among Hindus, illiteracy, poverty, political unrest, language differences, and the fact that nursing has been looked upon as servant's work.

Since Independence day 1947, many changes have taken place and the attitude towards nursing is changing. More women are being educated and many are taking up nursing as their profession.

We have very little information about medicine and nursing in India until the 15th century, when Vasco da Gama came to India. He set up trading posts on the west coast. Franciscan, Dominican and Jesuit missionaries came to minister to the sick and needy. The Portuguese set up European type of dispensaries at Goa and Madras and physicians from Europe were invited to India. One of these, Garcia da Orta, in 1550 wrote "Simples Drugs of India".

Military Nursing

Military nursing was the earliest type of nursing. In 1664, the East India Company helped to start a hospital for soldiers at Fort St George, Madras. Later, acivilian hospital was built and the medical staff, appointed by the East India Company, served in both hospitals. In 1797, a Lying-in-Hospital was built and in 1854 the government sanctioned a training school for midwives. In 1861, through the efforts of Miss Nightingale, reforms in military hospitals led to reforms in civil hospitals. Efforts were made to provide health services for the people of India. This laid the foundation for public health nursing.

Nursing in the military hospitals was of poor quality carried on by male orderlies and menial staff. In 1871 the Government General Hospital, Madras undertook a plan to train nurses. Nurses were brought from England to be in-charge and the first six students were those who had previously received their diploma in midwifery. Later this plan was reversed. General training was taken first followed by a course in midwifery.

In Bombay, among the one of the earliest hospitals is the Jamsetjee Jeejeebhoy group, the first of which was opened in 1843. Another hospital which was to play an important part in the development of modern nursing in India was the Pestani Hormusji Cama Hospital for women and children, which was founded in 1883 but not opened until 1886.

Provision for the nursing care of patients in these early hospitals was very limited. In the JJ Group, nursing was done by medical students and menials until 1868 when the government invited the Sisters of the Community of All Saints to come from England and take over the work of nursing. Their work was appreciated and the need for training nurses was felt. At this time, it was difficult to get nurses. There were only a few Anglo-Indian and Indian Christian girls working in mission hospitals. The sisters of all saints took the first steps to establish a training school for nurses in this hospital. In 1891, Bai Kashibai Ganpat was the first Indian nurse to come for training. Training was at first two years but became three years when the Bombay Presidency Nursing Association was established in 1909.

An outstanding graduate of the JJ Group of hospitals was Miss TK Adranvala. After her graduation, she worked as a ward sister, then became assistant Matron under the sisters and finally, superintendent of the hospitals. She held this position until she was asked to accept the position of Nursing Superintendent and Nurse adviser to the Government of India. She remained in this position until retiring in 1966. She continues active participation in nursing as a WHO representative in Nepal. Miss Adranvala has worked very hard to raise the status of the nursing profession in India. She has given much of her time to the interests of the TNAI having held the office of president for two terms and that of treasurer until she was released at her own request. The nursing profession in India is fortunate to have had such a capable person as Miss Adranvala as its representative in the World Health Organization. She is highly respected by all and many seek her wise counsel.

Mission Hospitals

Mission Hospitals were the first to begin the training of Indians as nurses, very gradually overcoming the prejudices of parents against sending their girls for a training which was felt to be beneath the dignity of decent educated girls. Religion prevented Hindu and Muslim girls from joining at all and so only Christian girls could be trained at first. But for many years, even they felt nursing was an inferior profession.

In the beginning there was no uniformity of courses or educational requirements. About 1907-1910 the North India United Board of Examiners for Mission Hospitals was organized and set up rules for admissions and standards of training and conducted a public examination. On 24th May 1909 the Indian Medical Mission Association granted the Nursing Diploma after examining student by Central Board for Nurses' Training Schools in South India. A few years later the Mid-India and the South India Boards of Nurse examiners were similarly set up. These are Examining Boards of the Nurses' League of the Christian Medical Association of India. The name of the South India Board was changed to 'The Board of Nursing Education, Nurses' League of Christian Medical Association of India branch in 1975.

The Dufferin Fund

Until the late 19th century there were no women doctors and therefore, no care for women except in mission hospitals. This fact was brought to the attention of Queen Victoria. At this time, Lady Dufferin was coming out to India with her husband who was on government service. Queen Victoria instructed Lady Dufferin about the need for medical care for women and children in India and asked her to take a special interest in this problem. Lady Dufferin wrote to her friends and influential people to get financial aid. Thus, in 1885, Lady Dufferin was responsible for starting the 'National Association for supplying Medical Aid by Women to Women of India'. This is commonly called the Dufferin Fund and continues to provide medical education for women, to train nurses and midwives for hospitals and private work, and to improve medical facilities for women.

Between 1890 and 1900, many schools under either missions or government were started in various parts of India. The directors fo these schools were English or American. Each school sets up its own pattern of training familiar to the director. There was a need for systematic training of nurses like that given in the Nightingale School in England. Thus it was, that in 1886, money from the Dufferin Fund was made available for this purpose. Miss Atkinson, a Nightingale nurse, was brought out from England to Bombay to set up and be the superintendent of the First Modern Training School for Nurses in India. The school was established in the Cama Hospital for Women and Children in 1891. It began with a one year course but by 1995 it had been extended to three years.

The leaders of nursing in India realized that more and better qualified teachers and ward supervisors were needed if standards were to be maintained and nursing was to advance. Hence, courses were set up in several places to give Indian nurses an opportunity to prepare themselves for responsible positions in hospitals and schools of nursing. Post-certificate courses were first offered in nursing administration, supervision and teaching. These originated at the College of Nursing, New Delhi; the College of Nursing, CMC Hospital, Vellore and the Government General Hospital, Madras.

The first four year basic bachelor degree programmes were established in 1946 at the Colleges of Nursing in Delhi and Vellore. This programme is now offered in a number of other colleges.

In 1963, the School of Nursing in Thiruvananthapuram instituted the first two year post-certificate bachelor degree programme. Other schools have begun this programme since that time.

In recent years, as higher education for nurses has developed around the world, courses in India have developed so that the nurse can specialize in almost any subject and continue education through the level of the Master's degree. The first Master's degree course, a two-year postgraduate programme was begun in 1960 at the College of Nursing in Delhi (Now Rajkumari Amrit Kaur College of Nursing, New Delhi. In 1970, many colleges of nursing were started and offering PCBSc Nursing and Basic BSc Nursing courses in various parts of India. In Karnataka, Bangalore University instituted PhD programme for nurses in 1991. The author of this book is the first person to get Doctoral degree in Nursing in the State of Karnataka.

AUXILIARY NURSING

The use of auxiliary nursing personnel to ease the shortage of professional nurses had been common in some countries when it was first put into practice in India. A two-year programme for the Auxiliary Nurse-Midwife was first established in 1951 at St Mary's Hospital, Tarn Taran in Punjab state. By 1962, there were 263 courses being offered in India. The auxiliary nurse midwife is prepared to practise elementary nursing and full midwifery. She functions primarily in the community rather than the hospital. The practice of the auxiliary nurse-midwife has helped to improve the amount of care given to the patient as well as the health teaching given to the public. In 1977 the ANM course was completely revised by the Indian Nursing Council and expanded to include sociology health education and communication skills and subjects necessary to equip the multipurpose health worker/ANM to serve effectively as a primary health care worker in the community. Such workers are key persons for achievement of the goal of 'Health for all by 2000 AD" to which we in India are committed.

Textbooks

One of the handicaps in the development of nursing schools was the lack of textbooks. In other countries books had been written by doctors and nurses. Some of these were translated into the vernacular for the early schools and colleges. Many English and American textbooks are being used in the schools today. There is a great need for textbooks which have been written by Indian nurses. A beginning had been made in this work and the first Textbook for Nurses in India was printed by the South India Examining Board of the Nurses' League of the

Christian Medical Association of India in 1941. The Nurses' League has also directed the publishing of a Textbook for Auxiliary Nurse-Midwives, first printed in 1967. This book was completely revised and published in two volumes in 1985 as a Textbook for the Health Worker (ANM) to meet the needs of the health worker. Several manuals related to the basic sciences and nursing have been published by other professional nursing bodies. Although progress has been made in the publication of textbooks by the nurses of India, there remains a wide area of subjects which have not been touched upon and the general need for more and varied textbooks continues. Since a few nursing educator started writing texts on Nursing, to quote, Late Dr (Mrs) Kasturi Sunder Rao wrote text on 'Community Health Nursing, and a few Bombay-based Nurses made an effort to write guides and two books on Nursing. In later part of 1990s onwards the author of this book also has written on 'Nursing Research' (1998), Community Health Nursing (1998), Nursing Administration (2000), Nursing Education (2003), Fundamentals of Nursing (2002) Medical Surgical Nursing (2003), Pediatric Child Health Nursing (2004), Midwifery and Reproductive Health Nursing (2006), Psychiatric Mental Health Nursing (2006), Nursing Theories (2007), on the basis of present needs in Indian context and started revision of earlier text and Essential series of all the books also availble are written by author.

Nursing education in India began with very brief periods of training as mentioned in the first part of this chapter. Orderlies and midwives were often chosen for this and were given a period of two to six months of closely supervised practical experience in general nursing, then called 'sick nursing'. This was training in the hospital, and certificates were given after completion of a training.

The basic Program for combined general nursing and midwifery developed rapidly after 1871. The need for theory as well as practical experience was felt. The training for general nursing was extended to two years and then three years before the student went on for midwifery training. The present basic program for nursing education throughout India consists of a three and half year program in general nursing and six to seven months in midwifery. Uniformity of training is maintained by recognition of schools which meet the standards and requirements given by the Indian Nursing Council. The basic certificate program now includes all areas of nursing as integrated community health nursing.

Now, most of the states in India started basic BSc Nursing, Postcertificate BSc Nursing and MSc Nursing degree courses in their related universities. And also there is Doctoral degree course in nursing leading to PhD in nursing.

REGISTRATION OF NURSES

As training for nurses, midwives, and health visitors progressed, the need for legislation to provide basic minimum standards in education and training was felt. It was also felt that registration would give greater professional status. For some years, nurses struggled to obtain proper examinations and examiners and registration for nurses. In 1926 Madras State formed the first Registration Council. While most states now have a recognized Registration Council, all do not. It is now possible for the students of all schools in India to be registered in one of the State Registration Councils.

The Indian Nursing Council

The Indian Nursing Council Act was passed by an ordinance on December 31st 1947. The council was constituted in 1949. The purpose of the council is to co-ordinate activities of the various State Registration Councils, to set up standards for nursing education and to make sure these standards are carried out. Before this time, nurses registered in one state were not necessarily recognised for registration in another. The condition to mutual recognition by the State Nurses Registration Council called reciprocity was possible only if uniform standards of nursing education was maintained. Therefore, the INC was given authority to prescribe curricula for nursing education in all of the states. At the same time, it was given authority to recognize programmes of nursing education or refuse recognition. The Indian Nursing Council is not itself a registering body nor examining body but it can enforce its standards by recognizing or refusing to recognize schools. And now almost all the states of India has their State Nursing Council for example, Karnataka State Nursing Council, etc.

Community Health Nursing

In India community health nursing had its beginning when the terrible conditions under which children were born were recognized as a cause for the high civilian mortality rate. It was realized that the untrained dais who attended women during delivery must be given training. This was not an easy job as the dais were unwilling to be trained and the patients were very willing to accept the old customary methods and could see no need to change. The first attempts to train dais were carried out by missionaries as early as 1886. In 1900, Lady Curzon brought about the establishment of the Victoria Memorial Scholarship for the purpose of improving safe delivery practices. The need for training a better type of midwife was felt. In this, Madras State led the way when they passed the Madras Registration of Nurses and Midwives Act of 1926.

Slowly the need for trained personnel for maternal and childhealth, as part of community health nursing was felt. To supply this need a Health School for the training of health visitors was started in Delhi in 1918. This has now become the Lady Reading Health School.

A further step forward was taken in 1948, when community health nursing was integrated in the basic programme of the new degree courses which were started at the College of Nursing, Delhi and the School of Nursing, CMC Hospital, Vellore under the University of Delhi and Madras respectively.

Since 1953, a post-certificate course in community health nursing has been given at the All India Institute of Hygiene and Public Health in Calcutta. In 1960, a course was established by the Lady Reading Health School in Delhi. Several other schools now offer this programme.

To prepare more community Health nurses, in 1957 the Government of India selected ten schools of nursing and gave assistance so that they could integrate community health nursing into their basic course. Since that time, recognition of a programme of basic nursing education required that community health nursing be integrated into the basic course. Thus, all professional nurses today can function in the hospital and the community at the level of a staff nurse.

Various international organizations, such as WHO, UNICEF and Colombo Plan have assisted by supplying trained personnel and equipment to help in the training of students in the rural field, maternity work and paediatrics.

THE NURSE'S RESPONSIBILITY FOR THE FUTURE OF NURSING

Throughout this study of nursing we have seen nursing advance from the kindly ministrations of a mother or a neighbour to the highly organized service of today. In the beginning individuals were inspired to help one another in distress. This essential care or service still remains but time has brought about changes in our ideas regarding nursing. Today we are not only relieve and give comfort but help our patients to live upto their optimum health. The new emphasis is on health nursing-nursing the mind, the family as a whole and as part of the community with the nurse as the health teacher.

Growing specialisation in medicine is resulting in a trend towards increased specialisation in nursing. The development of new tests and diagnostic procedures, new medicines and new equipment make specialisation even more necessary as the amount of scientific knowledge needed for a certain speciality becomes greater. Developments in other professions also influence trends in the nursing profession. As other members of the health team become more available and more highly specialized, the work of the nurse is changing towards more specific nursing functions. It has also added to the number and kind of professional relationships which must be maintained by the nurse. The power of spiritual factors is becoming of increasing interest as reports of the healing power of spiritual activity such as meditation is receiving more attention. Just as advances in technology tend to take the nurse away from the bedside and a direct relationship with the patient, so these developments are showing the need for a deeper therapeutic relationship between the nurse and the patient. The future will demand a balance of these factors in order to meet the total health needs of the individual and the community. Future trends are likely to show an effort to make this balance.

Many trends leading to professionalism are taking place because of the untiring efforts of nurses dedicated to achieving the aim of becoming a profession. In 1970, WHO recognized Nursing as a profession. It has often been a difficult struggle requiring real courage and vision by nursing leaders in the face of serious obstacles. Today nurses enjoy many rights and privileges, though desired standards are still not achieved in all areas, because nursing leaders have struggled to achieve them. Nurses who are going to be the future leaders have to carry on this work of greater achievement through growing amounts of writing and research.

Nursing today provides an ever widening scope of opportunity for service. With present trends leading towards greater opportunities, varieties of services and growing social and professional recognition, it should be exciting and challenging for nurses to know that all nurses members of this profession since they fulfill the criteria of the profession. (for further details please read the authors text on "NURSING ADMINISTRATION", 3rd Edition).

Medical Surgical Nursing is commonly defined as the nursing care of adults with suspected or diagnosed pathology of physiological function. It encompasses such a large scope that the trend is to subdivide medical-Surgical, Oncological (cancer) nursing, and only recently have the other specialties been developed.

Currently, all basic nursing programs prepare nurses to practice medical-surgical nursing. Advanced preparation at the master's and doctoral levels is necessary if the nurse wishes to devlop expertise and acquire in-depth knowledge in particular aspects or subdivisions of the specialty. These specialties would include intensive care units, the emergency room.

Medical-surgical nursing is the area of practice concerned with the care of adults with predicted or exisiting physiologic alterations, trauma, or disability. It is the backbone of modern nursing and the practice foundation of virtually all health care institutions.

Traditionally medical-surgical nursing was not considered a specialty area. Rather, practices with a focus on a specific type of health problem within the area of medical-surgical nursing were considered specialties. These included cardiovascular, perioperative, neurologic, gynecologic, infection control and emergency nursing, and practices limited to problems such as wound care, burns, hypertension and diabetes. Today this view has changed. Medical-surgical nursing is now formally recognized as a specialty in its own right, and the focused practice areas are seen as subspecialties.

Formal recognition as a specialty means that a practice area meets the criteria for specialty status, which were published in the document titled "Recognition of a Specialty Approval of Scope" Statements and Acknowledgement of Nursing practice Standards (ANA).

The criteria are that the practice area must:
- Be clearly defined and subscribe to the overall purposes and functions of nursing
- Define itself as nursing
- Adhere to the overall licensure requirements of the profession
- Be national or international in scope
- Be able to identify a need and demand for itself
- Have a well-derived knowledge base particular to the practice of the specialty
- Be organized and represented by a national specialty association
- Be concerned with phenomena within the discipline of nursing
- Have defined competencies for the area of specialty practice
- Have existing mechanisms for supporting, reviewing and disseminating research to support its knowledge base
- Have continuing education programs that prepare nurses in the specialty
- Include a substantial number of nurses who devote most of their practice to the specialty.

The nursing profession has adopted standards of practice that describe the responsibilities for which are accountable. All nurses, regardless of education, Standards of Clinical Nursing Practice to guide their practice. This broad set of standards has two components: standards of care and standards of professional performance. The nursing process and competent level of nursing care are the foundation of the standards of care. The standards of professional performance address expected quality of care, performance appraisal, education, collegiality, ethics, collaboration, research, and resource utilization. Each standard has measurement criteria to demonstrate competent practice.

The Academy of Medical Surgical Nurses, founded in 1991, is an international organization dedicated to fostering excellence in medical-surgical nursing practice. Its mission is to "enhance the clinical expertise, professionalism, and leadership of nurse's caring for adults in hospitals, the community, and long-term care."

CONCEPTS OF HEALTH AND ILLNESS

Health is a state of well-being of individual and community. So it can be examined at individual or community level. For individual the term 'health' refers to the optimal functioning of the individual, absence of disease, illness, impairment or injury. In the context of the community it refers to various objective measures of health, health status or health indices like incidence of, and prevalence of disease applied to different segments of population. Defining good health is difficult, because each person has personal concept of health.

The definition of health range on a continuum from the absence of diseases to optimal functioning to utopian ideals of complete state of physical, mental, emotional, spiritual and social well-being.

About 500 BC, **Pericles** defined 'health' as "That state of moral, mental and physical well-being which enables a person to face any crisis in life with the utmost grace (of God) and facility."

HS Hayman defines health as a state of feeling sound in body, mind and spirit, with a sense of reserve power. This perception, if health is based on normal functioning of the body's physiological process, understanding the principles of healthful living and attitude that regards health not only as a means of survival and self-fulfilment in itself, but as means to a creative social adjustment and a richer, fuller life as measured in constructive service to mankind.

H Blum defines 'health' as the person's capacity to function in a way to maximise potential, to maintain a balance appropriate to age and social needs, to be reasonably free of gross dissatisfaction, discomfort, disease or disability, and to behave in ways that promote survival as well as self-fulfilment or enjoyment.

- Health is the condition of being sound in body, mind or spirit especially freedom from physical disease or pain (Webber).
- Health refer to a "soundness of body or mind; that condition in which its functions are duly and efficiently discharged (Oxford English Dictionary).
- Health is a condition or quality of the human organism expressing the adequate functioning of the organising the given conditions, genetic and environmental.
- Health is a modus vivendi enabling imperfect men to achieve a rewarding and not too painful existence while they cope with an imperfect world.

R Dubiois views 'health' as adaptation a function of adjustment. He believes an (WHO's) utopian state of health can never be reached because the person can never be so perfectly adapted to the environment that life will not involve struggle, failure and suffering. Humans can adapt to environmental conditions or change the environment but each new adaptation produces new problems that demand new solution.

"Health is the achievement of a state of harmony between man's internal and external milieu" (Liverpool School of Tropical Medicine).

F and E Rathbone formulates health as a wholeness of function, movement towards self actualisation, relating to effective, creative use of potential, realistic interpretation of experiences and co-ordination of attitudinal, physiological and behavior adaptations.

Imogene King defined 'health' as a dynamic state in the life cycle of an organism that implies continuous adaptation to stresses in the internal and external environment through optimum use of one's resources to achieve maximum potential for daily living.

According to **S Perkin** "health is a state of relative equilibrium of body form and functions which results from its successful, dynamic adjustment to forces tending to disturb it. It is not passive interplay between body substance and forces infringing upon it, but an active response of the body forces working towards adjustment.

Health is wellness of an individual. According to **Dunn** the term 'high level wellness' implies well-being in degree or level.

High level wellness for the individual is defined as an integrated method of functioning which is oriented towards maximising the potential of which the individual is capable. It requires that an individual maintains a continuous balance and purposeful direction within the environment whereby he is functioning.

WHO defines "Health as state of complete physical, mental, social and spiritual well-being and not merely absence of disease."

This definition is positive and includes more than physical health, it infers that health is an absolute or ultimate state. But all individuals cannot achieve the same level of health because of innate differences, some of us are born with severe physical and mental limitations. So according to WHO, the complete well-being for all is unattainable goal. Hence, the US President's Commission stated, "health means an optimum state of physical, mental and' social well-being."

Terris M, a famous epidemiologist believes the WHO definition should be re-worded as "Health is a state of physical, mental and social well-being and ability to function and not merely the absence of 'illness' or infirmity." Thereby replacing 'disease' by illness and excluding 'complete' as health is not an absolute. The addition of "and ability to function" is necessary, as a definition of health requires both objective and subjective components. The objective component being the "ability to function," the subjective being "feeling of well-being."

A singular definition, and one which returns more to Pericles' version is that of the Liverpool School of Tropical Medicine: "Health is the achievement of a state of harmony between man's internal and external milieu."

However, WHO's definition has the following characteristics that promote a more positive concept of health.
- A concern for the individual as a total system.
- A view of health that identifies internal and external environment.
- An acknowledgement of the importance of an individual's role in life.

Health is a changing, evolving concept that is basic to nursing. For centuries, the concept of disease was the yardstick by which health was measured. Now there has been an increasing emphasis on health. Health is very difficult to define. There is no consensus about any definitions of health. There is no consensus about any definitions of health. There is knowledge of how to attain a certain level of health, but health itself cannot be measured.

Health is described in various sources as a value judgment, a subjective state, a relative concept, a spectrum, a cycle, a process, and as an abstraction that cannot be measured objectively. In many definitions physiological and psychological components of health are dichotomised. Other subconcepts that might be included in definitions of health include environmental and social influences (economical or financial), freedom of pain or disease, optimum capability, ability to adapt, purposeful direction and meaning in life, and harmony, balance, or sense of well-being.

Historically, health and illness were viewed as extremes on a continuum, with the absence of clinically recognisable disease being equated with the presence of health. In 1974 World Health Organization defined health in terms of total well-being and discouraged the conceptualisation of health as simply the absence of diseases. At the time, some considered this definition impractical; some viewed it as a possible goal for all people, while others consider complete well-being unobtainable. However this definition of health includes three characteristics of basic to a positive concept of health:
- It refers concern for the individual as a total person rather than a merely the sum of various parts.
- It places health in the context of environment.
- It equates health with productive and creative living.
- The harmonious balance of the state of physical, mental, social and spiritual well-being of the human individual integrated into his health and constitutes health.

The state of positive health implies the notion of "perfect functioning" of the body and mind. It conceptualise health **biologically** as a state in which every cell and every organ is functioning at optimum capacity and in perfect harmony with the rest of the body; **psychologically**, as a state in which the individuals feels a sense of perfect well-being and of mastery over his environment; **socially**, as a state in which the individual capacity for participation in the social system are optional, and spiritually, as state in which the individual which reaches out and strives for meaning and purpose in life.

The concept of perfect positive health cannot become a reality because man will never be so perfectly adapted to his environment that his life will not involve struggle, failure, and suffering positive health will therefore, always remain a mirage because every thing in life is subject to change. So health is a dynamic state of physical, mental, social, and spiritual well-being of an individual, not merely an absence of disease or infirmity.

More contemporary definitions of health have emphasized the relationship between health and wellness. Although health may be viewed as a static state of being at any given point of time, **wellness** is the process of moving toward integration of human functioning; maximisation of human potential; self-responsibility for health; greater awareness of self-satisfaction; and wholeness in body, mind and spirit.

ILLNESS, SICKNESS AND DISEASE

Illness is a highly personal state in which the person feels unhealthy or ill. Illness may or may not be related to disease. An individual could have a disease, for example, a growth in the stomach, and not feel ill. Parsons defines illness as "a state of disturbance in the normal functioning of the total human individual, including both the state of the organism as a biological system, and of his person and social adjustments."

Sickness is a status or social entity that is usually associated with disease or illness but can occur independently of them. When a person is defined as sick, several dependent behaviors are accepted that otherwise might be considered unacceptable. Bauman found that people use three distinct criteria to determine whether they are ill:
1. The presence of symptoms, such as elevated temperature or pain.
2. Their perceptions of how they feel; for example, good, bad, sick.
3. Their ability to carry out daily activities, such as job or schoolwork.

Disease can be described as an alteration in body functions resulting in a reduction of capacities or a shortening of the normal life span. Disease may further be described as *acute* or *chronic, communicable, congenital, degenerative, functional, malignant, psychosomatic,* or *idiopathic.* Intervention by physicians has the goal of eliminating or ameliorating disease processes. Primitive people thought disease was caused by "forces" or spirits. Later, this belief was replaced by the single causation theory. Increasingly, a number of factors are considered to interact in causing disease and determining the individual's response to treatment.

The causation of disease is called its etiology. A description of the etiology of a disease includes the identification of all causal factors that act together to bring about the particular disease. For example, the tubercle bacillus is designated as the biologic agent of tuberculosis. However, other etiologic factors, such as age, nutritional status, and even occupation, are involved in the development of tuberculosis and influence the course of infection.

Risk factors are situations, habits, or other phenomena that increase a person's vulnerability to illness or injury. Risk factors can be categorized into five interrelated areas: genetic makeup, age, physiologic factors, lifestyle, and environment: Examples of each follow:
- *Genetic makeup*: A person with a family history of diabetes mellitus or cancer is at risk of developing the disease later in life.
- *Age*: The risk of birth defects and complications of pregnancy increases after age 35; the risk of communicable disease is higher in school age children; and the risk of cardiovascular disease increases with age for both sexes.
- *Physiologic factors*: Pregnancy places the fetus and mother at increased risk of disease; obesity increases the risk of heart disease.
- *Lifestyle or health habits*: Overeating increases the risk of heart disease; smoking increases the risk of lung cancer; poor nutrition leads to several deficiencies; promiscuity increases the risk of sexually transmitted disease; excessive use of alcohol increases the risk of accident, liver disease, and disability; unabated stress increases the risk of accidents and illness; and certain activities such as skiing or mountain climbing increase the risk of injury.
- *Environment*: Exposure to specific hazards, such as asbestos, rubber, and plastic, increases the risk of certain kinds of cancer; unclean, overcrowded living conditions predispose people to infections and other communicable diseases; air, water, and noise pollution all increase susceptibility to illness.

All of these risks present challenges to health care workers, especially nurses, in terms of prevention. Measures to enhance health include maintaining ideal body weight; eating regular meals with few snacks; elimination of cigarette smoking; moderation of alcohol consumption; safety measures, such as using seat belts, to prevent accidents and injuries; and periodic screening for such health problems as cancer.

Health field concept view, all causes of death and disease have four contributing elements: (a) human biologic factors, such as genetic makeup and age; (b) behavioral factors or unhealthy lifestyles; (c) environmental hazards; and (d) inadequacies in the health care system. Using these four elements as a framework, a group of experts devised a method to assess the relative contributions of each of these elements to the ten leading causes of death. The results indicated that approximately 50% of deaths were due to unhealthy behavior or life-style; 20% to human biologic factors; 20% to environmental factors; and 10% to inadequacies in health care. These results have implications for nursing; the most important is that a substantial number of deaths could be avoided by efforts directed at health promotion and illness prevention.

Traditionally, medical practitioners have dealt with disease at a subsystem level. Subsystems are those aspects of the body subsystemed in the larger system of the whole body. A subsystem may be a cell, an organ, or an organ system. Only recently medical practitioners started looking at the person as an entity, or whole. Nurses, by contrast, have traditionally viewed the person as an entity, taking a holistic view of people. Nursing practice today is based on the multiple causation theory of health problems. Unemployment, pollution, lifestyle, and stressful events, while not disease, may all contribute to illness. These can be considered suprasystem problems, i.e., problems stemming from systems in which the individual is a subsystem. Thus, the concept of illness must include all aspects of the total person as well as the biologic and genetic factors that contribute to disease. Illness, then, is influenced by a person's family, social network, environment, and culture.

ILLNESS BEHAVIOR STAGES

Illness behavior is "any activity, undertaken by a person who feels ill, to define the state of his health and to discover a suitable remedy." Illness behavior depends on the way in which the person perceives illness, and it is selectively affected by multiple modifiers of patterning. For example, age, gender, occupation, socioeconomic status, religion, ethnicity, psychological stability, personality, education, meaning attached to symptoms, methods of coping with anxiety, attitude toward self, prior health-illness experiences, availability of resources, and degree, type, and duration of current stress situations are all factors that may be related to illness behavior.

Various scientists have described the stages of illness. By knowing these stages and the illness behaviors that accompany them, nurses can better understand their clients' behavior and determine ways to assist them. Illness behavior is "any activity undertaken by a person who feels ill, to define the state of his health and to discover a suitable remedy." How people behave when they are ill is affected by many variables, such as age, sex, occupation, socio-economic status, religion, ethnic origin, psychologic stability, personality, education and modes of coping. Such man describes five stages of illness as given below:

Symptom Experience Stage

The symptom experience stage is the transition stage during which people come to believe something is wrong. Either a significant person mentions that they look unwell, or people experience some symptoms, which can appear insidiously. The symptom experience stage has three aspects:

1. The physical experience of symptoms (e.g., pain or elevated temperature)
2. The cognitive aspect (the interpretation of the symptoms in terms that have some meaning to the person)
3. The emotional response (e.g., fear or anxiety).

During this stage, unwell persons usually consult others close to them about their symptoms or feelings. People validate with their spouses or support persons that the symptoms are real. At this stage, sick persons sometimes try home remedies, such as laxatives or cough medicines.

Assumption of the Sick Role

The second stage signals acceptance of tile illness. At this time, individuals decide that their symptoms or concerns are sufficiently severe to suggest that they are sick. Some people seek professional help quickly; others continue self-treatment, often following the suggestions of family and friends.

In this stage, sick people are usually afraid, but they now accept that they are ill even though they may not be able to accept the possible reasons. In conferring with people close to them, sick people seek not only advice but also support for the decision to give up some activities and, for example, stay home from work.

At the end of this stage, sick people experience one of two outcomes. They may find that the symptoms have changed and that they feel better. If family members support the perceptions of such persons, they are no longer considered or consider themselves sick. Then the recovered persons resume normal obligations, such as returning to work or attending a school concert.

If, however, the symptoms persist or increase and if lack of improvement is validated by the family or significant others, then sick people know they should seek some treatment. The choice of a treatment plan is often affected by the known available alternatives and previous experience.

Medical Care Contact Stage

Sick people seek the advice of a health professional either on their own initiative or at the urging of significant others. When people go for professional advice they are really asking for three types of information:
1. Validation of real illness
2. Explanation of the symptoms in understandable terms
3. Reassurance that they will be all right or prediction of what the outcome will be.

If the health professional does not validate illness, people have two recourses: to return to normal activities or to seek other advice. If the symptoms disappear, people often perceive that they really are not ill. If symptoms continue, people usually return to the health professional or go to a second person for care. People who are repeatedly told that they are not ill, may seek out quasi practitioners as a last resort to alleviate the perceived symptoms. Some people will go from health professional to health professional until they find someone who provides a diagnosis that fits their own perceptions.

Most people also want an understandable explanation of their symptoms. When symptoms are not explained, people may assume the health professional does not believe them or perhaps that they are imagining the symptoms. Overly technical explanations, however, often confuse and frighten people.

People often experience anxiety about seeking help with health problems. Even minor symptoms can be construed as serious. Therefore, clients need reassurance that they will be cured. Even when this reassurance cannot be given, most people want to know the likely outcome.

Dependent Patient Role Stage

When a health professional has validated that the person is ill, the individual becomes a client, dependent on the professional for help. During this stage, sick people may or may not be reluctant to accept a professional's recommendations. They may vacillate about what is best for them and alternately accept and reject the professional's suggestions. People vary greatly in the degree of ease with which they can give up their independence, particularly in relation to life and death. Role obligations—such as those of wage earner, father, mother, student, baseball team member, or choir member—complicate the decision to give up independence.

It is also common for the client and the health professional to hold different notions of the nature of the illness, unless complete and open communication exists. During this stage, a nurse can often provide information that may allay some fears and/or provide data that support the person. Misconceptions can result from limited information, which clients interpret in the light of their experiences. For example, a woman may be told by a physician that there is a small encapsulated growth in the right groin and that surgical removal is advised. If the woman's mother died after being told she had a growth in her breast, that person may assume that she also will die.

Most people accept their dependence on the physician, although they retain varying degrees of control over their own lives. For example, some people request precise information about their diseases, their treatment, and the cost of treatment, and they delay the decision to accept treatment until they have all this information. Others prefer that the physician proceed with treatment and do not request additional information.

During this period, sick people often become more passive and accepting. They require a predictable environment in which people are genuinely concerned about them. In addition to being concerned about themselves, some sick people regress to an earlier behavioral stage in their development. As a result, they may have fewer coping mechanisms (physical and emotional adaptive or defensive abilities). Frequently reactions are related to previous experiences and to misconceptions about what will happen.

People have varying dependence needs. For some, illness may meet dependence needs that have never been met and thus provide satisfaction. Other people have minimal dependence needs and do everything possible to return to independent functioning. A few may even try to maintain independence to the detriment of their recovery.

Recovery or Rehabilitation Stage

During this fifth stage, the client learns to give up the sick role and return to former roles and functions. For people with acute illnesses, the time as an ill person is generally short, and recovery is usually rapid. Thus, most find it relatively easy to return to their former lifestyles. People who have long-term illnesses and who must make adjustments in lifestyle may find recovery more difficult. Recovery is particularly difficult for people who have to relearn skills such as walking or talking.

During this stage, readiness for social functioning may not coincide with physical readiness. People may be physically able to go out to dinner but find that functioning socially is still too stressful or they may find that they have the desire to perform activities but not the strength. Nurses can help clients function with increasing independence by planning with them those functions they can accomplish by themselves and those with which they need assistance. It is also important for nurses to convey an attitude of hope and to support the client's return to health.

SICK ROLE BEHAVIOR

Sick role behavior is "the activity undertaken by those who consider themselves ill, for the purpose of getting well." Parsons describes four aspects of the sick role:

1. Clients are not held responsible for their condition.
2. Clients are excused from certain social roles and tasks.
3. Clients are obliged to try to get well as quickly as possible.
4. Clients or their families are obliged to seek competent help.

Many Indians believe that illness, though undesirable, is beyond a person's control and that individuals are not responsible for incurring an illness. Some subcultures view illness as punishment from God, and therefore consider the infirm responsible for their illnesses, because of their sins. This folk belief persists to some degree in Indian society. A client may say something like, "What have I done to deserve this?" This remark reflects a sense that illness is a punishment. Today, because of the recognition that lifestyle contributes to illness and disease, some people-for example, the cardiac client who smokes or the overweight person who develops diabetes-are being held increasingly responsible for developing some illnesses.

Nurses can help clients by providing factual information and by not judging the client. It is important to encourage behaviors that promote health and not to reinforce behaviors that may have helped bring about an illness.

The sick person is usually excused from some normal duties. Social pressures on the sick and people's expectations of the sick usually depend on the prognosis and the severity of the illness. People who are severely ill and whose prognosis is poor or uncertain are permitted more dependence than people who are less seriously ill. People who are not seriously ill and whose prognosis is good are more likely to be encouraged to fulfill personal and social responsibilities. The person with a cold may still be expected to give a scheduled speech or to take an examination. People who are chronically ill may be permanently exempted from some duties or activities by society.

Some people may express feelings of guilt because they are unable to fulfill their normal responsibilities. Nurses can express support to clients who cannot fulfill their perceived roles and help them substitute other appropriate activities, when desirable. For example, a young father who cannot play ball with his son may be able to help his son build a model airplane, thereby fulfilling the father's role in another way.

Another aspect of the sick role is the obligation of the person to get well as quickly as possible. The sick role is a dependent one, at least in some respects. The person who fears dependence may be threatened by assuming a sick role and having to seek help. This individual might ignore advice despite the most serious consequences. Some people, however, find dependence gratifying, some clients find dependence so satisfying that they perpetuate the sick role and do not try to get well or continue to complain of symptoms even after they are physically well. Some people in the dependent stage also find it satisfying to control others through excessive demands. With exceptions, people usually try to get well as quickly as possible.

Nurses can help clients assume a dependence appropriate to their developmental status and health. Part of the nurse's function is to reinforce both dependence and increasing independence at the appropriate times. For example, a man who is acutely ill may have to be shaved by the nurse; however, once he is stronger the nurse can assist him by providing shaving supplies and later complimenting him on his appearance.

An essential aspect of the sick role is seeking competent help. This presupposes that competent help is available to the client. It should also be recognized that the client's notion of competent help may be different from the general population's. For example, a man with a whiplash injury may become dissatisfied with his physician's treatment because of his slow recovery and may go to a healer who uses hypnotism. Or a domineering, talkative woman may reject advice to see a therapist and decide instead to join a cult of young people, considering the members of the cult competent help.

Nurses need to encourage some people to obtain competent heir from health professionals. Nurses who are aware of the health facilities available in a community can assist people to obtain care. People may require considerable support before seeking assistance because, for example, they fear the health problem might be serious or they believe competent help might not be available. A nurse's function in these instances is to provide accurate information about available health facilities while recognizing clients' beliefs and their right to hold them.

EFFECTS OF HOSPITALIZATION

Normal patterns of behavior generally change with illness; with hospitalization, the change can be even greater. Hospitilization usually disrupts a person's privacy, autonomy, lifestyle, rules, and finances.

Loss of Privacy

When a client enters a hospital or nursing facility, the loss or privacy is instantly obvious. Privacy has been described as a comfortable feeling reflecting a deserved degree of social retreat. Its dimensions and duration are controlled by the individual seeking the privacy. It is a personal internal state that cannot be imposed from without.

People need varying degrees of privacy and establish boundaries for privacy; when these boundaries are crossed, they feel invaded. Hospital personnel sometimes show little concern for clients' privacy. Clients are asked to provide information that often they consider private; they may share a roam with strangers; and their health is frequently discussed with many health professionals.

The boundaries of privacy are highly individual. The adult who lives alone may he used to privacy while eating, sleeping, and reading. A child from a large family may be accustomed to sharing these activities with others. It is important for nurses to ascertain what privacy means to the individual and try to support accustomed practices whenever possible.

Altered Autonomy

Autonomy is the state of being independent and self-directed without outside control. People vary in their sense of autonomy; some are accustomed to functioning independently in most of their life activities, while others are more accustomed to direction from others. An example of the Basanth is a writer who lives alone and works independently. By contrast, a wife in a patriarchal home may be accustomed to having decisions made by her husband and receiving direction from him.

Hospitalized people frequently give up much of their autonomy. Decisions about meals, hygienic practices, and sleeping are frequently made for them. This loss of individuality is often difficult to accept, and the client may feel dehumanized into "just a piece of machinery." Nurses have a major responsibility to humanize care by learning about the client as a person and by individualizing nursing care plans.

Altered Lifestyle

Hospitalization marks a change in life style. Many hospitals determine when people wake up and when they sleep. The woman who normally rises at 8:00 am and the man who usually works until 11:00 pm must change their habits. Food in a hospital is usually mass produced, and individual differences in taste are not always accommodated. Occasionally hospitals have relatively large populations from a particular culture and make special food arrangements. However, individual preferences are not always met.

Nurses can help clients adapt to life in a hospital in several ways:
- Providing explanations about hospital routines.
- Making arrangements wherever possible to accommodate the client's life-style, such as providing a bath in the evening rather than in the morning.
- Encouraging other health professionals to become aware of the person's life-style and to support healthy aspects of that life-style.
- Reinforcing desirable changes in practices with a view to making them a permanent part of the client's life-style.

Economic Burden

Hospitalization often places a genuine financial burden on clients and their families. Even though many people have health insurance, it may not reimburse all costs; in addition, many lose wages while they are hospitalized. Nurses can be aware of these costs and provide care that is as economical as is safely possible; for instance, they can use only the minimum supplies necessary for safe care. In some agencies, nurses may initiate referrals to the social service department to assist clients in making arrangements to address the financial burdens imposed by hospitalization. When this is not an independent nursing function, the nurse should consult with the client's physician to obtain such a referral.

EFFECTS OF ILLNESS ON FAMILY MEMBERS

A person's illness affects not only the person who is ill but also the family or significant others. The kind of effect and its extent depend chiefly on three factors: (a) which member of the family is ill, (b) how serious and long the illness is, and (c) what cultural and social customs that family follows.

The changes that can occur in the family include the following:
- Role changes
- Task reassignments
- Increased stress due to anxiety about the outcome of the illness for the client and conflict about unaccustomed responsibilities
- Financial problems
- Loneliness as a result of separation and pending loss
- Change in social customs.

Each member of the family is affected differently depending upon which member of the family is ill, because each plays a different role in the family and supports the family in different ways. Parents of young children, for example, have greater family responsibilities than parents of grown children.

The degree of change that family members experience is often related to their dependence on the sick person. For example, when a child is ill, there are few changes other than added responsibilities directly related to the child's illness. When the mother is ill, however, many changes are often necessary because other family members must assume her functions.

Sick Elderly Persons

When an elderly person is ill, a son or daughter often assumes the role of parent to the elderly person, providing housing, meals, and assistance with daily needs over a prolonged time. In other words, the parent-child roles are frequently reversed. This role reversal may be only temporary and may end when the illness ends, or it may become permanent.

The whole family, particularly the spouse of the sick person, experiences stress and concern about the outcome of the illness. Usually, the sick person's spouse feels a pending loss or separation most keenly. After a marriage of 50 at 60 years, elderly people may find it difficult to envisage what life will be like without a husband or wife. Younger persons in the family may deal with serious illness in an elderly person by stating, "He has led a good life" or "She had so much pain the past years." In this way, the young prepare themselves for that person's death. This same reasoning is rarely applied to a child or younger adult who is ill.

When an elderly person is ill, adult sons and daughters may face conflicting responsibilities. A daughter who lives some distance away needs to maintain her job and look after her own family, but at the same time her parents need her in another city. How often should she visit? How should she fulfill her responsibilities? These questions pose problems for many families today who live far apart.

The financial problems of the sick elderly can be a major problem for a family as well as a community. Because illness in this age group tends to be chronic, the costs of illness are often considerable. The greatest change in life-style is that the family must now allot time for hospital visits to the elderly relative.

Sick Parents

When the sick person is a parent, the degree to which the family experiences change is related to the responsibilities the individual has and the number and age of dependents in the person's care. For example, when a father is ill for a long time, his roles are usually taken over by other members of the family, frequently the mother. Such tasks as doing chores in the house or attending a child's basketball games, for example, are either reassigned or not performed at all. Anxiety of family members about the outcome of a parent's illness is usually high, especially if the parent is a wage earner. The implications to the family of prolonged illness or death are great in almost all areas of living because of the needs of the dependents.

Prolonged illness of the mother can have equally serious consequences. Often the children do not understand why their mother is in the hospital, and they may feel lonely and unwanted. Sometimes the mother's functions are taken over by grandparents or by aunts and uncles as well as by the father. When a young mother has a serious illness of unknown outcome, the father and family face worrisome problems of how to manage over a long period of lime. Most arrangements have financial implications and involve role changes for the father and children. In this situation, the father must become both father and mother and give up many of his normal social activities. The children may also need to assume more housekeeping functions.

Sick Children

Because a child is dependent on parents for so many daily needs, both sick children and their families may need to make fewer role adjustments than sick adults and their families. Task reassignments are also generally minimal. Sometimes a younger sibling takes over a paper route for a sick brother or sister, and other members of the family share the sick child's chores.

INFECTION AND INFLAMMATION

Infection

"Infection is a dynamic process involving invasion of the body by pathogenic micro-organisms and reaction of the tissues to organisms and their toxins." Contamination is mere presence of organism at any site without invasion and without features of inflammation.

Process of Nosocomial (hospital) infection results from the transmission of pathogens to a previously uninfected patient from a source in the hospital environment which is also a cross infection. The pathogens may also come form the patient himself (autoinfection). He may be a carrier of the pathogen or may become contaminated with virulent hospital strains during stay in the hospital. Nosocomial infections are iatrogenic when the source is the attending physician or surgeon and the team or measures adopted viz. frequent or prolonged use of supportive procedures such as indwelling venous or urinary catheters, tracheostomy tubes, and equipments for respiratory care. Nosocomial infection increases morbidity, mortality, stay and expense of the patient and worriers of the relatives.

A surgical infection is an infection which requires surgical treatment of surgical treatment and essentially is a wound infection.

Causative Agent

A variety of organisms may be responsible for wound infections. Pathogenic bacteria infecting wounds are:
- ***Aerobic bacteria:***
    - Gram-positive cocci—*Streptococci*, and *Staphylococci*.
    - Gram-positive bacilli—*C. diphtheriae*.
    - Gram-negative bacilli—*B. pyoscyaneus, E. coli, B. proteus*.
- ***Anaerobic bacteria:***
    - Gram-positive cocci—*Streptococci*.
    - Gram-positive bacilli—*Clostridia tetani, Clostridia welchii, Clostridia botulinum*, etc.
- ***Microaerophilic bacteria:*** *Streptococci*.

The micro-organisms commonly encountered in surgical infections are staphylococci, streptococci, clostridia, bacteroides, and the enteric bacteria.

Sources of Infection

The sources of bacteria which may come in contact with the wounds are:
- The air and dust.
- The nose, throat, mouth, skin of surgeon and the team.
- The skin and other focal septic sources of the patient.
- Materials used for toileting or dealing with the wound or in the operation field viz., instruments, swabs, threads, dressings, etc. In traumatic wounds the source of infecting bacteria are patient's skin or clothing or foreign body. In surgical wound the infection begins in the operation room, the sources being poor aseptic technique (including sterilization), excessive tissue trauma, incomplete hemostasis, etc.

Mode of entry: Sexual or close contact, skin to skin contact, parenneral fluid, through oral and respiratory passage, etc.

Effects of Infection

Mode of Entry: The injurious effect of infection is due to the released toxins by bacteria. They may be either exo or endotoxins. Exotoxins are specific soluble diffusible proteins produced by gram-positive bacteria during the growth of organism, e.g., *Clostridia* group, *Streptococci, Staphylococci, C. diphtheriae, Shigella dysenteriae, Endotoxins* are produced by the organisms and are kept inside the body. These are liberated after their death, e.g., *Salmonella typhi, E.coli,* bacteroides. Most of the common pathogenic organisms produce endotoxin.

All these toxins have both toxicogenic action and property of inducing production of antibody in the host. When these toxins are isolated and toxic property is destroyed they can be used to produce antibodies in the host after destroying their toxic property only. These are called toxoids. The effects of toxins may be local or general.

Effects: Local effects are due to (i) increased vascularity, (ii) vascular thrombosis, (iii) tissue oedema, (iv) fibrinolysis, (v) duppuration and (vi) necrosis.

The general effects are due to bacteremia, toxaemia, septicaemia or pyaemia.

Inflammation

"It is the reaction which occurs in immediate response to irritation or injury usually manifested locally." The aim is to neutralize or remove the irritant.

The classical features of inflammation are redness, swelling, heat, pain, and *impairment or loss of function* of that part.

Fever and chills indicate septicaemia, while elevated pulse rate is a sign of a toxic state.

Leukocytosis accompanies an acute bacterial infection more often than a viral infection. The more severe the infection the greater is the leukocytosis. In most infections the total leukocyte count is only slightly or moderately elevated.

Some common surgical infections and conditions:

Cellulitis is a nonsuppurative inflammation of the subcutaneous tissue.

Lymphangitis is an inflammation of lymphatic pathway. This is usually visible as erythematous streaking of the skin in fair complexion subject and is commonly seen in infection by haemolytic streptococci.

Erysipelas is an acute spreading cellulites and lymphangitis, usually caused by haemolytic streptococci which gain entrance through a break in the skin.

An abscess is a localized collection of pus surrounded by an area of inflamed tissue. A furuncle or boil is an abscess in a sweat gland or hair follicle.

Impetigo is an acute contagious skin disease characterized by the formation of intraepithelial abscesses.

A ***curbuncle*** is a multilocular suppurative condition in the subcutaneous tissues. The nape of the neck, dorsum of trunk, hands and digits are common sites. It is also called infective gangrene. This is commonly seen in diabetic persons.

Most abscesses are caused by pyogenic cocci. Commonest is *Staphylococcus aureus.*

Bacteremia is defined as presence of bacteria in the circulating blood.

Septicaemia is the condition in which bacteria multiply in the blood stream, e.g., Salmonella, E. coli, Ps. pycocyneus, streptococci, staphylococci, proteus, etc.

Pyaemia is when pyogenic micro-organisms are carried in the blood stream in the form of bacterial emboli or as infected clots to different parts of body where these initiate multiple focal abscesses.

In *toxaemia* toxins are circulating in the blood, e.g., in diptheria, tetanus and dysentery.

ASEPSIS

Asepsis can be defined as exclusion of organisms from coming in contact with the wound or operation field. It is basis of modern surgery. *Louis Pasteur is called the father of aseptic surgery* as he was the first to discover presence of microbes in the air and contamination by them.

- *Medical asepsis*: Those practices by which spread of infection from a diseased person is prevented. All articles coming in contact with the patient are rendered free form pathogenic organisms but are not necessarily sterile.
- *Surgical asepsis*: Indicates that all objects coming in contact with the patient are absolutely free from all organisms pathogenic and non-pathogenic, including sporebearers.

Sepsis: It denotes presence of infection.

Antisepsis is killing of all organisms already present in the wound. *J Lister* first started antiseptic measures by disinfection of sewage, etc. with carbolic acid and is *called the father of antiseptic surgery.*

For carrying out proper asepsis and antisepsis several rituals have to be observed.

Methods of Asepsis

- Designing of operation theatre: It should be air-conditioned, dustless, well ventilated with planned circulation of air. Regular cleaning and disinfection of wall. Separate septic and aseptic operation theatres and standardized operation theatre complex.
- Movements in operation theatre: should be restricted.
- Over crowding in operation theatre has to be avoided.
- Nasal carriers should be detected and are not allowed to enter operation theatre.
- Surgical team should no handle infected wound, burns or colostomy wound before going for an operation.
- Proper cleaning (including paring of nails) or surgical team and putting on sterilized gowns, masks, caps, gloves, etc.
- Proper preparation of the patient (vide pre-operative prep).

- Sterilisation of instruments.
- Sterilisation of drugs as and when necessary.

Methods of Antisepsis
- Local treatment of wound – by cleaning, debridement, excision, application of medicines in the form of powder, drugs, lotion, ointments, packs, drainage, etc.
- General – Administration of drugs viz., antibiotics, chemotherapy (bactriostatic or bactericidal), etc.

Sterilisation

Sterilisation is killing of al sorts of micro-organisms including bacteria, viruses, spirochaete, fungi, parasites and spores.

Disinfection – is killing of all organisms except spores.

Disinfectant – is a chemical substance of germicidal nature used to kill pathogenic micro-organisms of inanimate objects.

Antiseptic – is also a chemical agent but differs from disinfectant in a sense that these inhibit growth of micro-organisms so long they are in contact with them.

Methods of Destruction of Bacteria

All pathogenic organisms can be destroyed by any of the following methods as given below:

Natural Method

Sunlight: The heat of sunlight have a drying or dehydrating effect on the organisms which enables it to destroy the germs. This method is not effective unless the contaminated articles are exposed for 2-3 days continuously and hence is not usually applicable.

Physical Method
- Dry heat:
  - Electric (hot air oven) – By special electric ovens in the form of hot air at 121°C for 6 hours (commercial). Materials – Glasswares, vaselin, fats, talc, oils, carbon steel materials.
  Linen, rubber or plastic articles are not sterilized in this method.
  - *Flaming* – Contaminated noninflammable articles are sometimes disinfected by smearing with methyllated spirit and then flaming. This method destroys only surface bacteria and can be used in case of grave emergency or when no other way of disinfection is possible, e.g., tray, blunt instruments.
  - *Burning or incineration* – Contaminated articles of *highly infectious diseased patients* are burnt to kill the micro-organisms and prevent spread of infection, e.g., mattress, pillow, bed linens used by tetanus or gas gangrene patient.
- *Moist heat:*
  - *Boiling* – This is one of the commonest method of destruction of micro-organisms. In this, bacteria are killed within 5 to 30 minutes, e.g., syringe. Almost all instruments except sharp, rubber goods, silk, nylon, etc.
  - *Chemical method* – Chemical substances, called disinfectants are also used to kill pathogenic organisms. The stronger the chemical the lesser is the time required for disinfection. Common disinfectants are Lysol, carbolic acid, formalin.

The choice and action of disinfectants depend on:
- The type of article to be disinfected, e.g., metal, rubber, or linen.
- The nature and strength of agent used and its effect on the qualities, e.g., effet of Lysol 1:20 and carbolic 1:40 and its stability in the presence of organic matter.
- Time required for disinfection by the chemical to act effectively.
- Nature of solvent used and its temperature.
- Nature of contamination, the number and virulence of organisms.
- The cost of the chemical to be used.

For practical purposes – Two common methods are there for sterilization – chemical and heating. A combination of pressure and heat is undertaken for a special advantage that pressure increases heat and power of penetration is more. The different methods are briefly tabulized.

Autoclaving – For materials that will stand up to heat and moisture. In this method with increased pressure, temperature of water can be raised. This the most reliable method because of the power of penetration, microbiologic efficiency, easy control, and economy. 15lb pressure per sq. inch for 15–45 minutes at 121°C destroys al forms of organisms.

Materials sterilized – Almost all materials except glass wares, vaseline, fats, talc, oils, etc.

There are two types:
1. Those with gravity displacement of air.
2. Those with high vacuum sterilizer.

Steam with – Formaldehyde at subatmospheric pressure sterilization is done at a temperature below 90°C at 10 lbs pressure for 10 mts. All spores are killed when formaldehyde vapour is used. It is a modified autoclave system.

Pasteurisation – Is the method where materials are sterilized in thermostatically controlled water bath at 75–80°C for 10 minutes, e.g., Endoscope.

Irradiation – Gamma ray is used for sterilization in industry – Irradiation is from a cobalt 60 source or electron bormbardment from a linear accelerator.

Mateials sterilized – viz. disposable hospital supplies, plastic, syringes, sutures-catgut, etc.

Ethylene oxide gas – for heat labile article – This is also commercial.

Materials – delicate surgical instruments with optical lenses, plastic parts of heart lung machine, etc.

Chemicals – common solutions used are iodine, Lysol, carbolic acid, hibitane, cetrimide 1%, 2% glutaraldehyde.

Materials

- For sterilization of living tissues catguts, etc.
- Sharp instruments in pure Lysol for half an hour, etc.

ROLE OF NURSES IN SURGICAL SETTINGS

General Pre-Operative Nursing Care

This is preparing a patient for a surgical procedure. The pre-operative period is the time during which a person is prepared for surgery. This period varies in length and depends on the patient's condition. Surgery is a traumatic event for most patients. The better the patient is prepared and instructed for surgical procedure the easier is his post-operative course and the shorter is the convalescence.

Psychological consideration: Surgery is viewed as a crisis in life. Emotional responses to surgery may be manifested in various ways. Some patients may be talkative, some withdraw and some other may show non-adoptive responses. After assessing the patient carefully, appropriate nursing intervention can be planned.

A complete assessment of health status is a part of a preparation for surgery.

- *The patient's age*: The young and old are less able to cope with stresses.
- *Nutritional, water and electrolyte status*: Surgical risk is increased when the patient is malnourished and dehydrated.
- *The presence of previous pathological condition*: The nurse should observe the signs of disease.
- *Special conditions affecting the surgical risk*:
  – Obesity – The surgical risk is higher than the patient with normal weight.
  – Acute infection – An acute infection anywhere in the body requires a delay in surgery in most instances to help prevent post-operative complications.
  – Drug therapy – The drugs which have profound effect are hypoglycaemic, hypotensive, psychic, anticoagulants, steroids, etc. Continued use of anticoagulants may cause serious haemorrhage. Steroids also have serious effects on surgical patients.
  – Addiction – Alcoholism – Withdrawal symptoms may develop when a patient suddenly is deprived of alcohol during the surgical experience. In smoking post-operative pulmonary complications are more.
  – Wasting diseases – In diabetes mellitus the stress accompany the surgery may increase the need for insulin.
  – Skin disease at the operative site should be treated prior to operation.

Nursing Intervention

The most important part in pre-operative management is health teaching. Teaching should include sharing information about purposes of various types of care the patient receives pre-operatively and post-operatively.

- *Diaphragmatic breathing.* This causes deep breathing and helps the patient ventilate thoroughly. It is carried out as follows:
  – The patient lies on low Fowler's position, flexing knees and placing his hands over his lower rib cage and on sides of the abdomen.
  – The patient exhales thoroughly, his ribs move downward with exhalation.
  – Then he takes deepest breath.
  – The patient holds the breath for 3–5 seconds after inhaling deeply.
  – Then he exhales through pursed lips holding in a manner as though he will whistle taking double the time to inhale action. The patient is helped to practice this breathing twice a day for at least 15 times in each sitting.
- *Coughing:*
  – The patient lies in Fowler's position or a side-lying position.
  – The patient's hands are placed on the incision area to splint the surgical wound.
  – The patient takes a deep diaphragmatic breath.
  – After inhalation the patient is asked to make two strong coughs while keeping the mouth open, tongue extended and hands in position.
  – The patient then takes another deep breath and gives two more strong coughs.
  – The patient pratices coughing at least two or three times a day.
- *Moving in bed:* The patient is placed on back and is asked to flex on knee to about 45° to 90° and holding this position for a few seconds to extend the leg. This is done alternately. These exercise are repeated four to five times every 3–4 hours.
- *Legal considerations:*
  – The patient is placed must be told about the operative procedures, risk, possible complications and what disfigurement can occur.
  – He should be informed what expect during post-operative period.
  – Operative consent is to be taken from the patient, in the presence of witness. Parents or a guardian must sign for minor.
- *Psychological preparation of the patient and family:* Most of the patients fear for surgery. Common fears include fear of death, unfavourable diagnosis,

disablement which may bring disruption in family lift, etc. There is worry about anaesthesia, loss of self control and financial and employment limitations.
- The nurse should have knowledge of the type of surgery the patient is to undergo to guide for preparing the patient both psychologically and physically.
- The patient is to be given opportunity to discuss his fear and concern. It also includes listening to what is being said as well as nonverbal communication. Touch when used appropriately conveys the message of showing an interest in what the patient is experiencing.
- It is important to consider each patient as an individual person. Each will respond emotionally to a surgical experience in his own way.
- The nurse should also prepare family members for the special equipment needed in the care of the patient. She should offer emotional support to family members.
  * Regular bath with soap or cleaning after admission.
  * Maintenance of oral and general hygiene.
  * Any infective fever should be treated.
  * Bowel should move regularly.
  * Fluid intake should be plenty. When necessary glucose drinks in large amount, e.g., in jaundice.
  * Adequate diet followed by light diet in evening before operation and nothing by mouth on the day of operation is the standard method unless ordered specially
  * Tranquiliser on the night before operation.
  * Infants, children are old-age require special care. Infant and children are susceptible to infection; they tolerate fluid and electrolyte imbalance badly and they may have congenital disorders. The elderly are prone to have pulmonary, cardiovascular, urinary and liver disorders which should be taken care of.
  * Pre-operative antibiotic administration to prevent risk of post-operative infection.
- *Preparation of the patient immediately pre-operatively:*
  - Skin preparation at the site of surgery – The area of the skin prepared is larger than the immediate area around the incision to reduce the chance of infection. Where applicable the hair in the operative area is shaved. Sterile dressing may be applied to the cleaned and shaved area.
  - Administration of a cleansing enema as ordered because a full colon can cause contamination during surgery. The patient may have an involuntary bowel movement if the lower intestinal tract is not emptied while he is being anaesthetized.
  - Checking of the vital signs. Any abnormality of vital sign should be reported promptly. Surgery may need to be cancelled if abnormalities are present.
  - Removing of patient's valuables such as rings and wrist watch. Removing of dentures, contact lenses, artificial limbs and eyes, wigs, hair pin, clips and coloured nail polish. Braiding the long hair and putting on the hospital's cloth.
  - The patient should void urine before going to operation theatre.
  - Administration of the pre-operative medication at the time ordered.
  - Completing the patient's record.
  - Helping to move the patient in stretcher after checking the patient's identity.
  - Accompanying the patient to the operative room and handing over the patient and records to be operation room nurses.
  - Special preparations are given as ordered for some surgical conditions viz. cardiothoracic surgery, urosurgery, etc.

Preparation of Bad Risk Patients

This includes those patients who have:
- Malnutrition
- Vitamin deficiency
- Anaemia
- Hypoproteinaemia
- Fluid and electrolyte intake
- Obesity
- Cardiac and respiratory diseases
- Wasting diseases, e.g., diabetes, tuberculosis, cirrhosis of liver, rheumatic arthritis.

These should be treated as far as practicable.

General Postoperative Nursing Care

- *Preparation of patient's room*: Recovery room should be in the same floor. The furniture should be so arranged that stretcher on which patient is transported can be moved near the patient's bed.

  Preparation of the operation bed is done with clean linens. All equipments that may be necessary should be available viz. oxygen, suction machine, sphygmomanometer, infusion fluids and shock blocks, airway, emergency medicines, etc.
- *Maintenance of pulmonary ventilation*: The patient should be in a position so that he can breath normally with full use of all portions of his lungs and that vomitus, blood and mucus can drain and will not be aspirated. They lying position on the side is preferred after the airway has been removed to facilitate drainage from mouth and nose.
- *Maintenance of circulation and prevention of shock*: As soon as the nurse is certain that the patient's airway is clear, she should check the blood pressure and pulse. The blood pressure, pulse and respiration are usually taken every 15 minutes for first 2 hours, then every half

hour for another 2 hours and eventually every 4 hours until further orders. The rate, volume and rhythm of the pulse should be carefully observed and character and rate of respiration noted. A rapid thready pulse with sudden drop of blood pressure may indicate haemorrhage or circulatory failure. The surgeon should be notified immediately. Oxygen may be given to increase its concentration in the available circulating blood

- *Protection from injury*: Following anaesthesia, side rails are usually placed on the bed and are left until the patient is fully awake. Hot water bottles, heating pads or heat lamps must be used with care while the patient is unconscious. When infusions are given, the patient's arm should be secured on an arm board so that needle is not dislodged. The patient should be turned frequently and placed in good body alignment to prevent:
  - Nerve damage from pressure and
  - Muscle and joint strain due to lying in the same position for a long period of time.
- *Facilitate breathing and prevent hypostatic pneumonia*: Frequent changing of position. Raise the head end of the bed as soon as the systolic BP rises to 100 mm of Hg. Steam inhalation every 6 hourly.
- The nurse must check for soakage or bleeding. She should also look for tubes of any kind and connect them in drainage system as ordered.
- *Maintenance of fluid and electrolyte balance*: An adult requires about 2.5 litres and as much salt as contained in 1 pint of normal saline and 70 g. of protein in 24 hours. This salt should be maintained when IV infusion is given.
- There should be complete and accurate intake/output charting in the post-operative period. All fluids, medications and treatments that the patient received during this time must be recorded so that there will be no duplication.
- The nurse can ascertain the return of reflexes and consciousness of the patient by asking him his name and others. The patient may be returned to his room as soon as his blood pressure is stable, he is breathing freely, not vomiting and fully awake.
- Retention of urine is a usual complain after perineal, rectal or hernia operation. An indwelling catheter pre-operatively introduced is safe, otherwise if conservative measures fail a self retaining catheter should be indwelled.
- *Vomiting*: This may occur after general anaesthesia. In abdominal operation if Ryle's tube is there suction prevents vomiting. Otherwise if needed may be introduced later. In other operations usually vomiting tendency passes off. Anitiemetics may be necessary.
- *Oral hygiene*: This is important to prevent parotitis, gingivitis, bad odour, etc.
- *Diet*: It is advised depending on abdominal or extra-abdominal operations. In abdominal operations only water is first allowed till flatus is passed. In other water is first allowed till flatus is passed. In other conditions fluid is allowed after some definite period.
- *Bowel*: No purgative is advised in abdominal operations. Suppositories in some cases viz. appendicectomy and enema in selected cases viz., after cholecystectomy are advised after 4th or 5th day usually. In extra-abdominal operations it is usually not a problem.
- *Ambulation*: Nowadays, early ambulation is advised. This helps psychological, physical and physiological improvement.
- *Wound care*: Usually dressing is changed when a drain has been left or there is wound infection. Otherwise it is changed during stitch removal.

INTENSIVE CARE UNIT

ICCU and Role a Nurse in that Special Unit

ICCU is the acronym for Intensive Coronary Care Unit. The meaning of "Intensive" is close and maximum care to selected needy patients to overcome the crisis by watching the vital signs on the monitors and managing accordingly to save a life and to prevent further complication.

Physical Setup of ICCU

The bed strength of ICCU depends on the hospital's policy. The ideal setup should be oval shaped so that all the patients can be watched from the central monitoring system. All the beds should have glass partition covered with curtains.

Bright lights should be avoided except in emergency. Attractive light, blue curtains can be used. In any case and quiet atmosphere should prevail in ICCU.

The nurse patient ratio should be 1:1, means one nurse for one patient. One doctor should be on duty round the clock in ICCU.

The nurses or doctors who are working in ICCU should not use outside shoes. Slippers should be provided. Masks should be used.

Each patient should have one bedside monitor which should be connected to the central monitoring system in the centre of the ICCU.

The central monitoring system should have –
- Monitoring scope or TV screen where all patients can be monitored together.
- Arrhythmia monitor – any type of arrhythmia can be monitored and recorded.
- Telemetry system of monitoring is the use of battery powered ECG transmitters that do not require direct connection of the patient to the oscilloscope.

Telemetry monitoring equipment is used in the ICCU as well as in the general medical surgical units for the ambulatory patients, hence the need for nurses to acquire some basic skills in rhythm interpretation.

A friendly behavior towards the patient and their relatives is required.

Types of Patients Admitted in ICCU

- *Cardiac:*
  - Acute myocardial infarction.
  - Congestive cardiac failure, left ventricular failure.
  - Pulmonary oedema.
  - Heart block.
  - After cardiovascular surgery.
- *Others:*
  - Some post-operative patients with respiratory failure or shock of grave concern.
  - Poisoning patients with respiratory failure.
  - Some patients after neuro-surgical operations.
  - Patients with cardiac arrest due to any cause.

Role of Nurse in ICCU

The nurse who is posted in ICCU, must have some knowledge of normal cardiac rhythm and cardiac arrhythmia for proper treatment and management.

- *Functions of nurses in ICCU*:
  - Monitoring of cardiac activity.
  - Meeting need for oxygen – By giving oxygen inhalation, keeping the airway clean, taking care of respirators, taking care of the tracheostomy tubes.
  - Vital signs – Like regular checking of pulse, temperature and kidney function.
  - Intake and output chart – To make sure of heart and kidney function.
  - Proper medication – In time and correct dose recording on the nurses chart.
  - Rest for the patient – mental and physical by ensuring calmness of the unit, comfortable bed, etc.
    Mental rest – by medicines or injections.
  - Special diet – Diet is very important – light and easily digestable diet to prevent extra burden on the heart.
  - Lab. Investigations – Both general and special tests of blood, urine, stool, skiagram.
  - Elimination – To keep bowel regular to avoid discomfort by giving mile laxatives, etc.
  - General physical care – Like backcare, mouth care, sponging, etc.
  - Ambulation – Doctors will instruct about the ambulation and gradual ambulation of the patient must be done.
  - Daily reporting and recording of the patients condition, medication, rhythm strip, etc. must be done so that the progress or deterioration can be determined.
  - Proper identification of complication and treatment.
- *Care of the operative wound if there be any.*

Wound and Its Healing

Wound may be defined as distruption or break in the continuity of epithelial tissue. It may be revealed on the surface, i.e., external or may be concealed (e.g., wound of a peptic ulcer). In common practice wound means external or visible wounds caused by injury.

Causative Factors

Commonly wound may be caused by trauma, inflammation, pressure (decubitus ulcer), diseases (ulcerative colitis), chemicals (corrosive), extensive heat, etc.

Effects

Temporary loss of functions of all or part of the organ, haemorrhage, setting up of local and general inflammatory response, death of cells (necrosis), infection.

Types

- *Depending on cause wounds are broadly classified as follows*:
  - Incised – Interruption of tissue is made with sharp cutting instrument, e.g., knife, blade, edges of paper. The edges of this type of wounds are straight. So they can be brought in close approximation and healing is better. All operative wounds are incised wounds. If proper care is taken before making the wound and afterwards it heals well.
  - Lacerated – Usually disruption of tissue occurs by trauma with jagged irregular edged machinery, vehicle accident, teeth or claws of animal. Skin margin is irregular. Visible bleeding is less but chances of getting contamination is very high. It is difficult to suture and takes more time to heal.
  - Punctured – A deep narrow wound resulting from injury by a pointed instrument. Though the external opening of the wound is very small but internal tissues at variable depth can be injured.
  - Contusion – Interruption in the continuity of a tissue is caused by trauma with a blunt object or blow or fall on a blunt object. Skin is not split and bruising of the surrounding tissue occurs. Underlying structures are likely to be damaged, e.g., in crush injury.
  - Abrasion – In this type superficial layer of skin gets scraped off as a result of sliding, fall or friction. A raw tender area results which can get infected very easily.
  - Penetrating – Wound results from bullet or a stab. As the bullet penetrates and enters deep cavities it

injuries internal organs followed by bleeding and infection. There may be point of entrance and point of exit. When both of them are there they are called perforating.
- *Depending on state of contamination*:
  – Aseptic wound
  – Potentially infected wound
  – Infected wounds.

Complications

- Shock – This varies in degree according to the size and number of wounds, amount of blood loss general condition and age of the patient.
- Haemorrhage.
- Infection – Septic fever is caused by the absorption of the bacterial toxins from an infected wound and is characterized by a persistent high temperature and other local and general symptoms of acute inflammation.
- Aseptic traumatic fever – is due to absorption of ferment liberated from extravasated blood. The temperature may rise to 100° to 101°F on the second day after injury or operation but usually subsides within 48 hours.
- Traumatic delirium – Delirium may occur in alcoholic subjects after injury or operation.

Healing of Wound

Healing means replacement of lost tissue by viable tissue. Replacement may be by repair or regeneration. Usually two types are considered:

1. *Healing by first intention or primary union*: This occurs in clean wound where there is no loss of tissue and minimum space is there between margins, e.g., incised wound.

   Healing takes place with minimum granulation tissue and minimum scar. This is achieved by proper asepsis, no soiling, no tension, thorough haemostasis and proper apposition of different layers.

   Acute inflammation set within first 24 hours. Plasma or serum exudation occurs into the wound which gets solidified and glues the edges together. The fibrin of the solidified plasma becomes infiltrated with fibroblasts which is due course gives rise to immature fibrous tissues. Appearance of collagen fibrils occur within 4–5 days after injury. Adjacent capillaries supply fresh blood. The immature fibrous tissue becomes organized and epithelia grow from the edges of the skin or mucus membrane migrate and cover the surface.

2. *Healing by second intention or secondary healing*: When, there is loss of tissue to great extent or a gap is there between edges granulation tissue develops from the side and bottom of the wound and gradually the cavity or gap is filled up. Copious discharge or pus formation may be there. This needs to be drained and healing starts after all discharges have been drained. The wound is filled scab forms and epithelium grows from margin underneath the scab. There is organization of the clot. This is followed by wound contraction by progressive fibrosis and cicatrisation of the fibrosed scar.

   Healing by secondary suture–Occasionally called healing by third intention. When wounds are grossly infected and primary sutures are without any effect or sutures have been applied late a secondary suture is necessary.

Factors Affecting Healing (Table 1.1)

Favourable Factors

- Accurate apposition under aseptic conditions and rest to the pat.
- Aseptic wound produced by sterilized instruments, e.g., at operation.
- Proper sterilization all materials used.
- Aseptic and antiseptic measures for the wound and surrounding tissue specially skin.
- Proper haemostasis.
- Provision for exit of collection (if any) by drainage tube or sheet.
- Dressing of the wound to prevent contact with air or clothing.
- Application of heat to the part to improve circulation.
- Elevation of the part to promote venous return.
- Nutritious diet.
- Prophylactic antibiotics.
- Correction of any persistent general or local cause.

Retarding Factors

- *General*: Old age, anaemia, hypoprotenaemia, cachexia, poor general health, wasting diseases viz. diabetes mellitus, use of steroids and anti-coagulants, immuno compromised patient and patient with hepatic and renal dysfunction.
- *Local*
  – Defective operative technique.
  – Contamination of the wound, defective closure and drainage of the wound.
  – Ischaemia of the part, local malignancy, tissue tension, presence of foreign body, lack of rest.

Common Sources of Wound Infection

In Operation Theatre

- Lack of knowledge regarding asepsis.
- Infected surgeon, nurse and technician.
- Dust and foreign materials on OT furniture (inadequate) carbolization.

Table 1.1: Factors affecting wound healing.

Factors	Rationale	Nursing Interventions
Age of patient	• The older the patient, the less resilient the tissues	• Handle all tissues gently
Handling of tissues	• Rough handling causes injury and delayed healing	• Handle tissues carefully and evenly
Hemorrhage	• Accumulation of blood creates dead spaces as well as dead cells that must be removed. The area becomes a growth medium for organisms	• Monitor vital signs. Observe incision site for evidence of bleeding and infection
Hypovolemia	• Insufficient blood volume leads to vaso-constriction and reduced oxygen and nutrients available for wound healing	• Monitor for volume deficit (circulatory impairment). Correct fluid replacement as prescribed
Local factors Edema	• Reduces blood supply by exerting increased interstitial pressure on vessels	• Elevate pate; apply cool compresses
Inadequate dressing technique		
• Too small	• Permits bacterial invasion and contamination	• Follow guidelines for proper dressing technique
• Too tight	• Reduces blood supply carrying nutrients and oxygen	
Nutritional deficits	• Protein-calorie depletion may occur. Insulin secretion may be inhibited, causing blood glucose to rise.	• Correct deficits; this may require parenteral nutritional therapy • Monitor blood glucose levels • Administer vitamin supplements as prescribed
Foreign bodies	• Foreign bodies retard healing.	• Keep wounds free of dressing threads and talcum powder from gloves
Oxygen deficit (tissue oxygenation insufficient)	• Insufficient oxygen may be due to inadequate lung and cardiovascular function as well as localized vasoconstriction	• Encourage deep breathing, turning, controlled coughing
Drainage accumulation	• Accumulated secretions hamper healing process	• Monitor closed drainage systems for proper functioning • Institute measures to remove accumulated secretions
Medications		
• Corticosteroids	• May mask presence of infection by impairing normal inflammatory response	• Be aware of action and effect of medications patient is receiving
• Anticoagulants	• May cause hemorrhage	
• Broad-spectrum and specific antibiotics	• Effective if administered immediately before surgery for specific pathology or bacterial contamination. If administered after wound is closed, ineffective because of intravascular coagulation	
Patient overactivity	• Prevents approximation of wound edges • Resting favors healing	• Use measures to keep wound edges approximate: taping, bandaging, splints • Encourage rest
Systemic disorders • Hemorrhagic shock • Acidosis • Hypoxia • Renal failure • Hepatic disease • Sepsis	• These depress cell functions that directly affect wound healing	• Be familiar with the nature of the specific disorder. • Administer prescribed treatment. Cultures may be indicated to determine appropriate antibiotic
Immunosuppressed state	• Patient is more vulnerable to bacterial and viral invasion; defense mechanisms are impaired	• Provide maximum protection to prevent infection. • Restrict visitors with colds; institute mandatory hand hygiene by all staff
Wound stressors • Vomiting • Valsalva maneuver • Heavy coughing • Straining	• Produce tension on wounds, particularly of the torso	• Encourage frequent turning and ambulation and administer antiemetic medications as prescribed • Assist patient in splinting incision

- Inadequate masking of nose and mouth, use of soiled clothing and shoes by operating team (improper cleaning of clothes), inappropriate scrub up.
- Improper cleaning of skin and improper draping.
- Long exposure and subsequent drying of skin edges and wound surface during an operation.
- Trauma to tissue by excessive clamping and manipulation, excessive handling and testing of suture materials.
- Prolonged hypotension during and soon after surgery due to poor tissue perfusion.

In the Ward

- Breaking principles of surgical asepsis while caring a wound.
- Lack of personal hygiene.
- Cross infection from other patients, relatives, doctors, nurse, etc.
- Injudicious use of antibiotics.
- Use of contaminated articles, use of same article for many patient.
- Inappropriate care for drainage bottle, etc.

Common Organisms of Wound Infections

A surgical wound may get infected by any of the following organisms–*Staphylococus, Streptococus-haemolytic* or non-haemolytic, *Clostridia, Pseudomonus, E. Coli,* etc.

Most common is *Staphylo. aureus* – which are found on the skin and live and grow in sweat and sebaceous glands. *Staphylo albus* – are responsible for stitch abscess. *Streptococci* do not cause wound infection normally. But accidental wound might get infected by haemoloytic streptococci. The most dangerous organisms which might cause wound infection are clostridia which cause gas gangrene or tetanus.

Symptoms and Signs of Wound Infection

- *Local*: Pain and tenderness, warmth, erythema, edema and often purulent discharge.
- *General*: Fever tachycardia, leucocytosis. Patient may be in a toxic state.

Methods to Reduce Wound Infection

Certain measures if adopted in time brings down rate of wound infection to a great extent. The nurse has an important role in reducing rate of infection.

- *The medical measures:*
  - To improve general health by nutritious diet, vitamins.
  - To treat preoperative infection.
  - To use antibiotics.
- Nursing measures are to be adopted at three levels: Preoperative, operative and post-operative.
  1. *Preoperative measures*
     - To encourage patient and relatives for short hospitalization.
     - To ensure that co-existant infection is treated before operation.
     - Limited shaving.
     - Shaving is to be done on the previous night usually.
     - Repeated antiseptic cleaning.
     - Prophylaxis antibiotic according to doctor's order.
  2. *Operative measure*
     - Meticulous cleaning and asepsis.
     - Proper carbolization of OT including furniture, machine, floor.
     - Adequate scrub up and use of properly clean, ironed clothings and shoes.
     - To ensure that no powder remains on gloves.
     - Proper draping and less handling of suture material.
     - Prompt assistance so that operation time is minimized
     - Proper haemostasis.
  3. *Postoperative measure*
     - Proper care of wound maintaining strict asepsis.
     - Daily observation of the wound with or without dressing.
     - Maintain personal hygiene, early ambulation, adequate fluid intake and nutritious diet.
     - Hyperbaric oxygen.
     - Wound drainage and debridement.

CHAPTER 2

Management of Common Signs and Symptoms

MANAGEMENT OF FLUID AND ELECTROLYTE BALANCE

Introduction

A fluid medium is essential for normal body function. It is the most vital and at the same time the most abundant component of the human body. Life depends upon a constant source and regulation of fluid in the body. Without fluid there would be no form of life.

Electrolyte balance is closely related to fluid balance. The fluid disturbance or electrolyte disturbance leads to fatality. Fluid deprivation brings about death more early than food deprivation.

Distribution of Fluid

The fluid is distributed in the body in three compartments that are separated by semipermeable membrane. This is roughly distributed as follows:

Intracellular fluid is within the cell and interstitial fluid surrounds all living cells and allows for diffusion of nutrients, electrolytes, water, hormones, oxygen and waste products. Intravascular fluid is within the blood vessels.

Normal Control of Body Fluid

Fluid intake: The body receives water from two sources:
- Exogenous – as drinks or wish solid foods.
- Endogenous – released during the metabolic oxidation.

The total fluid intake per day	
Water intake	1300 cc
Water from solid food	1000 cc
Water produce from internal metabolic oxidation	300 cc
Total	**2600 cc per 24 hours**

Total fluid (40 litres)
- Intracellular (25 litres)
- Extracellular (15 litres)
  - Interstitial space (10.0 litres)
  - Intravascular space (5.0 litres)

Fluid loss: Daily fluid loss of an average adult taking normal amount of fluid is usually through various sources as follows:

1. Lung — 400 cc
2. Kidney — 1500 cc
3. Skin — 600 cc (may be 1000 cc in hot climate)
4. Bowel — 100 cc
5. Negligible amount along saliva and tears --------------------

Total: 2600 cc per 24 hours

The fluid loss in babies and growing children are proportionately greater than that of an adult. Kidneys of an infant do not conserve water as effectively as the kidneys of an infant do not conserve water as effectively as the kidneys of adults. In older child and adult if the body needs water the pituitary antidiuretic hormone promotes its reabsorption from the renal tubules and excessive fluid intake is eliminated through the kidneys. If large quantity of fluid is taken rapid absorption of fluid into the plasma compartment takes place. Blood volume may be temporarily increased as well as an increase in cardiac output. There is rapid adjustment to the increased fluid.

The normal daily replacement of water equals the normal daily loss. Since daily turnover of water of a body is more than half of his extracellular fluid volume, it is essential that his fluid losses be replaced at once.

Body Electrolyte Component

All body fluids contain chemical compounds. Chemical compounds in solution may be classified as electrolytes or non-electrolytes. An electrolyte is a substance which when dissolves in water splits into separate electrically charged particles known as ions. Positively charged ions are called cations and negatively charged ions are called anions.

They are follows:

Cations	*Anions*
Sodium (Na^+)	Chloride (Cl^-)
Potassium (K^+)	Bicarbonate (HCO_3^-)
Calcium (Ca^{++})	Phosphates ($HPO_4^-, H_2PO_4^-$)
Magnesium (Mg^{++})	Sulphates (SO_4^-)

They are important in maintenance of acid base balance and help to control body water volume. Identical electrolytes are in three fluid compartments but the concentration of the various electrolytes in each compartment varies markedly.

In general higher the concentration of the ions the more active is the solution. Some electrolytes ionize freely and provide high concentration of ions and are known as strong electrolytes. Some others maintain a reserve of neutral molecules in the solution. These are known as weak electrolytes.

In health the ratio of cations to anions in each of the body fluids and concentration of the various ions in these fluids is relatively constant. Electrolytes move more readily between interstitial and intravascular fluid than between the intracellular and interstitial fluids.

Electrolyte loss is mainly through the kidneys. Besides this, smaller amount of loss is through the skin, lungs and bowel. The kidneys selectively excrete electrolytes, retaining those needed for normal body fluid composition. Hormones influence the selective function of kidney.

A well balanced diet contains all the substances need to maintain electrolyte balance. Any excess of electrolytes ingested will be excreted by the kidneys.

Responsibilities of a Nurse in Maintaining Fluid and Electrolyte Balance

Important nursing functions include:
- Assisting the doctor in evaluating patients fluid and electrolyte status.
- Helping in prevention of fluid and electrolyte imbalance by replacement therapy and relief of symptoms.
- Recognition and reporting early symptoms of fluid and electrolyte imbalance.
- To keep a fluid balance chart.

Determination of Fluid and Electrolyte Balance

Every patient who are receiving IV fluids should have a chart of fluid intake and output. This record should be accurate. It is critically studied to determine whether there is the expected ratio between intake and output or there is excess or deficit. Any marked change in ratio should be reported to the doctor.

Fluid given by any route should be spaced throughout the twenty-four hours period. Not only does this practice help to maintain normal body fluid levels but it provides for better regulation of the electrolyte balance by the kidney and prevents the end product of metabolism and toxic materials from being excreted in concentrated form. In this way the danger of renal damage, formation of calculi and irritation of the lower urinary tract are reduced. In addition fluid spacing prevents overloading of the circulation.

The intake record should show the type and volume of all fluids the patient has received and the route by which they are administered. The time should be noted. The output record includes urinary output, vomiting, gastric suction and drainage from any body cavity or wound. Blood loss from any part of the body should be measured carefully.

Though diaphoresis is difficult to measure yet careful note of heavy perspiration and its duration should be recorded (accurate recording of body temperature helps the doctor to determine how much fluid the patient needs). Since, fluid loss through the skin and lungs increases the temperature rises.

Daily weight record is a good indication of the onset of dehydration or of the accumulation of fluid. The patient must be weighed on the same time and each day with the same clothings.

Prevention of Electrolyte and Fluid Imbalance

- *Oral rehydration therapy*: The best way to restore water and electrolytes to the body is to give them by mouth. Oral rehydration therapy is based on the observation that glucose given orally enhances the intestinal absorption of salt and water and is capable correction the electrolyte and water deficit. The composition of oral fluid as suggested by WHO is as follows:

Sodium chloride (table salt)	3.5 g
Potassium chloride	1.5 g
Sodium citrate	2.9 g
Glucose (dextrose)	20.0 g
Potable water	1 liter

  Oral rehydration mixture are now free available. The contents of the packet are dissolved in one litre of drinking water and should be used within 24 hours.
- *Parenteral*: If oral route is not possible then the commonest method of replacement is by intravenous infusion. In case of infant it may be given into subcutaneous tissue if venous route is not possible. Concentrated solution of glucose should always be given IV in small amounts at time and slowly because they will pull fluid from the body to dilute themselves. Normal saline solution may cause fluid to diffuse from the tissues to equalize the concentration of salt in the fluid compartments. If any of these concentrated solutions flow quickly into the vascular system pulmonary oedema can develop rapidly. The initial signs of pulmonary oedema are bounding pulse, engorged peripheral veins, hoarseness, dyspnoea, chest pain, cough, etc.

Common Solution Used Parenterally

- Glucose 5% in distilled water is often used to maintain fluid intake or to re-establish blood volume.
- 4.3% dextrose and 0.18% saline may be used as Dextrose-saline. It is isotonic.
- Isotonic solution of sodium chloride (0.9%) usually is given to re-establish the blood volume.
- One-sixth molar lactate solution may be used when sodium but not chloride needs replacement.
- Balance solution containing several electrolytes may be used. Ringer's lactate solution, Hartmann's solution. Darrows solution are examples.

Recognition of Various Common Conditions

- *Water depletion (dehydration):* Occurs due to diminished intake, severe diarrhea, vomiting, intestinal obstruction.
  Features: (a) Thirst; (b) Weakness, exhaustion; (c) Low urine volume; (d) Dry wrinkled skin and mouth; (e) Vertigo; (f) Sunken eyes; (g) Mental confusion, delirium; (h) Coma
- *Water intoxication (water excess):* Occurs when excessive amount of water is given orally, intravenously or by other routes.
  Features: (a) Drowsiness, weakness; (b) Headache; (c) Giddiness, nausea, vomiting; (d) Breathlessness; (e) Abdominal cramps; (f) Confusion; (g) Pitting oedema (late); (h) Pulmonary oedema; (i) Convulsion and coma; (j) Low serum sodium concentration.
- *Hyponatraemia (low sodium-ion in plasma):* Common causes are intestinal obstruction, severe diarrhea, dysentery, cholera, ulcerative colitis, bilious, pancreatic or intestinal fistula.
  Features: (a) Headache; (b) Nausea and vomiting; (c) Muscular cramp, convulsion; (d) Weakness (e) Abdominal cramps; (f) Less sweating; (g) Sunken eyes; (h) Loss of elasticity of skin; (i) Cold extremities; (j) Fall of BP.
- *Hypernatraemia (Sodium excess):* When excess of normal saline or hypertonic saline has been given IV.
  Features: (a) Puffiness of face, weakness; (b) Accumulation of fluid in the various serous sacs and pitting oedema; (c) In infancy – increased tension in anterior fontanelle, oedema and increase in the number of urination.
- *Hypokalaemia (Postassium depletion):* Observed in ulcerative colitis, intestinal fistula, when intravenous alimentation is continued for more than 72 hours, in diabetic coma treated by insulin, in prolonged saline infusion together with nasogastric aspiration.
  Features: (a) Lethargy, drowsiness, slurred speech (b) Anorexia; (c) Constipation; (d) Polyuria due to incontinence; (e) Muscular weakness; (f) Mental confusion; (g) Distension of the abdomen; (h) Shock; (i) Weakness of heart muscles causing circulation to slowed down which may lead to cardiac arrest.
- *Hyperkalaemia (Potassium excess)* viz. in renal failure.
  Features: (a) Nausea; (b) Weakness of the muscles; (c) Colic; (d) Spasticity of muscles due to overstimulation, skeletal muscle spasm; (e) Irrigular and slow heart beat due to overstimulation of cardiac muscle; (f) Sudden cardiac arrest.
- *Metabolic alkalosis (bicarbonate excess)* – accompanies with electrolyte imbalance.
  Features: (a) Slow and shallow breathing; (b) Tetany; (c) Convulsion; (d) Confusion; (e) Coma.
- *Metabolic acidosis (bicarbonate deficit),* viz. in renal failure, shock.
  Features: (a) Dyspnoea, tiredness, weakness; (b) Deep and periodic breathing; (c) Stupor; (d) Coma.

MANAGEMENT OF FEVER

Fever is an abnormally high body temperature, usually accompanied by shivering, headache and in severe instances, delirium.

The normal temperature in the closed mouth lies between 36.0°C to 37.5°C (98.8-99.5°F) when the body is at rest. Skin temperature is usually lower than that of deeper structures of the body. The rectal temperature is higher by 0.3-0.6°C (0.6-1.2°F) and the axillary temperature is 0.5-1°C lower than the oral temperature.

Pyrexia or fever is an elevation of body temperature above normal.

- Low pyrexia 99°F - 101°F or 37.2°C-38.3°C.
- Moderate pyrexia 101°F-103°F or 38.3°C–39.4°C.
- High pyrexia 103°F-105°F or 39.4°C-40.5°C.
- Hyperpyrexia 105°F-40.6°F and above.

Fever is a disturbed condition of the body which accompanies a rise in temperature. Fever or pyrexia present when the body temperature is raised above normal. In healthy persons the body temperature remain very constant around 98.4°F (36.9°C) although a slight swing of 0.5°F (0.3°C) above or below this figure may be normal in some people.

The temperature of the body is the balance between the heat production by means of the general metabolism of various bodily functions and heat loss through skin, lungs and exertion. The heat regulating center in the brain is responsible for the constant level of the body temperature in health.

In infection, fever is one of the most constant and reliable signs. It is probably caused by the toxic products produced by the infecting organisms.

Acute diseases, particularly infections may result in a rise of temperature. Such a condition is called pyrexia. Psychological upset such as fear or anger and hot atmospheric conditions may produce slight rise of temperature. A lowered body temperature is called hypothermia. This condition is commonly seen in elderly people in the winter season and may be caused by cold, damp accommodation, poor diet, inadequate clothing and too little exercise. Newborn babies are also susceptible to hypothermia.

Etiology

Common Causes of Pyrexia

- Bacterial or virus infections, e.g., diseases such as typhoid fever, lobar pneumonia
- Foreign protein, e.g., inoculations with serum or vaccine
- Injury of any type and inflammation

- Sunstroke
- Cerebral haemorrhage
- Any acute infectious disease, e.g. typhoid, bronchopneumonia, viral pneumonitis, encephalitis, tonsilitis
- Malaria
- Measles
- Severe dehydration
- Severe salt depletion
- Rheumatic heart disease
- Diarrhea
- Head injury
- Alcohol intoxication.

Clinical Manifestations

- Skin is hot and dry, urine scanty and highly colored and often contains albumen
- Pulse is bounding and full at first and later becomes weak and rate increased
- Respiration rate is increased in proportion to the increase in temperature and pulse
- Mouth is dry, the tongue coated and there may be nausea and vomiting
- Loss of appetite and the patient may be usually constipated
- There may be headache, irritations, restlessness and in high pyrexia, delerium and coma may occur.

Signs and Symptoms of Pyrexia

- Onset of fever is sudden or gradual according to cause
- Loss of appetite, often nausea and vomiting are associated symptoms
- Headache accompanied by restlessness and delirium
- Malaise and sometimes pain all over the body
- Constipation or diarrhoea
- Photophobia
- Convulsion
- The skin is red, hot and dry
- Pulse and respiration rate is increased. In a few cases, like typhoid pulse rate is not increased
- The output of urine is decreased.

Although fever is an essential part of the defence mechanism, most doctors advise that a patient with a temperature over 38°C (100.4°F) should stay in bed since his respiratory and pulse rate are increased. Because headache and irritability often accompany severe systemic infection with high fever, the room should be kept quiet and glaring light dimmed. The patient should be encouraged to sleep. A warm sponge bath, back rub and a smooth bed may help to induce sleep. Bath is needed since more body waste may be excreted through increased perspiration. To prevent drying of the mucous membrane of the mouth and nose, vegetable oil may be used to lubricate the lips and nose, patient is encouraged to clean the mouth and to take generous amount of fluids.

In fever associated with infection, toxins are often excreted through kidneys, more fluid than usual is evaporated by perspiration from the skin and by rapid respiration, more fluids are needed for accelerated metabolism. Therefore, an adult patient is urged to take 2500 to 3000 ml of fluid per day. In addition to water, fluids high in calories and containing vit. C, protein, salts and potassium, if not contraindicated by the disease, should be taken by the patient because they help to supply the body's metabolic an electrolyte needs. Solid food usually are not palatable to the patient with fever, but may be given if desired. At any cost, adequate rest and additional fluid intake are inevitable for the patient with fever.

Nursing Management

The nursing management of the patient with fever includes the following:

- **Isolation:** Isolation procedure is necessary only if the fever is due to some infections diseases. The fundamental aim of isolation is to prevent the spread of infection to others including nurse herself. The patient is nursed in a separate isolation cubicle. In some cases barrier nursing is implemented in a general ward selecting a corner bed near a window and separated by a screen with all precautions to prevent the spread of infection.
- **Rest:** In all cases of fever except in very mildest the patient is kept in bed because making a person to lie on bed is the only possible way of ensuring rest. The room should be well ventilated without draught. Proper ventilation prevents the risk of infection as well as add comfort to the patient. Temperature of the room most comfortable (5° to 19°C).

  Clothes should be loose garments. Position depends upon the nature of illness. If the lungs are likely to be affected upright position and if the heart is likely to be involved semirecumbent position is used. The urgency of further rest depends on the cause of the fever. Any special reason for adoption of specific position and the wishes and comfort of the patient should be considered and the congestion of the lungs by the sameness of position should be prevented.

  Rest both physical and mental is essential for the patients. So quietness with minimum disturbances is provided. Frequent disturbing of patients for doing nursing procedures and other various medications are disturbing and preventing rest to patient. As these are all essential for the cure of disease, it should be carried out in proper times but the maximum amount of rest and quietness should be provided and especially during sleep.
- **Sleep:** Sleeplessness or insomnia is frequently present in fever or illness. Anxiety or worry about his illness, stay in the somewhat frightening surroundings of the

hospital, or many other such feelings will be the cause for insomnia. Every word or actions of the nurse or doctor near the patient will be observed suspiciously. So a cheerful countenance, sympathy and reassurance of the nurse may allay the anxiety and ensure mental rest and sleep.

Nursing measures to induce sleep such as wiping the perspiration, changing the dress, straightening the bed linen, offering bedpan or urinal, providing additional blankets, giving the drinks at bed time, shading the bright light, meeting spiritual need, carrying out the treatment before sleep, using comfort devices, proper ventilation, avoiding draughts, relieving pain if any, solving problems before night, reducing fever by nursing measures, etc. should be adopted.

In addition to the above measures to relieve the physical causes of insomnia, symptoms such as cough and dyspnea in respiratory and circulatory diseases, indigestion, constipation or hunger pains in gastrointestinal diseases, pruritus in jaundice or skin disease may all interfere with sleep. These symptoms may be relieved by specific measure. Or, sedatives may be ordered for simple reasons of insomnia after trying the nursing measures.

- **Diet:** A suitable diet in fever is most important because such patient will have little or no appetite and yet adequate nourishment should be given to supply the bodily needs and to replace the wear and tear and to compensate the fluid loss through sweating. In the first few days of fever, fluids or semisolid foods, at least 4 to 5 pints of fluid should be given daily such as fruit juices, weak tea, cocoa, etc. milk is the most valuable food and easily assimilated. Pure milk, Custards, Bournvita, Horlicks, Ovaltines, etc. with or without milk are suitable. If pure milk is difficult to digest, citrated milk (60 mg of sodium citrate to each ounce of milk) is useful. Carbohydrate in the form of glucose, ordinary cane sugar, syrup, honey or as chocolate is of particular value in fever as it supply energy and easily digested.

As soon as possible, after acute stage, the patient should be given egg, fish, meat and fruits in palatable form to maintain adequate nutrition. Particularly in long-term illness, proteins should not be withheld for long, as they are essential to replace the wear and tear.

The type of food needed to fever patients is important. So also, a suitable type of food, even should be served as frequent small feeds. Otherwise overloading digestion may give rise to flatulence, epigastric pain and abdominal distension, producing respiratory and cardiac embarrassment and such abdominal distension, will interfere with his rest and sleep. The patients own appetite is a good guide to the amount of food required.

Also, the food should be served in an attractive manner to help the patient to increase the appetite, not to waste the food and to take and digest sufficient nourishment. In fever caused by certain particular illness, specific diets are essential with special items.

- **Skin and pressure areas:** In case of high fever, usually there is severe sweating which needs frequent change of clothes. As sweating is very distressing and produce insomnia, tepid sponging with water at a temperature of 70° to 80°F (21° to 27°) is good and conductive to sleep and help to reduce temperature.

Particular attention to the pressure areas of patients with prolonged confinement to bed especially with elderly people and frequent change of position is important because they are prone to develop pressure sores. Avoiding creases in bedsheet and providing comfortable mattress are essential details. Rubber mattress is very useful. The presence of any paralysis or incontinence calls for extra-attention to prevent developing pressure sores.

- **Attention to the mouth:** With fever of any degree, the mouth is usually dry and liable to become infected resulting stomatitis. So careful routine cleansing of the mouth is done at specific times during day and swabbing with suitable solutions is best. But swabbing should be done gently as too vigorous swabbing will only do more damage. Suitable solutions for cleansing the mouth are soda bicarbonate, dilute lemon juice or glycothymoline. Adequate administration of fluid is one essential way of ensuring a clean mouth. Juices or citrus fruits will increase the salivary secretions and keep the mouth clean and prevent drying of mucous membranes of the mouth.

- **Incontinence:** In long-term illness especially in elderly people, incontinence of urine an stool needs special attention to prevent the development of pressure sores. Again, incontinence may be caused by an overflow resulting from retention of urine. So a distended bladder should be watched for and catheterization with strict aseptic precaution should be done if the nursing measures fail to make the patient void. In persistent incontinence, a retention catheter may be provided with drainage bottle or with frequent releasing of the same.

- **Constipation:** Constipation is a constant feature in acute feverish illness. It will cause distension and discomfort to the patient. It must be treated and prevented. Purgatives like senokot and cascera or glycerine suppositories or an enema may be ordered according to the condition of the patient. If a patient is on fluid diet, bowel is not be opened daily and excessive purgation will be distressing to fever patients. Some patients are prone to constipation and used to regular purgatives. The nurse must ascertain form the patient

the name of the usual purgative he takes and it should be given in consultation with the doctor.
- **Prevention of venous thrombosis:** In patients with prolonged confinement to bed, thrombosis in the deep veins of the legs and pelvis is a danger due to sluggish circulations and trauma. In deep venous thrombosis a clot may break off, travel to the lungs, and cause pulmonary embolism which is fatal. So the limbs are moved actively and passively at intervals to prevent thrombosis and embolism and to prevent the joints becoming fixed with prolonged recombency especially in elderly people.
- **Rigors:** A rigor in the course of an illness is most frightening to the patient. So reassurance is important. The patient should be kept warm and adequately covered. Additional warmth may be given by the careful application of hot water bottle before sweating starts. When perspiring, tepid sponging will be necessary. Special nursing care of patient with rigor should be implemented.
- **Delirium:** Constant and skilled attention is necessary in all delirious patients. These patients are extremely restless and often try to get out of bed which may have serious effect. The nurse must try to restrain him with minimum force and extreme tact. In febrile delirium, cold compress to the forehead is often useful and soothing. Bed boards suitably padded to prevent injury may be needed. In most cases sedatives such as chloral hydrate, paraldehyde, compose or barbiturates may be ordered. In severe cases hyocine or morphine by inspection may be given.

  In all cases of delirium, utmost skill of the nurse is required to ensure the adequate fluid intake of the patients. Elderly patients who are liable to become delirious when seriously ill require special care in the matter of fluid intakes. But delirium developed due to high fever is relieved when the fever is reduced. So measures to reduce the fever should be resorted in such occasions.
- **Administering of antipyretic drugs:** Antipyretic drugs such as salicylates in the form of aspirin, crossin, etc. are given to patients with fever to reduce the temperature owing to their action on heat regulating center. They relieve pain in the muscles and joints. But in strong concentrated form it is irritating to the mucous membrane of the stomach.

  Whatever is the antipyretic drugs ordered, it should be given properly and the nurse should know the dose, effects and toxic reaction of the same when it is administered. Most of the drugs have good and bad effects. These should be realized by the nurse and nursing action should be directed accordingly. Salicylates in different names with different trademarks are used as antipyretics for the patient with fever.

Different types of cold applications are also useful in reducing fever.

To sum up nursing measures of patient with pyrexia includes the following:
- A patient with high temperature should be kept in bed as long as fever persists. He may be permitted to get up to toilet only
- The room should be quiet and well ventilated, bright light should be avoided and the temperature is best kept between 60 and 65°F
- An infant or young child should be placed in railed cot
- Clothing should be light and loose
- The attendants must wash their hands in an antiseptic solution before and after nursing care of the patient
- Careful observation and nursing measure should be taken to relieve discomfort. The mouth and tongue should be cleansed with sodium bicarbonate and glycerin before and after each meal. Frequent cold bath may be needed as body wastes are excreted through increased perspiration
- To prevent drying of the mucous membranes of the mouth and nose, glycerin should be applied to lubricate anterior nasal passage and lips
- Back care with methylated spirit and powder and special attention for pressure points
- Four hourly temperature, pulse and respiration should be taken and recorded on the chart
- If constipation is troublesome, the bowel should be moved by simple enema or mild laxative if there is no contraindication. If urine becomes concentrated or less than 100 ml. Daily in an adult, plenty of fluids by mouth is to be given
- Hyperpyrexia is best treated by cold and tepid sponging, cold compress to the forehead, ice cap on the head or ice packing on the body when needed. Sometimes ice-cold rectal saline is also used as retention enema to reduce body temperature.

  Note: Hypothermia is now used widely for variety of illness when extremely high temperature occurs. Precaution should be taken for sudden lowering of temperature which may lead to shock. Hypothermia decreases the body's metabolic needs, lowers body temperature and inhibits growth of infection.
- A suitable diet in acute febrile condition is most important. Patient is seriously ill and inclined to take little food or has no appetite at all but adequate nourishment must be given to maintain the nutrition. In addition, owing to the excessive loss of fluid through the skin by evaporation and due to rapid respiration more fluid are needed for maintaining the metabolic processes. The adult therefore is usually urged to take 2500 to 3000 ml of fluid a day. Infant and children should be given smaller amount. In addition to water fluids with some caloric values and containing

vitamin C, protein, salt and potassium is preferred. If not contraindicated by the disease fluid should be taken by the disease fluid should be taken by the patient because they help to supply the body's metabolic and electrolyte needs. Solid food usually is not palatable to the patient with a fever but may be allowed if desired. The main diet is milk, but if there is any abdominal distention it is better to give skimmed milk or diluted milk. Water and sweetened fruit juice may be given freely. In addition to fluid and milk, carbohydrate is given to supply energy for the body in the form of glucose, honey, syrup or chocolate. As soon as possible further addition of semisolid diet must be made such as chicken broth, custard, cornflower, half boiled egg, soji, bread, etc. Solid food should not be added until the temperature has returned to normal.

Treatment of fever includes the following:
- Antipyretic drugs may be given for lowering the temperature orally or IM or rectally, e.g. aspirin, Paracetamol
- Antihistaminic drugs sometimes give relief to symptoms of "Cold" which is usually accompanied by fever
- Hypnotics and tranquilizers may be required to prevent restlessness or convulsion
- If nausea and vomiting accompany a generalized infection, food and fluid should be withheld for the time. Antemetics are often useful in relieving nausea. If fever is high and vomiting is frequent fluid may be given parenterally. Infants need fluid replacement much sooner than adults. Tea, broth and soda, biscuits and dry toast are usually retained best as nausea subsides
- Other specific drugs are used according to cause.

After the episode of high fever the patient usually should stay in bed until the temperature has been normal for twenty-four hours. After a high and prolonged fever most adults feel weak, perspire on physical exertion and become tired easily for several days and weak. The patient of any age should have extra rest and should eat food rich in protein and high in calories. Children and young adults usually recover much more rapidly than elderly persons. During recovery the patient of any age needs quiet recreational activities such as reading to help pass the time and visitors.

Conscious means aware of an responding to ones surroundings consciousness refer to the state of being conscious. The fact of awareness by the mind of itself and the world. The words related to consciousness are as follows:
- Normal consciousness is an awareness of the self and the environment
- Sleep is a state of physical and apparent mental inactivity from which the patient can be aroused to normal consciousness.
- Clouding of consciousness is a state of reduced awareness, inattention, and sensory perception and difficulty in following detachment. There is impaired spoken words
- Delirium is characterized by irrelevant talks, disorientation, fear, irritability and misperception of stimuli
- Stupor is the state of minimal mental and physical activity, the response to spoken words is either absent or slow. The patient responds inadequately only by vigorous and repeated stimuli
- Coma is a state of total unresponsiveness. There is complete absence of response to the external environment, needs and even to repeated nervous stimuli
- *Unconsciousness* is an abnormal state resulting from disturbance of sensory perception to the extent that the patient is not aware of what is happening around him. It may be momentary or prolonged to days or even months. Clinically the patient who does not respond to the spoken word is unconscious. But the degree varies.

Unconscious Patient

The comatose condition of the patient can be distinguished from lighter states of impaired consciousness or the semicomatose state, in that, in the latter the patient makes some response to spoken word. There are many degrees of coma.
- *Light coma:* This is spontaneous and evoked movement.
- *Deep coma:* The heart rate is slow. But the respiratory rate is fast and the depth increased.
- *Premoribund:* The rhythm is periodic. There is tracheal tug. Pulse is irregular. Blood pressure is rising.
- *Moribund:* Apnoeic respiration, pupils dilated and fixed, pulse fast, blood pressure falling.

The degree of unconsciousness or level of unconsciousness includes:
- *Excitatory type:* Patient does not respond to but disturbed by sensory stimuli, i.e. bright light, noise and sudden movement.
- *Somnolent:* Patient is extremely drowsy and will respond only if spoken to directly.
- *Stuporous:* Responds only to painful stimuli, i.e. pricking or pinching.
- *Deep coma:* Does not respond to any type of stimulus and his reflexes are gone.

Management of unconsciousness is a lack of awareness of one's environment and the inability to respond to external stimuli. Therefore, observation of the patients condition and care to prevent any complications are particularly important. If possible a nurse should be assigned "special" to the patient or alternatively he could be nursed to intensive care ward.

Etiology of Unconsciousness

Common causes of unconsciousness includes the following:
- *Infective:* (i) Meningitis, (ii) Cerebral abscess (from middle ear infection).
- *Traumatic:* (i) Head injury, (ii) Operation on the brain.
- *Neoplastic:* Innocent or malignant growth of brain.
- *Metabolic:* (i) Uraemia, (ii) Diabetic coma, (iii) Insulin coma, (iv) Overdose of certain drugs.
- *Degenerative:* Cerebral arteriosclerosis causing-Thrombosis, haemorrhage or hypertensive encephalopathy.
- *Poisoning:* (i) By anaesthesia, (ii) Snake bite, (iii) Drugs-Opium poisoning, alcohol poisoning, Barbiturate poisoning.
- *Cerebral anemia:* (i) Due to shock, (ii) Due to haemorrhage, (iii) Due to embolus (including air and fat embolus).
- Anaphylactic shock
- Hypopituitarism
- Stokes-Adams syndrome
- Cholemia
- Eclampsia

The common causes of unconsciousness (in children) includes the following:
- Purulent meningitis
- TB meningitis
- Head injury
- Hyperpyrexia
- Foreign body in respiratory tract
- Cerebral hemorrhage
- Intracranial tumor.

Nursing Management of Unconscious Patient

- **Aim:** The primary objective is preservation and prolongation of life. Treatment of airway obstruction, shock, or cardiorespiratory failure should be started before going into details of the cause of these disorders.
- **Maintenance of airway:**
  - Signs and airway obstruction: Stridor, respiration with effort, wheezing or cyanosis. A finger is to be swept deep into the oropharynx to remove clotted blood, mucus, vomitus, any loose teeth or dentures or any foreign body.
  - The patient is kept in semiprone position and should not lie or be restrained flat on his back in spread-eagle fashion. Spinal injury requires special consideration:
    * To maintain normal body function
    * To prevent complications

  Generally nursing management of unconscious includes the following:
- **Positioning of the patient:** The patient is nursed in the prone, lateral or Sim's position. An unconscious patient is not nursed on his back because there is a risk that he may inhale vomitus or secretions from his mouth and pharynx.
- **Airway:** An adequate airway must be maintained at all times. It may be necessary to hold the patients jaw forward.

  Garments must be loose to allow free movements of the chest and abdomen. Frequent suction is sometimes required to prevent the pooling of secretions in the patients pharynx. Sufficient ventilation should be provided.
- **Observation and charting:** A chart may be kept to note the patients level of consciousness, reaction to vocal stimulation, the size of pupils and their reaction to light. These observations if required, may be taken every half-hour or hour.

  Temperature, pulse and respiration may be recorded every two or four hours and sometimes more frequently, particularly when the patient has a head injury.

  A blood pressure chart is usually kept, the frequency depending upon the cause of unconsciousness.

  The occurrence of muscular spasms is recorded. The nurse should note the area affected and the duration of the fits.

  A urine analysis chart will be commenced for patients suffering from diabetes mellitus or renal failure.
- **Hygiene:** A mosquito net, provided the mesh is fine enough to observe the patients colour, is used to protect the patient from flies and mosquitoes.

  Sponging is performed as frequently as necessary. Tepid sponging may be required if the patient becomes febrile. When sponging the patient and giving pressure care, the limbs should be put through a full range of movements (passive physiotherapy). Passive physiotherapy for patients who remain unconscious for a long period helps to prevent stiffening of joints, muscular contractions and venous stasis.

  Mouth toilets are performed to prevent drying of the mucous membrane and formation of sordes.

  Eye toilets may be necessary to keep the lid margins free form discharge. The eyes must be kept closed to prevent drying of the conjunctiva and corneal ulceration.

  The doctor may order the instillation of sterile oily eye drops.
- **Care of pressure areas and the prevention of foot drop**

  The patient should, if possible, be nursed on a ripple mattress.

  The bed linen must be kept taut and dry.

  A bed cradle may be used to take the weight of the bedclothes.

Pillows protected by plastic covers may be used to separate the bony prominences between the knees and ankles.

The patients position should be changed every hour and pressure areas massaged every two hours. Any sign of reddening or injury to the skin must be reported and the treatment intensified.

Foot drop occurring during hospitalization can be prevented by careful nursing. The feet should be kept at right ankles to the legs. Foot drop is liable to occur if the bedclothes are tucked in, tightly, causing constant pressure over the toes and feet.

A foot board or pillow at the bottom of the bed may be used to prevent the pressure and weight of clothes on the feet.

Passive physiotherapy will help to keep the ankles and feet in good condition. Padded splints may be used to maintain the correct position. If splints are used they must be removed for pressure area, sponging and physiotherapy and then carefully replaced. The hands and wrists may also need splinting to prevent wrist drop.

- **Nutrition:** The diet must certain adequate supply of all the nutrients required for life. These may be supplied as intravenous fluids or gastric tube feedings. If gastric tube feedings are commenced, care is taken that a variety of fluids are given, e.g. high protein milk, drinks, fruit juices and also water. The patient must be well nourished and hydrated.
- **Elimination:** The patient is observed for any signs of urinary retention and constipation. Any signs or symptoms of either condition will be reported, e.g. the abdomen may be distended if there is urinary retention and frequently the patient becomes very restless.

    If the patient is constipated, a glycerine suppository may be ordered. However, a patient having a fluid diet will have very little faecal residue.

    Incontinence of urine may occur in which case a bedpan or divided mattress may be used for a female patient and for a male patient a padded urinal or other suitable appliances may be used. These must be inspected at least every two hours.

    If the patient has retention of urine, gentle pressure over the bladder region will be helpful in partially emptying the bladder. However, catheterization is generally necessary.

    Accurate recordings must be on the patients fluid balance chart and the patient must be closely observed.
- **Relatives:** The relatives and friends must be given special consideration as they may be distressed at the patients condition. The ward sister usually arranges an appointment for them with the medical officer so that they may be informed of the patients progress. The nurse may assist the relatives as follows:
    - Check the room and remove any unnecessary equipment before the visitors arrive.
    - Explain to the visitors any new piece of equipment there may be to prevent undue alarm.
    - Arrange for a member or the clergy to visit the patient, if the relatives request this.
- **Routine care of unconscious patient**
    - *Maintenance of an adequate airway:*
        - The unconscious patient must be nursed on one side – semiprone position to avoid any tendency of the tongue to fallback on the throat and to encourage secretions from the mouth, respiratory tract and oesophagus to drain outward by gravity. Extension of the head and elevation of the jaw will raise the tongue out of the posterior oropharynx.
        - If the patient is lightly comatose an indwelling airway tube may stimulate vomiting or an endotracheal tube may produce coughing. But in deeply comatose patient, a rubber or metal airway should remain in the mouth until the cough reflex returns. If this is insufficient an endotracheal tube should be inserted, or positive pressure ventilation should be started where applicable.
        - Cleansing the air passage with an electric sucker or gauze piece.
        - Patient is to be kept in steam tent to make the secretions less which should be cleaned off and on.
        - Tracheotomy may have to be done to provide an adequate airway (assisting doctor if needed). Proper care of tracheotomy tube and of the wound has to be taken as a routine.

            If there is cardiac arrest mouth-to-mouth ventilation and closed chest massage should be started immediately. Ventilation with an oral airway and a mask, if available is very effective.
    - *Control of hemorrhage:* From the scalp or other parts of the body is the next most important step. This can usually be done by a suitable piece of gauze placed over the wound and secured by firm bandage. This should immediately be followed up by examination of the rest of the body for injury and management.
    - *Maintenance of circulation:*
        - Circulation of blood is enhanced by muscle movement. The patient must not be left in a position that hampers circulation to any part of the body.
        - Position is to be changed every 2 hours.
        - Reddened area should be massaged gently.
        - Air pressure mattress is helpful in preventing the development of decubitus ulcer.

- *Moving and position:*
  * Turning sheet should be used in moving an unconscious patient.
  * To prevent foot drop—the foot is to be kept straightened in position against foot blocks.
  * Both hands are to be kept in position, the fingers are to be rested on the pillow.
  * The wrist is to be supported on the pillow to prevent wrist drop.
  * If the patient does not move, all extremities should be put through the complete range of joint motion at least twice every day.
  * Massage of extremities is essential to promote circulation and to prevent venous thrombosis.
- *Anticonvulsants:* During comatose condition a single convulsion may endanger patient's life. A nonhypnotic anticonvulsant like diphenyl hydration is useful.
- *Antibiotics:* Are necessary depending on infectious condition, injury, etc. Any suitable one should immediately be started with.

- **Immediate care after admission:** Complications arise from loss of sensation, from paralysis and from general lowering of metabolic activity. For these reasons during nursing management a close watch is to be kept on the above mentioned points. Observation should be every 15 minutes at first till condition shows signs of improvement.
  - The unconsciousness patient is placed in a clean railed cot.
  - The patient is kept in flat position, at first head turned to one side and neck is to be extended for better salivation and oxygenation.
  - Oxygen inhalation should be started immediately.
  - Pulse rate respiration rate and body temperature should be noted carefully.
  - A call book is to be send immediately to the house physician concerned indicating name, bed no., age, sex, time of admission, pulse, respiration, temperature, state of the patient and if possible the cause. Whether patient has passed urine and stool or has vomited, etc. and any treatment received outside or not should be noted.
  - After sending call book emergency tray is to be kept nearby which includes:
    * Physical examination set
    * Sterile Ryle's tube with syringe and specimen tube.
    * Catheterization set
    * Infusion set
    * Lumbar puncture set
    * Tracheostomy set
    * Sucker machine with sterile catheter
    * Injection tray with emergency drugs
  - If temperature is high – ice cap is to be applied over the head. If subnormal – patient is to be kept warm wrapped with blanket.
  - Close observation and individual nursing care is essential for such patient.
  - Assisting doctor during physical examination and treatment, e.g. lumbar puncture or gastric lavage or during catheterization.
- **Skin care**
  - Thorough bath with warm water is to be given daily.
  - The skin should be dried properly to stimulate circulation.
  - If the skin is too dry – lanolin or cold cream to lubricate.
  - Proper hair wash is to be given once in a week.
- **Mouth care or oral hygiene**
  - Proper mouth care is to be given at every two hours interval.
  - Artificial dentures should be removed and safely stored until the patient is fully conscious.
  - Mouth gag is to be used during mouth care.
  - Glycerine is to be applied over the tongue and lips because it has hygroscopic action.
  - Painting of gum with 2% Mercurochrome.
- **Eye care**
  - Eyes should be carefully inspected several times a day.
  - If corneal reflex is absent or if the lids are not completely closed they should be covered with an eye shield.
  - Sterile paraffin or 0.5 to 1% methyl solution should be dropped in each eye to protect the cornea from drying up by providing moisture and lubrication. Negligency may cause drying of the cornea followed by ulceration which may lead to blindness.
- **Food and fluids:** Nutrition is not a serious matter unless the state of unconsciousness lasts for more than three or four days. Metabolic activity is depressed in these patients and caloric requirement is therefore very low. On the other hand loss of consciousness may be associated with injury or other disorders which may themselves require administration of glucose, electrolytes, water, plasma or even blood.
  - Protein and carbohydrate should be administered by IV infusion but not fat.
  - To maintain all his nutritional needs nasogastric tube is used an small amount of liquid containing all essential foods are usually given 100 to 200 cc, 2-3 hourly.
  - Electric sucker is to be kept ready before feeding as there is chance of aspiration.
  - Before starting feeding, one should be sure that the tube is in position.

- Before and after feeding water should be given gently. Medicine may also be given slowly through the Ryle's tube.
- Proper intake and output chart must be maintained.

- **Hyperthermia**
  - If heat regulating center (hypothalamus) is disturbed patients temperature will suddenly rise.
  - Elevation of temperature is a sign of complication, i.e. pneumonia, wound infection, dehydration, uremia, etc.
  - If temperature is 38.4°C (101°F) bedclothes should be removed and antipyretics as advised should be given through tube or by injection.
  - Tepid sponge may be given according to doctors order.
  - If temperature is due to increased intracranial pressure lumbar puncture is also done several times.

- **Hypothermia:** The unconscious patient may have a temperature that is too low (due to depressed vital center).
  - This type of patient needs extra cover
  - Room heater may be used for such patient.

- **Problems of elimination:** Unconscious patient often has both urinary and faecal incontinence.
  - *Regarding bladder:* Foley's type of catheter should be introduced and left indwelled to control urinary incontinence, to prevent bed soiling and to keep intake-output chart. Proper aseptic technique has to be maintained to prevent complications.
  Continuous drainage is to be given.
  Proper care of the tube is to be taken.
  Bladder wash with acriffin solution 1: 10,000 with proper aseptic care.
  Urine has to be examined for sugar, acetone and albumin at every four interval when indicated.
  Report is to be given to doctor and to treat accordingly.
  Proper output is to be maintained.
  - *Regarding bowel:* (i) The unconscious patient usually is given an enema two or three days interval to help to prevent faecal incontinence.

    If nasogastric tube is present mild laxative such as milk of magnesia may be given.
  - *Care of vaginal discharge:* If patient has vaginal discharge it should be reported to the doctor. Sometimes cleansing douche is ordered.

    The patient who is menstruating will need private care every four hours.

- **Prevention of further accident or injury**
  - Precautions are to be taken to prevent accidents.
  - No external heat is to be used, e.g. hot water bag.
  - Padded side rails should be kept on both sides since patient might have convulsions.

  - The unconscious patient should be observed half hourly. If condition is critical he needs observation at every 15 min interval.
  - Paraldehyde 5 cc or sodium phenobarbitone 30 to 60 mg may be ordered. After sedation observation is essential for signs of depression of vital function.
  - Patient should not be kept isolated in a room.

- **Observation**
  - Pupillary reaction
  - Level of consciousness
  - Stiffness of neck
  - Condition of limb-flaccidity, etc.
  - Convulsion etc.

  These will help doctor for proper diagnosis and treatment.

  A rising blood pressure with slowing of pulse rate indicates increased intracranial pressure and it should be reported immediately.

  Any marked change of pulse, respiration or any increase or decrease of level of consciousness should be reported immediately.

- **Convalescence**
  - Patient may completely recover after being unconscious for several weeks.
  - Effort should not be made to arouse him until the level of consciousness has lightened.
  - During convalescence – definite rest periods should be planned each day.
  - Patient needs encouragement and security of knowing that family and friends are concern and interested in his/her recovery.
  - Observation should be made for development of any complication which should properly be dealt with.

    Patient will also need to be reoriented since the memory is usually failing for the time immediately before, during and after the period of unconsciousness.

Management of Pain

Pain is a complex, multidimensional phenomenon. Everyone has experienced some types or degrees of pain. Pain prompts people to seek health care more often than any other problem. Pain is one of the most common problems being faced by nurses when they are dealing with the patients. And also nurses are in an excellent position to work with the client in pain and to help the client overcome the pain. For which nurse has to gain more knowledge about pain and its management. The nurse has a responsibility to understand the experience of pain and to initiate measures that provide relief or help the client learn to cope. Because, the nurse spends more time with the patient in pain than any other health care professionals and has the opportunity to help relieve pain and its harmful effects. Some of the definitions enhance the nurse's ability to assess the client who is in pain by focusing on specific aspects of the pain experience.

Definitions of Pain

- Pain is defined by McCaffery as "whatever the person experiencing the pain says it is, existing whenever the person says it does". It is subjective experience with no objective measurement.
- The International Association for the Study of Pain (IASP) defined, "pain is an unpleasant sensory and emotional experience associated with actual or potential tissue damage or it is described in terms of such damage". Pain can be a major factor inhibiting the ability and willingness to recover from illness.
- Mount Castle defined pain as "that sensory experiences evoked by stimuli that injure or threaten to destroy tissue, defined introspectively by every man as that which hurts".
- Sternbach defined pain as "(i) an abstract concept which refers to a personal, private sensation of hurt; (ii) a harmful stimulus that signals current or impending tissue damage; and (iii) a pattern of responses to protect the organism from harm".

The nursing definition of pain is "whatever bodily hurt, he says it does". The cardinal rule in the care of patients with pain is that all pain is real, even if its cause is unknown.

Nature of Pain

As stated earlier pain is whatever the experiencing person says it is and existing whenever the person says or does. This statement/definition makes the client the expert about his or her own pain. Because clinical pain is subjective and no objective measures of it exists, the only people who can accurately define their own pain are experiencing that pain. Although it is subjective in nature, the nurse charged with accurately assessing and helping to relieve the client's pain. To help a client gain relief, that nurse must believe that the pain exists.

Pain is a protective physiological mechanism. A person with a sprained ankle avoids bearing full weight on the foot to prevent further injury. Pain is a warning that tissue damage has occurred. The client who is unable to feel sensation, such as one with spinal cord tumor, is unaware of pain inducing injuries. Pain is a leading cause of disability. As the average lifespan increase more people have chronic diseases in which pain is a common symptom. Additional medical advances have resulted in diagnostic and therapeutic measures that are uncomfortable. Nurses care daily for clients in pain.

Purpose of Pain

Pain serves as a protective mechanism. If a person touches a hot stove, the pain signal causes the person to pull the hand away immediately. The skin would be seriously burned if this did not happen.

Pain can be a diagnostic tool. The quality and duration of the pain give important clues in determining a client's medical diagnosis. For example, in acute appendicitis, the clinician looks for rebound tenderness (the pain increases when pressure is released) when palpating the abdomen. This particular type of pain helps confirm the diagnosis of appendicitis rather than other gastrointestinal disorders.

Physiology of Pain

The opioid system and the nonopioid system are the two known endogenous (developing within) analgesia systems in humans. The best known is the opioid system. It is mediated by *endorphins* (endogenous opiate-like substances). The nonopioid system is mediated by monoamine substances such as norepinephrine and serotonin.

When pain occurs, sensory input from injured tissue causes peripheral *nociceptors* (receptive neurons for painful sensations) and central nervous system (CNS) pain pathways to enhance future responses to pain stimuli. Long-lasting changes in cells within the spinal cord *afferent* (ascending) and *efferent* (descending) *pain pathways* may thus occur after a brief noxious stimulus.

Physiological responses (such as elevated blood pressure, respiratory rate, and pulse rate; dilated pupils; perspiration; and pallor) to even a brief acute pain episode will show adaptation within minutes to a few hours. The body cannot sustain the extreme stress response physiologically for more than short periods. The body conserves its resources by physiological adaptation: a return to normal or near normal blood pressure, respiratory rate, and pulse rate; pupil size; and dry skin with little evidence of poor perfusion, even with continuing pain of *the same intensity*.

Factors of Influencing Pain

Situation: The situation associated with the pain influence the person's response to it. A person's responses to pain experienced in a formal crowded situations may differ greatly from the responses were he or she alone or in a hospital.

Culture: Culture influences how people learn to react to expressing pain. People respond to pain in different ways. The nurse must never assume to know how clients will respond. However, an understanding of cultural background, socioeconomic status, and personal attitudes help the nurse more accurately assess pain and its meaning for clients. A young girl in a stoic culture may be allowed to cry because of pain whereas boys are not allowed to cry in some cultures.

Age: Age is an important variable that influences pain, particularly in children and older adults. Age may release a client from culturally imposed norms in relation to pain expression. Developmental differences found among these age groups can influence how children and older react to the pain experience. Young children have difficulty in understanding pain and the procedures nurses administer that may cause pain. Young children who have not developed vocabularies also have difficulty verbally describing an expressing pain to parents/caregivers. Cognitively toddlers are unable to recall explanations about pain or associate pain as experiences that can occur in various situation. Older people may assign different meanings to that pain. Pain is often thought by the elderly as natural manifestation of aging.

Sex: Gender may be an important influence in pain. In most cultures boys are expected to show less expression of pain than girls. As they grow older men are also expected to express less pain than women.

Meaning of pain: The meaning of a person's pain is a factor that influences his or her responses to pain. A person will perceive pain differently, if it suggests a threat, loss, punishment, or challenges. For example, a woman in labor perceives pain differently from women expressing pain from a recent back injury or pain caused by childbirth may be responded differently from pain caused by surgery. If the cause is unknown, more negative psychological factors use such as fear, anxiety, etc. come into play and the pain may be misinterpreted resulting in an inappropriate response. A client copes differently with pain, depending on its meaning.

Anxiety: The degree of anxiety the client is experiencing also may influence the client's response to pain. It is not possible to separate the mind from the body, so pain is always has both physiologic and psychological components. When anxiety is high pain is felt greater. Emotionally healthy persons are usually able to tolerate moderate or even severe pain than those whole emotions are less stable.

Fatigue: Fatigue heightens perceptions of pain. This intensifies pain and decreases coping abilities. Pain is often experienced less after a restful sleep than at the end of a long day.

Attention: The degree at which a client focuses on pain can influence pain perception. Increased attention has been associated with increased pain, whereas distraction has been associated with a diminished pain response. This concept is one that nurses apply in various pain relief measures such as relaxation, guided emergency and massage.

Previous experience: Each person learns from painful experiences. Previous experience does not necessarily mean that a person will accept pain more easily in the future. If a person has had frequent episodes of pain without relief or bouts of severe pain, anxiety or even fear may occur. In contrast if a person had repeated experience of pain, may be better prepared to tolerate or take necessary actions to relieve pain to some extent.

Coping style: The experience of pain can be lonely, when client experiences pain in health care setting such as hospitals, the loneliness can be unbearable. Frequently client feels a loss of central pain and an inability to control their environments or the outcome of events coping style thus influences the ability to deal with pain.

Family and social support: Parents and attitudes of significant others also affect pain response. People in pain often depend on family members for support, assistance or protection. An absence of family members or friends can often make the pain more stressful. For children presence of parents is very essential.

Types of Pain

There are different ways to define types of pain, which include according to onset, duration, severity, modes of transmission, location, causation and causative force. The examples of which are as follows:
- Onset or time of occurrence, e.g. postoperative pain
- Duration, e.g. chronic pain or acute pain
- Severity or intensity, e.g. severe, mild or scored (0 to 10 on a scale)
- Location or source, e.g. superficial, deep or central pain
- Causation, e.g. pain due to receptor stimulation or nerve damage, or psychophysiologic pain
- Causative force or agent, e.g. spontaneous, self inflicted or other pain

The common terms used to classify pain are as follows.

Noninvasive Interventions

Noninvasive relief measures consist of cognitive behavioral strategies and physical modalities that use cutaneous stimulation. These treatments can be used to supplement pharmacological therapy and other modalities to control pain. Clients and their families can also be instructed to utilize these treatments at home and in inpatient settings.

Cognitive-behavioral interventions: The cognitive-behavioral interventions influence the cognitive and the motivational-affective components of pain perception. These methods cannot only help influence the level of pain, but also help the client gain a sense of self-control.

Trusting nurse-client relationship: Establishing a therapeutic relationship is the foundation for effective nursing care. The clients most likely to be comfortable are those who trust their nurses to be there, to listen, and to act.

Relaxation: Relaxation techniques (a variety of methods used to decrease anxiety and muscle tension) result in decreased heart rate and respiratory rate, and decreased muscle tension. The body's response to pain is almost "tricked" into reversing itself when relaxation exercises are implemented.

Relaxation exercises help reduce pain by decreasing anxiety and decreasing reflex muscular contraction. There are a wide variety of relaxation techniques, including focused breathing, progressive muscle relaxation, and meditation. Simple techniques should be used during episodes of brief pain (e.g. during procedures) or when pain is so severe that the client is unable to concentrate on complicated instructions.

To teach simple relaxation techniques, the nurse can instruct the client to: (i) take a deep breath and hold it; (ii) exhale slowly and concentrate on going limp; and (iii) start yawning. The yawning triggers a conditioned response in the client (i.e. the body associates yawning with relaxation and will relax when the client yawns). The technique can be enhanced if the nurse starts yawning. It is so contagious that even the client compromised by severe pain will usually start yawning with the nurse.

A more complex technique is *progressive muscle relaxation*, a strategy in which muscles are alternately tensed and relaxed. This type of technique is especially useful for clients who do not know what muscle relaxation feels like. By purposely contracting and releasing the muscle groups, the client is able to compare the difference and identify feelings of relaxation. Meditative relaxation techniques are also available, including audiotapes sold in most bookstores.

Relaxation is a learned response. The more frequently the client practices these techniques, the more skilled the body will be in learning to relax. Ideally, the best time to teach the client these methods is when pain is controlled or before the pain occurs (e.g., in the preoperative period).

Reframing is a technique that teaches clients to monitor their negative thoughts and replace them with more positive ones. For example, teach a client to replace an expression such as, "I cannot stand this pain, it's never going away", with one such as, "I've had similar pain before, and it's gotten better".

Distraction: Distraction focuses one's attention on something other than the pain, therefore placing pain on the periphery of awareness. Successful or distraction does not eliminate the pain; it makes it less troublesome. The main disadvantage of distraction is that as soon as the distractive stimuli stop, the pain returns in full force. For this reason, the most appropriate use of distraction techniques is for the relief of brief, episodic pain. It can be effective for procedural pain or the period between administration of an analgesic and the onset of the drug. Examples of distraction include the following:
- Active listening to recorded music (have the client tap fingers in rhythm to the beat)
- Reciting a poem or rhyme (children do this well)
- Describe a plot of a novel or movie
- Describe a series of pictures

Guided imagery: Guided imagery uses one's imagination to provide a pleasant substitute for the pain. It incorporates features of both relaxation and distraction. The client imagines a pleasant experience, such as going to the beach or the mountains. The experience should use all five senses to fully involve the client in the image.

The images chosen need to be ones that are pleasant for the client. Describing an ocean cruise would not be appropriate for a person who becomes seasick.

Humor: The old saying, "Laughter is the best medicine," carries some truth to it. Although there is nothing very funny about pain, laughing has been shown to provide pain relief. The act or laughing can cause distraction from the pain, induce relaxation by taking deep breaths and releasing tension, release endorphins, and provide a pleasant substitute for pain. This technique can be implemented by encouraging the client to watch humorous movies, read funny books, or listen to comedy routines. Because different people see humor in different types of situations, be sensitive to what the client views as funny.

Biofeedback: Biofeedback is a method that may help the client in pain to relax and relieve tension. Individuals learn to influence their physiological responses to stimuli and thus alter their pain experience.

Cutaneous stimulation: The technique of cutaneous stimulation involves stimulating the skin to control pain. It is theorized that this technique provides relief by stimulating nerve fibers that send signals to the dorsal horn of the spinal cord to "close the gate". The main advantage of these therapies is that many techniques are easy for the nurse to implement and easy to teach the client and family to perform. They are not usually meant to replace analgesic therapy, but to complement it.

Hot and cold application: In addition to stimulating nerves that can block pain transmission, superficial heat application increases circulation to the area, which promotes oxygenation and nutrient delivery to the injured tissues. It also decreases joint and muscle stiffness. Heat is contraindicated in cases of acute injury because it can increase the initial response of edema. It is also contraindicated in rheumatoid arthritis flare-ups and over topical applications of mentholated ointments. Heat treatments should be limited to 20- to 30-minute intervals because maximum vasodilatation occurs in that time.

Teach the client or family that hot or cold applications:
- Must have at least one layer of towel between the heating or cooling device and the skin.
- Should be placed on the skin only for short periods.
- Should not be applied to tissue that has been exposed to radiation therapy.

Cryotherapy (cold applications) induces local vasoconstriction and numbness, therefore altering the pain sensations. It is contraindicated in any condition where vasoconstriction might increase symptoms (e.g., peripheral vascular disease). For best results, cold therapy should be limited to 20- to 30-minute intervals. Either heat or cold can be used as cutaneous stimulation unless one is specifically contraindicated. Cold often provides faster relief. If the client has used heat or cold before, incorporate the modality that the client believes will be the most effective. Combining the two might provide better relief. An example of this would be to apply a hot pack for 4 minutes, followed by an ice pack for 2 minutes, repeated four times. In a hospital setting, a physician order is required for this therapy.

Acupressure and massage: One of the first responses to pain is to rub the painful part. People seem to instinctively understand the pain-relieving aspects of this intervention. In addition to blocking the pain transmission through nerve stimulation, massage can also promote relaxation. Acupressure is a type of massage that consists of continuous pressure on or the rubbing of acupuncture points. It is based on the same principles as acupuncture, but needles are not used. Massage also provides a form of nonverbal communication that can be therapeutic on its own.

Mentholated rubs: Ointments or lotions containing menthol are thought to provide relief by providing a counter irritation to the skin. The menthol gives the client the perception that the temperature of the skin has changed (becoming either warmer or cooler). This alters the sensation of pain or provides a distraction from the pain. Client response varies to mentholated rubs: some gain effective relief, but others have poor results. Their use is contraindicated on broken skin, on mucous membranes, or if pain increases.

Transcutaneous electrical nerve stimulation: Transcutaneous electrical nerve stimulation (TENS) is the process of applying a low-voltage electrical current to the skin through cutaneous electrodes. This modulates pain transmission, as do other cutaneous stimulation methods, but also distracts the client from pain. Research supports the effectiveness of using TENS for the relief of postoperative pain. It has also been used successfully in many pain syndromes (e.g. chronic low-back pain, menstrual cramps, temporomandibular joint (TMJ) syndrome, phantom limb pain, and others). It is administered by specially trained health professionals, usually a physical therapist. Other modalities of pain management should not be abandoned while a trial of TENS occurs.

TENS Contraindications
- No electrodes should be placed in the area over or surrounding demand cardiac pacemakers.
- No electrodes can be placed over the uterus of a pregnant woman.

Exercise: Exercise is an important treatment for chronic pain because it helps mobilize joints, strengthens weak muscles, and helps restore balance and coordination. Do not use passive range of motion if it increases discomfort or pain. Immobilization is frequently used to stabilize fractures or for clients with episodes of acute pain. Prolonged immobilization can lead to muscle atrophy and cardiovascular conditioning.

Psychotherapy: Psychotherapy may be beneficial to some clients, particularly those:
- Who are clinically depressed
- Who have a history of psychiatric problems
- Whose pain is difficult to control.

Some psychotherapists use *hypnosis* (altered state of consciousness when a person is more receptive to suggestion) to help clients alter pain perception. Hypnosis can be effective but should be used only by specially trained professionals.

Positioning: The final noninvasive technique is proper positioning and body alignment. Moving the client with the least possible stress on joints and skin will minimize exposure to painful stimuli. This includes supporting joints appropriately and maintaining wrinkle-free sheets.

Invasive Interventions

Invasive interventions are meant to complement behavioral, physical, and pharmacological therapies in those clients who do not obtain relief from those measures alone (AHCPR, 1994). Invasive measures are indicated primarily for chronic cancer pain and in some cases of chronic benign pain. These procedures are usually tried only when noninvasive measures have been attempted first with poor results.

Nerve block: Neural blockade is the process of injecting a local anesthetic or neurologic agent into the nerve. An anesthetic agent may be injected to act as a diagnostic tool in order to identify the nerves involved in a pain syndrome. A neurolytic agent is a chemical agent that causes destruction of the nerve and, therefore, creates an interruption in the pain signal.

Neurosurgery: Neurosurgical measures for pain control include neurostimulation procedures and destructive or ablative procedures. Neurostimulation procedures involve the implantation of electrical stimulation devices that send impulses to different parts of the nervous system. Some of these devices stimulate areas of the brain: others stimulate the spinal cord. Relief is thought to be provided by blocking the afferent fiber input at the spinal cord level or by stimulating release of endorphins using the body's ability to modulate pain.

Destructive or ablative procedures are used to destroy part of the nervous system that conducts pain. By interrupting the pain signal, it is prevented from reaching the cortex where realization of pain occurs. These procedures are reserved for clients with terminal illness.

Radiation therapy: Radiation can be used as a palliative measure for pain relief in clients with cancer. It can relieve both metastatic pain and pain caused by tumors at the primary cancer site. It enhances other pain management strategies, such as analgesic therapy, because it is aimed specifically at the cause of the client's pain. When administered for pain relief, the smallest dose of radiation is utilized to minimize side effects.

Acupuncture: Acupuncture is the insertion of small needles into the skin at specific (hoku) sites. The sites are chosen after the practitioner takes a detailed history and uses traditional Asian diagnostic techniques. The needles used for acupuncture have rounded ends that enter the skin without cutting the tissue. The practitioner may twirl or vibrate the needles manually or electrically. It is important that the nurse keep an open mind when the client chooses this therapy, or the client may be reluctant to discuss its use.

Evaluating pain management interventions is ongoing, focusing primarily on the client's subjective reports. Objective data to evaluate pain management include the following:
- Continuing use of pain assessment tools
- Client's facial expression and posture
- Presence (or absence) of restlessness
- Vital sign monitoring

Pain may be defined as "an unpleasant sensory and emotional experience associated with actual or potential tissue damage", and "whatever the client says it is, existing whenever the client says it does".

The gate control theory proposes that several processes (sensory, motivational-affective, and cognitive) combine to determine how a person perceives pain.

Assessment of pain helps establish a baseline of data and helps evaluate the effectiveness of the interventions.

Factors influencing pain perception include age, previous experience with pain, and cultural norms.

The subjective data to gather include location of pain, onset and duration, quality, intensity (on a scale of 0 to 10), aggravating and relieving factors, and how pain affects the activities of daily living.

Guidelines for Individualizing Pain Therapy

When providing pain relief measures, the nurse chooses therapies suited to the client's unique pain experience, McCaffer (1979) suggests nine useful guidelines for pain therapy. The following guidelines are eleven which include nine.

Establish a relationship of mutual trust: Always believe the client and try to convey concern. An adversial relationship between nurse and client lessens the effectiveness of pain therapies.

Use different types of pain relief measures: Using more than one therapy has an additive effective reducing pain. In addition, the character of pain may change throughout the day, requiring several different therapies.

Provide pain relief measures before pain becomes severe: It is easier to prevent severe pain than to relieve it after it exists. Giving analgesics half an hour before, client must walk or perform an activity is an example of controlling pain early.

Consider the client's ability or willingness to participate in pain relief measures: Some client cannot actively assist with pain therapy because of fatigue, sedation or altered level of consciousness. However, there are variations of pain-relief measures that require little effort, such as relaxation exercises in bed or listening to music as a distraction. The nurse will not relieve pain by forcing an unwilling patient to participate in therapy.

Choose pain-relief measures on the basis of the client's behavior reflecting the severity of pain: It would be a poor judgment to administer a patient narcotic if a client has only mild pain. The nurse carefully assesses the client's comments and behavior before choosing pain therapy. Some clients acquire relief from severe pain after using only mild analgesics. Only the client can determine the potency of an effective therapy.

Use measures that the client believes are effective: The client is the expert of pain. The client may have ideas about measures to use (e.g. rubbing lotion on a swollen finger) and times to use them will make pain therapy successful.

If a therapy is ineffective at first, encourage client to try again before abandoning it: Often, anxiety or doubt prevents a therapy from relieving pain, or the measure may require adjustment or practice to become effective. The nurse should be patient and understanding in helping the client learn to use measures that do not afford immediate relief.

Keep an open mind about what may relieve pain: New ways are often found to control pain. There is still much to be learned about the pain experience. Rejecting nonconventional therapies leads to mistrust. The nurse should se to it that sure all therapies are safe.

Keep trying: The nurse can easily become frustrated when efforts at pain relief fail. The nurse should not abandon the client when pain persists but reassess the situation and consider alternative therapies.

Protect the client: A pain therapy should not cause more distress than the pain itself. The nurse always observes the efforts response to therapy. The nurse's aim is to relieve pain without disabling the client mentally, emotionally or physically.

Educate the client about the pain: When possible, the nurse should explain the cause of the pain, time of occurrence, duration and quality and ways to gain relief. Education promotes the prevention of pain.

The basic nursing responsibility is protecting the client from harm. One simple way to promote comfort is

by removing or preventing painful stimuli. The following measures can be performed by the nurse to assist in pain control:
- Tighten and smooth wrinkled bed linen
- Reposition drainage tubes/ other objects on which patient is lying
- Place warm bath blankets for coolness
- Loosen constricting bandages (unless specifically applied as a pressure dressing)
- Change wet dressings
- Position the client in an anatomical alignment
- Check temperature of hot or cold applications including bath water
- Lift client on bed–do not pull. Patient up in bed; handle gently
- Position patient correctly on bed pain
- Avoid exposing skin or mucous membrane to irritants (e.g. diarrheal stool, wound drainage)
- Prevent urinary retention by keeping Foley's catheters patent and free-flowing
- Prevent constipation with fluids, diet and exercises.

Nurse's Role in administration of analgesics: The nurse spends the most time with the client in pain and is the team member who most often assesses the effectiveness of pain control interventions. When analgesics are prescribed, the nurse often has choices of drug, route, and interval. For example, the postoperative client may have the following orders:
- Morphine 10-15 mg IM or IV q2-4h pm severepain
- Vicodin i-ii tabs q3-4h pm moderate pain

When this client complains of pain, which analgesic should the nurse administer? Which route? Which dose? How frequently? The nurse has a large responsibility in making these decisions but also has autonomy in making these decisions. Each nurse may make a different decision, often based on the nurse's own biases.

The responsibilities of the nurse in administering analgesics includes:
- Determine whether to give the analgesic, and if more than one is ordered, which one.
- Assess the client's response to the analgesic, including assessing the effectiveness in pain relief and occurrence of any side effects.
- Report to the physician when a change is needed, including making suggestions for changes based on the nurse's knowledge of the client and pharmacology.
- Teach the client and family regarding the use of analgesics.

Invasive Interventions

The drugs used to relieve pain work by altering pain sensation, depressing pain perception or modifying the patient's response to pain as the nurse has considerable control over and responsibility for the effective use of medicines to reduce pain, knowledge of the drugs used in pain control, their routes of administration and side effects are needed. Examples of analgesic are of four types as follows:

1. Non-narcotic analgesics
   - Acetaminophen (Tylenol, Danol)
   - Acetylsalicylic acid (Aspirin)
   - Choline magnesium trisalicylate (tritisate)
2. NSAIDs
   - Ibuprofen (Brufen)
   - Naproxen (Naprosyn)
   - Indomethacin
   - Tolmetin
   - Piroxicam
3. Narcotic analgesics
   - Meperidine
   - Methylmorphine (Codiene)
   - Morphine sulfate (Morphine)
   - Fentany (Sublimaze)
   - Butorphanol (Butarin)
   - Hydromorphene HCl
4. Adjuvants
   - Amitriptyline
   - Hydroxyzine
   - Caffeine
   - Chloropromozine
   - Diazepam

There are four types of analgesic as mentioned below which include: (i) non-narcotic analgesics; (ii) NSAIDs; (iii) opioids and (iv) adjuvants or coanalgesics. Non-narcotic and NSAIDs provide relief for mild and moderate pain.

Principles of administering analgesics: Principles should be applied in the administration of analgesics, no matter which one is given.

Establishing and maintaining a therapeutic serum level is important. Peaks and valleys often occur when analgesics are administered in the traditional PRN (as needed) manner. When the dose is administered on an intermittent schedule, a larger dose is often required, causing the client to have a peak serum drug level in the sedation range. The client must wait for the return of pain before requesting the next dose of analgesic. Depending on the length or time it takes to obtain the medication and, once taken, to re-establish an adequate blood level, there could be a period of up to an hour or so without adequate pain control.

Preventive approach: Pain is much easier control if treated when it is anticipated or at a mild intensity. Once pain becomes severe, the analgesics ordered may not be effective enough to relieve it. Many clinicians still teach their clients to wait to take medication until they are sure they really need it. This practice leads to uncontrolled pain. There are two ways the preventive approach may be implemented:

1. *ATC (around the clock):* When pain is predictable, for example, the first few days following surgery or with chronic cancer pain, the medication is administered on a scheduled basis. This prevents the peaks and valleys of serum drug level that can lead to oversedation or toxicity and recurrence of pain, respectively. If the analgesics are ordered by the physician to be given PRN, it can still be a nursing measure to administer the drugs ATC, as long as they are given within the time constraints of the order.
2. *PRN (Latin for pro re nata,* which means "as required"): Pain is not always predictable: therefore PRN dosing may be required. For some clients this may be used in addition to scheduled dosing for "breakthrough" pain (pain that surpasses the level of analgesia, or pain relief without anesthesia, that the steady level of analgesics is providing). Examples of this include a cancer client on prolonged-release morphine who needs extra analgesics to participate in activities such as shopping or receiving visitors. Another example would be the orthopedic client who is receiving regularly scheduled analgesics for postoperative pain who needs additional pain relief for therapy sessions. In order to implement the preventive approach with PEN dosing, the medications should be given as soon as the pain appears, or when it is anticipated to begin.

CHAPTER 3

Nursing Management of Respiratory Problems

INTRODUCTION

The act of breathing involves two interrelated processes, ventilation and respiration–ventilation is the movement of air into and out of lungs. Respiration refers to the exchange of oxygen and carbon dioxide across cell membrane. The primary purpose of the respiratory system is gas exchange, which involves the transfer of oxygen and carbon dioxide between the atmosphere and blood. The respiratory system is divided into two parts, i.e. the upper respiratory tract and lower respiratory tract. The upper respiratory tract includes the nose, pharynx, adenoids, tonsils, epiglottis, larynx and trachea. The lower respiratory tract consists of bronchi, bronchioles, alveolar ducts and alveoli. With the exception of the right and left main stem bronchi, all lower airway structures are contained in the lungs. The right lung is divided into three lobes—upper, middle and lower and the left lung into two lobes—upper and lower. The structure of the chest walls (ribs, pleura, muscle of respiration) are also essential to respiration.

NURSING ASSESSMENT OF RESPIRATORY SYSTEM

Respiratory assessment should be tailored to the individual's health status. The most common symptoms or reasons, a person seeks health care include dyspnea, cough, sputum production, hemoptysis, wheezing or chest pain. Upper airways symptoms may include obstruction of noses, nasal discharge, sinus pain, sore throat or hoarseness.

Dyspnea

Dyspnea means breathlessness, but the terms used to describe difficult or labored breathing observable by others. It may cause other problems such as constipation or poor nutrition, as well as psychosocial problem related to poor self-esteem or changes in lifestyle. Individuals experiencing pulmonary dysfunctions, such as breathlessness, tend to perceive their illness in terms of its impact on their ability to carry-out activities of daily living. Which includes:

- Bathe, dress and groom
- Perform chores or hobbies
- Walk or exercise
- Get to the bathroom
- Prepare meals and rest
- Maintain family and social relationships
- Getting into home or climbing stairs
- Maintain employment
- Sleep
- Perform scanality
- Attend activities away from home.

Analysis of dyspnea according to its time and characteristics.

- *Timing:* Chronic or acute, episodic or paroxysmal, onset, duration and frequency.
- *Characteristics:*
  - Perceived severity
  - Phases of respiratory cycle—inspiratory, expiratory, throughout cycle.
- *Other symptoms related to dyspnea:*
- *Associated factors:*
  - Time of day
  - Seasonal or weather changes
  - Environmental irritants
  - Anxiety
  - Body position—paroxysmal nocturnal dyspnea (PND). Sudden onset while sleeping in recumbent position.
    - Orthopnea: Breathlessness on assuming recumbent position.
  - Activity.

Cough

Coughing has two main functions. It protects the lungs from aspiration and it helps propel foreign matter and excess mucus up through the airways. The individual can describe the cough in terms of timing and characteristics as follows:

- *Timing:* Chronic, acute, paroxysmal (periodic forceful episode difficult to control) onset (gradual or sudden).
- *Characteristics:*
  - Perceived severity
  - Pattern, occasional, upon rising, with activity (talking, exercising, eating).
- *Quality:*
  - Productive, non-productive
  - Dry progression to productive
  - Barking
  - Hoarse
  - Hacking

- *Other symptoms:*
  - Chest tightness
  - Fever, coryza
  - Choking.

Sputum Production

The mucous blanket lines the epithelial layer of the trachobronchial tree and cleanses it of inhaled particles and debris. Mucus is produced by the globet cells and submucosal glands. The cilia propel the mucous (which contains foreign particles, pus, blood and debris) upward toward the pharynx where it is coughed up, suctioned or swallowed. Normal sputum is clear and thin and average 100 ml/day. However, individuals with pulmonary disease often have sputum associated with these conditions making it important to assess the baseline super characteristics, describes as thick, viscous (gelatanious) tenacious (sticky), frothy, mucoid (colorless, clear, non-infectious watery, mucopurulent, and casts (from bronchioles, rubbery).
The mucopurulent sputum may be:
- *Creamy yellow: Staphylococcal pneumonia.*
- *Green: Pseudomonas pneumoniae*
- *Current jelly: Klebsiella pneumoniae.*
- *Rusty: Pneumococcal pneumonia.*
- *Pink frothy: Pulmonary edema*

The quantity of amount of sputum may be teaspoon, tablespoon or cups used as a measurement.

Hemoptysis

Hemoptysis is the coughing up of blood or blood-tinged sputum. It may contain air bubbles. The source of bleeding may be from anywhere in the upper or lower airways or from the lung parenchyma. Blood that originates in the GI tract and is coughed up as dark brown or resembling coffee grains in appearance termed as "hematemesis". It is usually never frothy, may be mixed with food particles, pH acidic dark-red or coffee colored. Bleeding from the nares (epistaxis) should be assessed as a cause for coughing up blood or vomiting of blood.

In hemoptysis, blood is usually frothy, pH alkaline, bright red. The coughing up of 400-1600 ml of blood in 24 hours period is considered massive and severe, needs immediate medical attention.

Wheezing

Wheezing is a continuous high-pitched, whistling sound produced when air passes through narrowed or obstructed airways. It is generally occurring during expiration, however, wheezing can be heard throughout respiratory cycle. Wheezing is usually heard with a stethoscope; however, wheezing may be audible to the person or heard by others in close proximity to the person. An analysis of this symptom should include factors that can cause bronchospasm and produce wheezing such as asthma, exposure to physiological irritants, stress, anxiety. Snoring or stridor cloud snoring may be experienced.

Chest Pain

Chest pain can result from several conditions. Chest pain may be cardiac origin. The chest pain of pulmonary origin can originate from the chest wall. Parietal pleura or lung parenchyma. The characteristics of pulmonary chest pain are:
- Pain from the chest wall is well-localised, constant ache increasing with movement. It may be due to trauma, cough and herpes zoster.
- Pain is parietal pleura is a sharp, abrupt onset, increasing with inspiration or with sudden ventilatory effort (cough, sneeze) unilateral.
- Pain from lung parenchyma is dull, constant poorly localised in benign pulmonary tumors and carcinoma; well-localised sharp, sudden onset in pneumothorax; sudden onset, increasing stabbing pain on inspiration, may radiate in cases of pulmonary embolus and infarction.

In addition to review of symptom or reason the person is seeking health care, the person should be interviewed about risk factors associated with respiratory dysfunction, including smoking, past pulmonary illnesses or exposure to respiratory infections, predisposition to genetic disorders, exposure to environmental irritants (dust, fume, gases, etc.) and the psychosocial effects of respiration disorders.

The emotional responses include anxiety, depression, hostility, fear or panic, etc. and ask the person's problems with swallowing and ambulating as well as neuromuscular diseases.

The common abnormalities of the thorax and lungs found by physical examinations are as follows:

Inspection

- *Pursed-lip breathing:* Is an exhalation through mouth with lips pursed together to slow exhalation. As seen in COPD, asthma suggests increasing breathlessness. Strategy taught is slow expiration, decrease dyspnea.
- *Tripod position:* Inability to be flat, i.e. leaning forward, with arms and elbows supported on overbed table. Seen in COPD, asthma in exacerbations, pulmonary edema, indicates moderate to severe respiratory distress.
- *Accessory muscle use:* In intercostal retractions neck and shoulder muscles are used to assist breathing. Muscles between ribs pull in during respiration. Due to COPD, asthma in exacerbation–secretion retention, indicate severe respiratory distress, hypoxemia.
- *Splinting:* A voluntary decrease in tidal volume to decreased pain on chest expansion. It is due to thoracic or abdominal incisions, chest trauma, plurasy.
- *Increased:* Anterioposterior (AP) chest diameter equal to the lateral, slope of ribs more horizontal (90°) or

spine. One to COPD, asthma, cystic fibrosis, lung hyperinflation, advanced age.
- *Tachypnea:* Increased rate of 20 breaths/minute, > 25 breath/minute in elderly. Due to fever, anxiety, hypoxemia, restrictive lung disease. Magnitude of increasing above normal rate reflects increased work of breathing.
- *Kussmaul's respiration:* Regular rapid and deep respirations are due to metabolic acidosis. Increase in rate aids body in CO_2 excretion.
- *Cyanoses:* Refer to a bluish color of skin best seen in earlobes, under eyelids or nailbeds. It is due to decreased oxygen transfer of lungs, decreased cardiac output, nonspecific unreliable indicator.
- *Clubbing of fingers:* Refer to increased depth, bulk, sponginess, of distal digit finger. It is due to chronic hypoxemia, cystic fibrosis, lung cancer, bronchiectasis.
- *Abdominal paradox:* An inward (rather than normal outward) movement of abdomen during inspiration. It is due to insufficient and ineffective breathing pattern–nonspecific indicator of severe respiratory distress.

Palpation

- Tracheal deviation is a leftward or rightward movement of trachea from normal midline position. It is nonspecific indicator of change in position of mediasternoid structure, medical emergency if caused by tension pneumothorax.
- Altered tactile fremitus is increased or decreased in vibrations. It is due to increased in pneumonia, pulmonary edema; decreased in pleural effusion, atelectic area, lung hyperinflation, absent in pneumothorax, large atelectasis.
- Altered chest movements, i.e. unequal or equal but diminished movement of two sides of chest with inspiration.
Usually unequal movement caused by atelectasis, pneumothorax, pleural effusion, splinting, equal but diminished movement caused by barrel chest, restrictive disease and neuromuscular disease.

Percussion

- Hyper-resonance is loud, laver-pitched sound over areas that normally produces a resonance sound. It is due to lung hyperinflation (COPD), lung collapse (pneumothorax), air trapping (asthma).
- Dullness is medium-pitched sound over areas that normally produce a resonant sound. It is due to increased density (pneumonia, large atelectasis). Increased fluid pleural space (pleural effusion).

Auscultation

- Fine crackles are series of short explosive, high-pitched sounds heard just before the end of inspiration: result of rapid equalisation of gas pressure when collapsed alveoli or terminal bronchioles suddenly snap open similar sound to that made by rolling hair between fingers just behind ear. Can be heard in fibrosis (asbestos interstitial edema, early pulmonary edema), alveolar filling (pneumonia), loss of lung volume (atelectasis), early phase of congestive heart failure.
- Coarse crackles are series of short, low-pitched sounds caused by air passing through airway intermittently occluded by mucus unstable bronchial wall of fold of mucosa, evident on inspiration and at times, expiration; similar sound to bowling quality with more fluid. These can be heard in congestive heart failure, pulmonary edema, pneumonia with severe congestion, COPD.
- Rhonchi are continuous rumbling, snoring, or rattling sounds from obstructions of a large airways with secretions most prominent on expiration; change often evident after coughing or suctioning. These are heard in COPD, cystic fibrosis, pneumonia, bronchietasis.
- Wheezing are continuous musical sound of constant pitch: result of partial obstruction of larynx or trachea. It is due to epiglottis, vocal cord edema after extubation, foreign body.
- Absent breath sounds, no sound evident over entire lung or area of lung. It is due to pleural effusion, main stem bronchi, obstruction, large atelectasis, pneumonectomy, lobectomy.
- Pleural friction rub is cracking or grating sound from roughened inflamed surfaces of the pleura rubbing together, evident during inspiration. It is due to pleurasy, pneumonia, pulmonary infarction.
- Bronchophony, whispered pectoriloquy a spoken or whispered syllable more distinct than normal on auscultation as in pneumonia.
- Egophony is a spoken "e" similar to "a" on auscultation because of altered transmission of voice sounds seen in pneumonia, pleural effusion.

DIAGNOSTIC STUDIES OF RESPIRATORY SYSTEM

Blood Studies

- Hemoglobin test reflects amount of hemoglobin available for combination with oxygen. Venous blood is used. The normal level of adult man is 135-180 g/dl (13.5-18 g/l) = Normal level of adult woman is 12-16 g/dl (120-160 g/l). The nursing responsibilities during the procedure is to explain the procedure and its purpose. No special care is required.
- Hematocrit test reflects ratio of red blood cells to plasma increased hematocrit (polycythemia) found in chronic hypoxemia. Venous blood is used. Normal for adult man is 40-54 percent and woman is 38-47 percent. The nursing responsibility is as in HB%.

- Antitrypsin assay is valuable in the identification of individuals with the genetic abnormality that leads to emphysema. This is a globulin that inhibits certain enzymes. The normal values of α1-antitrypsin assay.
  MM genotype: 2.1-3.8 u/ml
  M2 phenotype: 1.05-2.1 u/ml
  22 phenotype: 0.5-0.7 u/ml
  The nursing care includes as in hemoglobin. No food or fluid restrictions are necessary.
- *Complete blood count:* The normal counts of RBCs in male 4.6-6.2 million/D. 4.2-5.4 million/L in females. The normal level of WBC $4.0-11.0 \times 10^3$/L.
- *Arterial blood gases (ABGs):* Arterial blood is obtained through puncture of radial or femoral artery or through arterial catheter. ABGs are performed to assess acid-base-balance, ventilation status, need for oxygen therapy, change in oxygen therapy, or change in ventilation settings. Continuous ABG monitoring is also possible via a sensor or electrode inserted into the arterial catheter.

  Nursing responsibility in this test, thus includes. Explain the purposes of the test and its procedure to the patient in using oxygen (percentage, L/min). Avoid changing it for 20 minutes before obtaining sample. Assist with positioning (e.g. palm up, wrist slightly hyperextended if radial artery is used). Collect blood into heparanised syringe. To ensure accurate results, expel all air bubbles, and place sample in ice, unless it will be analysed in less than 1 minute. Apply pressure to artery for 5 minutes after specimen is obtained to prevent hematoma at the arterial puncture site.

  The normal values, parameters of ABGs are:
  - *Acid-base-balance* measured as pH (hydrogen ion concentration. Normal 7.35-7.45. Alkalemia increased 7.45. Acedemia decreased 7.35.
  - *Oxygenation* PaO_2 (partial pressure of dissolved O_2 in blood. Normal 80-100 mm Hg. Hyperoxemia 100 mm Hg, hypoxemia – 80 mm Hg.
  - *Ventilation* SaO_2 percentage of O_2 bound hemoglobin. $PaCO_2$ partial pressure of CO_2 dissolved in blood. The normal SaO_2 is 95-98 per cent. The normal $PaCO_2$: 35-45 mm Hg. Hypercapnia 45 mm Hg. Hypocapnia –35 mm Hg.
- *Oximetry:* Test monitors arterial or venous oxygen saturation device attached to the ear lobe, finger or nose for SPO_2 monitoring or is contained in a pulmonary artery catheter for SVO_2 monitoring. Oximetry is used for continuous monitoring in ICUs, inpatient and outpatient sortings and exercise testing.

  The nursing responsibilities include, applying probe to finger, forehead, earlobe or bridge of nose. When interpreting SPO_2 and SVO_2 values, first assess patient status and presence of factors that can alter accuracy of pulse oximeter reading. For SPO_2, these include motion, low perfusion, bright lights, use of intravascular dyes, acryling nails, dark skin colour. For SVO_2, these include change in O_2 delivery or O_2 consumptions. For SPO_2 notify physician of ± 4 percent change from baseline or decrease to less than 90 percent. For SVO_2 notify physician of ± 10 percent change from baseline or decrease to less than 60 percent.

Sputum Analysis

The nursing responsibilities include explain purposes. Some tests require specimens, collected in consecutive days usually 4 ml of sputum is sufficient. Coughing upon awakening is more likely to result in collecting sputum and not saliva. Instruct individual to rinse the mouth with water, demonstrate effective deep breathing and coughing, have individual practice deep breathing and coughing, instruct individual to notify staff as the specimen is collected. Following are different tests and nursing care.

Culture and Sensitivity

Single sputum specimen is collected in a sterile container. For diagnosing bacterial infection, select antibiotic and evaluate treatment. Here instruct patients on how to produce of good specimen for Gram stain test as given below if patients cannot produce specimen bronchoscopy may be used.

Gram Stain

Staining of sputum permits classification of bacteria into gram-negative and gram-positive types. Results guide therapy until culture and sensitivity results are obtained. Here nurse instructs patient to expectorate sputum into the container after coughing deeply. Obtain sputum in early morning because secretions collect during night. If unsuccessful try increasing oral fluids, intake unless fluids are restricted. Collect sputum in sterile container (sputum trap) during suctioning or by aspirating secretions from the trachea. Send specimen to laboratory promptly.

Acid-fast Smear Culture

Test is performed to collect sputum for acid-fast bacilli (AFB). A series of three early morning specimen is used. Nursing responsibility as in Gram stain and cover specimen and send to laboratory for analysis.

Cytology

In this single sputum specimen is collected in special container with fixative solution. Purpose is to determine presence of abnormal cells that may indicate malignant condition. The nurse should send specimens to laboratory promptly and take measure in other tests.

Radiological Studies

Chest X-ray

Test is used to screen, diagnose, and evaluate change. Most common views are posteroanterior and lateral. In this, nurse instructs patient to undress to waist, put on gown, and remove any metal between neck and waist.

Computed Tomography (CT)

Test is performed for diagnostic of lesions difficult to assess by conventional X-ray studies, such as those in the hilum, mediastenum, and pleura. Images show structures in cross-section. Nursing care is same as for chest X-ray.

Magnetic Resonance Imaging (MRI)

Test is used for diagnosis of lesions difficult to assess by CT scan (e.g. lung apex near the spine). Here, nurse explains purpose, takes measures as in chest X-ray and instructs the patient to remove all metal (e.g. jewellery, watch) before test. It takes about an hour.

Ventilation/Perfusion (V/P) Lung Scan

Test is used to identify areas of the lung not receiving air flow (ventilator) or blood flow (perfusion). It involves injection of radioisotope and inhalation of small amount of radioactive gas (Xenon). A gamma detecting device is used to record radioactivity. Ventilation without perfusion suggests pulmonary embolus. The nursing measures are as for chest X-ray. Also check for dye allergy. Obtain an accurate weight so that the dosage of radioactive agent can be calculated. No special care or precaution is needed afterwards (post test) because the gas and isotope transmit radioactivity for only brief interval.

Pulmonary Angiogram

Study is used to visualize pulmonary vasculature and locate obstructions or pathologic conditions such as pulmonary embolus. A radio-opaque dye is injected, usually through a catheter into the pulmonary artery or right side of the heart. Nursing measures same as chest X-ray. Know that dye injection may cause flushing, warm sensation, and coughing. Check pressure dressing site after procedure. Monitor blood pressure, pulse rate and circulation distal to injection site. Report and record significant changes.

Positron Emission Tomography (PET)

Test is used to distinguish benign and malignant lung nodules. It involves IV injection of a radioisotope with short half-life. Nursing measures same as V/P.

Endoscopic Examination

Bronchoscopy

This study is typically performed in outpatient procedure room. Flexible fiberoptic scope is used for diagnosis, biopsy, specimen collection, or assessment of changes. It may also be done to suction mucous plugs or to remove foreign objects. In this examination, the nurse instructs patient to be on NPO status for 6-12 hours. Obtain signed permit (consent). Give diazepam if ordered by physician before procedure to aid relaxation. After procedure, keep patient NPO until gag-reflex returns and monitor for laryngeal edema. If biopsy was done, monitor for hemorrhage and pneumothorax.

Mediastinoscopy

Test is used for inspection and biopsy of lymph nodes in mediastinal area. Nurse prepares patient for surgical intervention, obtains signed permit. Afterwards monitor as for bronchoscopy.

Biopsy

In lung biopsy specimen may be obtained by transbronchial or open-lung biopsy. This test is used to obtain specimens for laboratory analysis. Nursing measures same as bronchoscopy.

Others

Thoracentesis

Test is used to obtain specimen of pleural fluid for diagnosis, to remove pleural fluid or to instill medication. The physician inserts a large bore needle through chest wall into pleural space. Chest X-ray is always obtained after procedures to check pneumothorax. Nursing responsibility includes explaining procedures to patient and obtain signed permit prior to procedure. Position patient upright, instruct not to talk or cough, and assist during procedure. If large volume of fluid is removed, monitor for decrease in shortness of breath, send labelled specimen to laboratory.

Pulmonary Function Test

It is used to valuate lung function. It involves use of a spirometer to diagram air movement as patient performs prescribed respiratory manoeuvres. Nurse has to avoid scheduling immediately after meals times. Avoid administration of inhaled bronchiodilator for 6 hours before procedure.

Explain procedure to patient. Provide rest after procedure.

ACUTE BRONCHITIS

Bronchitis is an inflammation of the lower respiratory tract that is usually due to infection and occurs most frequently in patients with chronic respiratory disease. Bronchitis can be acute or chronic bronchitis.

Acute bronchitis is an inflammation of the bronchi and usually the trachea (tracheobronchitis).

Etiology

Acute bronchitis occurs most often in persons with chronic lung disease. It also occurs as an extension of the

URI in persons without underlying any lung disease, and is therefore communicable. It may be caused by physical and chemical agents such as dust, smoke, or volatile fumes. As air pollution increases, the incidence of acute bronchitis increases.

Acute bronchitis is typically viral, but bacterial pathogens such as *Streptococcus pneumoniae* and *Haemophilus influenzae* may also cause bronchitis, either primary or secondary infections which includes:
- *Viruses:* Rhinovirus, adenovirus, influenza A and B, parainfluenza virus and respiratory syncytial virus (RSV).
- *Bacteria*: *Streptococcus pneumoniae, Haemophilus influenzae, Moraxella catarrhalis, Bordetella pertussis, Mycoplasma pneumoniae, Chlamydia pneumoniae.*

Pathophysiology

As a part of the inflammatory process, there is increased blood flow to the affected area, causing an increased in pulmonary secretions. A painful cough with sputum productions, low-grade fever, and malaise are common symptoms. The patient may have pain beneath the sternum caused by inflammation of the tracheal wall. Bronchitis without tracheitis never seen, and tracheobronchitis is more appropriate term for this condition. Symptoms usually last 1 for 1 to 2 weeks but may continue for 3 to 4 weeks. Rhonchi and wheezes heard on chest examination. If symptoms worsen and there is a high fever, shortness of breath, pleuritic chest pain (pain on inspiration) rapid respirations and rales or sign if consolidation on physical examination of the chest, pneumonia suspected.

Management

Treatment of acute bronchitis is mainly supportive and includes the following:
- Codeine or dextromethorphan is prescribed for nocturnal cough.
- Bronchodilator therapy is prescribed for patients who are wheezing and for those whose peak expiratory rate prolonged, e.g., albuterol, or ipratropium.
- Decongestants and antihistamines are used sparingly, if at all, because they tend to dry secretions and make them more difficult to remove.
- Oral fluids intake of 2 to 3 litre per day is encouraged if there is no contraindications to it.
- Aspirin helps to reduce fever and alleviate some of the symptoms and inflammation.
- Patients who are smokers are urged to quit.
- Antibiotics are usually not prescribed unless there is evidence of bacterial infections.
- Rest is encouraged to give the body a chance to heal.

Nursing care is supportive and is directed towards helping the patient with prescribed therapy and avoiding future infections. Emphasis on assisting the patient to cough effectively, assisting with comfort, assisting with activities of daily living and teaching the patient and family.

To produce an effective cough, a deep inspiration must be followed by maximal expiratory effort against a closed glottis. This results in a tremendous increase in intrathoracic pressure. As glottis opens, mucus and inhaled particles are forced out of the airways at a high velocity. Persistent coughing can be annoying and tiring to the patient and those around him or her. Complications of persistent coughing includes, insomnia, exhaustion vomiting, urinary incontinence, rib or muscle trauma, pneumothorax, and fainting. If cough persists, give cough medication as prescribed. A semi-Fowler's position or high-Fowler's position usually facilitates breathing. Provide for good drainage of trachobronchial secretions and give antibiotics as ordered and assist in ADL.

PNEUMONIA

Pneumonia or pneumonitis is an acute inflammation of the lung tissue (lung parenchyma).

Etiology

Pneumonia is resulting from inhalation or transport via the bloodstream of infectious agents or noxious fumes or from radiation treatment. Pneumonia is classified according to whether infection was acquired in the community or in the hospital. Thus pneumonia is classified as "community acquired pneumonia (CAP) or hospital acquired pneumonia (HAP). HAP is also called nosocomial pneumonia. The causes of pneumonia are as follows.
- Community-acquired pneumonia caused by:
  - *Streptococcus pneumoniae*
  - *Haemophilus influenzae*
  - *Mycoplasma pneumoniae*
  - Respiratory viruses
  - *Chlamydia pneumoniae*
  - *Legionella pneumophila*
  - Oral anaerobes
  - *Moraxella catarrhalis*
  - *Staphylococcus aureus*
  - *Nocardia*
  - Enteric aerobic gram-negative bacteria (e.g. *Klebsiella*)
  - Fungi
  - *Mycobacterium tuberculosis.*
- Hospital-acquired pneumonia caused by:
  - *Pseudomonas aeruginosa*
  - *Enterobacter*
  - *Escherichia coli*
  - *Proteus*
  - *Klebsiella*

- *Staphylococcus aureus*
- *Streptococcus pneumoniae*
- Oral anaerobes.

The risk factors which predispose to pneumonia are:
- Smoking
- Air pollution
- Altered consciousness: Alcoholism, head injury, seizures, anesthesia, drug overdose
- Tracheal intubation (endotracheal intubations, tracheostomy)
- Upper respiratory tract infection
- Chronic diseases: Chronic lung diseases, diabetes mellitus, heart disease, uremia, cancer
- Immunosuppression
  - Drugs (carciosteroids, cancer chemotherapy, immunosuppressive therapy after organ transplant)
  - HIV
- Malnutrition
- Inhalation of aspiration of noxious substances
- Debilitating illness
- Bedrest and prolonged immobility
- Altered oropharyngeal flora.

The risk factors for hospital-acquired pneumonia are:
- Residence in an ICU
- Mechanical ventilation (those who required 48 hours or more ventilation)
- Endotracheal intubation or tracheostomy
- Recent surgery
- Debilitation, i.e. malnutrition
- Invasive devices
- Neuromuscular disease
- Depressed level of alertness
- Aspiration
- Antacid use
- Age 60 or older
- Prolonged hospital stay
- Any serious underlying disease.

Pathophysiology

Normally, the airway distal to the larynx is sterile because of protective defence mechanisms. These mechanisms include:
- Filtration of air
- Warming and humidification of inspired air
- Epiglottis closure over the trachea
- Cough reflex
- Mucociliary escalator mechanism
- Secretion of immunoglobulin A
- Alveolar macrophages.

Pneumonia results in inflammation of lung tissue. Depending on the particular pathogen and the hosts' physical status, the inflammatory process may involve different anatomical areas of the lung parenchyma and the pleurae. The normal function of respiratory system and primary pathophysiology and clinical manifestation are as follows:

- Normally 'mucociliary system' cleanses inhaled air by trapping particles. In pneumonia, hypertrophy of mucous membrane lining lung, resulting in hypersecretions leads to increased sputum production and cough:
  - Anerobic - Foul-smelling, sputum
  - *Klebsiella* - Current Jelly color
  - *Staphylococcus* - Creamy yellow
  - *Pseudomonas* – Green
  - Viral/mucopurulent

  And bronchospasms from increased secretions, leads to localised or diffuse wheezing dyspnea.

- Generally 'alveolocapillary membrane' exchanges oxygen-carbon dioxide. In pneumonia, there is increased permeability resulting in excess fluid in interstitial space, shows consolidation (in chest X-ray films) localised/bacterial; diffuse/viral, and also there is decreased surface area for gas exchange leads to hypoxaemia.

- Normally pleura maintains close approximation of lungs and chest wall; minimizes friction during lung expansion and contraction. In pneumonia there is inflammation of the pleura which shows, chest pain, especially on inspiration, pleural effusion, dullness on percussion, decreased breath sounds and decreased vocal fremitus.

- Normally respiratory muscle expands and contracts chest wall and thus pleura and lungs. In pneumonia there is hypoventilation and respiratory acidosis (in presence of underlying disease) leads to decreased chest expansion and hypercapnoea and low arterial blood pH.

- The lung defense system protects normally sterile lung from invasion. In pneumonia there is bacteremia, shows elevated blood cell counting; leukocytes (15,000 to 25000/mm), neutrophilia and tachypnoea and fever.

In pneumococcal pneumonia there is congestion, red hepatisation and gray hepatisation.

Clinical Manifestation

CAP has been traditionally thought to present any two syndromes; typical and atypical, although the distinctions are not clear.

Typical pneumonic syndrome is characterised by sudden onset of fever, chills, cough productive of purulent sputum, and pleuritic chest pain (in some cases). On physical examination signs of pulmonary consolidations such as dullness, percussion, increased fermitus, bronchial breath sounds, and crackles may be found. In elderly or debilitated patient, confusion or stupor may be predominant. Usually two types of pneumonia caused by *S. pneumoniae* and *H. influenzae*.

The atypical syndrome is characterised by a more gradual onset dry cough, and extrapulmonary manifestation such as headache, myalgia, fatigue, sore throat, nausea, vomiting and diarrhea. On physical examination, crackles are often heard. This type of classically produced by *Mycoplasma, pneumoniae* and *Legionell Chlamydia pneumoniae*. Viral pneumoniae are characterised by an atypical presentation with chills, fever, dry non-productive cough and extrapulmonary symptoms. Most of the pneumoniae run uncomplicated. If occurs, the complications are pneumonia including pleurisy, pleural effusion, atelectasis, delayed resolution, lung abscess, empyema, pericarditis, arthritis, meningitis and endocarditis.

Management

History, physical examination and chest X-ray often provide enough information to take management decisions without costly laboratory tests. Diagnostic tests include:
- Chest X-ray film to confirm consolidation and distribution and pleural effusions.
- Sputum studies for culture and sensitivity if unable to obtain specimen by usual means, may use,
  - Transtracheal aspiration,
  - Bronchoscopy with aspiration, biopsy or bronchial brushings.
- Arterial blood gas studies or pulse oximetry.
- Hematology: WBC count, cole agglutinin and compliment fixation for viral studies.
- Thoracentesis to obtain pleural fluid specimen if pleural effusion is present.

The possible nursing diagnosis on the basis and assessment will be:
- Airway clearance, ineffective r/t decreased energy, fatigue, tracheobronchial inflammation.
- Impaired gas exchange r/t alveolar capillary membrane changes altered oxygen delivery.
- Pain r/t pleural inflammation, coughing paroxysms.
- Rest for infection r/t compromised lung defense system.
- Knowledge deficient r/t condition, treatment.
- Anorexia r/t infection process-sputum production.
- Altered nutrition/body requirement r/t increased metabolic needs.

Prompt treatment with the appropriate antibiotic almost always cures bacterial and mycoplasmal pneumonia. In uncomplicated cases, the patient responds to drug therapy within 48 to 72 hours. Indications for improvement including decreased temperature, improved breathing, and reduced chest pain.

Abnormal physical finding lasts for more than 7 days. The nursing intervention includes.
- Maintaining effective airway clearance
  - Monitor for increased respiratory distress
  - Assist patient to cough effectively
  - If unable to clear down airway, suction airway using sterile technique
  - Assist with nebuliser therapy
  - Administer bronchiodilator as ordered. Monitor for side effects and response to therapy
  - Change position frequently to assist in mobilising secretions
  - Ensure fluid intake adequate to thin secretions.
- Facilitate breathing: Help the patient breathe deeply and expand the chest to increase ventilation.
  - Place the patient in position to facilitate breathing, usually upright or semiupright position.
  - A pillow may be placed lengthwise at the patient's back to provide support and thrust thorax slightly towards allowing free use of the diaphragm.
  - The patient who must be upright to breathe may find it restful to place head and arms on a pillow placed on an overbed table.
  - For the patient with severe hypoxemia, side rails should be in place. The patient can use them to assisting about in bed.
  - Some patients who breathe best when sitting up in a large armchair while leaning on a smaller chair. Placed in front of that. This chair is blocked to prevent it from slipping.
  - Assist with ADL pacing activities to prevent fatigue and respiratory distress.
- Administration of medication and treatment
  - Before starting prescribed antibiotic, collect sputum for culture and blood for culture if ordered.
  - Maintain antibiotic blood levels by giving antibiotic at scheduled time.
  - Give medication prescribed to relieve pain. Codeine may be ordered because it is less likely to inhibit cough reflex than more potent narcotics.
  - Begin oxygen therapy.
- Administering oxygen therapy
- Promoting comfort
  - Place in position of comfort, Preferably head of bed elevated 45 to 90 degrees.
  - Assess character and location of chest pain.
  - Administer analgesic for chest pain e.g. acetylsalicylic acid, acetaminophen and codeine.
  - Splint chest with hands when patient coughs.
  - Administer frequent mouth care. Protect lips and nares with lubricants.
  - Keep patient warm and dry and avoid chilling.
- Preventing spread of infection.
  - Standard precautions are used.
- Facilitating learning: The major teaching emphasis is on prevention.
  - Assess patient's understanding of pneumonia with questions concerning such information on how pneumonia is transmitted and risk factor.
  - Teach proper handling of secretions. Cover nose and mouth with tissue when coughing or sneezing.

- Discard tissues in paper or plastic bag for disposal. Expectorate into specimen container provided.
- Stress importance of handwashing after coughing, sneezing and expectorating.
- Reinforce importance and follow-up care.
- Reinforce the need for immunization, i.e., inlfuenza vaccine and pneumococcal vaccine. Pneumonia polysaccharide vaccine is given only every 3 to 5 years.
- Promoting adequate hydration and nutrition
  - Encourage oral fluids. If patient is receiving IV fluids, monitor rate. Observe for signs of fluid volume deficit or excess.
  - Ask patient what foods he or she would like to eat.
  - Offer small, frequent feedings.
  - Encourage high-carbohydrate and high-protein foods.

TUBERCULOSIS

Tuberculosis is an infectious disease caused by mycobacterium tuberculosis. It usually involves the lungs, but it also occurs in the kidneys, bones, adrenal glands, lymph nodes and meninges and can be disseminated throughout the body.

Etiology

Mycobacterium tuberculosis, a gram-positive, acid-fast bacillary, is usually spread via air-borne droplets, which are produced when the infected individual coughs, sneezes or speaks. Once released into a room, the organisms are dispersed and can be inhaled. Brief exposure to a tubercle bacilli rarely causes an infection. Rather it is more commonly spread to the individual who has had repeated close contact with an infected person. It is not highly infective and transmitted. It usually requires close, frequent or prolonged exposure. The disease cannot be spread by hands, books, glasses, dishes or other fomites.

Pathophysiology

When an individual with no previous exposure to TB (negative tuberculin reactor) inhales a sufficient number of tubercle bacilli into the alveoli, tuberculosis infection occurs. The body's reaction to the TB bacilli depends on the susceptibility of the individual, the size of the dose and the virulence of the organisms. Inflammation occurs within the alveoli (parenchyma) of the lungs, and natural body defenses attempt to counteract the infection.

When the bacilli is inhaled, they pass down the bronchial system and implant themselves on the respiratory bronchioles or alveoli. The lower part of the lungs are usually the site of initial bacterial implantation. After implantation, the bacilli multiply with no initial resistance from the host. The organisms are engulfed by phagocytosis (initially neutrophils and later macrophages) and may continue to multiply within the phagocytes.

Macrophages ingest the organism and present the microbacterial antigens to the T cells. CD4 cells secrete lymphokine than enhance the capacity of the macrophages to ingest and kill bacteria. Lymph nodes in the hilar region of the lung become enlarged on their filter drainage from the infected site. The inflammatory process and the cellular reaction produce a small, firm, white nodules called the 'primary tubercle'. The centre of the nodules contain tubercle bacilli cells gather around the centre and usually the outer portion becomes fibrosed. Thus, blood vessels are compressed, nutrition of tubercle is impaired, and necrosis occurs at the centre. The area becomes walled off by fibritic tissue, and the centre gradually becomes soft and cheesy in consistency. This later process is known as "Caseation necrosis". This material may become calcified (calcium deposits) or it may liquify (liquification necrosis). The liquified material may be coughed up, leaving a cavity or hole in the parenchyma of the lung. This cavity or cavities are visible on chest X-ray films and results in the diagnosis of cavitary disease. The only X-ray evidence of TB infection is a calcified nodule known as "Ghon's tubercle". Ghon's tubercle is referred to as the "primary complex". When a tuberculosis lesion regresses and heals, the infection enters a latent period in which it may persist without producing a clinical illness. The infection may develop into clinical disease if the persisting organism begins to multiply rapidly, or it may remain dormant. If the initial immune response is not adequate, control of the organisms is not maintained and clinical disease results. Certain individuals are at a higher risk for clinical disease including those who are immunosuppressed, e.g. HIV, cancer, person who received chemotherapy or corticosteroid therapy or have diabetes mellitus. Dormant but viable organism persists for years. Reactivation of TB can occur if the host defense mechanisms become impaired.

Clinical Manifestation

In the early stages of TB, the person is usually free of symptoms. Many cases, if it is found that incidentally when routine chest X-rays are taken, especially in older adults. Systemic manifestation may initially consist of fatigue, malaise, anorexia, weight loss, low grade fever (especially in late afternoons) and night sweats. The weight loss may not be excessive until late in the disease and is often attributed to overwork or other factors. Irregular menses may also be present in premenopausal women.

A characteristic pulmonary manifestation is cough that becomes frequent and produce mucoid or macopurulent's sputum. Chest pain characterised as dull or tight may also be present. Hemoptysis is not a common finding and is usually associated with more advanced cases. Sometimes TB has more acute, sudden manifestation, the patient has high fever, chills, generalised of the like symptoms, pleuritic pain and a production of cough.

The complication of TB are miliary tuberculosis, pleural effusion, TB pneumonia, involvement of other organs, e.g., bone, kidney, brain, etc.

Management

This will be diagnosed by taking prompt health history and physical examination. The diagnostic studies of TB include:

- Tubercular skin testing, montoux test.
- Chest X-rays.
- Bacteriological studies–sputum smear, sputum.
- WBC Serologic test by ELISA (enzyme-linked immunosorbent assay).
- CSF.

The common drugs used for management of tuberculosis are described in **Table 3.1**.

Table 3.1: Anti-tubercular drugs.

Drug	Mechanism of action	Side effects	Dose	Management in case of toxicity
Isoniazid (both oral and injectable)	It is both bacteriostatic and bactericidal drug	• Hepatotoxicity • Peripheral neuropathy • Rash and fever • Acne • Anemia • Arthritis • SLE like syndrome • Optic neuropathy, seizures and psychiatric symptoms	• Usual dose 300 mg (5 mg/kg) in adults. In children: 10–15 mg/kg with maximum of 300 mg • For intermittent therapy, a maximum dose of 900 mg twice or thrice a week is used with vitamin B_6	• Limit alcohol consumption • Monitor SGPT and hepatitis syndrome • Stop the drug at first symptom of hepatitis (nausea, vomiting, anorexia and flu-like symptoms) • Concomitant administration of vitamin B_6 reduces the incidence of peripheral neuritis, optic neuritis and seizures • Nowadays all oral packs of anti-tubercular drugs incorporate vitamin B_6
Rifampicin (oral)	• It has both intra-cellular and extra-cellular bactericidal activity, i.e., blocks RNA polymerase • It is also effective against a wide spectrum of gram-negative organisms	• Hepatotoxicity • Rash • Flu-like syndrome • Red orange colored urine • Drug interaction	Adults: 450-600 mg (10 mg/kg) daily or twice a week Children: 10–20 mg/kg	• Limit alcohol consumption • Monitor SGPT and hepatitis symptoms • Reassure the patient that dark urine is due to drug itself • Stop the drug if symptoms of hepatitis or jaundice develop
Pyrazinamide (oral)	Bactericidal drug, used in short-course therapy for tuberculosis. It has excellent CSF penetration, hence a preferred drug in tubercular meningitis	• Hepatotoxicity • Hyperuricemia • Polyarthralgias	Adults: 2 to 2.5 g daily (15 to 30 mg/kg)	• Monitor SGPT and hepatitis symptoms • Limit the dose to 15-30 mg/kg • Monitor uric acid levels in patients of gout or renal failure
Ethambatol (oral)	Bacteriostatic against rapidly growing mycobacterium	• Retrobulbar optic neuritis (dose related) • Hyperuricaemia (rare)	Adults: 15 mg/kg as a single dose daily. **For retreatment** 25 mg/kg daily for 2 months, then 15 mg/kg daily. **For intermittent therapy** 50 mg/kg twice a week	• Avoid in children due to its visual toxicity • Use the lowest dose 15 mg/kg/day • Monitor visual acuity (eye chart) and red-green color vision (ishihara color chart/book) monthly. Stop the drug at the first change in vision
Streptomycin, amikacin, capreomycin	These drugs inhibit bacterial protein synthesis (bactericidal) for rapidly dividing extracellular mycobacteria. These drugs poorly diffuse into CSF	• Ototoxicity • Renal toxicity • Less common are, i.e. peri-oral paresthesias, eosinophilia, rash and drug fever	Adults: 0.5 to 1.0 g (10–15 mg/kg) daily or five times a week. Children: 20–40 mg/kg with a maximum of 1.0 g/day	• Limit the dose and duration of therapy as far as possible • Avoid daily therapy in old persons (> 60 years) • Monitor blood urea and serum creatinine levels • Ask daily for symptoms of ototoxicity, i.e. tinnitus, vertigo, dizziness and decreased hearing • Perform audiometry if possible before and during the course of therapy if needed • Stop the drug at first development of adverse effect

- *Isoniazid (INH)*: Interferes with DNA metabolism and tubercle bacilli. It is bactericidal, penetrates all body tissues and fluids, including CSF. The side effects include peripheral nueritis, hepatotoxicity, hypersensitivity (skin rash, arthralgia, fever), optic neuritis, vit B6 neuritis. INH metabolizes primarily by liver and excretion by kidneys, pyridoxine (vit B6) administration during high dose therapy as prophylactive measure, use as single prophylactic agent. For active TB in individuals whose PPD converts to positive, ability to cross blood-brain barrier. Avoid alcohol and antacids during therapy. Daily alcohol intake interferes with metabolism of isoniazed and increases risk of hepatitis, antacids containing alluminium hydroxide also interferes with absorption of INH.
- Rifampicin has broad spectrum effects, inhibits RNA polymerase of tubercle bacillus. It is bactericidal, penetrates all body tissues, including CSF. It is most commonly used with INH, low incidence of side effects, suppression of effects of birth control pills, possible orange urine. The other side effects may develop are hepatitis, febrile reactions, thrombocytopenia (Rare) GI disturbance, peripheral neuropathy, hypersensitivity, hepatotoxicity increases when given with INH. During its therapy, urine, sweat, tears may turn orange temporarily decrease effectiveness of oral contraceptives, anticoagulants, corticosteroids, barbiturates, hypoglycemics and digitalis.
- Ethambutal inhibits RNA synthesis and a bacteriostatic for the TB bacilli and does not penetrate all body fluids except CSF. The common side effects are skin rash, GI disturbance, malaise, peripheral neuritis, and optic neuritis. It has no significant reaction with other drugs. Should be given with food. Periodic checking of vision needed. It is most commonly used as substitute drug when toxicity occurs with Refampicin and INH.
- Streptomycin inhibits protein synthesis and is bactericidal. Poor penetration into body tissues and CSF. The side effects of streptomycin and INH include (eighth cranial nerve damage streptomycin vestibular or occular) damage often irreversible, nephrotoxicity and hypersensitivity. It should be used cautiously in older adults those with renal disease and pregnant women; must be given parenterally. During its use patient should be monitored monthly for kidney function, vestibular function with caloric stimulation test, and hearing with audiogram.
- Pyrazinamide is bacteriostatic or bacteriocidal depending on susceptibility of mycobacterium (exact mechanism not known). Usual side effects of fever, skin rash, hyperuricemia, jaundice (rare) hepatitis, arthrolgia, GI irritation. High rate of effectiveness when used with streptomycin or capreomycin.

In addition, ethionamide, capromycine, kanamycin and para-amino salicylic acid (PAS), cycloserine (seromycin) and used as second line of drugs for TB treatment.

A problem with antituberculosis therapy is the length of time medication must be taken. In the past, 18 to 26 months was the usual period of time required for individuals to adhere to the medical regiment. Shorter courses of therapy (6 to 9 months) have been shown to be effective. Now three options for treatment are available. Regimen option for the initial treatment of tuberculosis include:

- *Option 1*: Four drug regimen consisting of isoniazid, rifampicin, pyrazinamide and either ethambutol or streptomycin. Therapy may be given daily or 2–3 times weekly if DOT (directly observed therapy). Ethambutol or streptomycin may be discontinued if susceptibility to isoniazid or rifampicin is documented. Pyrazinamide should be discontinued after 8 weeks. The total duration of the therapy should be at least 6 months and at least 3 months after sputum culture converts to negative. Fixed dose combination of all these drugs are available to simplify therapy.
- *Option 2*: Daily isoniazid, rifampicin, pyrazinamide and streptomycin or ethambutol for 2 weeks followed by DOT twice weekly administration of the same drugs for 6 weeks followed by rifampicin for 16 weeks.
- *Option 3*: DOT 3 times/weekly administration of isoniazid, rifampicin, pyrazinamide, and ethambutol or streptomycin for 6 months.

For TB with HIV infection cases, option 1, 2, 3 can be used, but treatment regimens should continue for a total of 9 months and at least 6 months beyond culture conversion.

Medical therapy is the primary treatment of tuberculosis, but surgery may be used to remove residual pulmonary lesions and patients. The surgical procedures then are used include wedge resection, segmental resection, lobectomy, etc.

A well-balanced diet containing the essential food groups, with a vitamin supplement is recommended. Those who are poorly nourished or underweight may benefit from six small feedings of high-calorie, high protein foods daily rather than three meals.

The major nursing responsibility is to teach the patient about TB and how it is transmitted. Preventing contamination of air with tubercle bacilli is accomplished by treating the patient antituberculosis drugs and teaching the patient to cover the nose and mouth with tissues when sneezing and coughing. Advise the patient, he must take antituberculosis drugs as prescribed and drugs are always taken as combination of at least four drugs initially and drugs must be taken uninterruptedly.

To improve airway clearance, the patient is taught to sit upright in a chair or bed. If the patient is confined to bed at home, he or she may find it helpful to sit on the side of the bed with the feet on a chair. The patient may be taught to take two or three deep breaths, cover the mouth with tissues and then cough. Using this method when coughing decreases fatigue because it requires less expenditure of energy than does repeated ineffective coughs. Many patients can cough most effectively when the mouth is moist and sips of water or a warm beverage such as tea or coffee can be encouraged before coughing.

For patients with thick tenacious sputum, fluid intake is encouraged to thin the secretions and make them easier to expectorate. Water is considered by many experts to be the most effective sputum liquifying agent.

To reduce fear about the disease and what lifestyle changes it will require, patients are encouraged to ask questions about anything they do not understand or anything that concerns them. The nurse who sits while talking with the patients signals them he or she will take the time to listen to the patient. All questions should be answered as completely as possible, supplying information appropriate to the patient's educational level and ability to comprehend what is being taught. Written materials with diagram and drawings that reinforce what is being taught are helpful. The materials are given to the patient for use later on.

Nurses and other health care workers need to know the protective measures they can use when caring for patients who have a positive TB smear or culture.

BRONCHIECTASIS

Bronchiectasis is a disorder characterised by permanent, abnormal or irreversible dilation of the bronchial tree or one or more large bronchi.

Pathophysiology

When infection attacks the bronchial lining, inflammation occurs, and an exudate forms. The progressive accumulation of secretions obstructs the bronchioles. The obstructed bronchioles then breakdown, and ciliated columnar epithelium is replaced by non-ciliated cuboidal epithelium and sometimes fibroitic tissue, resulting in localised areas of dilations or saccules. The pathologic changes result in dilation and destruction of the elastic and muscular structures of the bronchial wall.

There are two pathological types of bronchiectasis, i.e. saccular and cylindrical. Saccular bronchiectasis occurs mainly in large bronchi and is characterised by cavity-like dilations. The affected bronchi end in large sacs. Cylindrical bronchiectasis involve medium-sized bronchi that are mildly to moderately dilated. Fusiform bronchiectasis occurs mainly in large bronchi and is characterized by cavity-like dilations. The affected bronchi end in large sacs cylindrical bronchiectasis involves medium sized bronchi that are mildly to moderately dilated. Fusiform bronchiectasis a subtype of cylindrical tends to involve more 'pouching' of the bronchi. The explosive force of the bronchioles is diminished and they may remain filled with exudate. Only forceful coughing and postural drainage will empty them. Almost all forms of bronchiectasis are associated with bacterial infections and viral infections (adenovir, influenza).

Clinical Manifestations

The condition may develop so gradually that the person is unable to tell when the symptoms first began. Signs and symptoms of bronchiectasis vary with the severity of the conditions and may include the following:

Signs

- Cyanosis
- Clubbing of fingers
- Find crackles and coarse Rhonchi
- Dull or flat sound over the areas of mucus plugs
- Increased vocal and tactile fermitus over the middle and lower lobes
- Decreased diaphragmatic excursion, and
- Paroxysms of coughing on rising in morning and when lying down.

Symptoms

- Severe coughing productive of copious amounts of purulent sputum
- Hemoptysis
- Dyspnea
- Fatigue and weakness
- Loss of appetite and weight loss.

The diagnostic studies used to diagnose bronchiectasis are chest X-ray, bronchography, sputum examination and CT scanning.

Management

Treatment of bronchiectasis includes:
- Administration of antibiotics on the basis of sputum culture results.
- Administering of bronchodilator, mucolytic agents and expectorants.
- Postural drainage to assist in mobilizing secretions to larger airways where they can be coughed up.
- Bronchoscopy to remove thicker secretions.
- Maintaining good hydration to liquify secretion.
- Maintaining good general hygiene including oral hygiene may contribute to relief symptoms.
- Adequate rest, diet, exercise and diversional activities.
- Avoiding superimposed infections such as colds.
- Individual should reduce exposure to excessive air pollutants and irritants, avoid cigarette smoking and obtain pneumococcal and influenza vaccinations.

Surgical resection of the parts of the lungs, necessary when signs and symptoms of bronchiectasis persists despite medical therapy. The goal of surgery is to preserve as much functional lung as possible. Therefore, segmentectomy or lobectomy is given priority.

EMPYEMA

Empyema is pus within a body cavity most often the pleural cavity. It usually occurs after pleural effusion secondary to other respiratory diseases such as pneumonia, lung abscess, TB and fungal infections of the lung and also after thoracic surgery or chest trauma.

Clinical Manifestation

The patient with a lung infection or chest injury may develop empyema and should be observed closely for the following signs and symptoms of empyema:
- Cough (usually nonproductive)
- Dyspnea
- Tachypnea
- Tachycardia
- Elevation of temperature
- Unilateral chest expansion
- Malaise
- Decreased appetite.

The diagnosis can usually be made from the signs and symptoms and the medical history, but it is confirmed by a chest X-ray film that demonstrates the presence of a pleural exudate. A thoracentesis is performed to obtain sample of the pus for culture and sensitivity studies and to relieve the patient's respiratory symptoms.

Management

The aim of treatment of empyema is to obliterate the pleural space by draining the empyema cavity completely. The cavity can be drained in the following ways.
- Initial treatment is often daily thoracentesis with aspiration of the cavity and instillation of antibiotics into the pleural space. Oral or IV antibiotics may also be given.
- If the cavity cannot be evacuated within a few days and if the lung fails to re-expand to obliterate then space surgery is necessary. The types of surgery depends on the situation and may include:
  - Closed chest drainage
  - Rib resection
  - Decortication and
  - Thoracoplasty

Nursing depends on the type and effectiveness of the procedure and the patient's symptoms. Some patients require oxygen therapy. Bed rest and coughing and deep breathing exercises may be indicated to improve ventilations. In some cases, the patient will go through several treatments before the empyema in space is closed. This can be frustrating, and the patient can become very discouraged. A major nursing role is to support the patient and family during the various procedure.

LUNG ABSCESS

Lung abscess is a pus-containing lesion of the lung parenchyma that gives rise to a cavity. The cavity is formed by necrosis of the lung tissue.

Etiology

In many cases, the causes and pathogenesis of lung abscess are similar to those of pneumonia. The more common contributing factor to a lung abscess is aspiration of material into the lungs. Risk factors for aspiration include alcoholism, seizure disorder, drug overdose, general anaesthesia, and cerebrovascular accidents. Most of the lung abscesses are caused by infectious agents, i.e. *Klebsiella*, *S. aureus*, anaerobic bacilli. Lung abscess also can result from hematogenously spread lung infarct secondary to pulmonary embolus, malignant growth, TB and various fungus and parasitic diseases of the lung.

Pathophysiology

The areas of the lung most commonly affected are the atypical segments of the lower lobes and the posterior segments of the upper lobes. Fibrous tissues usually form around the abscess in an attempt to wall it off. The abscess may erode into the bronchial system, causing the production of foul smelling sputum. It may grow towards the pleura and cause pleuritic pain. Multiple small abscesses can occur within the lung.

Clinical Manifestation

The onset of a lung abscess is usually insidious, especially if anaerobic organisms are the primary cause. A more acute onset occurs with aerobic organisms. The most common manifestation is cough-producing, purulent (often dark brown) that is foul-smelling and foul tasting. Hemoptysis is common especially at the time that an abscess ruptures into a bronchus. Other common manifestations are fever, chills, prostration, pleuritic pain, dyspnea, cough and weight loss. History may reveal a predisposing condition such as alcoholism, pneumonia or oral infections.

Physical examination of the lungs indicate the dullness to percussion and decreases breath sounds on auscultation over the segment of lung involved. There may be transmission of breath sounds to the periphery if the communicating bronchus becomes patent and drainage of the segment begins. Crackle may also be present. Oral examination often reveals dental caries, gingivitis and peridontal infection.

Complication can occur include chronic pulmonary abscess, haemorrhage from abscess erosion into blood vessels, brain abscess, bronchopleural fistula, and empyema.

Management

Diagnosis is made on the basis of physical examination, chest X-ray, sputum culture and sensitivity. Prolonged administration of antibiotics (6 to 8 weeks). Penicillin is the choice antibiotics. Recently, clindamycin or metronidazole in combination with penicillin are used.

The patient should be taught how to cough effectively. Chest physiotherapy and postural drainages are helpful. Frequent mouth care (every 2 to 3 hours) is needed to relieve the foul smelling odor and taste from the sputum. Diluted hydrogen peroxide and mouthwash are often effective. Rest, good nutrition, adequate fluid intake are all supportive measures to facilitate recovery. If dentition is poor and dental hygiene is not adequate and the patient should be encouraged to obtain dental care.

Surgery is indicated but occasionally may be necessary if re-infection of a large cavity lesion occurs.

OCCUPATIONAL LUNG DISEASES

Occupational or environmental lung diseases result from inhaled dust or chemicals. The duration of exposure and the amount of inhalant have a major influence on whether the exposed individual will have lung damage. Another factor is the susceptibility of the host.

Etiology

Many pulmonary diseases are believed to be caused by substances inhaled in the work place. Occupational lung disease are more common in:
- Blue-collar workers than white collar workers.
- Industrial areas than in rural areas.
- Small and medium-sized business than in larger industrial plants.

In some instances it is debatable whether a person's lung disease is clearly occupation specific. This is true in cases of bronchitis, asthma, emphysema, or cancer, because all of these conditions can be caused or aggravated by several factors found in many different occupations and by non-occupational factors such as smoking and air pollution.

Types

Occupational lung disease can be divided into several categories. The major ones are:
- The pneumoconiosis (black lung disease)
- Asbestos-related lung diseases
- Hypersensitivity diseases including occupational asthma allergic alveolitis
- Byssinosis (brown lung disease).

Pathophysiology

The pathophysiology, clinical manifestation and prevention of some common occupational diseases are as follows:

- Pneumoconiosis also known as 'dust in the lungs' is called by inhalation and retention of dust particles. Examples of this condition are: Silicosis, asbestosis and Byssinosis.
  - Silicosis caused if inhaled silica dust, most common form seen in miners, foundry workers, and others who inhaled relatively low concentration of dust for 10–20 years.

    In this dust accumulation is tissue or tissue reaction with whorl-shaped nodules throughout lungs. In complicated silicosis there is progressive massive fibrosis throughout lungs decreased lung function and cor pulmonale. In acute silicosis, there is inflammatory reaction within alveoli, diffuse fibrosis. Rapid progression to respiratory failure. The clinical manifestation will include, breathlessness, weakness, chest pain, productive cough with sputum, dies of cor pulmonale and respiratory failure. The preventive measures include dust control and improved ventilation can reduce dust levels. Sand blasters in enclosed spaces can use special suits and breathing apparatus. The complicated progressive massive fibrosis shortens life-span.
- Asbestos-related lung disease: Asbestos caused lung cancer, malignant mesothelioma of pleura and periosteum, cancer of the larynx, and certain gastrointestinal cancer, also cause asbestosis of fibrotic lung disease.

    Fibrosis caused by asbestos called asbestosis, asbestos fibers, accumulated around terminal bronchioles, surrounds fibers with iron rich tissue, forming asbestos body with characteristic picture on X-ray, more asbestos bodies as more fibers are inhaled, after 20-30 years of exposure fibrosis begins in lungs, interstitial fibrosis develops. Pleural plaques, which are calcified lesions develop on pleura. Dyspnea, basal crackles, and decreased vital capacity, are early manifestation. The complications include diffused interstitial pulmonary fibrosis. Lung cancer especially in cigarette smokers, mesothelioma (cancer affecting pleura and peritonial membrane).

    Treatment with radical pleurectomy and pneumonectomy survival only for 1–2 years. Preventive measures include enforcement for regulations governing mining milling and use of asbestos. Protective masks must be used when working with asbestos.
- Hypersensitivity diseases fall into occupational category when can occur in bronchi, bronchioles or alveoli, coarse dust causes bronchial reactions, fine dust previous small airway and alveolar reactions.
  - In occupational asthma, hypersensitivity reaction mediated by histamine bronchoconstriction and increased mucus production repeated attacks

if cause unrecognised and asthma is untreated, may lead to permanent obstructive lung disease; asthmatic response that is well established can be provoked by other factors (i.e. house dust, cigarette smoke) and by fatigue, breathing cold air and coughing where wheezing is major symptom. It can be prevented by total elimination of antigen, desensitization not successful.

- In farmer's lung (hypersensitivity pneumonitis or allergic alveolitis), alveoli are inflamed, inundated by WBCs, sometimes filled with fluid, if exposure infrequent or level of dust low, symptoms are mild, and treatment not sought, chronic form develops over a period of time eventually fibrosis occurs, and fibrosis may be so well established that it cannot be arrested.

  Symptoms begin some hours after exposure to offending dust and include fatigue, shortness of breath, dry cough, fever, and chills. Symptoms may be severe enough to require emergency treatment and hospitalization; acute attacks treated with steroids, recovery may take 6 weeks and patient may have residual lung damage, real cure is permanent separation of patient and antigen.

  Preventive measures include properly dried and stored farm products (hay, straw, sugar cane) do not cause allergic alveolitis. Presumably fungi only grow in moist condition.

- Byssinosis (Brown lung disease) is occupational disease. Occurs in textile workers; mainly in cotton workers but also afflict workers in flax and hemp industries; cause is found in bales of raw cotton.

  In this, chronic bronchitis and emphysema develop in time. Constriction of bronchioles in response to something in crude cotton. Symptoms of asthma and allergy persists long, there is exposure to cotton antigen.
  Clinical manifestations that develop are tightness in chest on returning to work after a weekend away (Monday fever), strong relationship between amount of dust inhaled and symptoms. Persistent of symptom increases tightness of chest with chronic bronchitis and emphysema, person leaves industry as respiratory cripple.

  The preventive measures include—dust control measures, pretreating bales of cotton by washing with steam and other agents may inactivate causative agent, try to detect persons who are likely to become sensitized to cotton dust and keep them out of high risk areas.

Management

Medical therapy of these patients depend on the patient's signs, symptoms and complications. The major role of nurses is to be knowledgeable about the cause and prevention of occupational lung diseases, so that appropriate information and teaching can be presented to community. The best approach to management is to try to prevent or decrease environmental and occupational risks. Well-designed effective ventilation system can reduce exposure to irritants, wearing mask is appropriate in some occupations. Cigarette smoking must be avoided.

Early diagnosis is essential if the disease process is to be halted. The best treatment is to decrease or stop exposure to the harmful agents. Some places of employment at which there is a known risk of lung disease may require periodic test.

X-rays and pulmonary function studies for exposed employees. There is no specific treatment for most environmental lung diseases. Treatment is directed towards symptomatic relief. If there is coexisted problem such as pneumonia, chronic bronchitis, emphysema, or asthma they are treated on providing nursing care accordingly.

LUNG CANCER

Cancer of the lung may be either metastatic or primary. Metastatic tumours may follow malignancy anywhere in the body. Metastasis forms the colon and kidney are common. Metastasis to the lung may be discovered before the primary lesion is known, and sometimes locations of the primary lesion may be found only at autopsy.

Etiology

Cigarette smoking as a chronic respiratory irritant is by far the major risk factor in the development of lung cancer. Heredity may play a role in both the tendency to smoke and the predisposition to develop lung cancer. Another possible risk factor is pre-existing pulmonary disease such as TB, pulmonary fibrosis, bronchiectasis and COPD.

Pathophysiology

The pathogenesis of primary lung cancer is not well understood. Usually cancers originate from the epithelium of the bronchus (bronchogenic). They grow slowly and it takes 8 to 10 years for a tumor to reach 1 cm in size, which is smallest detactable lesion on an X-ray. Lung cancer occurs primarily in the segmental bronchi or beyond and have a preference for the upperlobes of the lungs. Pathologic changes in the bronchial system show non-specific inflammatory changes with hypersecretions of mucus, desquamation of cells, reactive hyperplasia of the basal cells, and metaplasia of normal respiratory epithelium to stratified squamous cells. Lung cancers metastasize primarily by direct extension and via the blood circulation and the lymph system. The common sites for metastatic growth are the liver, brain, bones, scalene lymph nodes and adrenal glands.

Certain lung cancers cause the paraneoplastic syndrome, which is characterised by various manifestations caused by certain substances (e.g. hormones, enzymes and antigens) produced by the tumor cells. Small cell lung cancer most commonly is associated with it.

Clinical Manifestation

Lung cancer is clinically silent for most individuals for the majority of its course. The clinical manifestations of lung cancer are usually non-specific and appear late in the disease process. A patient's signs and symptoms depend on several factors including location of the lesion. Signs and symptoms of lesion in the bronchus and lung include:
- Approximately 10 per cent of patients are asymptomatic and cancer is identified on routine chest X-ray film.
- Approximately 75 percent have a cough.
- Approximately 50 percent have a haemoptysis.
- Shortness of breath and a unilateral wheeze are common.

Peripheral lesions that perforate into pleural space shows extrapulmonary intrathoracic signs and symptoms. These include:
- Pain on inspiration
- Friction rub
- Pleural effusion
- Edema of face and neck when superior vena cava is involved
- Fatigue, and
- Clubbing fingers

Later manifestations include non-specific system and symptoms such as anorexia, fatigue, weight loss, nausea and vomiting. Hoarseness may be present as a result of involvement of the recurrent laryngeal nerve. Unilateral paralysis of the diaphragm, dysphagia and superior vena cava obstruction may occur because of the intrathoracic spread of the malignancy.

Management

Diagnosis may be confirmed by taking accurately the:
- Health history and physical examination
- Chest X-ray to depict tumor
- Sputum in cytologic study—for examining bacteria and cancer cells
- Bronchioscopy
- CT scan
- MRI
- Positron emission tomography (PET)
- Spirometry (preoperative)
- Mediastinoscopy
- Pulmonary angiography
- Lung scan

Fine-Needle Aspiration

Surgical resection is usually the only hope for cure in lung cancer. The types of thoracic surgery and indications for their use are as follows:

- Exploratory thoracotomy is performed to confirm suspected diagnosis of lung or chest disease, especially carcinoma; to obtain a biopsy; being replaced by non-invasive procedure (Thoracoscopy).
- Pneumonectomy is removal of a lung, bronchogenic carcinoma when lobectomy will not remove all of lesion, tuberculosis when other surgery will not remove all of diseased lung.
- Pneumonectomy is lung reduction surgery to reduce lung volume and decrease tension on respiratory muscle in persons with emphysema.
- Lobectomy is removal of one lobe of lung, bronchogenic carcinoma confined to a lobe, bronchiectasis, emphysematous blebs or bullae, lung abscess; fungal infections, benign tumors, and tuberculosis.
- Bilobectomy in removal of two lobes from right lungs, bronchogenic carcinoma when lobectomy will not remove all of disease.
- Sleeve lobectomy in the resection of main bronchus or distal trachea with reanastomosis to a distal uninvolved bronchus, bronchogenic carcinoma to preserve functional parenchyma.
- Segmental resection is known as segmentectomy, that is removal of one or more lung segments; bronchiectasis, lung abscess or cyst; metastatic carcinoma and tuberculosis.
- Wedge resection is a removal of pie-shaped section from surface of lung, well-circumscribed benign tumors, metastatic tumors or localised inflammatory disease, including TB.
- Decortication is removal of fibrinous peel from visceral pleura; chronic empyema.
- Thoracoplasty is removal of ribs, residual airspace after resectional surgery; chronic empyema space.

Radiation therapy is used as curative approach in the individual who has resectable tumor but who is considered a poor surgical risk. It is also used as palliative procedure to reduce distressing symptoms such as cough, hemoptysis, bronchial obstruction, and superior vena cava syndrome.

Chemotherapy may be used in the treatment of non-resectable tumors or as adjuvant therapy to surgery in non-small cell lung carcinoma.

Biologic therapy used as adjuvant therapy.

Phototherapy, i.e. laser surgery with use of the Nd:YAG also useful in some cases.

The best way to prevent lung cancer is to abstain from smoking. When it is confirmed, nurse has to assist in supporting the patient in all above stated procedures and take suitable nursing measures accordingly.

NURSING MANAGEMENT IN THORACIC SURGERY

Preoperative Care

Preoperative teaching is essential for patients who are undergoing thoracic surgery. The goal of teaching is

to prepare the patient for what he or she is expected to do postoperatively. The nurse who is caring for the patient is responsible for determining what the patient understands about the impending surgery and to be sure that preoperative teaching is completed. The points to be discussed in teaching include:
- Patient's knowledge of procedure
- Explanation of procedure is necessary, including intubation for anesthesia, site of incision and chest tube(s) and drainage system.
- Oxygen
- Blood administration and IV
- Pain medication, including PCA if used
- What the patient will be asked to do
  - Coughing and deep breathing
  - Arm exercise and
  - Ambulation.
- Where patient will be taken after surgery:
  - To recovery–how long
  - To ICU–for how long
- Where family can wait during surgery.

The other routines of preoperative care of any surgery has to be followed.

Postoperative Care

The care of the patient after thoracic surgery centres on promoting ventilation, and re-expansion of the lung by maintaining a clear airway, maintaining the closed drainage system, promoting nutrition, monitoring the incision for bleeding and subcutaneous emphysema.

In most of the hospitals, the patient is taken from the recovery room to the ICU. The immediate postoperative nursing cares are as follows:

Oxygen Therapy

Oxygen is attached to the endotracheal tube in the immediate postoperative period. After extubation, humidified oxygen is given by cannula, usually at 6 L/minute. Oxygen mask should not be used to avoid cough and to rouse secretion.

Hemodynamic Monitoring

The patient is usually attached to a cardiac monitor. A Swan-Ganz catheter and central venous pressure line are used for hemodynamic monitoring.

Position of the Patient in Bed

The patient is kept flat in bed or with head elevated slightly (20 degrees) until blood pressure is stabilised to preoperative levels. Once blood pressure is stabilised, the patient can usually breathe best in semi-Fowler's position with a pillow under the head and neck but not under the shoulders and back, because of the subscapular incision.

Monitoring Vital Signs

Vital signs are taken every 15 minutes until the patient is well recoverd from anesthesia, every hour until condition has stabilised, and then every 2 to 4 hours. Any deviation should be reported immediately to take suitable measures.

Initiating Coughing and Deep Breathing Exercises

The patient should be assisted to cough as soon as conscious and extubated. If blood pressure is stable, the patient is assisted to sitting position, and the incision is supported anteriorly and posteriorly by the nurse's hands. Firm, even pressure over the incisions with the open palm of the hands is most effective method. The nurse's head should be behind the patient when the patient is coughing. The patient is encouraged to breathe deeply, exhale and then cough. Sips of fluid especially warm ones such as tea or coffee often facilitate coughing. Deep breathing or coughing keep the airway patent, prevent atelectasis and facilitate re-expansion of the lung. Patient is assisted every 2 to 4 hours around the clock. When a patient is unable to cough effectively tracheobronchial suctioning is performed.

Promoting Abdominal Breathing

Abdominal breathing exercises are a valuable adjunct to the care of the patient with chest surgery, because it improves ventilation without increasing pain, assist in coughing more effectively.

Promoting Comfort by Pain Relief

Medication for pain should be given as needed and may be required as often as every 3 to 4 hours during the first 48 to 72 hours. PCA and epidural catheters are widely used for pain medication management. Usually morphine is ordered for pain. If medication for pain fails intercostal nerve block may be performed.

Promoting Arm Exercises

Passive arm exercises are usually started in the evening of surgery. The purpose of pulling the patient's arm through range of motion is to prevent restriction of function.

Promoting Nutrition

The patient is encouraged to take fluids postoperatively and to progress to general diet as soon as it is tolerated. Fluid helps liquefy secretions and make them easier to expectorate. A diet adequate in protein and vitamins (especially vitamin C) facilitates wound healing.

Monitoring the Incision for Bleeding or Subcutaneous Emphysema

The dressing is checked periodically for bleeding. Blood on the dressing is unusual and should be reported to the surgeon at once. The time and amount of blood are recorded in the patient's record. Air leak from the pleural space through the thoracotomy incision or around the chest tubes into the soft tissues indicates subcutaneous emphysema. The presence of air under the skin is readily detected and has been described as feeling like 'tissue paper' "rice krispies" under the skin.

Maintaining Chest Tube(s) and Drainage

All patients who have resectional surgery of the lung, except those having a pneumonectomy will require drainage of the pleural space by one or two chest tubes connected to closed drainage. Precautions to be observed with any type of closed drainage system are as follows:
- Monitor drainage system for tidaling (fluctuating) in one water seal chamber:
  - Be sure the patient is not lying on the tubes.
  - Check connections to be sure the chest tube system is intact.
  - Ask patient to cough or change position to see if tidaling is resorted.
  - Tidaling will stop when the lung is re-expanded.
- Never lift the closed drainage system above the level of the patient's chest, because this allows fluid to be pulled into the pleural space.
- Never clamp chest tubes without a written order from the surgeon because air (positive pressure) will be trapped in the pleural space, further collapsing the lung.
- A liter bottle of sterile water is kept at the bedside at all times. If the patient's chest drainage system cracks or breaks.
  - Insert patiently chest tube into the bottle of sterile water
  - Remove the cracked or broken system and
  - Obtain new system and connect it to patient's chest tube as soon as possible.
- If the patient's tube is accidentally pulled out of the chest (rarely occurs)
  - Apply gloves in accordance with body substance isolation policy
  - Pinch skin opening together with fingers
  - Apply occlusive dressing
  - Cover dressing with overlapping pieces of 2-inch tape
  - Call surgeon immediately

Chest tubes are removed when there is no tidaling of fluid in the water-sealed chamber and when X-ray films confirm the full re-expansion of the lung.

CHEST TRAUMA AND THORACIC INJURIES

Chest trauma is a major problem often seen in the casualty. Injury to the chest may affect the bony chest cage, pleura and lungs, diaphragm, or mediastinal contents.

Etiology

Injury to the chest are broadly classified into two groups—blunt and penetrating.
1. Blunt trauma or non-penetrating injuries damage the structures within the chest cavity without disrupting chest wall integrity. Blunt injury occurs when the body is struck by a blunt object, such as steering wheel. The external injury may appear minor but the impact may cause severe, life-threatening internal injuries such as ruptured spleen.
   - Blunt steering wheel injury to chest may lead to rib fracture, flail chest, pneumothorax, hemopneumothorax, cardiac contusion, pulmonary contusion, cardiac tamponade, great vessel tears.
   - Shoulder harness seat belt injury may lead to fractured clavicle, dislocated shoulder, rib fractures, pulmonary contusion, pericardial contusion, cardiac temponade.
   - Crush injury (e.g. heavy equipment, crushing thorax) leads to pneumothorax and hemopneumothorax, flail chest, great vessel tears and rupture, decreased blood returned with decreased cardiac output.
   - Countrecoup trauma—a type of blunt trauma, is caused by the impact of parts of the body against other objects. Examples are many head injuries caused by countrecoup trauma.

     The causes of blunt injuries are, motor vehicle accident, pedestrian accident, fall, assault with blunt object, crush injury, and explosion.
2. Penetrating trauma or injuries disrupt chest wall integrity and result in alteration in intrathoracic pressures. It occurs when a foreign body impales or passes through the body tissue, e.g. gunshot wound, stabbing, with knife, gunshot, stick, arrow and other missiles. Gunshot or stab wound to chest may lead to open pneumothorax, tension pneumothorax, hemopneumothorax, cardiac tamponade, esophageal damage, tracheal tear, great vessel tears.

Emergency care of the patient with chest trauma requires an accurate assessment of respiratory, cardiovascular and surface finding which include:
- Respiratory
  - Dyspnea, respiratory distress
  - Cough with or without hemoptysis
  - Cyanosis of the mouth, face, nail beds, mucous membrane
  - Tracheal deviation
  - Audible air escaping from the chest wound
  - Decreased breath sounds on side of injury
  - Decreased oxygen saturation, and
  - Frothy secretions.
- Cardiovascular
  - Rapid, thready pulse
  - Decreased blood pressure

- Narrowed pulse pressure
- Asymmetric blood pressure value in arms
- Distended neck veins
- Muffled heart sounds
- Chest pain
- Crunching sounds synchronous with heart sounds
- Arrhythmias.
• Surface findings
- Bruising
- Abrasions
- Open chest wounds
- Asymmetric chest movement
- Subcutaneous emphysema.

Nursing Intervention

The emergency care are:
• Ensure patient airway
• Administer high-flow O_2 with non-rebreather mask
• Establish IV access with two large-bore catheters. Begin fluid resuscitation as appropriate
• Remove clothing to assess injury
• Cover sucking chest wound with non-porous dressing taped on three sides
• Stabilize impaled objects with bulky dressings. Do not remove
• Assess for other significant injuries and treat appropriately
• Stabilise flail rib segment with hand followed by application of large pieces of tape horizontal across the flail segment
• Place patient in a semi-Fowler's position or position the patient on injured side if breathing is easier after Cervical spine injury has been ruled out.

An ongoing monitoring will include:
• Monitor vital signs, level of consciousness, oxygen saturation, cardiac rhythm, respiratory status and urinary output
• Anticipate intubation for respiratory distress
• Release dressing if tension pneumothorax develops after sucking chest wound is covered.

Thorax injuries range from single rib fracture to the life threatening tears of aorta, vena cava, and other major vessels. The most coronary thoracic emergencies are as follows:

RIB FRACTURES

Rib fractures are the most common type of chest injury (blunt injury), resulting from trauma ribs (4-9) 3rd to 10th are most commonly fractured because they are least protected by chest muscles. If the fractured rib is splintered or displaced, it may damage the pleura and lungs.

Ribs usually function at the point of maximum impact, but they may fracture at a site distant from impact. Rib fractures are caused by blows, crushing injuries, or strain caused by severe coughing or sneezing spells. When the rib is splintered or the fracture displaced, sharp fragments may penetrate the pleura and lungs, resulting in a hemothorax (blood in the pleural space) or pneumothorax (air in the pleural space) which are penetrating injuries.

Clinical manifestation of fractured ribs include:
• Pain at the site of injury, especially increasing on inspiration
• Localised tenderness and crepitus on palpation
• Splinting of chest and shallow breathing
Fractures are confirmed by chest X-ray.

The main goal in treatment is to decrease pain so that patient can breathe adequately to promote good chest expansion. Intercostal nerve blocks with local anesthesia (1% procaine) may be used to provide pain relief and analgesics is given to relieve pain so that the patient can be encouraged to breathe more rapidly.

The patient is observed for splinting of the chest and shallow breathing to which could lead to atelectasis. To improve breathing, the patient is placed in a position of comfort. Most of the patients are able to breathe best in Fowler's or semi-Fowler's positions.

The patient and family should be educated regarding:
• The patient should rest and do nothing strenuous for several days.
• The patient should take deep breath every hour.
• Narcotic drug therapy must be individualised and used with caution because these drugs can depress respiration.
• The pain is not relieved if analgesic call physician.
• If shortness of breath, sudden sharp chest pain, coughing up blood occurs, rush to casualty part of hospital.

FLAIL CHEST

Flail chest results from multiple rib fractures and thereby causing instability of the chest wall.

When multiple ribs or the sternum is fractured in more than one places, a portion of the chest wall becomes separated from the chest cage, resulting in a flail chest. The chest wall cannot provide the bony structures necessary to maintain Bellows action and ventilation. The affected (flail) area will move paradoxically the intact portions of the chest during respiration. During inspiration the affected portion is sucked in, and during expiration it bulges out. This paradoxical chest movement prevents adequate ventilation of the lung in the injured area. The underlying lung may or may not have a serious injury. Associated pain and any lung injury give rise to loss of compliance, will contribute to an alteration in breathing pattern and lead to hypoxemia. And may also develop hypercapnia and respiratory acidosis due to increased work of breathing.

Clinical Manifestations

- Severe chest pain
- Paradoxical breathing (asymmetrical chest movement)
- Oscillation of mediastinum
- Increasing dyspnea
- Rapid shallow respiration
- Accessory muscle breathing
- Restlessness
- Decreased breath sounds on auscultation
- Cyanosis
- Anxiety related to difficult breathing.

Management

- Stabilising the flail segment position end-expiratory pressure (PEEP) used with mechanical ventilation to improve oxygenation will maintain pressure in the lungs throughout the respiratory cycle.
- Provide supplemental oxygen: Monitor with pulse oximetry.
- Correct acid-base balance by mechanical ventilation
- Provide analgesic for pain control
- For severe pain, epidural anesthesia may be used
- Avoid fluid overload
- Patient should be confined to bed as he or she is on a ventilator.

PNEUMOTHORAX

A pneumothorax is a complete or partial collapse of a lung as a result of an accumulation of air in the pleural space. Pneumothorax may be closed or open.

Closed Pneumothorax

The common form is:

- Spontaneous pneumothorax, which is caused by rupture of small blebs on the visceral pleural space. The cause of the bleb is unknown. This condition occurs most commonly in male cigarette smokers between 20–40 years of age. The other causes include:
  - Injury to the lungs from mechanical ventilation
  - Injury to the lungs from insertion of a subclavian catheter
  - Perforation of esophagus
  - Injury to the lungs from broken ribs
- Receptive blebs or bullae in a patient with COPD (e.g., asthma).

Clinical Manifestation

Small or slowly developing pneumothorax may produce no symptoms, but in large or rapidly developing pneumothorax results in:

- Sharp pain on respiration
- Increasing dyspnea
- Increasing restlessness
- Diaphoresis
- Hypotension
- Tachycardia
- Absence of chest movement in affected side
- Hyperresonance on affected side (to percussion).

Management of closed pneumothorax will include:

- Observation on outpatient basis
- Giving supplemental oxygen
- Needle aspiration of air from pleural space, if present, insertion of chest catheter connected to a flutter valve or closed drainage system (suction or vented drainage).

Open Pneumothorax

Open pneumothorax occurs when air enters the pleural space through an opening in the chest wall. For example, gunshot or stab wound to chest in surgical thoracotomies. A penetrating chest wound is often referred to as a "sucking chest wound, because each time the person inspires, air is sucked into pleural space". In which, sucking sounds at wound site with respiration and tracheal deviation (trachea moves towards unaffected area during inspiration and returns towards midline) inspiration are the clinical manifestations.

This will be managed by occlusion of open wound and use other measures as in closed pneumothorax.

Tension Pneumothorax

Tension pneumothorax may result from either in open or a closed pneumothorax. It occurs when air enters the pleural space on inspiration but cannot leave it on expiration. Although usually a result of a closed pneumothorax, a tension pneumothorax can be caused by a penetrating chest injury. The accumulated air builds up positive pressure in the chest cavity resulting in the following:

- Lung collapse on the affected side.
- Mediastinal shift towards the unaffected side.
- Compression of mediastinal contents (heart, great vessels) resulting in decreased cardiac output and decreased venous return.

The clinical manifestation, tension pneumothorax will include:

- Severe dyspnea
- Agitation
- Trachea deviated from midline toward unaffected lung mediastinal shift
- Jugular venous distention
- Absence of chest movement on affected side
- Hypotension, tachycardia
- Breath sounds absent on affected side
- Hyperresonance on affected side
- Diminished heart sounds
- Shock
- Subcutaneous emphysema
- Ineffective ventilation.

Tension pneumothorax is a medical emergency because both the respiratory and circulatory systems are affected. If the tension of the pleural space is not relieved, the patient is likely to die from inadequate cardiac output or marked hypoxemia. Nurses are now being trained to insert large bore needle and chest tube into the chest walls to release the trapped air. Tension of pneumothorax usually occurs during mechanical ventilation or resuscitative efforts. Since it is the emergency defect in chest wall, covered with a sterile dressing, and insertion of chest tube connected to a flutter valve or closed drainage system.

Hemothorax

Hemothorax is an accumulation of blood in the intrapleural space. It is frequently found in association with open pneumothorax. It may be due to chest trauma, lung malignancy, complication of anticoagulative therapy, pulmonary embolus, and tearing of pleural adhesions.

The clinical manifestations are: If it is small, mild tachycardia, and dyspnea, air present. If it is large, respiratory distress may be present, which include shallow, rapid, respiration, dyspnea and air hunger. Chest pain or cough with or without hemoptysis. No breath sounds heard on auscultation.

If tension pneumothorax develops, feature of these also develop as a clinical manifestation.

Treatment of hemopneumothorax depends on air severity of the pneumothorax and the nature of the underlying disease. An emergency management will include chest insertion, auto-transfusion of collected blood, treatment of hypovolemia as necessary. Repeated spontaneous pneumothorax may need to be treated surgically by a partial pleurectomy, stapling or laser pleurodesis to promote adherence of the pleurae to one another. The injection of doxycycline (dry) an irritating agent can be used for pleurodesis.

Nursing intervention for closed, tension and open pneumothorax are as follows:

- *Closed pneumothorax* patient if he or she admitted performing the following:
  - Place the patient in semi-Fowler's position
  - Administer oxygen
  - Obtain thoracentesis tray and closed drainage equipment.

  For outpatients or for patients after chest tube removal, instruct the patient to:
  - Report any increased dyspnea to physician
  - Avoid strenuous exercises or activity that increases rate and depth of breathing
  - Avoid holding breath
  - Follow physician's instructions about resuming normal activity.

- *Tension pneumothorax* is life-threatening event; imperative that intervention be carried immediately to relieve increased intrapleural pressure; intervention same as those listed CP and performed the following:
  - Monitor vital signs frequently
  - Observe for cardiac dysrhythmias
  - Palpate for subcutaneous emphysema in upper chest and neck
  - Use same discharge instruction as in CP (above).

- *Open pneumothorax* performed the following:
  - Occlude wound on the non-porous covering
  - Same intervention as CP (closed pneumothorax)
  - Same discharge instruction as CP.

PLEURAL EFFUSION

The pleural space lies between the lung and chest wall and normally contains a very thin layer fluid. Pleural effusion is a collection of fluid in the pleural space. It is not a disease but rather a sign of a serious disease. Pleural effusion is frequently classified as transudative or exudative according to whether the protein content of the effusion is low or high, respectively. A transudate occurs primarily in noninflammatory conditions and is an accumulation of protein-poor, cell-poor fluid. Transudative pleural effusions (also called hydrothoraces) are caused by (1) increased hydrostatic pressure found in heart failure (HF), which is the most common cause of pleural effusion, or (2) decreased oncotic pressure (from hypoalbuminemia) found in chronic liver or renal disease. In these situations, fluid movement is facilitated out of the capillaries and into the pleural space.

An exudative effusion is an accumulation of fluid and cells in an area of inflammation. An exudative pleural effusion results from increased capillary permeability characteristic of the inflammatory reaction. This type of effusion occurs secondary to conditions such as pulmonary malignancies, pulmonary infections, pulmonary embolization, and GI disease (e.g., pancreatic disease, esophageal perforation).

The type of pleural effusion can be determined by a sample of pleural fluid obtained via thoracentesis (a procedure done to remove fluid from the pleural space). Exudates have a high protein content, and the fluid is generally dark yellow or amber. Transudates have a low protein content or contain no protein, and the fluid is clear or pale yellow. The fluid can also be analyzed for RBCs and WBCs, malignant cells, bacteria and glucose.

An empyema is a pleural effusion that contains pus. It is caused by conditions such as pneumonia, TB, lung abscess, and infection of surgical wounds of the chest. A complication of empyema is fibrothorax, in which there is fibrous fusion of the visceral and parietal pleurae.

Clinical Manifestations

Common clinical manifestations of pleural effusion are progressive dyspnea and decreased movement of the chest wall on the affected side. There may be pleuritic pain from the underlying disease. Physical examination of the chest will indicate dullness to percussion and absent or decreased breath sounds over the affected area. The chest X-ray will indicate an abnormality if the effusion is greater than 250 ml. Manifestations of empyema include the manifestations of pleural effusion, as well as fever, night sweats, cough, and weight loss. A thoracentesis reveals an exudates containing thick, purulent material.

If the cause of the pleural effusion is not known, a diagnostic thoracentesis is needed to obtain pleural fluid for analysis. If the degree of pleural effusion is severe enough to impair breathing, a therapeutic thoracentesis is done to improve breathing and to remove fluid for analysis.

A thoracentesis is performed by having the patient sit on the edge of a bed and lean forward over a bedside table. The puncture site is determined by chest X-ray, and percussion of the chest is used to assess the maximum degree of dullness. The skin is cleaned with an antiseptic solution and anesthetized locally. The thoracentesis needle is inserted into the intercostal space. Fluid can be aspirated with a syringe, or tubing can be connected to allow fluid to drain into a sterile collecting bottle. After the fluid is removed, the needle is withdrawn, and a bandage is applied over the insertion site. Usually only 1000 to 1200 ml of pleural fluid are removed at one time. Because high volumes are removed, rapid removal can result in hypotension, hypoxemia, or pulmonary edema. A follow-up chest X-ray should be done to detect a possible pneumothorax that could have been induced by perforation of the visceral pleura. During and after the procedure, vital signs and pulse oximetry are monitored, and the patient should be observed for any manifestations of respiratory distress.

Management of Pleural Effusion

The main goal of management of pleural effusions is to treat the underlying cause. For example, adequate treatment of HF with diuretics an sodium restriction will result in decreased pleural effusions. The treatment of pleural effusions secondary to malignant disease represents a more difficult problem. These types of pleural effusions are frequently recurrent and accumulate quickly after thoracentesis. Chemical pleurodesis may be used to sclerose the pleural space and prevent reaccumulation of effusion fluid. Although doxycyline (Vibramycin) and bleomycin (Blenoxane) have been used for sclerosing with good results, talc appears to be the most effective agent for pleurodesis. Thoracoscopy can be used to perform talc pleurodesis after inspection of the pleural space. After instillation of the sclerosing agent, patients may be instructed to rotate their positions to spread the agent uniformly throughout the pleural space. The decision to rotate the patient from side to side to back depends on physician preference and the patients ability to tolerate turning. Chest tubes are left in place after pleurodesis until fluid drainage is less than 150 ml/day and no air leaks are noted. A more rapid completion of the pleurodesis procedure, in less than 24 hours, is reported in the literature with good results, and this limited admission for symptomatic malignant effusions may become more frequent.

Treatment of empyema is generally with chest tube drainage. Appropriate antibiotic therapy is also needed to eradicate the causative organism. A condition called trapped lung can occur with effusions and empyemas. This is a fibrous peel around the pleura that can cause pulmonary restriction. A decortication surgical procedure to remove the pleural peel may need to be performed.

The other conditions of lungs briefed here as pleurisy and atelectasis.

Pleurisy (pleuritis) is an inflammation of the pleura. The most common causes are pneumonia, TB, chest trauma, pulmonary infarctions, and neoplasms. The inflammation usually subsides with adequate treatment of the primary disease. The pain of pleurisy is typically abrupt and sharp in onset and is aggravated by inspiration. The patients breathing is shallow and rapid to avoid unnecessary movement of the pleura and chest wall. A pleural friction rub may occur, which is the sound over areas where inflamed visceral pleura and parietal pleura rub over one another during inspiration. This sound is usually loudest at peak inspiration but can be heard during exhalation as well.

Treatment of pleurisy is aimed at treating the underlying disease and providing pain relief. Taking analgesics and lying on or splinting the affected side may provide some relief. The patient should be taught to splint the rib cage when coughing. Intercostal nerve blocks may be done if the pain is severe.

Atelectasis is a condition of the lungs characterized by collapsed, airless alveoli. The most common cause of atelectasis is airway obstruction that results from retained exudates and secretions. This is frequently observed in the postoperative patient. Normally the pores of Kohn provide for collateral passage of air from one alveolus to another. Deep inspiration is necessary to open the pores effectively. For this reason, deep-breathing exercises are important in preventing atelectasis in the high-risk patient (e.g., postoperative, immobilized patient).

PULMONARY EMBOLISM

Pulmonary embolism (PE) is the blockage of pulmonary arteries by a thrombus, fat or air embolus, or tumor tissue.

The word embolus derived from a Greek word meaning "plug" or "stopper". A pulmonary embolus consists of material that gains access to the venous system and then to the pulmonary circulation. The material eventually reaches a section of the pulmonary arterial vessels, where it lodges, thus obstructing perfusion.

Most pulmonary emboli arise from thrombi in the deep veins of the legs. Other sites of origin include the right side of the heart (especially with atrial fibrillation), the upper extremities (rare), and the pelvic veins (especially after surgery or childbirth). Lethal pulmonary emboli most commonly originate in the femoral or iliac veins. Emboli are mobile clots that generally do not stop moving until they lodge at a narrowed part of the circulatory system. The lungs are an ideal location for emboli to lodge because of their extensive arterial and capillary network. The lower lobes are most frequently affected because they have a higher blood flow than the other lobes.

Thrombi in the deep veins can dislodge spontaneously. However, a more common mechanism is jarring of the thrombus by mechanical forces, such as sudden standing, and by changes in the rate of blood flow, such as those that occur with the valsalva maneuver. The majority of patients with PE due to deep vein thrombosis (DVT) have no leg symptoms at the time of diagnosis.

In addition to dislodged thrombi, less common causes of PE include fat emboli (from fractured long bones), air emboli (from improperly administered IV therapy), bacterial vegetations, amniotic fluid, and tumors. Tumor emboli may originate from primary or metastatic malignancies.

The most common risk factors for PE are immobilization, surgery within the last 3 months, stroke, history of DVT, and malignancy. The Nurse's Health Study reported an increased risk of PE in women associated with obesity, heavy cigarette smoking, and hypertension. More than 95% of pulmonary emboli arise from thrombi in the deep veins of the lower extremity. Generally the DVTs that are below the knee have not been considered a risk factor for PE since they rarely migrate to the pulmonary circulation without first extending above the knee. Upper extremity DVT occasionally occurs in the presence of central venous catheters or cardiac pacing wires. These cases may resolve with removal of the catheter. The highest rate of DVT is seen in spinal cord injury patients.

Clinical Manifestations

The signs and symptoms of PE are generally subtle and nonspecific, making diagnosis difficult. The classic triad of dyspnea, chest pain, and hemoptysis occurs in only about 20% of patients. The most common manifestations of PE are anxiety and the sudden onset of unexplained dyspnea, tachypnea, or tachycardia. A mild to moderate hypoxemia with a low $PaCO_2$ is a common finding. Other manifestations are cough, pleuritic chest pain, hemoptysis, crackles, fever, accentuation of the pulmonic heart sound, and sudden change in mental status as a result of hypoxemia.

Massive emboli may produce sudden collapse of the patient with shock, pallor, severe dyspnea, hypoxemia, and crushing chest pain. However, some patients with massive PE do not have pain. The pulse is rapid and weak, the BP is low, and ECG indicates right ventricular strain. When rapid obstruction of 50% or more of the pulmonary vascular bed occurs, acute cor pulmonale may result because the right ventricle can no longer pump blood into the lungs. The mortality rate of persons with massive PE and shock is approximately 33%.

Medium sized emboli often cause pleuritic chest pain, dyspnea, slight fever, and a productive cough with blood streaked sputum. A physical examination may reveal tachycardia and a pleural friction rub. Small emboli frequently are undetected or produce vague, transient symptoms. The exception to this is the patient with underlying cardiopulmonary disease, in whom even small- or medium-sized emboli may result in severe cardiopulmonary compromise. However, repeated small emboli gradually cause a reduction in the capillary bed and eventual pulmonary hypertension. An ECG and chest X-ray may indicate right ventricular hypertrophy secondary to pulmonary hypertension.

Complications

Pulmonary infarction (death of lung tissue) is most likely when the following factors are present: (1) occlusion of a large or medium-sized pulmonary vessel (>2 mm in diameter), (2) insufficient collateral blood flow from the bronchial circulation, or (3) pre-existing lung disease. Infarction results in alveolar necrosis and hemorrhage. Occasionally the infracted tissue becomes infected, and an abscess may develop. Concomitant pleural effusion is frequently found.

Pulmonary hypertension occurs when more than 50% of the area of the normal pulmonary bed is compromised. Pulmonary hypertension also results from hypoxemia. As a single event, an embolus does not cause pulmonary hypertension unless it is massive. However, recurrent small to medium sized emboli may result in chronic pulmonary hypertension. Pulmonary hypertension eventually results in dilation and hypertrophy of the right ventricle. Depending on the degree of pulmonary hypertension and its rate of development, outcomes can vary, with some patients dying within months of the diagnosis and others living for decades.

Diagnostic Test

A ventilation perfusion lung scan is the most frequently used test to aid in the diagnosis of PE. The lung scan has two components and is most accurate when both are performed:

- Perfusion scanning involves IV injection of a radioisotope. A scanning device detects the adequacy of the pulmonary circulation
- Ventilation scanning involves inhalation of a radioactive gas such as xenon. Scanning reflects the distribution of gas through the lung. The ventilation component requires the cooperation of the patient and may be impossible to perform in the critically ill patient, particularly if the patient is intubated.

D-dimer testing may be recommended when a PE is initially suspected. D-dimer is a degradation product rarely found in healthy individuals. However, levels of D-dimer are elevated in any condition involving degradation of fibrin (infection, cancer, surgery, heart failure). They are elevated 8 times higher in venous thromboembolism. When D-dimer levels are normal (< 250 mcg/L), it is highly unlikely that the patient has a PE. Thus a normal or near normal D-dimer level can rule out a PE. In the event that the D-dimer levels are elevated, a noninvasive venous study is indicated to look for a DVT as the likely source of a PE. If a DVT is located by venous ultrasound, the index of suspicion for PE is very high and anticoagulant treatment should be initiated immediately. Patients with an elevated D-dimer level but normal venous ultrasound need an elevated D-dimer level but normal venous ultrasound need a lung scan or spiral CT scan.

If the lung scan is inconclusive, pulmonary angiography is recommended. Pulmonary angiography is an invasive procedure that involves the insertion of a catheter through the antecubital or femoral vein, advancement to the pulmonary artery, and injection of contrast medium. This allows visualization of the pulmonary of contrast medium. This allows visualization of the pulmonary vascular system and location of the embolus.

The use of computed tomography (CT) has revolutionized the diagnosis of PE. A spiral (or helical) CT scan, a noninvasive diagnostic test, may also be used to diagnose PE. Conventional CT scans rotate a frame 360 degrees in one direction, stop, make an image (called a slice), and then spin back in the opposite direction to make another slice after again stopping. The spiral CT scan is able to continuously rotate while obtaining slices and does not have to start and stop between each slice. This allows visualization of entire anatomic regions such as the lungs. The data can be computer reconstructed to allow for a three-dimensional picture of the area being imaged and assist in emboli visualization.

ABG analysis is important, but not diagnostic. The PaO_2 is low because of inadequate oxygenations secondary to an occluded pulmonary vasculature. The $PaCO_2$ is usually low because of hyperventilation. The pH remains normal unless respiratory alkalosis develops as a result of prolonged hyperventilation or to compensate for lactic acidosis caused by shock. Abnormal findings are usually reported on the chest X-ray (atelectasis, pleural effusion) and the ECG (ST segment and T wave changes), but they are not diagnostic for PE. Serum troponin levels are elevated in 30 to 50% of patients with PE, and, although not diagnostic, they are predictive of an adverse prognosis. Serum b-type natriuretic peptide (BNP) levels, while not diagnostic, may be helpful in identifying the severity of the clinical course.

Management of Pulmonary Emboli

When the diagnosis of PE has been made, treatment should be instituted immediately. The objectives of treatment are to (1) prevent further growth or multiplication of thrombi in the lower extremities, (2) prevent embolization from the upper or lower extremities to the pulmonary vascular system, and (3) provide cardiopulmonary support if indicated.

Conservative therapy: Supportive therapy for the patients cardiopulmonary status varies according to the severity of the PE. The administration of supplemental O_2 by mask or cannula may be adequate for some patients. Oxygen is given in a concentration determined by ABG analysis. In some situations, endotracheal intubation and mechanical ventilation may be needed to maintain adequate oxygenation. Respiratory measures such as turning, coughing, and deep breathing are necessary to prevent or treat atelectasis. If symptoms of shock are present, vasopressor agents may be necessary to support the systemic circulation. If heart failure is present, diuretics are used. Pain resulting from pleural irritation or reduced coronary blood flow is treated with opioids, usually morphine.

Drug therapy: Properly managed anticoagulant therapy is effective in the treatment of many patients with PE. Although unfractionated heparin has been traditionally used for PE, low-molecular-weight heparin (e.g., enoxaparin [Levenox]) is becoming more commonly used in the treatment of PE. Warfarin (Coumadin) should be initiated within the first 24 hours and is typically administered for 3 to 6 months. Factor Xa inhibitors and direct thrombin inhibitors are also being used in the treatment of PE.

The dosage of heparin is adjusted according to the activated partial thromboplastin time (APT), while warfarin dose is determined by the international normalized ration (INR). Frequent changes and titrations of heparin doses are needed initially in order to obtain a therapeutic apt level. The heparin works to prevent future clots, but does not dissolve existing clots. Anticoagulant therapy may be contraindicated if the patient has blood dyscrasias, hepatic dysfunction causing alteration in the clotting mechanism, injury to the intestine, overt bleeding, a history of hemorrhage stroke, or neurologic conditions.

Fibrinolytic agents, such as tissue plasminogen activator (tPA) or alteplase (Activase), dissolve the pulmonary embolus and the source of the thrombus in the pelvis or deep leg veins, thereby decreasing the likelihood of recurrent emboli. Indications for thrombolytic therapy in PE include hemodynamic instability and right ventricular dysfunction.

Surgical therapy: If the degree of pulmonary arterial obstruction is severe and the patient does not respond to conservative therapy, an immediate embolectomy may be indicated. Pulmonary embolectomy, a rare procedure, has a 50% mortality rate. Preoperative pulmonary angiography is necessary to identify and locate the site of the embolus. When a pulmonary embolectomy is performed, the patient also has placement of a vena cava filter.

To prevent further pulmonary embolization, an inferior vena cava (IVC) filter may be warranted. This device prevents migration of large clots into the pulmonary system, is easily and safely placed percutaneously, is biocompatible, and does not require the patient be anticoagulated. It can be used for patients who have an absolute contraindication to anticoagulant therapy. In addition, it may be used as a prophylactic measure for patients at high risk of PE (e.g., those with spinal cord injury or cor pulmonale). The complications associated with this device are rare and include misplacement, migration, and perforation. The spinal cord injury patient with an IVC filter cannot have assisted cough ("quad cough") to mobilize secretions since the quad cough procedure can displace the filter.

Nursing Interventions

Nursing measures aimed at prevention of PE parallel those for prophylaxis of deep vein thrombosis.

Acute intervention: The prognosis of a patient with PE is good if therapy is promptly instituted. The patient should be kept on bed rest in a semi-Fowler's position to facilitate breathing. An IV line should be maintained for medications and fluid therapy. The nurse should know the side effects of medications and observe for them. Oxygen therapy should be administered as ordered. Careful monitoring of vital signs, cardiac dysrhythmia monitoring, pulse oximetry, ABGs, and lung sounds is critical to assess the patients status. Laboratory results are monitored to assure normal ranges of aPPT and INR. Nursing care includes assessing for the complications of anticoagulant therapy (e.g., bleeding, hematomas, bruising) and PE (e.g., atelectasis, pneumonia). The nursing care plan includes interventions related to immobility and fall precautions.

The patient is usually anxious because of pain, sense of doom, inability to breathe, and fear of death. The nurse carefully explains the situation and provide emotional support and reassurance to help relieve the patients anxiety.

The patient affected by thromboembolic processes may require psychologic and emotional support. In addition to the thromboembolic problems, the patient may have an underlying chronic illness requiring long-term treatment. To provide supportive therapy, the nurse must understand and differentiate between the various problems caused by the underlying disease and those related to thromboembolic disease. Patient teaching regarding long-term anticoagulant therapy is critical. The anticoagulant therapy continues for at least 3 to 6 months; patients with recurrent emboli are treated indefinitely. Warfarin blood levels are initially drawn monthly, and patients may have follow-up appointments at a nurse-managed anticoagulation clinic to monitor their medication and adjust dosages.

Long-term management is similar to that for the patient with DVT. Discharge planning is aimed at limiting progression of the condition and preventing complications and recurrence. The nurse must reinforce the need for the patient to return to the health care provider for regular follow-up examination.

PULMONARY HYPERTENSION

Pulmonary hypertension is elevated pressures resulting from an increase in pulmonary vascular resistance to blood flow. The disease commonly presents with shortness of breath and fatigue. Pulmonary hypertension can occur as a primary disease (primary pulmonary hypertension) or as a secondary complication of a respiratory, cardiac, autoimmune, hepatic, or connective tissue disorder (secondary pulmonary hypertension).

Primary Pulmonary Hypertension

Primary pulmonary hypertension (PPH) is a severe and progressive disease. PPH is characterized by mean pulmonary arterial pressure greater than 30 mmHg with exercise in the absence of a demonstrable cause. Until the last decade, this disorder was rapidly progressive with right-sided heart failure and death. The median survival if untreated was 2.8 years. Epoprostenol (Flolan) therapy, introduced in the 1990s, greatly survival rates. Unfortunately, the disease remains incurable despite these advances.

Etiology

The exact etiology of PPH is unknown. It is rare and potentially fatal disease. PPH has been linked to the use of fenfluramine in the drug Fen-Phen, which was used as an appetite suppressant to treat obesity. The drug was withdrawn from the market in 1996. PPH affects more women than men; the mean age at diagnosis is 36 years old. It may have a genetic component as the incidence is higher in families.

Pathophysiology

Normally the pulmonary circulation is characterized by low resistance and low pressure. In pulmonary hypertension, the pulmonary pressures are elevated. Until recently the pathophysiology of PPH was poorly understood. Recently it was discovered that a key mechanism involved in PPH is a deficient release of vasodilator mediators from the pulmonary epithelium, with a resultant cascade of injury. Vasoconstriction, remodeling of the walls of the pulmonary vessels, and thrombosis in situ are the three elements that combine to cause the increased vascular resistance. The remodeling process is a complex set of events involving endothelial cell injury that results in intimal/medial wall thickening.

Clinical Manifestations

Classic symptoms of pulmonary hypertension are dyspnea on exertion and fatigue. Exertional chest pain, dizziness and exertional syncope are other symptoms. These symptoms are related to the inability of cardiac output to increase in response to increased oxygen demand. Eventually, as the disease progresses, dyspnea occurs at rest. Pulmonary hypertension increases the workload of the right ventricle and causes right ventricular hypertrophy (a condition called cor pulmonale) and eventually heart failure. A chest X-ray generally shows enlarged central pulmonary arteries and clear lung fields. An enlarged right heart may be seen. Echocardiogram usually reveals right ventricular hypertrophy. The mean time between onset of symptoms and the diagnosis is 2 years. By the time patients become symptomatic, the disease is already in the advanced stages and the pulmonary artery pressure is 2 to 3 times normal.

Management of Primary Pulmonary Hypertension

PPH is a diagnosis of exclusion. All other conditions must be ruled out. Diagnostic evaluation includes ECG, chest X-ray, pulmonary function tests, echocardiogram, and spiral CT. Cardiac catheterization is done to measure pulmonary artery pressure, cardiac output, and left ventricular filling pressure. Early recognition of pulmonary hypertension is essential to interrupt the vicious cycle responsible for the progression of the disease.

Although there is no cure of PPH, treatment can reliever symptoms, increase quality of life, and prolong life. Diuretic therapy relieves dyspnea and peripheral edema and may be useful in reducing right ventricular volume overload. Anticoagulation therapy is recommended for patients with severe pulmonary hypertension to prevent in situ thrombus formation and venous thrombosis. Warfarin is given to keep the INR in the 2 to 3 range. Hypoxia is a potent pulmonary vasoconstrictor, and use of low-flow oxygen provides symptomatic relief. The goal is to keep oxygen saturation at ≥ 90%.

Vasodilator therapy is used to reduce right ventricular overload by dilating pulmonary vessels and reversing remodeling. Some patients with pulmonary hypertension can be effectively managed with calcium channel blocker therapy, such as sustained-release nifedipine (Procardia) or diltiazem (Cardizem).

Epoprostenol (Flolan) has revolutionized the management of PPH. It is a prostacyclin that promotes pulmonary vasodilation and reduces pulmonary vascular resistance. Continuous epoprostenol has been shown to result in significant improvement in clinical symptoms and long-term survival. It is now the treatment of choice for selected patients who are unresponsive to calcium channel blockers. Its administration requires the placement of an indwelling central line catheter and continuous infusion pump. The patient and the family must be trained to use the portable intravenous infusion pump, mix medications, manage the central line, and monitor for complication. The half-life of the drug is less than 6 minutes. If the central line is disrupted, stopped, or dislodged for any reason, clinical deterioration from abrupt withdrawal of epoprostenol can occur. This is a serious event with potential rebound pulmonary hypertension and clinical deterioration developing within minutes. The patient will have signs and symptoms of right sided heart failure, including dyspnea, cyanosis, cough, syncope, and weakness. If the patient loses significant weight, the dosage, which is weight based, may become excessive. Symptoms of overdose include flushing, hypotension, and tachycardia. The major problems have been infectious related to vascular access and broken central lines.

Epoprostenol has been successful in improving the quality of life of patients with PPH. The drug was developed as a bridge to lung transplantation but is now a standard of care. Although the patient and family teaching is extensive, the patient on continuous epoprostenol therapy can be successfully managed with an interdisciplinary health care team.

Treprostinil (Remodulin), a prostacyclin, is used a continuous subcutaneous injection. It causes vasodilation of the pulmonary arterial system and inhibits platelet aggregation. The subcutaneous route had drawbacks, including needles that could dislodge and infusion site pain and reactions. The drug has recently been approved for continuous intravenous use. This drug is stable at room temperature and has a longer half-life than epoprostenol. It may be a reasonable alternative to epoprostenol for some patients.

Bosentan (Tracleer), a form of prostacyclin, is the only oral vasodilator currently approved for the treatment of pulmonary hypertension. It is an active endothelin receptor antagonist and works by blocking the hormone endothelin, which causes blood vessels to constrict. Monthly liver function tests are needed since there is a risk of hepatotoxicity. Sildenafil (Revatio) is an oral phosphodiesterase inhibitor that prolongs the vasodilatory effect of nitric oxide and appears to be as effective in decreasing pulmonary vascular resistance. It should not be taken by patients using nitrates because severe hypotension may develop. Iloprost (Ventavis) is inhaled form of prostacyclin in an aerosolized preparation. It is taken 6 to 9 times a day using a disk inserted into a nebulizer. Because of the risk of orthostatic hypotension, iloprost should not be taken by patients with low systolic blood pressure (<85 mm Hg). Beraprost (an oral formulation of prostacyclin) is undergoing clinical trials for the treatment of early stage pulmonary hypertension.

Surgical interventions for pulmonary hypertension include atrial septostomy (AS), pulmonary thromboendarterectomy (PTPE), and lung transplantation. AS involves the creation of an intra-atrial right to left shunt to decompress the right ventricle. It is indicated for a select group of patients awaiting lung transplantation. PTE may provide a potential cure for those patients suffering from chronic thromboembolic pulmonary hypertension. It is only recommended for patients with operable sites where the emboli can be surgically removed by embolectomy.

Lung transplantation has been the mainstay of treatment for pulmonary hypertension for those patients who do not respond to drug therapy and progress to severe right sided heart failure. Recurrence of the disease has not been reported in individuals, who have undergone transplantation. A patient education and support website for pulmonary hypertension is located.

Secondary Pulmonary Hypertension

Secondary pulmonary hypertension (SPH) occurs when a primary disease causes a chronic increase in pulmonary artery pressures. Secondary pulmonary hypertension can develop as a result of parenchymal lung disease, left ventricular dysfunction, intracardiac shunts, chronic pulmonary thromboembolism, or systemic connective tissue disease. The specific primary disease pathology can result in anatomic or vascular changes causing the pulmonary hypertension. Anatomic changes causing the increased pulmonary vascular resistance include (1) loss of capillaries as a result of alveolar wall damage (e.g., COPD), (2) stiffening of the pulmonary vasculature (e.g., pulmonary fibrosis connective tissue disorders), and (3) obstruction of blood flow (chronic emboli).

Vasomotor increases in pulmonary vascular resistance are found in conditions characterized by alveolar hypoxia. Hypoxia causes localized vasoconstriction and shunting of blood away from poorly ventilated alveoli. Alveolar hypoxia can be caused by a wide variety of conditions. It is possible to have a combination of both anatomic changes and vasomotor constriction. This is found in the patient with long-standing chronic bronchitis who has chronic hypoxia in addition to loss of lung tissue.

The symptoms can reflect the underlying disease, but some are directly attributable to SPH, including dyspnea, fatigue, lethargy and chest pain. The initial physical findings can include right ventricular hypertrophy and signs of right ventricular failure (increased pulmonic heart sound, right sided fourth heart sound, peripheral edema, hepatomegaly). Diagnosis of SPH is similar to that of PPH. Treatment of SPH consists mainly of treating the underlying primary disorder. When irreversible pulmonary vascular damage has occurred, therapies used for PPH are initiated. The efficacy of treatment for pulmonary hypertension has been primarily evaluated for PPH, and there are limited data on the effectiveness of these therapies for SPH. Epoprostenol is used in the management of SPH. More studies are ongoing into effective therapies for SPH.

COR PULMONALE

Cor pulmonale is enlargement of the right ventricle secondary to diseases of the lung, thorax, or pulmonary circulation. Pulmonary hypertension is usually a pre-existing condition in the individual with cor pulmonale. Cor pulmonale may be present with or without cardiac failure. The most common cause of cor pulmonale is COPD. Almost any disorder that effects the respiratory system can cause cor pulmonale.

Clinical Manifestations

Clinical manifestations of cor pulmonale include dyspnea, chronic productive cough, wheezing respirations, retrosternal or substernal pain, and fatigue. Chronic hypoxemia leads to polycythemia and increased total blood volume and viscosity of the blood. (Polycythemia is often present in cor pulmonale secondary to COPD). Compensatory mechanisms that are secondary to hypoxemia can aggravate the pulmonary hypertension. Episodes of cor pulmonale in a person with underlying chronic respiratory problems are frequently triggered by an acute respiratory tract infection.

Management

The primary management of cor pulmonale is directed at treating the underlying pulmonary problem that precipitated the heart problem. Long-term low flow O_2 therapy is used to correct the hypoxemia and reduce vasoconstriction in chronic states of respiratory disorders. If fluid, electrolyte, and acid-base imbalances present, they must be corrected. Diuretics and a low sodium diet will help decrease the plasma volume and the load on the heart. Bronchodilator therapy is indicated if the underlying respiratory problem is due to an obstructive disorder. Digoxin use is controversial. However, studies have confirmed a modest effect of digoxin on the failing right ventricle in chronic cor pulmonale. Other treatments include those for pulmonary hypertension, such as vasodilator therapy, calcium channel blockers, and anticoagulants. Theophylline may help due to its weak inotropic effect on the heart. When medical treatment fails, lung transplantation is an option for some patients.

Chronic management of cor pulmonale resulting from COPD is similar to that described for COPD. Continuous low flow O_2 during sleep, exercise, and small, frequent meals may allow the patient to feel better and be more active.

LUNG TRANSPLANTATION

Lung transplantation has become an important mode of therapy for patients with a variety of end-stage lung diseases. A variety of pulmonary disorders are potentially treatable with some type of lung transplantation. Improved patient selection criteria, technical advances, and better methods of immunosuppression have resulted in improved survival rates. Four types of transplant procedures are available: single lung transplantation, bilateral lung transplantation, heart-lung transplantation, and transplantation of lobes from a living related donor. Indications for lung transplantation:

- α1-antitrypsin deficiency
- Bronchiectasis
- Cystic fibrosis
- Emphysema
- Idiopathic pulmonary fibrosis
- Interstitial lung disease
- Pulmonary fibrosis secondary to other diseases (e.g., sarcoidosis)
- Pulmonary hypertension.

Single-lung transplantation involves an incision on the side of the chest. The opposite lung is ventilated while the diseased lung is excised. The lung is removed and the donor lung implanted. Three anastomoses are done: the bronchus, pulmonary artery, and pulmonary veins. In a bilateral lung transplantation, the incision is made across the sternum and the donor lungs are implanted separately. A median sternotomy incision is used for a heart-lung transplant procedure. Chest tubes are placed around the donor lungs to help them re-expand with air. Lobar transplantation from living donors is reserved for candidates who urgently need transplantation and are unlikely to survive until a donor becomes available. The majority of these transplant recipients are patients with cystic fibrosis, and their parents or relatives are donors.

Patients being considered for lung transplantation need to undergo extensive evaluation. The candidate for lung transplantation should not have a malignancy or recent history of malignancy (within the last 2 years), renal or liver insufficiency, or HIV. Typically patients wait an average of 12 to 18 months for a donor lung.

The candidate and the family undergo psychologic screening to determine the ability to cope with a postoperative regimen that requires strict adherence to immunosuppressive therapy, continuous monitoring for early signs of infection, and prompt reporting of manifestations of infection for medical evaluation. Many transplant centers require preoperative outpatient pulmonary rehabilitation to maximize physical conditioning.

Early postoperative care includes ventilatory support, fluid and hemodynamic management, immunosuppression, detection of early rejection and prevention or treatment of infection. Pulmonary clearance measures, including aerosolized bronchodilators, chest physiotherapy, and deep-breathing and coughing techniques, minimize potential complications. Maintenance of fluid balance is vital in the postoperative phase.

Lung transplant recipients are at high risk for bacterial, viral, fungal, and protozoal infections. Infections are the leading cause of death in the early period after the transplant. Gram-negative bacterial pneumonia is common. Among potential causes of viral infections, cytomegalovirus (CMV) is the most important in lung transplantation patients, usually seen 4 to 8 weeks postoperatively. Clinical manifestations of CMV infection include fever, bone marrow suppression, hepatitis, enteritis, and pneumonitis. Aspergillus is the most common fungal infection.

Immunosuppressive therapy usually includes a three drug regimen of cyclosprine or tacrolimus, azathioprine (Imuran) or mycophenolate mofetil (CellCept), and prednisone. However, because of an array of potential adverse effects and drug interactions, there are limitations to immunosuppressive therapy. Drug levels are monitored on a regular basis. Lung transplant recipients are usually maintained on higher levels of immunosuppressive therapy than other organ recipients.

Acute rejection is fairly common in lung transplantation and can be seen as soon as 5 to 7 days after surgery. It is characterized by low grade fever, fatigue, and oxygen desaturation with exercise. Accurate diagnosis is by transtracheal biopsy. Treatment is high doses of corticosteroids administered IV for 3 days. In patients with persistent or recurrent acute rejection, other strategies may include antilymphocyte antibodies or changing maintenance immunosuppressive drugs.

Bronchiolitis obliterans (an obstructive airway disease causing progressive occlusion) is thought to be a manifestation of chronic rejection in lung transplant patients. The onset is often subacute, with gradual onset of progressive obstructive airflow defect, including cough, dyspnea and recurrent lower respiratory tract infection. Treatment involves optimum maintenance immunosuppression.

Discharge planning begins in the preoperative phase. Prior to discharge, the patient needs to be able to perform self-care activities, including medication management and activities of daily living, and to accurately identify when to call the transplant team physician. Patients are placed in an outpatient rehabilitation program to improve physical endurance. Home spirometry has been useful in monitoring trends in lung function. Patients are taught to keep medication logs, laboratory results, and spirometry records. The average lung transplant patient takes 13 medications (range, 5 to 24) a day. After discharge, the patients are followed by the transplant team for transplant related issues. The patients return to their primary care team for their health maintenance and routine illnesses. As transplant procedures become more frequent, transplant patients will return to hospitals for other routine procedures. Coordination of care between the transplant team, primary care team, and inpatient teams is essential for ongoing successful management of these patients.

PULMONARY CONTUSION

A penetrating injury may cause contusion of the lung or pleura. Pulmonary contusion usually results from sudden compression followed by rapid compression of the thoracic cavity, causing blood to extravasate into pulmonary tissue.

The contusion is usually self-limiting because the pulmonary vasculature is a low pressure system. However, extensive contusion can precipitate pulmonary edema with resultant hypoxemia, hypercapnea, and respiratory acidosis.

Clinical Manifestation

Pulmonary contusion may vary from total absence of symptoms to the full spectrum of symptoms associated with non-cardiogenic pulmonary edema. Signs and symptoms (some of which may be delayed) include the following.
- Increasing dyspnea
- Tachypnea
- Increasing restlessness
- Crackles notes on auscultations, and
- Hemoptysis.

Management

Medical treatment of pulmonary contusion depends on the severity of the injury. Treatment may vary from outpatient monitoring to intubation and mechanical ventilating support when pulmonary edema present. The nursing care includes the following:
- Administer analgesic as ordered every 3 hours
- Monitor for fluid overload
  - Keep accurate records of all intake and output
  - Monitor vital signs every 30 minutes. Report increased pulse and respiration, and
  - Monitor breath sound every 30 minutes.
- Monitor ventilating status
  - Check for signs of respiratory distress–dyspnea, increased inspiration, changes in breath sound,
  - Check ABG results.
- Monitor for sign of symptom of flail chest
- Support patient to stay in bed until physical status is stabilised
  - Stay with patient, listen to patients concerned–explain what is planned, and
  - Assist with ADL
- Teach patient/family how to support pulmonary contusion.

CHRONIC BRONCHITIS

Chronic bronchitis is defined by the presence of chronic productive cough for minimum of 3 months per year for at least 2 consecutive years in patients in whom other causes have been excluded, it is characterised by physiologically by hypertrophy and hypersecretion of the bronchial mucous glands and structural alterations of the bronchi and bronchioles.

Etiology

Chronic bronchitis is caused by the inhalation of physical or chemical irritants or by viral or bacterial infections. The most common inhaled irritant is cigarette smoke (heavy cigarette smoking).

Pathophysiology

In chronic bronchitis, there is pathologic changes in the lung consisting of:
- Hyperplasia of mucus secreting glands in the trachea and bronchi,
- Increase in globlet cells
- Disappearance of cilia
- Chronic inflammatory charges and narrowing of small airways, and
- Altered functions of alveolar macrophages, leading to increased bronchial infections.

Frequently airways are colonised with micro-organisms. Infection occurs when the organisms increase. Most common infecting agents are S. *pneumoniae* and *H. influenzae*. Excess amounts of mucus are found in the airways and sometimes may occlude small bronchioles and scarring the bronchiole wall may occur chronic inflammation in the primary pathologic mechanism involved in causing the changes characteristics of chronic bronchitis.

Clinical Manifestations

The earliest symptom in chronic bronchitis is usually a frequent, productive cough during most winter months. It is often exacerbated by respiratory irritants and cold, damp air. Bronchospasm can occur at the end of paroxysms of coughing. Frequent respiratory infections are other common manifestation. Somewhat later, dyspnea on exertion may develop. Unfortunately a patient often attributes chronic cough to smoking rather than lung disease, thus delaying initiation of treatment. In addition, the patient may not be aware of the cough because he/she becomes accustomed to it.

Hypoxemia and hypercapnea result from hypoventilation caused by increased airway resistance. The bluish red colour of the skin results from polycythemia and cyanosis. Polycythemia develops as a result of increased production of red blood cells secondary to the body's attempt to compensate for chronic hypoxemia. Hemoglobin concentration may reach 200 g/L. Cyanosis develops when there is at least 5 g/dl or more of circulating unoxygenated hemoglobin.

The complication of chronic bronchitis are cor pulmonale, acute exacerbation of chronic bronchitis, and acute respiratory failure, peptic ulcer, and GERD, and pneumonia.

Management

Diagnostic studies of COPD include:
- Chest X-ray film, typical finding in chronic bronchitis and increased bronchovascular markings.
- Sputum studies for culture and sensitivity. Neutrophils and bronchial epithelial cells usually occurs in chronic bronchitis.
- ABG
- ECG
- Exercise testing with oximetry (if indicated)
- EEG or cardia nuclear scan (if indicated).

The primary goal of care for COPD patients are to:
- Improve ventilation
- Promote secretion–removal
- Prevent complication and progression of symptoms
- Promote patient comfort and participation in care, and
- Improve quality of life as much as possible.

Medical therapy of chronic bronchitis are depends on symptoms. Pulmonary function tests results in ABG findings. Therapy may include all or some of the modalities outlined here are as follows:
- Supportive measures: Education of patient and family about the following:
  - Avoidance of cigarette smoke
  - Avoidance of other inhaled irritants
  - Avoidance of persons with upper respiratory infections
  - Control of environmental temperature and humidity
  - Proper nutrition, and
  - Adequate hydration.
- Specific therapy: Medication such as
  - Bronchiodilator—α antitrypsin replacement for those with levels
  - Antimicrobials—ampicillium or another broad-spectrum antibiotic
  - Corticosteroids—to alleviate acute symptoms: e.g., prednisone
  - Digitalis—to treat LVF if present.
- Respiratory therapy in aerosol therapy used to deliver bronchiodilator, through metered cartridge device with spacer at rest.
  - Oxygen therapy for patients who are unable to maintain PaO_2.
- Relaxation exercises
  - Meditation for relax
- Breathing retraining
- Rehabilitation.

EMPHYSEMA

Emphysema is defined pathologically by destructive changes in alveolar walls and enlargement of air spaces distal to the terminal non-respiratory bronchioles. It is characterised physiologically by increased lung compliance, decreased diffusing, capacity and increased airway resistance.

Etiology

The cause of emphysema is not known. However, evidence suggests that proteases released by polymorph nuclear leukocytes or alveolar macrophages are involved in the destruction of the connective tissue of the lungs. Cigarette smoking, infections, ambient air pollution and heredity (AAT-a, antitrypsin) are the other causes of emphysema.

Pathophysiology

Emphysema is a condition of the lungs characterised by abnormal permanent enlargement of the airspaces distal to the terminal bronchioles, accompanied by destruction of these walls and without obvious fibrosis. Structural changes include:
- Hyperinflation of alveoli
- Destruction of alveolar walls
- Destruction of alveolar capillary walls
- Narrowed tortuous, small airways
- Loss of lung elasticity.

There are two types of emphysema centrilobular and panlobular. In centrilobular emphysema the primary area involvement is the central part of the lobula. Respiratory bronchioles enlarge, the walls are destroyed, and the bronchioles become confluent, chronic bronchioles associate with centrilobular types.

Panlobular emphysema, involves distentions and destruction of the whole lobule. Respiratory bronchioles, alveolar ducts and sacs and alveoli are all affected. There is a progressive loss of lung tissue and decreased alveolar-capillary surface area. Severe panlobular emphysema/ usually found in persons with alpha-antitrypsin (AAT) deficiency.

Clinical Manifestation

An early symptom of emphysema is dyspnea, which becomes progressively more severe. The patient will first complain of dyspnea on exertion that progresses to interfering with ADL to dyspnoea at rest. Minimal coughing is present, with no sputum or smell amounts of mucoid sputum. As more alveoli becomes over distended increasing amount of air are trapped. This causes flattened diaphragm and an increased anteroposterior diameter of the chest, forming the typical barrel chest.

Effective abdominal breathing decreased. The person becomes more of chest breather, relying on the intercostal and accessory muscles. Hypoxemia may be present. The person is characteristically thin and underweight. The person may suffer from protein-caloric malnutrition. Later clubbing finger may develop. The complications as in chronic bronchitis.

Management of emphysema same as in chronic bronchitis. Nursing intervention for persons with chronic bronchitis and pulmonary emphysema are also the same, which include administration of medication such as digitalis and diuretics as prescribed, improving gas exchange, oxygen therapy, improving efficiency for breathing pattern (pursed lip-breathing, forward-leaving position, abdominal breathing and exercise, pulmonary physiotherapy, segmental postural drainage), improving airway clearance, improving nutrition, preventing infection, preventing fluid volume excess, assisting with breathing in rest, assisting with central of environment, and mounting temperature and humidity, etc.

Teach the following:
- Progressive relaxation exercise:
  - Contract each muscle to a count of 10 and then relax it.
  - Do exercises in quiet room while sitting or lying in a comfortable position.
  - Do exercises for relaxing muscle, if desired.
  - Have another person serve as a "coach" by giving command to contract specific muscles, count to 10 and relax muscle.
  - The following are the examples of exercises helpful to some person with (COPD)
    * Raise shoulders, shrug them, and relax for 5 seconds, then relax them completely.
    * Make a fist of both hands. Squeeze them lightly for 5 seconds and relax them completely.
- Meditation exercises:
  - Sit or lie quietly with eyes closed and attempt to relax all muscles beginning with feet and moving upward.
  - Breathe in through the nose slowly (may help to count slowly to 4 on inhalation) and exhale slowly through pursed lips (mentally count to 6) with a natural rhythm, relaxed and peaceful (this can be coached or performed without assistance).
  - Survey the body points of tension, consciously relax the tense areas. The body is peaceful and relaxed.
  - Continue breathing as above. Aware of the feeling of well-being throughout your body. This can be used for 10 to 20 minutes or after 5 minutes go to step 5.
  - Listen for (or visualize) a special relaxation sound (or image). Listen to it closely (or visualise) all the while breathing as above.
  - At this point, positive suggestion can be used, for example, I am in control of my body. When I find myself getting tense, I can take moment to stop and breathe in all the air that I need and let the tension flow away.
  - After mental suggestion, continue breathing easily and slowly come back to normal alert to mental state.
  - Meditation can be used at any time to induce relaxed state of mind (e.g. to promote sleep).

While taking care of the person with COPD, nurse has to take the following areas should be addressed in a typical teaching programme for persons with chronic bronchitis or emphysema.

- Patients should be able to explain in lay terms, the basic functions and pathology of their lungs.
- Avoidance of respirative irritants and maintenance of a proper environment should be emphasised to people with COPD. Inhaled irritants (especially cigarette smoke) pose a serious threat to these persons. Steps the patient can take to reduce or avoid exposure to these irritants.
  - Stop smoking. The nurse should be familiar with community programmes and give a list of them to the patient, to involve in it.
  - Ask other persons not to smoke in the patient's room. Inhalation of secondary smoke can exacerbate symptoms.
  - Pay heed to announcement on radio and TV warning of pollution alert. Do not go outside during an alert.
  - Use an air-conditioner or HEPA filter or electrostatic filter to remove particular matter from air.
    * Keep filters clean and follow manufacturers' directions for use.
    * Use an activated charcoal filter if offending odours or gas pollutants are a problem.
  - Avoid abrupt environmental temperature or humidity changes, because they can increase sputum production and cause bronchospasms.
    * Use an airconditioner in hot weather
    * Use a face mask when going out in cold weather
    * Use a dehumidifier or humidifier as appropriate to maintain a humidity of 30 to 50 per cent.
  - If air travel is required, check with physician about need for suplemental oxygen.

- Avoid large crowds, especially during known influenza.
  * Avoid contact with people who have an upper respiratory infection
  * Receive influenza and pneumonia immunisation.
- The patient should be able to explain the following aspects of the home medication or treatment regimen.
  - State name, dose, action and side effects of each infection.
  - Explain how and where to use medication ordered on an as needed basis (e.g., bronchodilators, antibiotics, steroids, antacids).
  - Describe how to obtain and maintain any needed equipment or supplies (e.g. oxygen, nebulizers, humidifiers, aerosols IPPB machines and syringes medications).
- The patient should demonstrate how to carry out the specific home exercise programme:
  - Specific exercises to be completed
  - Frequency of exercise
  - Monitor physical response to exercises, such as heart rate increase, increase respiratory rate, or perceived fatigue.
- The patient should be able to list the names and telephone numbers of the appropriate support services.

ASTHMA

Asthma is an inflammatory disease characterised by hyper-responsiveness of the airways and periods of bronchospasm, resulting in intermittent airway obstruction. The onset of asthma is sudden, contrary to the slow, insidious progression of symptoms seen in chronic bronchitis and emphysema.

Etiology

Asthma is caused by increased responsiveness of the trachea and bronchi to various stimuli that cause narrowing of the airways and difficulty in breathing. The common factors triggering an asthma attack include:
- Environmental factors
  - Change in temperature especially cold air and
  - Change in humidity; dry air.
- Atmospheric pollutants
  - Cigarette and industrial smoke, ozone, sulphur dioxide, formaldehyde.
  - Exhaust fumes, oxidants, aerosol sprays.
- Strong odours, perfumes.
- Allergen inhalation.
  - Feathers, animal danders, dust mites molds allergens.
  - Foods treated with sulfites, beer, wine fruit juices, snack foods salads, potatoes, shellfish, fresh and dried fruits) and metabisulfites, bisulfites, tartrazines.
- Exercise and cold, dry air
- Stress or emotional upset
- Infection: Vital upper respiratory infection, sinusitis
- Medications: Aspirin and NSAIDs, β-blockers (including eyedrops of glaucoma)
- Enzymes: Including those in laundry detergents
- Occupational exposure: Metal salts, wood and vegetable dust, industrial chemicals and plastics
- Chemicals, toluene and others used in solvents, paints, rubber and plastics
- Hormones, menses
- Gastro-esophageal reflex (GER).

Pathophysiology

The mechanism that induces asthma remains unknown. There are two types of asthma. Extrinsic (atopic) and intrinsic (non-atopic).

Extrinsic asthma results from an inflammatory response of the airway caused by mast cell activation, eosinophil infiltration, and epithelial slughing. An attack is triggered by environmental allergen (dust, pollen, molos, animal dander and foods). An initial encounter with an allergen stimulates plasma cells to produce antigen-specific IgE, antibodies that bind mast cells in airways. When exposed to the allergen IgE antigen binding causes mast cell deregulation and release of inflammatory mediators. The result is an intense inflammatory response in the airways.

Intrinsic asthma occurs in adults 35 years of age in older, the asthma attack is often severe. Factors that precipitate attacks include respiratory tract infections, drugs (aspirin, β-adrenergic antagonism), environmental irritants, (occupational chemicals) air pollutions, cold, dry, air, exercise and emotional stress. Chemical mediator, interacts with the autonomic nervous systems causing inflammation and bronchoconstriction.

An asthmatic attack results from several physiological alterations, include altered immunological response increased airway resistance, increased lung compliance, impaired mucociliary function, and altered carbon dioxide exchange.

The primary pathophysiologic process in asthma is chronic inflammation, which leads to airway hyper-responsiveness (hyperreactivity) and acute airflow limitation. Exposure to allergens or irritants initiates the inflammatory cascade. A variety of inflammatory cells are involved in asthma. Examples of inflammatory cells in asthma are mast cells, macrophages, eosinophils, neutrophils, T and B lymphocytes, and epithelial cells of the airways.

As the inflammatory process begins, mast cells (found beneath the basement membrane of the bronchial wall) degranulate and release multiple inflammatory mediators. Common inflammatory mediators are leukotrienes, histamine, cytokines (e.g., interleukins 4 and 5), prostaglandin's, and nitric oxide. Some inflammatory mediators have effects on the blood vessels, causing vasodilation and increasing capillary permeability. Some mediators result in the airways being infiltrated by eosinophils, lymphocytes, and neutrophils. The resulting inflammatory process results in vascular congestion; edema formation; production of thick, tenacious mucus; bronchial muscle spasm; thickening of airway walls; and increased bronchial hyperresponsiveness. This whole process is sometimes referred to as the *early-phase response* in asthma. Clinically it can occur within 30 to 60 minutes after exposure to the allergen or irritant.

Symptoms can recur 4 to 10 hours after the initial attack because of eosinophil and lymphocyte activation and further release of more inflammatory mediators. The epithelial cells also produce cytokines and other inflammatory mediators. This delayed response is called the *late-phase response* in asthma. Only about 30 to 50% of patients experience this delayed response. It can be more severe than the early-phase response and persist for 24 hours or more. It is characterized by a self-sustaining cycle of inflammation. Airflow may be limited from the swelling of the airways with or without bronchoconstriction. Corticosteroids are effective in treating this inflammation.

Untreated inflammation can lead to long-term damage that is irreversible. Chronic inflammation resulting in structural changes in the bronchial wall is known as remodeling. The bronchial smooth muscle hypertrophies and collagen is deposited in the airway walls. The mechanisms responsible for remodeling are thought to be related to chronic or recurrent inflammation of the airways. The combination of damage to the epithelium of the airways, prolonged repair of the epithelium, fibrosis, and increased types of fibroblasts are central to remodeling. The airway smooth muscles hypertrophy and mucus secreting cells undergo hyperplasia in remodeling. There is some evidence that remodeling can occur even in mild asthma of recent onset, but it can be prevented by early introduction of inhaled corticosteroids.

Hyperventilation occurs during an asthma attack as lung receptors respond to increased lung volume from trapped air and airflow limitation. Decreased perfusion and ventilation of the alveoli and increased alveolar gas pressure lead to ventilation perfusion abnormalities in the lungs. The patient will be hypoxemia early on with decreased $PaCO_2$ and increased pH (respiratory alkalosis) as he or she is hyperventilating. As the airflow limitation worsens with air trapping, the patient works much harder to breathe. The $PaCO_2$ will normalize as the patient tires, and then it will rise to produce respiratory acidosis, which is an ominous sign signifying respiratory failure.

Alterations in the neural control of the airways also occur in asthma. The automatic nervous system, consisting of the parasympathetic and sympathetic systems, innervates the bronchi. Airway smooth muscle tone is regulated by the parasympathetic nervous system via the vagus nerve. Afferent and efferent impulses are conducted through the vagus nerve to the medulla and back to the lungs. When airway nerve endings are stimulated by mechanical or chemical stimuli (e.g., air pollution, cold air, dust, allergens), increased release of acetylcholine causes bronchoconstriction.

Clinical Manifestations

Asthma is characterised by an unpredictable and variable course. It causes recurrent episodes of wheezing, breathlessness, chest tightness, and cough, particularly at night and in the early morning. An attack of asthma may have an abrupt onset or it may be more gradual. Attacks often occur at night may last for a few minutes to several hours. In between, the patient may be asymptomatic with normal and abnormal pulmonary function. However, in some persons, compromised pulmonary functions may result in a state of continuous asthma and chronic debilitation characterised by irreversible airway disease.

The characteristic clinical manifestation of asthma are wheezing cough, dyspnea, and chest tightness after exposed to a precipitating factor or trigger. Expiration may be prolonged.

Instead of normal inspiratory-expiratory ratio of 1:2 it will be prolonged to 1:3 or 1:4. Normally the bronchioles constrict during expiration. However, as a result of bronchospasm, edema and mucus in the bronchioles, the airways become narrower than usual. This takes longer for the air to move out of the bronchioles. This produce the characteristic wheezing, air trapping and hyperinflation.

The signs and symptoms associated with asthma are correlated with normal lung functions and underlying pathophysiological origins (see aetiology). The character of asthmatic attacks can vary on a continuum from chronic or acute mild intermittent attacks to life threatening status asthmaticus. Severe acute asthma can result in complication such as rib fractures, pneumothorax, pneumomediastinum, atelectasis, pneumonia and *status asthmaticus*.

Status asthmaticus is a severe, life-threatening asthma attack that is refractory to usual treatment and places the patient at risk for developing respiratory failure. The causes of which include viral illnesses, ingestion of aspirin or other NSAIDs, emotional stress, increase in environmental pollutants or other allergen exposure, abrupt discontinuation of aerosal medication and ingestion of beta adrenergic blocking agent. In this exhaustion, diminished breath sounds, intubation and mechanical ventilation, complications of status asthmaticus include pneumothorax, pneumomediastenum, acute cor pulmonale with RVF and severe respiratory muscle fatigue leading to respiratory arrest. Death from status asthmaticus is usually the result of respiratory arrest or cardiac failure.

Management

The objective of medical management of asthma are to promote normal functioning of the individual, prevent recurrent symptoms, prevent severe attacks and prevent side effects of medication. The chief aim of various medication is to afford the patient immediate, progressive ongoing bronchial relaxation.

One approach to treat an acute asthmatic attack is as follows:

- Inhalation of beta-agonist such as albuterol sulphate (pro-ventil, ventalin), salmeterol (Serolvent), or metaproterenol sulphate in normal saline. Which stimulates beta 2-receptors in bronchial smooth muscle resulting in smooth muscle relaxation. It starts to act in 10 minutes, effects last 4-6 hours. Here, the nurse has to monitor vital signs, lung sounds, and peak expiratory flow rate (PEFR) before and after treatment. If this is not successful: Go for the following:
- Methylprednisoline IV loading dose 2 mg/kg or about 125 mg 6th hrs/then 60-125 mg 6th hourly for 48 hours total or until patient is stable, which reduces inflammation and edema of airway and decreases hyperactivity of airway. The benefits seen within 6 hours full effect in 6-8 hours.

  When patient is stabilised, change IV to 60 mg oral prednisoline by mouth daily or every other day. The oral prednisoline should be tapered off by 7-10 days, Taper 60 mg over 2 days, 40 mg over 2 days, 30 mg over 2 days and 10 mg over 2 days.
- Nebulized atrophine sulphate may be tried, or aminophylline may be given IV a pump is used for better control of infusion which relax bronchial smooth muscle.

Loading dose of aminophyllin 4 to 6 mg/kg over 15 to 30 minutes and then continuous infusion of 0.45 to 0.70 mg/kg/hour. Patients who have been taking aminophyllin at home will be placed on continuous IV therapy. Rate of infusion is 10-20 mg/ml. Too rapid infusion may cause severe hypotension, premature ventricular contractions, and cardiac arrest.

Here, the nurse has to monitor heart rate and rhythm closely, and report any change immediately to the concerned. Theophylline metabolised by the liver. For persons with liver disease, small doses are used. Patient taking cemitidene, erythromycin or ciprofloxacin require smaller doses. Smokers and those taking phenytoin require larger doses to maintain blood level.

Other common medications for asthma are as follows:

- NSAIDs such as cromolyn, nedocromil, administered through metered dose inhaler (MDI) or nebulizer, decreases airway inflammation and irritation, headache, bad taste in mouth.
- Corticosteroids (dexamethosone, triamcinolene acetonide, Flunisolid, fluticasone) administered through MDI has an anti-inflammatory action. Side effects are sore throat, hoarseness, cough, oral thrush.
- Leukotriene inhibitors/receptor antagonists such as zafir-lukast, zilenton, are anti-inflammatory used orally. Adverse effects include headache, nausea, diarrhoea, dizziness, myalgia, fever, dyspepsia, elevated glanine aminotransferase level.
- Theophylline can be administered orally or parenterally. It is long acting, "bronchiodilator". Side effects are nausea, vomiting, stomach cramps, diarrhea, headache, muscle cramps, tachycardia, irritability, restlessness, serum blood levels should be checked for therapeutic range.
- Anticholinergics (spray) administered through MDI or nebulizer, or nasal spray. It is short-acting bronchiodilator. Side effects are nervousness, dizziness, headache, palpations, blurred vision, nausea, GI distress and dry mouth.
- Beta-2-agonist such as salmeterol administered through MDI. It is long-acting bronchiodilator; may lead to adverse effects—headache, tremor, tachycardia, palpations, naso-pharyngitis, stomachache, cough, rash.

When administering the above drugs, nurse has to monitor the responses and side effects of the medication and act accordingly. And when using a metered dose inhaler (MDI) the nurse has to teach the patient as follows:

- Inhale through nose, then slowly exhale
- Place inhaler 1 to 2 inches off the mouth
- Press down inhaler while simultaneously inhaling one puff deeply. Breath in air from around the mouth piece while inhaling.
- Hold breath for 5 to 10 seconds to allow medication to reach lung.
- Repeat second puff if one is ordered.
- If any untoward effects, stop administering of MDI.

CYSTIC FIBROSIS

Cystic fibrosis is an autosomal recessive, multisystem disease characterised by altered function of the exocrine glands involving primarily the lungs, pancreas, and sweat glands. Abnormally thick, abundant secretions from mucus glands can lead to a chronic, diffuse, obstructive pulmonary disorder in almost all patients.

Etiology

Cystic fibrosis is an autosomal recessive disease resulting from mutations in a gene located on chromosome 7. The most common mutations in the CF gene is known as the CF transmembrane regulator (CFTR). The primary defect in the CF is abnormally regulated chloride channel activity. This defect alters ionic transport of sodium and chloride across epithelial surfaces. The high concentration of NaCl in the sweat of the patients with CF results from decreased chloride reabsorption in the sweat duct. The basic pathophysiologic mechanism is obstruction of exocrine gland duct with thick viscous secretions that adhere to the lumen of the ducts. The glands distal to the duct eventually undergo fibrosis.

Pathophysiology

Cystic fibrosis is an exocrine gland disease involving various systems, i.e., pulmonary, pancreatic/hepatic, GI, reproductive obstruction of the exocrine glands duct or passage ways occurs in nearly all adult patients with CF. Exocrine gland secretions are known to have a decreased water content, altered electrolyte concentration and abnormal organic constituents (especially no mucus glycoproteins), however, the specific biochemical or physiological defect that leads to obstruction is not known.

The following physiological alterations are found in adults with CF include:
- Pulmonary damage
- Gastrointestinal and pancreatic involvement
- Glucose intolerance.

Clinical Manifestations

The specific clinical manifestation by symptoms are:
- Pulmonary signs and symptoms of CF includes:
  - Chronic productive cough and/or recurrent bronchitis or pneumonia
  - Crackles and rhonchi decreased pulmonary compliance, digital clubbing, and
  - Shortness of breath and dyspnea on exertion, wheezing, and weight loss occurs with respiratory complication and usually indicate need for vigorous therapy.
- Gastrointestinal signs and symptoms include the following:
  - Frequent, bulky, greasy stools
  - Weight loss
  - Cramps and abdominal pain should arouse suspicion of obstruction
- Glucose intolerance signs and symptoms include:
  - Polyuria, polydipsia, polyphagia
  - Absence of ketoacidosis even with above signs.

Normally mucus production by goblet cells lubricate airways and entraps foreign particles. In CF, excessive amounts of mucus production leads to increased cough and mucus production, inflammation of small airways causing hyperinflation of alveoli give rise to fatigue, shortness of breath, chronic bacterial infections leading to fever, fatigue, shortness of breath, and eroding of a major blood vessel and secondary infection may lead to hemoptysis.

Management

The goals of medical management of CF are to minimize bronchial plugging and to inhibit bacterial colonisation. Measures to minimize bronchial plugging include:
- Chest physiotherapy with chest percussion and postural drainage are performed for 20 minutes two or three times daily and some time much more frequently.
- Administer dornase-alfa 2.5 mg ampule in compressed air-driven nebulizer for reducing visco-elasticity of CF secretion.
- Mucolytic agents may be ordered to thin secretions.
- Humidification of air, according to some physicians
- Antibiotics for infection.

Nursing measures include preventing pulmonary infections, care of hemoptysis, care of pneumothorax and care of cor pul-monale diet, activity and regimen.
- Prevention of pulmonary infection can be made best by:
  - Vigorous postural drainage and percussing
  - Room humidification if ordered
  - Aerosols with a bronchodilator, and
  - Monitoring for infection and take suitable measure accordingly.
- Nursing care and medical care during hemoptysis include:
  - Elevate head of bed 45 to 90 degrees
  - Turn patient's head to left side to facilitate expectoration of blood
  - Provide clean basin frequently so that patient is not made more anxious by amount of blood
  - Measure amount of hemoptysis and record time and amounts
  - Postural drainage and percussion are contraindicated if haemoptysis present
  - Vitamin K as ordered by mouth or subcutaneously to check bleeding
  - Stay with the patient until bleeding has subsided and made comfortable to less fearful, and
  - Bronchioscopy with endobronchial tamponade may be successful.
- Care of pneumothorax includes proper care for chest tube connected to closed drainage system and other measure used in pneumothorax
- Care of cor pulmonale includes supplement oxygen, long-term diuretic therapy. Digoxin if or as ordered by the physician
- Promoting adequate nutrition supplemental fat soluble vitamins and multivitamins and vitamin E. Pancreatin enzyme supplemented
- Patient should be encouraged to be upright position as a tolerated
- Patient and family educated about taking care of CF cases.

RESPIRATORY FAILURE

Acute respiratory failure (ARF) is used to describe any rapid change in respiration resulting in hypoxemia, hypercapnia, or both. ARF can be classified as hypoxemia or hypercapnia.

Hypoxemic respiratory failure is also related to an oxygenation failure, because the primary problem is inadequate O_2 transfer. This can be defined as a PaO_2 of 60 mm Hg or less when the patient is receiving an inspired O_2 concentration of 60 per cent or greater.

Hypercapnic respiratory failure is also referred to as ventilatory failure because the primary problem is insufficient CO_2 removal. It is defined as a $PaCO_2$ above normal (> 45 mm Hg) in combination with acidemia (pH < 7.35).

Etiology

Many disorders can lead to or associated with respiratory failure which can be divided into pulmonary and nonpulmonary diseases.
- Pulmonary disorders
  - Severe infection
  - Pulmonary edema
  - Pulmonary embolus
  - COPD - Chronic obstructive pulmonary disease
  - CF - Cystic fibrosis
  - ARDS - Acute respiratory distress syndrome
  - Cancer
  - Chest trauma (flail chest)
  - Severe atelectasis
  - Airway compromise, secondary to trauma, infection or surgery
- Non-pulmonary disorders
  - CNS disturbance secondary to drug overdose, anaesthesia, head injury
  - Neuromuscular disorders i.e., Guillain-Barré syndrome, myasthenia gravis, multiple sclerosis, poliomyelitis, muscular distrophy, spinal cord injury.
  - Postoperative reduction in ventilation following thoracic and abdominal surgery.
  - Prolonged mechanical ventilation.

Pathophysiology

The respiratory system is made up of two basic parts, the gas exchange organ (Lung) and the pump (the respiratory muscles and the respiratory control mechanism). Any alteration in the function of gas exchange unit or pump can result in respiratory insufficiency or respiratory failure. Regardless of the underlying condition, the resultant events or processes that occur in respiratory failure are the same. With inadequate ventilation, the arterial oxygen falls and tissue cells become hypoxic. Carbon dioxide accumulates, leading to a fall in pH and respiratory acidosis.

Lung or gas exchange unit respiratory failure is usually seen in person with underlying primary pulmonary disease such as COPD. In this situation respiratory failure as a result of pathology directly affects the respiratory unit.

Pump failure is associated with extrapulmonary disorders that may precipitate respiratory failure. In this situation the underlying disorder decreases the ability of lungs to move oxygen and carbon dioxide into and out of the lungs by altering either the central ventilatory control mechanism (e.g., drug overdose) neuromuscular function (e.g., Gullain-Barré syndrome) or chest wall movement (flail chest).

Acute respiratory failure is defined by predetermined physiological criteria, i.e., sudden onset of the following:
- PaO_2 50 mm Hg or less (measured in room air)
- $PaCO_2$ 50 mm Hg or more
- pH 7.35 or less

Clinical Manifestations

The sign and symptoms associated with hypercapnia, hypoxemia and respiratory acidosis are:
- Headache
- Irritability
- Increasing somnolence coma
- Asterixis (flapping tremor)
- Cardiac dysrhythmias
- Tachycardia
- Hypotension
- Cyanosis.

Management

The management of respiratory failure includes the following.
- Medical therapy is based on degree of severity.
  - Severe acute respiratory failure, focus on immediate oxygenation and ventilation.
  - Less severe acute respiratory failure: underlying cause determined and treated concurrently while treating hypoxemia and hypercapnia.
- Clinical evaluation
  - Diagnosis studies include—ABGs, chest X-ray film, bedside pulmonary spirometry, sputum for culture and sensitivity.
  - Treatment includes
    - Oxygen therapy.
    - Ventilation: may require intubation and mechanical ventilatory supports.
    - Treatment of underlying causes.

Nursing care includes improving gas exchange, ventilatory support, mechanical ventilation, improving airway clearance, improving breathing pattern, improving cardiac output, maintaining adequate nutrition, health promotion and prevention.

CHRONIC OBSTRUCTIVE PULMONARY DISEASE

Chronic obstructive pulmonary disease (COPD) is a preventable and treatable disease, state characterized by airflow limitation that is not fully reversible. The airflow limitation is usually progressive and associated with an abnormal inflammatory response of the lungs to noxious particles or gases, primarily caused by cigarette smoking. Although COPD affects the lungs, systemic consequences also develop.

The term chronic obstructive pulmonary disease encompasses two types of obstructive airway diseases, chronic bronchitis and emphysema. *Chronic bronchitis* is the presence of chronic productive cough for 3 months in each of 2 consecutive years in a patient in whom other causes of chronic cough have been excluded. Emphysema is an abnormal permanent enlargement of the air spaces distal to the terminal bronchioles, accompanied by destruction of their walls and without obvious fibrosis. Only about 10% of patients with COPD have pure emphysema. Patients with COPD may have a predominance of one of these conditions, but in reality it is often difficult to determine because the conditions unusually coexist. COPD is discussed in this session as one disease state from the standpoint of pathophysiology and management.

Patients with COPD may have asthma, and some patients with asthma may go on to develop fixed or irreversible airflow obstruction. It may be nearly impossible to differentiate asthma from COPD, especially if the individual has a history of cigarette smoking.

Etiology

Cigarette smoking: The major risk factor for developing COPD is cigarette smoking. It is still a major public health concern, especially among young people. Nearly all first time use of tobacco occurs before high school graduation, and each day 2000 teens will become regular, daily smokers, with one third of them eventually dying because of a smoking-related disease. Clinically significant airway obstruction develops in approximately 15 to 20% of smokers. Cigarette smoking remains the most preventable cause of premature death. In addition to being linked with COPD and lung cancer, cigarette smoking has also been implicated as a factor in cancers of the mouth, pharynx, larynx, esophagus, pancreas, kidney, stomach, colon, cervix, uterus, and bladder. When cigarettes are smoked, tar is inhaled, which contains approximately 4000 chemicals. Over 60 carcinogens have been isolated from cigarette smoke, including cyanide, formaldehyde, and ammonia. Nicotine is probably not a carcinogen, but it has other deleterious effects. It acts by stimulating the sympathetic nervous system, resulting in increased heart rate, increased peripheral vasoconstriction, increased BP, and increased cardiac workload. Nicotine also decreases the amount of functional hemoglobin and increases platelet aggregation. These effects of nicotine compound the problems in a person with coronary artery disease.

Cigarette smoke has several direct effects on the respiratory tract. The irritating effect of the smoke causes hyperplasia of cells, including goblet cells, which subsequently result in increased production of mucus. Hyperplasia reduces airway diameter and increases the difficulty in clearing secretions. Smoking reduces the ciliary activity and may cause actual loss of ciliated cells. Smoking also produces abnormal dilation of the distal air space with destruction of alveolar walls. Many cells develop large, atypical nuclei, which are considered a precancerous condition. After a short time of smoking, changes in small airway function can develop. In the early stages these changes are mostly inflammatory with mucosal edema and an influx of inflammatory cells. In later stages, however, thickening of the airway wall occurs by a remodeling process related to tissue repair and the inability of cilia to clear mucus, thus resulting in accumulation of inflammatory exudates in the airway lumen. Quitting smoking can prevent or delay the development of airflow limitation or reduce its progression.

Carbon monoxide (CO) is a component of tobacco smoke. CO has a high affinity for hemoglobin and combined with it more reality than does O_2, thereby reducing the smokers O_2-carrying capacity. The smoker inhales a lower percentage of O_2 than normal, resulting in less O_2 available at the alveolar level. The hearts need for O_2 is increased because of the stimulatory effect of nicotine on the sympathetic nervous system. Because the bloods O_2-carrying capacity is reduced, the heart must pump more rapidly to adequately supply tissues with O_2. CO also seems to impair psychomotor performance and judgment.

Passive smoking is the exposure of nonsmokers to cigarette smoke, also known as environmental tobacco smoke (ETS) or secondhand smoke. In adults, involuntary smoke exposure is associated with decreased pulmonary function, increased respiratory symptoms, and severe lower respiratory tract infections such as pneumonia. ETS also is associated with increased respiratory symptoms, and severe lower respiratory tract infections risk for lung cancer and nasal sinus cancer. The cardiovascular system is affected by ETS with increased heart rate and blood pressure and decreased levels of high-density lipoproteins (HDLs).

Occupational chemicals and dusts: If a person has intense or prolonged exposure to various dusts, vapors, irritants, or fumes in the workplace, COPD can develop independently of cigarette smoking. If the person smokes, the risk of COPD increases. Exposure to these irritants causes the airways to be hyper responsive.

Air pollution: High levels of urban air pollution are harmful to persons with existing lung disease. However, the effect of outdoor air pollution as a risk factor for COPD appears to be small compared to the effect of cigarette smoking. Another risk factor for COPD development is fossil fuels that are used for indoor heating and cooking. Many women, particularly because of cooking with these fuels in poorly ventilated areas.

Infection: Infections are a risk factor for developing COPD. Severe recurring respiratory tract infections in childhood have been associated with reduced lung function and increased respiratory symptoms in adulthood. Recurring infections impair normal defense mechanisms, making the bronchioles and alveoli more susceptible to injury. The person with COPD is prone to acute exacerbations of the disease, with 50% to 75% of cases thought to be caused by bacteria. These respiratory infections subsequently intensify the pathologic destruction of lung tissue and the progression of COPD. The most common causative organisms are *Haemophilus influenzae, Streptococcus pneumoniae,* and *Moraxella catarrhalis.*

Heredity: α1-Antitrypsin (AAT) deficiency is the genetic risk factor that leads to COPD. AAT deficiency, an autosomal recessive disorder, accounts for 1 to 2% of COPD cases. Also known as α1-protease inhibitor, AAT is a serum protein produced by the liver and normally found in the lungs. Severe AAT deficiency leads to premature bullous emphysema in the lungs found via radiologic testing. Normally AAT inhibits the lysis of lung tissues by proteolytic enzymes from neutrophils and macrophages. Emphysema occurs because of the AAT deficiency. Lower levels of AAT result in insufficient inactivation and subsequent destruction of lung tissue. Smoking greatly exacerbates the disease process in these patients.

The level of AAT is controlled by a pair of autosomal co-dominant genes. Low levels of AAT are related to homozygosity for the deficiency gene (ZZ), intermediate levels to heterozygosity (MZ), and normal values to homozygosity for the normal gene (MM). In the recessive gene homozygous group (ZZ), many individuals may have relatively normal lung function, especially those who never smoked. However, those with ZZ have the most severe disease. Clues to AAT deficiencies are the onset of symptoms often occurring by age 40, minimal to no tobacco use, and family history of emphysema. Chronic lever disease as an infant or adult with increased liver enzyme tests may also be seen. The people with this type of emphysema are primarily of northern European origin. A simple blood test can determine low levels of AAT. Those with borderline or low levels can then be genetically tested. IV administered AAT (Prolastin) augmentation therapy is approved for persons with AAT deficiency. The infusions are administered weekly. Its effectiveness in slowing the progression of the disease continues to be evaluated.

Aging: Some degree of emphysema is common in the lungs of the older person, even a nonsmoker. Aging results in changes in the lung structure, the thoracic cage, and the respiratory muscles. As people age there is gradual loss of the elastic recoil of the lung. The lungs become more rounded and smaller. The number of functional alveoli decreases as a result of the loss of the alveolar supporting structures and loss of the intraalveolar septum. These changes are similar to those seen in the patient with emphysema. Clinically significant emphysema, however, is usually not caused by aging alone. Thinner alveolar walls contribute to loss of alveolar septal tissue and alveolar capillaries. With fewer capillaries available for gas exchange, arterial O_2 (PaO_2) levels decrease from 80 mm Hg at 20 years of age to 65 to 70 mm Hg by 70 years of age.

Thoracic cage changes result from osteoporosis and calcification of the costal cartilages. The thoracic cage becomes stiff and rigid, and the ribs are less mobile. The shape of the rib cage gradually changes because of the increased residual volume (RV), causing it to expand and become rounded. Decreased chest compliance and elastic recoil of the lungs caused by aging affects the mechanical aspects of ventilation and increases the work of breathing. Changes in the elasticity of the lungs reduce the ventilatory reserve, and ability to clear secretions decreases with age.

Pathophysiology

COPD is characterized by chronic inflammation found in the airways, lung parenchyma (gas exchanging surfaces of the lungs [respiratory bronchioles and alveoli]), and pulmonary vasculature). The pathogenesis of COPD is complex and involves many mechanisms. However, the primary process is inflammation. The inflammatory process starts with inhalation of noxious particles and gases (e.g. cigarette smoke, air pollution). The predominant inflammatory cells, macrophages and lymphocytes (primarily CD8 cells), increase and release inflammatory mediators—including leukotrienes, interleukins and tumor necrosis factor. These mediators cause damage to the lung tissue. Later, neutrophils infiltrate into the lungs and release more inflammatory mediators. The airways become inflamed, resulting in increased numbers of enlarged goblet cells. This results in excess mucus production (or chronic bronchitis). Peripheral airways (small bronchi and bronchioles with internal diameter < 2 mm) undergo repeated cycles of injury and repair of the airway walls with resultant structural remodeling. Increased collagen and scar tissue formation in the walls cause fibrosis.

Destruction of the lung parenchyma in COPD patients results in emphysema with significant loss of attachments, which could be likened to rubber bands connecting airways and keeping the airways open. With loss of attachments ("rubber bands"), the peripheral airways collapse. One type of emphysema, called centrilobular, involves dilation and destruction of the respiratory bronchioles and is the most commonly seen in upper lobes in mild disease. The pathologic changes may occur throughout the lungs in severe disease and the pulmonary bed may also be destroyed. The second type of emphysema involves destruction of the alveolar ducts, alveolar sacs, and respiratory bronchioles and is called *panlobular*. It is most prominent in the lower lobes and is seen with α1-Antitrypsin deficiency. Destruction of the lung parenchyma is thought to be due to an imbalance of proteinases/antiproteinases. This occurs as a consequence of inflammation, but there can be a genetic basis to the proteinase imbalance. Individuals have elastin, which provides the structural makeup of the connection tissue of the alveolar wall. In a healthy person, proteinases (elastase is the main component) in the parenchyma function to break down the alveolar walls (elastin). Normally, proteinase inhibitors (called α1-antitrypsin [AAT]) prevent this destructive process. In smokers the numbers of neutrophils, macrophages, and other inflammatory cells are increased and with the inflammatory process overwhelm the body's normal AAT defense. Therefore there is destruction of the basic elastin structure of the parenchyma. In addition, inflammatory cells in COPD release a variety of inflammatory mediators such as leukotrienes and interleukins. In the genetic form of emphysema there is a deficiency of AAT, and an imbalance of proteinases/antiproteinases occurs. As the disease progresses, these microscopic lesions may progress to bullae in the lung parenchyma or blebs in the visceral pleura. These anatomic changes can be likened to a balloon that has been blown up too many times. Bullae and blebs are areas with greatly reduced diffusion of gases as the alveolar capillary bed is destroyed.

In COPD, as the supporting structures of the lung are destroyed, there is no pull or traction on the walls of the bronchioles. Like air being blown into a paper bag, air goes into the lungs easily but is unable to come out on its own; it remains in the lung. Thus the bronchioles tend to collapse (especially on expiration) and air is trapped in the distal alveoli. This trapped air in the lungs gives the patient the typical barrel-chested appearance. In COPD the lungs can be inflated easily but can only partially deflate.

Pulmonary vascular changes can begin early in the disease. Inflammatory cells infiltrate the smooth muscle of the blood vessels causing thickening as the disease advances. Because of the loss of alveolar walls and the capillaries surrounding them, the amount of surface area that is available for diffusion of O_2 decreases. The patient with COPD compensates for this problem by increasing the respiratory rate to increase alveolar ventilation. Typically, the patient does not have difficulty with hypoxemia at rest until late in the disease. However, hypoxemia may develop during exercise, and the patient may benefit from supplemental O_2. Air can move into the lungs, thus there is ventilation. However, because of the anatomic changes noted previously, perfusion of gases is affected, and thus there is a ventilation/perfusion imbalance. Hypercapnia and respiratory acidosis do not develop until late in the disease process. In severe cases, collagen deposition in the vessels along with emphysematous destruction of the capillary bed occurs, leading to pulmonary hypertension and cor pumonale; the prognosis is poor.

These changes in the lungs result in the following characteristic disease manifestations: mucus hypersecretion, dysfunction of the cilia, airflow limitation and hyperinflation of the lungs, gas exchange abnormalities, pulmonary hypertension, and cor pulmonale. Mucus hypersecretion and dysfunction of cilia lead to chronic cough and sputum production. Inability to expire air (largely irreversible) is the main smaller airways and is due to remodeling. Because of the loss of alveolar walls and attachments, the elastic recoil of the lung is decreased. Recoil is also affected by the influx of inflammatory cells and exudates in the bronchi together with hyperinflation of the lungs.

COPD has been shown to have systemic effects with inflammation (oxidative stress and inflammatory cells) and skeletal muscle wasting. Cigarette smoking begins the process of inflammation via oxidative stress, but inflammation appears to be sustained years after smoking ceases. This mechanism is being investigated. These effects limit the exercise abilities of the patient and worsen the prognosis.

Clinically it is common to find a combination of emphysema and chronic bronchitis in the same person, often with one condition predominating. Patients with COPD may also have asthma, and if they experience poorly reversible airflow limitation, the symptoms may be indistinguishable from COPD, but clinically are treated as asthma. Pathologically, the types of inflammatory cells are quite different between COPD and asthma.

Clinical Manifestations

Clinical manifestations of COPD typically develop slowly around 50 years of age after 20 pack years of cigarette smoking. A diagnosis of COPD should be considered in any patient who has symptoms of cough, sputum production, or dyspnea, and/or a history of exposure to risk factors for the disease. An intermittent cough, which is the earliest symptom, usually occurs in the morning with the expectation of small amounts of sticky mucus resulting from bouts of coughing. Patients usually seek medical help when they have an acute respiratory infection, with dyspnea being the main concern.

Dyspnea is often progressive, and usually occurs with exertion. However, patients may dismiss the importance of this symptom as they rationalize, "I'm just getting older". They change behaviors to avoid dyspnea, such as taking the elevator. Gradually the dyspnea interferes with daily activities, such as carrying grocery bags, and they cannot walk as fast as their spouse or peers.

In late stages of COPD, dyspnea may be present at rest. As more alveoli become over distended, increasing amounts of air are trapped. This causes a flattened diaphragm and an increased anterior-posterior diameter of the chest, forming the typical barrel chest. Effective abdominal breathing is decreased because of the flattened diaphragm from the over distended lungs. The person becomes more of a chest breather, relying on the intercostal and accessory muscles. However, chest breathing is not efficient breathing.

The language that patients use to describe the dyspnea may be a key to determining that the etiology is respiratory rather than other causes such as heart failure. Patients with dyspnea because of COPD (compared to heart failure) often say, "My breath does not go out all the way". They may also use words such as "heaviness", "gasping", and "increased effort to breathe" to describe the dyspnea.

The cough initially may be intermittent. Later it is present every day, but is seldom present during the night. There are ranges in the amount of sputum produced. It is difficult to quantify the amount of sputum produced because many people swallow it, particularly women. In some people the cough may be nonproductive.

Wheezing and chest tightness may be present, but may vary by time of the day or from day to day, especially in patients with more severe disease. The wheeze may arise from the laryngeal area, or wheezes may not be present on auscultation. Chest tightness, which often follows activity, may feel similar to muscular contraction.

During physical examination a prolonged expiratory phase of respiration, wheezes, or decreased breath sounds are noted in all lung fields. The patient may need to breathe louder than normal for auscultated breath sounds to be heard. The anterior-posterior diameter of the chest is increased ("barrel chest") from the chronic air trapping. The patient may sit upright with arms supported on a fixed surface such as an overbed table (*tripod position*). The patient may naturally purse lips on expiration (pursed-lip breathing) inspiration. Edema in the ankles may be the only clue to right-sided heart involvement.

Over time, hypoxemia (PaO_2 <60 mm Hg or O_2 saturation <88%) may develop with hypercapnia (PaO_2 >45 mm Hg) later in the disease. The bluish-red color of the skin results from polycythemia and cyanosis. Polycythemia develops as a result of increased production of red blood cells as the body attempts to compensate for chronic hypoxemia. Hemoglobin concentrations may reach 20 g/dl (200 g/L) or more. Cyanosis develops when there is at least 5 g/dL (50 g/L) or more of circulating unoxygenated hemoglobin.

As noted previously, it is sometimes quite difficult for the health care provider to distinguish COPD from asthma. However, there are some clinical features that are different.

Classification of COPD: COPD should be considered in any person with an exposure to risk factors such as cigarettes and/or environmental or occupational pollutants and/or chronic cough and dyspnea. The diagnosis is confirmed by spirometry. COPD can be classified as at risk, mild, moderate, severe, and very severe. The FEV1/FEV <70% establishes the diagnosis of COPD, and severity of obstruction (as indicated by FEV1) determines the stage of COPD. The management of COPD is primarily based on the patient's symptoms, but the staging provides a general guideline for the type of interventions.

Complications of COPD

Cor pulmonale: Cor pulmonale is hypertrophy of the right side of the heart, with or without heart failure, resulting from pulmonary hypertension. It is caused by diseases affecting the lungs or pulmonary blood vessels. Cor pulmonale is a late manifestation of chronic pulmonary heart disease. The patient benefits most when a diagnosis of pulmonary heart disease can be made early so therapy can be instituted. In patients with severe COPD, 40% demonstrate cor pulmonale, and the prognosis is poor. In COPD there may be an anatomic reduction of the pulmonary vascular bed as seen in emphysema with bullae. These patients would have increased pulmonary resistance.

Normally the right ventricle and pulmonary circulatory system are low pressure systems compared with the left ventricle and systemic circulation. When pulmonary hypertension develops, the pressures on the right side of the heart must increase to push blood into the lungs. Eventually, right-sided heart failure develops.

The clinical manifestations of chronic pulmonary heart disease and cor pulmonale are related to dilation and failure of the right ventricle with subsequent intravascular volume expansion and systemic venous congestion. Dyspnea is a usual symptom, and is associated with hypoxemia and hypercarbia. Lung sounds are normal or crackles may be heard in the bases of the lungs bilaterally. Heart sound changes include accentuation of the pulmonic component of the second heart sound, right-sided ventricular diastolic S3 gallop, and a loud pulmonic component of S2 along the left sternal border. ECG changes include increased P wave amplitude (P pulmonale), a tendency for right axis deviation, and incomplete right bundle branch block. Overt manifestations of right-sided heart failure may develop, which include distended neck veins (jugular venous distention), hepatomegaly with right upper quadrant tenderness, ascites, epigastric distress, peripheral edema, and weight gain.

Management of cor pulmonale includes continuous low-flow O_2. Long-term O_2 therapy improves survival of hypoxemic patients, especially when used >15 hours per day. Vasodilator therapy has not demonstrated sustained benefit and is not recommended on a routine basis. Although the use of digitalis is not indicated for right-sided heart failure, it may be used, but serum creatinine and blood urea nitrogen (BUN) are needed to monitor renal function as diuretics can cause volume depletion. Electrolytes must be monitored to assess for hypokalemia, which can predispose to dysrhythmias.

Exacerbations of COPD: Exacerbations of COPD are signaled by a change in the patients usual dyspnea, cough, and/or sputum that is different from the usual daily patterns. These flares require changes in management. Patients have an increase in dyspnea, sputum volume, and/or sputum purulence. They may also have nonspecific complaints of malaise, insomnia, fatigue, depression, confusion, decrease in exercise tolerance, increased wheezing, increased cough, or fever without other causes.

As the severity of COPD increases, exacerbations of COPD are associated with poorer outcomes. Exacerbations of COPD may be treated at home or in the hospital intermediate care unit or intensive care unit, depending on the severity. The primary causes of exacerbations of COPD are tracheobronchial infection and air pollution. Bacteria account for 33 to 75% of the cases of infection. The most common organisms causing exacerbations are *H. influenza, M. catarrhalils*, and *S. pneumoniae*. Other causes of COPD exacerbations include viruses.

Medications used to decrease airway resistance during exacerbations of COPD are bronchodilators and oral systemic corticosteroids. If a patient has clinical signs of airway infection (e.g. increased volume and change in color of sputum and/or fever, especially in the severe stages of COPD with more than three to four exacerbations per year), antibiotic treatment is usually used. Therapies used to treat exacerbations of COPD in the hospital are similar to home management, except supplemental oxygen therapy titrated by ABG measurement may be used. Attempts are made to use noninvasive mechanical methods (e.g., intubation). Teaching the patient and family early recognition of signs and symptoms of exacerbations is important to promote early treatment to prevent hospitalization and possible respiratory failure.

Acute Respiratory Failure: Patients with severe COPD who have exacerbations are at risk for the development of respiratory failure. Frequently, COPD patients wait too long to contact their health care provider when they develop fever, increased cough and dyspnea, or other symptoms suggestive of exacerbation of cor pulmonale may also lead to acute respiratory failure. Discontinuing bronchodilator or cortisoteroid medication may also precipitate respiratory failure. The use of β-adrenergic blockers (e.g., propranolol [Inderal]) may also exacerbate acute respiratory failure in the patient with a reversible component to the COPD. However, cardio selective β-adrenergic blockers (e.g. atenolol, metoprolol) should not be withheld from patients with mild to moderate diseases because they do not produce clinically significant problems with respiration.

The indiscriminate use of sedatives, benzodiazepines, and opioids, especially in the preoperative or postoperative patient who retains CO_2, may suppress the ventilatory drive and lead to respiratory failure. The person with COPD who retains CO_2 should be treated with low flow rates of O_2 with careful monitoring of ABGs to avoid hypercarbia to ensure that adequate oxygenation occurs, and to monitor for acidosis. It has been thought that high flow rates of O_2 depress the respiratory center and that the patients respirations will diminish or cease. However, it is vital to provide adequate oxygen while assessing the ABGs, rather than not providing O_2 because of the fear of CO_2 narcosis.

Surgery or severe, painful illness involving the chest or abdominal organs, may lead to splinting and ineffective ventilation and respiratory failure. To prevent postoperative pulmonary complications, careful preoperative screening, which includes pulmonary function tests and ABG assessment, is important in the patient with a heavy smoking history and/or COPD.

Peptic ulcer and gastroesophageal reflux disease: The incidence of peptic ulcer disease is increased in persons with COPD. The person for this occurrence is partly explained by hypersecretion of gastric acid resulting from increased arterial CO_2 and decreased arterial O_2 tension. This occurs only in patients who chronically retain CO_2. The ulcers are more commonly in the duodenum rather than stomach and do not cause pain. It is important to test gastric aspirates and feces for occult blood.

Gastroesophageal reflux disease (GERD), which may or may not be associated with a hiatal hernia, occurs frequently in patients with COPD and may aggravate respiratory symptoms. The reflux and accompanying heartburn may be aggravated or even precipitated by theophylline or β2-adrenergic agonists. However, patients with severe COPD and GERD have also been found to have asymptomatic GERD.

Depression/Anxiety: Patients with COPD experience, many losses as the disease progresses over time. They can feel helpless with low self-esteem and unable to vent their emotions for fear of compromising their breathing. The reported prevalence of depression in COPD varies, but may be four times more frequent in COPD than in the general population. Anxiety can complicate respiratory compromise and may precipitate dyspnea and hyperventilation. When a person is exceptionally dyspnic, particularly if it occurs suddenly, the person becomes anxious and tries to breathe faster, thus affecting his or her oxygenation status. Proper screening for anxiety and depression by health care providers is needed for a proper diagnosis.

After diagnosis, treatment consists of cognitive and behavioral psychotherapy and/or pharmacotherapy. Selective serotonin reuptake inhibitors (SSRIs) are often used for both depression and anxiety. Buspirone, which is one medication used to treat anxiety, has few if any respiratory depression effects. Benzodiazepines are avoided because they may depress the respiratory drive and may be habit forming. The nurse should explore the psychologic realm of the patient's disease and the impact it has on the patient's quality of life. Providing sufficient time for nursing interventions during an acute exacerbation is important to help reduce anxiety. When the patient becomes anxious because of dyspnea, the use of pursed-lip breathing and short-acting bronchodilators may be appropriate.

Diagnostic Studies

The diagnosis of COPD is confirmed by pulmonary function tests. Goals of the diagnostic workup are to confirm the diagnosis of COPD via spirometry, evaluate the severity of the disease, and determine the impact of the disease on the patient's quality of life. These factors enable the health care provider to design an individualized treatment plan. In addition to pulmonary function tests, other diagnostic studies are performed. Chest X-rays taken early in the disease are seldom diagnostic unless bullous disease is present. Patient may have significant airflow limitation as demonstrated by spirometry but not chronic cough. Most patients seek medical help because of dyspnea that starts affecting their daily activities. Later in the disease the findings presented in may be present.

A history and physical examination are extremely important in a diagnostic workup. Pulmonary function studies are useful in diagnosing and assessing the severity of COPD. Usually spirometry is ordered before and after bronchodilation. The most significant findings are related to increased resistance to expiratory airflow. Typical findings include the following:
- Reduced FEV1, FEF25%-75% FEV1/FVC ratio, diffusing capacity for carbon monoxide
- Increased residual volume, functional residual capacity (FRC)

When the FEV1/FVC ratio is less than 70%, it suggests the presence of obstructive lung disease. The value of FEV1 in milliliters can provide a guideline to determine the severity of the patients lung disease and the degree of disease progression.

The body mass index (BMI) and degree of dyspnea are useful in predicting outcomes, such as survival. Current practice guidelines recommend that the BMI and dyspnea be evaluated in all patients. BMI is obtained by dividing weight (in kilograms [kg]) by height (in square meter [m^2]). A BMI below 21 kg/m^2 is associated with an increase in mortality rate. Functional dyspnea can be assessed with the Medical Research Council Dyspnea Scale from level 0 (no trouble with breathlessness except with strenuous exercise) to level 4 (too breathless to leave the house or breathless when dressing or undressing).

ABGs are usually assessed in the sever stages and monitored in patients hospitalized with acute exacerbations. In the later stages of COPD, typical findings are low PaO_2, elevated PaO_2, decreased or low-normal pH, and increased bicarbonate (HCO_3) levels. In the early stages there may be normal or only slightly decreased PaO_2 and a normal PaO_2. A 6-minute walk to determine O_2 desaturation that occurs with exercise. An ECG may be normal or show signs indicative of right ventricular failure (e.g., low voltage, right-axis deviation, cor pulmonale). An echocardiogram or gated pool nuclear blood study can be used to evaluate right-sided ventricular and left ventricular function. Sputum for culture and sensitivity may be obtained, if the patient is hospitalized for an acute exacerbation and has not responded to empiric therapy with antibiotics.

MANAGEMENT OF COPD

The primary goals of care for the COPD patient are to (1) prevent disease progression, (2) reliever symptoms and improve exercise tolerance, (3) prevent and treat complications, (4) promote patient participation in care, (5) prevent and treat exacerbations, and (6) improve quality of life and reduce mortality risk. The majority of patients are treated as outpatients. They are hospitalized for exacerbations of COPD and potential complications when respiratory failure, pneumonia, and failure and/or cor pulmonale are also present. Environmental or occupational irritants should be evaluated for their possible negative effect, and ways to control or avoid them should be determined. For example, aerosol hair sprays and smoke-filled rooms should be avoided. The patient with COPD is extremely susceptible to pulmonary infections. The patient with COPD should have a vaccination with influenza virus vaccine yearly and with pneumococcal vaccine. Pneumucoccal revaccination is recommended once if the patient is ≥ 65 years of age, the vaccination was ≥ 5 years previously, and the patient was <65 years of age at the time of the primary vaccination.

Exacerbations of COPD should be treated as soon as possible especially if the patient is in the severe stages of COPD. Often the best indication of the presence of a bacterial infection is the increasing quantity, viscosity, or purulence of sputum. Some patients are given a prescription for 7 days to 10 days supply of antibiotics and are instructed to begin taking them at the first signs of change in sputum. The most common antibiotics given for outpatients are macrolides (e.g., azithromycin [Zithromax]), doxycycline and newer cephalosporins (e.g., cefpodoxime [Vatnin]). Amoxicillin may be used, but patterns of antibiotic resistance are limiting its use. If the patient has failed prior antibiotic therapy or is hospitalized, common antibiotics are amoxicillin/clavulanate (Agumentin), or respiratory fluoroquinolones (e.g. levofloxacin [Levaquin]).

Smoking Cessation

Cessation of cigarette smoking in all stages of COPD is the single most effective and cost-effective intervention to reduce the risk of developing COPD and stop the progression of the disease. After discontinuation of smoking, the accelerated decline in pulmonary function slows and pulmonary function usually improves. Normally individuals after age 35 lose approximately 20 to 25 ml (as measured by FEV1) of lung function per year as measured by spirometry. Persons with COPD who continue to smoke lose approximately 50 ml per year. With the cessation of smoking, the loss can fall to almost nonsmoking levels at 35 ml per year. Thus the sooner the smoker stops, the less pulmonary function is lost and the sooner the symptoms decrease, especially cough and sputum production.

Drug Therapy

Medications for COPD can reduce or abolish symptoms, increase the capacity to exercise, improve overall health, and reduce the number and severity of exacerbations. Presently no drug modifies the decline of lung function with COPD. Bronchodilator drug therapy relaxes smooth muscles in the airway and improves the ventilation of the lungs, thus reducing the degree of breathlessness. Although patients with COPD do not respond as dramatically as those with asthma to bronchodilator therapy, a reduction in dyspnea and an increase in FEV1 are usually achieved. The inhaled route of medication is preferred and given on a pm or regular basis. Medications are given in a stepwise fashion.

Bronchodilator medications commonly used are β2-adrenergic agonists, anticholinergic agents, and methylxanthines. The choice of bronchodilator depends on the availability and the patient's response. However, when the patient has mild COPD or intermittent symptoms, a short-acting bronchodilator is used as needed. Short-acting bronchodilators increase exercise tolerance. Albuterol or ipratropium (Atrovent) may be used as single agents, but combining bronchodilators improves their effect and decreases the risk of adverse effects, compared with the use of a single agent. As a single agent, ipratropium (Atrovent) is superior to albuterol because the only side effect is usually dry mouth.

These two agents can be nebulized together (DuoNeb) or delivered by one MDI (Combivent).

As symptoms persist or moderate stages of COPD develop, a long-acting bronchodilator is used in addition to a short-acting bronchodilator. Salmeterol (Serevent) is a widely used long-acting β-2-adrenergic agonist, and unlike in drug therapy for asthma, it can be used in COPD as monotherapy. Formoterol (Foradil) is another long-acting β2-agonist.

Titropium (Spiriva), a long-acting anticholinergic, can be used for daily therapy of bronchosapsm, and dyspnea in COPD. Tiotropium also improves bronchodilation, results in less dyspnea, improves quality of life, and deceases the number of COPD exacerbations when compared with ipratropium (Atrovent). Tiotropium is the first inhaled drug for COPD to be dosed once a day.

The use of long-acting theophyline in the treatment of COPD is controversial because it interacts with many drugs. Although it has some action as a mild bronchodilator in the patient with partial reversibility of airflow obstruction, its main value may be to improve contractility of the diaphragm and decrease diaphragramatic fatigue.

Inhaled corticosteroid therapy may be beneficial for patients with moderate-to-severe COPD. However, inhaled corticosteroids (ICS) do not appear to help patients with mild COPD. ICS combined with long-acting β2-adrenergic agonists (e.g., fluticasone/salmeterol [Advair]) are more effective than the single drug therapy. Oral corticosteroids should not be used for long-term therapy in COPD.

O_2 Therapy

O_2 therapy is frequently used in the treatment of COPD and other problems associated with hypoxemia. Long-term O_2 therapy (LTOT) improves survival, exercise capacity, cognitive performance, and sleep in hypoxemic patients. O_2 is a colorless, odorless, tasteless gas that constitutes 20.95% of the atmosphere. Administering supplemental O_2 raises the partial pressure of O_2 (PO_2) in inspired air. Used clinically it is considered a drug. For reimbursement purposes, it is considered durable medical equipment, which Medicare covers when certain clinical criteria are met (i.e., the patients O_2 saturation needs to be $\leq 88\%$, $PaO_2 \geq 55$ mm Hg).

Indications for Use: Goals for O_2 therapy are to reduce the work of breathing, maintain the PaO_2, and/or reduce the workload on the heart, keeping the $SaO_2 > 90\%$ during rest, sleep and exertion, or $PaO_2 > 60$ mm Hg. O_2 is usually administered to treat hypoxemia caused by (1) respiratory disorders such as COPD, pulmonary hypertension, cor pulmonale, pneumonia, atelectasis, lung cancer, and pulmonary emboli; (2) cardiovascular disorders such as myocardial infarction, dysrhythmias, angina pectoris, and cardiogenic shock; and (3) central nervous system disorders such as overdose of opioids, head injury, and disordered sleep (sleep apnea).

Methods of administration: The goal of O_2 administration is to supply the patient with adequate O_2 to maximize the O_2-carrying ability of the blood. There are various methods of O_2 administration. The method selected depends on factors such as the fraction of inspired O_2 (FIO_2) required by the patient and delivered by the device, the mobility of the patient, humidification required, patient cooperation, comfort, cost, and available financial resources.

O_2 delivery systems are classified as low- or high-flow systems. Most methods of O_2 administration are low-flow devices that deliver O_2 in concentrations that vary with the person's respiratory pattern. In contrast, the Venturi mask is a high-flow device that delivers fixed concentrations of O_2 independent of the patient's respiratory pattern. With the Venturi mask, O_2 is delivered to a small jet (Venturi device) in the center of a wide-based cone. Air is entrained (pulled through) openings in the cone as O_2 flows through the small jet. The mask has large vents through which exhaled air can escape. The degree of restriction or narrowness of the jet determines the amount of entrainment and dilution of pure O_2 with room air, and thus the concentration of O_2 delivered can be precise. Mechanical ventilators are another example of a high-flow O_2 delivery system. Because room air is mixed with O_2, in low-flow systems, the percentage of O_2 delivered to the patient is not as precise as with high-flow systems.

Humidification and nebulizers: O_2 obtained from cylinders or wall systems is dry. Dry O_2 has an irritating effect on mucous membranes and dries secretions. Therefore it is important that O_2 be humidified when administered, wither by humidification or nebulization. A common device used for humidification when the patient has a catheter, cannula, or low-flow mask is a bubble through humidifier. It is a small jar filled with sterile distilled water that is attached to O_2 source by means of a flow meter. O_2 passes into the jar, bubbles through the water, and then goes through tubing to the patient's catheter, cannula, or mask. The purpose of the bubble-through humidifier is to restore the humidity conditions of room air. However, the need for bubble-through humidifiers at flow rates between 1 and 4L per minute is dependent on patient preference.

Another means of administering humidified O_2 is via a nebulizer. It delivers particulate water mist (aerosols) with nearly 100% humidity. The humidity can be raised by heating the water, which increases the ability of the gas to hold moisture. Heated (98.6F [37°C]) and humidified (100%) gas is required when the upper airway is bypassed in acute care. however, patients with established tracheotomies do not always require 100% humidity. When nebulizers are used, large-size tubing should be employed to connect the device to a facemask or T bar. If small-size tubing is used, condensation can occlude the flow of O_2. Vapotherm can deliver high flows (15 to 20 L/min) of warm humidified air (either sterile air or O_2) to the patient through a nasal cannula or transtracheal cannula using technology to warm and saturate the gas stream.

Complications

Combustion: O_2 supports combustion and increases the rate of burning. This is why it is important that smoking be prohibited in the area in which O_2 is being used. A "No Smoking" sign should be prominently displayed on the patient's door. The patient should also be cautioned against smoking cigarettes with O_2 cannula in place.

CO_2 Narcosis: The two chemoreceptors in the respiratory center that control the drive to breathe respond to CO_2 and O_2. Normally, CO_2 accumulation is the major stimulant of the respiratory center. Over time some COPD patients develop a tolerance for high CO_2 levels (the respiratory center loses its sensitivity to the elevated CO_2 levels). Theoretically, for these individuals the "O_2 drive" to breathe is hypoxemia. Thus there has been concern regarding the dangers of administering O_2 to COPD patients and reducing their drive to breathe. This has been a pervasive myth but is not a serious threat. In fact, not providing adequate O_2 to these patients is much more detrimental. Although O_2 administration should be titrated to the lowest effective dose, many patients who have end-stage COPD require high flow rates and higher concentrations for survival. They may, in fact, exhibit higher than normal levels of CO_2 in their blood, but this is of little concern. What is important is careful, ongoing assessment when providing O_2 to these patients, monitoring both physical and cognitive effects of O_2.

It is critical to start O_2 at low flow rates until ABGs can be obtained. ABGs are used as a guide to determine what FIO_2 level is sufficient and can be tolerated. The patients mental status and vital signs should be assessed before starting O_2 therapy and frequently thereafter.

O_2 Toxicity: Pulmonary O_2 Toxicity may result from prolonged exposure to a high level of O_2 (PaO_2). The development of O_2 toxicity is relatively rare, but is determined by patient tolerance, exposure time, and effective dose. High concentrations of O_2 damage alveolar-capillary membranes inactivate pulmonary surfactant, cause interstitial and alveolar edema, and decrease compliance. These individuals develop acute respiratory distress syndrome (ARDS). Prevention of O_2 toxicity is important for the patient who is receiving O_2. The amount of O_2 administered should be just enough to maintain the PaO_2 within a normal or acceptable range for the patient. ABGs should be monitored frequently to evaluate the effectiveness of therapy and to guide the tapering of supplemental O_2. A safe limit of O_2 concentrations has not yet been established. All levels above 50% and used for longer than 24 hours should be considered potentially toxic. Levels of 40% and below may be regarded as relatively nontoxic and may not result in development of significant O_2 toxicity if the exposure period is short.

Absorption atelectasis: Normally, nitrogen, which constitutes 79% of the air that is breathed, is not absorbed into the bloodstream. This prevents alveolar collapse. When high concentrations of O_2 are given, nitrogen is washed out of the alveoli and replaced with O_2. If airway obstruction occurs, the O_2 is absorbed into the bloodstream and the alveoli collapse. This process is called absorption atelectasis.

Infection: Infection can be a major hazard of O_2 administration. Head nebulizers present the highest risk. The constant use of humidity supports bacterial growth, with the common infecting organism being *Pseudomonas aeruginosa*. Disposable equipment that operates as a closed system should be used. There should be a hospital policy stating the required frequency of equipment changes based on the type of equipment used at that particular institution.

Chronic O_2 Therapy at Home: Improved survival occurs in patients with COPD who receive long-term O_2 therapy (LTOT) (> 15 hours/day) to treat hypoxemia. The improved prognosis results from preventing progression of the disease and subsequent cor pulmonale. The benefits of long-term O_2 therapy include improved mental acuity, lung mechanics, sleep, and exercise tolerance; decreased hematocrit; and reduced pulmonary hypertension. Some patients believe they will become "addicted" to O_2 and are very reluctant to use it. They need to be educated that it is not "addicting" and that it needs to be used for the prescribed times during the day because of the positive effects on the heart, lungs, and brain. The need for LTOT should be evaluated when the patient's condition has stabilized. The goal of O_2 therapy is to maintain SaO_2 > 90% during rest, sleep and exertion.

Short-term home O_2 therapy (1 to 30 days) may be indicated for the patient in whom hypoxemia persists after discharge from the hospital. For example, the patient with underlying COPD who develops a serious respiratory infection may continue to have clearing of the infection after completion of antibiotic therapy and discharge from the hospital. This patient may demonstrate continued hypoxemia for 4 to 6 weeks after discharge. It is important to measure the patient's oxygenation status by ABGs 30 to 90 days after an acute episode to determine if the O_2 is still warranted.

Patients whose disease is stable with a PaO_2 of 55 mm Hg or less (Corresponding to an SaO_2 of 88% or less) should receive LTOT. A patient whose PaO_2 is between 55 and 60 mm Hg (SaO_2 89% and who exhibits signs of tissue hypoxia, such as cor pulmonale, erythorcytosis, peripheral edema from right-sided heart failure, or impaired mental status, should also receive LTOT. Desaturation only during exercise or sleep suggests consideration of O_2 therapy specifically under those conditions. Patients may receive O_2 only during exercise and/or sleep. The need for O_2 during these periods should be evaluated with a 6-minute walk test or overnight oximetry. Sleep disordered breathing may be seen in some of these patients, and they will require a full sleep study.

Periodic reevaluations are necessary for the patient who is using chronic supplemental O_2. Generally the recommendation is that the patient should be reevaluated every 30 to 90 days during the first year of therapy and annually after that, as long as the patient remains stable.

Nasal cannulas, either regular or the O_2-conserving type, are usually used to deliver O_2 from a central source in the home. The source may be a liver O_2 from a central source in the home. The source may be a liquid O_2 storage system, compressed O_2 in tanks, or an O_2 concentrator or extractor, depending on the patients home environment, insurance coverage, activity level, and proximity to an O_2 supply company. The patient can use extension tubing without adversely affecting the O_2 flow delivery to increase mobility in the home. Small, portable systems, such as liquid O_2 may be provided for the patient who remains active outside the home.

Home O_2 systems are usually rented from a company that sends a respiratory therapist to the patient's home. The therapist teaches the patient and family how to use the O_2 system, how to care for it, and how to recognize when the supply is running low and needs to be recorded. A patient and family teaching guide for the use of O_2 at home is presented.

The patient who uses home O_2 should be encouraged to remain active and to travel normally. If travel is by automobile, arrangement can be made for O_2 to be available at the destination point. O_2 supply companies can often assist in these arrangements. If a patient wishes to travel by bus, train, or airplane, the patient should inform the appropriate people when reservations are made that O_2 will be needed for travel. If there is a potential for the patient to become hypoxic, oxygen needs for flying can be determined via a hypoxia inhalation test or through a mathematical formula. Patients on LTOT should be instructed to increase the O_2 flow by 1 to 2 L/min during the flight. Those with resting PaO_2 of 70 mm Hg are likely to be safe to fly without O_2. However, they may become hypoxemic as PaO_2 may fall an average of 25 mm Hg. If patients have other comorbidities, such as certain cardiac disease or anemia, they may also become hypoxemic. Patients should be warned that walking along the aisles on an airplane cabins are pressurized to an elevation of 7000 or 8000 feet, the patient who uses supplemental O_2 should have it provided during flight. The airline's O_2 system must be used. Patients may not use their own O_2 system during flight because it is not properly pressurized. Airlines allow patients to bring their O_2 system to be carried in the reservoirs (liquid or tank) must be empty and the valves left open. Some patients may need to avoid prolonged exposure to high elevations during travel unless they are instructed by their health care provider regarding adjustments in their O_2 flow to attempt to compensate for attitude.

Surgical therapy for COPD: Three different surgical procedures have been used in sever COPD. One type of surgery is lung volume reduction therapy (LVRS). The goal of therapy is to reduce the size of the lungs by removing about 30% of the most diseased lung tissue so the remaining healthy lung tissue can perform better. The rationale for this type of surgery is that by reducing the size of the hyperinflated emphysematous lungs, there is decreased airway obstruction and increased room for the remaining normal alveoli to expand and function. The procedure reduces lung volume and improves lung and chest wall mechanics. There are different types of LVRS. In one approach a median sternotomy is performed and parts of each lung are removed and tissue reattached using a stapling device. Another approach is a video-assisted thoracoscopy that can be performed unilaterally or bilaterally. In this approach either a stapling or laser procedure can be done, or they can be done together. The most common postoperative complication is pneumonia. Another technique for LVRS is a minimally invasive technique via a bronchoscope. In certain patients LVRS has been shown to improve breathing, lung capacity, and quality of life. However, it does not cure COPD. It is best used for patients with upper lobe emphysema. However, hospital costs of LVRS are high and it is still considered experimental.

The second surgical procedure is bullectomy. This procedure is used for patients with emphysematous COPD who have large bullae (>1 cm). The bullae are usually resected via thoracoscope. In certain patients this procedure has resulted in improved lung function and reduction in dyspnea.

The third surgical procedure is lung transplantation. COPD patients are the largest group of patient on waiting lists for lung transplantation. Although single-lung transplant is the most commonly used technique because of a shortage of donors, bilateral transplantation can be performed. In some cases LVRS is a bridge until transplantation. In appropriately selected patients with very advanced COPD, lung transplantation improves functional capacity and enhances quality of life. However, rejection and effects of immunosuppressive therapy remains an obstacle.

Respiratory and physical therapy: Respiratory therapy (RT) and physical therapy (PT) rehabilitation activities are performed by respiratory therapists or physical therapists depending on the institution. RT and/or PT activities include breathing retraining, effective cough techniques, and chest physiotherapy. RT is responsible for aerosol-nebulization therapy.

Breathing Retraining: The patient with COPD develops an increased respiratory rate with a prolonged expiration to compensate for the obstruction to airflow resulting in dyspnea. In addition, the accessory muscles of breathing in the neck and upper part of the chest are used excessively to promote chest wall movement. These muscles are not designed for long-term use, and as a result the patient experiences increased fatigue. Breathing exercises may assist the patient during rest and activity (e.g., lifting, walking, stair climbing) by decreasing dyspnea, improving oxygenation, and slowing the respiratory rate. The main types of breathing exercises commonly taught are (1) pursed-lip breathing and (2) diaphragmatic breathing.

The proposed rationale for using pursed-lip breathing (PLB) is to prolong exhalation and thereby prevent bronchiolar collapse and air trapping. Often instinctively patients will perform this technique. The patient should be taught PLB before, during, and after any causing dyspnea or tachypnea. The patient is taught to inhale slowly through the nose and then to exhale slowly through pursed lips, almost as if whistling. Exhalation should be at least three times as long as inhalation. It is helpful to have the nurse demonstrate the breathing exercises so the patient can imitate the action. The following techniques can be used to teach PLB:

- Blow through a straw in a glass of water with the intent of forming small bubbles.
- Blow at a lit candle enough to bend the flame without blowing it out.
- Steadily blow a table-tennis ball across a table.
- Blow a tissue held in the hand until it gently flaps

Patients should be taught to use "just enough" positive pressure with the pursed lips because excessive resistance may increase the work of breathing. The issue of whether and how extensively PLB affects dyspnea is still questioned, but current evidence seems to support the use of PLB to improve the breathing of patients with COPD.

Diaphragmic (abdominal) breathing focuses on using the diaphragm instead of the accessory muscles of the chest to (1) achieve maximum inhalation and (2) slow the respiratory rate. To date, evidence from controlled studies does not support the use of diaphragmic breathing in patients with COPD patients. For patients with severe COPD, diaphragmatic breathing may result in hyperinflation because of increased fatigue and dyspnea and abdominal paradoxic breathing (the inward movement of the abdomen and the outward movement of the upper chest during inspiration) rather than with normal chest wall motion (the outward movement of the abdomen and upper chest simultaneously during inspiration).

PLB slows the respiratory rate and is much easier to learn than diaphragmatic breathing. In the setting of extreme acute dyspnea when the patient is hospitalized for infection or heart failure, it is more important to focus on helping the patient slow the respiratory rate by using the principles of PLB.

PLB is simple and easy to teach and learn. PLB should be practiced for 8 to 10 repetitions three or four times a day. PLB gives the patient more control over breathing, especially during exercise and periods of dyspnea.

Effective coughing: Many patients with COPD have developed ineffective coughing patterns that do not adequately clear their airways of sputum. In addition, they fear they may develop spastic coughing, resulting in increased dyspnea. Huff coughing is an effective technique that the patient can be easily taught. The main goals of effective coughing are to conserve energy, reduce fatigue, and facilitate removal of secretions.

Chest physiotherapy: Chest physiotherapy (CPT) is indicated in the patient with (1) excessive bronchial secretions who has difficulty clearing secretions with expectorated sputum production greater than 25 ml per day, (2) evidence or suggestion of retained secretions in the presence of an artificial airway, or (3) lobar atelectasis caused by or suspected of being caused by mucous plugging.

Chest physiotherapy consists of percussion, vibration, and postural drainage. Percussion and vibration are manual or mechanical techniques used to augment postural drainage. Postural drainage uses the principle of gravity to assist in bronchial drainage. Percussion and vibration are used after the patient has assumed a postural drainage position to assist in loosening the mobilized secretions. Percussion, vibration, and postural drainage may assist in bringing secretions into larger, more central airways. Effective coughing is then necessary to help raise these secretions. After each drainage position change, the patient should be given time to cough and deep breathe. These techniques are individualized based on the patient's pulmonary condition and response to the initial treatment. Sometimes it takes several hours after CPT for secretions to be expectorated. It is important to evaluate CPT for both its effectiveness and relief of the patient's symptoms. CPT should be performed by an individual who has been properly trained. Complications associated with improperly performed CPT include fractured ribs, bruising, hypoxemia, and discomfort to the patient. CPT may not be beneficial and may be stressful for some patients. Some patients may develop hypoxemia and bronchospasms with CPT.

Percussion: Percussion is performed in the appropriate postural drainage with the hands in a cuplike position. The hands are cupped, and the fingers and thumbs are closed. The cupped hand should create an air pocket between the patient's chest and the hand. Both hands are cupped and used in an alternating rhythmic fashion. Percussion is accomplished with flexion and extension of the wrists. If it is performed correctly, a hollow sound should be heard. The air-cushion impact facilitates the movement of thick mucus. A thin towel should be placed over the area to be percussed, or the patient may choose to wear a T-shirt or hospital gown. The patients face should be in clear view when percussing. In case a mucous plug occludes the airway and the patient is unable to speak. Percussion should not be performed over the kidneys, sternum, spinal cord, bony prominences, or may tender or painful area. Other contraindications to percussion include hemoptysis, carcinoma, and induced bronchospasm. Commercial devices that percuss are available if the patient lives alone and has no one to help with the therapy.

Vibration: Vibration is accomplished by tensing the hand and arm muscles repeatedly and pressing mildly with the flat of the hand on the affected area while the patient slowly exhales a deep breath. Isometric contractions of the arms and hands are also appropriate. The vibrations facilitate movement of secretions to larger airways. Mild vibration is tolerated better than percussion and can be used in situations where percussion may be contraindicated. Commercial vibrators are available for hospital and home use.

Postural drainage: The lungs are divided into five lobes, with three on the right side and two on the left side. There are 18 segments in the lungs, which can be drained by 18 positions shows the modified postural drainage positions most often used in clinical practice. The purpose of various positions in postural drainage is to drain each segment toward the larger airways. The postural drainage positions are determined by the areas of involved lung, which are assessed by chest X-rays, percussion, palpation, and auscultation. Aerosolized bronchodilators and hydration therapy are frequently administered before postural drainage. The chosen postural drainage position is maintained for 5 to 15 minutes or during percussion/vibration. The degree of slope can be obtained with pillows, blocks, books, or a tilt board.

The frequency and choice of postural drainage, positions depend on the location of retained secretions and patient tolerance to dependent positions. A common order is two to four times a day. In acute situations, postural drainage may be performed as frequently as every 1 to 2 hours. The procedure should be planned to occur and be completed at least 1 hour before meals or 3 hours after meals.

If a patient has difficulty in assuming various positions, adaptations will be needed to reduce the angle or length of time of the procedure. A side-lying position can be used for the patient who cannot tolerate a head down position. There are also beds on the market that can rotate and percuss in various postural drainage positions. Some positions for postural drainage (e.g., Trendelenburg) should not be performed on the patient with trauma, hemoptysis, heart disease, or head injury, and in other situations where the patient's condition is not stable.

Flutter Mucus Clearance Device

The Flutter mucus clearance device is a handheld device that is shaped like a small, fat pipe. It provides expiratory pressure (PEP) treatment for patients with mucus-producing conditions. The Flutter has a mouthpiece, a high-density stainless steel ball, and a cone that holds the ball. When the patient exhales through the Flutter, the steel ball moves, which causes vibrations in the lungs and loosens mucus. It helps move mucus up through the airways to the mouth where the mucous can be expectorated. Although the Flutter valve is mostly used in patients with cystic fibrosis, it has been effectively used in patients with excessive secretions with COPD and bronchiectasis.

High-Frequency Chest Compression (ThAIRapy Vest)

High-frequency chest compression uses an inflatable vest (ThAIRapy vest) with hoses connected to a high-frequency pulse generator. The pulse generator delivers air to the vest, which vibrates the chest. The high-frequency air waves clear all lobes of the lungs. The vest has been found to be more effective than conventional CPT in clearing mucus, and it can be done without the aid of another person. The unit weighs only 30 lb and is quiet. It comes in its own suitcase and is portable.

Acapella

Acapella is a small handheld device that combines the benefits of both PEP therapy and airway vibrations of the Flutter valve to mobilize pulmonary secretions. It works by using oscillating vibrations that travel to the lung, shaking free mucous plugs that the patient can then cough up. It can be used in virtually any setting, as the patients are free to sit, stand, or recline. It improves clearance of secretions, is easier to tolerate than CPT, takes less than half the time of conventional CPT sessions, and facilitates opening of airways.

Aerosol Nebulization Therapy

Medications for COPD patients are most often delivered via metered-dose or dry powder inhalers. This is the preferred delivery route, although devices that deliver a suspension of fine particles of liquid in a gas, called nebulizers, may also be used to deliver medications to the COPD patient. Nebulizers are usually powered by a compressed air or O_2 generator. At home the patient may have an air-powered compressor, in the hospital, wall O_2 or compressed air is used to power the nebulizer.

Aerosolized medication orders must include the medication, dose, diluent, and whether it is to be nebulized with O_2 or compressed air. Medication is nebulized or reduced to a fine spray, and depending on several factors, including droplet size, it can be inhaled into the patients tracheobronchial tree. The advantage to aerosol-nebulization therapy is that it is easy to use. Medications that are routinely nebulized include albuterol and ipratropium.

The patient is placed in an upright position that allows for most efficient breathing to ensure adequate penetration and deposition of the aerosolized medication. The patient must breathe slowly and deeply through the mouth and hold inspiration for 2 to 3 seconds. Deep diaphragmatic breathing helps ensure deposition of the medication. The patient is instructed to do normal breathing in between these large forced breaths to prevent alveolar hypoventilation and dizziness. After the treatment the patient should be instructed to cough effectively. Postural drainage and CPT are ideally done after bronchodilator medications are given.

A disadvantage of nebulizer equipment use is the potential for bacterial growth. Because home nebulization is used for the patient with COPD, it is important for the health care professional in the hospital and home care setting to review cleaning procedures for home respiratory equipment with the patient. A frequently used, effective home-cleaning method is to wash the nebulizer daily in soap and water, rinse it with water, and soak it for 20 to 30 minutes in a 1:1 white vinegar-water solution followed by a water rinse and air drying. Commercial respiratory cleaning agents may also be used if directions are followed carefully. Cleaning the nebulizer in the top shelf of an automatic dishwater saves time, and the hot water destroys most organisms.

Nutritional Therapy

Weight loss and malnutrition are commonly seen in the patient with severe emphysematous COPD. The cause of this weight loss is not entirely known but is likely multifactorial. Eating becomes an effort because of dyspnea and O_2 desaturation, especially in the later stages COPD. Patients may require more caloric expenditure than calories ingested. A full stomach presses up on the flattened diaphragm, causing increased dyspnea and discomfort. It is difficult for some patient to eat and breathe at the same time; therefore inadequate amounts of food are eaten. Also large amounts of energy are expended to breathe and maintain even normal activities. Therefore weight loss and muscle wasting are likely. Excessive weight loss is also related to increased energy inflammatory processes occurring in the lung, which may lead to a cachectic state.

The patient with COPD should try to keep body mass index (BMI) between 21 and 25 kg/m^2. Being either overweight or underweight can be problem with COPD. However, a reduced BMI or weight loss is associated with poor outcomes in acute exacerbations and increased morbidity and mortality rates in COPD patients.

To decrease dyspnea and conserve energy, the patient should rest for at least 30 minutes before eating, use a bronchodilator before meals, and select eat five to six small, frequent meals to avoid feelings of bloating and early satiety when eating. Liquid, blenderized, or commercial diets may be helpful. Foods that require a great deal of chewing should be avoided or served in another manner (e.g., grated, pureed). Cold foods may give less of a sense of fullness than hot foods. Exercises and treatments should be avoided for at least 1 hour before and after eating. The exertion involved in the preparation and eating of food is often fatiguing. The use of frozen foods and a microwave oven may help conserve the patient's energy in food preparation. The patients dentition should be assessed because broken, missing teeth or loose dentures make eating more difficult. Activity such as walking or getting out of bed during the day can stimulate the appetite and promote weight gain. Many patients with COPD have feelings of bloating and early satiety when eating. This sensation can be attributed to swallowing air while eating, side effects of medication (especially corticosteroids and theophylline), and the abnormal position of the diaphragm relative to the stomach in association with hyperinflation. Intestinal gas–forming foods should be avoided, such as cabbage, Brussels sprouts, and beans.

Underweight patients with emphysematous COPD have a greater than normal nutritional requirement for protein and calories. They may need 25 to 45 kcal/kg and 1.2 to 1.9 g of protein per kilogram diet is recommended and can be divided into five or six small meals a day. High-protein, high-calorie nutritional supplements can be offered between meals. Ice cream added to these supplements can help increase calories. Drinking skim or 1% milk rather than whole milk may cause less mucus production. Nonprotein calories should be divided evenly between fat and carbohydrate while not overfeeding the patient. In most cases just getting the patients to eat adequate amounts of any foods can be difficult. The oral anabolic steroid, oxandrolone (Oxandrin), has shown promise in helping patients gain weight and improve muscle strength. Megestrol (Megace) has also been used to stimulate and increase appetite. If the patient has O_2 prescribed, use of supplemental O_2 by nasal cannulas while eating may also be beneficial, because eating expends energy. Fluid intake should be at least 3 L per day unless contraindicated for other medical conditions, such as heart or renal failure. Fluids should be taken between meals (rather than with them) to prevent excess stomach distension and to decrease pressure on the diaphragm. Sodium restriction may be indicated if there is accompanying heart failure.

Nursing Diagnoses

Nursing diagnoses for the patient with CF include, but are not limited to, the following:
- Ineffective airway clearance related to abundant, thick bronchial mucus, weakness, and fatigue
- Ineffective breathing pattern related to bronchoconstriction, anxiety, and airway obstruction
- Impaired gas exchange related to recurring lung infections
- Imbalanced nutrition: less than body requirements related to dietary intolerances, intestinal gas, and altered pancreatic enzyme production

Planning

The overall goals are that the patient with CF will have:
- Adequate airway clearance
- Reduced risk factors associated with respiratory infections
- Adequate nutritional support to maintain appropriate BMI
- Ability to perform ADLs
- No complications related to CF
- Active participation in planning and implementing a therapeutic regimen

Nursing Implementation

The nurse and other health professionals can assist young adults to gain independence by helping them assume responsibility for their care and for their vocational or school goals. An important issue that should be discussed is sexuality. Delayed or irregular menstruation is not uncommon. There may be delayed development of secondary sex characteristics such as breasts in girls. The person may use the illness to avoid certain events or relationships. The healthy person may hesitate to make friends with someone who is sick. Other crises and life transitions that must be dealt with in the young adult include building confidence and self-respect on the basis of achievements, persevering with employment goals, developing motivation to achieve, learning to cope with the treatment program, and adjusting to the need for dependence if health fails. Disclosing the CF diagnosis to friends, potential spouses, or employers may pose challenges emotionally and financially.

The issue of marrying and having children is difficult. Genetic counseling may be an appropriate suggestion for the couple considering having children. Most men with CF are sterile. Women with the disease may have difficulty becoming pregnant. In addition, any children produced will either be carriers of CF or have the disease. Another concern is the shortened life span of the parent with CF, and the parent's ability to care for the child must be taken into consideration.

Acute intervention for the patient with CF includes relief of bronchoconstriction, airway obstruction, and airflow limitation. Interventions include aggressive CPT, antibiotics, O_2 therapy, and corticosteroids in severe disease. Good nutrition is important to support the immune system. Advances in long-term vascular access (e.g. implanted ports) have made IV access and administration of medication much easier. This has also eased the transition for IV treatment at home.

CPT is the mainstay of intervention for ineffective airway clearance for these patients. Home management of cystic fibrosis includes an aggressive plan of postural drainage with percussion and vibration, use of mucus-clearing devices and techniques (discussed earlier in the chapter), aerosol-nebulization therapy, and breathing retraining. The patient is taught controlled coughing techniques, deep-breathing exercises, and progressive exercise conditioning such as a bicycling program.

The family and the person with CF have a great financial and emotional burden. The cost of drugs, special equipment, and health care is often a financial hardship. Because most CF patients live to childbearing age, family planning and genetic counseling are important. The burden of living with a chronic disease at a young age can be emotionally overwhelming. Community resources are often available to help the family. In addition, the cystic fibrosis foundation can be of assistance. As the person continues toward and into adulthood, the nurse and other skilled health professionals should be available to help the patient and family cope with complications resulting from the disease.

CHAPTER 4

Nursing Management of Digestive Disorders

INTRODUCTION

The gastrointestinal (GI) system, also termed as the digestive system and alimentary canal, consists of the GI tract and its accessory organs. The GI tract or alimentary canal is a hollow muscular tube that extends from mouth to the anus. Its principal function is to provide the body with fluid, nutrients, and electrolyte. This is accomplished through the processes of ingestion (taking food), digestion (breakdown of food) and absorption (transfer of food products into circulation). Another main function of the GI system is the storage and final excretion of the solid waste products of digestion, i.e. elimination.

The GI system consists of the GI tract, and its associated organs and glands, which includes mouth, esophagus, stomach, small intestine, large intestine, rectum, and anus. The associated organs are the liver, pancreas, and gallbladder. Proper functioning of the GI system is essential to the maintenance of proper nutrition and health. Psychological or emotional factors such as stress and anxiety influence GI functioning in many persons. Stress may be manifested as anorexia, epigastric and abdominal pain or diarrhea. However, GI problems should never be solely attributed to psychological factors. Organic and psychologically-based problem can exist independently or concurrently. Physical factors such as dietary intake, ingestion of alcohol, and cafeine-containing products, cigarette smoking, and fatigue may affect GI function. Some organic diseases of the GI system such as peptic ulcer, ulcerative colitis may be aggravated by stress. These both physical and emotional factors affect the GI functions. So it is very essential for the nurses to understand the disorders of digestive system, because they will come across such clients, and to provide proper nursing services.

NURSING ASSESSMENT OF DIGESTIVE SYSTEM

Assessment of digestive system involves a detailed health history as well as a comprehensive physical examination of the oral cavity, abdomen, rectum and anus. And a review of the client's demographic data.

Demographic Data

A review of the patient's demographic data such as age, sex, culture, religion and occupation is helpful, when assessing GI system, because many GI disorders are associated with it. For example, many GI cancers occur more frequently in the elderly and in males, whereas others are more common in females. Sexual abuse may play role in GI problems in some women. Reproductive cycling in females contribute to other GI manifestations. Duodenal ulcers develop in younger adults, whereas gastric ulcers are more common in middle-aged and older adults.

Past Health History

The nurse collects data about previous hospitalizations, major illness, surgery, use of medications and allergies as a part of past health history.

- Informations should be gathered from the patients about the history or existence of the following diseases or problems related to GI functioning: Abdominal pain, gastritis, nausea, and vomiting, diarrhea, and constipation, hepatitis, colitis, peptic ulcer, abdominal distension, jaundice, anamia, haital hernia, gallbladder disease, dysphagia, heartburn, dyspepsia, changes in appetite, hematemesis, food intolerance, indigestion, excessive gas, bloating, melena, hemorrhoids, hernia, or rectal bleeding. In addition, nurse should ask whether the client currently has or previously had a change in bowel habits, GI bleeding, jaundice, ulcers, colitis, or unexplained weight loss or gain.

- The health history should include an assessment of the patient's past and current use of medications, particularly in relation to liver problems. Because many chemicals and drugs are potentially hepatotoxic (e.g., alcohol, arsenic, carbon tetrachloride, gold compounds, mercury, phosphorous, anabolic steroids, halothane, isoniazed, propylthiouracil, sulfonamides, thiazide diurectics, methotrexate, acetominephen). The nurse should ask the patient if laxatives or antacids are taken, including the kind and frequency. The use of prescription or over the counter appetite suppressant drug should be noted including name, duration, frequency and also any allergies to medication should be noted.

- Information should be obtained about the hospitalization for any problems related to the GI system, including abdominal surgery, rectal surgery, reasons for surgery, postoperative course and possible blood transfusion, etc.

- The nurse should also have the knowledge about the patient's health practices related to GI system, such as maintenance of normal body weight, attention to proper dental care, maintenance of adequate nutrition and effective elimination habits and patient should be asked about exposure to hepatotoxic chemicals and exposure to hepatitis or parasitic infection. And also patient should be assessed in relation to certain habits like consumption of alcohol and cigarette smoking, which may delay healing of ulcers and lead to liver problems.
- Thorough nutritional assessment is essential. The nurse should ask open-ended questions that will allow the patients to express beliefs and feelings about the diet. The nurse may need to ask the patient to do a 24 hours dietary recall to analyse the adequacy of diet and find out whether patient is taking adequate diet or not. The patient should be questioned about any changes in appetite food tolerance and weight. Anorexia and weight loss may indicate carcinoma. The nurse should ask the patient about allergies to any food and determine what GI symptoms show allergic response cause.
- A detailed account of the patient's bowel elimination pattern should be elicited. The frequency, time of the day, and usual consistency of stool should be noted. The use of laxatives and enema, including type, frequency, and results should be documented. Any recent changes in bowel pattern should be investigated.
- Activity and exercise may affect GI motility. Immobility is risk for constipation. So the patient's ambulatory status may be assessed to determine if the patient is capable of securing and preparing food. Any limitation in it should be noted.
- The patient should be asked if GI symptoms affect sleep or rest. For example, a patient with a hiatal hernia may be awakened because of burning pain, sleep may be improved by elevating the head of the bed for such patients. Hunger can prevent sleep and should be relieved by a light, easily digested snack unless contraindicated. A patient often has bed time ritual that involves the use of a particular food or beverages, e.g., warm milk, herbal tea, etc. should be noted.
- Cognitive-perceptual pattern, i.e. decrease in sensory adequacy can result in problems related to the acquisition, preparation and ingestion of food. For example, changes in taste or smell can affect appetite and eating pleasure. The nurse should assess the patient in this pattern to judge the effect of deficiencies on adequate nutritional intake and pain in another area that requires careful assessment related to its effect on GI system and nutrition. The possible effects of pain medication related to constipation, sedation and appetite suppressive should be assessed.
- Self-perception and Self-concept pattern should be assessed because many GI and nutritional problems can have a serious effect on the patient's self-perception, for example: (1) Overweight and underweight persons often have problems related to self-esteem and body image, (2) The altered physical changes often associated with liver disease can be problematic for the patient, e.g., jaundice, ascites.
- It is important that the nurse should be aware of the role-relationship pattern of patient. For example, problem related to the GI system such as: Cirrhosis, alcoholism, hepatitis, ostomies, obesity, and carcinoma can have a major impact on the patient's ability to maintain usual roles and relationships.
- It is also important that nurse should ask sensitive questions to determine sexuality-reproductive pattern of the patient, changes related to sexuality and reproductive status on result from problems of the GI system. For example, obesity, jaundice, anorexia, could decrease the acceptance of a potential sexual partner. Chronic alcoholism decreases meaningful sexual relationship. The presence of an ostomy could affect the patient's confidence related to sexual activity. Anorexia can affect the reproductive status of a female patient. Alcoholism can affect the reproductive status of both men and women.
- The nurse should try to determine the coping stress tolerance pattern of the patient, because GI symptoms such as epigastric pain, nausea, and diarrhea develop in many individuals in response to stressful or emotional situations. Some organic GI problems such as peptic ulcers are aggravated by stress. The nurse should also assess the value-belief pattern of the patients, i.e. the patient's spiritual and cultural belief regarding food and food preparations which helps for prescribing food and medication accordingly.

Physical Examination of Digestive System

The physical examination of the digestive system include examination of the oral cavity, abdomen, anus and rectum.

Oral cavity: Assessment of oral cavity involves inspection and palpation. The nurse puts on gloves, faces the client and begins by inspecting the lips. For observation of abnormalities of color, lesions, nodules and symmetry. The abnormalities of lips include pallor, or cyanosis, cracking ulcer, or fissure using a tonge blade. The nurse should inspect the buccal mucosa and not the color, any areas of pigmentation or any lesion. In assessing teeth and gums, nurse should look for caries, abnormal shape and position of teeth, and swelling, bleeding, discoloration or inflammation of gingivae. Any distinctive breath odor should be noted. The pharynx should be inspected for any abnormalities. Abnormalities of mouth include thrush, leukoplakia, white plaques with red patches, cancer sore, etc.

The nurse should palpate any suspicious area in the mouth such as ulcer, nodules, indurations and areas of tenderness should be palpated. It should be noted that if patient having any dentures or partial appliances should be removed when examining the oral cavity.

Abdomen

To assess the patient's abdomen, have the client lie in a supine position with the arms at the sides. Bending the knees slightly helps to relax the abdomen muscles. Begin in the patient's right lower quadrants and proceed in clockwise manner. When assessing the abdomen, the nurse proceeds the following sequence: Inspection, auscultation, percussion and palpation. The sequence may vary according to situations:

- *Inspection:* The nurse should inspect the abdomen for skin changes (color, texture, scars, striae, dilated veins, rashes and lesions), umbilicus (location and contour) symmetry, contour (flat, rounded, carved, concave, protuberant, distention), observable mass (hernias or other masses) and movement (pulsations and peristalsis).
- *Auscultation* of the abdomen begins by listening with the diaphragm of the stethoscope, which provides information on bowel and vascular sounds. The stethoscope is lightly pressed on the abdominal wall in all four quadrants. Begin in the right lower quadrant at the ilecaecal valve area because bowel sounds are normally present there. Normal bowel sounds occur 5 to 35 times per minute and sound like high-pitched clicks or gurgles. The nurse should listen for bowel sounds for 2 to 5 minutes. Bowel sounds cannot be described as absent until no sound is heard for 5 minutes in each quadrant. The frequency and intensity of the bowel sounds vary depending on the phase of digestion. Loud gurgles indicate hyperperistalsis termed as 'borborygoni (stomach growling). Terms used to describe bowel sounds include, present, absent, increased, decreased, high pitched, tinkling, gurgling and rushing.

  The nurse uses the bell of the stethoscope to auscultate vascular sounds. Three abnormal sounds should be listened for: A bruit, a venous hum, or a friction rub. The nurse listens over the aorta, renal arteries, and iliac arteries. A bruit is heard over the aorta which indicates presence of aortic aneurysm. A continuous venous hum heard in preumbilical area indicates engorged liver circulation. Friction rub indicates hepatic tumor or splenic infarction.
- *Percussion* of the abdomen is to determine the size and location of the abdominal organs and to detect fluid, air and masses. The nurse uses percussion in all four quadrants and compare sounds. Normally, percussion sounds over the abdomen are tympanic (high-pitched loud or musical over gas) or dull (thud-like sounds over fluid or solid organs).

To percuss the liver, the nurse should start below the umbilicus in the right midclavicular line and percuss lightly upward until dullness is heard, thus determining the lower border of liver dullness. After the lower border of the liver has been determined, the nurse should start the nipple line in the midclavicular line and percuss downward between ribs to the area of dullness indicating the upper border of the liver. The height or vertical space between two areas should be measured to determine the size of the liver. Dull sounds normally occur over the liver and spleen or a bladder filled with urine. Abnormal findings occur because of the presence of ascites or abnormal masses.

Interpretation of Common Finding of Inspection
- Scars on strials may be result of pregnancy, obesity, ascites, tumors edema, surgical procedure, or healed burned areas.
- Engorged veins may be caused by obstruction of vena cava or portal vein and circulation from abdomen.
- Skin color observe for evidence of jaundice, or inflammation (redness).
- Visible peristalsis may be caused by pyrolic or intestinal obstruction; normally peristalsis not visible except the slow waves in thin persons.
- Visible pulsation normally slight pulsation of aorta is visible to epigastric region.
- Visible masses and altered contour observe for hernia, distension of ascites, and obesity; instructing patient to cough may bring hernia 'bulge or elicit pain or discomfort' in the abdomen, marked concavity may be caused by malnutrition.
- Spider angioma appear on the upper portion of the body and blanch with pressure: Commonly result from liver disease.

Interpretation of Common Findings from Auscultation
- Absence from Sounds in 5 minutes may be due to peritonitis, paralytic ileus, pneumonia, and hypokalemia.
- Repeated, high-pitched sounds occurring at frequent intervals. Increased peristalsis heard in gastroenteritis, early pyloric obstruction, early intestinal obstruction, and diarrhea.
- Bruit presence of abnormal sounds (turbulence of blood flow through partially occluded or diseased aorta or renal artery).
- Hum and friction rub heard over liver and splenic areas, indicating an increased venous blood flow, possibly related to peritoneal inflammation.
- Palpation is of value in determining the outlines of the abdominal organs, determining the presence and characteristics of any abdominal masses, and identifying the presence of direct tenderness, guarding, rebound tenderness and muscular rigidity.

Light palpation is used to detect tenderness or cutaneous hypersensitivity, muscular resistance, masses, and swelling. The nurse uses the pads of the fingertips with the finger together, and press gently, depressing the abdominal wall about 1 cm. All quadrants are palpated using smooth movement.

Deep palpation is used to delineate abdominal organs and masses. The palmar surface of the fingers should be used to press more deeply. Again all quadrants should be palpated. When palpating masses, the nurse should note the location, size, shape and presence of tenderness. The patient's facial expression should be observed during these maneuver, because it will give non-verbal cues of discomfort or pain.

An alternate method for deep abdominal palpation is the two-hand method. One hand is placed on the top of the other. The fingers of the top hand apply pressure to the bottom hand. The fingers of the bottom hand feel for organs and masses.

To palpate nurse's left hand is placed behind the patient to support the right eleventh and twelfth rib. The patient may relax on nurse's hand. The nurse should press the left hand forward and place the right hand on the patient's right abdomen lateral to the rectus muscle. The fingertips should be below the lower border of liver, dullness and pointed towards the right costal margin. The nurse should gently press in and up. The patient should take deep breath with the abdomen so that liver drops and is in a better position to be palpated. The nurse should try to feel the lower edge as it comes down to the fingertips. The liver edge should be firm, sharp and smooth. Any abnormality should be noted.

To palpate spleen, the nurse moves to the left side of the patient. The nurse places the left hand under the patient and supports and presses the patient's left lower rib cage forward. The right hand is placed below the left costal margin and pressed it in towards the spleen. The nurse should ask the patient to breathe deeply. The tip or edge of an enlarged spleen will be felt by the fingertips. The spleen is normally not palpable.

Rectum and Anus

Examination of the anus and rectum is potentially embarassing and uncomfortable for the patient. The nurse uses a gentle approach and a matter-of-fact manner. The client's position depends on the circumstances of the examination. A female client may be examined while in the lithotomy position immediately following assessment of the genitalia, in the Sim's position or in a dorsal recumbent position. A male client may be examined in the Sim's position or while standing and leaning across the examination table, a position which facilitates palpation of the prostate gland.

Clients are draped accordingly. For the digital examination of the rectum the gloved lubricated index finger is placed against the anus while the patient strains (Valsalva maneuver). Then as the sphincter relaxes, the finger is inserted. The finger is pointed towards the umbilicus. The nurse should try to get the patient to relax. The finger inserted into the rectum as far as possible, and all surfaces are palpated. Nodules, tenderness or any irregularities should be assessed. A sample of stool can be removed with the gloved finger and should be checked for occult blood. Abnormal findings may include pruritus ani, coccygeal or pilonidal sinus, tract openings, fistulas, fissures, external haemorrhoids, rectal prolapse, and internal hemorrhoids, etc.

DIAGNOSTIC STUDIES IN DIGESTIVE SYSTEM

Number of examinations and tests performed for diagnosis of problems of the digestive system are both consuming and unpleasant. Several tests are intrusive procedures that are uncomfortable and embarassing for the patient which results in added stress for the patient. It remains the nurse's responsibility to meet the educational and psychological needs of the patient by answering questions concerning the test procedure, rationale for its use and specific test preparation in a caring manner.

Laboratory Tests

Numerous tests may be used as a part of the evaluation of the GI biliary, and exocrine pancreas function. The main blood and urine tests are as follows:

Blood Tests

- *Stomach gastrin test:* Gastrin is a gastric hormone that is a powerful stimulus for gastric acid secretion. Elevated levels are found in those with pernicious anemia and Zollinger-Ellison syndrome. The normal gastrin value is less than 200 dg/ml (200 mg/L)
- Helicobacter pylori detected in serum is a highly sensitive but less specific, indicator of an active infection. *H. pylori* infection predisposes to peptic ulcer disease.
- *Total bilirubin test:* Bilirubin is exerted in the obstruction in the biliary tract contribute primarily to a rise in conjugated (direct) values. The normal value 0.1 to 1.0 mg/dl, conjugaged 0.1–0.3 mg/dl, unconjugated 0.1–0.8 mg/dl.
- *Alkaline phosphate:* It is found in many tissues with high concentration in bone, liver and biliary tract epithelium. Obstructive biliary tract disease and carcinoma may cause significant elevations. The normal value is 30–85 1nu/ml.
- *Amylase:* It is secreted normally by the acinar cells of the pancreas. Damage to these cells or obstruction of the pancreatic duct causes the enzyme to be absorbed into the blood is significant quantities. It is a sensitive yet non-specific test for pancreatic disease. The normal value is 80–150 somogyl units.

- *Lipase:* It is a pancreatic enzyem normally secreted into the duodenum. It appears in the blood when damage occurs to the acinor cells. It is a specific test for pancreatic disease. The normal value 0-110 units/L.
- Calcium levels may be low in cases of severe pancreatitis or steatorrhea because calcium soaps are formed from the sequestration of calcium by fat necrosis. The normal value is 9.0-11.5 mg/dl.
- Total protein of blood includes albumen and globulin. Although primarily a reflection of liver function, serum protein level is also a meausre of nutrition. Malnourished patients have greatly decreased levels of blood protein. The normal protein is 6.8 g/dl (Albumin 3.2-4.5 g/dl, Globulin 2.3-3.4 g/dl).
- *D-xylose absorption test:* D-xylose is a monosaccharide that is easily absorbed by the normal intestine but not metabolized by the body. D-xylose is administered orally and assists in the diagnosis of malabsorption. Normally blood levels of 25-40 mg/dl 2 hr after ingestion.
- *Lactose tolerance test:* An oral dose of lactose is administered. In the absence of intestinal lactase, the lactose is neither broken down nor absorbed and plasma glucose levels do not rise. The test assists in the diagnosis of lactose intolerance. Normally rise in blood glucose level is more than 20 mg/dl.
- *CEA test:* Carcinoembryonic antigen is a protein normally present in fetal gut tissue. It is typically elevated in persons with colorectal tumours. It is useful in determining prognosis and response to therapy. The normal value is less than 5 mg/ml.

Urine Tests

- *5-Hydroxyindoleacetic Acid (5-HIAA):* Carcinoid tumors are serotin in secreting and are derived from neuroectoderm tissue, e.g., the appendix and intestine. These neurohormones are metabolised to 5-HIAA by the liver and excreted in urine. The normal value is 2–5 mg/2 hr.
- *Urine Bilirubin:* Bilirubin is not normally excreted in the urine. Biliary structure, inflammation, or stones may cause its presence.
- *Urobilinogen:* A sensitive test for hepatic or biliary diseases. Decreased levels are seen in those with biliary obstruction and pancreatic cancer. In 24-hour collection, urobilinogen is 0.2–1.2 units and 0.05–2.5 mg.
- *Urine Amylase:* Normally 10-80 amylase units/hour. A rise in levels usually minimises the rise in serum amylase. The level remains elevated for 7-10 days; however, which allows for retrospective diagnosis.

Stool Examination

Stool specimens are collected primarily for culture, determination of fat content, and examination for the presence of ova, parasites, and fresh or occult blood. Stools to be analyzed for the presence of bacteria, i.e. *Salmonella, Shigella, Staphylococcus aureus*. Detection of occult blood in the stool is useful in identifying bleeding in the GI Tract occult blood may be identified by one of the three tests—*guaiac test (hemoccult), benzidine*, or *orthotobrdine (occultest)*.

The color of the stool also indicates few cues for the following:
- Brown : Presence of fecal urobilinogen
- White : Barium
- Gray, tan (clay) : Lack of bile, biliary obstruction
- Black : Tarry-Upper GI bleeding. Dry-Rapid peristalsis with bile presence
- Green : Rapid peristalsis with bile presence

RADIOLOGICAL STUDIES

Upper GI or Barium Swallow

It is a X-ray study with fluoroscopy with contrast medium. This is used to diagnose structural abnormalities of the esophagus, stomach and duodenal bulb. The nurse's responsibility in this procedure includes:
- Explain procedure to patient and that patient will need to drink contrast medium and assume various positions on X-ray table.
- Keep patient NPO (nil per oral) for 8-12 hours before procedure.
- Tell the patient to avoid smoking after midnight, the night before the study.
- After X-ray test, take measures to prevent contrast medium impaction (fluids, laxatives).
- Tell patient that stool may be white upto 72 hours after test.

Small Bowel Series

In this contrast medium is ingested and flat film taken q 20 min until medium reaches terminal ileum. Here the nurse's responsibilities are as stated in barium swallow.

These procedures are used to identify esophageal and stomach disorder such as strid varices, polyps, tumors, hiatal hernia and peptic ulcers.

Lower GI or Barium Enema

It is fluoroscopic X-ray examination of colon, used contrast medium, which is administered rectally (enema). Double contrast or air contrast barium enema is test of choice. Air is infused after barium is evacuated. The nurse's responsibility in barium enema includes:
- Before the procedure, administer laxatives and enema until colon is clear of stool evening before procedure.
- Administer clear liquid diet evening before procedure.
- Keep patient NPO for 8 hours before test.

- Instruct patient about being given barium by enema.
- Explain that cramping and urge to defecate may occur during procedure and that patient may be placed in various positions on tilt table.
- After the procedure give fluids, laxatives or suppositories to assist in expelling barium.
- And observe stool for passage of contrast medium.

This procedure identifies polyps, tumors and other lesion in colon.

Oral Cholecystogram (Gallbladder Series)

It is X-ray examination visualizes gallbladder (GB) after radiopaque dye, such as iopanoic acid (Telepaque) has been ingested orally. It is used to determine the GB ability to concentrate and store dye and to observe the patency of the biliary duct system. It also may be used to detect gallstones, obstructions of the biliary tract, and other GB disorders. In this procedure, the nurse's responsibilities will include:

- Assess patient for sensitivity to iodine, (telepaque contains iodine).
- Administer radiopaque dye evening before test.
- Give 6 tablets (3q) 1q 5 minutes.
- Explain that patient may need 2 consecutive days of dye ingestion.
- Keep patient NPO after ingestion of dye.
- Observe for side effects of dye, such as nausea, vomitting, diarrhea.
- May give fatty test meal after X-ray test to check for GB emptying.
- Assess patient's medication for possible contraindications, precautions or complications with the use of dye.

Cholangiography

Cholangiogram: In the X-rays are used to visualize biliary duct system after IV injection of radiopaque dye, the nurse's responsibilities in the procedure will include:

- Keep patient NPO for 8 hours prior to procedure.
- Assess sensitivity to iodine dye.
- During injection of dye, assess for urticaria, extreme flushing and respiratory distress.
- Assess patient's medications for possibly contraindication, complications, with the use of dye. Percutaneous transhepatic cholangiogram. This is performed after local anesthesia. Liver is entered with long needles (under fluoroscopy) bile duct is entered, bile withdrawn and radiopaque dye injected. Fluoroscopy is used to determine filling of hepatic and biliary ducts. The nurse's responsibilities are:
- Observe patient for signs of hemorrhage or bile leakage.
- Assess patient's medications for possible contraindications precautions or complications with the use of dye. Surgical cholangiogram is performed during surgery on biliary structure such as gallbladder, contrast medium is injected into common bile duct. The nursing responsibilities are:
  - Explain the patient that anesthetic will be used.
  - Assess patient's medications for possible contraindications, precautions, or complications with the use of dye.

Ultrasound

This non-invasive procedure uses high frequency sound waves (ultrasound waves), which are passed into body structures and recorded as they are reflected (bounded). A conductive gel (lubricant jelly) is applied to the skin and a transducer is placed on the area. In these procedures nurses should be aware that patient's bowel must be cleaned, because of the presence of solid material in GI tract, causes change in reflected sounds and that ultrasound is not transmitted well through gas or air. Schedule test before upper GI or barium enema:

- Abdominal ultrasound study detects abdominal masses (tumors and cysts) and is also used to assess ascites.
- Hepatobiliary ultrasound study detects subphrenic abscesses, cysts, tumors, cirrhosis and is used to visualize biliary ducts.
- GB ultrasound study detects gallstones (high degree of accuracy) and can be used for a patient with jaundice, or allergic reaction to GB contrast media. The nurse's responsibilities include:
  - Administer clear liquids for 24 hours before examination.
  - Give laxatives evening before and cleansing enema morning of examination.
  - Keep patient NPO 8 hours prior to procedure.

Nuclear Imaging Scans

The purpose of nuclear imaging scans is to show size, shape, and position of organ. Functional disorders and structural defects may be identified. Radionuclide (radioactive isotope) is injected IV and a counter (scanning) device picks up radioactive emission, which is recorded on paper. Only tracer doses of radioactive isotopes are used. In these procedures, nurses use to:

- Tell patients that substances contain only traces of radioactivity and pose little to no danger.
- Schedule no more than one radionuclide test on the same day.
- Explain to patient need to lie flat during the scanning.
  - Gastric emptying studies: A Radionuclide study is used to assess ability of stomach to empty solids or liquids. In solid emptying study, egg white containing Tc 99m is eaten. In liquid emptying study, orange juice with Tc 99 m is drunk. Sequential

images from gamma camera are recorded q2 minutes for upto 60 minutes. Study is used in patients with emptying disorders from peptic ulcer, ulcer surgery, diabetes and gastric malignancy.
- Liver and spleen scan: Here patient is given IV injection of Tc 99m and positioned under camera to record distribution of radioactivity in liver and spleen. In normal person, intensity of liver and spleen images is equal. Test is useful in detecting hepatomegaly hepatocellular diseases, hepatic malignancy and splenomegaly.

Computed Tomography (CT)

Computed tomography (CT) is a non-invasive radiological examination combines special X-ray machine used for CT (exposures at different depth) with computer. This study detects mainly biliary tract, liver and pancreatic disorders. Use of contrast medium accentuates density differences and helps detect biliary problems. In this procedure, nurses are used to explain procedures to patient and determine sensitivity to iodine if contrast material is used.

Magnetic Resonance Imaging (MRI)

MRI is a non-invasive procedure using radiofrequency waves and a magnetic field. This procedure is used to detect hepatic metastasis, sources of GI bleeding, and to stage colorectal cancer. The nurse's responsibilities in MRI includes:
- Keep patient NPO for six hours prior to procedure.
- Explain procedure to patient.
- This procedure contraindicated in patient with metal implants (e.g., pacemaker), or who is pregnant.

ENDOSCOPIC EXAMINATION

Endoscopy refers to the direct visualization of a body structure through a lighted instrument (scope). Most of the GI tract can be visualised by endoscopy, especially with the flexible fibroptic scopes. The fiberscope is an instrument channel through which biopsy forceps and cytology brushes may be passed. Cameras may be attached and pictures taken. Endoscopy is frequently done in combination with the biopsy and cytologic studies. The major complication of GI endoscopy is perforations through the structure being scooped. All endoscopic procedures required informed, written consent.

Esophago-gastro-duodenoscopy

Esophago-gastro-duodenoscopy is a technique directly visualizes mucosal lining of esophagus, stomach and duodenum with flexible, fibroptic endoscope. Tests may use video imaging to visualize stomach motility, inflammations, ulcerations, tumors, varices, or Mallory-weiss tear may be detected. The nursing responsibility in this procedure includes:

- Keep patient NPO for 8 hours prior to the procedure.
- Make sure signed consent is on chart.
- Give preoperative medication if ordered (diazepam, midazolam, or meperidine).
- Explain to patient that local anesthetic may be sprayed on throat before insection of scope and that patient will be sedated during procedure.
- After procedure, keep patient NPO until gag reflex returns.
- Gently tickle back of throat to determine reflex.
- Use warm saline gargles for relief of sore throat.
- Check temperature q 15-30 minutes for 1-2-hours (sudden temperature spike is sign of perforation).

Colonoscopy

Study directly visualizes entire colon upto iliocecal valve with flexible fiberoptic scope. Patient's position is changed frequently during procedure to assist with advancement of scope to cecum. Test is used to diagnose inflammatory bowel disease, detect tumors, and dilate strictures. Procedure allows for removal of colonic polyps without laparotomy. The nursing responsibilities in this procedure will include:

- Before the procedure, keep patient on clear liquids 1-3 days.
- Keep patient NPO for 8 hours prior to procedure.
- Make sure signed consent is on chart.
- Administer laxatives 1-3-days before and enema night before.
- Explain to patient some information regarding insertion of scope as for sigmoidoscopy.
- Explain to patient that sedation will be given.
- Administer alternate preparation of 1 glass of golytely or colyte evening before (8 oz glass q 10 min).
- On morning of procedure, allow clear liquids.
- After the procedure, be aware that patient may experience abdominal cramps caused by stimulation of peristalsis because the patient's bowel is constantly inflated with air during procedure.
- Observe for rectal bleeding and signs of perforation (e.g., malaise, abdominal distentions).

Endoscopic Retrograde Cholangiopancreatography (ERCP)

In ERCP fiberoptic endoscope is inserted through the oral cavity into descending duodenum, then common bile and pancreatic ducts are cannulated. Contrast medium is injected into ducts and allows for direct visualization of structures. Technique can also be used to retrieve a gallstone from distal GBD, dilate structures, biopsy tumors diagnose pseudocysts. In this procedure, the nursing responsibilities will include the following:

- Before the procedure, explain procedure to patient including patient's role.

- Keep patient NPO 8 hours prior to procedure.
- Ensure consent form is signed.
- Administer sedation immediately before and during procedure.
- Administer antibiotics if ordered.
- After the procuedure, check vital signs.
- Check for signs of perforation or infection.
- Be aware that pancreatitis is most common complication.
- Check for return of gag reflex.

Peritoneoscopy (Laparoscopy)

Peritoneal cavity and contents are visualized with laparoscope. Biospy specimen may also be taken. Double puncture peritoneoscope permits better visualization of abdominal cavity, especially liver. This technique can climinate need for exploratory laparotomy in many patients. In this, following are the "nursing responsibilities".

- Make sure signed permit is on chart.
- Keep patient NPO 8 hr before study.
- Administer preoperative sedative medication.
- Ensure that bladder and bowel are emptied.
- Instruct patient that local anaesthesia is used before scope insertion.
- Observe for possible complications of bleeding and bowel perforation after the procedure.

LIVER BIOPSY

It is an invasive procedure; uses needle inserted between sixth and seventh or eighth and ninth intercostal spaces on the right side to obtain specimens of hepatic tissue. The nurse's responsibilities include:

- Check patient's coagulation status (PT, CT, BT) prior to procedure.
- Ensure patient's blood is typed and cross matched.
- Take vital signs as baseline data.
- Explain holding breath after expiration when needle is inserted.
- Ensure that informed consent has been signed.
- After the procedure, check vital signs to detect internal bleeding, q 15 min × 2, q 30 min × 4, q 1 hr × 4.
- Keep patient lying on right side for minimum 2 hours to splint puncture site.
- Keep patient on bed in flat position for 12-14 hours.
- Assess patient for complications such as bile peritonitis, shock pneumothorax.

PROBLEMS OF MOUTH

Ingestion is the process of taking food and fluids into the body via the GI tract. It begins in the mouth with mastication of food by teeth. Food then passes down the esophagus and into the stomach. It is important that sufficient nutrient is ingested to meet bodily requirements.

Oral problems, such as poor dental health, infections and inflammation and cancer interfere with ingestion.

Dental Problems/Tooth and Gum Disorder

Tooth decay is by far the most common problem affecting the teeth termed as "dental caries". It is the result of a pathological process that causes the gradual destructions of the enamel and dentin of the teeth. Caries development starts when 'plaque' builds up and adheres to the teeth. Plaque is a gelationous substance consisting of bacteria, saliva and epithelial cells.

Prevention is the most appropriate management of dental problem, which includes:

- Widespread fluoridation of water supplies reduces dental decay. Fluoride makes tooth enamel more resistant to acids and is commonly added to drinking water in many localities. It is widely available in toothpastes, dental rinses and mouthwashes.
- Early treatment of periodontal disease consists of scaling and root planning.
- Scaling is the removal of calculus and root planning is the smoothening of root surfaces. Gingivectomy and gingivoplasty may be necessary.

ORAL INFECTIONS AND INFLAMMATION

Any of the structures of the mouth may develop infections when oral infections and inflammations are present, they can severely or seriously affect the ability of the patient to adequately and comfortably ingest food and fluids by mouth. These infections are inflammations; may be specific mouth disease or they may occur in the presence are inflammation may be specific mouth disease or they may occur in the presence of some systemic disease such as leukemia or vitamin deficiency.

Pathophysiology

The structure of the mouth causes many ulcerative diseases to have similar signs and symptoms. The mucus throughout the mouth is thin, and evolving vesicles and bullae break open rapidly into ulcers. The ulcers are typically further traumatized by the teeth and can become readily infected by the abundant oral flora. Many of the causative organisms are the same on those that cause common skin infections. The common inflammation and infections of the oral cavity are as follows. With this etiology, there comes clinical manifestation and treatment.

- *Gingivitis:* Inflammation of the gingivae in the early form of periodontal disease. It may occur due to neglected oral hygiene, malocclusion, missing or irregular teeth, faulty dentistry, eating of soft rather than fibrous foods.

  The clinical manifestation include inflamed gingivae and interdental papillae, bleeding during toothbrushing, development of pus, formation of abscess with loosening teeth (Periodontitis).

Treatment include prevention through health teaching, dental care, gingival massage, professional cleaning of teeth, non-fibrous foods, conscientious brushing habits with flossing.

- *Vincent's angina* (Necrotizing ulcerative gingivitis, Trench mouth): It is an acute bacterial infection of the gingivae, caused by a tremendous proliferation of normal mouth flora, such as spirochetes and fusiform bacilli. It is commonly triggered by poor oral hygiene, nutritional deficiencies (B and C vitamins), alcoholism, infections, or immunocompromise.

  The clinical manifestations are, painful bleeding gingivae, eroding necrotic lesions of interdental papillae, ulceration than bleed, increased saliva with metallic taste, fetid mouth odor, anorexia, fever and general malaise.

  The nursing measure will include: advising the patient to take rest (physical and mental), avoidance of smoking and alcoholic beverages, advice soft nutritious diet, correct oral hygiene habits, topical application of antibiotics, mouth irrigations with H_2O_2 and saline solutions.

- *Oral candidiasis* (monilasis or thrush): is caused by an increase in the level of Candida albicans, a yeast-like fungus is normally found in the skin, GI tract, vagina and oral cavity. Overgrowth of the organism may result from antibiotic depletion of normal flora (prolonged high dose of antibiotics) or immunosupresors from steroid therapy, chemotherapy or HIV infections.

  The clinical manifestations are pearly, bluish white (creamy white) "milk-curd" membranous lesions on mucosa of mouth and larynx, sore mouth, yeasty halitosis. The conditions is painful and if widespread, can interfere with oral nutrition. When mucosa bleeds, and ulcerates when patches are scraped off.

  Treatments include nystatin, or amphotericin B as oral suspension or buccal tablets, good oral hygiene. Oral nystatin, ketoconazole, clotrimazole; amphotericin for the immuno-compromized person.

- *Herpes simplex stomatitis* (cold sore, fever-blister): It is an externally common viral infection that produces characteristic blisters commonly called 'cold sore' or fever blister. It is caused by herpes simplex virus, type I or II, predisposing factors of upper respiratory infections, excessive exposure to sunlight, food allergies, emotional tensions, onset of menstruation.

  The virus is harboured in a dormant state by cells in the sensory nerve ganglia. Reactivation of the virus can occur with emotional stress, fever, exposure to cold or ultraviolet rays. The lesion appears most commonly on the mucus membranous border junction of the lips in the form of small vesicles, which then erupt and form painful, shallow ulcers. Vesicle formation may be single or clustered. Painful vesicles and ulceration of mouth, lips or edge of nose; may have prodromal itching or burning, fever, malaise, lymphadenopathy may occur.

  Treatment is palliative, which include mild antiseptic mouthwash. Application of spirits of camphor, corticosteroid cream, viscous lidocaine, removal or control of predisposing factors, topical or systemic antiviral agents, e.g., acyclovir (zovirax) in severe cases.

- *Aphthous stomatitis* (Cancer sore): It is a recurrent and chronic form of infection secondary to systemic disease, trauma, stress or unknown causes. It produces well circumscribed ulcers on the soft tissues of the mouth, including lips, tongue, insides of the cheeks, pharynx and soft palate. Ulcers of the mouth and lips causing extreme pain, ulcers surrounded by erythematous base. Painful small ulceration on oral mucosa heals in 1 to 3 weeks.

  Treatment is palliative; includes mouthwashes, hydrocortisone, antibiotic ointment, fluocinonide (Lidex ointment in orabase), Corticosterdoid (topical or systemic) tetracycline oral suspension for children.

- Parotitis is an inflammation of the salivary or parotid glands. The viral inflammation known as "mumps" in children.

  Parotitis usually caused by staphylococcus species, *Streptococcus* species (occasionally). Acute bacterial parotitis typically occurs in debilitated or elderly patients in whom dehydration, minimal oral intake, or medication have resulted in chronic dry mouth. Poor oral hygiene also causes parotitis. Acute parotitis occurs in postoperation patient called "surgical mumps".

  The clinical manifestations are: Pain in the glands with an abrupt onset, i.e. pain in area of gland and ear, absence of salivation, purulent exudate from duct of gland, fever and swelling.

  Treatment includes application of heat and cold, frequent oral hygiene, adequate hydration, broad spectrum antibiotics, occasionally needed. Nursing measures are mouthwashes, warm compresses, preventive measures such as chewing gum, sucking on hard candy (Lemon drops) adequate fluid intake.

- Stomatitis is the inflammation of the mouth caused by trauma, pathogens, irritants (tobacco, alcohol) renal, liver and hematologic disorders, side effects of many cancer chemotherapeutic drugs.

  The clinical manifestation is excessive salivation, halitosis, sore mouth.

  Treatment includes, removal or treatment of cause, oral hygiene with soothing solutions, topical medication, soft, bland diet.

ORAL CANCER

Carcinoma of the oral cavity may occur on the lips or anywehre within the mouth which includes tongue, floor of the mouth, buccal mucosa, hard palate, soft palate, pharyngeal walls and tonsils.

Etiology

The development of oral cancer is clearly linked to a history of smoking and alcohol consumption and the risk increases strongly with heavy use. The exact cause of oral cancer is not clear, but there are number of predisposing factors which includes:
- Constant over-exposure to ultraviolet radiation from the sun, for cancer lips.
- Tobacco usage (smoking and chewing), i.e. pipe and cigarette smoking, snuff, chewing tobacco.
- Chronic alcohol intake (excessive use of alcohol).
- Chronic irritation (jagged tooth, ill-fitting prosthesis, chemical or mechanical irritants).
- Ruddy fair complexion leads to lip cancer.
- Syphilis, immunosuppression leads to lip cancer.
- Recurrent herpetic lesions.
- Poor oral hygiene.
- Hot and spicy foods or drinks.
- Malnutrition.
- Cirrhosis of the liver.
- Age over 45 years.
- Family history of oral cancer.

Pathophysiology

The vast majority of oral cancer arise from the squamous cells, which line the surface, oral epithelium, epidermoid, basal cell and other carcinoma may arise. The majority of tumors arise on the lateral or ventral surfaces of the tongue, although rarely on the dorsal surface, and commonly go unnoticed by the patients. A single ulcer is the typical pattern. The tongue has an abundant vascular supply and lymphatic drainage channels, and spread of the cancer to adjacent structures may be rapid. Metastasis to the neck has already occurred in 60% of patients at the time of the diagnosis is made. The mortality rate is high, early metastasis is rare, although rapid extension to the mandible or floor of the mouth is possible. Tumors that involve the parotid gland are usually benign, although those arising submaxillary glands have a high rate of malignancy and tend to grow rapidly.

Clinical Manifestations

Many oral cancers are asymptomatic in the early stages. The premalignant lesions of the oral cavity are:
- Leukoplakia—is a potentially precancerous, yellow-white or grey white lesions may occur in any region of mouth also called "white patch" or "smoker's patch". Leukoplakia is the result of chronic irritation usually from the smoking and Candida infection.
- The patch becomes keratonical (hard and leathery) is sometimes described as hyperkeratosis.
- Erythroplasia—is a red, velvety-appearing patch that is often indicative of early squamous cell carcinoma occur on the mouth or tongue. These may turn to malignant.

Cancer of the lip usually appears as an indurated, painless ulcer on the lip. The first sign of carcinoma of tongue is ulcer or area of thickening. Soreness or pain of the tongue may occur, especially on eating hot or highly-seasoned foods. Cancer lesions are most likely to develop in the proximal half of the tongue. Later symptoms of cancer of the tongue include increased salivation, slurred speech, dysphagia, toothache, and earache.

Approximately 30% of oral cancer present with an asymptomatic neck mass. Anyhow, the common clinical manifestation of oral cancer are as follows:
- Masses in the mouth or neck.
- Chronic ear pain.
- Enlarged lymph nodes (cervical nodes are commonly affected).
- Discomfort or burning.
- Ulcer on lateral or ventral surface of the tongue or elsewhere.
- Dysphagia.
- Visible lesions on lips or elsewhere.
- Presence of erythroplasia (bright red, velvety leisions).

Diagnostic Study

- Biopsy of the suspected lesion with cytologic examination. It may be used to evaluate lymph nodes, leukoplakia or erythroplasia.
- Ultrasonography is an excellent adjust to evaluate masses that are closed to the surface.
- Computed tomography (CT) scans may be used to evaluate deeper, less definite masses.
- Magnetic resonance imaging (MRI) is most useful in the effort to evaluate deep masses of the inconclusive structure.

Treatment

Treatment of oral cancer depends on the location and staging of the tumor. Early-stage cancer is usually treated by either radiation or surgery, depend upon the size and accessibility of the tumor. More invasive cancers may require both modalities and advanced cancers are treated palliatively.

Radiation Therapy for Oral Cancer

Early lesions are highly curable with radiation, if they are confined to the mucosa, and the use of radiation prevents widespread tissue destruction. Radiation may be delivered by external beam or through the insertion of needle. If both radiation and surgery are planned, the radiation therapy is usually administered after the surgery because irradiated tissue is more susceptible to infection and breakdown. Care of the patient with implanted radioactive needles in oral tissue includes the following:

- Implant care
  - Do not pull on the strings. Any movement could alter the placement or direction of the radiation or cause the needles to loosen.
  - Check needles-patency several times each day.
  - Monitor linens, bed areas, and emesis basin, for needles that may dislodge.
  - Ensure that a protective container is present in the room to contain any needles that might dislodge.
- Patient care
  - Be familiar with gentle oral hygiene q 2h while awake.
  - Encourage the patient to avoid hot and cold foods and beverages as well as smoking.
  - If the patient has dentures, encourage their removal at night, for comfort. Assess gums for irritations and bleeding whenever dentures are removed.
  - Provide viscous Lidocaine (Xylocaine) solution or lozenges as needed, when oral discomfort interferes with nutrition.
  - Provide the patient with an alternate means of communication, talking around implanted needles is usually difficult or impossible.
  - Assist the patient to implement the mouth care regimen prescribed by the physician.
  - The side effects of radiation therapy to the mouth and neck include mucositis, xerostomia, and dental decay should be reported and managed accordingly.

Surgical Management

Surgical management of oral cancers range from local excision of small tumors to expensive surgery for invasive tumors. Some examples are partial mandibulectomy, hemiglossectomy, resection of the buccal mucosa and floor of the mouth and radical neck dissection, etc. Chemotherapy and radiation therapy also may be used along with surgical measures wherever indicated in palliative purposes. Because of depression, alcohol or presurgery radiation treatment patient may be malnourished even before surgery and after the surgery also there may be chance to become malnourished. For which nurse must observe for tolerance of the feedings and adjust the amount, time and formula if nausea, vomiting, diarrhea or distension occurs. The patient usually instructed about the tube feedings. When the patient can swallow, small amount of water is given. Close observation for choking is essential. Suction may be necessary to prevent aspiration. While managing the patient undergoing for surgery for oral cancer, the nurse can follow the undermentioned guidelines for care:

- Preoperative
  - Clarify the patient's knowledge of changes expected after surgery.
  - Explain expected postoperative measures including suctioning, nasogastric tube, etc.
  - Provide opportunities for the patient to begin to express feelings about changes in body image.
- Postoperative

Monitoring

- Assess facial movement for facial nerve damage (if parotid gland excised); ask the patient to raise the eyebrows, frown, smile, show the teeth, pucker the lips.
- Assess the degree and character of drainage:
  - Amount of drainage and presence of blood should be mentioned.
  - Hemorrhage may occur with wide resection of tongue.

Maintaining an Adequate Airway

- Place the patient in sidelying position initially.
- Place the patient in Fowler's position when fully alert.
- Suction the mouth (except for lop surgery).
- Gauze wick may be used to direct salive into an emesis basin.
- Maintain patency of drainage tubes if used.

Promoting Oral Hygiene and Comfort

- Clean involved areas of the mouth with a cotton applicator moistened with H_2O_2 and saline.
- Mouth irrigations.
  - Use sterile equipment.
  - Use a solution of sterile water, diluted H_2O_2, normal saline, or sodium bicarbonate.
  - Avoid commercial mouthwashes.
  - Protect any dressings from getting wet.
  - A catheter may be inserted along the side of the cheek and the solution injected with gentle pressure; a spray may also be used.
  - Give analgesics as indicated (pain is not usually severe).

Promoting Nutrition

- Tube feedings will be used initially with hemiglossectomy.
- Oral fluids: Place in back of throat with asepto syringe or feeding up with attached tubing.
- Eating soft foods
  - Encourage the patient to feed self when possible.
  - Teach the patient to drink clear water after all meals to cleanse the mouth.

- Avoid using a fork, which may traumatize new tissue.
- Avoid very hot or cold foods (hot foods may irritate new tissue cold foods may cause facial pain or paralyze oral function.

Promoting Speech

- Limit patient's response intitially to yes or no, which can be answered by gestures.
- When ability speech returns, encourage patient to speak slowly.
- Listen carefully and validate communication before acting on requests.
- Speak in a soft, clear voice.
- Refer the patient to a speech therapist if needed.

Promoting Body Image

- Prepare all visitors for visible outcomes of surgery.
- Include the family in all teaching.
- Encourage the patient to ventilate feelings about changes.
- Encourage socialization with others.

Nursing Management of Oral Cancer

Nursing Assessment

Subjective and objective data should be collected as follows, The subjective data include:
- Important health information:
  - *Past health history:* Recurrent herpetic lesions, syphilis, exposure to sunlight.
  - *Medications:* Use of immunosuppressants.
  - Surgical or other treatment—Removal of prior tumors.
- Functional health patterns:
  - Health perception—health management: Use of alcohol and tobacco, pipe smoking; Poor oral hygiene.
- Nutritional metabolic: Reduction in oral intake, weight loss, difficulty in chewing, increased salivation, intolerance to certain foods and temperatures of foods.
- Cognitive-perceptual: Mouth or tongue soreness or pain, toothache, earache, neck stiffness, dysphagia, difficulty in speaking.

The objective data includes:
- Integumentary: Indurated, painless ulcer on lips painless neckmasses
- Gastrointestinal: Areas of thickening or roughness, ulcers, leukoplakia, or erythroplasia on the tongue, increased salivation, drooling, slurred speech, foul breath odor.

Nursing Diagnosis

Nursing diagnosis for the patients with oral cancer may include the following:

Altered nutrition: Less than body requirement related to oral pain, difficulty in chewing, and swallowing, surgical resection, and radiation therapy.
- Pain related to tumor and surgical radiation.
- Anxiety related to diagnosis of cancer, uncertain future, potential for disfiguring surgery, recurrence bronchoscopy.
- Ineffective individual coping related to body image change, smoking and alcohol cessation.
- Altered health maintenance related to lack of knowledge of disease process and therapeutic regimen, and unavailability of support systems.

Planning

The objective of oral cancer patient will include that the patient will:
- Have a patent airway.
- Be able to communicate.
- Have adequate nutritional intake to promote healing.
- Have relief of pain and discomfort.

Implementation

The nurse should take preventive measures such as:
- Teach clients to avoid excessive use of tobacco, alcohol, hot and spicy foods and drinks.
- Encourage use of sunscreen during exposure to sunlight.
- Screen smokers and drinkers of alcohol and teach them to stop smoking and to limit alcohol intake.
- Ensure that client fix broken teeth and improperly-fitting dentures.
- Teach persons at risk to observe for manifestation of cancer.
- Ensure that client's tumor is excised and followed with chemotherapy and radiation as indicated.
- Provide nutritional support with tube feedings or feedings through precaution endoscopic gastrostomy and gastrostomy tube.

Evaluation

The expected outcomes (objectives) that the patient with oral cancer will:
- Maintain airway.
- Be able to communciate.
- Have adequate nutritional intake.
- Have relief of pain and discomfort.

NAUSEA AND VOMITING

Nausea and vomiting are the most common symptoms of GI diseases, which most often occur together but may occur independently. They are part of the body's protective mechanisms and are usually a response to chemical, bacterial, or viral insults to the body's integrity. They are present in a wide array of disorders and if persistent can lead to serious consequences.

Nausea is a feeling of discomfort in the epigastrium with a conscious desire to vomit. Anorexia usually accompanies nausea and is brought on by unpleasant stimulation involving any of the five senses. Generally, nausea occurs before vomiting and is characterized by contraction of the duodenum and by slowing of gastric motility and emptying.

Vomiting is the forceful ejection of partially digested food and secretions from the upper GI tract. It occurs when the gut becomes overly irritated, excited, or distended. It can be a protective mechanism to rid the body of spoiled or irritating foods and liquids. Immediately before the act of vomiting, the person becomes aware of the need to vomit. The autonomic nervous system is activated resulting in both parasympathetic and sympathetic nervous systems, stimulation sympathetic activation produces tachycardia, tachypnea and diaphoresis. Parasympathetic stimulation causes relaxation of lower esophageal sphincter, an increase in gastric motility and a pronounced increase in gastric motility and a pronounced increase in salivation.

Vomiting is a complex act that requires coordinated activities of several structures, closure of the glottis, deep inspiration with contraction of the diaphragm in the inspiratory position, closure of the glottis relaxation of the stomach and lower esophageal spincter, and contraction of the abdominal muscles with increasing abdominal pressure. These stimulation activities force the stomach contents up through the esophagus into the pharynx and out of the mouth.

Etiology

Nausea and vomiting are the most common manifestations of the Gastrointestinal disorders. They are also found in a wide variety of conditions that are unrelated in GI disease. These include:
- Pregnancy.
- Infectious diseases.
- CNS disorders (e.g., meningitis, CNS lesion).
- Cardiovascular problem (e.g., digitalis, antibiotics).
- Metabolic disorders (e.g., uremia, diabetic acidosis, etc.
- Psychological factors (e.g., stress, fear, unpleasant nights and odors).

Pathophysiology

Nausea may be accompanied by weakness, hypersalivation, and diaphoresis. Gastric tone and peristalsis are typically slowed or absent. The neural pathways that control nausea are not well identified but probably are the same general pathways that control vomiting. The vomiting center is located in the medulla (brainstem) adjacent to the respiratory and salivary control centers and can be stimulated by the vagus nerve and sympathetic nervous system. Receptors can be found throughout the GI tract and internal organs that, when triggered by spasm or inflammation, can directly produce vomiting. Indirect stimulation can come from the chemoreceptor trigger zone (CTZ) which is located on the floor of the fourth ventricle and appears to act as an emetic chemoreceptor responding to chemical stimuli in the blood. A wide variety of medication and other substances can act on the CTZ in this manner. The CTZ also mediate the response to nonchemical stimuli such as radiation and motion sickness. There is a strong evidence that dopamine receptors in the CTZ play a role in mediating vomiting.

When nausea and vomiting are prolonged, dehydration can rapidly occur. In addition to water, essential electrolytes, (e.g. potassium) are also lost. As vomiting persists, there may be severe electrolyte imbalances, loss of extracellular fluids (ECF) volume, decreased plasma volume and eventually circulatory failure. Metabolic alkosis can result from loss of gastric HCL. When contents from the small intestine are vomited. Weight loss is evident in a short time when vomiting is severe. The threat of aspiration is constant concern when vomiting is severe.

Nursing Management

Nursing Assessment

The nurse has to obtain the important health information which include:
- Past health history: GI disorders, chronic indigestion, food allergies, pregnancy, infection, CNS disorders, recent travel, bulimia, metabolic disorders, cancer, cardiovascular disease, renal disease.
- Medications: Use of antiemetics, digitalis, opiates, ferrous sulphate aspirin, aminophylline, alcohol, antibiotics, general anesthesia, chemotherapy.
- Surgery of other treatment: Recent surgery.

And also functional health pattern like amount, frequency, character and color of vomitus, dry heaves, anorexia, weight loss, abdominal tenderness, weakness, fatigue, stress, fear, etc.

And also objective data include observing for lethargy, sunken eyeballs, pallor, dry mucous membrane, poor skin turgor, GI symptoms like amount frequency, character (e.g., projectile, or regurgitation) content (undigested food, bloody bile, feces) and color of vomitus (red, coffee ground, green-yellow) and decreased output of urine, concentrated urine to locate causes.

Nursing Diagnosis

- Selfcare deficiency related to fatigue and discomfort and prolonged nausea and vomitus.
- Altered oral mucous membrane related to persistent vomiting and inadequate oral hygiene.

- Vomiting related to multiple etiologies.
- Fluid volume deficient r/t prolonging.
- Anxiety r/t lack of knowledge of cause.
- Altered nutrition less than body requirements.

Planning

The overall goals of the patient with nausea/vomiting will
- Experience minimal or no nausea and vomiting.
- Have normal electrolyte levels and hydration status.
- Return to normal pattern of fluid balance and nutrition intake.

Nursing Implementation

The patient with nausea and vomiting should be managed with following guidelines for:

Safety and Comfort

- Keep head of the bed elevated and emesis basin handy.
- Protect airway with suction and positioning if patient is not alert.
- Provide frequent mouth care.
- Control sights and odors in room.
- Reduce anxiety if possible.
- Provide quiet or distraction on the basis of patient response.
- Modify environmental stimuli (cool cloth, dim light) and evaluate response.
- Provide ongoing patient support. Explore any strategies.

Diet Modification

- Maintain NPO if vomiting is severe.
- Explore use of clear liquids:
  - Serve liquid cool or room temperature.
  - Try effervescent drinks and evaluate effect.
  - Avoid fatty foods.
  - Avoid highly sweetened foods and milk products.
  - Encourage adequate, fluids to prevent dehydration.
  - Keep meals small, avoid overdistention.

Drugs/Medications (Table 4.1)

- Administer medication before vomiting occurs, if possible.
- Evaluate the patient response to medication.
- Maintain patient safety and assess for sedation or confusion.

Generally the drugs used for nausea and vomiting and their nursing intervention are as follows:
- *Antihistamines* are believed to act on neurons in the vomiting center and in the vestibular pathways. They are effective in motion sickness and morning sickness management, but have little known effect in GI disorders. These drugs cause drowsiness and sedation. The nurse has to monitor drowsiness and sedation and instruct patient to use caution with all activities that require alertness. Driving may be hazardous, so should be avoided. The example of antihistamine are buclizine hydrochloride, cyclizine hydrochloride, meclizine, promethazine (all generic names).
- *Antidopaminerics* are believed to act by antagonizing dopamine receptors in the CTZ. They also have antihistamine and anticholinergic effects. They are effective in managing mild symptoms and often first lane therapies. The examples of antidopamergics are prochlorperazine, ethylperazine, fluphenazine droperidol. The nursing measures in this therapy include:
  - Monitor severity of drowsiness and sedation.
  - Teach patient to avoid all hazardous activities and driving during use.
  - Avoid alcohol and sun exposure.
- *Anticholinergics* reduce neuron transmission and are useful in the management of motion sickness and postoperative nausea. But the common side effects of dry mouth, urinary retention and drowsiness limit their use. During use, nurse should instruct patient to apply dry surfaces behind the ear. Use in advance anticipated need, e.g., scopalamine (Transderm-Scop).
- *Benzyamides have* complex action in both CNS and GI tract and useful in preventing vomiting associated with anesthetics and chemotherapeutic agents.
  - Metadopramide stimulates gastric emptying.
  - Domoperidone does not cross blood-brain barrier.
  - Here nurse has to monitor side effects. Diarrhea and mild sedation.
- *Serotonin antagonists* like ondansetron (Zofran) and Granisertron bind serotonin receptor sites along GI tract and afferent nerves. They are useful in controlling severe chemotherapy induced and postoperative vomiting.
- *Cannabis derivatives* the antiemetic site of action is uncertain but the active ingredient in marijuana is often useful in controlling chemotherapy related nausea and vomiting. In such cases, the nurse has to instruct patient to alert on mood and behavioral changes. Drowsiness is common, so driving should be avoided. Avoid concurrent alcohol use while using this drug.

GASTROESOPHAGEAL REFLUX DISEASE (GERD)

Gastroesophageal reflux diseases (GERD) is not a disease but a heterogenous syndrome resulting from esophageal reflux. Most cases are attributed to the inappropriate relaxation of lower esophageal sphincter (LES) in response to unknown stimulus.

Table 4.1: Antimetic drugs.

Agent	Dose and route	Action	Uses	Side effects
Antihistaminics				
Diphenhydramine	25–50 mg, 4–6 hourly orally, can be used parenterally	These act on the neurons of vomiting centre and vestibular pathways (afferent limb of vomiting reflex)	Vomiting due to motion sickness, pregnancy, inner ear disease, uraemia and postoperative vomiting	Sedation, dizziness
Meclizine	25–50 mg orally/day			
Promethazine	25 mg 4–6 hours/orally, can be used parenterally			
Anticholinergics				
Scopolamine	1.5 mg/3rd day patch	These reduce neuron transmission in CTZ	Postoperative vomiting	Dry mouth, blurred vision, epigastric discomfort, constipation, urinary retention
Dopamine receptors inhibitors				
Phenothiazine (prochlorperazine)	25 mg suppository per rectum q 6 hours oral, is available as parenterally	These antagonise the dopamine receptors in CTZ and also have mild antihistaminic and anticholinergic effect	All types of vomiting except motion sickness and labyrinthine disease	Hypotension, extrapyramidal side effects, akathisia, drowsiness, anxiety, sedation
Droperidol	1–2.5 mg q 3–6 hours IV		Gastroparesis	
Metoclopramide	10–20 mg oral or IV 6 hourly			
Domperidone	20–40 mg orally 3–4 times a day, can be given parenterally			
Sedative				
Diazepam	2 to 5 mg q 4–6 hours orally or IV	These act on the vomiting centre and suppress vomiting	Psychogenic vomiting	Sedation
Lorazepam	1 to 3 mg q 4–6 hours orally or IV		Added to metoclopramide or steroids to control vomiting in cancer patients	
Serotonin receptors antagonists				
Dolastran	100 mg or 1.8 mg/kg IV or 200 mg oral	These block the serotonin receptors site throughout the GI tract and afferent nerves	Chemotherapy induced vomiting in combination with corticosteroids	Mild headache, diarrhea or constipation, transient rise in transaminases
Lorazepam	8 mg or 0.15 mg/kg infusion or 8 mg tds orally			
Corticosteroids				
Dexamethasone	8–20 mg IV 4–20 mg oral 40–100 mg IV	These are not antiemetic, but potentiate the effect of antiemetic when used with them	These are combined with metoclopramide to control vomiting due to cancer chemotherapy	Side effects are of corticosteroids
Methylprednisolone				
Antibiogtic				
Erythromycin	125 mg q 6 hours orally	It prevents gastroesophageal reflux	Gastroparesis	Abdominal cramps, bloating, nausea

Etiology

The common cause of GERD is Haital Hernia, the presence of which displaces the LES into the thorax and, number of environmental and physical factors have been identified that appear to influence the tone and contractility of the LES and these may play an etiological role in some cases of GERD. The pressure of the LES is lowered by fatty acids, chocolate, peppermint, cola, coffee and tea; nicotine, alcohol, drugs such as calcium channel blockers, the theophylline, and possible non-steroidal anti-inflammatory drugs (NSAID), elevated levels of estrogen and progestrone; and that conditions that elevate intra-abdominal pressure such as obesity, pregnancy or heavy lifting.

Pathophysiology

There are two zones of high pressure, one at each end of the esophagus, normally prevent the reflux of gastric contents. The zones maintain a constant pressure and relax only during swallowing. Although they are termed as LES, they are not really distinct anatomical structures. Esophageal reflux occurs when either gastric volume or intra-abdominal pressure is elevated or when LES tone is decreased. Periodic reflux occurs normally in most persons and is usually asymptomatic. The normal physiologic response to occasional reflux is immediate swallowing one or more rapid swallows induce peristatic contractions to clear the reflux and neutralize the acid with bicarbonate-rich saliva. However, the esophagus has only a limited ability to withstand the damaging effects of acid reflux and GERD will develop when frequent episodes of reflux breakdown the mucosal barrier and initiate an inflammatory response.

The degree of esophageal inflammation related to the number, duration and acidity or alkalinity of the reflux episodes. The effectiveness and efficiency of esophageal clearance also are important. Esophageal clearance is particularly important at night when the swallowing rate and salivation decrease by two thirds and recumbent position interferes with clearance. An inflamed esophageal gradually loses its ability to clear reflexed material quickly and efficiently, and the duration of each episode gradually lengthens. Hyperemia and erosion occur in the face of chronic inflammation. Minor capillary bleeding is common, although frank bleeding is rare. Repeated episodes of inflammation and healing can gradually produce a change in the epithelial tissue, which makes it more resistant to acid. Overtime, fibrotic tissue changes can also result in esophageal stricture, which can progressively impair normal swallowing.

Clinical Manifestations

- Heartburn is caused by irritation of the esophagus by the gastric secretion. It is a burning, tight sensation that appears intermittently beneath the lower sternum and spreads upward to the throat or jaw. It occurs following ingestion of substances that decrease LES pressure. It is relieved with milk, alkaline substance or water.
- Pulmonary symptoms including wheezing, hoarseness, coughing, (nocturnal cough), dyspnea are secondary to microaspiration of gastric contents into the pulmonary system.
- Gastric symptoms including early satiety, prostating bloating, nausea, and vomiting, are related to gastric stasis.
- Regurgitation is effortless return of material from stomach into esophagus or mouth, oftenly described as hot, bitter or sour liquid coming into the throat or mouth. This taste is perceived in the pharynx.
- Water brash a reflex, hypersecretion that does not have a bitter taste.
- Frequent belching and flatulence and feeling of lump in the throat or food stopping.
- Dysphagia difficulty in swallowing.
- Odynophagia painfull swallowing.
- Bleeching.

In addition GERD patients may experience complication of respiratory system—bronchospasm, laryngospasm, circopharyngeal system and other complications include:
- Esophageal stricture (due to repeated episodes),
- Esophageal metaplasia (Barretts esophagus),
- Pneumonia (due to aspiration of gastric contents to pulmonary system).

Management of GERD

Patients with GERD are rarely admitted to the acute care setting unless they require surgery or experience serious complications. The problem is self-managed in the outpatient setting. The goal of treatment is to decrease the incidence of reflux and eliminate the symptoms.

The diagnostic studies are performed to determine the causes are:
- Barium swallow for determining the protrusion of upper part of the stomach (gastric cardia).
- Radionuclide tests to detect reflux of gastric contents and the rate of esophageal clearance.
- Esophagoscopy—to detect the incompetence of LES and the extent of inflammation, potential scarring and strictures.
- Biopsy and cytologic tests to differentiate hiatal hernia, carcinoma and Barrett's esophagus.
- Esophageal motility (manometry) studies to measure pressure in the esophagus and GES.
- pH monitoring for presence of acid or alkaline. Pharmacologic management is focussed on improving LES function, increasing esophageal clearance, decreasing volume or acidity reflux, and protecting esophageal mucosa.

- Antacids are used to relieve heartburn by their neutralizing effect on hydrochloric acid. (For example, Gelucil, Maalox, Mylanta).
- Antacids plus alginic acid (Gaviscon) are used to neutralize gastric acid and reacts with sodium bicarbonate and forms a viscous solution that floats to the surface of the gastric contents and coats the esophagus acting on mechanical barrier to reflux.

  When client is an antacid and alginic acid, the nurse should evaluate the effectiveness of the drug, monitor frequency of use and monitor for constipation or diarrhea and assist patient to adjust product use as needed.

  Anti-secretory drugs, i.e. histamine (H2) receptors are used to reduce the gastric acid secretion and supports tissue healing which include ranitidine, cimetidine, famotidine, nizaoidine. During use of these, the nurse should instruct patient to take drugs with meals if ordered at intervals, and monitor for common side effects, fatigue, headache, diarrhea.
- Prokinetic drugs are used to increase LES pressure and enhance gastrointestinal motility, which includes cisapride (Propulsid). Here the nurse has to instruct patient to take drug no more than 15 minutes before eating and monitor levels of drugs that require useful titration.
- Proton pump inhibitors are used to inhabit enzyme system of gastric parietal cells and suppress gastric acid secretions by more than 90 percent. Here the nurse has to instruct patient to take the drug before meals and monitor for side effects, abdominal cramping, headache, diarrhea. For example, omeprazole, lansoprazole are PP inhibitors.

Surgical management: Antireflux surgery is usually performed in patient with severe GERD who do not respond to aggressive medical management which includes:
- Nissen fundoplication
- Hill gastropexy
- Belseys fundoplication
- Antireflux prosthesis.

Nursing Management

The nurse by using nursing process, assesses the client on the basis of clinical manifestation stated above and take body weight, ascultate for signs for reflux aspirates and observe for hoarseness or wheezing-day or night.

The nursing diagnosis are made from analysis of patient's data. The diagnoses are not limited to pain and knowledge deficit. The objectives of nursing care will include reports, minimal or no episodes of heart burn and list diet and life style changes. GERD is typically managed by using a combination of drug therapy, diet, and life style modification and assisting surgical therapies if needed.

The nurse discusses the medication regimen with the patient and ensures that written information about the safe use and expected side effects of all meciations is provided, and administer the ordered medication and observe for response and side effects; Antacids that contain aluminium tend to cause constipation, where as those contain magnesium tend to cause diarrhea. Several of the antacids are combination of aluminium and magnesium designed to minimize these effects. If the patient is taking bethenechol (cholenergic) side effects to observe for urinary urgency, increased salivation, abdominal cramping with darrhea, nausea, vomiting, and hypotension. Side effects of metadopramide (dopamine antogonist) a prokinetic drug includes restlessness, anxiety and insomnia. Side effects of sucralfate (acid-protective) include drowsiness, dizziness, nausea, vomiting, constipation, urticaria and rash.

When nursing the patient with GERD the nurse has to use the following. Diet and lifestyle modifications to manage the same:
- In relation to diet patient are encouraged to:
  - Eat 4-6 small meals daily.
  - Follow a low-fat, adequate protein diet.
  - Reduce intake of chocolate, tea and all foods and beverages that contain caffeine.
  - Limit or eliminate alcohol intake.
  - Eat slowly and chew food thoroughly.
  - Avoid evening snacking and do not eat for 2-3 hours before bed time.
  - Remain upright for 1-2 hours after meals when possible and never eat in bed.
  - Avoid any food that directly produces heart burn.
  - Reduce over all body weight if indicated.
- The nurse has to promote lifestyle of the patient by encouraging to:
  - Eliminate or drastically reduce smoking.
  - Avoid evening smoking, and never smoke in bed.
  - Avoid constrictive clothing over the abdomen.
  - Avoid activities that involve straining, heavy lifting or working in a bent-over position.
  - Elevate the head of the bed at least 6-8 inches for sleep using wooden blocks or a thick foam wedge.
  - Never sleep flat in bed.
- For prevention of GERD, the nurse should use the following teaching guidelines for patient and family.
  - Explain the rationale for a high-protein, low-fat diet.
  - Encourage the patient to eat small, frequent meals to prevent gastric distention.
  - Explain the rationale for avoiding alcohol, smoking (causes an almost immediate, marked decrease in LES pressure) and beverage that contains caffeine.
  - Instruct the patient not to lie down for 2 to 3 hours after eating, wear tight clothing around the waist, or bend over (especially after eating).

- Encourage the patient to sleep with head of bed elevated on 4-6 inch blocks (gravity fosters esophageal emptying).
- Teach regarding medication including rationale for their use and common side effects.
- Discuss strategies for weight reduction if appropriate.
- Encourage patient and family to share concerns about lifestyle changes and living with a chronic problem.

HIATAL HERNIA

Hiatal hernia is herniation of a portion of the stomach into the esophagus through an opening, or hiatus, in the diaphragm. It is also referred to as 'diaphragmatic hernia and esophageal hernia' (**Fig. 4.1A**).

Hiatal hernias are common in older adults and occur more frequently in women than in men. They are classified into two types (1) Sliding hiatal hernia and (2) Paraesophagical hiatal hernia.

- *In sliding:* The junction of the stomach and esophagus is above the hiatus of the diaphragm and a part of the stomach slides through the hiatal opening in the diaphragm. It "slides" into the thoracic cavity when the patient is supine and usually goes back into the abdominal cavity when the patient is standing upright (**Fig. 4.1B**).
- In paraesophageal or rolling, the esophagogastric junction remains in the normal position, but the fundus and the greater curvature of the stomach roll up through the diaphragm forming a pocket alongside the esophagus (**Fig. 4.1C**).

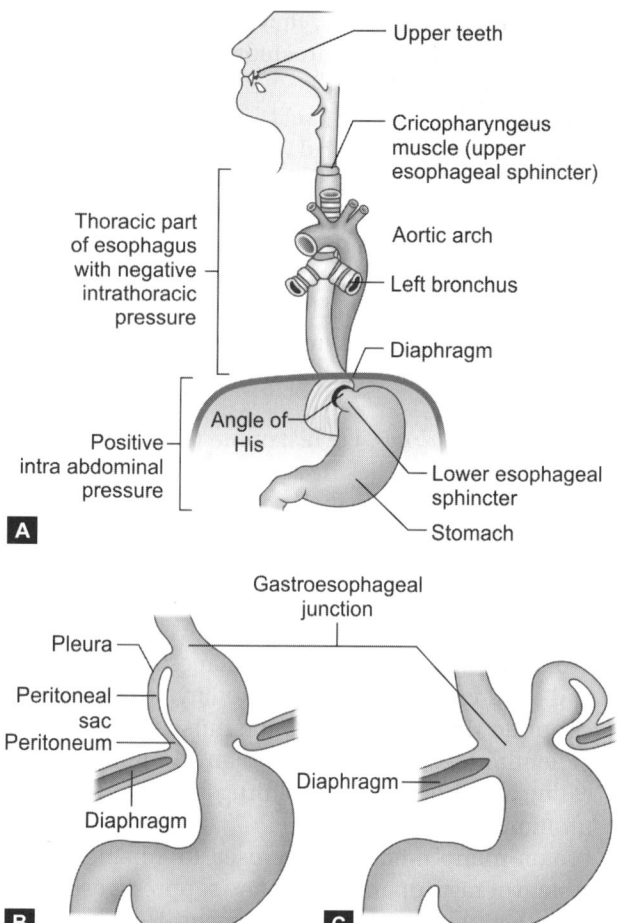

Fig. 4.1A to C: A. Normal esophagus; **B.** Siding hiatal hernia; **C.** Rolling or paraesophageal hernia.

Etiology

The actual cause of hiatal hernia is unknown. Many factors contribute to the development of hiatal hernia. Structural changes, such as weakening of the muscles in the diaphragm around the esophagogastric opening are usually contributing factors. Factors that increase intra-abdominal pressure, including obesity, pregnancy, ascites, tumors, tight corsets, intense physical exertions, and heavy lifting on a continued basis, may also predispose to development of a hiatal hernia. Other predisposing factors are increased age, trauma, poor nutrition, and forced recumbent position, as when a prolonged illness confines the person to bed. In some cases, congenital weakness is a contributing factor.

Pathophysiology

A hiatal hernia involves herniation of part of the stomach through weakness in the diaphragm. The resulting regurgitations and motor dysfunction cause the major manifestation of the hiatal hernia. With sliding hernias the problems are rarely anatomical. The problems relate directly to the functional consequences of chronic reflux. Reflux occurs from the ongoing exposure of the LES to the low pressure environment of the thorax where sphincter function is significantly impaired.

Reflux is rarely a concern with rolling hernias, because the LES remains anchord below the diaphragm. However, the anatomical risks of volvulus, strangulation and obstructions are high. In addition, venous obstruction in the herniated portion of the stomach causes the mucosa to become engorged and to ooze. Slow bleeding leads to the development of iron deficiency anaemia, but significant bleeding is rare.

Clinical Manifestation

Manifestation of hiatal hernia varies in kind and severity. In sliding hiatal hernia, clients may have heartburn 30 to 60 minutes after meals. In addition, reflux may result in substernal pain. The clients with a rolling hernia does not have manifestation of reflux but client may complain of a feeling of fullness after eating or have difficulty in breathing. Some clients experience chest pain similar to that of anginal pain. Pain is usually worse when the client assumes a recumbent position. Bending over may cause a severe burning pain which is usually relieved by sitting or standing. The other common factors of pain includes large meals, alcohol, and smoking. Nocturnal attacks are common especially if the person has eaten before going to sleep.

The complication that may occur with hiatal hernia includes problems such as hemorrhage from erosion, stenosis, ulceration of the herniated portion of the stomach, strangulation of the hernia, and regurgitation with tracheal aspiration. Severe chronic esophagitis may follow reflux problem.

Diagnostic Studies

A barium swallow is an important diagnostic measure that may show the protrusion of gastric mucosa through the esophageal hiatus in the patient with hiatal hernia. The other tests are similar that are performed in the GERD.

Management of Hiatal Hernia

Conservation therapy of hiatal hernia includes administration of antacids, and antisecretory agents, elimination of constricting garments, avoidance of lifting and straining, elimination of alcohol and smoking, and elevation of the head of the bed.

Elevation of the bed on 4 to 6 inch blocks assists gravity in maintaining the stomach in the abdominal cavity and also helps prevent reflux and tracheal aspiration. If obese, the client is encouraged to lose weight.

Surgical corrections of rolling hernias is mandatory because the risk of serous complications is significant. The objective of surgical interventions for hiatal hernia is to reduce reflux by enhancing the integrity of the LES. Surgical procedures are termed "Vulvoloplastics or antireflux" procedures. There are three slightly varied procedures namely:
1. The Hill gastropexy
2. The Nissen fundoplications
3. The Belseys fundoplication.

The diet and activities of hiatal hernia are as discussed in GERD.

Surgical Nursing Management of Hiatal Hernia

Preoperative teaching focus on instructing the patient in deep breathing, the correct use of an incentive spirometer and splinting the incision effectively, for coughing. The surgical approaches all involve the diaphragm, and pulmonary hygiene is essential in preventing respiratory complications. Individuals who are overweight are encouraged to lose weight if possible before surgery and smokers are encouraged to significantly reduce or eliminate their use of tobacco. The nurse also teaches the patient about nasogastric tube that will be inserted during surgery with open procedures and planned time frame for restarting oral feedings.

Postoperative care focuses on concern related to prevention of respiratory complications, maintenance of fluid and electrolytic balance, and prevention of infection. If thoracic approach is used, a chest tube is inserted. Assessment and management related to closed chest drainage are important. After surgical intervention, there should be no symptoms of gastric reflux. The patient should be instructed to report symptoms such as heartburn and regurgitation. A normal diet can be resumed within 6 weeks. The patient should avoid foods that are causing gas problems and should try to prevent gastric distension. Food should be thoroughly chewed.

ACHALASIA

Achalasia is a primary motility disorders of the esophagus, are conditions in which the normal function of the esophagus is disturbed which problem may be primary in the esophagus or secondary to another systemic disease (neuromuscular disorders, i.e. cerebrovascular accident, multiple sclerosis, myasthenia grans, amyotrophic lateral sclerosis, myopathic cranial nerve disease or traum 5th, 9th, 10th). The classic motility disorder is a failure of the esophageal muscle to relax in synchrony, which can result in mechanical or functional obstruction of good passage. Failure to close adequately after swallowing can also occur, resulting in chronic reflux or regurgitation. Esophageal spasm is common component of motility disorder and the spasm is usually intense enough to mimic angina.

As stated above Achalasia is the predominant primary disorder in which the lower esophageal muscles and sphncter fail to relax appropriately in response to swallowing.

Etiology

The cause of the achalasia is unknown, although a familial link is possible. It usually develops in early or middle adulthood and one-third of cases develop after age of 60 years and both sexes are affected equally.

Pathophysiology

Achalasia (cardiospasm) results from a neuromuscular defect that is localized in the inner circular muscle layer of the esophagus. Degeneration of ganglion cells causes both a failure of peristalsis and severe muscle spasm. Here the peristalsis of the lower third (smooth muscle) of the esophagus is absent.

Pressure in the LES is increased, along with incomplete relaxation of the LES. As the disease progresses, the portion of the esophagus around the constriction becomes dilated and the muscle walls hypertrophy. Obstruction of esophagus at or near the diaphragm occurs. Food and fluid accumulate in the lower esophagus. Although the severity of achalasia varies widely, the spasms may be so severe that little or no food can enter the stomach. In extreme cases, the esophagus may hold a liter or more food and fluid above the constricted area. The altered peristalsis is a result of impairment of the autonomic nervous system innervating the esophagus.

Chronic and progressively worsening dysphagia is the classic symptom and occurs more frequently with liquids. Spasm may be provoked by cold or hot liquids or foods and worsened by stress or overeating. Substernal chest pain (similar to pain of angina) occurs during or imemdiately after a meal. Halitosis and the inability to erucate are other symptoms. Another common symptom is regurgitation of sour tasting food and liquids especially when the patient is in horizontal position weight loss is typical. A foul mouth odor from retension of food and the esophagus may be a chronic problem.

Diagnostic Studies

The classic 'bird's beak narrowing plus dilation are readily observed with barium studies. Esophageal manometry reveals an elevated resting LES pressure, combined with diminished or absent peristaltic waves.

Management of Achalasia

Treatment of achalasia consists of dilation, surgery and use of drugs. All these therapies are directed at relieving the stasis caused by the increased LES pressure, non-relaxing LES, and aperistaltic esophagus. The aim of management is to relieve symptoms. Symptomatic treatment consists of semi-soft bland diet, eating slowly and drinking fluid with meals and sleeping with the head elevated.

Esophageal dilation (bougienage) is an effective treatment measure for many patients. Pneumatic dilation of LES with a balloon-tipped dilator passed orally is usually used. The commonly used dilators for pneumatic dilation are the Mosherbag, the Tucker mercury dilator, and Browne-McHardy dilator. They all depend on forcible expansion of a balloon in the LES. The forceful dilation does not restore normal esophageal motility, but it does provide for emptying of the esophagus into the stomach.

Surgical measures that may be necessary in the "Esophagomyotomy". In this procedure, the muscle fibers that enclose the narrowed area of the esophagus are divided. This allows the mucosa to pouch out through the division in the muscle layer to allow food to be swallowed without obstruction. Measure similar to this procedure is Heller's Myotomy (cardiomyotomy) which disrupts the LES in a similar manner and reduces LES Pressure. An antiregina procedure is frequently done with myotomy. This procedure can be performed laparoscopically, reducing the potential for postoperative complications.

Various classes of medications are used in the treatment of achalasia include anticholenergics and calcium channel blockers (e.g., nifedipine procardia), but none of them proved to be effective. Analgesics may be needed when pain is severe. Recent studies indicated that "botulinum toxin injection which relaxes esophageal muscle delivered endoscopically in the management of achalasia.

Health Education

The nurse works with the patient and family to explore diet and lifestyle modifications that will best control dysphagia, which is prominent in achalasia. Education begins with careful assessment of the scope and severity of dysphagia, which includes:

- Swallowing ability with liquids v/s solids.
- Response to foods of differing textures and temperature.
- Variability of the dysphagia (intermittant or constant).
- Response to stress, fatigue and other activities.
- Approaches used by the patient to manage the dysphagia and the degree of success.

The nurse encourages the person to experiment with various types and consistency of foods and meal sizes to evaluate their influence on swallowing. Small, frequent semi-soft meals, are usually best tolerated. Warm liquids are recommended, and extremes of temperature should be avoided because they usually worsen the spasm. The nurse also advises the patient to experiment with changing positions during eating. Some individuals can swallow more effectively if they arch their back. Use of the valsalva, a maneuver (bearing down with a closed glottis) while swallowing may help proper food beyond the LES. Nocturnal reflux of retained food and fluid presents a significant risk for aspiration. The nurse should instruct the patients to sleep on a foam wedge or with the head of the bed elevated. And suitable advices also should be given to the patient who has undergone surgical procedures.

ESOPHAGEAL CARCINOMA

Carcinoma of the esophagus is unique in its geographic distribution. Both benign and malignant tumors occur in the esophagus. Benign tumors are usually leiomyomas, and extremely rare and usually asymptomatic. They require no intervention unless symptoms necessitate local excision.

Malignant tumors of the esophagus are not common, but they assume increased importance because of their virulence.

Etiology

The cause of cancer of the esophagus is unknown. Possible predisposing factors are cigarette smoking, excessive alcohol intake chronic trauma, poor oral hygiene, and spicy foods. The most important risk factors include exposure to asbestos and metal and low intake of fresh fruits and vegetables.

Pathophysiology

Tumors may develop at any point along the length of the esophagus, but the majority occur in the middle and lower two-thirds of the esophagus. Squamous cell tumors have typically predominated. They tend to develop in the middle third and clearly related to the risk factors of smoking and alcohol use. Adenocarcinomas represent the remaining minority of tumors. These tend to develop in the lower third of the esophagus and may evolve from the Barret's epithelium. It is an acquired condition in which changes occur in response to acid irritation over a period of 1 to 2 years and its presence increases the risk of cancer.

Esophageal tumors of all types appear to emerge as a part of an initially slow process that begins with benign tissue changes. Local growth of the tumor is rapid, however, the early spread is common because of the rich lymphatic supply found in the esophagus. Tumors are characteristically intraluminal and ulcerating. With a tendency to encircle the esophageal wall, as well as extend upon down the length. The spread of cancer is by local invasion or through the bloodstream or lymphatics. Neoplasm of the upper and middle esophagus may extend into the pulmonary system and those of the lower esophagus into the diaphragm, vertebral or heart.

The common clinical manifestation of esophageal cancer are as follows:
- Early disease is largely asymptomatic.
- Gradually progressive dysphagia.
- Odynophagia—typically steady, dull, substernal pain.
- Regurgitation—foul breath, from retained food in esophagus.
- Heartburn, anorexia, weight loss.

The on set of symptoms is usually late in relation to the extent of the tumor. Progressive dysphagia is the most common symptom and may be expressed as a substernal feeling as if food is not passing. Initially the dysphagia occurs only with meat, then soft foods and eventually with liquids. Pain develops late and it is described as occurring in the substernal, epigastric, or back areas and usually increases with swallowing. The pain may radiate to the neck, jaw, ears, and shoulders. If the tumor is in upper third of esophagus symptoms such as sore throat, choking, and hoarseness may occur. Weight loss is fairly common. When esophageal stenosis is severe, regurgitation of blood-flecked esophageal contents is common.

The complication of the esophageal cancer will include the following:
- Hemorrhage may occur if the cancer erodes through the esophagus and into the aorta.
- Esophageal perforation with fistula formation into the lung or trachea may develop.
- Esophageal obstruction due to enlargement of the tumor.

Diagnostic Studies

- Barium swallow with fluoroscopy may demonstrate a narrowing of the esophagus at the site of tumor. Creater may be visible.
- Esophagoscopy with biopsy is necessary to make a definitive diagnosis of carcinoma by identification of malignant cells.
- Endoscopy—ultrasonography is also used to detect tumor invasion to muscle layer.
- Bronchoscopic examination may be performed to detect malignant involvements of the trachea.
- Computerized tomography scanning and magnetic resonance imaging are also used to assess the extent of disease.

Management

Treatment of esophageal cancer are based on the location and size of the tumor, degree of metastasis and the individual health status.

Non-surgical options are usually selected where the individual is unable or unwilling to undergo radical surgery. Surgery may not be performed if the patient is an older adult or in poor physical health. Palliative therapy consists of restoration of the swallowing function and maintenance of nutrition and hydration. Dilation, stent replacement or both can relieve obstruction. Laser therapy or vaporization with neodymium, yttrium aluminium-garnet (Nd:YAG) by means of endoscopy may be used in combination with dilation. Dilation is done with various types of dilators (celestin tube) to relieve dysphagia and allows for improved nutrition. Placement of a stent or prosthesis may help when dilation is no longer effective. The prosthesis are composed of silicone rubber or nylon-reinforced latex tubes with distal and proximal cellars.

Radiation therapy is the treatment of choice for palliation. It reduces tumor size and gives consistent long-term symptom relief. But it may lead to debilitating stricture or stenosis because esophageal tissue is extremely sensitive to radiation. The best results of esophageal cancer treatment have been obtained by the surgery and radiation.

Radical surgery is the only definitive treatment of esophageal cancer. The types of surgical procedures that can be performed are:
- Esophagectomy: Removal of part or all of the esophagues with the use of a dacrongraft to replace the resected pain.
- Esophagogastrostomy: Resection of a portion of the esophagus and anastomosis of the remaining portion of the esophagus.
- Esophagoenterostomy: Resection of a portion of the esophagus and anastomosis of a segment of colon to the remaining portion.

After surgery parenteral fluids are given. When fluids are allowed after bowel sounds have returned 30 to 60 ml water are given hourly with gradual progression to small, frequent, bland meals. The patient should be in an upright position to prevent regurgitation of the fluid. The patient is observed for signs of intolerance to the feeding or leakage of the feeding into the mediastinum. Symptom of leakage (pain, temperature, dyspnea) and food intolerance (vomiting and abdominal distension) should be monitored and suitable measures to be taken accordingly.

GASTRITIS AND DYSPEPSIA

Gastritis, an inflammation of the gastric mucosa, is one of the most problems affecting the stomach. The terms gastritis and dyspepsia are used in a highly non-specific manner by both lay persons and health care professionals. Gastritis refers to a diffuse of localized response of the gastric mucosa to injury or infection. The dyspepsia refers to a symptom complex of fullness, heartburn, bloating and possibly nausea that is typically experienced after eating and may not be accompanied to any histological changes in the stomach or duodenum.

Dyspepsia Syndrome

Dyspepsia syndrome: It is a syndrome of chronic dyspepsia, one of the most common GI complaints encountered in primary practice. The person experiences persistent or recurrent discomfort centered in the upper abdomen. There is no evidence of structural or biochemical abnormality and the cause is unknown. Study findings to date indicate that individual with dyspepsia syndrome have:
- Normal rates of acid secretion.
- Postprondial hypomotility and delayed gastric emptying, and 25 to 50 percent cases. Cause is unknown.
- Increased sensitivity of gastric distention, cause is unknown.
- No identified link with life stress or personality profiles.

Symptoms
- Epigastric discomfort or pain.
- Feeling of fullness or flatulence.
- Early satiety.
- Bloating or nausea.

Treatment of Dyspepsia Syndrome

There is no approved drug treatment, but
- Histamine receptor antagonists may be used for ulcer-like pain.
- Antacids may be used for occasional heartburn or bloating syndrome.
- Prokinetic agents (Cispride) are helpful in many cases.
- Diet and lifestyle changes are suggested will include:
  - Reducing dietary fat (it prolongs digestion, worsen bloating).
  - Avoiding foods that precipitate symptoms.

Gastritis may be acute or chronic and may be diffused or localized.

ACUTE GASTRITIS

Etiology of Acute Gastritis

Acute gastritis is short-term inflammatory process that can be initiated by numerous factors such as excess alcohol ingestion, drug effects (aspirin, NSAID, corticosteroids, etc.), severe physical stress or trauma, ingestion of caustic noxious substances, and bacterial contaminated water or food (*Staphylococcus, Salmonella* or *Staphylococci*).

Pathophysiology

Acute gastritis develops when the protective mechanism of the mucosa are overwhelmed by the presence of bacteria or irritating substances. In other words, gastritis occurs as the result of a breakdown in the normal gastric mucosal barrier. This mucosal barrier normally potects the stomach tissue from autodigestion by acid and the enzyme pepsia. When the barrier is broken, acid can diffuse back into the mucosa. This allows hydrochloric acid (HCl) to enter. The HCl acid stimulates the conversion of pepsinogen to pepsin and stimulates the release of histamine from mast cells. The combined results of these occurrences is tissue edema, disruption of capillary walls with loss of plasma into the gastric lumen and possible hermorrhage.

Regeneration of the gastric mucosa after injury is both prompt and efficient, however, and the disorder usually is self-limiting once the irritating agent is removed. The common symptoms of acute gastritis include anorexia, nausea, and vomiting, abdominal cramping or diarrhea, epigastric pain and fever. Painless GI bleeding, may occur and in persons using aspirin and NSAIDs.

Management

Acute gastritis cases are managed by removing the causative agent and supporting the patient while the mucosa heals itself. The person is usually put on nothing by mouth (NPO) status to support healing of the mucosa and then slowly advanced to liquids and a return to a normal diet. Antacids and histamine-2 (H2) receptor antagonists may be administered to reduce acid secretion and increase comfort. Temporary IV fluid and electrolyte replacement may be indicated in severe cases and the patient is monitored carefully for signs of bleeding.

The nurse also should give health instruction to prevent bacterial food-borne illness and concerning safe good handling and preparation. The nurse will educate the individual and family to take general measures to prevent food-related illness as follows:
- Wash hands before handling food.
- Do not thaw foods in the kitchen counter.
- Keep meats, fish, poultry, mayonnaise and cream-filled food, refrigerated.
- Wash hands and utensils after contact with raw meat or poultry.

- Never leave perishable foods unrefrigerated for more than 2 hours-less in hot weather.
- Use a meat thermometer when cooking large pieces of meat especially pork.
- Stuff poultry immediately before roasting (warm stuffing is a good medium for bacterial growth).
- Avoid slow cooling of meat and poultry.
- Freeze or refrigerate leftovers promptly.
- Can low-acid food (foods other than tomatoes or fruits) under pressure to prevent botulism.
- Discard any can that bulges.

CHRONIC GASTRITIS

Gastritis can occur from reflux of bile salts from the duodenum into the stomach as a result of anatomical changes following surgical procedures such as gastroduodenostomy and gastrojejunostomy. Prolonged vomiting may also cause reflux of bile salts, inflammation of the mucosal lining as a result of hypersecretion of HCl acid. The chronic gastritis can result from repeated episodes of acute gastritis.

Pathophysiology

Chronic gastritis is a separate clinical entity that can be further subdivided into Type A and Type B. Its presence is usually a sign of some underlying disease process.

- Type A is believed to be autoimmune in nature and involves all of the acid-secreting gastric tissue, particularly the tissue in the fundus. Circular antibodies are produced that attack the gastric parietal cells and eventually may cause pernicious anemia from loss of the intrinsic factor.
- Type B is related to the presence of *Helicobacter pylori* (*H pylori*). It primarily involves the antrum of the stomach. There is less reduction in the acid secretions, gastrin levels remain normal, and vitamin B12 absorption is rarely impaired. As the condition progresses, the mucosa increasingly atrophies, and acid secretion is reduced. The presence of *H pylori* has been correlated with the presence of other gastric disorders including gastric and duodenal ulcer and gastric cancer.

The clinical manifestation of chronic gastritis are similar to those described for acute gastritis. In addition eventually the body's storage of cobalmin (B12) in the liver is depleted and a deficiency state exists. Lack of this leads to deficiency of important vitamins which is essential for the growth and development of RBC results in development of anemia, i.e., cobalmin deficiency anemia.

Diagnostic studies include endoscopic examination with biopsy. Breath, urine, serum or gastric tissue biopsy tests are available for the determination of *H pylori*. CBC for presence of anemia, gastric analysis for presence of HCl acid and stool test for occult blood. Cytologic examination of carcinoma.

Management

The treatment of chronic gastritis focuses on evaluating and eliminating the specific cause (e.g., cessaction of alcoholic intake abstinence from drugs), currently double and triple antibiotic combinations are used to eradicate infection with *H pylori*. Original triple therapy consists of tetracycline + metronidaole + bismuth sub-salicylate × 14 days. New triple therapy includes amoxcilin + clarithromycin + omeprazole × 7 days.

For the patient with pernicious anemia, regular injection of cobalmin (vit. B12) are needed. An individualized bland diet and use of antacids are recommended.

UPPER GASTROINTESTINAL BLEEDING

Upper gastrointestinal bleeding is serious problem. The severity of bleeding depends on whether the origin is venous, capillary or arterial. The bleeding may be obvious or occult.

An obvious bleeding are:

- Hematemesis refers to bloody vomitus appearing as fresh, bright red blood or 'coffee ground' appearance (dark, grain-digested blood).
- Melena refers to a black, tarry stools (often foul smelling) caused by digestion of blood in the GI tract. The black appearance is from the presence of iron.
- Occult bleeding refers to small amount of blood in gastric secretions. Vomitus or stools not apparent by appearance detectable by guaiac test.

Bleeding from arterial source is profuse and the blood is bright red. It indicates that blood has not been contacted with gastric secretions. In contrast 'coffee ground' vomitus reveals that the blood and other contents have been in the stomach and have been changed by contact with gastric secretions. A massive upper GI bleeding is generally defined as a loss of more than 1500 ml of blood of 25 per cent of intravascular blood volume.

Etiology

The common causes of upper gastrointestinal bleeding includes:

- Drug induced: Some medications prescribed are self-administered and prolonged use causes bleeding which includes salicylates, corticosteroids, NSAIDS.
- Chronic esophagitis, Mallory-Weiss tear or syndrome, or esophageal varices, leads to upper GI bleeding.
- Peptic ulcer disease, stress ulcer, haemorrhagic gastritis, Ca. Polyps.
- Systemic diseases such as blood dyscrasias, leukemia and uremia.

Management

As the nurse begins care of the patient admitted with upper GI bleeding, a thorough and accurate assessment is made by taking important health information, including past health history. Use of medication as mentioned in the etiology and observe for signs of fever, shock, etc. Sometimes, patient experiencing upper GI bleeding may not be able to provide specific information about the cause of bleeding until the immediate physical needs are met.

An immediate nursing assessment should be performed while getting the patient ready for initial treatment. The assessment should include the patient's level of consciousness, vital signs, appearance of neck veins, skin color, and capillary refill. The abdomen should be checked for distension, guarding and peristalsis. Immediate determination of vital signs indicate whether the patient is in shock from blood loss and also provides a baseline blood pressure and pulse by which to monitor the progress of treatment. Signs and symptoms of shock include, low blood pressure, rapid, weak pulse increased thirst, cold, clammy skin, and restlessness. Vital signs should be monitored every 15 to 30 minutes and concerned doctor should be informed of any significant changes. Treatment of shock should be initiated promptly.

The patient should be approached in a calm and assured manner to help decrease the level of anxiety. Once an infusion has been started, the IV Line must be maintained for fluid or blood replacement. An accurate intake and output record is essential so that the patient's hydration status can be assessed. When the NG tube is inserted, the nurse pays her attention to keep it in proper position and observing the aspirate for blood. Care of nasogastric tube to be taken promptly.

Antacids are sometiems used after upper GI bleeding to reduce the acidity of gastric content. Anticipating the effect of prescribed preparations can be helped in providing better care. The expected outcomes of such bleeding cases will:
- Have no further GI bleeding.
- Have the cause of the bleeding identified and treated.
- Experience a return to a normal hemodynamic stage.
- Experience minimal or no symptom of pain or anxiety.

PEPTIC ULCER DISEASE (PUD)

Peptic ulcer is an erosion of the gastrointestinal (GI) mucosa resulting from the digestive action of hydrochloric acid (HCl) and pepsin. Any portion of the GI tract that comes into contact with gastric secretions is susceptible to ulcer development, including the lower esophagus, stomach, duodenum and margin of gastrojejunal anastomosis after surgical procedure.

Classification of PUD

Peptic ulcers can be classified as acute or chronic depending on the degree of mucosal involvement and gastric or duodenal according to the location:
- The acute ulcer is associated with superficial erosion and minimal inflammation. It is of short duration and resolves quickly when the cause is identified and removed.
- A chronic ulcer is one of long duration, eroding through the muscular wall with the formation of fibrous tissue. It is present continuously for many months or intermittently throughout the person's life time. A chronic ulcer is at least four times as common as acute erosion.

Gastric and duodenal ulcer although defined as peptic ulcer, are distinctly different in their aetiology and incidence, but generally treatment of all types of ulcer, is almost quite similar.

The differences between Gastric and Duodenal ulcers as given below:

Duodenal ulcer	Gastric ulcer
Lesion	
• Superficial; smooth margins round, oval, or cone shaped • Predominantly antrum, also in body and fundus of stomach	• Penetrating (associated with deformity of duodenal bulb from healing of recurrent ulcers • First 1–2 cm of duodenum
Gastric secretion incidence	

• Normal to decreased
  – Greater in women
  – Peak age fifth to sixth decade
  – More common in persons of lower socio-economic status and in unskilled labourers
  – Increased with smoking, drug and alcohol use
  – Increased with incompetent pyloric spincter
  – Increased with stress ulcers after severe burns, head trauma and major surgery
	• Increased
	  – Greater in men, but increasing in women in postmenopausal
	  – Peak age 35-45 years
	  – Associated with psychologic stress
	  – Increased with smoking, alcohol and drug use
	  – Associated with other disease, e.g., COPD disease hyperparathyroidism Zollinger-Ellison syndrome, chronic renal failure

Clinical manifestations	
• Burning or gaseous pressure in high left epigastrium and back and upper abdomen • Pain 1-2 hour after meals; if penetrating ulcer, aggravation of discomfort with food • Occasional nausea and vomiting, weight loss	• Burning, cramping, pressure like pain across midepigastrium and upper abdomen; backpain with posterior ulcers • Pain 2-4 hours after meals and midmorning, midafternoon, middle of night, periodic and episodic • Pain relief with antacids and food; occasional nausea and vomiting
Recurrence rate complications	
• High • Hemorrhage, perforation out-let obstruction, intractability	• High • Hemorrhage, perforation obstruction

Etiology

Peptic ulcers were once believed to be the direct result of acid over secretion in response to stressful events. This assumption is reflected in the traditional treatment, approaches, which emphasized acid neutralization and acid reduction. Although it is true that ulcers will not develop in the absence of acid, it is increasingly apparent that the primary etiological factors relate to:
- Infection by the organism *Helicobacter pylori (H pylori)* which produces a chronic gastritis.
- The side effects of NSAIDs administration. These factors target the mucosal defenses of the stomach and duodenum and can eventually lead to ulceration. The other factors are, like; decreasing or increasing of gastrical secretions lead to peptic ulcer.

Pathophysiology

The integrity of the gastric mucosa is maintained when a balance exists between the acid-secreting functions and mucosal protective functions of the stomach and duodenum. Peptic ulcers develop only in the presence of an acid environment. It has been well established that the patient with pernicious anemia and achlorhydria rarely has gastric ulcers. An excess of gastric acid may not be necessary for ulcer development. The typical person with gastric ulcer has normal to less than normal gastric acidity compared with person with a duodenal ulcer. However, some intraluminal acid does seen to be essential for gastric ulcer to occur.

The stomach is normally protected from auto-digestion by gastric mucosal barrier. Under specific circumstances, the mucosal barrier can be impaired and back-diffusion of acid can occur. When the barrier is broken, HCl acid freely enters the mucosa and causes injury to the tissue, this results in cellular destruction and inflammation. Histamine is released from the damaged mucosa, resulting in vasodilation and increased capillary permeability. The release of histamine is then capable of stimulating further secretion of acid and pepsin. Variety of agents are known to destroy the mucosal barrier, by generating ammonia in the mucus layer *H pylori* may create a chromic inflammation. Ulcerogenic drugs inhibit synthesis of mucus, e.g., aspirin cause abnormal permeability, e.g., prostaglandin, decrease the rate of mucous renewal (Corticosteroids), and destroy the broncosal barrier (Cytotoxic drugs). When the mucosal barrier is disrupted, there is compensatory increase in blood flow. This phenomenon can occur in several ways.

Clinical Manifestation

The clinical manifestation of gastric and duodenal ulcers (Fig. 4.2) may be completely symptomatic. Clinical manifestation associated with peptic ulcer disease are:

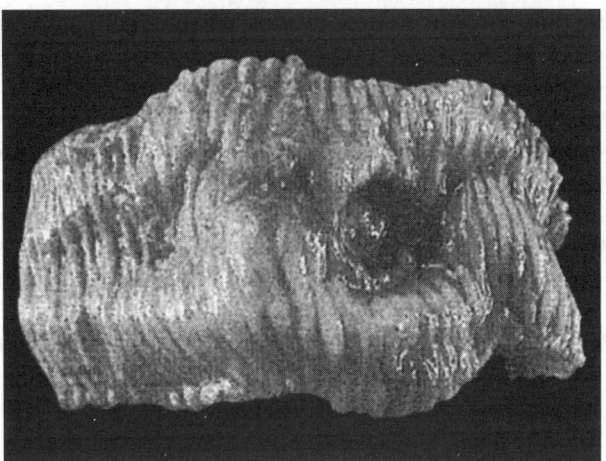

Fig. 4.2: Peptic ulcer of the duodenum.

Duodenal ulcer	Gastric ulcer
Pain	
• Episodic in nature lasting 30 minutes to 2 hours	• Dull epigastric location near midline
• Epigastric location near midline, may radiate around costal border to back	• Early satiety
• Described as gnawing, burning, aching	
• Occurs 1–3 hrs after meals and at night (12–3 AM)	
• Often relieved by food or antacid	• Not usually relieved by food or antacid

In both there is common manifestation including dyspepsia, syndrome, anorexia, weight loss. The complication of peptic ulcer are hemorrhage, perforation, gastrointestinal obstruction.

Diagnostic Studies

The diagnostic measures used to determine the presence and location of peptic ulcers are:

• Complete blood count	• Fibroptic endoscopy with biopsy
• Urinalysis	• Upper GI barium-contrast study
• Liver enzymes	• Gastric cytology
• *H pylori* testing of breath, urine, blood, stool	

Management

When the patient's clinical manifestations and health history suggest the diagnosis of a peptic ulcer and diagnostic studies confirm its presence, a medical regimen is instituted. The regimen consists of adequate rest, dietary modifications, medications, elimination of smoking and long-term follow up care:

- Adequate rest benefits the patient to elimination of stressors, help decrease the stimulus for overproduction of HCl acid.
- Dietary modification may be necessary so that foods and beverages irritating to the patient can be avoided or eliminated (alcohol and caffeine contents). A bland diet consisting of six small meals may be suggested.
- Smoking has an irritating effect on the mucosa, increases gastric motility, and delays mucosal healing. So it should be eliminated.
- Medications have major role in the treatment of peptic ulcers:
  - Antacids are weak bases that neutralize free hydrochloric acid to prevent irritation and permit mucosal healing.
  - Histamine receptor antagonists inhibit HCL secretion by binding to the H2 receptor on stomach cells and blocking, the release of histamine which is a secretogogue for HCl. Gastrict emptying is unaffected by their use, e.g., cimetidine, ranitidine, famotidine, nizatidine.
  - Bosom pump inhibitors more effective than H2 receptor antagonists, e.g., omeprazole, lansoprazole, pantaprazole.
  - Mucosol protective agents, sucralfate, misoprostol.
  - Antibiotic therapy is instituted for patients verified with *H. pylori*.

The nurse has to teach the following points for the patient and family members for self-care management, to the patients with peptic ulcer disease:

Medication (Table 4.2)
- Know the dosage, administration, action and side effects of all drugs in use.
- Take all the prescribed drugs, even when pain is relieved. It is essential to complete the full treatment.
- Keep antacids available for use as needed, but do not take them at the same time as H2 receptor antagonists. Antacids should be taken 1 to 3 hours after meals, at bed time and as needed for pain.
- Avoid the use of over-the-counter H2 receptor antagonists.
- Use acetaminophen for routine pain relief during treatment if needed. Avoid the use of all NSAIDs including aspirin, ibuprofen.
- If the treatment of arthritis or other chronic illness require the ongoing use of NSAIDS, explore the use of misoprostol with health care provider.
- Know the symptoms of ulcer recurrence and report them promptly to the health care provider.

Diet
- Eat three balanced meals a day.
- Eat snacks between meals if this helps control pain.
- Avoid bed time snacking because it increases night time acid secretion.
- Eat slowly and chew food thoroughly. Do not overeat.
- Avoid any foods that increase discomfort.
- Avoid the use of alcohol during treatment if possible. Never drink alcohol on an empty stomach.

Table 4.2: Durgs used in treatment of peptic ulcer.

	Effective dose	Maintenance	Side effects
Drugs used for acid suppression			
H2-antagonists			
Cimetidine (not used nowadays)	400 mg/12 hourly or 800 mg at night	400 mg at night	Confusion, diarrhoea, drug interaction and androgenic effects
Ranitidine and nizatidine	150 mg/12 hourly or 300 mg at night	150 mg at night	Same but less common
Famotidine	20 mg/12 hourly or 40 mg at night	20 mg at night	Same but less common
Proton pump inhibitors			
Omeprazole Lansoprazole Pantoprazole Rabeprazole	20–40 mg once daily; 30 mg once daily; 40 mg once daily; 20 mg once daily	20 mg at night; 15 mg at night; Not recommended; Not recommended	Hypergastrinaemia, diarrhoea, drug interactions, headache and rashes
Drugs which enhance mucosal defence and prokinetics			
Colloidal bismuth	125 mg 6 hourly	Not recommended	Blackens tongue, teeth, bismuth, toxicity on prolonged use
Misoprostol	200 µg 6 hourly	200 µg 6 hourly	Abortifacient, contraindicated in women of child bearing age
Sucralfate	2 g 12 hourly	Not recommended	May bind certain drugs, cramps diarrhoea, extrapyramidal effects
Dompridone	10–20 mg 8 hourly	Not recommended	Hyperprolactinaemia and dystonia

Smoking

- Stop smoking if possible.
- Explore community support for smoking cessation or use of nicotine withdrawal patches.

Stress Reduction

- Participate in recreation and hobbies that promote relaxation.
- Participate in a moderate aerobic exercise program for promotion of well-being.
- Provide for increased rest during healing.

Explain the importance of reporting of any of the following:

- Increased nausea and/or vomiting.
- Increase in epigastric pain.
- Bloody emesis or tarry stools.

The nursing care plan of patient with peptic ulcer disease is as follows:

Surgical Management of Peptic Ulcer

When the medical therapy has been tried and proved unsuccessful the surgery is indicated. The following criteria are used as general indication for surgical intervention:

- Intractibility: Failure of the ulcer to heal or recurrence of the ulcer after therapy.
- History of hemorrhage or increased risk of bleeding during treatment.
- Prepyloric or pyloric ulcers, both have high recurrence rates.
- Concurrent conditions, such as severe burns, trauma, or sepsis.
- Multiple ulcer sites.
- Drug-induced ulcers, especially when withdrawal from the drug may put the person at risk.
- Possible existence of a malignant ulcer.
- Obstruction.

Usually the surgical procedure performed to treat ulcer disease are partial gastrectomy, vagotomy or pyloroplasty.

Partial gastrectomy with removal of the distal two-thirds of the stomach and anastomosis of the gastric stump to the duodenum is called "gastroduodenostomy" or Billroth's operation. Partial gastrectomy with removal of the distal two-thirds of the stomach and anastomosis of the gastric stump to the jejunum is called as "gastrojejunostomy" or Billroth's II operation. In both procedures the antrum and pylorus are removed, because the duodenum is bypassed. The Billroth's II operation is preferred to prevent recurrence of duodenal ulcers.

Pain R/T

- Increased gastric secretion.
- Decreased mucosal protection.
- Ingestion of gastric irritants

(As manifested by burning cramp-like pain in epigastrium and abdomen).

- Pain onset 1-2 hours after meals with gastric ulcer.
- Pain onset 2-4 hours after meals.

Verbalization of Satisfaction with Pain Control

- Determine pain characteristics from verbal description and physical assessment data.
- Administer antacids, H2 antagonists, PP inhibition, anticholinergic, protective agents on prescribed to reduce pain.
- Teach the patient to avoid smoking and ingesting spicy, hot or cold foods, coffee, tea, and cold drinks and alcoholic beverages to prevent increasing acid production.
- Teach patients stress reduction as relaxation results in decrease acid products and reduction in pain.

Ineffective Management of Therapeutic Regimen R/T

- Lack of knowledge of management of peptic ulcer.
- Not following treatment plan.
- Unwillingness to modify lifestyles.

As manifested by request question about home care, incorrect responses to questions about disease. Noncompliance with medical regimen.

Verbalization of plan to modify lifestyle and incorporate therapeutic regimen into lifestyle.

- Explain ulcer disease process at patient level to faster understanding.
- Help patient to identify stressors and initiate modification in daily routine as stress causes hypersecretion of HCl and pepsin which can alter mucosal barrier.
- Discuss diet plan and assist with implementation at home and in work setting.
- Explain rationale for the elimination of alcohol, spicy foods, coffee, tea and cola from diets.
- Explain harmful effects of smoking which directly irritates gastric mucosa.
- Inform patient what to do if symptoms related to ulcer recur to ensure early initiation of treatment.
  Pain related to acute exacerbation of disease process and inadequate comfort measures.

As manifested by verbalization of increase in pain, non-verbal indication of pain, e.g., moaning, crying, doubling up.

Expression of Satisfaction with Pain Management

- Encourage bed rest or light activity to conserve energy and promote comfort.
- Provide quiet, relaxed environment and limit visitors to decrease stress and other factors that increase secretion.
- Administer medication as ordered to relieve pain.
  Vomiting R/T acute exacerbation of disease process.

As manifested by increase in nausea and vomiting. Decrease in or absence of nausea and vomiting.
- Maintain NPO status to prevent irritation of GI mucosa.
- Maintain NG tube to suction to keep stomach empty and remove any stimulus for HCl acid and pepsin secretion.
- Check vomitus or aspirate for occult blood to assess hemorrhage.

Potential for hemorrhage R/T eroded mucus tissue.
- Monitor for signs of hemorrhage.
- Carry out medical and nursing interventions if hemorrhage occurs.
- Assess for evidence of hematemesis, bright red melena stool, abdominal pain or discomfort. Symptoms of shock to pain appropriate action.
- If ulcer is actively bleeding, observe NG tube aspirate or emesis for amount and color to assess degree of bleeding.
- Take vital signs every 15 to 30 minutes to determine hemodynamic status and an indication of shock.
- Maintain IV infusion line to provide ready access for blood and fluid replacement.
- If RBC infusion given, observe for transfusion reaction for appropriate action.

(Write the responses and progress of ulcers)

Vagotomy is the severing of the vagus nerve, either totally (truncal) or selectively at some point in its innervation to the stomach. In a truncal vagotomy the nerve is severed bilaterally in both the anterior and the posterior trunk.

Selective vagotomy consists of cutting the nerve at a particular branch of the vagus nerve, resulting in denervation of only a portion of the stomach, such as the antrum or the parietal cell mass.

Pyloroplasty consists of surgical enlargement of the sphincter to facilitate the easy passage of contents from the stomach. It is most commonly done after vagotomy or to enlarge an opening that has been constricted from scar tissue. A vagotomy causes decreased gastric motility. A pyloroplasty accompanying vagotomy increases gastric emptying.

The combination of a Billroth I or II operation with vagotomy has the advantage of eliminating the ulcer and the stimulus for acid secretion. Surgical removal of the antrum results in removal of the source of gastrin secretion. Vagotomy eliminates the stimulus of HCl acid and gastrin hormone secretion caused by vagal stimulation.

The postoperative complication of peptic ulcer surgery.

Dumping Syndrome

Dumping syndrome is the term used for a group of unpleasant vasomotor and gastrointestinal system that occurs after surgery. It is associated with meals having a hyperosmolar composition. The onset of symptoms occurs at the end of a meal or within 15 to 30 minutes after eating. The patient usually describes feeling of generalized weakness, sweating, palpitations and dizziness. These symptoms are attributed to the sudden decrease in plasma volume. The patients complain of abdominal cramps, borborygmi and the urge to defecate. In addition, diaphoresis, tachycardia, feeling of fullness or discomfort, nausea, diarrhea, may be present. These manifestations usually last for longer than an hour after meal.

For which, prevention is the key and its management which includes small frequent meals, moderate fat, high-protein diet, limited carbohydrates, no simple sugars, minimal liquids with meals, avoiding very hot or very cold foods and beverages, and rest on left side for 20-30 minutes after eating. Anticholinergic or antispasmodic medication are useful.

Postprandial Hypoglycemia

Postprandial hypoglycemia is considered a variant of the dumping syndrome, since it is the result of uncontrolled gastric emptying of a bolus of fluid high in carbohydrate into the small intestine. The bolus of fluid concentrated carbohydrate results in hypoglycemia and the release of excessive amounts of insulin into the circulation. The symptoms experienced are sweating, weakness, mental confusion, palpitations, tachycardia, and anxiety.

The immediate ingestion of sugared fluids or candy relieves the hypoglycemic symptoms.

Bile Reflux Gastritis

Bile reflux gastritis occurs when surgery that involves the pylorus. Prolonged contact with bile damage, the gastric mucosa may cause bile reflux gastritis. The symptoms associated with epigastric distress that increases after meals. Vomiting relieved the distress but only temporarily. The administration of cholestyramine (Questran) either before or with meals are helpful to relieve bile reflux gastritis.

CANCER OF THE STOMACH

Cancer of the stomach is the most common malignant disease more prevalent among the lower economic class primarily living in urban areas. The male:female ratio is about 2:1. Gastric Cancer is rare before the age of 40, and the incidence increases sharply with age.

Etiology

The cause of cancer of the stomach remains unknown yet it is highly erratic. Worldwide incidence pattern suggests the involvement of multiple environmental, genetic and possibly cultural factors. Diet and living conditions appear to be the most significant aspects in etiology and early life

exposure is critical. The risk factors of gastric cancer will include the following:
- Diet high in smoked preserved foods which contain nitrites and nitrates.
- Diet low in fresh fruits and vegetables.
- High nitrate content in the soil and water.
- Presence of chronic gastritis and achlorhydria.

Pathophysiology

Gastric cancers are virtually all primary adenocarcinoma that are derived from the epithelium. They have been found traditionally in the pyloric and antral regions, particularly along the lesser curvature. There are numerous ways to classify gastric cancers, which manifest in a variety of forms. Histologically, the cancer is classified as diffused or intestinal. The intestinal form is associated with the presence of intestinal metaplasia in the stomach. The diffuse forms have believed to begin locally in the mucosa and exhibit a long latency.

Gastric cancers may spread directly through the stomach wall into adjacent tissues; to the lymphates, to the regional lymph nodes of the stomach; to the esophagus, spleen, pancreas and liver or through the blood stream to the lungs or bones.

Involvement of regional lymph nodes occur early. Prognosis depends on the depth of invasion and extent of metastasis.

Gastric cancer has an insidious onset. It is accompanied by vague non-descript dyspeptic symptoms that overlap with multiple benign disorders, including non-ulcer dyspepsia and peptic ulcer.

The possible clinical manifestations of gastric cancer are:
- Dyspepsia: Early satiety, bloating, anorexia.
- Epigastric pain or burning (usually mild and relieved by antacids).
- Mild nausea.
- Weight loss (may be rapid and severe).
- Fatigue and weakness.
- Change in the bowel habits; constipation or diarrhea.
- Marked cachexia and a palpable mass in the abdomen.

Diagnostic Studies
- Biopsy
- Lab analysis of blood, stool, gastric secretion
- Endoscopy
- Blood chemistry studies
- Barium meal
- Carcinoembryonic antigen (CEA) test
- CT Scanning

Management

When the diagnosis of gastric malignancy has been confirmed, the treatment of choice is surgical removal of the tumor. The preoperative management of the patient with gastric cancer focuses on the correction of nutritional deficits, treatment of anemia, and replacement of blood volume.

The nursing care of the patient undergoing gastric surgery (a total gastrectomy for gastric cancer-total gastrectomy with esophagojejunostomy) are as follows.

Preoperative Care
- Teach deep breathing exercises.
- Explain special postoperative measures; nasogastric tube and parenteral fluids until peristalsis returns.

Postoperative Care
- Promote pulmonary ventilation
  - Position patient in mid or high Fowler's position.
  - Encourage patient to turn and breathe deep at least q2h (or more frequently until ambulating well); Splint or support incision with hands or folded towel during coughing if needed to clear secretions.
  - Provide adequate analgesics during first few days.
  - Patient-controlled analgesia (PCA) is effective.
  - Encourage ambulation.
  - Provide good mouth care until oral fluids can be resumed.
- Promote nutrition
  - Measure NG drainage accurately, monitor for blood in drainage. Do not irrigate or reposition tube unless ordered.
  - Monitor for signs of leakage of anastomosis (dyspnea, pain, fever) when oral fluids are resumed.
  - Add food in small amounts at frequent intervals until well tolerated.
  - Monitor for early satiety and regurgitation.
  - If regurgitation occurs, tell patients to eat less food at a slower pace.
  - Report signs of dumping syndrome to doctor (weakness, faintness, palpitations, diaphoresis, nausea and darrhea).
  - Monitor weight.
- Provide patient/family education
  - Gradually increase amount of food each meal until able to eat 3 to 6 meals per day if possible.
  - If discomfort occurs after eating, decrease size of meals and amount of fluids with meals; eat more slowly.
  - Avoid eating simple carbohydrates and concentrated sweets.
  - Avoid stress during and immediately after meals; plan a rest period after eating. Lie on left side.
  - Elevate the head when lying down (if cardia of stomach removed).
  - Monitor weight regularly.

- Report signs of complications: Vomiting after meals, increasing feeling of abdominal fullness or weakness, hematemesis, tarry stools and persistent diarrhea.

IRRITABLE BOWEL SYNDROME (IBS)

Irritable bowel syndrome (IBS) is a symptom of complex characterized by intermittent and recurrent abdominal pain associated with an alteration in bowel function (diarrhea and constipation). Other symptoms commonly found include abdominal distention, excessive flatulence, urge to defecate, and sensation of incomplete evacuation.

Etiology

The cause is unknown. Much more common in women. Related to stress and excessive intake of food. Often linked to a history of physical or sexual abuse. Onset typically during late adolescence to mid-thirties. Most frequently encountered GI condition in Medical practice.

Pathophysiology

Major findings are rarely present. Lab tests are typically normal but colon spasticity can be visualized by X-ray and endoscopy. Increased small bowel motility plus increased frequency and amplitude of large bowel contraction occurs. Symptom patterns include:
- Spastic colon: Colicky abdominal pain, periodic constipation and diarrhea.
- Painless urgent diarrhea after meals.

Management

Treatment involves lifestyle modification and supportive care, i.e. Diet modification includes avoiding rich fatty foods, gas producing foods, gastric stimulants (alcohol and smoking) using medication such as bulk forming, antispasmodic, antidiarrheal and motility agents. In addition, adequate rest, stress management and regular aerobic exercises are advised.

DIARRHEA

Diarrhea is not a disease but a symptom. It is commonly used to denote an increase in stool frequency or volume and an increase in the looseness of stool. Diarrhea may be acute or chronic. Acute diarrhea, most commonly results from infection diarrhea is considered chronic when it persists for atleast 2 weeks or when it subsides and returns more than 2 to 4 weeks after the initial episode. Chronic diarrhea is usually related to changes in the GI tract, that alter the fluid and electrolyte balance.

Etiology

Causes of diarrhea can be divided into the general classification of decreased fluid absorption, increased fluid secretion, motility disturbances or a combination of them. The causes of diarrhea are:
- Decreased fluid absorption
  - Oral intake of poorly absorbable solutes (e.g., Laxatives)
  - Maldigestion and malabsorption
    - Mucosal damage: Tropical sprue, Crohn's disease, radiation injury, ulcerative colitis, ischemic bowel disease.
    - Pancreatic insufficiency.
    - Intestinal enzyme deficiency (e.g., Lactase)
    - Bile salt deficiency.
    - Decreased surface area eg. intestinal resection).
- Increased fluid secretion
  - Infections: Bacterial endotoxin (e.g., cholera, *E coli*, *Shigella*, *Salmonella*, *Staphylococcus*, *Clostridium*, *Campylobacter jejuni*).
    - Viral agents (Rotavirus, HIV).
    - Parasitic agents, *Giardia lamblia*, *Cryptosporidium*, *Trichinella*, hookworm).
    - Drugs: Laxatives, antibiotics, suspension or elixirs containing sorbitol (e.g., acetaminophen).
    - Hormonal: Vasoactive intestinal polypeptide (VIP) secretion from adenoma of the pancreas, gastrin secretion caused by Zollinger-Ellison syndrome, calcitonin secretion from carcinoma of thyroid.
  - Tumor: Villus adenoma.
- Motility disorders
  - Irritable bowel syndrome
  - Diabetic enteropathy
  - Visceral scleroderma
  - Carcinoid syndrome
  - Vagotomy.

The risk factors of acute diarrhea are:
- Recent travel to developing nations.
- Outdoor camping.
- Ingestion of raw meat, seafood, or shellfish.
- Eating at banquets, restaurants, picnics, or fast food centers.
- Day care placement of employment.
- Residence in institutions, nursing homes, prisons or mental institutions.
- Prostitution.
- Intravenous drug abuse.

Pathophysiology

Large-volume diarrhea is caused by hypersecretion of water and electrolytes by the intestinal mucosa. This secretion occurs in response to the osmotic pressure exerted by non-absorbed food particles in the chyme or from direct irritation of the mucosa. Peristalsis increased, and the transit time through the intestine is significantly decreased. Increased peristalsis may result from inflammation as mucosal cells hypersecrete water in the presence of infectious organisms. Diarrhea may be accompanied by severe abdominal cramping, tenesmus (persistent spasm) of the anal area, abdominal distension and borborygmus (loud bowel sounds).

Fluid and electrolyte imbalances can quickly result from diarrhea, depending on its severity. Mild diarrhea in adults can lead to losses of sodium and potassium (causing metabolic alkalosis). Severe diarrhea causes dehydration, hyponatremia, hypokalemia, and metabolic acidosis (from the loss of large amounts of bicarbonate). Malnourished or elderly persons tolerate severe diarrhea less well than do younger or well-nourished persons. Persistent diarrhea also readily leads to skin breakdown in the perianal region.

Clinical Manifestations

Bacterial or viral infection of the intestine may result in explosive water diarrhea, tenesmus (spasmotic contraction of anal sphincter with pain and persistent desire to defecate) and abdominal cramping pain, perianal skin irritation may also develop. Systemic manifestations include fever, nausea, vomiting and malaise, blood and mucus may be present in the stool depending on the causative agent as given below:

Viral (Rotavirus Norwalk)

Onset is 18-24 hours and duration 24-48 hours shows signs and symptoms include explosive, water diarrhea, nausea, vomiting and abdominal cramps.

Bacterial

- *Escherichia coli*: Onset 4 to 24 hours duration 3-4 days, signs and symptoms are four or five loose stools per day, nausea, malaise, low-grade fever.
- Enterohemorrhagic *E coli*: Onset 4-24 hours, duration 4-9 days signs and symptoms are bloody diarrhea, severe cramping, fever.
- *Shigella*: Onset 24 hours duration 7 days, signs and symptoms are watery stool containing blood and mucus, tenesmus, urgency severe cramping and fever.
- *Salmonella*: Onset 6-48 hours duration 2-5 days. Signs and symptoms are watery diarrhea, nausea, vomiting, abdominal cramps and fever.
- *Campylobacter species*: Onset 24 hours duration less than 7 days. Signs and symptoms are profuse watery diarrhea, malaise, nausea abdominal cramps, low-grade fever.
- *Clostridium perfringens*: Onset 8-12 hours duration 24 hours. Signs and symptoms are watery diarrhea, abdominal cramps, vomiting.
- *Clostridum difficile*: Onset 4 days after start of antibiotics, duration 24 hours. It is associated with antibiotic treatment, symptoms range from mild, watery diarrhea to severe abdominal pain, fever, leukocytosis and leukocytes in stool.

All these are treated with proper antibiotics and antidiarrheal drugs.

Parasitic

- *Entamoeba histolytica leads to amebiasis*: Onset 4-day duration weeks to months. Here ingested cyst releases active trophozite that invades and ulcerates intestinal mucosa. It can migrate to liver and cause abscesses. Clinical manifestations are: Abdominal cramping, frequent soft stools with blood and mucus (in severe cases watery stools), flatulence, distention fever, leukocytes in stool and reappearance of symptoms. It is treated by metronidazole for 5-10 days often in combination with other amebicides.
- *Giardia lamblia leads to Giardiasis*: Here infested cyst releases active trophozoite that infects the small intestine and onset is 1-3 weeks and duration is a few days to 3 months shows sudden onset, malodorous, explosive, watery diarrhea, abdominal cramping and bloating, malabsorption in severe cases. Treatment self-limiting in 2-6 weeks but may recur. Quinacrine (Atabrin or flage for at least 2-10 cases).
- *Cryptosporidium leads to cryptosporidiosis*: The parasite is present in birds, fish, cattle, sheet and spread by person to person contact and contaminated water. In which organism is ingested and primarily affects the small intestine. It can affect the entire GI tract in immunocompromised persons. It causes massive watery diarrhea, which exceeds 4L/day, if persistent malabsorption may develop-nausea and fatigue, abdominal cramps, weight loss in AIDS for which no effective therapy is available. Supportive treatment, replacement of fluid and electrolyte.
- *Trichinella spiralis causes trichinosis*: It is due to ingestion of undercooked pork and pork products. In which larvae of round worms infect the meat and mature in the intestine. Larvae are then released into blood and lymphatics and pass into striated muscle of the host where they encyst. Early state symptoms include nausea, anorexia, cramping and diarrhea, muscle pain and fever develop in 2-8 weeks can involve jaw, eyes diaphragm and heart, for which only symptomatic treatment can be available. Use of mebondazole or thiabendazole is helpful.

Diagnostic Studies

Accurate diagnosis and management require a thorough history, physical examination and when indicated Lab tests.

Management

The management of diarrhea involves the prevention of fluid and electrolyte imbalance, controlling the symptoms and treating the underlying cause if possible. Aggressive rehydration with oral replacement solutions is used if the person is alert and able to take oral fluids. Solutions such as the WHO solution, pedialyte, resol, and rehydralate are preferred to fruit juices, soda or even gatorade because they have balanced electrolyte composition plus glucose. Clear liquids are provided along with diets low in fiber but rich in sodium and glucose. Oral rehydration therapy with available standard ORS can be instituted.

The use of antidiarrheal agents are variable. Common medication for treatment of acute diarrhea are:

Local Acting

- Bismuth sub-salicylate (Pepto Bismol) mechanism not known may bind bacterial toxin.
- Kaolin and pectin (Kao pectate) which soothes the intestinal mucosa and increases absorption of water, nutrients and electrolytes.

These are in liquid form. So shake well before using. Bismuth product may turn the stool black. No significant side effects with Kaolin and pectin.

Systemic Acting Drugs

Include loperamide (imodium, tincture of opium (Paregoric), Diphenoxylate hydrochloride with atrophine (Lomotil). These drugs act systematically to reduce peristalsis and GI motility. Be aware that these drugs are part of the narcotic family; potential for addiction exists with paregoric. Loperamide has few side effects and no associated physical dependence. Lomotil has a low potential for dependency. So, monitor patient response, can enhance bacterial invasion and prolong excreation of the pathogen. Monitor for narcotic side effects-CNS depression or respiratory depression.

FECAL INCONTINENCE

Fecal incontinence or the involuntary passage of stool may be due to multiple causes.

Etiology

The causes for the fecal incontinence are:

Traumatic

- Obstetric
- Post-surgical
- Hemorrhoidectomy
- Anterior resection
- Fistulectomy
- Anorectal surgery
- Spinal cord injury

Neurologic

- Stroke
- Tumor
- Degenerative diseases
- Iatrogenic drug intoxication
- Multiple sclerosis
- Diabetes mellitus
- Dementia

Inflammatory

- Infections
- Trauma
- Radiation

Other

- Pelvic floor relaxation
- Perineal descent
- Loss of elasticity of rectum
- Decreased sphincter tone (age relaxation)
- Rectal prolapse
- Focal impaction
- Diarrhea
- Medications.

Pathophysiology

Normally fecal contents pass from the sigmoid colon into the rectum, causing rectal distention. Sensory (stretch) receptors in the muscles surrounding the rectum provide the sensation of rectal filling. This causes a reflex relaxation of the internal anal sphincter and contraction of the external anal sphincter. Sensory receptors in the epithelium of the anal canal can usually distinguish among solid, liquid, and gas. The combination of contraction of the abdominal muscles, relaxation of the pelvic muscles, squatting (which straightens the anorectal angle) and voluntary relaxation of the external anal sphincter allows for elimination of feces.

Management

The diagnosis and effective management of fecal incontinence require a thorough health history and physical examinations with appropriate diagnostic studies (as per causes stated above.) The nurse should identify normal bowel habits and current symptoms, including frequency and nature of the stools. The nursing diagnosis of the patient with fecal incontinence are:

- Impaired skin integrity r/t incontinence of stool and irritation in perianal area.
- Social isolation r/t embarrassment and odor.
- Self-esteem disturbance r/t inability to manage bowel evacuation independently.

  The overall goal is that patient with fecal incontinence will have normal bowel control.
    - Maintain perianal skin integrity
    - Not suffer any self-esteem problem.

Preventions and treatment of fecal incontinence may be managed by implementing a bowel-training program.

The patient should be put on a bedpan, assisted to a bedside commode, or walked to the bathroom at a regular time daily to assist with re-establishment of bowel regularity. Bowel training is the major approach used with patients who have cognitive and neurological problems resulting from stroke or other chronic diseases. If a person can sit on a toilet, it may be possible to achieve automatic defecation, when a pattern of consistent timing, familar surroundings, and controlled diet and fluid intake can be achieved. This approach allows many patients to defecate predictable and remain continent throughout the day. Surgical correction is possible for small groups of patients whose incontinence is related to structural problems of the rectum and anus. Perianal pouching is an alternative in the management of fecal incontinence. Pouching provides skin protection and fecal containment as well as comfort and dignity. Since odor is a problem; deodorant spray and room deodars can be used.

CONSTIPATION

The term 'Constipation' refers to an abnormal infrequency of defecation or the passage of abnormally hard stools or both. It may be defined as a decrease of frequency of bowel movement from what is "normal" for the individual, hard, difficult-to-pass stools, a decrease in stool volume, and retention of feces in the rectum.

Etiology

Frequently constipation may be due to insufficient dietary fibers, inadequate fluid intake, medication use, and lack of exercise. It may be due to sociocultural beliefs. Chronic laxative abuse, and multiple organic causes as given below:
- Colonic disorders
  - Luminal or extra-luminal obstructing lesions
  - Inflammatory strictures
  - Volvulus
  - Intussusception
  - Irritable bowel syndrome
  - Diverticular disease
  - Rectocele.
- Drug induced
  - Antacids (calcium and aluminium)
  - Antidepressants
  - Anticholinergics
  - Anticonvulsives
  - Antipsychotics
  - Antihypertensives
  - Barium sulfate
  - Iron supplements
  - Bismuth
  - Calcium supplements
  - Laxative abuse.
- Systemic disorders
  - Metabolic disorders: Diabetes mellitus, hypothyroidism, pregnancy, hypercalcemia, hyperparathyroidism.
  - Collagen vascular disease: Scleroderma, amyloidosis.
  - Neurogenic disorders:
    * Hirschsprung's megacolon
    * Neurofibromatosis
    * Autonomic neuropathy (pseudoobstruction)
    * Multiple sclerosis
    * Parkinson's disease
    * Spinal cord lesion or injury
    * Cerebrovascular accident.

Pathophysiology

Constipation may result from decreased motility of the colon or from retention of feces in the lesser portion of the colon or rectum. Dietary fiber increases the water content of the stool, and colonic motility is enhanced through the bacterial degradation of the fiber.

The longer the feces remain in the colon, the greater the amount of water reabsorbed and the drier the stool becomes. The stool is then more difficult to expel. Occassionally constipation is not detrimental to health, but habitual constipation leads to decreased intestinal muscle tone, increased use of valsalvas maneuver as the person bears down in the attempt to pass the hardened stool, and an increased incidence of hemorrhoids, in mass complication of chronic constipation. Diverticulosis is other complication.

The clinical manifestation of constipation are:
- Hard, dry stool
- Abdominal distention
- Decreased frequency of bowel movement
- Abdominal pain
- Straining
- Rectal pressure
- Tenesmus
- Increased flatulence
- Nausea
- Anorexia
- Headache
- Palpable mass
- Stool with blood
- Urinary retention
- Dizziness

Management of Constipation

A thorough history and physical examination should be performed, so that the underlying causes of constipation can be identified and treatment started. Usual diagnostic studies can be followed accordingly.

Most causes of constipation can be managed by/with the diet therapy including dietary fiber and fluid and an exercise program. Laxatives should always be used cautiously because with chronic overuse, they may become a cause of constipation (**Table 4.3**).

The common cathartic agents used in constipation are:
- Bulk forming agents absorb water, increase bulk, thereby stimulating peristalsis in which polysaccharides and cellulose derivatives mix with intestinal fluids, swell and stimulate peristalsis, e.g., psyllium, methyl cellulose. During its use, ensure adequate fluid intake to prevent impaction or obstruction. Take separately from presribed drugs to avoid problems with absorption.
- Emollients are stool softeners and lubricants, which lubricate intestinal tract and soften feces, making hard stools easier to pass, do not affect peristalsis, e.g., Docusate sodium, Docusate calcium. These docusate salts act as a detergent in the intestine, reducing surface tension, which facilitates the incorporation of liquid and fat, softening the stool. The preparations lose effectiveness with long-term use. Discontinue if abdominal cramping occurs.
- Lubricants, i.e. mineral oils, soften fecal matter by lubricating the intestinal mucosa, facilitating easy stool passage. Excessive use interfere with absorption of fat soluble vitamins A, D, E and K leading to deficiency. These mineral oils should not take with meals or drugs, because oils can impair absorption, swallow carefully to prevent lipid aspiration.
- Hyperosmolar laxatives like lactulose, polyethyline glysol, sorbitol, which nonabsorbable sugars are degraded by colonic bacteria and increase stool osmolarity. Fluid is drawn into the intestine, stimulating peristalsis. When these are used, adjust the dose and frequency of administration to control side effects and regulate defection. Monitor for fluid and electrolyte imbalance, if response is severe.
- Saline laxatives cause osmotic retention of fluid which distends the colon and increases peristalsis, e.g.,

Table 4.3: Laxatives.

Class and agent	Dose	Action	Side effects
Bulk forming, e.g.			
• Ispaghula husk • Methylcellulose	• 4–6 g/oral	• Increase stool bulk	• Obstruction, if taken without water, impaction at or above stricture
Stimulants			
• Bisacodyl • Castor oil • Phenolphthalein • Senna	• 5–15 mg/oral • 15–60 mL/oral • 30–270 mg/oral	• Contact laxatives • Increase motility and secretion • Stimulate motor activity	• Gastric irritation, malabsorption and rectal stimulation, skin rash, photosensitivity
Emollients			
• Docusate sodium	• 50–360 g/oral	• Surfactent action facilitates mixture of colonic contents to soften stool	• Skin rash
Lubricants			
• Mineral oil	• 15–45 mg/oral or as enema	• Penetrates and softens stools	• Malabsorption, lipid pneumonia
Osmotic			
• Magnesium salts, e.g., hydroxide • Lactulose or lactitol	• 5–15 g/oral • 15–60 mg/oral	• Osmotic effect • Degraded products like short-chain fatty acid stimulates stool osmolality	• Magnesium toxicity • Abdominal bloating
Others			
• Polyethylene glycol (used for bowel preparation before surgery) • Glycerine	• 2 L/oral • Suppository or enema	—	• Abdominal bloating
Suppositories			
• Bisacodyl and glycerin		• Local effect	
Enemas			
• Arachis oil, docusate sodium, hypertonic phosphate, sodium citrate		• Local effect	

magnesium citrate, Mg. sulfate, Mg. hydroxide. The liquids preparations are more effective than tablets. Take with full glass of water. Monitor for fluid and electrolyte imbalance if response is severe.
- Stimulants increase peristalsis by irritating colon wall and stimulating enteric nerves, e.g., cascara sagroda, senna, Bisa-codyl (Bulcolax), castor oil. Cramps and diarrhea can occur. Monitor for fluid and electrolyte imbalance if reaction is severe.

Nursing management should be based on the patient symptoms and the assessment of the patient. An important role of the nurse is teaching the patient the importance of dietary measures to prevent constipation. The following are teaching guidelines for the patient with constipation:
- Eat dietary fiber
  - Eat 20 to 30 grams of fiber per day. Gradually increase amount of fiber eaten over 1 to 2 weeks. Fiber softens hard stools and add bulk to stool, promoting, evacuation. Food high in fiber; Raw vegetable and fruits, beans.
- Drink fluids
  - Drink 3 quarts per day. Drink water or fruit juice, avoid coffee, tea and cola.
- Exercise regularly
  - Walk, swim, or bike at least three times per week.
  - Contract and relax abdominal muscles when standing or by doing sit-ups to strengthen muscles and prevent straining.
  - Exercises stimulates bowel motility and moves stools through the intestine.
- Set a regular time to defecate.
- Do not delay defecations
  - Respons to the urge to have bowel movement as soon as possible.
  - Delaying defecation results in hard stools and decreased 'urge' to defecate.
  - Water is absorbed from stool by the intestine over time.
  - The intestine becomes less sensitive to the presence of stool in the rectum.
- Record your bowel eliminating time: Develop a habit of recording when you have a bowel movement on your calender. Regular monitoring of bowel movement will assist in early problem identification.
- Avoid laxatives and enemas: Do not overuse laxatives and enemas as they can actually cause constipation. The normal motility of the bowel is interrupted and bowel movements slow or stop.

ACUTE ABDOMEN

The patient with an acute abdomen has an acute onset of abdominal pain requiring prompt decision-making. Many disorders must be ruled out before a diagnosis is confirmed.

Etiology

Causes of an acute abdomen are varied as follows:
- Abdominal penetrating trauma
- Acute ischemic bowel
- Appendicitis
- Bowel obstruction with perforation or necrosis
- Cholecystitis
- Crohn's disease
- Diverticulosis with peritonitis
- Foreign body perforation
- Gastritis
- Gastroenteritis
- Mesenteric adenitis
- Pancreatitis
- Pelvic inflammatory disease
- Perforated gastrointestinal malignancy
- Peritonitis
- Ruptured abdominal aneurysm
- Ruptured ectopic pregnancy
- Ruptured ovarian cyst
- Ulcerative colitis
- Uterine rupture
- Volvulus.

Clinical Manifestation

Pain is the most common presenting symptom. The patient also complains abdominal tenderness, vomiting, diarrhea, constipation, flatulence, fatigue, fever, and increase in abdominal girth.

Management

Assessment begins with a complete history and physical examination including rectal and pelvic examination. CBC, urinalysis abd. X-ray, ECG, pregnancy test (for ladies) are also performed to get some clue for causes of acute abdomen. An assessment finding will include:
- Diffuse, localized, dull, burning or sharp, abdominal pain and tenderness.
- Rebound tenderness
- Abdominal distention
- Abdominal rigidity
- Nausea, vomiting
- Diarrhea
- Hematemesis
- Melena.

In addition, signs and symptoms of hypovolemic shock:
- Decreased blood pressure
- Decreased pulse pressure
- Tachycardia
- Cool, clammy skin
- Decreased level of consciousness.

Acute abdomen requires an emergency management. The goal of which is to identify and treat the cause. Because

many causes of which do not require surgery. An initial intervention will include:
- Ensure patent airway
- Administer oxygen via nasal cannula or nonbreather mask.
- Establish IV access with large bore catheter and infuse warm normal saline or lactated Ringer's solution.

Insert additional large bore catheter if shock is present.
- Obtain blood for CBC; electrolytes.
- Anticipate order for amylase, pregnancy test, clotting studies and type and crossmatch as appropriate.
- Obtain urinalysis.
- Insert nasogastric (NG) tube as needed.
- Monitor vital signs, level of consciousness, O_2 saturation, intake and output.
- Assess quality and amount of pain.
- Anticipate surgical intervention.
- Keep NPO.

ABDOMINAL TRAUMA

Injuries to the abdominal area most often occur as a result of blunt trauma or penetration injuries. (i) Blunt trauma usually occurs due to falls, motor vehicle collisions, pedestrian event, assault with blunt object, crash injuries and explosions. (ii) Penetrating injuries are due to stab, knife, gunshot wounds and other reasons. Regardless of whether it is blunt or penetration injury, the result is often the same damage to/or alteration of the internal organs.

Common injuries of the abdomin includes lacerated liver, ruptured spleen, pancreatic trauma, mesenteric artery tears, diaphragmatic rupture, urinary bladder rupture. These injuries may result in massive blood loss and hypovolemic shock. Surgery (laparotomy) is performed as early as possible to repair the damaged organs and to stop bleeding. Common sequelae of intra-abdominal trauma are peritonitis and massive infection, particularly when the bowel is perforated.

Clinical Manifestations

The clinical manifestations of abdominal trauma are:
- Guarding and splinting of the abdominal wall.
- A hard, distended abdomen (indicating intra-abdominal bleeding).
- Decreased or absent bowel sounds.
- Contusions, abrasions or bruising over abdomen.
- Abdominal pain.
- Pain over the scapula caused by irritation of the phrenic nerve by free blood in the abdomen.
- Hematemesis of hematuria and so.
- Signs of hypovolemic shock.
- An ecchymotic discoloration around the umbilicus (collens sign) can indicate intra-abdominal or retroperitoneal hemorrhage.

Intraabdominal injuries are often associated with rib fractures, fractured femur, fractured pelvis, and thoracic injury. If any of these injuries are present, the patient should be observed for abdominal trauma.

Management

Routine diagnostic procedures include CBC, urinalysis, X-ray of abdomen, CT Scan and peritoneal lavage. For emergency management of the abdomenal trauma focuses on establishing a patent airway, and adequate breathing fluid replacement and prevention of hypovolemic shock. The nursing intervention will include:
- Ensure patent airway.
- Administer oxygen via non-breather mask.
- Control external bleeding with direct pressure or sterile pressure dressing.
- Establish IV access with large bore catheters and infuse warm normal saline or lactated Ringers solutions.
- Obtain blood for type and crossmatch and CBC.
- Remove clothing.
- Stabilize impaled objects with bulky dressing.
- Cover-protruding organs or tissue with sterile, saline dressing.
- Insert indwelling urinary catherter if there is no blood at the meatus, pelvic fracture, or boggy prostate.
- Obtain urine for urinalysis.
- Insert NG tube if no evidence of facial trauma.
- Anticipate diagnostic peritonial lavage.
- Monitor vital signs, level of consciousness, O_2 saturations and urine output.
- Maintain patient's warmth using blankets, Warm IV fluids or Warm humidified oxygen.

Regardless of the mechanism of injury, physical evidence of abdominal trauma in a patient who is hemodynamically unstable, mandates immediate laparotomy, for which routine preoperative procedure and postoperative intervention will be followed in addition to specific intervention.

APPENDICITIS

Appendicitis is an inflammation of the vermiform appendix, a narrow blind tube that extends from the inferior part of the ceacum usually just below the ileocecal valve.

Etiology

The most common causes of appendicities are obstructions of the lumen by a fecalith (accumulated feces), foreign bodies, tumor of the cecum or appendix, or intramural thickening caused by lymphoid hyperplasia.

Pathophysiology

The inflammatory process of the appendicitis can involve all or part of the appendix. Intraluminal pressure increases, leading to occlusion of the capillaries and venules and vascular endorgement. Bacterial invasion follows and microabscesses may develop in the appendiceal wall or surrounding tissue, which, unless treated, can progress to gangrene and perforation within 24 to 36 hours. If the inflammatory process develops fairly, slowly the infection may be successfully be walled off in a local abscess. In more rapidly developing cases, the risk of rupture and acute peritonitis is quite high.

Clinical Manifestations

The clinical manifestations of appendicits is abdominal pain that comes in waves. The pain is persistent and continuous, eventually shifting to the right lower quadrant and localizing at McBurney's point (located half way between the umbilicus and the right iliac crest). It typically begins with periumbilical pain, followed by anorexia, nausea, and vomiting. Further assessment of the patient reveals localized tenderness, rebound tenderness and muscle guarding. The patient usually prefers to lie still, often with right leg flexed. Low-grade fever may or may not be present, and coughing aggravates pain. Rovsing's sign may be elicited by palpation of the left lower quadrants, cauing pain to be felt in the right lower quadrant, complications of acute appendicites are performation, peritonitis and abscesses.

Management

The diagnosis of appendicits is made from the classic physical and laboratory indicators when they are present. The patient with abdominal pain is advised to see physician and to avoid self-treatment. Until then the patient is advised to take anything by mouth. (NPO) to ensure that stomach is empty in the event of surgery is needed. An icebag may be applied to the right lower quadrant to decrease the flow of blood to the area and impede the inflammatory process. Heat is never used because it may cause appendix to rupture.

Surgery is usually performed as soon as a diagnosis is made. Pre and postoperative nursing management is similar to that of patients after laparotomy or any surgical treatment. In addition, patient should be observed for evidence of peritonitis.

PERITONITIS

Peritonitis involves either a local or generalized inflammation of the peritoneum, the membranous lining of the abdomen, that covers the viscera. Peritonitis may be primary or secondary, aseptic or septic and acute or chronic.

Etiology

Primary peritonitis usually caused by bacterial infection, bloodborne organism, genital tract organism and cirrhosis with ascites. Whereas secondary peritonitis often results from trauma, surgical injury or chemical irritations, which includes ruptured appendix, perforated peptic ulcer, diverticulitis, pelvic inflammatory disease, urinary tract infections, or trauma, bowel obstructions and surgical complications.

Peritonitis may appear in acute or chronic forms, and trauma or rupture of an organ containing chemical irritants or bacteria, which are released into peritoneal cavity, e.g., gastric ulcer perforations and ruptured ectopic pregnancy. Bacterial peritonitis can be caused by a traumatic injury (e.g., gunshot wound ruptured appendix) or it can be secondary to other diseases or conditions (e.g., pancreatitis, peritoneal dialysis).

Pathophysiology

The peritoneal lining serves as a semipermeable membrane lining that allows the flow of water and electrolytes between the blood stream and peritoneal cavity. When peritonitis occurs, fluid can shift into the abdominal cavity at a rate of 300 to 500 ml/hr in response to acute inflammation. The inflammatory process also shunts extra blood to the inflamed areas of the bowel to contract the secondary bacterial infection and peristalsis typically ceases. The bowel increasingly becomes distended with gas and fluid. The circulatory fluid and electrolyte changes can rapidly become critical. Local reaction of the peritoneum include redness and inflammation and the production of large amounts of fluid that contains electrolytes and proteins. Hypovolemia, electrolyte imbalance, dehydration, and finally shock can develop. This loss of circulatory volume is proportional to the severity of peritoneal involvement. The fluid usually becomes purulent as the condition progresses and as the bacteria becomes more numerous. The bacteria also may enter the blood and cause septicemia.

Clinical Manifestation

Abdominal pain is the most common symptom of peritonitis. A universal sign of peritonitis is tenderness over the involved area. Rebound tenderness, muscular rigidity, and spasm are other major signs of irritation of the peritoneum. Abdominal distentions, or ascites, fever, tachycardia, tachypnea, nausea, vomiting, altered bowel habits may also be present. These manifestations vary depending on severity and acuteness of the underlying cause. Complications of peritonitis include hypovolemic shock, septicemia, intra-abdominal abscess, paralytic ileus, and organ failure.

Diagnostic Studies

- CBC
- Serum electrolytes
- Abdominal X-ray
- Abdominal paracentesis and culture of fluid
- CT Scan or ultrasound
- Peritonoscopy.

Management

The goal of management of peritonitis are to identify and eliminate the cause, combat infection, and prevent complications. Patients with milder cases of peritonitis or those who are poor surgical risks may be managed non-surgically. Treatment consists of antibiotics, NG suction, analgesics, and IV fluid administration.

Patient who requires surgery need preoperative preparation as described earlier. Those patients may need total parenteral nutrition (TPN) because of increased nutrition requirement. Postoperative nursing management is similar to that provided for any surgical patient who has undergone abdominal surgery.

DIVERTICULITIS

Diverticula are small outpouchings or herniation of the mucosal lining of the gastrointestinal track. Diverticulosis has been described as a disease of west because its higher incidence in developed countries. The incidence of the disease should wide geographic variation that are at least partly attributable to the quantity of non-absorbable dietary fiber. Low-fiber diets have been shown to increase intraluminal pressure in the bowel but aging also appears to change the composition of the bowel which decreases its tensile strength.

Pathophysiology

Diverticula tend to form at point in the colon wall where blood vessels penetrate the mucosal and muscular layers, creating points of relative weakness. The increased muscular contractions in the sigmoid colon that are generated to push stool in the rectum increase both the thickness of the muscle and the intraluminal pressure. The weaker connective tissue then herniates between the circular muscle and the intraluminal pressure, the weaker connective tissue then herniates between the circular muscle band and forms the diverticula.

Diverticulitis frequently develops in a single diverticulum in response to irritation initiated by trapped foecal material. Blood supply to the area decreases, and bacteria proliferates in the obstructed diverticulum. Perforation of the dome may occur, which, if small is usually quickly and effectively walled off. Large perforation may progress to abscess formation or general peritonitis. Generalized inflammation can result in thickening and scarring of the bowel wall.

Clinical Manifestations

Usually diverticular disease is asymptomatic, but mild inflammation can trigger a nonspecific bowel dysfunction that resolves in a matter of hours or days. The clinical manifestations of diverticulitis reflect the inflammation of the diverticula or the developments of complication. Cramps lower left quadrant abdominal pain accompanied by low grade fever in classic sign.

The pain is triggered by muscle spasms of the sigmoid colon and is acute and persistent in nature. Nausea, vomiting, and a feeling of bloating are also common. The inflammatory process also frequently involves the bladder and cause urinary symptoms. The development of abscess initiates the symptoms of localised peritonitis. Diverticular disease is one of the most common cause's of GI bleeding. Meckel's diverticulum is a congenital abnormality in which a blind tube, similar in structure to the appendix is present, which is usually open into the distal ileum near the ileocecal valve. The tube may be attached to the umbilicus by a fibrous band.

Management

The preliminary diagnosis of diverticulitis may be made from the history and presenting symptoms. CT scan, barium enema reveals presence of abscess and diverticular pouches respectively.

An episode of diverticulitis is managed by resting the bowel. Hospitalization may be required in acute episodes. The patient is given nothing by mouth and regimen of IV fluids, antibiotics, anticholinergic (Probanthine) is started to reduce bowel spasm. Mild cases managed at home environment. Acute diverticulitis usually subsides with conservative medical management. However, surgical intervention may be needed to deal with complications.

Nursing care during an acute episode is largely supportive and focussed on patient comfort. The nurse teaches rationale for bed rest and bowel rest and the role of there interventions play in bowel healing. The nurse monitors fluid and electrolytes balance and status of the pain. The patient is regularly assessed for complications. Asymptomatic diverticulosis is managed by prevention of constipation through the use of a high-fiber diet. Encourage mere fluid intake (2500 ml to 3000 ml/day). Diet modification may be made by allowing foods high in fiber with emphasis on cellulose and hemocellulose type (wheat, whole grain breads and cereals, peas, carrots, seedless grapes, lettuce, peaches, prunes) and avoiding foods containing nuts and seeds, or indigestible strings or threads (cucumbers, celery, tomatoes, corn pop, strawberries, rasoberries, pea-nuts and seeds). The patient is also encouraged to avoid activities that increase intra-abdominal pressure. Weight loss may be recommended in the attempt to lower the baseline levels of intra-abdominal pressure.

INFLAMMATORY BOWEL DISEASE (IBD)

Inflammatory is an umbrella term used to describe conditions that are characterised by bowel inflammation. Crohn's disease and ulcerative colitis are the two major forms of IBD. They have distinctly different pathological characteristics but share among overlapping features.

Etiology

Exact cause is unknown. The passive causes include:
- An infectious agent (bacteria, virus)
- An autoimmune reaction from the presence of immune-related disorder
- Food allergies
- Heredity.

ULCERATIVE COLITIS

Ulcerative colitis characterized by inflammation and ulceration of the colon and rectum. It may occur at any age but peaks between the ages of 15 and 25 years. There is a second, smaller peak onset between 50-80 years. It affects both sexes but has higher incidence in women.

Pathophysiology and ClinicaL Manifestation

The inflammation of ulcerative colitis is diffuse and involves the mucosa and submucosa. With alternate periods of exacerbations and remissions the disease is usually begun in the rectum and sigmoid colon and spreads up the colon in a continuous pattern. The mucosa of the colon is hyperemic and endematous in the affected area. Multiple abscesses develop in the crypts of the Lieberkühn (intestinal gland). As the disease advances the abscesses break through the crypts into the submucosa, leaving ulceration. These ulcerations also destroy the mucosal epithelium, causing bleeding and diarrhea. Losses of fluid and electrolytic occur because of the diseased mucosal surface area of absorption. Breakdown of cells results in protein loss through the stools. Areas of inflamed mucosa form pseudopolyps, tongue-like projection and the bowel lumen. Grannulation tissue develops and the mucosa musculature becomes thickened, shortening in colon.

Clinical Manifestations

- Anorexia, nausea, and weight loss.
- Weakness and malaise.
- Fever and leucocytosis (High fever and WBC more than 15000/mw suggest abscess).
- Iron deficiency anemia.
- Profuse diarrhea (15-20 stool/day).
- Stools containing blood, mucus and possibly pus.
- Abdominal cramping can be present before the bowel movements.
- Loss of fluid, sodium, calcium, potassium and bicarbonate.

The complications of ulcerative colitis be classified into those that are intestinal and those that are extraintestinal. Intestinal include hemorrage, strictures perforation, toxic megacolon and colonic dilation. An extraintestinal complication of ulcerative colitis are:
- Involvement of large joints, peripheral arthritis, ankylosing, spondylitis, sacroiliitis and finger clubbing.
- Skin erythema nodosum, pyoderma gangrenosum.
- Mouth Apthous ulcers.
- Eye-conjunctivitis, uveitis, episcleritis.
- Hepato-cholelithiasis, fatty liver, cirrhosis, cholangitis.
- Renal kidney stones, ureteral obstruction.

Diagnostic Studies

- Fiberoptic colonoscopy
- Sigmoidoscopy
- Barium enema
- CBC
- Stool for blood culture and sensitivity.

Management of Ulcerative Colitis

The goals of treatment are to rest the bowel, control the inflammation, combat infection, correct malnutrition, alleviate stress and symptomatic relief using drug therapy. The common drugs used for IBD are:

- Aminosalicylates (oral) are converted in colon to sulfapyridine and 5-amino salicylic acid, which may exert an anti-inflammatory effect, possibly through prostaglandin inhibition (e.g., azulfidine, oslazine, mesalamine). During this medications, nurse has to assess for allergy to sulfonamides or aspirins. Monitor for common side effects, anorexia, nausea, vomiting and headache and teach patients to take the drug in divided doses with full glass of fluid or with food. Maintain a liberal intake and report incidence of sit in rash or other adverse effects.
- Aminosalicylates (Rectal) has same actions as stated in oral. Drugs used are 'mesalamine' in suspension for retention enema and mesalamine suppository. Administer enema while patient is positioned on left side and teach patient to retain as long as possible.
- Corticosteroids (oral/IV) has potent systemic anti-inflammatory action, e.g., prednisolone/prednisone. During medication, teach patient to; take with food or fluid, monitor weight gain; assess for edema; Be alert to signs of infection and report promptly, discontinue drug. Maintain good personal hygiene and keep perianal area clean and dry.
- Corticosteroid (Rectal) has same effect in oral or IV, e.g.,, hydrocortisone intrarectal foam (Cort-foam), retentive enema (cortenema). Budesonide enema has rapid presystemic metabolism minimises absorption in addition to above actions. Hence, administer enema while patient is positioned on left side and teach patient to retain as long as possible. Other interventions as stated above, side effects should be less.
- Immunosuppressive agents have potent systemic suppressors of immune response; may take 4-6 months for full effect, e.g., mercaptopurine (parinethol), azathioprine (imuran). During these medications, teach patient to report any signs of infection; be alert

to easy bruising. Return for lab work as scheduled. Maintain liberal daily fluid intake with food or after meals. Another drug cyclosporine (Sandimmun) is oral solution. It may be mixed in glass and given with milk or orange juice at room temperature. Avoid refrigeration. Teach patient to monitor blood pressure; report hematuria or any change in urinary infection.

Surgical intervention may be selected for patients with incurable colitis whose disease cannot be satisfactorily controlled with standard medical management. This procedure is curative in nature and involves removal of the entire colon, i.e. Brook ileostomy, Dr Nils Kocks, continent ileostomy, Sleoanal anastomosis, or ileorectostomy, ileoanal resurr.

The drugs used are:
- Sulfasalazine
- Corticosteroids
- Immunosuppressive agents (6-MP, azathioprine)

The dosage and the routes of administration depend on the severity of the illness and the area involved. The elemental diet and parenteral nutrition may be used. Parenteral nutrition for severe cases, small bowel fistulas, small bowel syndrome. It is given to promote healing and reduce complications. The elemental diet provides a high caloric, high nitrogen, fat free, no residue sustrate that is absorbed in the proximal small bowel. Vitamin deficiency may develop. Vitamin B_{12} injection may be used.

Surgical intervention is avoided in Crohn's disease as much as possible because of recurrence of the disease process in same region is virtually inevitable.

The nurse should educate the patient and family to take care of the person with inflammatory bowel disease as given below.

Diet and Fluids
- Eat a high caloric and well-balanced diet.
- Avoid any food that increases symptoms (e.g., fresh fruits, and vegetables, fatty foods, spicy foods and alcohol).
- Assess the effect of dairy products on disease symptoms and limit use if appropriate.
- Take multivitamins/mineral supplements daily.
- Ensure a liberal fluid intake—2500–3000 ml per day. Drink electrol or other commercial products if tolerated during flare-ups, to replace lost electrolytes.
- Use salt liberally during disease flare ups.

Elimination
- Take medication as prescribed.
- Keep rectal area clean and dry; use analgesic rectal ointment or sitz baths for rectal discomfort.
- Consult with physician about the appropriateness of antidiarrheal agents or bulk laxatives when diarrhea is present.
- Monitor weight daily disease flare ups.

Rest and Coping
- Maintain a regular sleep schedule.
- Schedule daily activities to avoid fatigue, take rest periods as needed.
- Use relaxation strategies when stress levels rise.
- Discuss concern with family or support person.
- Attend local IBD support group if available.

CROHN'S DISEASE

Crohn's disease is a chronic, nonspecific inflammatory bowel disorder of unknown origin that can affect any part of the GI tract. It may occur at any age. But occurs most often between the age of 25 and 30 years. Both sexes are affected with slightly high incidence in women.

Pathophysiology

Crohn's disease can affect any part of the GI tract, but is most often seen in the terminal ileum, jejunum and colon. The inflammation involves all layers of the bowel wall (i.e. transmural). Area of involvements are usually discontinuous with segments of normal bowel occurring between diseased portions. Typically ulcerations are deep and longitudinal and penetrate between islands of inflamed edematous mucosa causing the classic cobblestone appearance. Thickening of bowel wall occurs as well as narrowing of the lumen with stricture development. Abscesses or fistula tract, that communicates with other loops of bowel, skin, bladder, rectum or vagina may develop.

Clinical Manifestation

The manifestations depend largely on the anatomical site of involvement, extent of the disease process and presence or absence of complications. The onset of Crohn's disease is usually insidious. With non-specific complaints such as diarrhea, fatigue, abdominal pain, weight loss, and fever. Fever diagnosis is difficult than ulcerative colitis. The principal symptoms are diarrhea and abdominal pain. Other manifestations include abdominal cramping, anal tenderness, abdominal distention, fever and fatigue. Extraintestinal manifestation such as arthritis, finger clubbing, may precede the onset of disease. As the disease progresses, there is weight loss, malnutrition, dehydration, electrolyte imbalances, anemia, increased peristalsis and pain around the umbilicus and right lower quadrant. The complications are fistulas, strictures, anal abscesses, perforation, toxic megacolon.

Diagnostic Studies
- Complete blood cell count
- Serum chemistries
- Stool for occult blood
- Barium enema of small and large intestine
- Procosigmoidoscope examination
- Sigmoidoscopy and colonoscopy with biopsy.

Management

The goal of management is to control the inflammatory process, relieve symptoms, correct metabolic and nutritional problems and promote healing. Drug therapy and nutritional support are the mainstays of treatment.

Health Maintenance

- Report signs requiring medical attention:
  - Change in pattern or severity of abdominal pain or diarrhea
  - Development of constipation
  - Change in stool character
  - Unusual discharge from rectum and
  - Fever
- Plan for regular follow-up care.

INTESTINAL OBSTRUCTION

Normal functioning of the small and large intestine depends on an open lumen for the movement of intestinal content, as well as adequate circulation and nervous innervation to sustain rhythmic peristalsis. Any factor or condition that either narrows the intestinal passage way or interfere with peristalsis can result in bowel obstruction.

Intestinal obstruction occurs when intestinal contents cannot pass through the GI tract, and it requires prompt treatment. The obstruction may either be partial or complete.

Etiology

The intestinal obstruction can be classified as mechanical and non-mechanical.

The causes of mechanical obstruction are:

- *Adhesions:* It may form after abdominal surgery for unknown reasons; perhaps related to inflammatory responses in the healing bowel. In some cases, the adhesion may become massive. The fibrous bands of scar tissue can loop over bowel segments, either causing the bowel to kink or compress the loop.
- *Hernias:* A hernia is a protrusion of an organ or structure from its normal cavity through a congenital or acquired defect usually in the muscle of the abdominal wall. Depending on its location, hernia may contain peritoneurymentum, a loop of bowel or a section of bladder. Inguinal and umbilical hernias usually result from congenital weakness of the muscle, whereas incisional hernias for usually complications of surgery. Hernia can result in bowel obstruction if the abdominal wall defect through which the hernia protrudes becomes so tight that the bowel segments become strangulated. The lumps or swellings may always be present or may have appeared suddenly after coughing, straining, lifting and other vigorous exertion.
- *Tumor:* Tumor mass will gradually restrict the internal tumours of the bowel as it enlarges. Eventually a fecal mass may be unable to pass through the constriction, leading to partial or complete obstruction.
- *Volvulus:* A twisting of the bowel upon itself, usually at least a full 180°, obstructing the intestinal lumen both proximally or distally, is called 'Volvulus'. The acute obstruction can quickly result in bowel infarction and can be life-threatening as a result of necrosis, perforation and peritonitis.
- *Intussusception:* Intussusception involves a telescoping of the bowel in itself. In invagination occurs with peristalsis and in the adult often is triggered by the presence of tumor mass. The bowel segment containing the mass is propelled by peristalsis and adjacent bowel segment. Constriction is immediate and strangulation of the trapped segment can develop.

The other possible causes of mechanical obstruction will include fecal impaction, gallstones and stricture resulting from the diverticulitis and IBD.

The causes of nonmechanical obstruction may result from a neuromuscular or vascular disorder.

- Paralytic ileus (or Adynamic ileus) results from a lack of peristaltic activity, usually as a result of neurogenic impairment. Ileus is a common temporary problem after abdominal surgery particularly if the bowel has been extensively handled. Other causes of paralytic ileus include inflammatory responses (e.g., appendicitis, pancreatitis), electrolyte abnormalities, and thoracic and lumbar spinal fractures.
- Vascular distinctions are rare and are due to an interference with the blood supply to a position of the intestines. The common causes are emboli; and atherosclerosis of mesenteric arteries, thrombosis of the mesenteric arteries.

Pathophysiology

Intestinal obstruction triggers a series of GI tract events whose clinical manifestation depends largely on the location of the obstruction and the degree of circulatory compromise. Normally 6 to 8 liters of fluid enters the small bowel daily. Most of the fluid is absorbed before it reaches the colon. Approximately 75 percent of the intestinal gas is swallowed air. Bacterial metabolism produce methane and hydrogen gases, fluid and intestinal content accumulates proximal to the intestinal obstruction. This causes distention and the distal bowel may collapse. The distention reduces the absorption of the fluids and stimulates intestinal secretion. As the fluid increases, so does the pressure in the lumen of the bowel. The increased pressure leads to an increase in capillary permeability and extravasation of fluids and electrolytes into the peritoneal cavity. Edema, congestion and necrosis from impaired blood supply and possible rupture of the bowel may occur.

The retention of fluid in the intestine and peritoneal cavity can lead to a severe reduction in circulating blood volume and result in hypotension and hypovolemic shock.

Vascular compromise is the most serious aspect of obstruction. Bowel ischemia breaks down the normal barrier to bacteria and the stagnant and distended bowel becomes increasingly permeable to bacteria. Organism can enter the peritoneal cavity and lead to peritonitis. Bacteria are normally sparse in the small bowel but accumulated rapidly during obstruction. *E. coli*, *Klebsiella* prevalent and the release of toxins can result in septic shock. The ischemic process can progress to gangrene and perforation. Submucosal hemorrhage and sloughing can also be a source of substantial blood loss.

Clinical Manifestation

The clinical manifestations of intestinal obstructions very based on the exact site of obstruction and include nausea, vomiting, abdominal pain, distention, inability to pass flatulence and constipation (fecal impaction secondary to constipation, colonar perforation).

Obstruction located high in the small intestine produces rapid onset, sometimes projective vomiting with bile containing vomitus. Vomiting from more distal obstruction of the small intestine is more gradual in onset. The vomitus may be orange brown and foul-smelling because of bacterial growth. Vomiting may be entirely absent in large bowel obstruction if the ileocecal valve is competent. Otherwise, the patient may eventually vomit faeculent material.

Abdominal pain is fairly universal symptom. Simple obstruction produce cramy and poorly localized pain. Its onset parallels the initial increase in peristalsis that raises intraluminal pressure in an attempt to clear the obstruction. Frequent loud, high pitched bowel sounds are often heard on auscultation. The pain typically lessens as the obstructions worsen. Smooth muscle atony decreases peristalsis and bowel sounds are diminished. The pain associated with bowel strangulation is constant and severe vomitings usually relieve abdominal pain in high intestinal obstruction. Persistent, colicky abdominal pain is seen with lower intestinal obstruction.

Abdominal distention usualy develops slowly although obstipation is common. Rising fever usually indicates the presence of dying bowel. Laboratory values typically reflect the progressive nature of the dehydration. There is decreased urine output, hemoconcentration, hypokalemia and hyponatremia.

Management

Intestinal obstruction is a potentially life-threatening condition. Assessment must begin with a detailed patient's history and physical examination. The type of location of obstruction usually causes characteristic symptoms. The nurse should determine the location, duration, intensity and frequency of abdominal pain and whether abdominal tenderness or rigidity is present. Onset, frequency, color, odor and amount of vomitus should be recorded. Bowel function, including passage of flatus should be determined. this should auscultate for bowel sounds and document character and location, irrespective the abdomen for scars, palpable mass, and distention, and observe for muscle guarding and tenderness. The usual diagnosis measures taken are abdominal X-rays, barium enema, as these given, e.g., clues for locating obstruction. Lab tests are also helpful, CBC, serum-electrolyte, amylase, BUN. The nurse should prepare the patient for such measures.

Treatment is directed towards decompression of the intestine by removal of gas and fluid, correction and maintenance of fluid and electrolyte balance, and relief or removal of the obstruction. NG or intestinal tube may be used to decompress the bowel. NG tubes should be inserted before surgery to empty the stomach and relieve distention. They are also used instead of nasointestinal tubes to treat partial or complete small-bowel obstructions. Intestinal tubes such as the Center or Miller-Abbot or Dennis tubes are passed into the small intestine. They are 10 feet (9300 cm) long and mercury-weighed. The patient should be monitored closely for signs of dehydrations and electrolyte imbalance. A strict intake and output record should be maintained. All vomitus and tube drainage should be included. IV fluids should be administered. Serum electrolyte levels should be monitored. A patient with high obstruction is more likely to have metabolic alkalosis. A patient with low obstruction is at greater risk of metabolic acidosis. The patient is often restless and constantly changes position to relieve the pain. Analgesics may be with held until the obstruction is diagnosed because they may mask other signs and symptoms and decrease intestinal motility. The nurse should provide comfort measures to promote a restful environment, and keep distraction and visitors to a minimum. Nursing care of the patient after surgery for an intestinal obstruction is similar to the care of the patient after laparotomy.

COLORECTAL CANCER

Colorectal cancer has been widely spread by the turn of the last millenmium. The causes of colorectal cancer remain unclear. Groups at high-risk of colorectal cancer have been identified are:
- Age (after 40 years) is a risk time for both men and women.
- Colorectal polyps.
- Chronic inflammatory bowel disease (H/o ulcerative colitis).
- Family history of colorectal cancer or adenomas.
- Previous history of colorectal cancer.

- History of genital or breast cancer (woman).
- High caloric, high fat or low-fiber diet.
- Cigarette smoking.
- Obesity (nature of the risk currently unknow).

Pathophysiology

Adenocarcinoma is the most common type of colon cancer. Most colorectal cancers appear to arise from adenomatous polyps. All tumors tend to spread through the walls of the intestine and into the lymphatic system. Tumors commonly spread to the liver because the venous blood flow from the colorectal tumor is through the portal vein. Since the cancer of the colon may spread by direct extension or through the lymphatic or circulatory systems it may seed at distant point in the peritonium or at distant points in the colon. The liver and lungs are the major organs of metastasis.

Clinical Manifestation

The clinical manifestation of the colon cancer varies with the location of the tumor. There are usually no early symptoms and the disease is often diagnosed incidentally. Cancer in distal colon and rectum typically produces symphony related to partial obstruction. The lesions are more likely to be annular, and they grow circumferentially, encircling the colon wall. The lumen becomes narrow and constricted. Obstruction occurs when formed stool is unable to pass through the narrowed lumen.

The patient may experience a change in bowel habits, a feeling of incomplete bowel emptying, or rectal bleeding. The clinical manifestation of bowel cancer are as follows:

- Frequently a symptomatic and diagnosed incidently.
- Symptoms of partial bowel obstruction:
  - Change in bowel habits, e.g., constipation or diarrhea
  - Pencil or ribbon shaped stool.
  - Sensation of incomplete bowel emptying.
- Gas or bloating
- Occurs blood in the stool or rectal bleeding
- Weakness, fatigue, malaise, anorexia and anemia.
- Weight loss usually accompany with metastasis.
- Abdominal pain (usually accompanies in larger lesions).

Diagnostic test: Rectal examination, sigmoidoscopy, colonoscopy, Barium enema, CBC, LFT, Ocult blood test, CEA test, CT scan and ultrasound.

Management

Prognosis and treatment correlates with pathological staging of the disease. Several methods of staging currently being used are:
- Duke's classification
- TNM classification.

Duke staging system for colorectal cancer.

A – Negative nodes, limitations of lesion to mucosa.
B1 – Negative nodes, extension of lesion through mucosa but still within the bowel wall.
B2 – Negative nodes extention through entire bowel wall.
C1 – Positive nodes, limitation of lesion to bowel wall.
C2 – Positive nodes, extension of lesion through entire bowel wall.
D – Presence of distant unresectable metastasis.

This staging is used to establish the appropriate level of intervention and treatment.

The most recent classifications of colorectal cancer is the tumor, node, metastasis, system which is based on pathologic assessment and includes data from the history and physical examination and presurgical and lab evaluation:

T – Primary tumors.
Tx – Primary tumour cannot be assessed.
T0 – No evidence of primary tumour.
Tis – Carcinoma in situ
T1 – Tumor invades submucosa.
T2 – Tumors invades muscularis propria.
T3 – Tumor invades through the msculari, propriat into the subserosa or into the non-peritonealized pericalic or perirectal tissue.
T4 – Tumour perforates the visceral peritoneum or directly invades other organs or structures.
N – Regional lymph node involvement.
Nx – Regional lymph node cannot be assessed.
No – No regional lymph node metastasis.
MI – Distinct metastasis.

After diagnosis has been confirmed, treatment may initiated by radiation and chemotherapy.

Radiation may be used preoperatively or as a palliative measure for patients with advanced lesions. It is primary objective is to reduce tumor size and provide symptomatic relief.

Chemotherpay is recommended when a patient has a positive lymph node at the time of surgery or has metastatic disease. No drug is available that can cure malignant colon or rectal tumors.

Surgery is the only curative treatment of colorectal cancer. Success of surgery depends on resection of the tumor with an adequate margin of healthy bowel and resection of the regional lymph nodes. The usual surgical procedure includes:

- Right hemicolectomy is performed when the cancer is located in the cecum, ascending colon, hepatic flexure, or transverse colon to the right of the middle artery. A portion of the terminal ileum, the appendix are removed, and an ileotransverse anastomosis is performed.
- A left hemicolectomy involves resection of the left transverse colon, the splenic flexure, the descending

colon, the sigmoid colon and the upper portion of the rectum and abdominal-perineal resection, laparoscopy colectomy is also performed. Pre and postoperative care are similar to that of any laparotomy within specific activities is initiated accordingly (See Ostomy Surgery).

OSTOMY SURGERY

An ostomy is a surgical procedure in which an opening is made to allow the passage of intestinal contents from the bowel to an incision trauma. The stoma which is the opening on the surface of the abdomen is created when the intestine is brough through the abdominal wall and sutured to the skin. It may be permanent or temporary. Fecal matter is diverted through the stoma to the outside of the abdominal wall.

- An ileostomy is opening from the ileum through the abdominal wall and is also referred to as a conventional or Brooke's ileostomy. It is most commonly used in surgical treatment of ulcerative colitis Crohn's disease and familial polyp.
- A cecostomy is an opening between the cecum and the abdominal wall. They are usually temporary most often used for fecal diversion before surgery or for palliation.
- A colostomy is an opening between the colon and abdominal wall. The proximal end of the colon is sutured to the skin. Temporary colostomy is usually performed to protect an end-to-end anastomosis after a bowel resection or in an emergency measure following bowel obstruction (e.g., malignant tumor), abdominal trauma (Gunshot wound) or a perforated diverticulum. Loop colostomy and double barrel colostomy are more commonly performed as temporary colostomy, but they may be permanent.

Preoperative Care

Preoperative care focuses on patient teaching. The nurse assesses the patient's knowledge and understanding of the proposed surgery and its outcomes. This inlcudes brief overview of GI tract structure and functioning and the nature of functioning of the ostomy. Emotional preparation for ostomy surgery is extremely important. The nurse encourages the pateint to verbalize feelings related to the radical change to body image and function. Validating the appropriateness of these concerns lays in the family for an effective working relationship with patient.

The patient may need to progress through the grieving process, and if the person is in the shock state, specific factual teaching may be ineffective. The nurse offers acceptance of all feelings and reinforces the importance of open communication.

The preparation phase may include nutritional support and possibly total parental nutrition (TPN), if the patient's nutitional state is inadequate for surgery. The patient should know what to except in the postoperative period. The nurse discusses the management of postoperative pain. The nature and apperance of all incisions and drains and the purpose of the NG tube and IV lines. Bowel cleansing is also performed and may include the use of enemas, laxatives, and antibiotics to reduce intestinal bacterial flora.

Postoperative Care

Postoperative nursing care should focus on assessing the stoma protecting the skin, selecting the pouch, and assisting the patient to adapt psychologically to a changed body. In addition, maintenance of fluid and electrolyte balance, stoma monitoring and managing the wound are important.

The following guidelines should be kept in mind while changing the ostomy pouch:
- Stoma measurement
  - Use the measuring guide and sample diameters and cut the ostomy appliances to fit pattern should be 1/8 to 1/4 inch larger than stoma.
  - Use the same procedure to prepare the skin barrier.
  - *Note:* The pouch opening is cut slightly larger than that of the skin barrier to prevent paper from cutting the stoma.
- Removing pouch
  - Empty drainable pouch to prevent spills.
  - Disconnect pouch from skin wafer if two-piece system is used.
  - Gently peel the wafer away from the skin beginning at the top.
- Skin care
  - Cleanse the skin with warm water and dry thoroughly. Use soap only stool adheres to skin. Rinse thoroughly with water.
  - Assess peristomal skin and stoma carefully for signs of irritation or infection.
  - Pat peristoma skin dry thoroughly.
- Applying new pouch
  - Center the pouch opening over the stoma. Ask patient to abdominal muscle to make application easier.
  - Gently press into place and hold for at least 30 seconds to seal special emphasis will be on ostomy skin care as follows:
  - When a pouch seal leaks, the pouch should be immediately changed, not taped. Stool held against the skin quickly results in severe irritation.
  - Pouches are removed gently, with one hand holding the skin in place to decrease pulling.
  - The skin should be gently but thoroughly cleansed, rinsed and patted dry.
  - Peristomal hair should be trimmed but not shaved to prevent folliculitis.

- A skin barrier should be used to protect the peristomal skin from liquid stools.
- A skin sealant should be used under all types.
- The patient should consult special nurse for specific care if available.

An ostomy irrigation is an enema given through the stoma to stimulate bowel emptying at a regular and convenient time for which the following guidelines are helpful.

- Assemble all equipment: Water container, irrigating sleeve and belt, skin care, items, new pouch system, ready for use.
- Remove old pouch and dispose.
- Clean the stoma and peristomal skin with water and assess.
- Apply the irrigating sleeve and belt. Place open end of sleeve in toilet.
- Fill irrigating container with 500 ml to 1000 ml of lukewarm tap water, and suspend container at shoulder height.
- Run water through the tubing to remove air.
- Gently insert the irrigating cone into stoma, and slowly start the flow of water. Catheters are inserted no more than 2 to 4 inches. Do not fork. If cramping occurs, stop the irrigation and wait.
- Allow approximately 15 to 20 minutes for stool to empty.
- Rinse sleeves, dry the bottom, roll it up and close off the end. Patient should go about regular activities for 30 to 45 minutes.
- Remove sleeve, clean stoma, and apply new pouch.
- Clean and store the irrigating equipment.

ANORECTAL DISORDERS

A variety of common disorders can affect the perianal area. Persons who experience anorectal disorders typically seek medical care for symptoms such as pain, tenderness, itching or the development of rectal bleeding. Many of them will be treated on outpatient basis. They include hemorrhoid, fissure, abscesses, fistula, pilonideal sinus.

Hemorrhoids are masses of dilated blood vessels that lie beneath the lining of the skin in the anal canal. They are dilated hemorrhoidal veins. They may be internal or external. Internal occurring about the internal sphincter, external occurring outside the external sphincter. Symptoms of hemorrhoids include bleeding, pruritus, prolapse and pain are common in all age groups.

Hemorrhoids affect the person of all ages, but they typically cause more problems with increasing age. Pregnancy is common condition for initiating or aggravating hemorrhoids. Other conditions associated with the development of hemorrhoids include obesity, congestive heart failure, and chronic liver disease which result in portal hypertension. These conditions are associated with persistent elevation in intra-abdominal pressure. Sedentary occupations that involve long period of sitting or standing also implicated though exact mechanism is unknown.

The diagnosis of hemorrhoids is done by inspection, digital examination, proctoscopy or examination with the flexible sigmoidoscopy.

Conservative management of hemorrhoids includes a high-fiber diet, bulk laxatives warm sitz baths, and gentle cleansing. A high fever diet and increased fluid intake prevent constipation and reduce straining, which allows engorgement of the veins to subside. Ointments such as Nupercaine, creams, suppositories and impregnated pads that contain anti-inflammatory agents, (hydrocortisone) or astrigent and anesthesia may be used to shrink the mucous membrane and relive discomfort. Stool softeners may be ordered to keep the stool soft and sitz bath may be ordered to relieve pain.

Application of ice packs for few hours followed by warm packs may be used for thrombosed hemorrhoids. If severe pain, bleeding or thrombosis are present, more definitive treatment may be indicated. A variety of options have been used over time including sclerotherapy, cryotherapy, binocular diathermy, rubber band ligation and surgical haemorrhoidectomy.

The following guidelines are helpful for persons undergoing anal/rectal surgery:

- Preoperative care
  - Bowel preparation is standard, but an enema may not be prescribed if rectal pain is acute.
  - Stool softeners may given to promote a soft stool before surgery.
- Postoperative care
  - Administer analgesics as prescribed, especially before initial defecation (considerable rectal discomfort may be present).
  - Provide emotional sport before and after first defecation.
  - Suggest side-lying position.
  - Provide sitz baths as ordered (monitor for hypotension secondary to dilation of pelvic blood vessels in early postoperative period).
- Promotion of elimination
  - Administer prescribed stool softeners.
  - Encourage patient to defecate as soon as the inclination occurs (prevents strictures and preserves normal anal lumen considerable anxiety is usually personal).
  - Monitor for hypotension, dizziness, and faintness during first defecation.
  - If an enema must be given, use small bore rectal tube.
- Patient teaching
  - Clean rectal area after each defecation until healing is complete (sitz bath is recommended).

- Avoid constipation with a high-fiber diet, high-fluid intake, regular exercise, and regular time for defecation.
- Use stool softeners until healing is complete.
- Seek medical consultation for rectal bleeding, suppurative drainage, continued pain on defecation, or continued constipation despite preventive measures.

Anal Fissure

An anal fissure or fissure in and around the anus is a skin ulcer or a crack in the lining of the anal walt that is caused by trauma or local infection. It is frequently associated with constipation and subsequent stretching of the anus from hard feces. The most common clinical manifestations are painful spasm of the anal sphincter and severe, burning pain during defecation. Some bleeding may occur and constipation resutls becasue of pain assocaited with bowel movements.

Conservative treatment consists of bowel regulations with mineral oil and stool softeners. Sitz bath and anal anesthetics suppositories (Anusol) are also ordered. Surgical treatment usually consists of excision of fissure. Postoperative care is similar to that of hemorroidectomy.

Anorectal Abscess

Anorectal abscesses are defined as undrained collections of perianal pus. They are due to perirectal infections in patient who have compromised local circulation or active inflammatory disease. The most common causative organism are *E coli, Staphylococci and Streptococci*. Clinical manifestation includes local pain, swelling, foul-smelling, drainage, tenderness and elevated temperature and sepsis can occur.

Surgical therapy consists of drainage of abscess of packing is used. It should be allowed to heal by granulation. The packing is changed every day and moist and hot compresses are applied to the area. Care must be taken to avoid soiling the dressing during urination and defecation. A low-residue diet is given. The patient may leave the hospital with area open. Teaching, should include wound care, the importance of sitzbath, thorough cleaning after bowel movement and periodic check-up.

Anorectal Fistula

An anorectal fistula is an abnormal tunnel leading out from the anus or rectum. It is a hollow tract leading through anal tissue from anorectal canal through skin near anus. It may extend to the outside the skin, vagina or buttocks. Anorectal fissures are complications of Crohn's disease. This condition often precedes an anorectal abscess.

Feces may enter the fistula and cause an infection. There may be persistent, blood stained, purulent discharge, or stool leakage from the fistula. The patient may have to wear a pad to prevent staining of clothes.

Surgical therapy involves a fistulotomy or a fistulectomy, Gauze packing is inserted and the wound is left to heal by granulation. Care is the same after hemorrhoidectomy.

Pilonidal Sinus

A pilonidal sinus is a small tract under the skin between the buttocks in the sacrococcygeal area. It is thought to be congenital origin. It may have several openings and is lined with epithelium and hair, thus the name pilonidal (a nest of hair).

The skin is moist and movement of the buttocks causes the short wiry hair to penetrate the skin. The irritated skin becomes infected and forms a pilonidal cyst or abscess. There are no symptoms unless there is an infection. If it becomes infected, the patient complains of pain.

The formed abscess requires incision and drainage. The wound may be closed or left open to heal by secondary intention. This wound is packed and sitz bath are ordered. Nursing care includes hot moist, heat application when an abscess is present. The patient is usualy more comfortable lying on the abdomen or side. The patient should be instructed to avoid contamination of dressing during urination or defecation and to avoid straining whenever possible.

JAUNDICE

Jaundice, a yellowish discoloration of body tissues, resulting from an alteration in normal bilirubin metabolism or flow of bile into the hepatic or biliary duct systems. It is a symptom which results, when the concentration of bilirubin level has to be approximately three times normal level (2 to 3 mg) for jaundice to occur. The three types of jaundice are classified in hemolytic, hepatocellular and obstructive.

- Hemolytic jaundice (prehepatic) is due to an increased breakdown of red blood cells which produces an increased amount of unconjugated bilirubin in the blood. The liver is unable to handle this increased load. Causes of this type include blood transfusion reaction, sickle cells crisis, and hemolytic anemia.
- Hepatocellular jaundice (hepatic) results from the liver's altered ability to take up bilirubin from the blood or to conjugate or excrete it. Both unconjugated and conjugated bilirubin serum levels increase. Because conjugated bilirubin is water soluble; it is excreted in the urine. The most common cause of this type are hepatitis, cirrhosis, and hepatocarcinoma.
- Obstructive jaundice (posthepatic) is due to impeded or obstructed flow of bile through the liver or biliary duct system. The obstruction may be intrahepatic or extrahepatic. Intrahepatic obstructions are due to swelling or fibrosis of the liver's caliculi and bile ducts. This can be caused by damage from liver tumors, hepatitis, or cirrhosis. Causes of extrahepatic

obstructions include common bile duct obstruction from a stone, sclerosing cholangitis and carcinoma of the head of the pancreas. Here moderate elevation is both conjugated and unconjugated bilirubin and urine bilirubin.

Jaundice is a major problem in patients with diffuse hepatocellular disorder, which includes hepatitis, cirrhosis and hepatic carcinoma.

HEPATITIS

Hepatitis is an inflammation of the liver. Although the term hepatitis is most often used in conjunction with viral hepatitis, the disease can also be caused by the bacteria or toxic injury to the liver. Although some differences exist in the pathological and clinical phenomena of viral, bacterial, and toxic hepatitis, the clinical management of the person with any of these types of hepatitis is quite similar.

Toxic Hepatitis

Since liver has a primary role in the metabolism of foreign substances, many agents including drugs, alcohol, industrial toxins and persons can cause toxic hepatism. Many health care workers are concerned about hepatic injury caused by adverse drug reactions from the drugs they handle.

Etiology

The agents that produce hepatic injury are categorized into two major groups: Predictable (intrinsic) hepatotoxins and non-predictable (idiosyncratic) hepatotoxins.

- Predictable hepatotoxic agents cause toxic hepatitis with predictable regularity and produce injury in a high percentage of persons exposed to them. Occurrence of toxic hepatitis is dose dependent. The predictable hepatotoxins are further divided into two subgroups—direct or indirect:
  1. The direct predictable hepatotoxin agents have direct effect on hepatic cells and organelles, producing structural changes that lead to metabolic defects. For example:
     - Carbon tetrachloride and other chlorinated hydrocarbon (Ind-toxin).
     - Yellow phosphorous (Industrial toxin).
     - Mushroom poisoning (Plant toxin).
  2. The indirect predictable hepatotoxins are mostly; Drugs such as ethanol, tetracycline, methotrexate, L-asparaginase, puromycin, 6-merca topurine, acetami-nophine, mictramycin, urethane, halothane, cholecystographic dyes, rifamycin B. These are agents which first interfere with normal metabolic function and this alteration in metabolic function produces structural change.
- Non-predictable hepatoxic agents produce hepatic injury only in unusually susceptible persons and in only a small percentage of persons exposed to them. Occurrence is not dose-dependent. These drugs such as phenytoin, PAS, INH, chlorpromazine and androgens and anabolic steroids, chlorpropamide, imipramine, methyldopa, monoamino oxidase (MAO) inhibitors, oral contraceptives, sulfanamides, allupurinol, clindamycin, erythromycin, esters, nitrofurantoin, oxacillin and oestrogen steroid.

Pathophysiology

The morphological changes produced in the liver by the toxin, depending on the specific hepatotoxin. For example, carbon tetrachloride, tetracycline, and ethanol cause fatty infiltration and/or necrosis, oral contraceptives, cholecystographic dyes and chloropromazine produces cholestasis and portal inflammation. The alterations may result in only minimal manifestations of altered liver function such as slightly-elevated serum enzymes or major manifestation associated with terminal liver failure.

Clinical Manifestation

Early manifestation includes anorexia, nausea, vomiting, lethargy, elevated ALT and AST levels. Later manifestations are hepatomegaly, hepatic tenderness, dark urine, elevated serum bilirubin level and urine bilirubin level.

Management

Proper attention is focussed on identifying the toxic agents and removing or eliminating it. Gastric lavage, and cleansing of the bowel may be indicated to remove the hepatotoxins from the intestinal tract. There are specific treatments for particular hepatotoxins (Follow as prescribed). In most instances of toxic hepatitis, medical treatment is supportive and focussed on particular manifestation such as treatment of cirrhosis, portal-systemic encephalophathy or accompanying renal failure. Nursing care includes maintaining fluid and electrolyte balance, promoting a well-balanced diet, when food and fluids are allowed, and promoting rest and treating complications.

Nurses also should teach patient's family to use only prescribed medication with precaution to the liver injury.

Viral Hepatitis

Viral hepatitis is by far the most important liver infections. The term viral hepatitis is used to refer to several clinically similar but etiologically and epidemiologically distinct infections.

Etiology

Viral hepatitis can be caused by one of the five major viruses A, B, C, D and E, i.e., HAV, HBV, HCV, HDV, HEV. Two other forms of hepatitis—hepatitis F and hepatitis G have been identified but occur rarely.

- HAV is a RNA virus transmitted through feco-oral route. Incubation period is 15-50 days (average 28 days). Crowded condition, poor personal hygiene, poor sanitation, contaminated food, milk water and shell-fish, persons with subclinical infections, infected food handlers, and sexual contacts are the sources of infection and spread of disease. Most infections during 2 weeks before onset of symptoms; infectious until 1-2 weeks after symptoms start.
- HBV is a DNA virus that is transmitted by percutaneous (IV drug use, accidental needle-strick punctures or permucosal exposure to infective blood, blood products, or per mucosal exposure to infectious blood, blood products or other body fluids (semen, vaginal secretions, saliva) Perinatal transmission is also possible. The source and spread of disease are caused by contaminated needle, syringes and blood products, sexual activities with infected partners and asymptomatic carriers, e.g., Tattoo/body piercing bite, most infections before and after symptoms appear for 4-6-months in carriers, it continues through patient's lifetime, incubation period is 45-18 days.
- HCV is RNA virus that is primarily transmitted percutaneously. Thus, the major risk factor for infection is direct percutaneous exposure such as injecting drugs, transfusion of blood products, hemodialysis, tattooing, high-risk sexual behavior, organ transplantation and exposure to blood and blood products by health workers. Less frequent routes are sexual and perinatal.
- HDV also called delta virus, is defective RNA virus that cannot survive on its own. So it can cause infections only together with HBV; routes of transmission same as for HBV. Blood is infectious at all stages of HDV infections. Incubation period is 2-26 weeks. Chronic carriers of HBV are always at risk.
- HEV is an RNA virus, that is transmitted by the feco-oral route. The most common mode of transmission is drinking contaminated water.
- HGV is an RNA virus which is found in some blood donors and can be transmitted by transfusion. It frequently coexists with other hepatitis virus, e.g., HCV.

Pathophysiology

Viral hepatitis causes diffuse inflammatory infiltrations of hepatic tissue with mononuclear cells and local spotty or single cell necrosis. The liver cells may be very swollen. With typical viral hepatitis, there is no collapse of lobules, no loss of lobular architecture, and minimal or no fibrosis. Inflammation degeneration and regeneration occur simultaneously, distorting the normal lobular pattern and creating pressure within and around the portal vein areas and obstructing the bile channels. These changes are associated with elevated serum transminase levels, prolonged prothrombin time and slightly elevated bilirubin level. The outcome of viral hepatitis is affected by such factors as the following:

- Virulence of the virus.
- Amount of hepatic damage sustained.
- Natural individual barriers to damage and disease of the liver such as immune status, nutritional status, and overall health of the individual.

Most patients recover normal level functions but the disease can progress to atypical life-threatening variants.

- Fulminant viral hepatitis—sudden, severe, degenerated and atrophy of liver, resulting in hepatic failure.
- Subacute viral hepatitis—severe, but slower degeneration of livers.
- Confluent hepatic necrosis—submassive or massive destruction of substantial groups of adjacent cell with necrosis of portions of a lobule (submassive) or entire lobule (massive), can result in chronic active disease or cirrhosis but most patients will recover.

Clinical Manifestations

The clinical manifestation of viral hepatitis may be classified into three phases (1) Preicteric or prodramal phase, (2) Icteric phase, (3) Posticteric phase or convalescent phase:

Preicteric	Icteric	Posticteric
Anorexia	Jaundice	Malaise
Nausea, vomiting	Pruritis	Easy fatigability
Right upper quadrant discomfort	Dark urine	Hepatomegally
Constipation or diarrhea	Bilirubinuria	
Decreased sense of taste and smell	White stool	
Malaise	Fatigue	
Headache	Continual hepatomegaly with tenderness	
Fever	Weight loss	
Arthralgia		
Urticaria		
Hepaticmegaly		
Splenomegaly		
Weight loss.		

Complications that can occur include chronic persistent hepatitis, chronic active hepatitis, fulminant viral hepatitis and cirrhosis of the liver.

Diagnostic Studies
- Liver function studies.
- Hepatitis serology.
    - HGs Ag
    - Anti-HBs
    - Anti-HBs, IgH and IgG
    - Anti-HAV, IgH and IgG
    - Anti-HCV.

Management

There is no specific treatment or therapy for viral hepatitis. Most patients can be managed at home. Emphasis on measures to rest the body and assist the liver in regenerating needs to be stressed. Adequate nutrients and rest seem to be more beneficial for healing and liver cell (hepatocyte) regeneration. Rest reduced the metabolic demands on the liver and promotes cell generation. The degree of rest depends on the severity of symptoms. Dietary emphasis is on a well-balanced diet that the patient can tolerate. A low fat, high carbohydrate diet may be better tolerated. Protein and sodium are restricted. Alcohol should be avoided.

Vitamin K is given if the prothromb in time is prolonged. Antihistamines are given for pruritus associated with jaundice, and antiemetics are given for nausea. Most patients of hepatitis are not hospitalized. Those requiring hospitalization include persons with serum bilirubin concentration 10 mg or greater than 10 times normal. In persons with fulminating hepatitis, hospitalization and bed rest are indicated. Unnecessary medication including sedatives are discontinued. Coagulation defects may be treated with administration of fresh frozen plasma. The patient's intake and output is carefully monitored, and intravenous fluid continuously. Electrolytes administered in vomiting and diarrhea may cause electrolyte imbalance, particularly hypokalemia.

Hepatitis A vaccine and immonologlobulins are used in the prevention of viral hepatitis. Hepatitis B vaccine and immunoglobulin is the first line of defence against hepatitis B.

The possible nursing diagnosis of viral hepatitis are:
- Fatigue r/t imbalance between energy level and demand, decreased rest, feeling of malaise.
- Activity intolerance r/t fatigue, weakness.
- Fluid volume deficit r/t vomiting, sweating, decreased intake, increased temperature.
- Infection (Risk for) r/t length of infectivity through blood and body fluids.
- Nutrition, altered r/t anorexia, inadequate intake, increased metabolic needs.
- Pain r/t arthralgia, pruritis, headache, abdominal tenderness.
- Health maintenance, altered r/t lack of knowledge, indifference to "safe sex" practice and needle.
- Skin integrity r/t jaundice, pruritis, scratching.
- Injury r/t altered clothing or prothrombic time.

Preventive Measures for Viral Hepatitis

All patients with hepatitis require precautions to prevent spread of virus. For patients with hepatitis A virus (HAV), the following transmission based precautions are necessary:
- Proper handwashing by patient and staff.
- Wearing gloves when handling feces and urine.
- Wearing a glove when soiling of uniform is likely.
- Cleansing the toilet daily and use private toilet.
- Having a private room (only if patient cannot take care of selfregarding proper disposal of urine and feces).
- Proper cleansing, bagging, and labelling of contaminated items such as bed linens and bedpan.
- Discarding contaminated items such as rectal thermometer.

For the patients with HBV, transmission-based precautions are used and include the following:
- Good handwashing by patient and staff.
- Wearing gloves when handling blood and body fluids.
- Wearing gown, goggles and/or mask when splattering of blood and body fluid is likely.
- Proper cleansing, bagging and labelling of contaminated equipment and linens.
- Proper disposing of needles or any items exposed to the patient's blood or body fluids.
- Careful labelling of blood specimen and protect personnel working with them.
- Avoiding contamination of open cuts and mucus membranes with patient's blood and body fluids.
- Teaching patients to avoid sexual contact until results of liver function tests have returned to normal.

Similar precaution is to be followed in other hepatitis. At times, the nurse in the hospital and particularly nurse in the community are also involved in identifying patient's contacts who will require prophylactic therapy.

CIRRHOSIS OF LIVER

Cirrhosis of the liver is the term applied to chronic disease of the liver characterised by diffuse inflammation and fibrosis resulting in drastic structural changes and significant loss of liver function in which extensive degeneration and destruction of the liver parenchymal cells. The liver cells attempt to regenerate but the regenerative process is disorganized, resulting in abnormal blood vessels and bile duct relationships from the fibrosis. The overgrowth of new and fibrous connective tissue distorts liver's normal lobular structure resulting in lobules of irregular size and shape with impeded vascular flow. Cirrhosis may be insidious and prolonged course.

Etiology and Pathophysiology

Cirrhosis of the liver can be classified in various ways. The major types of cirrhosis based on pathological classification are:
- Alcoholic Previously called "Laennecs Cirrhosis" also called portal or nutritional cirrhosis is usually associated with alcohol abuse or malnutrition. The first change in the liver from excessive alcohol intake is an accumulation of fat in the liver cells. Uncomplicated fatty changes in the liver are potentially reversible if the person stops drinking alcohol. If the alcohol abuse continues, widespread scar formation occurs in the liver (**Fig. 4.3**).
- Postnecrotic cirrhosis is a complication of viral toxic or idiopathic (autoimmune) hepatitis due to massive necrosis from hepatotoxins. Broad bands of scar tissue from within liver.
- Biliary cirrhosis is associated with inflammation of intrahepatic bile-ductules resulting in biliary obstruction in liver and common bile duct. Cholangitis (destruction of the intrahepatic bile ducts) of unknown etiology may occur. There is chronic impairment of bile drainage occurs. Liver is first large, then becomes firm and nodular, Jaundice is a major symptom. Pruritis, hypercholestremia, cholestasis (blockage of bile flow) and malabsorption are common manifestation due to diffuse fibrosis of liver.
- Cardiac cirrhosis results from long-standing, severe, right sided heart failure in patient with cor pulmonale, constrictive pericarditis and tricuspid insufficiency.
- Nonspecific metabolic cirrhosis are due to metabolic problems, infectious diseases, infiltrative diseases and GI diseases in which portal and liver fibrosis may develop, liver is enlarged and firm.

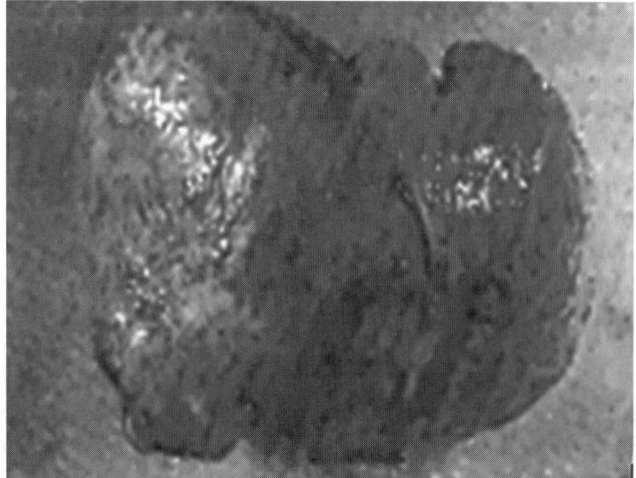

Fig. 4.3: Cirrhosis that developed secondary to alcoholism. The characteristic diffuse nodularity of the surface is due to the combination of regeneration and scarring of the liver.

Clinical Manifestation

The onset of cirrhosis is usually insidious. GI disturbances are common, early symptoms include anorexia, dyspepsia, flatulence, nausea and vomiting and change in bowel habits (constipation or diarrhea)–due to altered metabolism of carbohydrate, fats and proteins. Pain may be due to swelling and stretching of the capsule and spasm of biliary ducts, other symptoms include, fever, lassitude, slight weighlessness and enlargement of liver and spleen. Liver may be palpable. Later symptoms may be severe and result from liver failure and portal hypertension, jaundice, peripheral, edema, and ascites develop gradually. Other late symptoms are as follows:

Gastrointestinal	Hematologic
• Anorexia	• Anemia
• Dyspepsia	• Thrombocytopenia
• Nausea	• Leukopenia
• Vomiting	• Coagulation disorder
• Change in bowel habits	• Splenomegally
• Dull abdominal pain	
• Factor hepatitis	
• Esophageal and gastric varices	
• Hematemesis	
• Hemorrhoidal varices	
• Congestive gastritis	
Endocrine disturbance/ metabolic	**Cardiovascular**
• Potassium deficiency	• Fluid retention
• Hyponatremia	• Peripheral edema
• Hypoalbuminemia.	• Ascites
Integumentary/skin lesions	**Neurologic**
• Jaundice	• Hepatic encephalopathy
• Spider angioma	• Peripheral neuropathy
• Palmar erythema	• Asterixis
• Purpura	• Rynoductre
• Petechea	• Amenorrhea
• Caput medusae	• Testicular atrophy
	• Gynecomastia
	• Impotence.

The major complications of cirrhosis of liver are portal hypertension with resultant esophageal varices, peripheral edema and ascites, hepatic encephalopathy (coma) and hepatorenal syndrome.

Diagnostic Studies

- Liver function studies:
  - Alkaline phosphatase
  - Asparate aminotransferase (AST)

- Alumine aminotransferase (ALT)
- Serum glutamic pyruvic transaminase (SGPT)
- Y-glutamyl transferase
* Liver biopsy (percutaneous needle)
* Esophagogastroduodenoscopy
* Angiography
* Liver scan
* Serum electrolyte
* Prothrombin time
* Serum albumin
* CBC
* Stool for ocult blood
* Upper GI barium swallow.

Management

Although there is no specific therapy for cirrhosis, certain measures can be taken to promote liver cell regeneration and prevent or treat complications.

Rest is significant in reducing metabolic demands of the liver and allowing for recovery of liver cells. At various times, during the progress of cirrhosis the rest may have to take the form of complete bedrest. Avoidance of alcohol and aspirin and administration of B-complex vitamin are helpful.

For ascites, sodium restriction, diuretics and fluid removal are indicated. Administration of 3000-calories high carbohydrate, protein (depends on stage), low-fat diet, low sodium diet are advised. The diuretics used for ascites are spironolactone (Aidactine), amiloride (Midamor) triamferene (Dyrenium), Furosemide (Lasix). In some cases, paracentesis, or peritoneovenous shunts are indicated.

For Esophageal varices β-adrenorgic blockers, vasopressin are used. And endoscopic sclerotherapy or ligation, balloon tampanode, somatostatin, surgical shunting procedures, transjugular intrahepatic portosystematin shunt may be indicated accordingly.

For hepatic encephalopathy, sterilization of GI tract with antibiotics, and levodopa are used.

Nursing assessment will include eliciting complete history focussing on recent history of fever, infected weakness, fatigue, changes in the sclera, edema, itching, muscle wasting, use of alcohol, change in appetite, weight loss, anorexia, nausea, vomiting, indigestion, flatulence, abdominal tenderness, change in the movement of bowel and bladder, sexuality (erectile dysfunction decreased libido or changes in menstrual pattern assessing vital signs, other manifestation and the need for nursing management.

The usual nursing intervention of cirrhosis is supporting respiration (by using Fowler's position), controlling fatigue (with bedrest), maintaining fluid and electrolyte balance (IV or oral fluid if no restriction) helping the patient to avoid alcohol, preventing infection, preventing bleeding and falls, promoting nutrition, controlling pruritis, promoting positive self-esteem. The factors which are supposed to monitor in the person with cirrhosis are:

* Monitor urine and stool for blood.
* Check up patient's body daily for purpura, hematoma and petechea.
* Check mouth especially gums, carefully for signs of bleeding.
* Check vital signs at least every 4 hours.
* Monitor prothrombin time, portal thromboplastin, and thrombocyte count frequently.

Following are the guidelines for decreasing the risk of bleeding:

* Avoid all intramuscular and subcutaneous injections if possible.
* Use the smaller gauge needle possible while giving an injection.
* Apply pressure to injection site and venous puncture sites for at least 5 minutes and arterial punctures for 10 minutes.
* Give Vitamin K as ordered.
* Use or instruct patient to use a soft bristle tooth brush or cotton swabs for oral hygiene.
* Instruct patient to avoid foods (e.g., spicy, hot or raw) that can traumatize esophageal varices.
* Provide assistance to avoid falling.
* Make sure that room is free of clutters, that floors are dry, and shoes or slippers are worn to avoid injuries.

CHOLELITHIASIS

Gallstones can occur at anywhere in the biliary tree. The cholelithasis refer to stone formation in the gallbladder. Either acute or chronic inflammation termed as "Cholecystitis" can result precipitated by the presence of stones. When stones form in or migrate to the common bile duct the condition is termed as choledocholelithasis.

Etiology

Cholecystitis is most commonly associated with stones. When it occurs in the absence of stones it is thought to be caused by bacteria reaching gallbladder via the vascular or lymphatic route or chemical irritant in the bile. *E.coli, Streptococci,* and *Salmonellae* are common bacteria. Other causative factors include adhesions, neoplasms, extensive fasting, frequent weight fluctuations, anesthesia and narcotics.

The actual cause of cholelithiasis is unknown. It develops when the valarice that keeps cholestrol, bile salts and calcium in solutions is altered so that precipitation of these substances occurs. Conditions that upset this balance include infection and disturbance in the metabolism of cholestrol. A high percentage of gallstones are precipitated of cholestrol. Other components of bile that precipitates into stone are bile salts, bilirubin, calcium and proteins.

Stones sometimes are mixed. The risk factors for cholestrol gallstones are obesity, middle age, pregnancy, multiparity, use of oral contraceptives, rapid weight loss, diseases of the ileum and hypercholestrolemia.

Pathophysiology

Bile is primarily composed of water plus conjugated bilirubin, organic and inorganic ions, small amounts of proteins and three lipids bile salts, lecithin, and cholestetrol. When the balance of these three lipids remain intact, cholesterol is held in solution. If the balance is upset cholesterol can be precipitated. Cholesterol gallstone formation is enhanced by the production of a mucin glycoprotein, which traps cholesterol particles. Supersaturation of the bile with cholesterol also impairs gallbladder mobility and contributes to statis.

Cholestrol stones are hard, white or yellow-brown in color, radiolucent and can be quite large up to 4 cm. Black-pigmented stones form as the result of an increase of unconjugated bilirubin and calcium with a corresponding decrease in bile salts. Gallbladder motility may also be impaired. Brown stones develop in the intra and extrahepatic ducts and are usually preceded by bacterial invasion.

Clinical Manifestations

Manifestation of cholecystitis varies from indigestion and moderate to severe pain, fever and jaundice. Initial symptoms of acute cholecystitis include indigestion and pain and tenderness in the right upper quadrant (RUQ), which may be referred to the right shoulder and scapula. The pain may be accompanied by anorexia, nausea and possibly vomiting, restlessness and diaphoresis. Manifestation of inflammation are such as leukocytosis and fever.

Physical findings include RUQ tenderness and abdominal rigidity. Symptoms of chronic cholecystitis include history of fat intolerance, dyspepsia, heart burn and flatulence.

Cholelithiasis may produce severe symptom or non at all. The severity of symptoms depends on whether the stones are stationary or mobile and whether obstruction is present.

The clinical manifestations caused by obstructed blood flow are:
- Obstructive jaundice due to no bile flow into deodenum.
- Dark amber urine which forms when shaken are due to soluble bilirubin in urine.
- No urobilirubin in urine due to no bilirubin reaching small intestine to be converted to urobilirubin.
- Clay-colored stools urobilirubin.
- Pruritis due to deposition of bile salts in skin tissues.
- Intolerance for fatty foods—No bile in small intestine for fat digestion.
- Bleeding tendencies—Lack or decreased absorption of Vitamin K resulting in decreased production of prothrombins.
- Steatorrhea—No bile salts in duodenum, preventing fat emulsion and digestion.
- Billary colic—Murphy sign—i.e. Pain colicy and more flow steady. Complications of cholecystitis include subphrenic absess, pancreatitis, cholangitis (inflammation of bile ducts), biliary cirrhosis, fistulas, and rupture of gallbladder which can produce bile peritonitis.

Diagnostic Study

- Ultrasound
- Cholecystogram or IV cholengiogram
- Liver function studies
- WBC counts and
- Serum bilirubin.

Management

During an acute episode of cholecystitis the focus of treatment is on control of pain, control of possible infection with antibiotics and maintenance of fluid and electrolyte balance. Treatment is mainly supportive and symptomatic. conservative therapy includes:
- IV fluids.
- NPO with NG tube later progressing to low fat diets.
- Antiemetic to prevent nausea and vomiting.
- Analgesics to relieve pain (i.e. meperidine) as prescribed.
- Administration of Fat - soluble vitamins (A B E/C).
- Anticholenergic to decrease secretions which prevents biliary contraction.
- Antispasmodic counteracts smooth muscle spasm.
- Hydrocholetic drugs - Dehydrocholic acid, Florantyrone (Zanchal).
- Antibiotics.
- ETCEP with spincterotomy (Pillotomy).
- Cholestrol solvents.
- Extracorporeal shock-wave lithotripsy (ESWL).

The dissolution therapy incldues:
- Ursodeoxycholic acid (UDCA).
- Ursodial.
- Chenodeoxycholic acid (CDCA).
- Any medication prescribed by the physician.
  Surgical intervention for cholelithiasis is frequently indicated and may consider any one of the several procedures as follows:
- Cholecystectomy—Removal of gallbladder.
- Cholecystostomy—Incision of gallbladder for removal of stones.
- Choledocholithotomy—Incision to common bile duct for removal of stones.

- Cholicystogastrotomy—Anastomosis between stomach and gallbladder.
- Choledecysoduo—Anastomosis between denostomy gall bladder and duodenum to relieve obstruction to distal end of common bile duct.
- Laparoscopic—Removal of gallbladder cholecystectomy via Laproscopy using a dissecting laser.

The nurse has to follow the undermentioned guidelines for the patient undergoing open cholecysteatomy in addition to general guidelines.

Preoperative

Patient with complete preoperative preparations at home before their arrival on the day of surgery. The nurse will verify that the patient has had NPO and completed any required bowel preparation. Preoperative teaching includes:
- Teach patient the importance of frequent breathing and use of incentive spirometer because the high incision and RUQ pain predispose the patient to atelectasis and right lower lobe pneumonia.
- Explain the types of biliary drainage tubes which are anticipated if any.
- Teach the patient about the pain control plan to be used in the postoperative period.

Postoperative

- Place the patient in low-Fowler's position, assist to change position frequently.
- Urge patient to deep breathing at regular intervals (every 1 to 2 hrs) and to cough if secretions are present until ambulating well. Assist patient to effectively splint the incision. Encourage use of incentive spirometer.
- Give analgesics fairly liberally for the first 2 to 3 days.
- Use patient-controlled analgesia if possible. Meperidine has been the drug of choice because it is believed to minimize spasms in the bile ducts, but morphine is being used with increasing frequency.
- Maintain a dry, intact dressing, usually a drain is inserted near the stump of the cyst duct; Some serous fluid drainage is normal initially.
- Encourage progressive ambulation when permitted.
- Increase diet gradually to be regular with fat content as tolerated (appetite and fat tolerance may be diminished if there is external biliary drainage).

Biliary Drainage

- Connect any biliary drainage tubes to be closed gravity drainage.
- Attach sufficient tubing so the patient can move without restriction.
- Explain to patient the importance of avoiding kinks, clamping or pulling of the tube.
- Monitor the amount and color of drainage frequently, measure and record drainage at least every shift.
- Report any signs of peritonitis (abdominal pain, rigidity or fever) to the concerned doctor.
- Monitor color of urine and stools; stools will be grayish white, if the bile is flowing out a drainage tube, but the normal color should gradually reappear as external drainage diminishes and disappears.

PRIMARY SCLEROSING CHOLANGITIS (PSC)

Inflammation and scarring of the biliary tree occur more commonly as a result of gallstones and bile duct infection. Parasites are most common source of infections. When no cause for the bile duct injury can be found, the process is called ideopathic or primary sclerosing cholangitis. It has closest link with inflammatory bowel disease.

Pathophysiology

PSC causes changes in and around the large bile ducts from inflammation obstruction and intra and extrahepatic fibrosis. Strictures can usually be found in multiple locations. These strictures are short and diffusely distributed and alternate with normal or dilated segments of the ducts to create a bead-like appearance in X-ray. It is unusual for the gallbladder or cystic ducts to be involved.

Clinical Manifestation

Many patients are symptomatic in early stages. Others are seen with combination of fatigue, fever, jaundice, abdominal pain and weight loss. Persistent severe pruritis can be a particularly difficult aspect of the disease. Patient may experience recurrent attacks of cholangitis.

Diagnostic studies of other liver and biliary disorders.

Management

Drug therapy aimed at reducing biliary tree inflammation and preventing the scarring that leads to obstruction. The drug ursodeoxycholic acid has shown promise. surgical procedures other than transplant have been effective for diffuse disease. Endoscopic treatment to remove stones, relieve obstruction, dilate ducts, and place stout tubes in ongoing but primarily in the form of clinical trials.

The uncertain nature of PSC is one of its most difficult characteristics. Patients are instructed about the disease and its possible outcome and are prepared for the possibility of the eventual need for liver transplant. Persistent jaundice may negatively affect body image, and chronic severe pruritis may be a daily nightmare. Some patients are responding to cholestyramine resin (Drug), which theoretically binds the itching triggering elements in the bile. The nurse also suggests that patient experiments with common intervention that may lessen his/her itching. A low fat diet is recommended to patient who develops problems with diarrhea or steatorrhea and the fat restriction usually promptly corrects the problems. Fat soluble vitamin replacement is often needed.

The following strategies to control pruritis are helpful:
- Avoid irritating clothing (Wool or restrictive clothing).
- Use tepid water for bathing rather than hot.
  - Experiment with nonirritating soaps and detergents
  - Pat skin dry after bathing or showering; do not rub.
- Apply emollient creams and lotions to dry skin regularly.
- Avoid activities that increase body temperature or cause sweating.
- Experiment with treatments such as oatameal baths.
- Keep the fingernails short and consider use of cotton gloves at night to minimize skin damage from scratching.
- Use antipruritic medications as ordered.

ACUTE PANCREATITIS

Acute pancreatitis is an acute inflammatory process of the pancreas. The degree of inflammation varies from mild edema to severe Hemorrhage necrosis.

Etiology

Acute pancreatitis is most common in middle-aged men and women, but affects more men than women. Many factors can cause injury to the pancreas. The primary etiological factors are biliary tract disease and alcoholism. The other less common causes are:
- Acute pancreatitis include trauma (postsurgical, abnormal).
- Viral infections (mumps, coxsakie virus B).
- Pancreating duodenum ulcer.
- Abscesses.
- Cystic fibrosis.
- Kaposis sarcoma.
- Certain drugs (corticosteroids, thiazetic diurectics, oral contraceptives sulfanamide and NSAIDS).
- Metabolic disorders: (hyperlipidaemia, renal failure).
- After surgical procedure (of pancreas, stomach, duodenum and biliary tract).
- After ERCP.
- Idiopathic.

Pathophysiology

The most common pathogenic mechanism is believed to be autodigestion of the pancreas. The two major pathological varieties of acute pancreatitis are (1) acute intestinal form and (2) acute hemorrhagic form. Although either can be fatal, intestinal form is often a milder form. The defining characteristics of acute intestinal pancreatitis is a diffusely swollen and inflamed pancreas, which retains its anatomical features. There are minimal or no area of hemorrhage or necrosis in gland. The interstitial spaces becomes grossly swollen by extracellular edema and the ducts may contain purulent material. The acute hemorrhage disease presents with a different picture. The gland readily shows acute inflammation, Hemorrhage, and marked tissue necrosis. Extensive fat necrosis is present in patients with fulminant disease not just in the pancreas but throughout the abdominal and thoracic cavities and subcutaneous tissues. Necrosis of vessel can cause significant loss of blood and abscesses and infections form in areas of walled-off necrotic tissue. Systemic complications such as fat emboli, hypotension, shock and fluid overload are common.

The etiologic factors cause injury to pancreatic cells or activation of the pancreatic enzymes in the pancreas. Trypsionogen is an inactive proteolytic enzyme produced by pancreas. Activation of pancreatic enzymes before they reach the duodenum has long been recognized as a major component of the disease process. Enzyme activation overwhelms all of the normal protective mechanisms of the pancreas and initiates a massive attack on the pancreatic tissues. Pancreatic autodigestion is initiated. Other systemic effects of the activated enzymes include:
- Activation of complement and kinin-producing increased vascular permeability and vasodilation.
- Increased stickiness of the inflammatory leucocytes with formation of emboli, which plug the microvasculature.
- Initiation of consumptive coagulopathy, leading to disseminated intravascular coagulation.
- Increased permeability causing massive movement of fluids which leads to circulatory insufficiency.
- Release of myocardial-depressant factor, which further compromises cardiac function.
- Activation of the renin-angiotensin network, which impairs renal function in conjunction with circulatory insufficiency.

Clinical Manifestations

Pain

- Steady and severe in nature, excruciating in fulminant cases.
- Located in the epigastric or umbilical region, may radiate to the back.
- Worsened by lying supine; may be lessened by flexed knee, curved back positioning.

Vomiting

- Varies in severity but is usually protracted.
- Worsened by ingestion of food or fluid.
- Does not relive the pain.
- Usually accompanied by nausea.

Fever

Rarely exceeds 39°C.

Abdominal Findings

- Rigidity, tenderness, guarding.
- Distension.
- Decreased or absent peristalsis.

Additional Features of Fulminal Disease

- Symptoms of hypovolemic shock.
- Oliguria; acute tubular necrosis.
- Ascites.
- Jaundice.
- Respiratory failure.
- Grey Turner's sign (bluish discoloration along the flanks).
- Cullen's sign (bluish discoloration around the umbilicus).

(These signs indicate the accumulation of blood in these areas and represent the presence of hemorrhagic pancreatitis).

The significant local complications of acute pancreatitis are pseudocyst and absess. The main systemic complication as pulmonary (plueral effusion, atelectasis and pneumonia) and tetany and hypotension hypovolemia, hypoalbuminemia, leukocytosis, ARDS, GI bleeding, pseudocyst, hyperglycemia, hypocalcemia, and hyperlipidemia.

Diagnostic Studies

The primary diagnostic tests are serum amylase, lipase and urinary amylase level. Usually there is elevation. The secondary tests are blood glucose, (hyperglycemic due to impaired carbohydrate metabolism due to E-cell damage and release of glucagon). Serum calcium (hypocalcemia) and serum triglycerides (Hyperlipidemia) and also CTS, ERCEP.

Management

The main objective of the management of acute pancreatitis are: Relief of pain; prevention and alleviation of shock; reduction of pancreatic secretions, control of fluid and electrolyte imbalance, prevention and treatment of infections and removal of precipitatory cause for which the measures to be taken according to the following:

- Administer meparidin (analgesics) to relieve pain.
- NPO with NG tube to suction and reduce secretions.
- Cimetidine or rantidine IV.
- Administer antibiotics as prescribed.
- Lactated Ringer's solution for fluid and electrolyte valancy and bedrest and proper diet, good oral hygiene should be maintained and take measures to treat complications accordingly and teach patients to avoid alcohol.

CHRONIC PANCREATITIS

Chronic pancreatitis is progressive destruction of the pancreas with fibrotitic replacement of pancreatic tissue structure and calcification may also occur in the pancreas.

Etiology

Chrome pancreatic may follow acute pancreatitis. The two major types are chronic-obstructive pancreatitis and chronic-calcifying pancreatitis. Chronic obstructive pancreatis is associated with biliary disease. The most common cause is inflammation of the spincter associated with cholelithiasis. Cancer of the ampules of valex duodenum, or pancreas also can cause this type. The chronic calcifying pancreatitis, there are inflammation and sclerosis mainly in the head of the pancreas and around the pancreatic duct. It is associated with alcohol. These are also called "alcohol-induced pancreatitis".

Pathophysiology

The basic pathological change of chronic pancreatitis is destruction of the exocrine parenchymas and replacements with fibrous tissue. This process is associated with varying degrees of duct dilation. Scarring and fibritic changes may occur throughout the pancreas or be limited to the selected areas. Calcium salts may be deposited in both the ducts and the parenchyma, usually in areas of fat necrosis. Ductal obstructions occur secondarily. The factors which influence the solubility on the calcium-rich pancreatic secretions are not well-identified. As the process becomes increasingly severe the islets of Langerhans are also involved and destroyed.

Clinical Manifestation

As with acute pancreatitis, a major manifestation of the chronic pancreatic is abdominal pain. The patient may have episodes of acute pain, but it is usually chronic (recurrent attack at intervals of months or years). The attacks may become more and more frequent until they are almost constant, or they may diminish as the pancreatic fibrosis develops. The pain is located in the same area as in the acute pancreatitis, but it is usually described as heavy, gnawing feeling and sometimes a burning and cramp like. The pain is not relieved by food or antacids. The other manifestations are pancreatic insufficiency including malabsorption with weight loss, constipation, mild jaundice with dark urine, steatorrhea and diabetes mellitus. The steatorrhea may become severe with voluminous, foul, fatty stools. Urine and stools may be frothy. Some abdominal tenderness may be present.

Diagnosis: (Diagnostic studies as in acute pancreatitis).

Management

When the patient with chronic pancreatitis is experiencing an acute attack, the therapy is identical as that for acute pancreatitis. At other times, the focus is on prevention of further attacks, relief of pain, and control of pancreatic exocrine and endocrine insufficiency. It sometimes takes large, frequent doses of analgesics to relieve pain and diet, pancreatic enzyme replacement, and control of diabetes are measures used to control pancreatic insufficiency. The diet is a bland, low-fat, high-carbohydrate and high protein diet. The patient does not tolerate fatty, rich and stimulating foods and these should be avoided to decrease pancreatic secretions and demands on the pancreas. Alcohol must be totally eliminated. Antacids and anticholenising drugs may be given to decrease HCl acid. For diabetes insulin is giving as per instruction of the medical doctors. When pseudocysts or obstruction develops, surgery may be indicated and treated accordingly.

CHAPTER 5

Nursing Management of Cardiovascular Disorders

NURSING ASSESSMENT OF CARDIOVASCULAR SYSTEM (CVS)

Systematic cardiovascular assessment provides the nurse with baseline data useful in identifying the physiological and psychosocial needs of the patient and for planning appropriate nursing interventions to meet these needs.

A careful history and physical examination should help the nurse in differentiating symptoms that reflect a cardiovascular problem from problems of other body systems. Many illnesses affect the cardiovascular system directly or indirectly. The patient should be questioned about a history of chest pain, shortness of breath, alcoholism, or excessive drinking, anemia, rheumatic fever, streptococcal sore throat, congenital heart disease, stroke, syncope, hypertension, thrombophlebitis, intermittent claudications, varicositis and edema.

The classic symptoms of heart disease include dyspnea, chest pain, or discomfort, edema, syncope, palpitations and excessive fatigue. Cardiovascular function, which may be adequate at rest may be insufficient during exercise or exertion. Therefore, careful attention is directed to the effect of activity on the patient's symptoms.

Dyspnea

Dyspnea is an abnormally uncomfortable awareness of breathing, in which patient complains of shortness of breath. It is a subjective experience associated with anxiety and variety of disease processes.

- Exertional dyspnea: Dyspnea on exertion is a common symptom of cardiac dysfunctions. In the early stages of heart failure, dyspnea usually is provoked only by effort and is relieved promptly by rest. It is important to identify the amount of exertion necessary to produce dyspnea, because the lower the cardiac reserve (heart's ability to adjust and adapt to increased demands), lesser the effort is required to precipitate dyspnea.
- Orthopnea refers to dyspnea in the recumbent position. It is usually a symptom of more advanced heart failure that is exertional dyspnea. Patients insist that they require two or more pillows to sleep restfully. When the person assumes the recumbent position, gravitational forces redistribute blood from the lowest extremities and splanchnic bed increase venous return. The augmentation of intrathoracic blood volume elevates pulmonary venous and capillary pressures, resulting in a transient pulmonary congestion, orthopnea, (usually is relieved in less than 5 minutes after the patient sits upright).
- Paraxysmal nocturnal dyspnoea is also known as cardiac asthma, is characterized by severe attacks of shortness of breath that generally occur 2 to 5 hours after the onset of sleep. This condition is commonly associated with sweating and wheezing. Classically, the person awakens from sleep, arises and quickly opens with the perception of needing fresh air. These frightening attacks are precipitated by the same physiological mechanism that causes orthopnea. The diseased heart is unable to compensate for this increase in blood volume by pumping extra fluid into the circulatory system and pulmonary congestion results. Paraxysmal nocturnal dyspnea is relieved by sitting on the side of the bed or getting out of the bed. For relief of dyspnea, 20 minutes or more is needed. The cues to dyspnea are air hunger, especially after exertion, pillows or upright chair necessary for sleep.

Chest Pain

Although pain or discomfort in the chest is one of the cardinal symptoms of cardiac disorder, chest pain can be precipitated by various conditions. For example, chest pain may be caused by anxiety, ischemia, heart disease, acute dissection of the aorta, acute pericardia, pulmonary disorders, (pleurisy and pulmonary embolism) esophageal spasm, or reflux, and peptic ulcer disease. The cues for chest pain-related heart disorders are indigestion, burning, numbness, tightness or pressure in midchest, epigastric or substernal pain, radiating to shoulder, neck, and arms.

Syncope

Syncope is dyspnea as a generalized muscle weakness with an inability to stand upright, accompanied by loss of consciousness. The most common cause of syncope is decreased perfusion to the brain. Any condition that results in a sudden reduction of cardiac output (CO) and therefore reduced cerebral blood flow could potentially cause a syncopal episode. In patients with cardiovascular disorders, conditions such as orthostatic hypotension, hypovolemia, or variety of dysrhythmias may precipitate syncope.

Palpitation

Palpitation is a common subjective phenomenon defined as an unpleasant awareness of the irregular heart beat. It may be precipitated by a change in cardiac rate or rhythm, i.e. by an increase in myocardial contractivity. Patient may experience sensation of heart in throat or skipped beat, racing heart, and dizziness. Patients may describe that heart beat as "pounding", "racing" or skipping. Palpitation that occurs either during or after strenuous activity are considered physiological. Palpitations that occur during mild exertion may suggest the presence of heart failure, anemia or thyrotoxicosis. Other non-cardiac factors may precipitate palpitation include, nervousness, heavy meals, lack of sleep and a large intake of Caffene-containing beverage, alcohol or tobacco.

Fatigue

Fatigue refers to no energy, needs more rest than usual, normal activities result in tiring. Fatigue and lassitude have many causes, but it has direct consequence of heart failure. The exact physiological mechanism is not known. But probably, it is a consequence of an inadequate cardiac output. Such fatigue can occur during effort or at rest and generally worsens as the day progresses. Fatigue that occurs after mild exertion may indicate a low cardiac reserve if the heart is unable to meet even small increase in metabolic demand.

Dizzy

Dizzy, light headedness: Dizzy with change of position; woozy, unstable and weak.

Edema (Fluid Retention)

The cues for oedema are: Weight gain, bloated feeling, swelling, tightening of clothing, shoes no longer fitting comfortably, marks or identification left from constricting garments.

Tenderness in Calf of Legs

The cues for tenderness of calf of legs are—inability to bear weight, swelling of the involved extremity; inflamed warm skin over vein; distended, discoloured, tortuous veins in calves of legs, ache in lower extremities after standing for short periods.

PHYSICAL EXAMINATION

Physical examination of the CVS includes the standard assessment techniques of inspection, palpation, percussion and auscultations.

Inspection

Inspection of the patient includes skin color, neck vein distention, respiration, pulsations and clubbing and capillary refill. The inspection of the skin color, hair distribution and venous blood flow provide information about arterial blood flow. A person's normal color depends on race, ethnic background and lifestyle and is an indication of adequate cardiac output (CO) and circulation. Pallor may indicate anemia, hypoxia, or peripheral vasoconstriction. Cyanosis (cerebral), a bluish discoloration of the skin is most easily observed by examining the earlobes, the oral mucosa at the base of the tongue, legs and the nailbeds. Peripheral cyanosis results from low CO and generally is accompanied by decreased skin temperature and mottling. In contrast to central cyanosis, no cyanosis of the tongue is present. Central cyanosis is caused by low arsenal oxygen saturation, (ex. congenital heart defects). Skin color and the extremities also be assessed for noting any erythema or pigmentation changes as well as the shiny, or dry, scaly skin, which may indicate vascular disorders.

A general estimate of venous pressure can be obtained by observation of the neck veins. Normally, when a person is supine, the neck veins are distended. However, when the head of the bed is elevated to a 45 degree angle, the neck veins are collapsed. If jugular distention is present, assess the jugular venous pressure by measuring from the highest point of visible distention to the sternal angle. Measurements above 3 cm area considered elevated. The Jugular veins reflect venous tone, blood volume and right atrial pressure. Therefore, distended neck veins suggest increased venous pressure, which may be caused by right-sided heart failure, circulatory volume load, superior venacaval obstructions or tricuspid valve regurgitation.

The rate and character of the patients' respirations are important to assess. Normally an adult breathes comfortably at a rate of 12 to 20 times per minute. Particular attention is paid to the case of difficulty in breathing and patient's general demeanour.

Inspection of the anterior chest is best accomplished with the patient lying supine, either flat or with the head slightly elevated. Observe the pericardium for the apical inpulse, which is a pulsation of the chest wall caused by the forward thrustings of the left ventricle during systole. When visible, the apical impulse occupies the fourth or fifth intercostal space at or inside midclavicular line. The apical impulse was formerly known as the point of maximal impulse. The apical inpulse is not always visible, but it is palpable in about half of adults.

The nails are assessed for clubbing and capillary refill. The exact cause is unknown. However, clubbing of the finger in the fistulas with right to left shunting. Capillary filling or blanching (whitening) is an indicator of peripheral circulation to the fingers and toes and can be tested in all nailbeds. The examiner presses a thumbnail against the edge of a patient's finger nails or toe nail and quickly releases it and notes the blanching resposne and observes for the returning colour within three seconds.

Palpations

Palpations of the pulses in the neck and extremities also provides information on arterial blood flow. One method of evaluating arterial flow of the vascular system is to palpate the extremities simultaneously to determine skin temperature. A second method is to palpate the peripheral pulses, which are evaluated bilaterally on the basis of their absence or presence, rate, rhythm, amplitude, quality and equality. Each pulse, except the carotids should be palpated on the left and right sides simultaneously to evaluate the contralateral symmetry.

A scale may be used to document pulse volume or amplitude by rating on a scale of 0 to +4 as follows:

- 0 = Absent
- + = Palpable, but diminished
- ++ = Normal or average
- +++ = Full and risk
- ++++ = Full and bounding, often visible.

Several abnormalities may be detected during palpation of pulses.

- A hypokinetic (weak) pulse signifies a narrowed pulse pressure, that is decreased differences between systolic and diastolic pressure. It is usually produced by a low CO and is associated with often detected in such conditions as severe LVF, hypovolemia, or mitral and aortic valve stenosis.
- A hyperkinetic (bounding) pulse represents a widened pulse pressure. It is usually associated with increased left ventricular stroke volume and a decreased peripheral vascular resistance. This is found in hyperkinetic circulatory state caused by exercise, fever, anaemia or hyperthyroidism.
- Pulsus alternans is a condition in which the heart beats regularly, but the pulses vary in amplitude. It is caused by an alternating left ventricular contractile force and usually indicates severe depression of myocardial infarction, pulsus alternans can be detected by palpation and accurately by auscultation.
- Pulsus paradoxus signifies a reduction in the amplitude of the arterial pulse during inspiration. Variation in pulse strength can be palpated and also readily detected by sphygmomanometry. Pulsus paradoxus is a result of decreased left ventricular stroke volume and the transmission of negative intrathoracic pressure to the aorta. It may occur in conditions such as cardiac temponade and constrictive pericarditis and also COPD.

Edema is defined as an accumulation of fluid in the interstitial spaces. It may be localized to one particular body part, organ or tissue or that may be generalized distribution. An important indicator for cardiovascular function in the presence of absence of peripheral edema, especially in the feet, ankles, legs and the sacrum. This is caused by gravity flow or by interruption of the venous return to the heart as a result of constricting clothing or pressure on the veins of the lower extremities. Edema often disappears on elevation of the body part. In contrast, pitting oedema does not disappeear with elevation of the extremity of body part, and it may indicate fluid overload or pathological condition (e.g. congestive heart failure). Pitting oedema is present if an indication is left in the skin after a thumb or finger has been used to apply gentle pressure.

Percussion

The borders of the right and left sides of the heart can be estimated by percussion. The use of percussion for detecting cardiac enlargement generally has been replaced by chest X-ray which is much more accurate. The nurse stands to the right of the recumbent patient and percusses along the curve of the rib in the fourth and the fifth intercostal spaces (ICS), starting at the midaxillary line. The percussion note over the heart is dull in comparison with the resonance over the lung and is recorded in relation to midclavicular line. Cardiac dullness is the characteristics of cardiac hypertrophy.

Auscultation

The movement of the cardiac valves creates some turbulence in the blood flow. The vibration of the blood causes normal heart sounds. These sounds can be heard through a stethoscope placed on the chest wall. The first heart sound (S1) which is associated with the closure of the tricuspid and mitral valve (AV) has a soft "lubb" sound. S1 is longer and lower pitched than the second heart sound (S2). The second heart sound (S2) which is associated with the closure of the aortic and pulmonic (semilunar) valve, has a sharp "dubb" sound. The first and second heart sounds together are referred to as "lub-dub". S1 corresponds to the beat of the carotid pulse. As stated earlier S2 is caused mainly by the closure of the semilunar valves. S2 is usually loudest at the base of the heart and is described as shorter, higher pitched and "snappier" than S1. S1 signals the beginning of systole, S2 signals the beginning of diastole. The nurse should listen to the auscultatory areas in sequence with both the diaphragm and bell of the stethoscope.

The first and second heart sounds are heard best with diaphragm of the stethoscope because they are high-pitched.

Extra heart sounds (S3 or S4) if present, are heard best with the bell of the stethoscope because they are low-pitched. The nurse listens at the apical area with diaphragm of the stethoscope while simultaneously palpating the radial pulse. If fewer radial than apical pulse are counted, a pulse deficit is present. A patient with a pulse deficit should have the apical and radial pulse taken often to monitor this abnormality. A judgement about the rhythm (regular or irregular) is also made when listening at the apex.

Normally no sounds are heard between S1 and S2 during the periods of systole and diastole. Sounds that are heard during these periods probably represent abnormalities and should be described. An exception to this is normal splitting of S2, which is best heard at the pulmonic area during inspiration. Splitting of this heart sound can be abnormal if S1 is heard during expiration or if it is constant (fixed) during the respiratory cycle.

If an abnormal sound is heard, it should be documented. This description should include the timing (during systole or diastole), location (the site on the chest where it is heard the loudest), pitch (heard best with the diaphragm or bell of the stethoscope), position (heard best when the patient is recumbent, sitting, leaning forward, or in the left lateral cubitus position). Characteristic (harsh, musical, soft, short, long) and any abnormal findings (irregular cardiac rhythms or palpable chest wall heaves) associated with sound.

The abnormal sound, occurring during diastole and systole are classified as either murmurs or extra sound (S3 and S4). Murmurs are sounds produced by turbulent blood flow through the heart or the walls of large arteries. Most murmurs are the result of cardiac abnormalities, but some occur in normal cardiac structures. Murmurs are graded on six point scale of loudness and recorded as Roman numeral ratio, the numerator is intensity of the murmur and denominator is always VI which indicates the six-point scale sued.

DIAGNOSTIC STUDIES OF CVS

A number of diagnostic procedures add to the information obtained from the history and physical examination of the cardiovascular system. These procedures are usually classified as noninvasive or invasive. If only needle insertion for withdrawal of blood or injection of dye is used these studies are usually considered noninvasive. Catheter insertion for angiography is considered as invasive procedure. Certain responsibilities of the nurse remains the same regardless of whether patient is to undergo invasive or noninvasive procedure. First, the nurse must see that the procedure is scheduled and that any necessary preliminaries (e.g. special diets or changes in medication) are completed. Appropriate safety measures, such as the use of bedside rails after administration of preprocedure medicatioan or identification of patient allergies should be instituted. Comfort measures such as oral care before procedure are important. The nurse must also check to see to it that in obtaining consent the procedure should be explained skillfully, relieving the anxiety of patients and significant ones of the patient. These are the most common diagnostic measures to be carried out by nurses to assess the cardiovascular system and main nursing responsibility required for the same is presented as follows:

Chest X-ray

A radiograph of the chest may be taken to determine overall size and configuration of the heart in which patient is placed in two upright positions to examine the lung fields and size of the heart. The two common positions are anterior/posterior (AP) and left lateral. Normal heart size and contour for the individual age, sex and size are noted. Most abnormalities of heart size and calcification of the heart muscle, valves and great vessels can be detected with a standard posterior anterior and lateral view of the chest.

The nursing responsibilities include inquiring about the frequency of recent X-rays and possibility of pregnancy (of female). Provide lead shielding to the areas not being viewed, remove any jewellery or metal objects that may obstruct the view of the heart and lungs.

Cardiac Fluoroscopy

It facilitates the observation of the heart from varying view while the heart is in motion. Fluoroscopy can be used to detect ventricular aneurysms, monitor prosthetic valve movement, or assess the position of cardiac calcification during the cardiac cycle. Because of the radiational risk associated with fluoroscopy, most of them are not used in this procedure. Nursing responsibility is the same as for chest X-rays.

Electrocardiogram (ECG)

The ECG is a graphic representation of the electrical forces produced within the heart. The ECG is an essential tool for cardiac evaluation, but it must be combined with other data sources for an accurate diagnosis. An ECG may be normal even in the presence of heart disease. Conversely, abnormal variance may be seen in the ECG of a normal heart. The ECG may be used for a variety of diagnostic purposes as given below:
- Tachycardia, bradycadia, dysrhythmia.
- Sudden onset of dyspnea.
- Pain occurring in the upper portion of the trunk and in the extremities.
- Syncopical episodes.
- Shock state or coma.
- Preoperative status.
- Postoperative hypertention.
- Hypertension, murmurs, or cardiomegaly.
- Artificial pacemaker function.

In taking ECG, electrodes are placed on the chest and extremities, allowing the ECG machine to record cardiac electrical activity from different views by using standard 12-lead ECG machine. ECG can detect rhythm of heart, site of pacemaker, conduction abnormalities, position of the heart, size of atria and ventricles and presence of injury.

The nurse has to inform the patient step-by-step procedure and assures of its safe, painless nature and comfortability.

Instruct the patient to avoid moving to decrease muscle motion artifact.

Ambulatory ECG Monitoring

Holter Monitoring

It is used to obtain a continuous graphic tracing of patient's ECG during daily activities, in which recording of ECG rhythm for 24–48 hours and then correlating rhythm changes with symptoms recorded in diary. Normal patient activity is encouraged to stimulate conditions that produce symptoms. Electrodes are placed on chest and a recorder is used to store information until it is recalled, printed, and analysed for any rhythm disturbance. It can be performed on an inpatient or outpatient basis.

In this procedure, nurse has to prepare skin and apply electrodes as leads. Explain importance of keeping an accurate diary of activities and symptoms. Tell the patient that no bath or shower can be taken during monitoring. Skin irritations may develop from electrodes. Take care of it.

Stress Testing (ECG during Exercise)

It may be performed for a variety of reasons and often combined with ECG to obtain additional information about heart functions. Indications for performing a stress test are:

- Evaluation of the patient with symptoms suggestive of coronary artery disease.
- Determination of the patient's physical work capacity and aerobic capacity.
- Determination of the patient's functional capacity after a myocardial infarction and as an aid in planning and exercise rehabilitation program.
- Evaluation of the exercise induced dysrhythmias.
- Evaluation of the symptom-free person older than 40 years of age who is at risk for coronary artery disease.
- Evaluation of pharmacological intervention for dysrhythmias, angina or ischemia.

Various protocols are used to evaluate the effect of exercise tolerance on myocardial function. A common protocol uses 3 minutes, stages at speeds and elevation of the treadmill belt. Continued monitoring of vital signs and ECG rhythms or ischemic changes are important in the diagnosis of left ventricular function and coronary artery disease. An exercise bike may be used if the patient is unable to walk on the treadmill. Stress test is designed to progressively increasing myocardial oxygen demand. Some patients may experience untoward effects (ventricular tachycardia, change in systolic BP, chest pain, etc). So test may be terminated at any point of test.

Adequate preparation for stress testing is important. Although procedure is not painful. It can be fatiguing. Patient may become anxious because they will be exercising at a level that may produce symptoms such as dyspnoea, palpitations and chest pain. The nurse may review the purposes and method of stress testing and encourage the patient to do the following:

- Avoid coffee, tea and alcohol on the day of test.
- Avoid smoking and taking nitroglycerine during the 2 hours immediately before the test.
- Wear comfortable, loose fitting clothes (women should be advised to wear a brassiere for support).
- Wear sturdy, comfortable walking shoes.
- Consult the physician about taking any medication before the test.

And the nurse should:

- Instruct the patient about procedure and application of lead placements.
- Monitor vital signs and obtain 12-lead ECG before exercise, during each stage of exercise, and after exercise until all vital signs and ECG changes have returned to normal.
- Monitor patient's symptoms throughout procedure.

Transtelephonic Event Recorders

Allow more freedom than regular Holter Monitor. It records rhythm disturbances that are not frequent enough to be recorded in a 24 hour period. Some units have electrodes that are attached to the chest and have a loop of memory that captures the onset and end of an event. Other types are placed directly on patient's wrist, chest, or fingers have no loop memory, but records the patient's ECG in real time. Recordings are transmitted over the phone to a receiving unit, and the recordings are printed out for review. Tracings can then be erased and the unit can be reused.

The nurse has to instruct the patient in the use of equipment for recording and transmitting transient events. Teach the patient about skin preparation for lead placement or steddy skin contact for units not requiring electrodes. This will ensure the reception of optimal ECG tracings for analysis.

Sonic Studies

Echocardiogram (M-mode-two-dimensional)

Echocardiography uses ultrasound to assess cardiac structure and mobility noninvasively. It is useful in the diagnosis of a variety of cardiac conditions as follows:

- Abnormal pericardial fluid.
- Vulvular disorders including prosthetic valves.
- Ventricular aneurysms.
- Cardiac chamber size.
- Stroke volume and cardiac outputs.

- Some myocardial abnormalities, such as idiopathic hypertrophic subaortic stensosis (IHSS).
- Wall motion abnormalities.

In this, a small transducer is placed on the chest of the patient at the level of third or fourth intercostal space near the left lower sternal border. The transducer transmits high frequency sound waves then receives these waves back from the patient as they are reflected from different structures. The ultrasonic beam that is reflected back from the patient's heart produces "echoes" that are viewed as lines and spaces on an oscilloscope. These lines and spaces represent bone, cardiac chambers and valves, the septum and the muscle. A copy of echocardiogram is recorded on paper.

Here, the nursing responsibility is to place the patient in supine position on left side facing equipment. Instruct patient and family about procedure and sensations (pressure and mechanical movement from head of transducer). No contraindication to procedure exists.

Stress Echocardiogram

It is the combination of exercise, treadmill test and echocar diogram. Resting images of the heart are taken with ultrasound and then the patient exercises. Postexercise images are taken immediately after exercise (which 1 minute of stopping exercises). Differences in left ventricular wall motion and thickening before and after exercise is evaluated. Here, the nurse has to instruct and prepare patient for exercise treadmill. Make the patient aware that ultrasound is not harmful and the importance of speed in returning to examination table for imaging after exercise. Contraindication includes any patient unable to reach peak exercise.

Dobutamine Echocardiogram

It is used as a substitute for the exercise stress test in individual unable to walk on a treadmill. Dobutamine (a positive in-strophic agent) is infused IV and dosage is increased in 5 minutes intervals while echocardiogram is performed to detect wall motion abnormalities in each stage. In this, nursing responsibilities include—starting IV infusion, administering debutamine, monitoring vital signs before, during and after test until baseline is achieved. Monitor patient for signs and symptoms of distress during procedure.

Transesophageal Echocardiogram (TEE)

TEE allows high resolution ultrasonic imaging of the cardiac structure and great vessels via the esophagus. The clinical indications for TEE are:
- Mitral valve prosthetic dysfunction.
- Mitral valve regurgitation.
- Infective endocarditis.
- Congenital heart disease.
- Intracardial thrombi (especially left atrium and left atrial appendage).
- Cardiac tumor.
- Intraoperative assessment: left ventricle functions, adequacy of valve repair and replacement.

This technique uses a probe with an ultrasound transducer at the tip is swallowed. This procedure can be performed at the bedside without contrast dye. It is performed under local anesthetic and sedation. Usually the physician controls the angle of and depth of esophagus with transducer. As it passes down the esophagus, it sends back clear images of heart size, wall motion, valvular abnormalities, and possible source of thrombi without interference from lungs or chest ribs. A contrast medium may be injected IV for evaluating direction of blood flow if an atrial or ventricular septal defect is suspected. Doppler ultrasound and color flow imaging can also be used concurrently.

In this procedure, nursing responsibility will include the following:
- Instruct patient to be NPO for at least 6 hours before test.
- A tranquilizer will be given and throat locally anesthetized. So, if done as an outpatient, a designated driver is needed.
- Monitor vital signs and oxygen saturation levels and perform suctioning continually during procedure.
- Explain to patient the proper procedure for easy passage of transducer.
- Assist patient to relax.
- Patient may not eat or drink until gag reflex returns.

Scintigraphic Studies

Nuclear cardiological study involves IV injection of radioactive isotopes. Radioactive uptake is counted over the heart by scintillation camera. It supplies information about myocardial contractility, myocardial perfusion and acute cell injury. The common nuclear cardiological are as:

Thallium 201 Scan

Thallium 201 is injected IV and used to evaluate blood flow in different parts of heart. Cold spots correlate with area of infarction. For stress testing, IV thallium is given 1 minute before the patient reaches maximum heart rate on bicycle or treadmill. Patient is then required to continue exercise for 1 minute to circulate the radioactive isotopes. Actual scanning is done within 5-10 minutes after exercise. A second testing scan performed 2-4 hours later and compared to postexercise scan. Instruct patient to eat only a light meal between scans.

Dypyridomole Thallium Scan

As with thallium exercise test, depyridamole (Persantine) is also injected. This drug acts as a powerful vasodilator and will increase blood flow to well perfused coronary arteries. Scanning procedure is same as with thallium scan. In this, instruct the patient to hold all caffeine products for 12 hours before procedure.

Technetium 99 m Sestamibi Scan

In this technetium 99 m sestamibi is injected IV and taken up area of MI, producing hot spots. Maximum results are produced when performed 1–6 days after suspected MI waiting period after injection is 1-1/2–2 hours.

Blood Pool Imaging

In this technetium 99 m per technetate injected intravenously. Single injection allows sequential evaluation of heart for several hours. Study is indicated for patient with recent MI or congestive heart failure, especially if not recovering well. It can be used to measure effectiveness of various cardiac medications and can be done at the patient's bedside.

Posterior Emission Tomography (PET)

PET is a radionuclide-based imaging technique that uses short lived radionuclides as tracers to report both perfusion and metabolic events. Here, uses two radionuclides. Nitrogen-13-ammonia is injected intravenously and scanned to evaluate myocardial perfusion. A second radioactive isotope. Fluoro-18-1-deoxyglucose is then injected and scanned to show myocardial metabolic function. In the normal heart, both scans will match, but in an ischaemic or damaged heart, they will differ. The patient may or may not be stressed. A baseline resting scan is usually obtained for comparison. Here the nurse has to:
- Instruct the procedure.
- Explain that patient will be scanned by a machine and will need to stay still for a period of time.
- Patient's glucose level must be between 6 and 140 mg/dl. for accurate metabolic activity.
- If exercise included as part of testing, patient will need to be NPO and refrain from tobacco and caffeine for 24 hours prior to test.

In general, in all studies related to IV injection of isotopes, nurse has the responsibility to:
- Explain procedure to patient.
- Establish IV line for injection of isotopes.
- Explain that isotopes used in small diagnostic and will loss most of its radioactivity in a few hours.
- Patient's glucose level must be between 60 and 140 mg/dl, for accurate metabolic activity.
- If exercise is included as a part of testing, patient will need to be NPO and refrain from tobacco and caffeine for 24 hours prior to test.

In general in all studies related to IV injection of isotopes nurse has the responsibility to:
- Explain procedure to patient.
- Establish IV line for injection fo isotopes.
- Explain that isotopes are used in small diagnostic quantities and will lose most of their radioactivity in a few hours.
- Inform the patient that he or she will be lying down on back with arm extended overhead for period of time.
- Repeated scans are performed within a few minutes to hours after the injection.

Magnetic Resonance Imaging (MRI)

It is a noninvasive imaging technique which obtains information about cardiac tissue integrity, aneurysms, ejection factions, cardiac output, and patency of proximal coronary arteries. It does not involve ionizing radiations and is an extremely safe procedure. It provides images in multiple planes with uniformly good resolution. It has limited use in critical care patients, because of access and equipment problem. It cannot be used in persons with any implanted metallic devices. In this procedure, the nurses will explain the procedure to patient, inform the patient that the small diameter of the cylinder along with loud nose of the procedure may cease panic or anxiety. Antianxiety medications and music may be recommended.

Blood Studies

The important blood studies are followed in diagnosis are:
- Creatinine kinase (CK)
- CK-MB fraction
- AST (SGOT)
- Myoglobin
- Troponin
- Lactic dehydrogenase (LOH)
- Serum lipids: Cholestrol, Tryglycerides, Lipoproteins.
- Drug levels: Digoxin, quinidine, inderol (propronolol).

Cardiac Catheterization

It is an extremely valuable diagnosis tool used for obtaining detailed information about the structures and functions of the cardiac chambers, valves and coronary arteries. This diagnostic study involves insertion of catheter in the heart. Information can be obtained about O_2 saturation and pressure readings within chambers. Dye can be injected to assist in examining structure and motion of heart. Procedure is done by insertion of catheter into a vein for right-sided heart or an artery for left-sided heart.

The nursing responsibilities before procedure are:
- Obtain written permission.
- Withhold food and fluids for 6–18 hours before procedure.
- Give sedation, if ordered.
- Inform patient about use of local anesthesia, insertion of catheter and feeling of warmth and fluttering sensation of heart as catheter is passed.
- Note that patient may be instructed to cough or take a deep breathing when catheter is inserted.

- See that the patient is monitored by ECG throughout procedure.

After the procedure, nurse has the responsibility to:
- Assess circulation to extremity used for catheter insertion.
- Check peripheral pulses, color and sensation of extremity, every 15 minutes for 1 hour and then with decreasing frequency.
- Observe injection site for swelling and bleeding.
- Place sand bag over arterial site if indicated.
- Monitor vital signs.
- Assess for abnormal heart rate, arrhythmias and signs of pulmonary emboli (respiratory difficulty).

In addition to above diagnostic tests, the following should also be performed.
- Coronary angiography.
- Intracoronary ultrasound.
- Hemodynamic monitoring.
- Electrophysiology study.
- Peripheral arteriography and venography.
- Digital subtraction angiography and general routine blood tests, urinalysis, etc.

HYPERTENSION

Hypertension is defined as a consistent constant elevation of the systolic or diastolic pressure above 140/90 mm Hg. It is sustained deviation of blood pressure (BP). In adults, hypertension exists when systolic blood pressure (SBP) is equal to or greater than 140 mm Hg or diastolic blood pressure (DBP) is equal to or greater than 90 mm Hg for extended periods of time. The diagnosis of hypertension requires that elevated readings be present on at least three occasions during several weeks.

High blood pressure (HBP) means that the heart is working harder than normal, putting both the heart and the blood vessels under strain. HBP may contribute to myocardial infarctions, cerebrovascular accidents, (CVA), renal failure and atherosclerosis. Hypertension causes no symptoms to motivate a person to seek treatment. When symptoms do occur, they signify either secondary causes of hypertension or effects of sustained elevation of BP on target organs (coronary artery disease, left ventricular hypertrophy, cerebrovascular disease, peripheral vascular disease, or renal insufficiency).

Etiology

The etiology of hypertension can be classified as either primary (essential) or secondary.

Primary (essential) hypertension accounts for more than 90 percent of all cases and has no known cause, although it is theorized that genetic factor, hormonal changes, and alterations in sympathetic tone all may play a role in its development.

Although the exact cause is unknown, several contributing factors including increased SNS activity, overproduction of sodium retaining hormones and vasoconstrictors, increased sodium intake, more than ideal body weight, diabetes mellitus and excessive alcohol intake. The identified risk factors in primary hypertension are as follows:

- *Age:* Blood pressure rises progressively with advancing or increasing age—elevated BP is present in approximately 50 percent of people over 65 years of age, and with onset usually between the ages of 30 and 50 years.
- *Sex:* Hypertension is more prevalent in men and young adulthood and early middle age. After the age of 55, hypertension is more prevalent in women.
- *Race:* Incidence of HBP is twice as great in African-Americans as in Caucasians.
- *Family history:* Level of BP is strongly familial. Risk of hypertension increases for those with a close relatives having hypertension.
- *Obesity:* Weight gain is associated with increased frequency of hypertension. The risk is greater with central abdominal obesity.
- *Smoking:* Smoking greatly increases the risk of cardiovascular disease. Nicotine constricts blood vessels. Hypertensives who smoke are at even greater risk.
- *High salt diet:* Sodium causes water retention, increasing blood volume. Excessive dietary sodium intake can contribute to hypertension in some patients, and decreases the efficacy of certain antihypertensive medication.
- *Elevated serum lipids:* Elevated levels of cholesterol and triglycerides are primary risk factors in atherosclerosis. Narrowing of arteries increases blood pressure. Hyperlipidemia is more common in hypertensives.
- *Alcohol:* Alcohol increases plasma catecholamines. Excessive alcohol intake is strongly associated with hypertension. Hypertensives should limit their daily intake of ethanol to 1 Oz.
- *Sedantary lifestyles:* Regular physical activity can help control weight and reduce cardiovascular risk. Physical activity may decrease.
- *Diabetes mellitus:* Hypertension is more common in diabetics. Where hypertension and diabetes coexist, complications are more severe.
- *Socioeconomic status:* Hypertension is more prevalent in low socioeconomic groups and among the less educated.
- *Emotional stress:* Stress stimulates sympathetic nerve systems. People exposed to repeated stress may develop hypertension more frequently than others. People who become hypertensive may respond differently to stress from those who do not become hypertensive.

Secondary Hypertension

It develops as a consequence of a particular underlying disease or condition. It is elevated BP with a specific cause that often can be identified and corrected. This type of hypertension accounts for less than 5 percent of hypertension in adults but more than 80 percent of hypertension in children. If a person below the age of 20 or over the age of 50 suddenly develops hypertension, if it is severe, a secondary cause should be suspected. Clinical findings suggest that secondary hypertension include unprovoked hypokalemia, abdominal bruit, variable pressure with tachycardia, sweating and tremor, or family history of renal diseases. Causes of secondary hypertension include the following:

- Coarctation or congenital narrowing of the aorta.
- Renal disease such as renal artery stenosis parenchymal disease (glomerulonephritis, renal failure) and renovascular disease.
- Endocrine disorders such as pheochromocytoma (excessive secretion of catecholamines). Cushing syndrome (blood volume), hyperaldosteronism, primary aldosteronisms (increase in aldosterone causing sodium and water retention and increase blood volume).
- Neurologic disorders such as brain tumor, quadriplegia and head injury.
- Sleep apnea.
- Medications such as sympathetic stimulants (including cocaine) monamino oxidase inhibitors taken with tyramine containing foods, estrogen replacement therapy, oral contraceptive pills, and nonsteroidal anti-inflammatory drugs (NSAIDs).
- Pregnancy-induced hypertension cause is unknown, generalized vasospasm may be a contributing factor.

Pathophysiology

Blood pressure is the force exerted by the blood against the walls of the blood vessels and must be adequate to maintain tissue perfusion during activity and rest. The maintenance of normal BP and tissue perfusion requires the integration of both systemic factors and local peripheral vascular effects. Arterial BP (ABP) is primarily a function of cardiac output (CO) and systemic vascular resistance (SVR). The relationship is summarized by following equation

$$ABP = CO \times SVR$$

Cardiac output (CO) is the total blood flow through the systemic or pulmonary circulation per minute. CO can be described as the stroke volume amount of blood pumped out of the left ventricle per beat (approximately 70 ml) multiplied by the heart rate (HR) for one minute. Systemic vascular resistance (SVR) is the force opposing the movement of blood within the blood vessels. Radius of the small arteries and arterioles is the principal factor determining vascular resistance. A small change in the radius of the arterioles create a major change in the SVR. If SVR is increased and CO remains constant or increases ABP will increase.

The mechanism that regulates BP can affect either CO or SVR or both. Regulation of BP is a complex process involving nervous, cardiovascular, renal and endocrine functions. BP is regulated by both short-term (seconds to hours) and long-term (days to weeks mechanisms). Short-term mechanisms including autonomic nervous system and vascular endothelium, one active within a few seconds. Long-term mechanisms include renal and hormonal process that regulates arteriolar resistance and blood volume.

The regulation of blood pressure is a complex process involving renal control of sodium and water retention and nervous system control of vascular tone. The two primary regulatory factors are blood flow and peripheral vascular resistance refers to size of the peripheral blood vessels. The more constricted the vessel, the greater the resistance to flow and the more dilated the vessel, the lesser is resistance. As peripheral vessels become more constricted, the blood pressure becomes more elevated. Dilation and constriction of the peripheral blood vessels are controlled by primarily by the SNS in stimulated, catecholamines, such as epinephrine and nonepinephrine are released. These chemical causes increased vasoconstriction, increased cardiac output, and increased strength of ventricular contraction. Likewise, when the renin angiotensin system is activated, angiotensin causes vasoconstriction of the blood vessels. Long term vasoconstriction of renal vessels causes permanent renal damage and may lead to kidney failure. Other important organs such as the brain and heart also suffer long-term damage from untreated hypertension.

Clinical Manifestation

Hypertension is called the "Silent Killer", because it is a disease that usually occurs without any symptoms. It is frequently asymptomatic until it becomes severe and target organ disease has occurred. A patient with severe hypertension may experience a variety of symptoms secondary to effects on blood vessels in the various organs and tissues or to the increased work load of the heart. These secondary symptoms include fatigue, reduced activity tolerance, dizziness, palpitations, angina, and dyspnea. The most advanced disease may produce symptoms such as early morning headache, blurred vision, and spontaneous nose bleed, and depression. However, these symptoms are not more frequent in people with hypertension than in the general population.

The most common complications of hypertension are target organ disease occurring in the heart (hypertensive heart disease), brain (cerebrovascular disease), peripheral vasculature (peripheral vascular disease), kidney (nephrosclerosis) and eyes (retinal damages).

Diagnostic Studies

The initial diagnosis of hypertension is made on the basis of two or more elevated blood pressure readings, supine and sitting, obtained on at least two separate occasions. If the first two readings differ more than 5 mm Hg additional readings should be obtained. Postural changes in BP and pulse should be measured in older adults, people taking antihypertensive drugs and when orthostatic hypertension is suspected.

Specific diagnostic test will be ordered to rule out an underlying cause or evaluate the extent of organ damage. A comprehensive physical examination is performed, including careful evaluation of blood vessels of the retina and as typically supplemented with laboratory tests, that will evaluate the neurological, cardiovascular and renal system for evidence of target organ damage. The laboratory studies that are performed in a person with sustained hypertension, routine urinalysis, BUN and serum creatinine levels are used to screen for renal involvement.

Measurement of serum electrolytes, especially potassium levels is important to detect hyperaldesteronism. Fasting blood glucose level (diabetes) serum cholesterol and triglyceride level provide information about additional risk factors, that predispose to atherosclerosis. Complete blood count, serum chemistry, ECG to know cardiac status.

Management

The management of hypertension does not involve any specific treatment but management is usually improved when the patient is able to make targeted lifestyle adjustment that support the drug therapy. Two important measures are abstaining from smoking and stress reduction management. Smoking has a direct vasoconstrictive effect on the blood vessels and should be given up it at all possible costs. The role of stress is less clear but the use of relaxation and stress management strategies are often helpful in blood pressure control.

Lifestyle modifications should be used in all hypertensive patients either as definitive or adjunctive therapy. These modifications directed toward reducing BP and overall cardiovascular risk. Modifications include:
1. Dietary changes.
2. Limitation of alcohol intake.
3. Regular physical activity.
4. Avoidance of tobacco use (smoking and chewing).

Based on assigned risk group, lifestyle modifications are usually continued upto one year before drug therapy is used. Patients with hypertension are encouraged to develop a pattern of regular aerobic exercise, which may help control their hypertension and also contributes to weight loss and reduces cardiac risk factors. Patients are cautioned to avoid strenuous exercises, particularly activities involve heavylifting or the Valsalva's maneuver. Weightlifting should be avoided and sustained moderate exertion is preferable to bursts of efforts.

Drug Therapy (Table 5.1)

This is the primary treatment of essential hypertension. The drug currently available for treating hypertension have two main actions—reduction of ever and volume of circulating blood. The drugs used in the treatment of hypertension include diuretics, adrenergic (sympathetic) inhibitors, vasodilators, angiotensin inhibitors and calcium channel blockers. The details of medications used for hypertension are as follows:

Diuretics

Thiazide/thiazide-like Diuretics

Thiazide/Thiazide-like diuretics blocks or inhibits sodium reasorbtion in the distal convulted tubule, in the portion of ascending tubule; Water exerted with sodium, producing decreased volume. They will be increased in Na^+ and Cl. Initial decrease in ECF and sustained decrease in SVR lowers BP moderately in 2 to 4 weeks. The technical terms used for these drugs are bendroflumethiazide, bebzythiazide, chlorothiazide, cyclothiazide, hydrochlorothiazide, (Esidrex), hydroflumethazide indapamide, methyl chlorothiazide, metalazine, polythiazyde, quinethiazone and trichlomethiazide, Thiazides are ineffective in renal failure.

The side effects of thiazides are:
- Fluid and electrolyte imbalances: Volume depletion, hypocalemia, hyponatremia, hypercalcemia, hyperuricemia, metabolic alkalosis.
- CNS effects: Vertigo, headache, weakness.
- GI effects, anorexia, nausea, vomiting, diarrhea, constipation and pancreatitis.
- Sexual problems: impotence and decreased libido.
- Blood dyscreas and dermatologic effects; photosensitivity and skin rash.
- Decreased gluco-tolerance.

During this treatment nurses have to monitor the following:
- Check vital signs before administering in early days of treatment.
- Monitor lab value of electrolytes, particularly potassium.
- Monitor patient weight.
- Teach patients to:
  - Take drug early in the day.
  - Maintain liberal fluid intake.
  - Take drug with food if GI upsets occur.
  - Eat potassium-rich diet (e.g. fruits, legumes, whole grains, cereals and potato).
  - Expect an increased frequency and volume of urination.

Table 5.1: Antihypertensive drugs.

Site of action	Drug	Dosage	Indications	Contraindication/ cautions	Common side effects
Diuretics					
Antiadrenergic drugs					
Central	Clonidine	Oral: 0.05–0.6 mg twice daily	• Mild to moderate hypertension • Hypertension with renal disease	• Psychiatric disturbance • Sleep disorders	Postural hypotension, sedation, dry mouth, impotence, constipation, fluid retention, depression, sleep disturbance, rebound hypertension after abrupt withdrawal
	Methyldopa (also acts by blocking sympathetic nerves)	Oral: 250–1000 mg twice daily	• Mild to moderate hypertension • Drug of choice for hypertension in pregnancy	• Phoechromocytoma • Hepatic disease • During MAO inhibitor treatment	Postural hypotension, sedation, fatigue, diarrhoea, impaired ejaculation, fever, gynecomastia, lactation, positive Coomb's test, chronic hepatitis, ulcerative colitis, SLE like syndrome
Autonomic ganglia blocker	Trimethaphan	IV: 1–6 mg/min	Severe and malignant hypertension	Severe coronary artery disease, severe cerebrovascular insufficiency, diabetes on hypoglycemic therapy, glaucoma, prostatism	Postural hypotension, visual disturbance, dry mouth, constipation, urinary retention, impotence
Adrenergic nerve endings, e.g., adrenolytics	Reserpine	Oral: 0.05–0.25 mg daily	• Mild to moderate hypertension in young • Raynaud's phenomenon	Pheochromocytoma, peptic ulcer, depression, MAO inhibitor therapy	Depression, nightmares, nasal congestion, dyspepsia, diarrhoea, impotence
	Guanethidine	Oral: 10–15 mg day	Moderate to severe hypertension	Pheochromocytoma, coronary artery disease, cerebrovascular insufficiecny, MAO inhibitor therapy	Postural hypotension, bradycardia, dry mouth diarrhoea, impaired ejaculation, edema, asthma
	Phentolamine	Oral: 1–5 mg bolus	Suspected or proved pheochromocytoma	Severe coronary artery disease	Tachycardia, weakness dizziness, flushing
Alpha receptors blockers	Phenoxybenzamine	Oral: 10–50 mg once or twice a day	Proved phecoromocytoma		Postural hypotension, miosis, tachycardia, dry mouth, nasal congestion
	Prazosin	Oral: 1–10 mg twice a day	• Mild to moderate hypertension • Raynaud's phenomenon	Use with caution in elderly	Sudden syncope, headache, sedation, dizziness, tachycardia, dry mouth, fluid retention
Beta-blockers					
Alpha and beta receptor blockers	Labetalol	Oral: 100–600 mg twice a day; IV: 2 mg/min	Similar	Similar	Similar to beta blockers with more postural effects
Vasodilators					
Vascular smooth muscle	Hydralazine	Oral: 10–75 mg 4 times a day	As an adjuvant to treatment of moderate to severe hypertension	Systemic lupus erythematosus (SLE), severe coronary artery disease	Headache, tachycardia, angina, nausea, anorexia, vomiting, diarrhoea, SLE syndrome, rash edema

Contd...

Contd...

Site of action	Drug	Dosage	Indications	Contraindication/ cautions	Common side effects
	Minoxidil	Oral: 2.5–40 mg times a day	Severe hypertension	Severe coronary artery disease	Tachycardia, aggravation of angina, fluid retention, hair growth (hypertrichosis), coarsening of facial features, pericardial effusion
	Diazoxide	IV 1–3 mg/kg upto 150 mg rapidly	Severe to malignant hypertension	Diabetes, hyperuricemia, CHF	Hyperglycemia, hyperuricemia, fluid retention, apprehension, weakness, nausea, vomiting, diaphoresis, muscle twitching, cyanide toxicity
	Nitroprusside	IV: 0.5–8 (mg/kg/min)	Malignant hypertension		
Calcium channel blockers					
Angiotensin converting enzyme (ACE) inhibitors					
The drugs act by blocking the ACE, suppress the angiotensin II formation, thus, affect primarily renin-angiotensin aldosterone system	Captopril	Oral: 12.5–75 mg twice a day	• Mild to moderate hypertension • Renal artery stenosis (unilateral) • CHF refractory to digoxin and diuretics • Hypertension with renal failure (serum creatinine < 3.5 mg%) • Nephrotic syndrome to reduce albuminuria	• Renal failure (reduce the dose) • Bilateral renal artery stenosis • Pregnancy	Leukopenia, pancytopenia, hypotension, angiedema, cough, urticarial rash, fever, loss of taste, acute renal failure in bilateral renal artery stenosis, hyperkalemia
	Enalapril	Oral: 2.5–40 mg/day	-do-	-do-	Same as captopril but cough and angiedema can be more frequent. All are given once daily dose but side-effects are reduced, if given
	Fosinopril	Oral: 10–40 mg/day			
	Lisnopril	Oral: 5–40 mg/day			
	Ramipril	Oral: 2.5–20 mg/day			
	Perindopril	Oral: 2–4 mg/day			
Angiotensin receptor blockers (ARBs)					
They block angiotensin receptors	Losartan	Oral: 25–50 mg once or twice/day	• Mild to moderate hypertension • Renal hypertension	• Pregnancy • Bilateral renal artery stenosis	• Hypotension, acute renal failure in bilateral renal artery stenosis, hyperkalemia
	Irbesartan	Oral: 150–300 mg once or twice/day	• Diabetic nephropathy with hypertension	-do-	
	Telmisartan or olmesartan	20–40 mg once or twice/day	-do-	-do-	-do-

- Report the incidence of muscle weakness. Cramping, fatigue and nausea.
- Change positions slowly.

Loop Diuretics

It blocks sodium and water reabsorption in medullary portion of ascending tubule, cause rapid volume depletion. The drugs used are bumetanide, ethacrynic acid, furosemide (Lasix). The side effects are fluid and electrolyte imbalance as with thiazides except hypercalcemia, ototoxicity (hearing impairment, deafness, vertigo) that is usually reversible. Metabolic effects including hypeuricemia, hyperglycemia, increased LDL cholesterol and triglycerides with decreased HDL cholesterol. Nursing intervention are as same as with thiazides, but potassium loss can be severe. So, nurse has to monitor:

- Daily weight to assess response to treatment.
- Lab values for increase in uric acid and glucose BUN.

Potassium Sparing Diuretics

It inhibits aldosterone; sodium excreted in exchange of potassium. The drugs are amiloride, spironolactone, and triamaterine. The side effects are hyperkalemia, nausea, vomiting, diarrhea, headache, leg cramps and dizziness. Nursing intervention includes:

- Monitor lab value for potassium excess.
- Weigh patient daily.
- Teach patient to:
  - Expect an increased volume of urine.
  - Avoid potassium-rich foods.
  - Report any incidence of drowsiness or GI side effects.

Adrenergic Inhibitors

Centrally Acting Alpha Blockers

These activate central receptors that suppress vasomotor and cardiac centers causing decrease in peripheral resistance. They reduce sympathetic outflow from CNS and peripheral sympathetic tone produces vasodilation and decreases SVR and BP. Commonly used are cloridine, gunabenz, guantacine, methyldopa (Aldomat). The side effects of these drugs are—dry mouth, sedation, impotence, nausea, dizziness, sleep disturbance, nightmares, restlessness, and depression. There is symptomatic bradycardia in patient wth conduction disorder. In this, nursing intervention includes:

- Change position slowly.
- Teach patient to:
  - Change position slowly.
  - Avoid hot baths, steam rooms, saunas.
  - Use gum or hard candies to counteract dry mouth.
  - Be cautious in driving or operating machinery if drowsiness or sedation occurs.
  - Report any decline in sexual responsiveness.

Peripheral Acting Adrenergic Antagonists

It depletes catecholamine, in peripheral sympathetic postganglionic fibers and blocks norepinephrine release from adrenergic nerve endings. Usually used are guanadrel, guanethedine (ismelin) rauwolfin, serpentina, reserpine (texpasil). The side effects include marked orthostatic hypertension, diarrhea, cramps bradycardia, retrograde or delayed ejaculation, sodium and water retention sedation and inability to concentrate, depression, nasal stuffiness with reserpine. The nursing intervention is as with the above drug and report incidence of edema in hands and feet.

Beta Adrenergic Blockers

Beta adrenergic blockers block beta-adrenergic receptors of sympathetic nervous system, decreasing heart rate and blood pressure. Please note that beta-blockers should not be used in patients with asthma. COPD, CHF and heart block. Use with caution in diabetes and peripheral vascular disease. Commonly used beta-blockers are acebutolol, atenolol, betaxolol, carteolol, metaprolol, nadolol, petbutolol, pindolol, propranolol, timolol and essmolol. The side effects of these drugs are bronchospasm, atrioventricular conduction block, impaired peripheral circulation, nightmares, depression, weakness, reduced exercise capability. It can be included in exacerbate symptom of ischemic heart disease. The nursing intervention includes:

- Establish baseline vital signs and lab values before treatment.
- Check blood pressure and pulse before administration.
- Teach patients to:
  - Change position slowly.
  - Take drug as prescribed.
  - Avoid abruptly discontinuing the use.
  - Report any decline in sexual responsiveness.
  - Report incidence of fatigue, drowsiness, difficulty in breathing.
  - Be alert to the signs of hypoglycemia if diabetic drug masks the symptoms.

Combined Alpha and Beta-adrenergic Blockers

Labetalol is a common drug used as combined one. Action and nursing actions are as same as beta blockers.

Vasodilators

Vasodilators such as diazoxide, hydralazine, minoxidil, nitroglycerine (tridil) dilate peripheral blood vessels by directly relaxing vascular smooth muscle. These are usually used in combination with other antihypertensives as they increase sodium and fluid retention and cause reflex cardiac stimulation.

Diazoxide direct arterial vasodilation reduces SVR and BP. It is used intravenously for hypertensive crisis in hospitalized patients. It should be administered only into peripheral veins. The side effects include reflex sympathetic activation producing increased HR, CO and salt and water retention. Hyperglycemia is especially in type 2 diabetes.

Hydralazine has same effect as diazoxide; it should be given IV in hypertensive crisis in hospitalized patients. Also use two oral doses per day. The side effects are headache, nausea, flushing, palpitation bradycardia, angina, hemolytic anemia, vasculitis and rapidly progressive glomerulonephritis.

Minoxidil (Leniten) used in severe hypertension associated with renal failure. It may cause reflex tachycardia, fluid retention and ECG changes and tridol administered intravenously in case of hypertensive crisis with myocardial ischemia.

The nursing intervention during the use of vasodilator in hypertension clients are as follows:
- Check BP and pulse before each dose. Palpitation and tachycardia are common during first week of therapy.
- Teach patients to:
    - Change in position slowly because dizziness is common.
    - Avoid hot baths, steam rooms, saunas.
    - Take drug with meals.
    - Be prepared for nasal congestion and excess lacrimation.
    - Report incidence of constipation or peripheral edema.

Angiotensin Inhibitors

ACE (Angiotensin Converting Enzyme) Inhibitors

These inhibit conversion of angiotensin to angiotensin II, thus blocking the release of aldosterone, thereby reducing sodium and water retention commonly used are Benazepril, Captopril, Clazapril, Enlapril, Fosionopril, Lisionopril, Moexpril, Perindopril, Ramipril, Ouinapril, Trandolapril, Enalaprila (injectable). The side effects are hypotension, loss of taste, cough, hyperkalemia, acute renal failure, skin rash angioneurotic edema. The nursing interventions are:
- Monitor for first dose syncope in patients with CHF.
- Monitor renal function through lab work and potassium levels.
- Check BP before administering.
- Teach patient to change position slowly, report any incidence of fatigue, skin rash, impaired taste and chronic cough.

Angiotensin II Receptor Antagonist

It selectively blocks the binding angiotensin I to the angiotensin II receptors found in many tissues and vascular smooth muscle, which blocks its vasoconstrictive and aldosterone-secreting effects. The commonly used are Candisartan, Irbesartan, Losartan, Tasosartan, Valsartan. The side effects are hyperkalemia and decreased renal function. These drugs prevent action of angiotensin II and produce vasodilative and increasing salt and water excretion. The nursing intervention are as in ACE inhibitors.

Calcium Channel Blockers

Calcium channel blockers inhibit influx of calcium into muscle cells; act on vascular smooth muscles (primary arteries) to reduce spasms and promote vasodilation. Here it blocks movement of extracellular calcium into cells causing peripheral vasodilation and decreased SVR. The commonly used calcium channel blockers are Amlodipine, Diltiazem, Felodipine, Istadipine, Mibefradil, Nicrandipine, Nifedipine, Nisoldipine, Verapamol (Isoptin) and Verapanil SR. The side effects are nausea, headache, dizziness, peripheral edema, reflex tachycardia. Reflex disease in HR (with ditiacem), constipation (with verapamil). The nursing interventions include:
- Check vital signs before administering (bradycardia is common).
- Monitor renal and liver function tests.
- Teach patient to take drugs before meals, change positions slowly, report any incidence of peripheral edema, fatigue and headache.

In addition to the above, the patient and family especially the members who prepare the meals should be educated about sodium-restricted diet.

The primary nursing responsibilities for long-term management of hypertension are to assist the patient in reducing BP and complying with the treatment plan. Nursing actions include patient and family education, detection and reporting of adverse treatment effects, compliance assessments, enhancement and evaluation of therapeutic effectiveness. Patient education includes diet therapy, drug therapy, physical activity, home monitoring of BP (if appropriate) and avoidance of tobacco (if applicable). When presenting information to the patient or family, the nurse should do the following:
- Provide the numerical value of the patient's BP and explain that it exceeds normal limits.
- Inform the patient that hypertension usually asymptomatic and symptoms do not reliably indicate BP levels.
- Explain that long-term follow-up and therapy are necessary.
- Explain that therapy will not cure but should control hypertension.
- Tell the patient that controlled hypertension is usually compatible with an excellent prognosis and a normal lifestyle.
- Explain to the patient about dangers of uncontrolled hypertension.
- Be specific about the names, actions, dosages and side effects of prescribed medication.
- Tell the patient to plan regular and convenient times for taking medications.

- Tell the patient not to discontinue drugs abruptly because withdrawal may cause a severe hypertensive reaction.
- Tell the patient not to double upon doses when a dose is missed.
- Instruct the patient that if BP increases, not to take an increased medication dosage before consulting a health care provider.
- Tell the patient not to take a medication belonging to someone else.
- Make aware the patient that side effects of medication often diminish with the passage of time.
- Tell the patient to consult the health care provider about changing drugs or dosage if impotence or other sexual problems develop.
- Tell the patient to supplement diet with foods high in potassium (e.g. citrus fruits, and green leafy vegetables) if he/she is taking potassium-losing diuretics.
- Tell the patient to avoid hot baths, excessive amounts of alcohol, and strenuous exercises within 3 hours of taking medication that promote vasodilation.
- Explain to decrease orthostatic hypotension, the patient should arise slowly from bed, sit on side of bed for a few minutes, stand slowly, not stand still for a long time, do leg exercises to increase venous return, sleep with head of bed raised or on pillows, and lie or sit down when dizziness occurs.

CORONARY ARTERY DISEASE (CAD)

Coronary artery disease is a type of blood vessel disorder that is included in the general category of atherosclerosis. The term atherosclerosis is derived from two Greek words. 'Athero' meaning 'Fatty Mish' and 'Skleros' meaning "Hard". This word combination indicates that atherosclerosis begins as soft deposits of fat, that hardens with age. Atherosclerosis is often referred to as 'hardening of the arteries'. Although this condition can occur in any artery in the body, the atheromas (fatty deposits) have a preference for the coronary arteries. Patients with CAD often seek health care after experiencing angina or myocardial infarction (MI). Vascular diseases such as dysrhythmia, heart failure, and cardiomyopathy. All nurses need to be familiar with the management of coronary artery diseases.

Etiology

Atheroclerosis is the major cause of coronary artery diseases. It is characterized by a focal deposit of cholesterol and lipids, primarily within the wall of the artery. Many risk factors have been associated with CAD are:
- *Age and gender:* Incidence of CAD occurs in men between 35 to 45 years age. After the age of 65 incidence of men and women equalizes; although there is evidence suggesting that more women are being seen with CAD earlier because of increased stress, increased smoking, presence of hypertension and use of birth control pills. For both decrease in elasticity of arteries with age. Estrogen in females lowers serum cholesterol.
- *Heredity:* Genetic predisposition is an important factor in the occurrence of CAD, but exact mechanism is not yet known.
- *Diabetes:* Incidence of CAD is two-three times more in diabetes. This may be due to elevated levels of circulating insulin helps to form atheroma and damaged arterial intima and insulin also modifies lipid metabolisms.
- *Hypertension:* Hypertension affects the ability of blood vessels to constrict or dilate. Decreased elasticity of blood vessels, tearing affect on arteries, and increased resistance of ejection of ventricular volume may lead to CAD.
- Smoking and tobacco use.

The unifying factor promoting CAD is nicotine. Nicotine has the following physiological effects and may cause CAD:
- Decreased high-density lipoproteins (HDL).
- Displacement of oxygen from hemoglobin.
- Increased catecholamine in response to nicotine, increasing heart rate and blood pressure.
- Increased platelet adhesiveness.
- Accelerates atheroma formation.
- Accelerates atheroma formation.
- Coronary spasm.
- *Sedentary lifestyle:* This alters lipid metabolism and decrease in HDLS. Physical inactivity may lead to CAD.
- *Diet:* Dietary intake of more cholesterol and fat, provides more substance for lesion formation. Hypercholesterdemia, familial hyperlipidemia, increased levels of low density lipoproteins, and increasing atherogenesis.
- *Obesity:* Obese persons are more prone to diabetes, hypertension, and hyperlipidemias. In addition, they often demonstrate other behaviors such as sendentary lifestyles, that are known as risk factors for CAD.
- *Stress and behavior pattern:* Catecholamine, released during stress response, increases platelet aggregation and may also precipitate vasospasm. It was generally agreed that individuals with type 'A' behavior had a higher incidence of CAD than individuals who were more relaxed. The type 'A' personality characters include the following:
  - Perfectionistic
  - Always tense
  - Competitive
  - Unduly irritable
  - Aggressive
  - Obsessed with number of sale made, articles written
  - Constantly time oriented
  - Patients seen, forms completed

- Has hurry sickness
- Never says 'no'
- Holds in feelings
- Compulsive
- Never has leisure time
- Impatient
- Never takes a relaxing vacation or day offs.

There are three major clinical manifestations in coronary artery disease, which include angina pectoris, acute myocardial infarction and hidden cardiac death. They are stages of the continuum and CAD.

ANGINA PECTORIS

Angina pectoris is literally translated as pain (angina) in the chest (pectoris). Myocardial ischemia is expressed symptomatically as angina. More specifically, angina pectoris is transient chest pain caused by myocardial ischemia. It usually lasts for only few minutes (3 to 5 min), and commonly subsides when the precipitating factor (usual exertion) is relieved. Typical exertional angina should not persist longer than 20 minutes after rest and administration of nitroglycerine.

Etiology

Myocardial ischemia develops when the demand for myocardial oxygen exceeds the ability of the coronary arteries to supply it. The below given are the primary reasons for insufficient blood flow in narrowing of coronary arteries by atherosclerosis. Extracardiac factors may precipitate myocardial ischemia and anginal pain. They include:

- Physical exertion: Increases the heart rate (HR) Increasing heart rate decreases the time the heart spends in diastole, which is the time of greatest coronary blood flow. Walking outdoors is the most common form of the exertions that produce an attack. Isometric exertions of the arms as on raking leaves, painting or lifting heavy objects also causes exertional angina.
- Strong emotions stimulate the sympathetic nervous system and increase the work of the heart. This results in an increase in HR, BP and myocardial contractility.
- Consumption of heavy meal (especially if the person exerts afterwards) can increase the work of the heart. During the digestive process, blood is diverted to the GI system, causing a low flow rate in the coronary arteries.
- Temperature extremes it may be either hot or cold. Increases the workload of the heart (blood vessels constrict in response to the cold climate; blood vessels dilate and blood pools in the skin in response to a hot stimulus). Cold weather also causes increased metabolism to maintain internal temperature regulation.
- Cigarette smoking causes vasoconstriction and an increased HR because of nicotine stimulation of the catecholamine release. It also diminishes available oxygen by increasing level of carbon monoxide.
- Sexual activity increases the workload and sympathetic stimulation. In a person with severe CAD, the resulting extra workload of the heart may precipitate angina.
- Stimulants, such as cocaine, cause increased HR and subsequent myocardial demand. Stimulation of catecholamine release is the precipitating factor.
- Circadian rhythm have been related to the occurrence of the stable angina, unstable angina, MI and cardiac death. These manifestations of CAD tend to occur in the early morning after awakening.

Pathophysiology

Coronary artery disease refers to the development and progression of plaque accumulation in the coronary arteries. This process has three stages along the continuum viz., stable angina, unstable angina and myocardial infarction.

Normally the endothelium of the coronary artery allows for unrestricted blood flow to the myocardium. Any kind of trauma or irritant can disrupt this protective endothelium. The body's response to injury is a complex interplay of chemical mediators designed to protect the area. Endothelial injury causes the release of thromboxane, which minimizes the extent of injury through local vasoconstriction and by stimulating platelet aggregation. The intima releases prostacyclin in response to the effects of thromboxane. Prostacycline works to restore equilibrium through local vasodilation and by opposing platelet aggregation. With repeated injury, the deteriorated intima cannot produce enough prostacycline and platelet aggregation forces predominate.

Platelets and accumulating monocytes release powerful growth factors into the arterial wall. These factors stimulate the proliferation and migration of medial smooth muscle cells into the intima. This structural changes cause an increased permeability of the vessel wall to the cholesterol. The accumulation of cholesterol produces a fatty streak that protrudes into the lumen of the artery. Smooth muscle cells and fibrous tissue form a fibrous cap over the fatty streak. The fatty streak continues to grow, invading both the intima and media. Involvement of the media affects the ability of the vessel wall to vasodilate and vasoconstrict. The artery may continue to maintain the supply of oxygen and nutrients to the myocardium as long as the blockage is less than 70 percent of the arterial lumen. Concomitant conditions such as anemia, smoking and hypovolemia further compromise the delivery of oxygen to the myocardium.

The presence of risk factors accelerate atherogenesis, thereby decreasing oxygen supply. Risk factors can also increase the myocardium's demands for oxygen. The demand of the myocardium for oxygen can be met only by an adequate blood supply. As long as supply is greater than or equal to demand, aerobic metabolism occurs. When demand is greater than that of supply, the myocardium must switch to anaerobic metabolism for nourishments. Anaerobic metabolism produces lactic acid which is believed to be responsible for ischemic anginal pain. The pain is the most common initial symptom of CAD. With stable angina the patient is usually experiencing a known threshold beyond which myocardial oxygen demand exceeds supply. Myocardial oxygen demand increases with any condition causing an increase in heart rate, an increase in resistance to ejecting blood volume, and an increase in myocardial size.

When atherosclerosis progresses beyond 70 percent, pressure within the lesion (plaque) can increase to the point of plaque rupture. Rupture of the fibrous cap exposes the inner plaque to the circulating blood. In an effort to heal, collagen accumulates, smooth muscle cells proliferate and clotting factors are activated. Aggregating platelets activate the coagulation system immediately to seal the rupture. With plaque disruptions stable angina becomes unstable angina. Risk factors like nicotine from tobacco use, increases platelet adhesion and increases the potential for clotting at the site of disruption. Catecholamines released during the stress response also increase platelet aggregation. The third stage that occurs is complete obstruction of the coronary artery with a fibrous cloth called coronary thrombosis or acute MI.

Clinical Manifestation

The following may occur with stable angina, unstable angina or acute MI.

- Chest pain or anginal equivalent (Jaw pain, left arm pain).
- Non-verbal indicators of pain: clutch, rub, stroke and the chest.
- Increase or decrease in heart rate.
- Dysrhythmias.
- Increase or decrease in blood pressure.
- Angina that occurs with predictable level of exertion (in stable angina).
- Angina not necessarily associated with activity and ST depression. (or unstable angina).

In addition to the unique feature of myocardial infarction which includes:

- Angina not relieved by rest or nitroglycerin therapy.
- Associated with symptoms: dizziness, dyspnea, nausea, vomiting feeling of impending doom.
- Altered neurological status, if decreased output.
- Rales, if decreased contractility creates left ventricular function.
- Presence of S3 or S4 gallop.
- Diminished pulses.
- Pallor.
- ECG ST elevation, Q-waves, J-wave abnormalities.
- Elevated ESR.

Management

When a patient has a history indicating coronary artery disease, thorough physical examination should be carried out and physician may order several diagnostic studies, which the nurse has to promptly attend and assist. Those studies include chest X-ray, ECG, serum enzyme level [creatinine kinase (CK)-lactic dehydrogenase (LDH)] cardiac troponin, serum lipid level. Exercise stress test. Nuclear imaging studies, Position emission tomography (PET), coronary angiographic studies and echocardiography.

Nursing assessment made on the basis of present subjective and objective data. Nursing diagnosis for the patient with angina may include chest pain, anxiety, decreased cardiac output, activity intolerances related to myocardial ischemia. The main nursing objectives for the patient with angina are pain assessment, evaluation of treatment and reinforcement of appropriate therapy. Because chest pain may be caused by many factors other than ischemia (e.g. pericarditis, valvular disease, pulmonary artery stenosis, MI, congestive cardiomyopathy). It is important to have a clear understanding of the patient's chest pain.

The nurse should determine whether breathing in or out of changing positions makes the patients chest pain better or worse. Anginal pain does not vary with body positions or respiration. In contrast, the pain is deep or superficial, mild or intense, diffuse or localized. Cardiac pain usually is deep or intense and diffuse. The patient may rub the entire chest to explain as to where the pain is occurring. If the nurse is present during anginal attack, the following measures should be taken:

- Administration of oxygen.
- Determination of vital signs.
- 12-Lead ECG.
- Prompt pain relief Ist with a nitrate followed by narcotic analgesic if needed.
- Physical assessment fo the chest.
- Comfortable positioning of the patient.

The patient will more likely appear distressed and have pale, cool, clammy skin. The blood pressure and heart rate will probably be elevated and an atrial gallop (S4) sound may be heard. If a ventricular gallop (S3) is heard, it may indicate LV decompensation. A murmur may be heard during an anginal attack secondary to ischemia of a papillary muscle. The murmur is likely to be transient and abates with the cessation of symptoms. Supportive and realistic assurance and a calm, soothing manner help reduce the patient's anxiety.

The patient should be instructed in the proper use of nitroglycerine tablets. Nitrates decrease myocardial oxygen demand by venodilate (decrease preload), peripherally vasodilated (decrease after load), increase myocardial oxygen supply and coronary vasodilate. Nitroglycerine should be easily accessible to the patient at all times. However, patients should be taught not to carry nitroglycerine in their pockets because heat from the body can cause loss of potency of the tablet. For protection from degradation. It should be kept in a tightly closed dark glass bottle. The patient should be instructed to place a nitroglycerine tablet beneath the tongue and allow it to dissolve. This should cause a fizzing or slightly warm feeling locally. The patient should be warned that heart rate may increase and pounding headache, dizziness, or flush may occur. The patient should be cautioned against quickly rising to standing position, because postural hypertension may occur after nitroglycerine ingestion. If pain has not been relieved after 5 minutes ask him/her to repeat the dose, but not to exceeded three tablets. If pain persists after three doses, the patient should be referred to seek immediate proper medical attention **(Table 5.2)**.

The patient should be reassured that a long, productive life is possible even with angina. The patient should be educated regarding coronary artery disease and angina, precipitating factors, risk factors and medication. Educating the patient and family about diet that are low in sodium and reduced in saturated fat may be appropriate. Maintaining ideal body weight is important in controlling angina because weight above the level increase myocardial workload, and may cause pain. Several small meals in place of three meals per day may be suggested. Application of topical nitrates over the chest may be taught to patient.

Nursing Management

Nursing diagnosis will be made thorough nursing assessment by asking the patient to describe the anginal attack (when, where, how often, how long, and other associative symptoms and signs), family history, previous history and their habits, etc. The main nursing diagnosis which needs nursing interventions are:

- Pain related to an imbalance in O_2 supply and demand.
- Decreased cardiac output related to reduced preload, overload, contractility and HR secondary to the hemodynamic effects of drugs.
- Anxiety related to chest pain, uncertain prognosis and threatening environment.

    In addition, control of angina pectoris is achieved through the:
    - Review information on low-fat/low cholesterol diet with patient.
    - Inform patient of available cardiac rehabilitation programs, that offer structured classes on exercise, smoking cessation and weight control.

Table 5.2: Commonly used nitrates.

Drugs	Usual dose	Side effects
Sublingual nitroglycerine	0.3–0.6 mg	Headache, flushing, dizziness, tachycardia, hypotension
Isosorbide dinitrate (short-acting)	80–120 mg	Flushing, headache, dizziness, tachycardia, GI upset and sleep disturbance, methemoglobinemia, cyanosis
Transdermal nitroglycerin (skin patch)	0.4–1.2 mg/hr for 12–24 hr	-do-
Isosorbide-5 mononitrate (long-acting)	20–30 mg bid or 40 mg od	-do-

- Avoid excessive caffeine intake (coffee, cola drinks) that can increase the heart rate and produce angina.
- Avoid the use of alcohol or drink only in moderation.
- Avoid use of 'diet pills', nasal decongestants or any over the counter medication that can increase the HR or stimulate HBP.

MYOCARDIAL INFARCTION

Myocardial infarction occurs when ischemic intracellular changes become irreversible and necrosis results. Angina as a result of ischemia causes reversible cellular injury, and infarction in the result of sustained ischemia causing irreversible cellular death.

Pathophysiology

Cardiac cells can withstand ischemia condition for approximately 20 minutes before cellular death (necrosis) begins. Contractile function of the heart stops in the area of myocardial necrosis. The degree of altered function depends on the area of the heart involved the LV. A transmural MI occurs when the entire thickness of the myocardium in a region involved. A subendocardial MI (non-transmural) exists when the damage has not penetrated through the entire thickness of the myocardial wall. Infarction is described as the area of occurrence, as anterior, inferior, lateral, or posterior wall infarctions, common combination and anterolateral or anterioseptal MI. An inferior MI also called diaphragmatic MI. The location and area of the infarct correlates with the part of the coronary circulation involved. The degree of pre-established collateral circulation also determines the severity of infarction. The clot extends into lumens, completely obstructs lumen. Complete obstruction of the coronary artery with the fibrous clot is termed as coronary thrombosis or coronary occlusion. Coronary occlusion creates a rapid series of physiological events. The first of these events is immediate myocardial ischemia distal to the occlusion. Ischemia alters the integrity and permeability of the myocardial cell membranes to vital electrolytes. This instability depresses myocardial contractility and predisposes the patients to sudden death from dysrhythmias.

The body responses to cell death is inflammatory process within 24 hours, leukocytes infiltrate the area. Enzymes are released from the dead cardiac cells and important diagnostic indicators of MI.

Clinical Manifestation

- Chest pain very severe immobilizing chest pain not relieved by rest or nitrate administration is the hall-mark of MI. This pain is usually described as a heaviness, tightness, or constrictions. Common locations are substernal or retrosternal, radiating to the neck, jaw and arms or to the back. It may occur when patient is active, or at rest, awake or during sleep and it commonly occurs at early morning hours. It lasts for 20 minutes or more.
- Nausea and vomiting as a result of vasovagal reflexes initiated from the area of the infarcted myocardium.
- Sympathetic nervous system stimulation is increased due to release of increased catecholemine (norephinephrine) and epinephrine leads to ashen cool and clammy skin (cold sweats).
- Fever: The temperature may increase upto 38°C.
- Cardiac vascular manifestation includes elevated BP and HR. Later, BP may drop as decreased cardiac output, urinary output may be decreased. Crackles may be noted in the lungs. Later hepatic engorgement and peripheral edema occurs which indicates cardiac failure.

In addition, following complications may develop:
- Arrhythmias (Abnormal wave)
- Congestive heart failure.
- Cardiogenic shock.
- Papillary muscle dysfunction.
- Ventricular aneurysm.
- Pericarditis.
- Dressler's syndrome.
- Right ventricular infarction.
- Pulmonary embolism.

Difference between angina and myocardial infarction shown in **Table 5.3**.

Management

Common diagnostic parameters used to determine whether a person has sustained an acute MI include: (1) The patient's history of pain. Risk factors and health history, (2) 12-lead ECG. Consistent with acute MI. (ST-T wave elevated by greater than 1 mm or more in two continuous leads and (3) Serious measurement of myocardial serum enzyme and comparison of the pain with angina as given below:

Acute nursing interventions for patient with MI are best done in a specialized unit (ICCU). Such nursing includes the initial ICCU stay for 1 to 2 days and the rest of hospitalization for 4 to 6 days. Priorities for nursing intervention in the initial stage of recovery after MI includes pain assessment and relief, physiologic monitoring, promotion of rest and comfort, alleviation of stress and anxiety and understanding of the patient's emotional and behavioral reactions. In initial stages, of emergency management, the nursing responsibility includes:
- Ensure patent airway.
- Administer oxygen by nasal cannula or non-rebreather mask.
- Insert two IV catheters.
- Obtain 12-lead ECG.
- Determine location of pain—assess severity using pain scale (0-10).
- Medicate for pain as ordered (e.g. morphine, nitroglycerin).
- Identify underlying rhythm.
- Obtain cardiac enzyme levels.
- Assess need for thrombolytic therapy as appropriate.
- Administer asprin and beta-adrenergic blockers for cardiacrelated chest pain unless contraindicated.

Ongoing monitoring by nurses include the following:
- Monitor vital signs, level of consciousness, cardiac rhythm, and O_2 saturation.
- Monitor pain and remedicate as needed.
- Reassure patient.
- Anticipate need for intubation if respiratory distress is evident.
- Prepare for CPR, defibrillation, transcutaneous pacing, or cardioversion and nurses should keep in mind that common medication used for coronary artery disease and nursing intervention during their administration as follows:
  - Antiplatelet agents (asprin, ticlopidine) inhibits platelet aggregation: Aspirin should be prescribed unless a true hypersensitivity reaction is present or the patient has a severe risk of bleeding.
  - Nitrates (Isosorbide denitrate, Isosorbide mononitrate, nitroglycer): Nitrate decreases myocardial oxygen by venodilate, peripherally vasodilate, increase myocardial oxygen supply and coronary vasodilate. Patient should be lying or sitting with administration of sublingual nitrates. Intravenous nitroglycerin is titrated to relief of symptoms or limiting side effects such as headache or systolic BP less than 90 mm Hg. IV preparations are usually replaced with oral or topical preparation when the patient has been symptom-free for 24 hours. Cautiously use with known aortic stenosis. Anticipate headache develop within 24 hours. A nitrate-free interval of 6 to 8 hours may improve responsiveness to therapy.

Table 5.3: Difference between angina and myocardial infarction.

Angina	Myocardial infarction
Precipitating factors	
• Stress, either physiologic (exertion or psychology)	• Exertion or rest
• Digestion of heavy meal	• Physical or emotional stress
• Valsalva's maneuver during micturation or defecation	• Often no precipitation factors are associated with angina
• Extremity of weather	
• Hot baths or showers	
• Sexual excitation	
Location	
• Midanterior chest	• Midanterior chest
• Substernal	• Substernal
• Abdominal with radiation to neck, back arms, fingers	• Diffuse
• Diffuse, no easily located	• Radiation to neck and jaw or down left arm or both arms to fingers
Description	
• Deep sensation of tightness or squeezing feeling	• Severe pressure, squeezing or heaviness with a report of such severe pain that the patient would rather than experience pain again
• Mild to moderate in severity or pressure	
• Similar attack each time	• Residual 'soreness' of thoracic arc
• Twinges or dullness in several days following MI	
Onset and duration	
• Gradual or sudden onset	• Sudden onset
• Usual duration of 15 minutes or less (usually less than 30 minutes)	• Duration of 30 min to 2 hours
• Relief by nitroglycerine	• No relief from rest or nitroglycerine
Associated clinical manifestations	
• Apprehension	• Apprehension
• Dyspnea	• Nausea and vomiting
• Diaphoresis	• Dyspnea
• Nausea	• Diaphoresis
• Desire to void	• Extreme fatigue
• Belching	• Dizziness or faintness (after abatement of pain)

Topical nitrates must be cleaned from the skin surface before applying new dose. Appropriate areas of application include any hair-free area, preferably in noticeable areas when the initial dose is being determined. Application areas should be rotated. Gloves should be worn when applying topical preparation.

- Beta blockers (Atenolol, metoprolol, timlol, esmolol, propranolol): Beta blocker decreases myocardial oxygen demand by decreasing contractility, slow heart rate, slow impulse conduction, decreased BP. They also increase myocardial O2 supply, slow heart rate, thereby increasing diastolic filling time and coronary perfusion and decreases incidence of morbidity and mortality after MI. IV Metoprolol is given in 5 mg increments over 1 to 2 minutes. Other beta blockers may be prescribed IV instead metoprolol. All IV preparations are followed by oral preparations after patient is stabilized. Monitor for atrioventricular block including PR interval, symptomatic bradycardia hypotension, left ventricular failure (rales, decerease CO) and brock spasm. Beta 1 cardio selective agents are the profound drugs. Beta 2 agents should be avoided in patients with respiratory or peripheral vascular disease. Target heart rate for betablockade is 50 to 60 beats per minute.
- Calcium channel blockers (Amidolpin, dilitiagen, verapanil, nifedepin) which decrease myocardial oxygen demand and increase in myocardial oxygen

supply by inhibiting the influx of calcium through the slow calcium channels. Heart rate decreases and conduction through the AV node slows (decreases demand indirectly increases supply). Inhibition of calcium influx into the arterial cell also promotes vasodilation of peripheral arteries (decreased demand) and coronary arteries (increased supply). They often prescribed when vasospasm is considered as the part of the pathology or if significant hypertension exists. Monitor for symptomatic bradycardia, prolonger PR intervals, advanced heart blocks, hypotension, congestive heart failure and peripheral edema.

- Heparin (intravenous) prevents propagation of established thrombus by rapidly inhibiting thrombin. Nursing intervention here includes that heparin PTTs should be measured 6 hours after any change in dose. Dose is weight based. Therapeutic levels should be maintained between 1.5 and 2.5 times patient's control. Hemoglobin, hematocrit, and platelets should be followed for heparininduced thrombocytopnea. Recurrent ischemia, active bleeding and hypotension may signify subtherapeutic or supratherapeutic dosages should be evaluated immediately.

- Thrombolytics (Streptokinase, tissue plasminogen activator). They are given in acute myocardial infarction to activate plasmin for lysis of obstructive clots specific, therefore, systemic lysis may occur. Patients must be carefully screened before administration of thrombolytic agents. The nurse monitors for reperfusion, reocclusion and bleeding complications with thrombolysis administration. Interventions are directed towards preventing bleeding complications.

- Morphine sulphate blunts the deleterious consequences of sympathetic stimulation with pain, and vasodilates creating decreased preload. Here, nurse should establish baseline vital signs, level of consciousness and orientation. Monitor for hypotension, respiratory depression changes in level of consciousness. Doses are usually given in increments of 2 to 5 mg.

- Oxygen increases arterial O_2 saturation. Monitor for adequate arterial oxygenation with finger pulse oximetry. Maintain saturation level by about 90%.

- Cholesterol lowering agent (Atorvastatin, Lovastatin, Pravastatin, Simvastatin, Cremfibrozil, Nicotinic acid) they reduce the substance for lipid deposition in the coronary artery. Side effects vary with drug class. Insolence of side may limit the usefulness of certain medications. Lipid levels should be obtained at regular intervals to monitor for success in effecting charges. Patients must be educated that cholesterol lowering agents do not substitue for dietary modification.

- Angiotensin-converting enzyme inhibitor (Captabril, Enalapril, Beneapril, Lisinopril, Posinopril). They decrease afterload and preload, thereby decreasing the workload of the heart. This prevents remodelling of the left ventricle (Remodelling refers to hypertrophy of the unaffected left ventricle to compensate for the infarcted area). Long-term consequences of remodelling are increased oxygen demand and heart failure. During their administration, nurse monitors for adverse affects: angioneurotic edema, cough, hypotension, hyperkalemia, pruritic rash, renal failure. First dose requires taking BP before and 30 minutes after administration. NPO (Nil per orally) in coronary artery diseases may be treated with following procedures:
  - Intra-aortic balloon (IABP).
  - Percutaneous transluminal coronary angioplasty (PTCA).
  - Intracoronary stunting.
  - Coronary artery bypass graft (CABP).

Health teaching for patients with coronary artery disease include use and storage of nitroglycerin in case of angina and guidelines for sexual activity after MI, risk factors, modification and resumption of activities.

- Use and storage of nitroglycerin:
  - Sit or lie down at onset of angina/chest pain.
  - Place tablet under the tongue and allow tablet to dissolve, don't chew.
  - If pain not relieved within 5 minutes, take a second tablet. A third tablet can be used after an additional 5 minutes if pain persists. Continuing pain after 3 tablets and 15 minutes indicate need to receive immediate medical attention.
  - Tablet will cause tingling sensation under the tongue.
  - Rest for 15 to 20 minutes after taking nitroglycerin to avoid faintness.
  - A tablet with the physician's permission may be taken 10 minutes before an activity known to trigger an anginal attack.
  - Anticipate the occurrence of hypotension, tachycardia, and headache in response to the medication. Headache may persist for 15 to 20 minutes after administration.
  - Keep a record of number of anginal attacks experienced, the number of tablets needed to obtain pain relief and precipitating factors if known.
  - Carry tablets for immediate use if necessary. Do not pack in luggage when travelling.
  - Keep tablets in tightly closed original container. Tablets need to be protected from exposure to light and moisture.

- Tablet should be stored in a cool dry place.
- Check expiry date on prescription. Tablet should be discarded after 6 months once the bottle has been opened. Plan for replacement of supply.
- Risk factor modification:
  - Provide specific instruction on smoking cessation, daily exercise and diet modification.
  - Consider referral to a smoking cessation program or outpatient cardiac rehabilitation program.
  - Encourage adherence to a diet low in calories saturated fats and cholesterol.
  - Discuss the benefits of stress management techniques in decreasing negative effect on oxygen demand. Refer to individual or group counseling as needed.
- Resumption of activities:
  - Provide specific instructions on activities that are permissible and those that should be avoided.
  - Discuss resumption of driving and return to work.
  - Discuss guidelines for resuming sexual relations (e.g. 2 weeks for low risk patients to 4 weeks for Post CABG patients) as given below:
  - During sex, your heart beats should be about 117 per minute.

Stages of Sexual Response

- *Arousal:* Flushed, breathing and heart rate increase, BP goes up slightly.
- *Plateau:* Increase in respiration, BP and heart rate.
- *Orgasm (15 to 20 seconds):* Pulse may reach 150 beats per min. BP reaches 160/90.
- *Resolution:* Return to resting state within second; angina or palpations are most likely to occur during resolution.

General Guidelines for Sexual Activity in MI

- Sexual foreplay at a relaxed pace allows your heart rate and BP to increase more slowly.
- Hugging, stroking, and touching are safe ways to get back in touch with your partner.
- Talk with your partner. Express your feelings.
- Extramarital affairs or sex with new partner may produce more stress.
- Avoid positions for sex that require you to support yourself on your arms for a long time.
- Have a sex in a pleasant, comfortable environment.
- Do not take very hot or cold baths or showers before or after sex.
- Be rested before sex.
- Do not have sex after a heavy meal or drinking alcohol.
- If you have any question about side effects of any drug, do not stop taking the drug, but talk to your health care provider.
- Masturbation and manual or oral stimulation are not harmful to your heart. Anal intercourse may lead to an irregular heartbeat. Avoid this choice unless you clear it with your health care professional.

Treatment of MI

The treatment of MI is aimed at the following:

- Protection of ischemic and injured heart tissue to preserve muscle function.
- Reduce the infarct size and prevent death.
- Early restoration of coronary blood flow by innovation modalities,
- Use of pharmocologic agents to improve oxygen supply and demand, reduce and/or prevent dysrhythmias, and inhibit the progression of coronary artery disease.
- Endogenous catecholamines release during pain imposes an increased workload on the heart muscle, thus causing an increase in oxygen demand.

Thus, the treatment modalities will include:

- The patient should be admitted in ICU of the hospital.
- The patient is given resuscitation, if required and oxygen inhalation for respiratory distress. Good oxygen therapy improves oxygenation to ischemic heart muscle.
- The patient is given analgesic to control pain. An opiate analgesic therapy includes:
  - Morphine is used to relieve pain, improve cardiac hemodynamics by reducing preload, and after load, and to provide anxiety relief. Those who are allergic to morphine; meperdine may be given to avoid respiratory depressions.
  - Nitroglycerin may be administered IV (severe cases) sublingual or paste, to promote venous (low dose) and arterial (high dose) relaxation as well as relaxation of coronary vessels and prevention of coronary spasm.
  - Benzodiazepine (Diazapam) are also used with analgesics to reduce anxiety.
- In addition, following drugs will be used for MI:
  - Thrombolytic agents such as tissue plasminogen activator (Activase), Streptokinase (Streptase), and Urokinase (Abbokinase) are used to re-establish blood flow in coronary vessels by dissolving obstructing thrombus through IV or intracoronary.
  - Along with thrombolytic agents, anticoagulants are also useful for patients who are in situations like prolonged bedrest, pulmonary embolism, deep vein thrombosis, mural thrombi, cardiogenic shock and atrial fibrillation, e.g. Heparine by subcutaneously and every 8 hours.
  - Beta-adrenergic blocking agents (e.g. metaprolol as prescribed) are used for the purpose of limiting the extent of cardiac damage and to improve

oxygen supply and demand, decrease sympathetic stimulation to the heart, promote blood flow in the small vessels of the heart, and antidysrhythmic effects.
- For control of arrhythmia, hypokalemia if present, is corrected, and the patient is given lignocaine (xylocaine) as prescribed. Lignocaine decreases ventricular irritability, which commonly occurs in postmyocardial infarction.
- Calcium channel blockers also may be used to improve the balance between oxygen supply and demand by decreasing heart rate, blood pressure and dilating coronary vessels.
- In cases of sinus bradycardia, hypotension or syncope, the patient is given atropin sulphate 0.3 mg by IV and repeated if necessary.
- If the hypotension is severe due to arrhythmias, treatment is with direct current shock. In cases of ventricular fibrillation, treatment given with direct current shock. If it fails cardiac massage, alternating with direct mouth-to-mouth resuscitation is given until defibrillator is available. The patient is also given IV infusion of 8.4 percent solution of sodium bicarbonate, 50-100 ml. Thereafter, lignocain IV and follow-up as prescribed by the physician.

Nursing Management

- The patient is kept in rest with restriction of patients' physical activity and is advised to avoid alcohol and for abstinence from smoking (if they are in that habit). Once the acute phase is over, the patient can gradually increase physical activity and it is usually taking 6 weeks time to resume normal life.
- In nursing assessment the nurse should gather information regarding patient's chest pain, its nature, intensity, onset and duration, location and radiation and also precipitating and aggravating factors (any maneuvers and medications alleviating pain).
    - and also observe other symptoms experienced associated with pain, i.e. diaphoresis, facial pallor, dyspnea, guarding behaviors, rigid posture, weakness, and confusion.
    - and also previous health status, current medication, allergies, (opiate analgesics, iodine, Shellfish) recent trauma or surgery, aspirin ingestion, peptic ulcers, fainting spells, drug and alcohol use and also any significant ones.
- The probable nursing diagnoses will be:
    - Pain related to an imbalance in oxygen supply and demand.
    - Anxiety related to chest pain, fear of death, threatening environment.
    - Decreased cardiac output related to impaired contractility.
    - Activity intolerance related to insufficient oxygenation to perform ADL and deconditioning effects of bedrest.
    - Risk for injury (bleeding) related to dissolution of protective clot.
    - Altered tissue perfusion (Myocardial), R/T coronary restenosis and extension of infarction.

SHOCK

Shock is defined as a complex, life-threatening condition (or syndrome) characterized by inadequate blood flow to the tissues and cells of the body (Rice 1991). In other words, it is a failure of the circulatory system to maintain adequate perfusion of vital organs. Various disorders leading to inadequate tissue perfusion. This inadequate oxygenation results in anaerobic cellular metabolism and accumulated waste products in cells. If the condition is untreated, cell and organ death occurs.

Adequate blood flow to the cells and tissues require the following components:
- An adequate cardiac pump,
- An effective vasculature or circulatory system and
- Adequate blood volume.

If one of these components is impaired, blood flow to the tissues will be threatened or compromised. Inadequate blood flow to the tissues results in inadequate oxygen and nutrients to the cells, cellular starvation, cell death, organ failure and eventual death (if not treated). Thus, shock is a clinical syndrome resulting in decreased blood flow to body tissues, causing cellular dysfunction and eventual organ failure. Regardless of the cause of shock the end result is inadequate supply of oxygen and nutrients to body cells from impaired tissue perfusion.

Shock affects all body systems. It may develop rapidly or slowly depending on the underlying cause. During shock the body struggle to survive, calling on all its homeostatic mechanisms to restore blood flow and tissue perfusion. Shock may occur as a complication of many disorders and therefore all patients have the potential to develop shock.

Shock is a complex clinical syndrome that may occur at any time and in any place. It is a life-threatening condition often requiring team action by many health care providers including nurses, physicians, laboratory technicians, etc.

Shock causes thousands of deaths and unknown number of permanent injuries every year. Because shock is potentially lethal, it is essential that nurses are able to identify clients at risk of developing shock, recognize the early assessment finding indicating shock, and initiate appropriate interventions before shock ensues. In order to recognize the development of shock, it is important for the nurses to understand the process taking place in the body.

Classification of Shock

There have been many attempts to classify shock, but none of these have been total satisfaction. Here, one classification suggested by many is that it is based on a consideration of defects in the three primary mechanisms responsible for adequate circulation:
- Defect in vascular tone, i.e. distributive shock.
- Defect in the ability of the heart to act as a pump, i.e. cardiogenic shock.
- Defect in the intravascular volume, i.e. hypovolemic shock.

Distributive Shock

Distributive or vasogenic shock occurs when there is a maldistribution of the blood volume in the vasculature. It is due to changes in blood vessel tone, that increases the size of the vascular space without an increase in the circulating blood volume. This results in relative hypovolaemia (total fluid volume remains the same but is redistributed). Vasogenic shock is further divided into three types, i.e. anaphylactic, neurogenic and septic shock.

1. Anaphylactic Shock

It is a severe hypersensitivity reaction resulting in massive systemic vasodilation. The precipitating factors of this anaphylactic shock will include drugs (penicillin), insect bites/stings, contrast media, blood transfusions, anesthetic agents, foods and vaccine. Anaphylactic shock is an acute and potentially life-threatening allergic reaction. It is an immediate hypersensitive reaction characterized by dilatation of arterioles and capillaries and increased capillary permeability causing microvascular leakage throughout the body. Anaphylactic shock can result in respiratory failure as a result of laryngeal edema or severe bronchospasm and circulatory failure resulting from vasodilatation.

2. Neurogenic Shock

Neurogenic shock is an uncommon and often transitory disorder, is caused by massive vasodilatation as a result of loss of sympathetic vasoconstrictor tone in the vascular smooth muscle and impairment of autonomic function. The massive vasodilatation causes pooling of blood in the venous vasculature, decreased venous return to the heart, decreased cardiac output, and eventually inadequate tissue perfusion. Typically, the patient in neurogenic shock which develop hypotension, and bradycardia. There are several precipitating factors that can lead to neurogenic shock, which includes injury and disease to the spinal cord; spinal anesthesia, deep general anesthesia or epidural block; and vasomotor center depression due to severe pain, drugs, hypoglycemia and emotional stress.

3. Septic Shock

Septic shock is due to a release of vasoactive substances. It is more commonly caused by gram-negative bacteria, although many patients with septic shock never have positive blood culture. Septic shock can also occur secondary to staphylococcal, streptococcal, fungal and protozoal infections. The causes of septic shock will include:
- Infections, e.g. urinary tract, respiratory tract, post-abortion, postpartum, caused by invasive procedures, and indwelling lines and catheter.
- Compromised patients including older adults, patients with chronic diseases (Diabetes, Cancer and AIDS), patients receiving immonosuppressive therapy, and malnourished or debilitated patients.

Cardiogenic Shock

Cardiogenic shock often referred to as "Pump failure" occurs when heart can no longer pump blood efficiently to all parts of the body and when cardiac output is decreased. There is no decreased intravascular volume or vasodilatation of the vascular space. Cardiogenic shock is the usual result of left ventricular dysfunction. However, the right ventricle also may be involved. The ventricles are the pumping chambers of the heart and when either one fails, blood backs up into the systemic circulation. Left ventricular dysfunction causes blood to back up into pulmonary system causing pulmonary congestion and decreased cardiac output to the systemic cirulation. A vicious cycle develops as the SVR increases in response to the decreased cardiac output. The failing heart has to pump harder against this higher systemic resistance.

Cardiogenic shock occurs when the heart has an impaired pumping ability, it may be of coronary or non-coronary origin. It is due to inadequate pumping action of the heart, because of primary cardiac muscle dysfunction or mechanical obstructions of blood flow caused by myocardial infarction (MI). Valvular insufficiency is due to disease or trauma, cardiac dysrhythmias, or an obstructive condition such as pericardial temponade or pulmonary embolus, pericardial disease, tension pneumothorax, autovalvular damage and pulmonary embolism.

Hypovolemic Shock

Hypovolemic shock occurs when there is disease in the intravascular volume. It is due to inadequate circulating blood volume resulting from hemorrhage with actual blood loss, burns with a loss of plasma proteins and fluid shifts to dehydration with a loss of fluid volume. Hypovolemic shock is the most common type of shock and develops when the intravascular volume decreases to the point where compensatory mechanisms are unable to maintain organ and tissue perfusion. The precipitatory

factors of hypovolemic shock as already stated above, to be specific, are given below:
- External fluid losses are due to:
  - Hemorrhage, (most common cause).
  - Burns.
  - Excessive use of diuretics.
  - Loss of GI Fluid (vomiting, diarrhea, fistulas, nasogastric suctioning).
  - Diabetes insipidus.
  - Diabetic ketoacidosis.
  - Profound diaphoresis.
- Internal fluid shifts.
  - Pooling of blood in the interstitial spaces (ascits, peritonitis and intestinal obstruction).
  - Internal bleeding (fracture of long bones, ruptured spleen, hemothorax, severe pancreatitis, femoral arterial puncture or catheters in patient on anti-coagulant therapy).

Pathophysiology of Shock

Shock is a dynamic event in which several different processes may be occurring at the same time. In addition, patient may progress towards death or towards normal homeostatic functioning over widely varying time periods. The shock syndrome can be divided into four stages:
1. Initial stage.
2. Compensatory stage
3. Progressive stage
4. Irreversible or refractory stage.

Although there are no clear cut divisions between the stages, in order to understand the pathophysiology of the shock syndrome, these stages are helpful.

Initial Stage

During the initial stage, there will be no clinical sign or symptoms, however, changes are occurring at the cellular level. When body cells lack an adequate blood supply and an adequate supply of oxygen, the ability to metabolize energy is impaired. Energy metabolism occurs within the cell where nutrients are chemically broken down and stored in the form of adenosine triphosphate (ATP). Cells use this stored energy to perform necessary functions such as active transport, muscular contraction and biochemical synthesis as well as specialized cellular function such as the conduction of electrical impulses. ATP can be synthesized aerobically or anaerobically. Aerobic metabolism yields far greater amounts of ATP per mole of glucose than aerobic metabolism and therefore, is a more efficient and effective means of producing energy. Additionally, anaerobic metabolism results in the accumulation of the toxic end product, lactic acid which must be removed from the cell and transported to the liver for conversion into glucose and glycogen.

In shock, the cells lack adequate blood supply and are deprived of oxygen and nutrients, therefore, they must produce energy through anaerobic metabolism. This results in low energy yields from nutrients and an acidotic intracellular environment. The cell swells and its membrane becomes more permeable allowing electrolytes and fluids to seep from and into the cell. The sodium-potassium pump becomes impaired. Cell structures (mitochondria and lysosomes) are damaged and death of the cell results.

Compensatory Stage

The compensatory stage is the reversible stage in which compensatory mechanisms are effective in maintaining adequate perfusion to the vital organs. In this stage, most of the metabolic needs of the body continue to be met. Here, regardless of the cause of shock, the body attempts to compensate for a decrease in tissue perfusion in a variety of ways. First, a decrease in arterial pressure causes a similar decrease in capillary hydrostatic pressure. When the hydrostatic pressure no longer exceeds the colloidal osmotic pressure, fluid moves from the interstitial space to the intravascular space. This process is sometimes called "auto-transfusion". It may add sufficient volume to the vascular space to maintain normal arterial pressure without the help of other compensatory mechanisms.

A reduction in mean arterial pressure will inhibit baroreceptor activity, resulting in stimulation of the vasomotor center in the medulla, causing activation of the sympathetic nervous system and release epinephrine. Stimulation of alpha adrenergic receptor causes selective peripheral vasoconstriction. Blood flow to the heart and brain is maintained, whereas the blood flow to the kidneys and skin is decreased. Beta-adrenergic receptors' stimulation causes a mild increase in heart rate and force of contraction, resulting in an increased cardiac output. This sympathetic stimulation causes dilatation of the coronary arteries, resulting in an increase in oxygen to the myocardium, which now has an increased oxygen demand as a result of increase in heart rate and contractability.

The decrease in the blood flow to the kidneys stimulates the release of rennin into the blood. In the blood-stream, renin activates angiotensinogen to produce angiotensin I, which then circulates to the lungs where it is converted to angiotensin II. Angiotensin is a strong vasoconstrictor resulting in arterial and venous constriction. The net result is increased venous return to the heart and an increase in blood pressure. Angiotensin also simultaneously stimulates the adrenal cortex to release aldosterone, which results in sodium reabsorption by the kidneys. The increased reabsorption raises the serum osmolarity and stimulates the release of ADH. The action of ADH results in increased water reasorption by the kidneys, increased blood volume and increased venous return to the heart. Thus, venous return is increased by the combination of autotransfusion, vasoconstriction and hormonal changes. Increased venous return, as well as increased heart rate and myocardial contractility caused by beta-adrenergic receptor stimulation result in increased cardiac output, maintenance of blood pressure, and adequate tissue perfusion.

The clinical manifestation of the compensatory stage may be subtle and can be overlooked. One of the most reliable signs of this stage is the patient's level of consciousness. Subtle changes in sensorium, usually in the form of restlessness, irritability or apprehension are frequently observed and are primarily caused by hypoxia of brain cells. Sedation at this time is contraindicated because it will mask important neurologic signs. Pupil size may not be an accurate indicator of the degree of shock, because drugs such as atrophine and morphine will cause dilatation or constriction of the pupil.

During this stage, the resting supine, blood pressure may be slightly elevated, slightly decreased or normal for the patient. For this reason, blood pressure may not be useful indicator at this stage. Orthostatic hypotension (a decrease in at least 15 mm Hg when a patient is raised from a flat position to an elevation of 90 degrees or standing) is significant and indicated absolute or relative volume depletion.

The heart rate in this stage is moderately increased. The pulse may be bounding or thready, depending on the stroke volume and the degree of peripheral vasoconstriction. Respirations increase in rate and depth in an attempt to compensate for tissue hypoxia, resulting in respiratory alkalosis. Urine output may begin to decrease, because of reduced renal perfusion as a result of vasoconstriction. Because of extravascular volume, depletion, the patient complains thirst. In addition, thirst may be caused by decreased secretion of saliva secondary to peripheral vasoconstriction. Vasoconstriction in the skin will result in cool and pale extremities. An exception is septic shock, in which skin may be warm and dry. The body temperature at this stage will be slightly decreased except in septic shock, in which, it may be elevated. Bowel sounds will often be hypoactive because of decreased peristalsis as a result of reduced blood flow to the gastrointestinal system.

Progressive Stage

In this stage of shock, compensating mechanisms are becoming ineffective and may even be detrimental to the patient.

Aggressive management is necessary at this stage to reverse the shock stage.

When shock is not detected and the precipitating cause is not corrected during the earlier stages, a massive sympathetic nervous system occurs. Profound vasoconstriction of most vascular beds occurs with some peripheral vessels possibly becoming totally occluded. Renal ischemia leads to activation of the renin-angiotensin mechanism, causing even more pronounced vasoconstriction. Despite the attempt of the body to increase cardiac output by increasing the heart rate and myocardial contractility, there is a net decrease in cardiac output. The decreased cardiac output and profound vasoconstriction leads to tissue hypoxia which causes the cells to undergo anaerobic metabolism. A byproduct of anaerobic cellular metabolism is lactic acid production. Metabolic acidosis results from the accumulation of lactic acid and impaired renal excretion of acids. As the shock stage progresses, the rise in the lactic acid level will often correlate with the severity of the shock state. Acidosis has a direct depressant effect on cardiac function by impairing calcium metabolism within myocardial cells.

Associated with the sympathetic nervous system response is the secretion of large amounts of catecholamines from the adrenal medulla. Catecholamines enhance the cellular metabolism of the brain and heart. Catecholamines also stimulate the liver to undergo glycogenolysis, releasing its glycogen stores in the form of glucose. In addition, the pancreatic release of insulin is suppressed. Therefore, the brain, which does not require insulin for glucose utilization, has large quantities of glucose available for metabolism.

The clinical manifestation of progressive stage of shock includes the patient demonstrates listlessness, apathy and confusion. In addition a decreased response to painful stimuli may be observed. When the blood pressure begins to fall, the patient is no longer in compensatory shock. Regardless of the previous blood pressure, a systolic pressure below 80 mm Hg should be regarded as a danger signal. It is important to remember that a hypertensive patient does not often initially display a pressure this low. A guide for determining hypotension is a reduction in blood pressure greater than 25 percent of the baseline for the patient. In addition to hypotension, a narrowed pulse pressure (difference between systolic and diastolic BP) is often present. This finding indicates decreased stroke volume from a decrease in systolic pressure and a normal or elevated diastolic pressure. Since cuff pressures are likely to be inaccurate during this stage of shock because of the severe peripheral vasoconstrictions, intra-arterial monitoring may be used to provide more reliable pressure readings.

Tachycardia is evident during this stage of shock, and the pulse in older adults and patients who are receiving beta-adrenergic blocking drugs may be an exception and show like heart rate change. Respirations increase in rate in an attempt to compensate for tissue hypoxi a and metabolic acidosis. However, the respirations become more shallow as the patient begins to tire and weaken. Urine output decreases and fall below 0.5 ml/kg/hr. indicating inadequate renal perfusion, which can lead to renal failure. The lips and mucosa are dry, and the patient may continue to complain of thirst. The skin is cold, pale and clammy with slow capillary refill noted. There may be cyanosis caused by tissue hypoxia. Body temperature is usually subnormal.

Irreversible or Refractory Stage

Irreversible or refractory stage of shock is the stage during which compensatory mechanisms are either nonfunctioning or totally ineffective. Cellular necrosis and multiple organ dysfunction syndrome (MODS) may occur. Attempts to restore the blood pressure have failed and death is imminent.

As shock progresses, the sympathetic nervous system activity can no longer compensate to maintain homeostasis. Thus, one of the major compensatory mechanisms has failed. There is pooling and sludging of blood because of the lack of vasomotor tone. Thrombosis of small blood vessels also occurs. Tissue hypoxia resulting from peripheral vasoconstriction and decreased cardiac output makes it necessary for cells to metabolize anaerobically. The accumulation of lactic acid and other acid metabolities in the body's tissues contribute to cell death. The acid environment also causes increased capillary permeability, allows fluid and plasma proteins to leave the vascular space. Because the venous end of the capillaries remains constricted and the arterial end is dilated, blood pools in the capillary bed. This also causes further peripheral vasoconstrictions and a vicious cycle of decompensation ensues.

As shock progresses, hypotension and the resulting tachycardia decrease coronary blood flow leading to myocardial depression, which further decreases cardiac output. Cerebral ischemia occurs. The body cannot maintain vasoconstriction for long with the vicious cycle repeating itself. Consequently, failure of the medullary vasomotor center occurs, which results in loss of sympathetic tone. The result is respiratory or cardiac arrest and death.

The clinical manifestation of this stage includes all body systems, especially the cardiovascular system, show evidence of decompensation. The patient is usually unconscious and may be unresponsive to all stimuli. The systolic blood pressure continues to fall and may not respond to therapeutic measures to raise it. The diastolic pressure blood pressure falls toward zero. The heart rate becomes progressively slower. The pulse is weak, and a pulse deficit may be present. Cardiac dysrythmias may develop because of an ischemic myocardium and increased serum potassium levels from the release of potassium from the dead cells.

Because of the respiratory center depression, there are likely to be slow shallow respirations with an irregular rhythm and sometimes Cheyne-Stokes respirations. If the patient is in an ICU, intubation and mechanical ventilation will usually be used. Damage to the pulmonary endothelial cells increases capillary permeability and interstitial and alveolar edema and hemorrhage an impaired gas exchange may occur. The resulting hypoxemia and respiratory acidosis will further decrease tissue oxygen delivery.

Ischemia of the intestinal mucosa also increases permeability, allowing bacteria and their toxins to enter the blood stream and causing sepsis. Renal ischemia may result in acute tubular necrosis with altered fluid and other metabolic disturbances. Urine output is minimal, and there may be a considerable in serum creatinine and BUN level, indicating some degree of acute renal failure.

The skin is cold and clammy, with a significant decrease in temperature (except in septic shock). Cyanosis may be present and is usually observed in the lips, mucous membranes, and nailbeds. However, it may be more obvious in the palms, soles and palpebral conjunctiva (inside the eyelids) of dark skinned patients.

Infection, acute tubular necrosis, acute respiratory distress and disseminated intravascular coagulation are the common complications of shock.

Management of Shock

It is difficult to know when shock actually exists and when therapy should begin. Treatment should generally be instituted for shock whenever at least two of the following three conditions occur.
- Systolic BP 80 mm Hg or less.
- Pulse pressure of 20 mm Hg or less.
- Pulse rate of 120 or more.

Pulse pressure is calculated by substracting diastolic BP from systolic BP. Normally pulse pressure is between 30 and 50 mm Hg.

Emergency Management

Emergency care of the patient in shock is important and may increase greatly the patient's chances of survival. For example, emergency management of hypovolemic shock is as follows:

The possible causes of hypovolemic shock are major traumas resulting in multiple or serious injuries that are associated with blood or fluid loss, esophageal varices, postoperative bleeding, etc.

The possible assessment findings are:
- Decreased level of consciousness.
- Restlessness, anxiety and weakness.
- Rapid, weak and thready pulse.
- Hypotension.
- Cool and clammy skin.
- Tachypnea, dyspnea or shallow irregular respirations.
- Extreme thirst.
- Nausea, vomiting.
- Chills.
- Feeling of impending doom.

Nursing intervention will:
- Establish and maintain airway; anticipate need for intubation if respiratory distress is evident.
- Administer high flow humidified oxygen (100 percent) by non-rebreather mask.
- Maintain cervical spine precautions if indicated.
- Monitor vital signs, level of consciousness and cardiac rhythm.
- Establish IV access with two large gauge catheters and administer IV fluids.
- Assess for external bleeding sites and apply pressure dressings. Use of pneumatic antishock garment (PASG) to control bleeding if indicated.
- Assess for life-threatening injuries (e.g. hemothorax, cardiac tamponade liver laceration and pelvic fractures).
- Insert an indwelling catheter and nasogastric tube if indicated.

Therapeutic Management

Whenever possible, the patient should be treated in an ICU and should receive continuous ECG monitoring. A general goal is to keep the mean arterial BP greater than 60 mm Hg.
- Establishment of patent airway.
- Management of shock begins by ensuring that the patient has an adequate airway. Maintaining clients' airway is vital to the treatment of shock. In all types of shock, supplemental oxygen is administered to protect against hypoxemia. Oxygen can be delivered via nasal cannula, mask highflow nonrebreathing mask, endotracheal tube.
- *Fluid replacement:* In shock, various fluids are given to correct specific problems such as electrolyte or protein deficiencies or other defects of the blood, including acidosis and hyponatremia. However, in treating hypovolemic shock, the immediate result of therapy seems to depend less on the type of fluid administered for fluid replacement than on the amount of fluid administered. Because shock (except cardiogenic) almost always involves as a decreased effective circulating blood volume, the cornerstone of shock therapy is expansion of that volume by the IV administration of appropriate fluids either crystalloids, colloids or blood products or combinations. At least two large-gauge IV catheters should be inserted immediately before severe vasoconstriction access and intravenous access becomes difficult.

Crystalloids are electrolyte solutions that are either hypotonic, hypertonic or isotonic relative to plasma. However, in the critically-ill patient, approximately two-thirds of the volume will diffuse out of the vascular space because of the increased permeability and reduced oncotic pressure. Therefore, large amount of crystalloids are needed for adequate volume replacement. Because of the expansion of the interstitial space following large amounts of crystalloid administration, the development of systemic edema is common. The common crystalloids are 0.9 percent Saline. Ringer's lactate (Isotonic); hypertonic saline 3 percent, i.e. D5 NS (Hypertonic) 45 percent NS, 33 percent NS D5W (hypotonic).

Colloids are primarily remaining in the intravascular space because of the size of the molecules. The osmotic pressure of these solutions draws fluid into the intravascular space expanding the intravascular volume. Colloids are extremely effective volume expanders. However, none is ideal. Each colloid has significant toxicities that must be considered. Colloids are used in the treatment of shock when plasma protein loss is excessive as in burn shock and peritonitis. If needed, packed cells are administered as soon as possible after they have been typed and crossmatched.

Pharmacologic Management

The primary purpose of drugs used in the treatment of shock is correction of the poor tissue perfusion. These drugs are administered intravenously. They are as follows:
- Sympathomimetic drugs are drugs that mimic the action of the sympathetic nervous system. The effects of these drugs are mediated through action on the alpha-adrenergic, or beta-adrenergic receptors. The various drugs differ in their alpha and beta effects. Debutamine, dopamine, epinephrine (adrenaline), isoproterenol, levarenol, meteraminol, methaximine, and phenylephrine are examples of sympathomimetric drugs. Many of them (epinephrine and norepinephrine) can cause peripheral. Vasoconstriction drugs are referred to as 'Vasopressor drugs'.
- Vasodilators some patients in shock show evidence of excessive vasoconstriction and poor perfusion in spite of volume replacement and normal high systemic pressures. An excessive constriction can reduce blood flow. In such cases vasodilators are used. The common vasodilators are nitroglycerin, sodium nitroprusside, phentolamine and morphine sulphate.
- Corticosteroids have several effects that may assist the client in neurogenic shock after the spinal cord injury. IV corticosterroid therapy may be helpful in anaphylactic shock. Steroids may prevent the delayed symptoms that are thought to be caused by the release of chemical mediators. The common steroids used are dexamethesone, hydrocortisone and methylprednisolone. They inhibit inflammatory process, stabilizes lysosomal membranes, reduces capillary permeability, reduces release of chemical mediators in the septic process, and promotes sodium retention.
- Antibiotics are essential when shock is due to infection. If septic shock, it is suspected that a blood specimen

for culture and sensitivity is taken once and broad spectrum antibiotics are started even though the specific infections organism is not identified.

Nutritional Management

During the acute phase of shock syndrome, the patient receives nothing by mouth because of gastrointestinal tract is not adequately perfused. As recovery begins, nutrition plays an important role in limiting morbidity. Since anorexia is almost universally present, parenteral or enteral feeding is often used. Enteral tube feeding via a feeding pump is commonly the initial method of supplying nutrition. Parenteral feeding is generally adopted only if tube feeding is contraindicated or if they fail to meet the patient's caloric requirements.

Nursing Management

In shock, patient's condition can change rapidly, frequent nursing assessment is essential. Documentations of progress and response to intervention needs to be concise, yet convey the patient's status minute by minute.

The first step in assessing a person in shock via general overview, giving attention as necessary to the ABCs (airways breathing and circulation). Once the airway is patent, air exchange is adequate, a pulse is present and cervical spine is immobilized (if it is trauma). Perform rapid cursory initial head-to-toe physical assessment. The initial assessment goal is to identify major problems and gross abnormalities. Give further detailed attention to specific injuries or problems after shock is stabilized with the use of physical assessment skills, the nurse has to make following observations:

- Airway patency: Presence of noisy respirations and obstructions.
- Breathing respiratory rate and efforts.
- Respiratory pattern: Chest wall expansion; Chest wall bulges or deflates. Tachypnoea, wheezing, crackles, absence of breath sounds, coughing (anaphylaxis) and choking.
- Circulation: Pulse, blood pressure, skin colour, and temperature. Tachycardia, hypotension, weak thready pulse, flat neck vein and fullness of jugular vein engorgment (JVE).
- Heart sounds: abnormal heart sounds and dysrythmias.
- Level of consciousness: Orientation X3 (Person, place, time) ability to move extremities, sensation in all extremities, hand grasps, response to verbal and painful stimuli, pupil size and reaction to light; presence of abnormal posturing; restlessness, anxiety, altered orientation, lethargy, stupor, coma and so on to evaluate neurologic function.
- State of hydration and perfusion of skin: (e.g. capillary refill time less than 3 seconds) condition of mucus membrane, sclera, and conjunctive presence of pallor cool, moist skins or warm, flushed skin (Septic and anaphylactic shock) cyanosis (Later shock) uriticaria, rash and angioedema (anaphylic shock).
- Position of trachea: tracheal deviation may indicate tension pneumothorax.
- Presence, location, intensity, duration of pain, what relieves the pain.
- Abdominal distension, rigidity, vomiting, hyperactive or diminished bowel sounds.
- Circumference of abdomen and or extremities.
- Peripheral pulses.
- Presence of incerations, contusions, ecchymoses, petechiae, purpura (also check bruising over flank area).
- Bone deformities.
- Presence of medical alert tags or bracelets.

Nursing Diagnoses

The possible potential nursing diagnoses for patient in shock are:
- Ineffective airway clearance.
- Ineffective breathing pattern.
- Impaired gas exchange.
- Altered tissue perfusion: cerebral, cardiopulmonary, renal, GI, peripheral.
- Decreased cardiac output.
- Fluid volume deficit.
- Altered nutrition: less than body requirement.
- Constipation.
- Activity intolerance.
- Impaired physical mobility.
- Sensory/perceptual alteration, visual, auditory, kinetic, olfactory, tactile gestating,
- Sleep patten disturbance.
- Impaired or risk for skin integrity.
- Self care deficit, bathing, grooming, dressing, toileting.
- Body image disturbance.
- Self esteem disturbance.
- Altered role performance.
- Personal identity disturbance.
- Anxiety, fears, pain and spiritual distress.
- Anticipatry grievance.

Planning

Nursing care of the client with shock is complex. Frequent reassessment of the client and nursing activities are essential because the client status often changes rapidly. Specific nursing and medical intervention vary according to individual needs and the setting in which care is delivered. However, these common objectives of the care of the client with shock are:
- Return of tissue perfusion and cellular function to normal.
- Meeting metabolic demands.
- Preventing further injury.
- Effective coping by the client and significant others.

Nursing Intervention

In terms of the patient's cardiovascular status, the recommended position for the treatment of shock (after the chest-X-Ray have ruled and neck and spine injury) is supine with the legs elevated to an angle of 45 degrees. The trunk should be horizontal, the head at the level of chest and the knees straight. This Trendelenburg (head down) position should be avoided in shock because it may:

- Initiate aortic and carotic sinus deflexes, causing impaired cerebral blood flow and decreased jugular venous flow.
- Cause the abdominal organs to press against diaphragm, thus limiting respiratory excursion and possibly contributing to respiratory distress.
- Decrease filling of the coronary arteries causing myocardia ischemia.
- Cause an increase in intracranial pressure in the presence of head injury.

This modified Tredelenburg's position promotes increased venous return from the lower extremities without compressing abdominal organs against diaphragm.

CARDIOGENIC SHOCK

Cardiogenic shock occurs when the heart muscle loses its contractile power. It is a grave condition resulting from sudden and complete loss of cardiac function.

Etiology

Absence or inadequate contraction causing cardiac arrest occurs mainly due to: Ventricular fibrillations and occasionally due to ventricular systole. The condition may also result from circulatory collapse with sudden hypotension as in syncope, vasomotor collapse, profound hyperthermia, CNS damage, hypovolemic shock, severe hemorrhage, septicemia, and accidents such as drowning and electrocution. It also occurs from drug or anaesthetic overdose and from cardiac catheterization. Extensive damage of the left ventricle due to myocardial infarction commonly initiates a perpetuating 'shock cycle'.

Pathophysiology

Pathological changes occur according to predisposing factors. An impaired contractility causes a marked reduction in cardiac output. This decreased cardiac output results in a lack of blood and oxygen. The lack of blood and oxygen to the heart muscles results in continued damage to the heart muscle, a further decline in contractile power and a continued inability of the heart to provide blood and oxygen to the vital organs. At the end-stage, cardiomyopathy, severe valvular dysfunction, and ventricular aneurysm also precipitate cardiogenic shock.

Clinical Manifestation

- Confusion, restlessness, mental lethargy due to poor perfusion of brain.
- Low systolic pressure (HP 80 mm Hg or dp mm Hg less than previous level).
- Oliguria—urine output less than 30 ml per hour for at least 2 hours, due to decreased perfusion of kidney, oliguria may lead to acute tubular necrosis.
- Cold, clammy skin—The onset is sudden or gradual, but it presents with pale, cold, sweaty skin (due to blood is shunted from the peripheral circulation to perfuse vital organs).
- This condition may give rise to hypotension, tachycardia and heart sound may be difficult to analyse as sinus tachycardia is more than 100 per minute.
- Weak thready, peripheral pulses, fatigue, hypotension are due to inadequate cardiac output.
- There may be peripheral vasoconstriction leading to peripheral cyanosis or gangrene.
- There will be dyspnea, tachypnea, cyanosis due to increased left ventricular pressures resulting in elevation of left atrial and pulmonary pressure, causing pulmonary congestion.
- There may be dysrythmias due to lack of oxygen to heart muscle and sinus tachycardia as a compensatory mechanism for decreased cardiac output. There may be Cheyne-Stokes respiration, confusion, irritability and an impairment of continuousness.
- Chest pain due to lack of oxygen and blood to heart muscle.
- There may also be progressive acidosis, visual and cerebral impairment while the cardiac arrhythmias may be intractable.
- If late, there may be permanent cerebral damage or loss of peripheral tissue even after recovery.
- Hypoxemia is common particularly when there is pulmonary edema.
- Neurologic impairment, respiratory distress, renal failure, multi-organ dysfunction syndrome and death are the complications of cardiogenic shock.

Diagnosis

Diagnosis of the condition is made on clinical grounds PCWP, 18 mm Hg or greater, chest X-ray (Pul. Vascular congestion). Abnormal laboratory value such as BUN, creatinine and liver enzymes.

Medical Measures

- Use of cardiac glycosides (Digoxin) and positive inotropic drugs (dopamine to stimulate cardiac contractility as prescribed).
- Use of vasodilators to decrease workload of heart and temporary cardiac output.

- Use of vasopressors (sometimes it requires).
- Use of diuretics to decrease total body fluid volume and to relieve systemic and pulmonary congestion.
- Introducing counterpulsation therapy.
- Cardiopulmonary bypass.
- Left ventricular assisting device.
- Emergency cardiac surgery.

Nursing Management

The nurses should make continuous nursing assessment which includes:
- Identify patients at risk for development of cardiogenic shock.
- Assess the early symptoms that are indicative to shock, restlessness, confusion, increasing heart rate, decreasing pulse pressure.
- Observe the presence of pulses alternansm (LHF), decreasing urine output, weakness, fatigue, etc.
- Observe the presence of central and peripheral cyanosis.
- Observe the development of edema.
- Identify signs and symptoms indicative to myocardial infarctions.
- Identify patient's and significant other's reaction to crisis situation.

The probable nursing diagnosis may be:
- Decreased cardiac output related to impaired contractility due to extensive heart muscle damage.
- Impaired gas exchange related to pulmonary congestion due to elevated left ventricular pressure.
- Altered tissue perfusion (renal, cerebral, cardiopulmonary gastrointestinal, and peripheral) related to decreased blood flow.
- Anxiety related to ICU and threat to death.

Nursing intervention: The condition urgently calls for identification of the primary cause and immediate management. The patient is protected from unnecessary disturbance and is maintained adequate airway. The patient is also given oxygen inhalation and small doses of morphine (IV) for anxiety and pain. For further details please see "nursing care plan".

HEART FAILURE

Heart failure occurs when the myocardium is unable to maintain a sufficient cardiac output to meet the metabolic needs of the body. This condition results from systolic dysfunction or diastolic dysfunction.
- Systolic dysfunction results from inadequate pumping of blood from the ventricle. The decrease in pumping power results in a decreased cardiac output. Any process that alters myocardial contractility can produce systolic dysfunction.
- Diastolic dysfunction (stiff heart syndrome) occurs when the ventricle does not fill adequately during diastole. Inadequate filling decreases the amount of blood in the ventricle for cardiac output. Systolic function is often normal or augmented.

Etiology of HF

The incidence of heart failure increases with advancing age and coronary artery disease. An increase in the number of survivors of MI is in part responsible for the increasing number of patients with heart failure. Additional predictors of heart failure include diabetes, cigarette smoking, obesity and elevated total cholesterol-to-high density lipoprotein cholesterol ratio, and abnormally high or low hematocrit level and proteinuria.

The common causes for chronic and acute heart failure (CCF) are as follows:

Chronic	Acute
Coronary artery disease	Acute myocardial infarction
Hypertensive heart disease	Arrhythmias
Rheumatic heart disease	Pulmonary emboli
Cor pulmonale	Thyrotoxicosis
Cardiomyopathy	Hypertensive crisis
Anemia	Rupture of papillary muscle
Bacterial endocarditis	Ventricular sepral defect

The common causes for systolic and diastolic dysfunctions are as follows:

Systolic	Diastolic
Coronary artery disease	Coronary artery disease
Hypertension	Hypertrophy
Metabolic disorders	Fibrosis of advanced age constrictive pericarditis
Myocarditis	Myocarditis
Alcohol	Hypertension
Cocaine	Aortic stenosis
Cardiac valve diseases	Ventricular remodelling
Dilated cardiomyopathy	Collagen diseases
	Cardiomyopathy

Congestive heart failure may be caused by any interference with normal mechanisms regulating cardiac output. Cardiac output depends on preload, afterload, myocardial contractility, heart rate and metabolic state of the individual. Any alteration in these factors can lead to decreased ventricular function and the resultant of manifestations of CCF; there are some precipitating causes for heart failure. The common precipitating causes for CCF and their mechanism are as follows:
- *Anemia:* Decreases oxygen carrying capacity of the blood, stimulating increase in cardiac output to meet tissue demand.

- *Infection:* Increases oxygen demand of tissues stimulating increase in cardiac output.
- *Thyrotoxicosis:* Increases the tissue metabolic rate, accelerating heart rate and workload of the heart.
- *Hypothyroidism:* Indirectly predisposes to increase atherosclerosis, severe hypothyroidism decreases myocardial contractility.
- *Arrhythmias:* May decrease cardiac output and increase workload and oxygen requirement of myocardial tissue.
- *Bacterial-endocarditis:* Increases metabolic demands and oxygen requirements.
- *Valvular dysfunction:* Causes stenosis and regurgitation.
- *Pulmonary embolism:* Increases pulmonary pressure and exerts a pressure load on right ventricle, leading to right ventricle hypertrophy and failure.
- *Pulmonary disease:* Increases pulmonary pressure and exerts a pressure level on the right ventricle, leading to RVH failure.
- *Paget's disease:* Increases work load of the heart by increasing the vascular bed in skeletal muscle.
- *Nutritional deficiencies:* May decrease cardiac function by decreasing myocardial muscle mass and contractility.
- *Hypovolemia:* Increases preload and causes volume load on right ventricle (RV).

Classification of Heart Failure

In addition to above types of heart failure, heart failure can be classified as follows:

Left-sided v/s Right-sided Heart Failure

- In left-sided heart failure, left ventricle cardiac output is less than volume received from the pulmonary circulation; blood accumulates in left ventricle, left atrium and pulmonary circulation.
- In right-sided heart failure, right ventricle cardiac output is less than volume received from the peripheral venous circulation, blood accumulates in RA, RV and peripheral venous system.

Forward v/s Backward Failure

- In forward failure, decreased cardiac output results in inadequate tissue perfusion.
- In backward failure, blood remains in ventricle after systole, increasing atrial and venous pressure; rise in venous pressure forces fluid out of capillary membrane into extracellular spaces.

High-output v/s Low-output Failure

- High output failure occurs in response to conditions that cause the heart to work harder to supply blood; the increased oxygen demand can be met only with an increase in cardiac output; systemic vascular resistance decreases to promote cardiac output.
- Low output failure occurs in response to high blood pressure of hypovolemia which, results in impaired peripheral circulation and peripheral vasoconstriction.

Acute v/s Chronic Failure

- Acute failure occurs in response to a sudden decrease in cardiac output which results in rapid decrease in tissue perfusion.
- So chronic failure, body adjusts to decrease in cardiac output through compensatory mechanisms which results in systemic congestion.

Recently New York Heart Association classified heart failure as follows:

- *Class I:* No symptoms tolerate ordinary physical activity.
- *Class II:* Comfortable at rest, ordinary physical activity results in symptoms.
- *Class III:* Comfortable at rest, less than ordinary physical activity results in symptoms.
- *Class IV:* Symptoms may be present at rest, symptoms with any physical activity.

Pathophysiology

In most cases heart failure begins with left ventricular systolic dysfunction. Ventricular failure can be described as:

- A defect in systolic functions that results in impaired ventricular emptying; or
- A defect in diastolic function that causes an impairment in ventricular filling.

It is now recognized that patients with heart failure actually comprise three distinct groups:
1. Those with failure of systolic ejection;
2. Those with abnormal resistance to diastolic filling;
3. Those with mixed systolic and diastolic dysfunction.

- Systolic failure is the most common cause of heart failure. It is a defect in the ability of the cardia myofibrils to shorten, which decreases the muscles' ability to generate enough pressure to eject blood forward through the high-pressure aorta. Inability to move blood forward through the aorta results in:
    - A decreased left ventricular ejection traction (LVET).
    - An acute increase in left ventricular endodiastolic pressure (LVEDP).
    - An increase in fluid accumulation in the pulmonary vascular bed (pulmonary congestion).

    Systolic failure is due to impaired contractile function (MI), increased after local (HBP) or mechanical abnormalities (valvular disease).
- Diastolic failure is not a disorder of contractility, but of relaxation and ventricular filling. In fact, there is

normal or hyperdynamic systolic function. Diastolic failure is characterized by high-filling pressure and the resultant venous engorgement in both the pulmonary and systemic systems. The diagnosis of diastolic failure is made on the basis of the presence of pulmonary congestion and pulmonary hypertension in the setting of a normal ejection pattern.

- Systolic and diastolic failure of mixed origin is seen in disease state such as dilated cardiomyopathy (DCM), a condition in which poor systolic function is further compromised by dilated left ventricular walls that are unable to relax. This patient often has extremely poor ejection tractions, high pulmonary pressures and biventricular failures.

Heart failures can have an abrupt onset as with acute MI or it can be an insidious process resulting from slow progressive changes. The overloaded heart resorts to certain compensatory mechanisms which include:
- Ventricular dilation.
- Ventricular hypertrophy.
- Increased sympathetic nervous system stimulation, and
- Hormonal response.

Dilation is an enlargement of the chambers of the heart. It occurs where pressure in the heart chambers, usually, the left ventricle is elevated over time. The muscle fibres of the heart stretch and thereby increase that contractile force. Initially this increased contraction leads to increased cardiac output and maintenance of arterial blood pressue and perfusion. Therefore, dilation is an adaption mechanism to cope with increasing blood volume. Eventually this becomes inadequate because the elastic elements of the muscle fibres are overstretched and overstrained.

Hypertrophy is an increase in the muscle mass and cardiac wall thickness in response to overwork and strain. It occurs slowly because it takes time for this increased muscle tissue to develop. It generally follows persistent or chronic dilation and then further increases the contractile power of the muscle fibers. This will lead to an increase in cardiac output and maintenance of tissue perfusion. However, hypertrophic heart muscle has poor contractility.

Sympathetic nervous system activation is often the first mechanism triggered in low cardiac output. It is a least effective compensatory mechanism, because there is inadequate stroke volume and CO. There is increased sympathetic nervous system activation resulting in the increased release of epinephrine and norepinephrine. This results in an increased heart rate. Myocardial contractility and peripheral vascular constrictions. This improves CO. However, later, it leads to worsening the ventricular performance with overlooked volume due to peripheral vascular conditions.

Hormonal responses—as the CO falls, blood flow to the kidneys decreases, causing decreased glomerular blood flow. This is interpreted by the juxtaglomerular apparatus in the kidney as decreased volume. The decrease in renal blood flow activates the renin-angiotensin system to correct a perceived hypovolemia. Angiotensin causes the adrenal cortex to release aldesterone which causes sodium retention and increased peripheral vasoconstriction, which increases asteral blood pressure. The posterior pituitary senses the increased osmotic pressure and it secretes ADH, which increases water absorption in renal tubules causing water retention and therefore increased blood volume. Therefore, the blood volume is increased in a person who is already volume overloaded.

Clinical Manifestations of Heart Failure

Classic symptoms of heart failure include dyspnea with exertion, orthopnea, nocturnal dyspnea, a dry, hacking cough, and unexplained fatigue. When volume overload contributes to pathology, the following additional symptoms occur—rales, a third heart sound, peripheral edema, unexplained weight gain, jugular venous distention, hepatic engorgements, ascites and worsening dyspnea. Compensatory mechanism accounts for many of the clinical signs and symptoms of heart failure.

The more common symptoms as well as symptoms encountered with progressive heart failure are as follows:
- Respiratory symptoms
  - Dyspnea.
  - Orthopnea.
  - Paroxysmal noctural dyspnea.
  - Persistent hacking cough.
  - Alternating periods of apnea and hyperapnea.
  - Rales (Crackles).
- Cardiovascular symptoms
  - Angina.
  - Jugular venous distention.
  - Tachycardia.
  - Decrease in systolic blood pressure with increase in diastolic pressure.
  - S3 and S4 heart sounds.
- Gastrointestinal symptoms
  - Enlargement and tenderness in the right upper quadrant of abdomen.
  - Ascitis.
  - Nausea.
  - Vomiting.
  - Bloating.
  - Anorexia.
  - Epigastric pain.
- Cerebral symptoms
  - Altered mental status (confusion, restlessness).
- Generalized symptoms
  - Fatigue.
  - Decrease in activity intolerance.

- Edema (Peripheral pitting).
- Weight gain.
- Psychosocial
  - Anxiety.

The clinical manifestations specific to right-sided and left-sided heart failure are as follows:

- Right-sided heart failure.
  Signs
  - Right ventricle heaves.
  - Murmurs.
  - Peripheral edema.
  - Weight gain.
  - Edema of dependant body part (sacrum, anterior tibias, pedal edema)
  - Ascitis.
  - Anasarea (Massive generalized body edema).
  - Jugular venous distension.
  - Hepatomegaly (Liver engorgement).
  - Right-sided pleural effusion.

  Symptoms
  - Fatigue.
  - Dependent edema.
  - Right upper quadrant pain.
  - Anorexia and GI bloating.
  - Nausea.

- Left-sided heart failure
  Signs
  - Left ventricle heaves.
  - Cheyne-Stokes respirations.
  - Pulsus alternans (alternating pulses: strong, weak).
  - Increased heart rate.
  - PMI displaced inferiorly and posteriorly (LV hypertrophy).
  - Decreased PaO_2, slight increased $PaCO_2$ (poor oxygen exchange).
  - Crackles (Pulmonary edema).
  - S3 and S4 heart sounds.

  Symptoms
  - Fatigue.
  - Dyspnea (Shallow respiration upto 32-40/m).
  - Orthopnea (Shortness of breath in recumbent position).
  - Dry, hacking cough.
  - Pulmonary edema.
    - Nocturia.
    - Paroxysmal nocturnal dyspnea.

Management of Heart Failure

Along with other team members, nurses assess the health status of the patient with heart failure by identifying the clinical manifestations particularly paroxysmal nocturnal dyspnea, orthopnea, new-onset of dyspnea on excretion, fatigue, lower extremity edema, persistent cough and recent weight gain and records, and perform physical assessment which includes third heart sound, respiratory distress, pulmonary rales, elevated jugular venous pressure, increased in daily weight without increased intake, abdominal distension, cool extremities and decreased pulse, alteration in level of consciousness and decreased urine output.

In addition, nurses also assist in diagnostive test such as ABGs, serum chemistries, liver profile, chest X-ray, hemodynamic monitoring, Twelve-lead ECG and monitor echocardiogram, nuclear imaging studies and cardiac catheterization.

Nursing diagnosis are determined from analysis of patient's data. The possible nursing diagnosis will include:

- Decreased cardiac output r/t alteration in preload, afterload or inotropic changes in heart.
- Impaired gas exchange r/t alveololar-capillary membrane changes.
- Fluid volume excess r/t imbalance between O_2 supply and O_2 demand.
- Hopelessness r/t failing or deteriorating physiological changes.

The objectives of nursing intervention will be:

- Improving cardiac output.
- Improving gas exchange.
- Restoring fluid volume balance.
- Improving activity tolerance.
- Supporting the patient experiencing hopelessness, and
- Educating the patient and family regarding care.

The guidelines for taking care of the person with heart failure are as follows:

- Support oxygenation
  - Administer oxygen by nasal cannula at 2 to 6 L/min. for oxygen saturation greater than 90 percent.
  - Give oxygen as needed for dyspnea.
  - Patient should be well supported in a semi-Fowler's position.
  - Encourage use of incentive spirometry fourth hourly.
- Balance rest and activity.
  - Reinforce importance of conservation of energy and planning for activities that avoid fatigue.
  - Encourage activities within prescribed restriction; monitor for intolerance to activity (dyspnea, fatigue, increased pulse rate doesn't stabilize).
  - Assist with ADL as necessary; encourage independence within patient's limitations.
  - Provide diversional activities that assist in conservation of energy.
  - Provide calm and quiet environment.
- Perform head-to-toe assessment in each shift, including assessment of lab. values, daily weight, and intake and output.

- Provide skin care, particularly over edematous areas; use prophylactic measures to prevent skin breakdown.
- Assist in maintaining an adequate nutritional intake while observing prescribed dietary modifications (offer small meals with supplements).
- Monitor constipation, give prescribed stool softeners.
- Give prescribed medications and monitor for adverse effects.
- Provide patient and family with opportunities to discuss their concerns and time to learn about the diagnosis and plan of care.

Role of Nurses in Medication

Nurses are also responsible for educating the patient as well as family regarding the care of the person with heart failure which include:

- Monitor for signs and symptoms of recurring heart failure and report these signs and symptoms to the primary provider.
  - Weight gain of 1 to 1.5 kg (2 to 3 lb).
  - Loss of appetite.
  - Shortness of breath.
  - Orthopnea.
  - Swelling of ankles, feet or abdomen.
  - Persistent cough.
  - Frequent night-time urination.
- Avoid fatigue and plan activity to allow for rest periods. Incorporate ADL, occupational activity and sexual activity into daily routine by pacing activities.
- Plan and eat meals within sodium restrictions.
  - Avoid salty foods.
  - Avoid drugs with high sodium content (e.g. some laxatives and antacids, Alee-seltser) read the labels.
  - Eat several small meals rather than three large meals per day.
- Take prescribed medications.
  - If several medications are prescribed, develop a method to facilitate accurate administration.
  - Digitalis: Check own pulse rate daily; report a rate of less than 50/min to primary provider and signs and symptoms of toxicity.
  - Diuretics:
    - Weigh self daily at same time of day.
    - Eat foods high in potassium and low in sodium (such as oranges, bananas) if on potassium-depleting diuretics.
  - Vasodilators:
    - Report signs of hypotension (light-headedness, rapid pulse, syncope) to physician.
    - Avoid alcohol when taking vasodilators.
- Adopt healthy lifestyle choices; daily routines; develop support groups; smoking cessation; alcohol intake limited to not more than one drink per day and minimize risk of infections.
- Comply with follow-up appointment.

Thorough evaluation also needed for follow-up scheme.

CARDIAC DYSRHYTHMIAS

Arrhythmias are abnormal cardiac rhythms also called as dysrhythmias. The ability to recognize arrhythmias is an essential skill for the nurse. Cardiac monitoring is now used in a wide range of hospital and clinical settings. Prompt assessment of an abnormal cardiac rhythm and patient response to the rhythm is critical.

Cardiac tissue has those properties which enable the conduction system to initiate an electrical impulse that is transmitted through the cardiac tissue stimulating muscle contraction. The four properties are:

1. Automaticity, i.e. ability to initiate an impulse spontaneously and continuously.
2. Contractility, i.e. ability to respond mechanically to an impulse.
3. Conductivity, i.e. ability to transmit an impulse along a membrane in an orderly manner.
4. Excitability, i.e. ability to be electrically stimulated.

The conduction system of the heart is made up of specialized neuromuscular tissues located throughout the heart. A normal cardiac impulse begins in the sinoatrial (SA) node in the upper right atrium. It is transmitted over the atrial myocardium via Bachman's bundle and internodal pathways to the atrioventricular (AV) node. From the AV node, the impulse spreads through the bundle of His and down the left and right bundle branches, emerging in the Purkinje's fibers, which transmit the impulse to the ventricles. A rhythm is classified as 'normal' when it meets the following criteria in ECG:

- Presence of one upright and consistent-appearing P wave before each QRS complex, all PR intervals between 0.12 and 0.20 seconds.
- The PR intervals are consistent and the heart rate is between 60 and 100 beats per minute.

Conduction to the point just before the impulse leaves the Purkinje's fibers take place within the time of the PR intervals of the ECG. When the impulse emerges from the Purkinje's fibers, ventricular depolarization occurs, producing mechanical contraction of the ventricles and QRS complex on the ECG. Rates of conduction system are:

- SA node 60-100 times/min.
- AV junction 40-60 times/min.
- Purkinje's fibers 20-40 times/min.

The autonomic nervous system plays an important role in the rate of impulse formation, the speed of conduction, and the strength of cardiac contraction. The components of the autonomic nervous system that affect the heart are this right and left vagus nerve fibres of the parasympathetic nervous system and fibers of the sympathetic nervous system. Stimulation of the vagus nerve causes a decreased rate of firing of the SA node, slaved impulse condition of the

AV node and decreased force of cardiac muscle contraction. Stimulation of the sympathetic nerves that supply the heart has essentially the opposite effect on the heart.

Etiology

Cardiac arrhythymias are the result of alterations in impulse formation or propagation. Arrhythmias are often classified by the anatomical site of the dysfunction. For example, sinus dysrhythmias and atrial dysrhythmias. Common causes of arrhythmias include underlying cardiac disease, sympathetic stimulation, vagal stimulation, electrolyte imbalances and hypoxia, which are due to:
- Drug effects of toxicity.
- Myocardial cell degeneration.
- Hypertrophy of cardiac muscle.
- Emotional crisis.
- Connective tissue disorders.
- Alcohol.
- Metabolic conditions (e.g. thyroid dysfunction)
- Coffee, tea, tobacco.
- Electrolyte imbalances.
- Cellular hypoxia.
- Edema.
- Acid-base imbalance.
- Myocardial ischemia.
- Degeneration of conduction system.

Pathophysiology

Alterations in impulse formation and propagation arise from one of the three pathophysiological processes: altered automaticities, altered conduction resulting in delays or blocks and re-entry mechanisms.

Altered Automaticity

Automaticity is the ability to depolarize spontaneously without external stimulation, it is a property that normally confineds to the cells of the SA node. The SA node usually depolarizes at a faster rate than other potential pacemaker cells because of the steep slope of phase 4, allowing sinus cells to reach threshold at faster rate. A variety of conditions can alter the automaticity of SA node and produce faster or slower than usual heart rates. Vagal stimulation will decrease this slope, resulting in a slower heart rate. Sympathetic stimulation and hypoxia will steepen phase 4 resulting in faster heart rates. If the phase-4 depolarization is found, the AV node or ventricular condition system increases, enhanced automaticity is said to exist. Some causes for enhanced automaticity are hypoxia, catecholamines, hypokalemia, hypocalcemia, atrophine, trauma and digital toxicity.

Even cells that do not normally have automaticity may develop abnormal automaticity if the resting membranes potential or threshold potential is altered, increasing the threshold slows the heart rate because it then takes longer to reach threshold. If the resting membrane potential is made, less negative automaticity will increase because it is easier to reach threshold. Altered automaticity may be a consequence of ischemia, infarction, hypokalemia, hypocalcemia or cardiomyopathy. This abnormality is not easily impressed by the activity of the faster pacemakers.

Altered Conductivity

When the rate of amplitude of depolarization decreases, conduction also decreases. Electrolyte imbalances affect the rate of depolarization by altering the resting membrane potential. Hypokalemia causes the resting membrane potential to be positive, decreasing the rate of depolarization and slowing conduction. Any condition decreases the amplitude of the action potential such as ischemia, hypercalemia, or calcification of the conducting figures can cause cardiac conduction disturbances. Abnormality in conduction occur anywhere in the conduction system, including the SA node, the AV node, and the bundle branches. The severity of impaired conduction ranges from a slight delay to complete cessation or block of impulse transmission.

Re-entry

Re-entry occurs when an impulse is delayed within a pathway of slow conduction, long enough that the impulse is still viable when the remaining myocardium repolarizes. The impulse then re-enters surrounding tissue and produces another impulse. This typically occurs when two different pathways share an initial and final segment. The first impulse travels down the faster pathway, leaving behind its refractory trail. Should a second, early impulse follow, it will be blocked because that path is re-fractory. The second impulse then enters the slow pathway and can return retrograde through the fast path, initiating a circuitous pattern.

Clinical Manifestation

In most cases with arrhythmias are asymptomatic as long as cardiac output meets the body's metabolic demands. The clinical manifestations associated with most arrhythmias directly relate to decrease in cardiac output from slow or fast heart rates. Significant changes in heart rate may not allow adequate time for the ventricles to fill and empty. The clinical manifestation includes:

General

- Palpitations (racing heart, skipped beats)
- Anxiety.
- Fatigue.

Altered Cardiac Output

- Pallor
- Confusion

- Cool and clammy skin
- Dizziness
- Cyanotic
- Weakness
- Shortness of breath
- Presyncope
- Rales
- Syncope with loss of consciousness
- Decreased blood pressure
- Chest pain
- Atrial thrombi (may dislodge to causes systemic emboli).

Management

The diagnosis of arrhythmias begins with the 12-lead ECG. Each arrhythmia exhibits characteristic changes in the ECG tracing. A systematic approach to analyzing the ECG rhythm helps distinguish the different dysrhythmias. The systematic interpretation of ECG tracing are:

- Rale (atrial and ventricular).
- Rhythm (atrial and ventricular).
- Presence or absence of P waves.
- PR inteval 0.12-0.20 seconds.
- QRS complex 0.06-0.12 seconds
- QT internal less than 0.55 seconds.
- Interpretation.

Please note that normal sinus rhythm has an atrial (P) and ventricular (QRS) rate of 60 to 100 beats per minute, a regular rhythm (consistent PP and RR intervals) and a P wave before every QRS.

The other diagnostic tests used in the assessment of arrhythmias include signal-averaged electrocardiomyography, ambulatory holter monitoring and electrophysiological studies.

Medical and nursing management of arrhythmias focuses on alleviating symptoms from altered cardiac output and eliminating or reversing the aetiology. Arrhythmia occurring in out-of-hospital setting and present problems of management. Determination of the rhythm by cardiac monitoring is a high priority. Emergency management of arrhythmias indicated where arrhythmias may be due to hypoxia, shock, poisoning, drug ingestion, myocardial infarction, CCF, conduction defects, pulmonary disorders near-drowning, electrolyte imbalances, metabolic imbalances, and electric shock.

During this assessment findings will be:
- Irregular rate and rhythm, palpitations.
- Chest, neck, shoulder or arm pain.
- Dizziness, syncope.
- Dyspnea.
- Extreme restlessness.
- Decreased level of consciousness.
- Feeling of impending doom.
- Numbness, tingling of arms.
- Weakness and fatigue.
- Cold and clammy skin.
- Diaphoresis.
- Pallor.
- Nausea and vomiting.
- Decreased blood pressure.
- Decreased oxygen saturations.

The nursing intervention will include initially:
- Ensure patient airway.
- Administer O_2 via nasal cannula or non-breather mask.
- Establish IV access.
- Apply cardiac electrodes.
- Identify underlying rhythm.
- Identify ectopic beats.

Ongoing monitoring includes:
- Monitor vital signs, level of consciousness, O_2 saturation and cardiac rhythm.
- Anticipate need for intubation if respiratory distress is evident.
- Prepare to initiate CPR, defibrillation or both.

Management of specific arrhythmias according to their types are as follows with their descriptions:

Sinus Bradycardia

Sinus bradycardia is characterized by atrial and ventricular rates less than 60 beats per minute. It is a normal sinus rhythm in aerobically trained athletes and in other individuals during sleep. It occurs in response to carotid sinus massage Valsalva's maneuver, hypothermia, increased intraocular pressure, increased vagal tone, and administration of parasympathomimetic drugs. It can be associated with hypothyroidum, increased intracranial pressure, obstructive jaundice and inferior wall MI.

ECG shows the P wave precedes each QRS complex and has normal encounter and a fixed interval. The clinical significance of sinus bradycardia depends on how the patient tolerates hemodynamically. Hypotension with decrease CO (cardiac output) may occur in some circumstances. An acute MI may predispose the heart to escape arrhythmias and premature beats.

Treatment consists of administration of atrophane (anticholenergic) or isoproterenol is usually effective in increasing HR.

Sinus Tachycardia

Sinus tachycardia is characterized by an atrial and ventricular rate of 100 beats per minute or more (upper limit 150/m). It is associated with physiologic stressors such as exercise, fever, pain, hypotension, hypovelemia, anxiety, anemia, hypoxia, hypoglycemia, myocardial ischemia, CCF and hyperthyroidism. It can also be occured by using of drugs such as epinephrine, non-epinephrine, caffeine, atropine theophylline, nifedipine, hydralozine and ingestion of alcohol, caffeine and tobacco.

ECG shows P wave is normal, precedes each QRS complex and has a normal contour and a fixed interval. It is normal, but HR greater than 100 beat/minute. The clinical significance depends on the patient tolerance on increased heart beat. The patient may complain of palpitations of no symptoms or has symptoms and dizziness and hypotension. In the patient with compromised myocardium, and tachycardia may cause decrease in CO with resultant lightheadedness, chest pain and heart failure.

Treatment is determined by underlying causes. Sinus tachycardia can usually be slowed with digoxin, beta blockers if necessary.

Sinus Dysrhythmia

Sinus dysrhythmia is the most common arrhythmia. It is typically found in young adults and elderly persons. It is an irregular rhythm in which PP intervals are accompanied by changes in RR intervals. The cyclic pattern of changing PP or RR intervals correlates with the pattern of inspiration and expiration. During inspiration, the intervals shorten as the heart rate increases. Conversely, intervals lengthen during expiration. This condition cannot be treated unless the bradycardia phase is marked, causing symptoms that can be treated with administration of atropine.

Sick Sinus Syndrome (SSS)

SSS is one type of tachycardia—bradycardia syndrome, which is characterized by the presence of bradycardia with intermittant episodes of tachydysrythmias. The episode of tachydysrythmia often is followed by a long pause before returning to sinus bradycardia. Complication of this inefficient rhythm includes heart failure and CVA resulting from thromboembolism. This condition is associated with ischemia degeneration of SA node, in which (SSS) some patient remian free of symptoms or complain only palpitations. For the patient with severe symptoms, the heart rhythm is stabilized with a permanent implantable pacemaker for the slow phase and administration of digoxin or beta blockers to control the ventricular rate of the tachycardia phase.

Sinus Exit Block and Sinus Arrest

Sinus exit block occurs when an impulse originates in the SA node but is blocked immediately. No P wave or QRS complex is generated resulting in a long pause. The next impulse occurs in a time interval representing the normal PP interval. Sinus arrest infers that the SA node never fired; therefore, there is no P or QRS complex. The next impulse is asynchronous to the normal PP interval.

This condition may occur as a result of medication such as degoxin hypoxin, myocardial ischemia and damage or injury to the SA node. The patient is symptomatic from a decrease in cardiac output the pauses or long or frequent. The patient may feel palpitations from the strong stroke volume that accompanies the next beat after the pause. When the patient is symptomatic, atropine may be administered to increase the HR and CO. Definitive therapy includes the insertion of permanent pacemaker.

Premature Atrial Contraction or Beat (PAC or PAB)

PAC or PAB is a contraction originating from an ectopic focus on the atrium in a location other than the sinus node. It originates in the left or right atrium and travel across the atria by abnormal pathway creating a distorted P wave. In normal heart, PAC can result from emotional stress or the use of caffeine, tobacco or alcohol. PAC also occurs in disease state such as infection, inflammation, hyperthyrodism COPD, heart disease (AHD), valvular diseases and others.

ECG shows HR variation with the underlying rate and frequency of PAC and the rhythm is irregular. The P wave has a different contour from that of a normal P wave. It may be notched to have negative deflection or it may be hidden in the preceding T wave. The PR interval may be shroter or stronger than a normal PR interval originating from the sinus node. But it is within normal limits. The QRS complex is usually normal. A PAC may be a prelude to supraventricular tachycardia.

Treatment depends on the patient's symptoms, withdrawal of sources of stimulation warranted. Drugs such as digoxin, quinidine, procaimide, flecanamide and betablocker are used.

Wantering Atrial Pacemaker (WAP)

WAP occurs when at least three ectopic sites create the impulse for the cardiac rhythm. ECG shows P waves of different shapes and PR intervals of different lengths. The impulse can originate from the area around the AV node creating inverted P waves from retrograde conduction. Impulses from this lower area may also cause stimulation of the atria at the same time or after the ventricles. The P wave that appear buried in the QRS or occur inverted after the QRS.

WAP usually signifies underlying heart disease or drug toxicity. The patients are asymptomatic unless the HR increases or decreases enough to affect cardiac output. The nurse mentions for changes in the rhythm and in the patient's symptoms. Then treat accordingly.

Atrial Tachycardia or Paraxysmal Supraventricular Tachycardia (PSVT or PAT)

PSVT or PAT in an arrhythmia originating in an ectopic focus anywhere above the bifurcation of the bundle of HIS. Paroxysmal refers to an abrupt onset and termination. Termination is sometimes followed by a brief period of asystole. Some degree of AV block may be present.

In the normal heart, paroxysmal atrial tachycardia (PAT) or PSVT is associated with overexertion, emotional stress, changes in position, deep inspiration and stimulant such as tobacco, or caffeine. It is also associated with RHD, Woff-Parkinson-White (WPW) syndrome, CAD or cor pulmonale. Transient episodes of PAT may occur in children and young adults in the absence of heart disease.

ECG in PAT, heart rate is approximately 150 to 250 (ranges from 100 to 300) per minute and rhythm is regular. The P waves are present, but may be hidden in the preceding T waves and has an abnormal contour. The PR interval may be prolonged, shortened or normal and QRS complex may have a normal or abnormal contour. The clinical significance of PAT depends on symptoms and heart rate. The prolonged episodes and HR greater than 180 beats/mib may precipitate a decreased CO with hypotension and MI.

Treatment includes vagal stimulation and drug therapy. Vagal stimulation induced by carotid massage or Valsalva's maneuver may be used to treat PAT. Administration of adenosine (Adenocard) intravenously is most commonly used to convert PSVT to a normal sinus rhythm. If the rate is unresponsive to adenosine, verapamil, digoxin, dilitrazen, or beta blockers may be effective.

Atrial Flutter

Atrial flutter is an atrial tachyarrhythmia identified by recurring regular, sawtooth-shaped flutter waves. It rarely occurs in normal heart. In disease state, it is associated with CAD, hypertension, mitral valve disorders, pulmonary embolus, cor pulmonale, cardiomyopathy, hyperthyroidism and use of drugs such as digitalis, quinidine, and epinephrine and surgical procedures.

Atrial flutter can be best visualized in leads II, III, and AVF and V on the 12-lead ECG. It is usually associated with a slower ventricular response, because of the refractory characteristic fixed ratio of flutter waves to QRS complexes. The P wave is represented by saw-tooth waves, the PR intervals are variable, and QRS complex is normal in contour. Atrial rate is 250 to 350 beats/minute. High ventricular rates associated with atrial flutter can decrease CO and cause serious consequences such as heart failure.

Treatment includes electrical cardioversion may be used to convert the atrial flutter to sinus rhythm in an emergency situation. Drugs used include verapamil, dilitizem, digoxin, soralol, propafenone, quinidine, procainamide and beta blockers. Ibutilide is effective at terminating atrial flutter in a closely-monitored situation and is used intravenously. Radiofrequency catheter abalation is increasingly being used as curative therapy of atrial flutter.

Atrial Fibrillation

Atrial fibrillation is the most rapid atrial dysrhythmia characterized by a total disorganization of atrial electrical activity without effective atrial contraction. Atrial fibrillation may be paroxysmal and transient or chronic. Generally associated with underlying heart disease and typically with pericarditis, thyrotoxicosis, cardiomyopathy, CAD, HHD, Rh, mitral valve disease, cardiac surgery, heart failure and excessive alcohol intake (holiday heart), gastroenteritis and stress.

The ECG demonstrates baseline fibrillatory wave or undulations of variable contour at a rate of 300 to 600 per minute. Atria depolarizes chaotically at rates of 350 to 600 per minute. The baseline is composed of irregular undulations without definable P waves. The QRS complex is usually normal, but the ventricular rhythm is irregularly irregular (**Fig. 5.1A**).

Because of ventricular rhythm irregularity and the loss of synchronous atrial contractions (atrial kick), CO is decreased. Symptoms include fatigue, dyspnea and dizziness. Thrombi may form in the atria and cause emboli, which may lodge in the pulmonary or peripheral blood vessels. The goal of treatment is to prevent complications through control of the ventricular rate and restoration of normal sinus rhythm (NSR). The risk of emboli may necessitate long-term anticoagulation in some patients. Drugs used to control fast ventricular rates include diliitazem, digoxin and beta blockers.

Premature Junctional Beat (PJB)

PJB arises from an ectopic focus either at the junction of atrial and AV nodal tissue or at the junction of AV nodal tissue and bundle of HIS. If the PJBs arise from the first junction, the P wave will be inverted and premature and will precede the QRS complex. In the second case, the P wave is either hidden in the QRS or is inverted and follows the QRS. The abnormal timing and the inversion of the P wave are caused by depolarization of the atria in a retrograde fashion. The QRS is normal, but the PR interval is less than 0.12 second.

PJB mainly occurs in normal heart. They also may result from digitalis toxicity, ischemia, hypoxia, pain, fever, anxiety, nicotine, caffeine, or electrolyte imbalance. Treatment when needed is directed towards correcting the underlying cause.

Junctional Arrhythmias

Junctional arrhythmias refer to an arrhythmia which originates in the area of AV node. The PJB is one among junctional arrhythmia. Other junctional arrhythmia include junctional escape rhythm (JER), accelerated junctional rhythm (AJR) and junctional tachycardia (JT). JER is often associated with the aerobically trained person who has sinus bradycardia, which may occur with acute MI and dysfunction of SA node. AJR and JT is observed with acute MI digital toxicity and acute Rh, fever during open heart surgery.

Treatment according to the patient tolerance of the rhythm and the patient's clinical condition. Inderol, cardizem and phenytoin are used.

Premature Ventricular Contraction/Beat (PVC/PVB)

PVC or PVB is contraction originating in an ectopic focus in the ventricles. They are associated with stimulants such as caffeine, alcohol aminophylline, epinephrine, isoproterenol and digoxin. They are also associated with hypokalemia, hypoxia, fever, exercise and emotional stress diseases associated are MI, CHF, CAD and mitral valve prolapse (MVP).

PVC is the premature occurrence of a QRS complex, which is wide and distorted in shape compared with a QRS complex initiated from the supraventricular tissue. The QRS complex is usually wider than 0.12 seconds, and the T wave is generally large and opposite in direction to the major deflection of the QRS complex. Retrograde conduction may occur and the P wave may be seen following the ectopic beat. PVC that are initiated form different foci appear different on contour from each other called multifocal PVCs. When every other beat is a PVC, it is called "ventricular bigeming" **(Fig. 5.1A)**. When every third beat is PVC, it is called "ventricular trigeming" two consecutive PVCs are "Couplets". Three consecutive PVCs are called "TRIPLETS". Ventricular tachycardia occurs when there are three or more consecutive PVCs. When a PVC falls on the T wave of preceding beat, the R on T phenomenon occurs and is considered to be dangerous because it may precipitate ventricular tachycardia or ventricular fibrillation.

ECG finding shows HR variation according to intrinsic rate and a number of PVCs rhythm is irregular because of premature beat. A retrograde P wave is possible. The P wave is rarely visible and is usually lost in the QRS complex of PVC. The PR interval is not measurable. The QRS complex is wide and distorted in shape, more than 0.12 second **(Fig. 5.1B)**.

PVCs are usually a benign finding in the patient with a normal heart PVCs may reduce the CO and precipitate angina and heart failure. PVCs in ischemic heart disease or acute MI represents ventricular irritability. They may also occur as "reperfusion arrhythmias after lysis of a coronary artery clot with thrombolytic therapy in acute MI or following plaque reduction from percutaneous transluminal coronary angioplasty (PTCA).

For treating PVCs, lidocaine is the drug of choice, with an initial IV bolus of 1 to 1.5 mg/kg following by a second bolus of 0.5 to 1.5 mg/kg and continuous lidocaine infusion of 2 to 4 mg/minute. Procainamide in the second drug of choice if lidocaine is ineffective.

Ventricular Tachycardia

If the SA node and AV junction fail to initiate impulses, a ventricular pacemaking cell will automatically begin to initiate impulses at a rate of 20 to 40 beats per minute. This is known as "idioventricular rhythm". P-waves when seen are not associated with the ventricular rhythm. The QRS complex is greater than 0.12 wide and bizzarre. If the rate of ventricular initiated rhythm increases, to 40 to 100 beats per minute, it is known as an "accelerated idioventricular rhythm (AIVR). AIVR may be seen in hypoxin, in digital toxicity, as complication of acute MI and as reperfusions dysrhythmia after thrombolytic therapy.

Ventricular tachycardia (VT) may be sustained (lasting longer than 30 seconds) or non-sustained (lasting 30 seconds or less). VT is associated with acute MI, CAD, significant electrolyte imbalance (Eg. K) cardiomyopathy MVP, long QT syndrome, and coronary reperfusion after therapy.

ECG shown ventricular rate 110 to 250 beats per minute. Rhythm may be regular or irregular. ECG may be taken when a run of three or more PVCs occur. The QRS complex distorted in appearance, with a duration exceeding 0.12 seconds and with the ST-T direction pointing opposite to the major QRS deflection. It occurs when an ectopic focus or foci fire repetitively and the ventricle takes control as the pacemaker. The ventricular rate is 110 to 250; the RR interval may be regular or irregular. AVdissociation may be present, with P waves occurring independently of the QRS complex. VT may cause a severe decrease in CO as a result of ventricular diastolic filling times and loss of atrial contraction. The result may be pulmonary edema, shock and decreased blood flow to the brain. It should be treated immediately **(Fig. 5.1C)**.

Treatment includes, if the patient is hemodynamically stable lidocaine bolus administration. If lidocaine is ineffective, IV procainamide may be tried. The third drug of choice is bretylium IV at a dose of 5 mg/kg for several minutes and increased to 10 mg/kg at 15 to 30 minutes (not to exceed 30 to 35 mg/kg). A continuous infusion of bretylium (1 to 2 mg/min) may be started.

Torsades De Pointes

Torsades de pointes, a variation of ventricular tachycardia, can also progress a ventricular fibrillation if not managed appropriately. It is otherwise known as polymorphic ventricular tachycardia. It is a type of VT characterized by a QRS contour that gradually changes into polarity over a series of beats. It usually occurs when QT prolongation is present.

Magnesium sulphate infusion is the drug of choice for torsade de pointes. Other drugs can be used, are isoproterenol or lidocaine infusion if hemodynamic state is stable. If the patient is unconscious or hemodynamically unstable, immediate cardioversion starting initially with 50 Joules. A defibrillator is used in the synchronized mode of cardioversion.

Ventricular Fibrillation (VF)

VF is a severe derangement of the heart rhythm characterized on the ECG by irregular undulations of

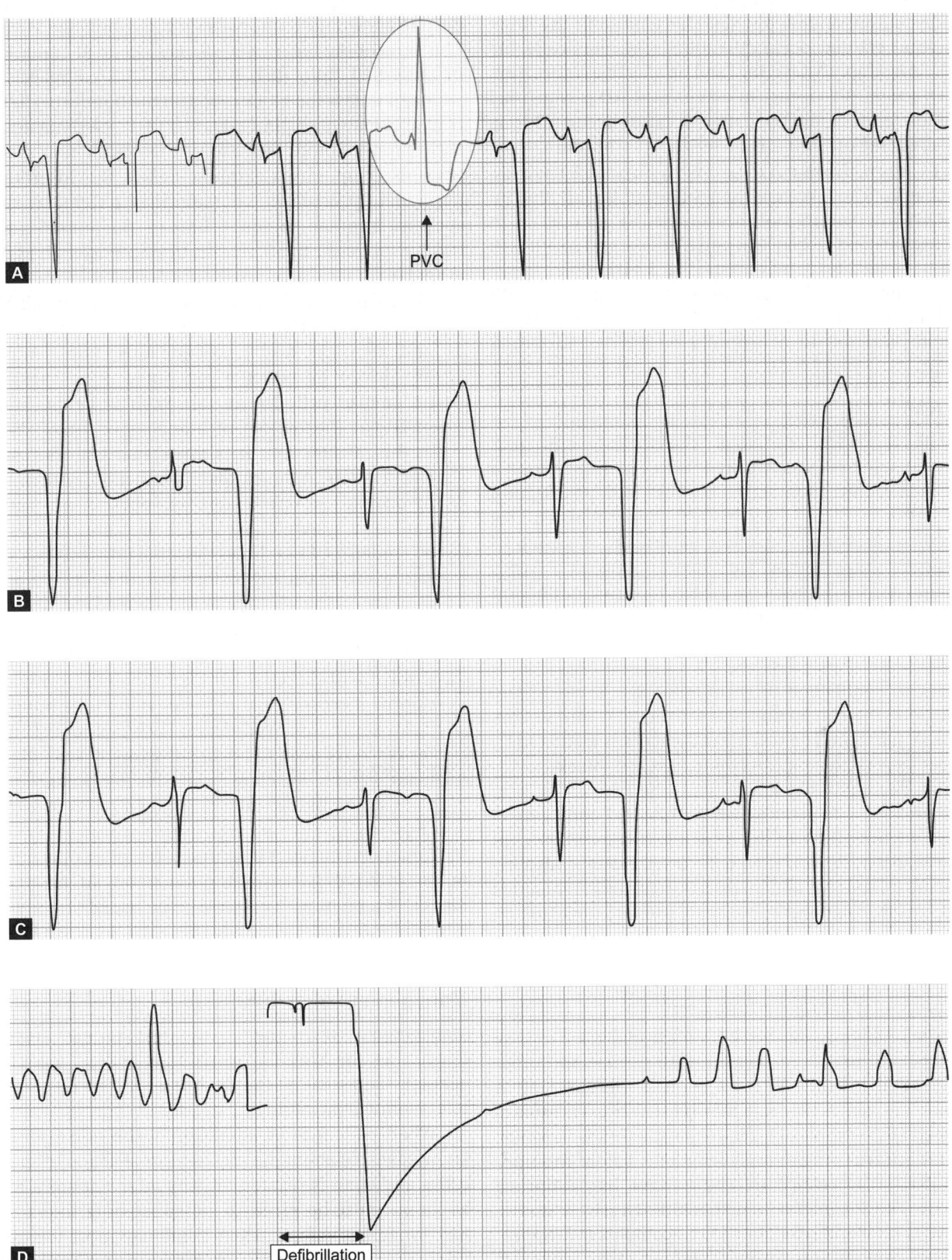

Figs. 5.1A to D: A. Normal Sinus rhythm with premature ventricular contraction; B. Ventricular bigeminy; C. Ventricular tachycardia; D. Ventricular fibrillation with defibrillation

varying contour and amplitude. This represents the firing of multiple ectopic foci in the ventricle. Mechanically, the ventricle is simply "quivering" and no effective contraction or CO occurs. VF occurs in acute MI, CAD, myocardial ischemia and cardiomyopathy. It also occurs during cardiac pacing or cardiac catheterization procedure.

ECG shows HR is not measurable. Rhythm is irregular and chaotic. The P wave is not visible and the PR interval and QRS interval are not measurable. VF may result in unconsciousness, absence of pulse, apnea, and seizures, if not intervened, death may occur **(Fig. 5.1D)**.

Treatment consists of immediate initiation of CPR and initiation of advanced cardiac life support (ACLS) measures with the use of defibrillation and definitive drug therapy.

Asystole

Asystole represents the total absence of ventricular electrical activity. Occasionally P waves can be seen. No ventricular contraction occurs because of depolarization does not occur. This is a lethal arrhythmia that requires immediate treatment. Asystole is usually a result of advanced cardiac disease. Treatment consists of CPR with initiation of ACLS measures which includes intubation and IV therapy with epinephrine and atrophine.

Atrioventricular Block (AV Block)

A block to conduction of an impulse may occur at any point along the conduction pathways. One common area in the AV junction. The severity of the block is identified by degrees i.e., first, second, and third degree AV blocks.

- First degree AV block is present when the PR interval is prolonged to greater than 0.20 second, indicating a conduction delay in the AV node. It is usually found in association with rheumatic fever, digitalis toxicity, acute inferior MI and increased vagal tone. When this occurs in isolation, the patient is asymptomatic and no treatment is needed **(Fig. 5.2A)**.
- Second-degree AV block may be divided into two categories. Type I (Mobitz I or Wenckabach phenoma) and Type II (Mobitz II) **(Fig. 5.2B)**.

Type I AV block may result from use of digoxin or beta blockers, and may be associated with cardiac and other diseases that can slow AV conduction. In this atrial rate is normal, but ventricular rate may be slower as a result of dropped QRS complexes. Ventricular rhythm is irregular. The PR interval progressively lengthens before the nonconducted P wave occurs. The P wave has a normal contour. The PR interval lengthens progressively until a P wave is nonconducted and a QRS complex is dropped. The QRS complex has a normal contour of the patient in symptomatic atropine it is used to increase heart rate or temporary pacemaker may be needed (for MI).

Type II AV block is less common but more serious. It is characterized by nonconducted sinus impulses despite constant PR intervals for the conducted P waves. The nonconducted P waves may occur at random or in patterned ratio (2:1, 3:1). The QRS complexes are widened unless the block is within the bundle of His type II blocks may occur in CAD, MI, RHD, cardiomyopathy and chronic fibrotic disease of the conduction system. For this temporary treatment before the insertion of permanent pacemaker, i.e. temporary pacemaker drugs such as atropine, epinephrine, or dopamine can be tried to increase heart rate until pacemaker therapy is available.

- Third degree AV block is a complete heart block. Here all the sinus atrial impulses are blocked and the atria and ventricle beat independently. The ventricles are driven by either a junctional or a ventricular pacemaker cell. The usual lesion is in the bundle of His or the bundle of branches but may also be at the AV junction. It is associated with fibrosis or calcification of the cardiac conduction system, CAD myocarditis, cardiomyopathy, open heart surgery and some systemic diseases such as amyloidosis and scleroderma. ECG shows the atrial rate usually a sinus rate which is usually a sinus rate of 60 to 100 beats/min artery. The ventricular rate depends on the site of block. The P wave has normal contour. The PR interval is variable and there is no relationship between the P wave and the QRS complex. The QRS complex is normal if escape rhythm is initiated in the bundle of his or above. The third-degree AV block almost always results in reduced CO with subsequent ischemia and heart failure. Syncope from this block may result from severe bradycardia or even episodes of asystole **(Fig. 5.2C)**.

Treatment includes insertion of temporary pacemaker or an external pacemaker applied on an emergency basis in a patient with acute MI. The use of drug include atropine, epinephrine and dopamine to increase HR and support BP prior to pacemaker insertion.

Management of Arrhythmias

Management of patient with arrhythmias includes diagnosing the specific arrhythmia and its associated aetiology and treating the disorders with medications or interventional procedures.

When patient is on medication, the nurse must be knowledgeable about the mechanism of action of specific drugs and their associated nursing interventions. Careful attention must be given to potential drug interactions and synergetic effects when combination of therapy is used. The metabolism and excretion of medications may be impaired in the elderly and in patients with decreased perfusion to the kidney and liver. The nurse must be aware of new agents approved for the management of cardiac arrhythmia and how to monitor their safe use.

Nursing Management of Cardiovascular Disorders

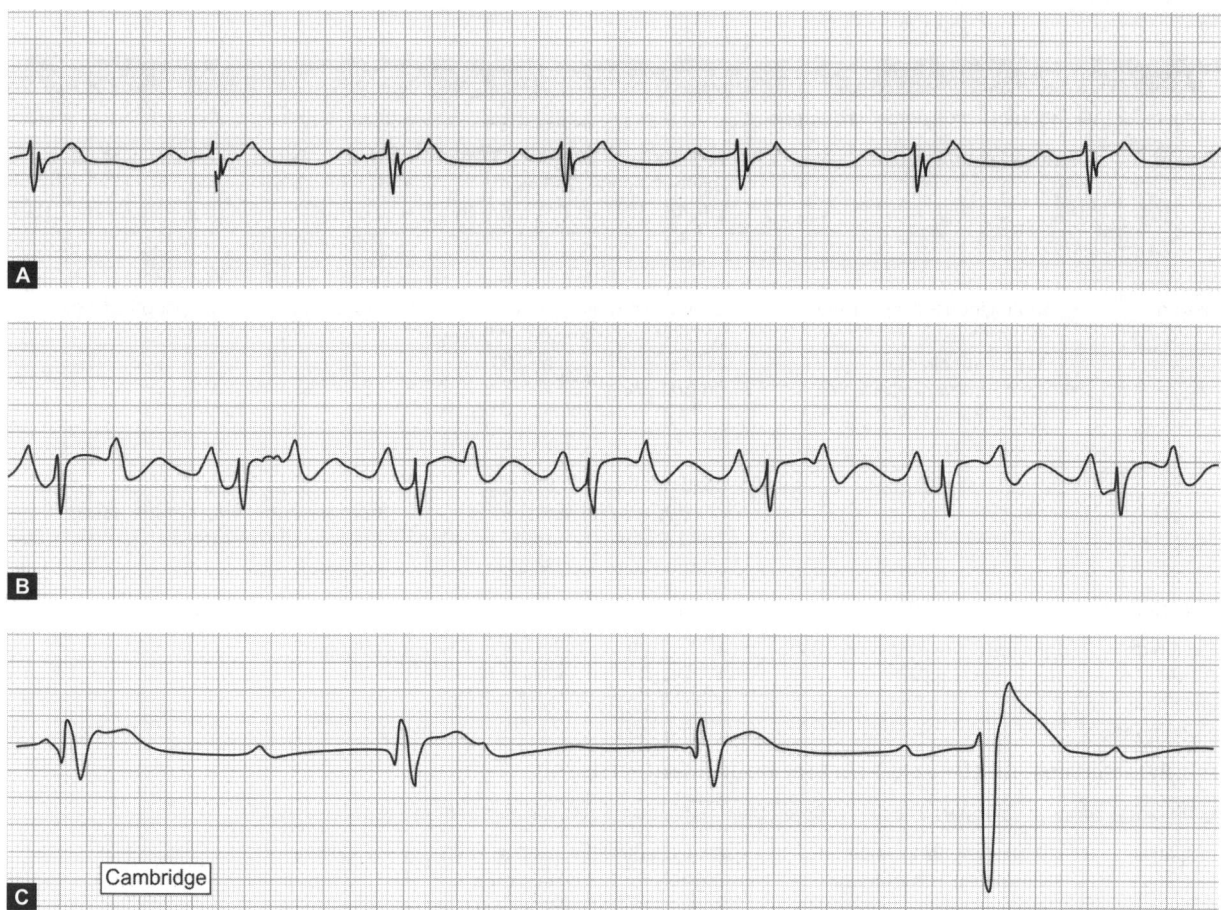

Figs. 5.2A to C: A. First-degree AV block; B. Second-degree AV block (Mobitz 1); C. Third-degree AV block

Nursing management of the patient experiencing arrhythmia include interventions to decrease oxygen demand. The nurse spaces activities and encourages frequent rest periods. While medication therapy is being adjusted, patients are on continuous monitoring (telemetry). Rhythms are documented every 4 to 8 hours and as needed. Skin care is provided to minimize the irritation of monitoring electrodes.

Drugs used in arrhythmias **(Table 5.4)**.

The nurse must be alert to changes in a patient's rhythm. Assessment for changes in the cardiac output are documented. Emergency drugs should be available

Table 5.4: Antiarrhythmic drugs.

Drugs	Uses	Doses	Side effects
Class I: Block NA+ channels			
IA. Reduce V_{max} and prolong action potential duration			
Quinidine	• VT and SVT; APC/VPC • PSVT, atrial fibrillation	200–600 mg every 4–6 hourly until reverted, then 200–300 mg 6–8 hourly depending on the condition	• Nausea, vomiting abdominal pain • Hepatitis • Hemolytic anemia, agranulocytosis, thrombocytopenic purpura • Bradycardia, hypotension • Allergy, rash, angioneurotic edema, flushing • Cinchonism, e.g., impaired hearing
Procainamide	• Same as above • Arrhythmias associated with anaesthesia and surgery	250–1000 mg every 3–6 hourly orally	• Same as above • May induce lupus like syndrome

Contd...

Contd...

Drugs	Uses	Doses	Side effects
IB. Do not reduce V_{max} shorten action potential duration			
Mexiletine	Ventricular arrhythmias	200–400 mg tid upto 1200 mg/day/oral or 200–250 mg IV infusion at a rate of 1 mg/min	• Nausea, vomiting, constipation • Bradycardia, hypotension • Confusion, convulsions, ataxia and CNS disturbance • Hepatitis, blood dyscrasias
Phenytoin	• Digital induced ventricular arrhythmias • As an antiepileptic • For neuropathic pains, e.g. trigeminal neuralgia, diabetic neuropathy	Oral: 100 mg bid or tid IV: Dilantinisation 500–1000 mg as IV drip followed by 100 mg tid orally or IV	Read side effects in antiepileptic drugs
Lidocaine	Ventricular arrhythmias	Loading dose: 1–1.5 mg/kg IV push, may be repeated as 0.5–1.5 mg/kg IV after 5–15 minutes followed by drip	• Nervousness, dizziness, blurred vision, tremors, numbness, tinnitus, nausea, vomiting • Bradycardia, hypotension, cardiovascular collapse
IC. Reduce V_{max} primarily, slow conduction and can prolong refractoriness			
• Elecainide • Others, e.g. encainide, eropafenone	Supraventricular and ventricular arrhythmias, e.g., VT	• 50–100 mg 12 hourly orally • 25–50 mg 8 hourly orally • 150 mg tid orally (upto 300 mg tid)	Proarrhythmic
Class II: Beta blockers—read beta blockers. They are discussed in Table 5.1			
Class III: Drugs block K⁺ channels, block multiple phases of action potential and prolong repolarisation			
Amiodarone	• Potentially life-threatening ventricular arrhythmias unresponsive to conventional therapy • Supraventricular arrhythmias, e.g., AV nodal, AV reentry, junctional tachycardia, atrial flutter and fibrillation	Oral: Loading dose 800 to 1600 mg/day for 1–3 weeks, then 600–800 mg/day for 4 weeks then 400 mg/day IV for VT: 15 mg/min as infusion for 10 minutes followed by 1 mg/min for 6 hours for the next several days as necessary	• Liver toxicity • GI symptoms • Pulmonary fibrosis • Photosensitivity • Hypothyroidism or hyperthyroidism • Disorders of thyroid function, e.g. hyper and hypothyroidism • Cardiac toxicity, e.g. bradycardia, ventricular tachyarrhythmias • Neuropathy
Bretylium tosylate	• Life-threatening ventricular arrhythmias unresponsive to conventional drugs • Drug-resistant ventricular tachyarrhythmias	VF: 5 mg/kg IV (diluted both 50–100 mL of 5% dextrose) push; if no response, then 10 mg/kg IV push (diluted with 50–100 mL of dextrose) then maintain infusion at 1–2 mg/min (do not exceed 30–35 mg/kg/day)	• Orthostatic hypotension • Nausea, vomiting • Increased salivation and parotid pain
Sotalol	Ventricular tachyarrhythmias	Oral: 80 bid to 320 mg/day	Side effects of beta-blockers
Class IV: Calcium channel blockers—read the text (discussed in) Table 5.1			
Other antiarrhythmics			
Adenosine: It slows the conduction through AV node and accessory pathways	• Narrow QRS complex paroxysmal supraventricular tachycardia (PSVT) • Used for pharmacological stress testing	IV: 6 mg IV push over 1–3 seconds (follow with 20 mL NS flush), if no response in 1–2 min; then 12 mg repeat IV push	• Flushing; dyspnoea, headache, chest pressure • Hypotension • Bradycardia and conduction disturbance

and intravenous access should be ensured. Ancillary equipment such as defibrillators, oxygen suction and temporary pacemaker should be readily available and in good working condition.

Interventions such as cardioversion defibrillation, coronary ablation, pacemaker therapy, automatic implantable cardioverterdefibrillators, and CPR are also part of the managements of patients with arrhythmias.

INFLAMMATORY HEART DISEASE

Pericarditis

Pericarditis is an inflammatory process of the visceral or parietal pericardium (inflammations of the pericardial sac). It can be acute or chronic and can spread from or to the myocardium.

Etiology

Pericarditis can occur as a result of bacterial, viral or fungal infection. The causes of pericarditis are as follows:

Infections

- Viral causes including Coxsakie virus B, Coxsakie virus A, adenovirus, mumps, Epstein-Barr, varicella Zoster and hepatitis B.
- Bacterial causes including pneumococci, staphylococci, streptococci septicemia from gram-negative organisms and tuberculosis.
- Fungal causes including histoplasma, candida species, infections such as toxoplasmosis and lyme disease.

Non-infections

- Uraemia.
- Acute MI.
- Neoplasms such as lung cancer, breast cancer, Hodgkin's disease and lymphoma.
- Trauma after thoracic surgery, pacemaker insertion and cardial diagnostic procedures.
- Radiation.
- Dissecting aortic aneurysm.
- Myxedema

Hypertensive or Autoimmune

- Delayed post-myocardial-pericardial injury.
- Post-myocardial infarction syndrome (Dresslers).
- Post-pericardiotomy syndrome.
- Rheumatic fever.
- Drug reactions (e.g. Procainamide and hydralazine).

Pathophysiology

In acute pericarditis, the membranes surrounding the heart become inflamed. The inflamed membrane rub against each other and produces the classic pericardial friction rub of pericarditis. The friction rub sounds scratching and harsh on the auscultation and lasts throughout systole and diastole. The patient complains of severe precardial chest pain, which may closely resemble that of acute MI. The pain intensifies when the person is lying supine and decreases with sitting. The pain also intensifies when the patient breathes deeply. Patient shows other signs and symptoms.

Chronic pericarditis can be constrictive or adhesive. It usually begins with an initial episode of acute pericarditis (often secondary to neoplasia, radiation, previous surgery, or idiopathic causes) and is characterized by fibrin deposition with clinically undetected pericardial effusion. Organization and resorption of the effusion slowly follows with progression towards the chronic stage of fibrous scarring, thickening of the pericardium from calcium deposition, and eventual obliteration of the pericardial space. The fibrositic, thickened and adherent pericardium encases the heart, thereby, impairing the ability of the atria and ventricles to stretch sufficiently during diastolic filling.

Clinical Manifestations

In acute pericarditis, patient may complain chest pain, dyspnea and a pericardial friction rub. The intense, plueritic chest pain is generally sharpest over the left precardium or retrosternally but may radiate to the trapezius ridge and neck (mimicking angina) or sometimes to the epigastrium or abdomen (mimicking abdominal or other non-cardiac pathologic condition). The pain is aggravated by lying supine, deep breathing, coughing, swallowing and moving the trunk and is eased by sitting up and leaning forward. The dyspnea accompanying acute pericarditis is related to the patients' need to breathe in, rapid, shallow breaths to avoid chest pain and may be aggravated by fever and anxiety. The pericardial rub is a scratching, grating, high-pitched sound believed to arise from friction between the roughened pericardial and epicardial surface. It is best heart with stethoscope.

The two major complications of acute pericarditis induced are pericardial effusion and cardiac tamponade. The accumulation of fluid within the pericardial sac is called "Pericardial effusion". The fluid may be serous, purulent, or hemorrhagic. Serous effusion usually accompany heart failure. Purulent effusions indicate underlying disorders such as tuberculosis or neoplasm. Hemorrhagic effusions most often occur from trauma, aneurysm, rupture, coagulation abnormalities. Large effusions may compress adjoining structures. Pulmonary tissue compression can cause cough dyspnea and tachypnea. Phrenic nerve compression can induce hiccups and compression of the laryngeal nerve may result in hoarseness. Heart sounds are generally distant and muffled, although BP is maintained by compensatory mechanism.

The cardiac tamponade develops as the pericardial effusion increases in size compensatory mechanism ultimately fail to adjust to the decreased cardiac output.

This can lead to cardiac failure, shock and death. The signs and symptoms of cardiac temponade include
- Decrease in systolic BP.
- Narrowing pulse pressure.
- Pulses Paradoxus (Greater than 10 mm Hg).
- Increase in venous pressure and distention of neck veins.
- Tachycardia.
- Tachypnea.
- Possible friction rub.
- Muffled heart sounds.
- Low voltage EGG.
- Rapid enlargement of cardiac heart on chest X-Ray.
- Peripheral cyanosis.
- Anxiety.
- Chest pain.

The chronic pericarditis patient may complain of dyspnea and fatigue and exhibits symptom of heart failure as a result of diminished ability of the heart pump.

Management of Acute Pericarditis

To diagnose, careful history and physical examination are needed. In addition, auscultation of chest, EGG, Chest X-Ray, echocardiography, pericardiocentesis, CT scan, nuclear scan of the heart are useful. The management includes:
- Treatment of underlying disease.
- Bedrest.
- Aspirin.
- NSAIDs (Non-steroid anti-inflammation drug)
- Corticosteroids.
- Pericardiocentesis (for large pericardial effusion or cardiac temponade)

In chronic pericarditis, removal of the pericardium may be necessary to restore cardiac function.

The management of the patient's pain and anxiety during acute pericarditis are primary nursing considerations. Assessment and careful observation of pain and attending to it are important and also monitor the anxiety level and take anxiety-reducing measures in addition to regular treatment including care of surgical patients.

In addition, the nurse teaches the patient and their significant others about the nature of the disease and the purposes and correct use of all medications. She teaches measures to decrease fatigue and provides information on how to minimize the risk of complications. The nurse also provides an overview of the signs and symptoms of recurrent pericarditis that would need to be promptly reported to the health care provider.

MYOCARDITIS

Myocarditis, a focal or diffuse inflammation of the myocardium that causes an infiltrate in the myocardial interstitium and injury to an adjacent myocardial cells.

Etiology

Myocarditis may be primary with an unknown etiology or secondary from an identifiable cause such as drug sensitivity or toxicity, connective tissue disease, sarcoidosis, or infection. The inflammation process often develops secondary to infective endocarditis. Myocarditis may be acute or chronic. It has been associated with variety of a etiologic agents including viruses, bacteria, rickettsia, fungi, parasites, radiation and pharmacological and chemical factors. Viral infection is the most common cause. It includes viruses like coxsackievirus B, coxsackievirus A, echovirus, poliovirus, influenza A and B, rubella, mumps, rabies, Epstein-Barr, hepatitis and HIV.

The pathophysiologic mechanisms of myocarditis are poorly understood because there is usually a period of several weeks after the initial infection before the development of manifestations of myocarditis. Immunologic mechanisms may play a role in the development of myocarditis. The majority of infections are benign, self-limiting, and sub-clinical although viral myocardium in infants and pregnant women may be virulent.

Clinical Manifestation

During the acute viral phase, symptoms are flu-like and include fever, lymphadenopathy, pharyngitis, myalgia and gastrointestinal complaints. Hepatitis, encephalitis, nephritis and orchitis also can occur. The clinical manifestations for patient with myocarditis are variable ranging from a benign course without any overt manifestations to severe heart involvement of sudden death:

Usually early cardiac manifestations appear 7 to 10 days after viral infection and include pericardial chest pain with an associated friction rub because pericarditis often accompanies myocarditis. Cardiac signs (S3 Crackles, jugular venous distention and peripheral edema) may progress to CHF including pericardial effusion, syncope, and possibly ischemic pain. ECG changes include ST segments, elevation and QT interval prolongation.

Management

Diagnosis can be made through as in pericarditis. In addition, histologic confirmation of myocarditis through endomyocardial biopsy (EMB). The patient with myocarditis are treated with bedrest and digitalis to prevent heart failure and cardiogenic shock. Immunosuppression may be beneficial in reducing inflammation and preventing irreversible myocardial damage. Medical therapy also includes treatment of underlying disease with antibiotics, conventional therapy for CHF and management of arrhythmias.

Nursing care includes ongoing monitoring of the patients, physiological status. Patients are commonly anxious about the sudden onset of heart disease and its implications for the future. The nurse provides emotional support and encourages verbalizations of feelings. If EMB is performed, postbiopsy nursing care focuses on the potential for injury that can occur, such as haematoma or bleeding at the connulation site, cardiac tamponade or pneumothorax. Any alteration should be referred to the physician concerned immediately. Vital signs are monitored closely to assess for continual hemodynamic stability. Monitoring for heart failure is an important consideration. Measure to decrease cardiac workload include frequent rest periods, provisions for a quiet environment, and the use of semi-Fowler's position. The patients and their family members significant and others were educated regarding the disease. The nurse encourages slow progression of activities with frequent rest periods and the use of medication with instructions.

INFECTIVE ENDOCARDITIS

Infective endocarditis previously known as bacterial endocarditis is an infection of the endorcardial surface with microorganism, present in the lesion. The endocardium, the inner layer of the heart, is contagious with the valves of the heart. Therefore, inflammation from infective endocarditis usually affects the cardiac valves.

Infective endocarditis classified as subacute and acute. The subacute form has a longer clincial course of more insidious onset with less toxicity, and the causative organisms usually of low virulence. In contrast, the acute form has a shorter clinical course with more rapid onset, increased toxicity and more pathogenic causative organism.

Etiology

Etiologic organisms associated with infective endocarditis includes:
- Streptococci
  - Alpha and hemolytic streptococci
  - Enterococci
  - *Streptococcus bovis* and
  - *Streptococcus pneumoniae.*
- Staphylococci
  - *Staphylococcus aureus*
  - *Staphylococcus epidermidis.*
- Gram-negative bacteria
  - *Escherichia coli*
  - *Klebsialla* and
  - *Pseudomonas.*
- Polymicrobic endocarditis.
  - *Staphylococcus agalaective* and methicillin susceptible *Staphylococcus aureus.*
  - *Pseudomonas aeruginosa*, hemolytic streptococci and micrococcus.
- *Haemophilus*
- *Actinobacillus*
- *Cardiobacterium*
- *Eikenella*
- *Kingella.*

The predisposing conditions to the development of infective endocarditis are as follows:
- Cardiac conditions:
  - Rheumatic heart disease.
  - Aortic valve leaflet abnormalities.
  - Mitral valve prolapse with murmur.
  - Cyanotic congenital heart disease.
  - Prosthetic valve.
  - Degenerative valvular lesions.
  - Prior endocarditis.
  - Morjan's syndrome.
  - Asymmetric septal hypertrophy.
  - Idiopathic hypertrophic subsolesions.
- Non-cardiac diseases:
  - Associate risks.
  - Intravascular devices (leading) bacteraemia.
- Procedure:
  - Associated risks.
  - Intravascular devices (leading to nosocomial bacteraemia.
  - Procedures that require endocarditis antibiotic prophylaxis.

The patient populations at risk for infective endocarditis are:

High Risk
- Prosthetic heart valves.
- Previous history of endocarditis.
- Complex congenital cyanotic heart disease.
- Surgically constructed systemic pulmonary shunts or conduits.

Moderate Risk
- Patent ductus arteriosus.
- Ventricular septal defect.
- Primum atrial septal defect.
- Coarctation of aorta.
- Acquired valvular dysfunction.
- Hypertrophic cardiomyopathy.
- Some clinical presentation of mitral valve prolapse.

Pathophysiology

A damaged cardiac valve or a ventricular septal defect produces turbulent blood flow, which allows bacteria to settle on the low pressure side of the valve or defect. The hallmark of endocarditis is the "Platletfibrin-bacteria mass" on the value called a vegetation. The organism surround the heart valve become embedded on the valve matrix, and result in vegetative, the primary lesions of the infective endocarditis consist of fibrin, leukocytes, platelets, and microbes that adhere to the valve surface or endocardium. The loss of portions of these friable types of vegetation into the circulation results in embolization. Systemic embolization occurs from left sided heart vegetation, progressing to organ (particularly brain, kidneys and spleen) and limb infarction. Right sided heart lesions embolize to the lungs. If the vegetative emboli enter organs, abscesses may form.

The infection may spread locally to cause damage to the valves or to their supporting structures. The resulting valvular incompetence and eventual invasion of the myocardium in the infectious disease result in CHF, generalized myocardial dysfunction and sepsis.

Clinical Manifestations

The onset of SBE (Subacute Bacterial Endocarditis) is gradual and the patient reports malaise and general achiness. Low grade fever is usually present, although a high fever usually occurs with *S. aureus*, infection. The other non-specific manifestations that may accompany fever include chills, weakness, malaise, fatigue, and anorexia. Arthralgia, myalgia, backpain, abdominal discomfort, weight loss and headache, clubbing of fingers may occur in SBE.

Vascular manifestation's infective endocarditis includes splinter hemorrhages (black longitudinal streaks) that may occur in nail beds. Petechiae may occur as a result of fragmentation and microembolization of vegetative lesions and are common in the conjunctiva, the lips, the buccal mucosa, the palate, and over the ankles, the feet and the antecubital and popleteal areas oslers nodes (painful, tender, red or purple peasize lesions) may be found in fingertips or toes. Janeway lesions (flat painless, small red spots) may be found on the palms and soles. Fundoscopic examination may reveal haemorrhagic retinal lesions called Rohith's spots.

Auscultation reveals murmurs over the affected area and clinical manifestations secondary to embolizations in various body organs may also be present, if embolization of organs and cardinal symptom are as follows:
- *Spleen:* Sharp left upper quadrant pain and splenomegaly, local tenderness and abdominal rigidity.
- *Kidney:* Pain in the flank, hematuria and azotaemia.
- *Peripheral:* Blood vessel of arms and legs may cause gangrene.
- *Brain:* Hemiplegia, ataxia, aphasia, visual changes. LOC changes.
- *Pulmonary:* Occurs in right sided endocarditis emboli

Management

For diagnosis obtaining the patient's recent health history is very important particularly inquiry regarding any recent dental urologic, surgical or gynecologic including normal or abnormal obstetric delivery, heart disease diagnostic procedures, infection of skin and respiration or urinary origin are helpful.

In addition to thorough physical examination and routine diagnostic procedures, useful are blood culture and sensitivity, WBC count with differential rheuma old factor, urin analysis, chest X-Ray, ECG, echocardiography and cardiac catheterization.

The major aim of the therapy is to eliminate all micro-organisms from the vegetative grown and prevent complications. The therapy includes:
- Appropriate antibiotic therapy.
- Antipyretics.
- Rest.
- Repetitions of blood cultures and sensitivity tests.
- Surgical valvular repair or replacement (for severe valvular damage).

The nurse teaches the patient to avoid excessive fatigue and to stop activity immediately if chest pain, dyspnea, light headedness, or faintness occurs. Patients should avoid others with infections. The nurse instructs the patient to inform all primary care providers including physicians, and dentists about history of infective endocarditis, so that appropriate antibiotic therapy can be administered prior to intrusive procedure. American Heart Association recommended following antibiotic prophylaxis of infective endocarditis:
- For dental, oral, respiratory tract or esophageal procedure, if Streptococcus viridans is a pathogen, the antibiotic choice will be:
  - Amoxicillin 2 g 1 hr before procedure, alternative if unable to take oral or if allergic to penicillin.
  - Ampicillin IV.
  - Clindamycin, oral or IV.
  - First-generation Cephalosporins - Cefazin. IV Azithromycin or Clarithromycin.
- For genitourinary and nonesophageal GI, procedures if pathogens is entered coccus faecalis, antibiotic choice will be parenteral Ampicillin or Amoxicillin, IV/IM Gentamicin IV Nafcillin, IV Vancomycin (for *Staphylococcus*).

In addition, the patient should brush with soft-bristled toothbrush and floss regularly to protect the gums and or event caries. Good dental hygiene is of utmost importance in decreasing the risk of recurrent infective endocarditis.

Problems

- Activity intolerance related to imbalance between oxygen supply and demand.
- Ineffective management, R/T Therapy.
- Pain related to arthralgia. Myalgia and embolization.
- Altered health maintenance.
- Emboli R/T dislodging vegetation and immobility.
- Anxiety R/T Critical illness.

RHEUMATIC HEART DISEASE

Rheumatic heart disease is an acute inflammatory reaction involving all layers. The resulting damage to the heart from Rh fever is termed "Rheumatic heart disease" a chronic condition characterized by scarring and deformity of heart valves.

Etiology

Rheumatic fever almost always occurs as a delayed sequela (usually after 2 to 3 weeks) of a group A-beta-haemolytic streptococcal infection of the upper respiratory system. In addition socioeconomic factors, familial factors and presence of an altered immune response have a predisposing role in the development of rheumatic fever.

Pathophysiology

The inflammation of rheumatic heart disease may involve:
- The lining of the heart or endocardium (endocarditis) including the valves, resulting scarring, distortion and stenosis of the valves.
- The heart muscle (myocarditis)
- The outer covering of the heart (Pericarditis), where it may cause adhesions of surrounding tissues.

Clinical Manifestations

The development of symptoms of chronic rheumatic heart disease depends on the involvement of the particular part of the heart.

Management

Careful history and physical examination are needed to diagnoses rheumatic heart disease. In addition, ASO titre (Antistreptolysin Otiter) ESR, C-reactive protein, throat culture, WBC count, RBC parameter, chest-X-ray, echocardiography and ECG are useful to identify RHD.

Prophylactic penicillin is prescribed during acute episodes of rheumatic fever and for several years thereafter lifelong antibiotic prophylaxis may be necessary for persons with significant rheumatic heart disease. Corticosteroids may be prescribed during acute rheumatic fever to decrease the cardiac inflammation. If congestive heart failure occurs, bedrest, sodium and fluid restrictions, diuretics, and inotrope usually are prescribed. Antipyretics are also used cautiously.

The nurse emphasizes to the patient and family the importance of rest and adequate nutrition. Additional education to be given as in cardiac diseases.

VALVULAR HEART DISEASE

The heart contains two atro-ventricular valves, the mitral and tricuspid, and two semilunar valves, the aortic and the pulmonic which are located in four strategic locations to control unidirectional blood flow. Types of valvular heart diseases are defined according to the valve or valves affected and the two types of functional alterations, stenosis and regurgitation.

Mitral Stenosis

Mitral stenosis occurs when the blood flow from the left atrium to the left ventricle during ventricular diastole (Ventricular filling) is impeded due to thickening or fibritic changes in the mitral valve.

Etiology

The primary cause is rheumatic fever and carditis, which causes an inflammatory process of the mitral valves chordae tendineae or commissures (leaflets). Less common causes include bacterial vegetation, thrombus formation, calcification of the mitral annulus and atrial myexema (tumor).

Pathophysiology

In mitral stenosis, the mitral valve leaflets become thickened and fibrotic from scar tissue formation and calcification. As the valve leaflets become stiff and fosed, the valve lumen progressively narrows and becomes immobile. In addition, the chorda tendinea may shorten and thicken. The mitral value of orifice may decrease in size from its normal 4 to 6 cm to less than one cm. With progressive mitral stenosis, left atrial pressure elevates as a result of incomplete emptying of the left atrium. Sustained elevated left atrial pressure causes the myocardium to compensate with left atrial dilation and hypertrophy. In addition, high pressures in the left atrium lead to elevated pulmonary venous capillary and arterial pressures. Eventually sustained elevation of the left atrial pressure can produce pulmonary hypertension and subsequent right ventricular hypertrophy. With the increased pressure in the pulmonary vasculature, leakage of fluid across the pulmonary pillary membrane into the lung enterstitium can be produced pulmonary edema. Persons with mitral stenosis also have reduced cardiac output and increases cardiac arrhythmias (atrial fibrillation), later this may allow thrombus formation and arterial embolization to vital organs.

Clinical Manifestations

The most common cause rheumatic fever. In addition there will be fatigue, weakness. The primary symptoms include dyspnea, an exertion orthopnea, paroxysmal nocturnal dyspnea, predisposing causes to respiratory infections, haemoptysis, pulmonary hypertension and edema. These symptoms may be precipitated by emotional stress, respiratory infections, sexual intercourse or atrial fibrillation. Later neural deficits only associated with emboli (haemiparesis) CVA, ascites, hepatic angina with hepatomegaly, chest pain, palpitations (AF) diastolic murmurs accentuated first heart sound, opening snap. If not treated and right ventricular failrue occurs leads to jugular vein distentions, pitting edema and hepatomegaly.

Management

Diagnosis of mitral stenosis is established by the clinical symptoms such as an opening snap (best heard at the apex with stethoscope diaphragm) and a low-pitched, rumbling diastolic murmur (best heard at the apex with the stethoscope bell) results from increased velocity of blood flow. If valve calcified no murmur, heard. ECG echocardiogram and cardiac catheterization are also helpful in diagnosis of mitral stenosis.

Mildly symptomatic patient with mitral stenosis are treated with diuretics, and digitalis is used to control heart rate in the event of atrial fibrillations. Anticoagulation therapy is used to prevent embolization. Medical therapy includes antibiotic prophylaxis before dental and surgical procedures to reduce the risk of bacterial endocarditis. Mechanical enlargement of the mitral valve is indicated when the disease causes either loss of exercise capacity or pulmonary hypertension.

- Percutaneous valvuloplasty using baloon dilation provides a non-surgical alternative to repair of mitral stenosis.
- Surgical commissurotomy can also be performed while the valve leaflets remain mobile.
- Mitral valve replacement using open heart surgery.
- Cardiopulmonary bypass is performed when the valve is severely calcified.

Patient who experiences symptoms related to mitral stenosis are prescribed sodium-restricted diet to help prevent fluid retention, and progressive heart failure. Nursing interventions are taken accordingly.

Mitral Regurgitation

Mitral regurgitation (mitral insufficiency) occurs when the mitral valve fails to completely close during ventricular systole, and consequently some blood flows backward into the left atrium. Mitral regurgitation can be acute or chronic.

Etiology

The causes of mitral regurgitations are numerous and may be inflammatory, degenerative, infective, structural, or congenital in nature. The majority of cases may be attributed to chronic rheumatic heart disease, isolated rupture of chordae tendineae, mitral valve prolapse, ischeni papillary muscle dysfunction and infective endocarditis.

Pathophysiology

The regurgitant mitral orifice is parallel with aortic valve, so that burden imposed on the left ventricle and the left atrium are determined by the etiology, severity and duration of mitral regurgitation. In chronic regurgitation, volume overload on the left ventricle, the left atrium, and the pulmonary bed is created by the backward flow of blood from the left ventricle into the left atrium during ventricular systole, resulting in varying degrees of left atrial enlargement and left ventricular dilation. Acute mitral regurgitation does not result in dilation of the left atrium or left ventricle. Without dilation to accommodate the regurgitant volume, pulmonary vascular pressure rise ultimately, causing pulmonary edema.

Clinical Manifestation

The resultant clinical picture in acute M. regurgitation is that of pulmonary edema and shock. Patient will have thready, peripheral pulses and cool, clammy extremities. Auscultation findings of a new systolic murmur may be obscured by a low cardiac output.

Patient with chronic mitral regurgitation may remain asymptomatic for many years until the development of some degree of LVF. Initial symptoms include weakness, fatigue and dyspnea that gradually progress to orthopnea, paraxysmal nocturnal dyspnea, and peripheral edema, and brisk carotid pulse. Auscultatory findings reflect accentuated left ventricular filling leading to an audible third heart sound (S3) even in the absence of left ventricular dysfunction. The murmur is a loud pansystolic or holosystolic murmur at the apex radiating to the left axilla.

Management

The diagnosis of mitral regurgitation is made by auscultatory findings. Chest-X-ray reveals left atrial enlargement need occassional left ventricular dilation. ECG echocardiogram also is used for diagnosis. Definitive diagnosis is made through cardiac catheterization, which assess left ventricular function and the degree of regurgitation.

Patient with mild mitral regurgitation are generally managed medically. Acute mitral regurgitation need hospitalization and hemodynamic stabilization. As with other cardiac cases, management of heart failure, arrhythmias, and others by antibiotic prophylaxis, diuretics and digitalis are useful accordingly. The nursing care is also designed accordingly.

Mitral Valve Prolapse (MVP)

Mitral valve prolapse occurs when abnormalities in the mitral valve leaflets, cordae tindinea or papillary muscles allow prolapse of the mitral valve leaflets backward into the left atrium during ventricular systole. It is also known as Barlow's syndrome as well as a "floppy or billowing" mitral valve.

Etiology

The cause of MVP is unknown but related to pathogenic mechanisms of mitral valve apparatus. If incidence is possibly linked to an autosomal dominant inherited trait, and is associated with other inherited connective tissue disorders such as Marfan syndrome, Ehlers-Danlos syndrome and ostegenesis imperfecta. Other causes include endocarditis, CAD, myocarditis, cardiomyopathy, cardiac trauma and hyperthyroidism.

Pathophysiology

In mitral valve prolapse, the leaflets of mitral valve become enlarged or thickened, and the chordae tendineae may become elongated. These changes permit the valve leaflets to billow upward into the left atrium during ventricular systole. Depending on the degree of prolapse and integrity of the valve leaflets mitral regurgitation may occur. The subsequent pathophysiology parallels that of mitral regurgitation.

Clinical Manifestation

Many cases of MVP are symptomatic. Persons with symptomatic complain of palpitations secondary to arrhythmias and tachycardia, other systems include light-headedness, syncope, fatigue, lethargy, weakness, dyspnea, and chest tightness. In addition, hyperventilation, anxiety, depression, panic attacks and atypical chest pain may occur. Many symptoms are vague, and puzzling and are not necessarily degree of prolapse.

Management

MVP is diagnosed principally by echocardiography, although cardiac angiography may be used to confirm diagnosis. Individuals who experience palpitations require 24 hours ambulatory ECG monitoring to determine severity of arrhythmias.

Asymptomatic persons with MVP usually do not require treatment. Symptomatic persons may require medications for the arrhythmias. Beta blockers are the treatemnt of choice for managing palpitations and chest pain. The drug of choice is atenolol or propanolol. Antibiotic prophylaxis are used to prevent endocarditis. All persons with MVP need regular follow-up and should have an echocardiogram every few years to monitor disease, severity and progression.

Persons with MVP are encouraged to avoid caffeine which may exacerbate the incidence of tachycardia and atrial dysrhythmias.

Aortic Stenosis (AS)

Aortic stenosis occurs when the aortic valve leaflets become stiff, fused or calcified and impede blood flow from the left ventricle into the aorta during ventricular systole.

Etiology

Aortic stenosis is caused by congenital malformation of the aortic valve inflammatory heart disease (endocarditis) or degenerative disease (calcification). Hypertrophic cardiomyopathy leads to subvalvular lesion that may mimic aortic stenosis.

Pathophysiology

Aortic stenosis results in obstruction of flow from the left ventricle to the aorta during systole. The effect is concentric for left ventricular hypertrophy and increased myocardial oxygen consumption because of the increased myocardial mass. As the disease course progresses and compensatory mechanisms fail, reduced cardiac output leads to pulmonary hypertension.

Clinical Manifestation

The general symptoms is fatigue, dyspnea on exertions, syncope (especially on exertion), pain resembles angina pectoris, bradycardia, dysrhythmias (with heart failure). Systolic murmurs normal or soft S1, prominent S4 Crescendodecrescendo murmur.

Management

A diagnosis of aortic valve stenosis is made by clinical symptoms, clinical findings and diagnostic test. Test that help are ECG, chest X-ray echocardiogram, and cardiac catheterization. Percutaneous balloon valvuloplasty may be used to alleviate aorta stenosis. The definitive therapy for patients with aortic stenosis is valve replacement with a prosthetic aortic valve. In addition, measures to be taken to manage arrhythmias and heart failure. Nursing care is designed accordingly.

The diet of persons with aortic stenosis is unrestricted, unless heart failure is present, in which case the nurse instructs patient to restrict their daily intake of sodium and fluid. Activity level must be carefully monitored because patients are at risk for sudden cardiac death. Patients are cautioned against undue physical exertion or stress, which may precipitate heart failure or arrhythmias. Patients and families need ongoing teaching, and support effectively to manage this ongoing challange in their daily lives. The nurse also reminds patient of the seeking prophylactic antibiotic treatment against endocarditis before any invasive dental procedure or surgery.

Aortic Regurgitation

Aortic regurgitation occurs when an incompetent aortic valve allows blood to flow backward from the aorta into the left ventricle during diastole.

Etiology

Aortic regurgitation may result in a primary disease of the aortic valve leaflets, the aortic root, or both acute aortic regurgitation may be the result of a primary disease of the aortic valve leaflets, the aortic root, or both. Acute aortic regurgitation is caused by bacterial endocarditis, trauma or aortic dissection and constitute a life threatening emergency. Chronic aortic regurgitation is generally the syphilis, or chronic rheumatic conditions such as ankylosing spondylitis, or Reiter's syndrome.

Pathophysiology

The basic physiologic consequence of aortic regurgitation is retrograde blood flow from the ascending aorta into the left ventricle resulting in volume overload. The left ventricle initially compensates for chronic aortic regurgitation by dilation and hypertrophy. Myocardial contractility eventually declines and blood volume increases in the left atrium and pulmonary vasculature. Ultimately, pulmonary hypertension and right ventricular failure develops.

Clinical Manifestation

Patients with acute aortic regurgitation have sudden clinical manifestations of cardiovascular collapse. Abrupt onset of profound dyspnea, transient chest pain, progression to shock which need immediate medical attention.

Patient with chronic aortic regurgitation have pulses that are of the "water-hammer" or collapsing type with abrupt distension during systole and quick collapse during diastole (Corrigan's pulse). Pistolshot pulse sounds can be auscultated over the femoral arteries, and some persons demonstrate a typical head bobbing with each heart beat. Auscultatory findings include a soft or absent S1, presence of S3 or S4 and a soft decrescendo and highpitched diastolic murmur. A systolic murmur also can be heard i.e., systolic ejection click.

In chronic aortic regurgitation it appear symptomatic for many years and seen with external dyspnea, orthopnea, paroxysmal nocturnal dyspnea only after considerable myocardial dysfunction. Nocturnal angina with diaphoresis and abdominal discomfort may be present.

Management

The diagnosis of aortic regurgitation made by auscultative finding, regular chest X-ray, ECG, and echocardiogram digitalis and diuretic are helpful to persons with heart failure. Aortic valve replacement is indicated for symptomatic persons, after thorough diagnosis. The other measure as in other valvular diseases.

Tricuspid Valve Disease

Tricuspid stenosis is a restriction of the tricuspid valve orifice that impedes blood flow from the right atrium to the right ventricle during right ventricular diastole (filling). Conversely, tricuspid regurgitation involves an imcompetent tricuspid valve that allows blood to flow backward from the right ventricle to the right atrium during ventricular systole.

Etiology

Tricuspid stenosis is extremely uncommon and occurs almost exclusively in patient with rheumatic mitral stenosis. It is also seen in IV drugs users. Tricuspid regurgitation is usually the result of pulmonary hypertension or right ventricular dysfunction.

Pathophysiology

In tricuspid stenosis, right atrial outflow is obstructed, resulting in right atrial enlargement and elevated systemic venous pressures. Volume overload of the right atrium and ventricle occur in tricuspid regurgitation.

Clinical Manifestation

Tricuspid stenosis and regurgitation result in the backward flow of blood into the systemic circulation. Common manifestations are peripheral edema, ascites, and hepatomegaly. The murmur of stenosis is presystolic (Sinus rhythm) or midsystolic (AF) and pansystolic murmur may be heard in regurgitation. Both types of murmurs dramatically increased in intensity with inspiration.

Management

As in other valvular disease are according to underlying cause.

Pulmonary Valve Disease

Tricuspid and pulmonary valve disease all cause similar consequences to cardiac function. Pulmonic valve disease is an uncommon entity and in the case of pulmonary stenosis, it is always congenital. Pulmonary regurgitation as an isolated abnormality has a benign course but it generally is associated with disease of other valves.

To sum up, the management of valvular heart disease includes following measures.

- Diagnostic measures
    - History and physical examination
    - Chest X-ray
    - ECG
    - Echocardiography
    - Cardiac catheterization
- Nonsurgical measures
    - Prophylactic antibiotic therapy to prevent Rh. fever, Infective endocarditis.
    - Digitalis
    - Diuretics
    - Sodium restriction

- Anticoagulant agents-warfarin-dipyramidole
- Aspirin
- Antiarrhythmic drugs
- Oral nitrates
- Beta-adrenergic blockers
- Percutaneous transluminal balloon valvulopathy.
- Surgical measures
  - Valvuloplasty; repair of valve and suturing of torn leaflets.
  - Closed commissurotomy (Valvulotomy dilation of valve; repair of leaflet or commissure, fibrous band or ring).
  - Annuloplasty; repair of ring or annulus of incompetent or diseased valve.
  - Valve replacement.

CARDIAC SURGERY

Numerous diseases and conditions may create the need for cardiac surgery. The most common reason for an adult to undergo cardiac surgery is myocardial revascularization (CABG). In addition, patients undergo cardiac surgery for valve repair or replacement, repair of structural defects (acquired or congenital) implantation of devices and cardiac transplantation. The indication for cardiac surgery includes:

- Aneurysm of sinus of valsalva
- Constrictive pericarditis
- Congenital heart defects
- Coronary artery disease
- Dissecting aortic aneurysm
- Valvular insufficiency or stenosis
- Ventricular aneurysm
- Ventricular spetal defect
- Ventricular arrhythmias.

The indications for cardiac surgery and associated procedures are:
- Ischemic heart disease; coronary artery bypass graft. (CABP)
- Repair of structural abnormalities:
  - Valve repair
  - Atrial septal defect repair
  - Ventricular septal defect repair
  - Atrial tumor resection
  - Aortic aneurysm (thoracic) repair.
- Implantation of devices:
  - Automatic implantable cardioverter defibrillator
  - Ventricular assist device
  - Artificial heart chamber
- Transplantation: Replacement of diseased heart with healthy heart.

Cardiac surgery is classified either as an open heart surgery or closed heart surgery, depending on whether the heart is "Opened" during the course of the surgery. Cardiac surgery involving the repair of internal structural defects is open heart, whereas revascularization is a closed heart procedure.

Cardiac surgery today provides pain relief, improvement in lifestyle, and improved survival and for the patient undergoing open heart surgical treatment.

Nursing Management

Care of the person undergoing cardiac surgery involves multidisciplinary team approach utilizing the skills of a variety of health care professionals including nurses, physicians, nutritionists and others.

The nurse caring for the cardiac surgery patient provides individualized care that is appropriate for the patient's medical condition, health history and psychosocial history. Important goals for the preoperative period include obtaining an accurate and complete patient history, providing preoperative teaching to the patient and family about the planned surgery and preparation of patients physiologically and psychologically for surgery. The nurse has to take active part in or collect information by required preoperative diagnostic test such as chest X-ray, cardiac catheterization, coronary angiography, cardiography, stress testing and serum blood analysis as appropriate. A complete baseline database is documented before surgery. Baseline vital signs including apical and radial heart rates and bilateral arm blood pressure integrity of all pulses (both proximal and distal), neurological status, height, weight, nutritional status, elimination pattern and psychological status are assessed and recorded in the immediate preoperation period. Before surgery, patient continues their normal medical and activity routines. With the exceptions of the withholding aspirin for 1 to 3 days before the day of surgery. Patients remain NPO after midnight before surgery.

Nurse has the main responsibility to perform preoperative teaching to patient undergoing cardiac surgery, which includes the following:
- General information: Places of care during hospitalization
  - CCU or ICU after surgery.
  - Return to general patient care unit in 2 to 3 days.
  - Visiting hours and location of waiting rooms.
- Description of surgery:
  - Simple explanation of anatomy of heart and effect of the patient's cardiovascular disorder (eg. incompetent valve, CAD).
  - Explanation of surgical procedure including planned incision.
  - Definition of any unfamiliar terms: Bypass, extracorporeal.
  - Length of time and surgery: 2 to 4 hours.
  - Length of time until able to see family (1-1/2 to 2 hours after surgery).

- Preparation for surgery:
  - Shower or bath at night before surgery with special antimicrobial soap.
  - Surgical shave: Shaving the entire chest and abdomen, neck to groin and left mid-axillary line to right.
  - Legs shaved in saphenous vein grafts will be used.
  - Preoperative medication.
- Explanation of monitors:
  - Round patches on chest connected to cardiac monitor that record patient's heart beats.
  - Monitor makes beeping sound all the time.
- Explanation of lines:
  - Intravenous routes for fluid and medications.
  - Central venous line in neck or chest to monitor fluid status.
  - Pulmonary artery catheter in chest or neck to measure pulmonary pressure and monitor fluid status.
  - Plastic connector line to obtain blood samples without needle stick.
- Explanation of drainage tube:
  - Indwelling urinary catheter.
  - Chest tube: bloody drainage expected.
- Explanation of breathing tube:
  - Tube in windpipe connected to machine called ventilator.
  - Unable to speak with tube in place but can mouth words and communicate in writing.
  - Tube is removed when patient is awake and stable.
  - Secretions in lungs or tube removed by nurse using a suction catheter.
  - Food and oral fluids are not permitted until breathing tube is removed.
- Explanation and demonstration of activities and exercises:
  - Purpose of activity is to promote circulation, keep lungs clear, and prevent infection.
  - Activities include turning from side to side in bed; sitting on edge of bed. Sitting on chair at the night or morning after surgery.
  - Range of motion exercises.
  - Deep breathing using sustained maximal inspiration.
  - Tubes and lines will restrict movement to a certain extent but nurse assists.
- Relief of pain:
  - Some pain will be experienced, but it will not be excruciating.
  - Frequent pain medication will be given to relieve pain but patient should inform always when there is pain.

And following guidelines for care of the person who has undergone cardiac surgery.

- Monitoring of:
  - Cardiovascular
    * Blood pressure and pulse (rate, pulse devidit).
    * Pulmonary artery pressure (PAP). Pulmonary capillary wedge pressure. (PCWD), cardiac output (CO), central venous pressure (CVP) and left atrial pressure (LAP).
    * ECG for signs of arrhythmias.
    * Body temperature.
    * Skin color, temperature and capillary filling.
    * Signs of hypovolemic shock (decreased CVP, LAP and CO).
    * Signs of cardiac temponade (cessation of chest drainage) restlessness, increased CVP, PAP and LAP, tachycardial paradoxical pulse, narrowed pulse pressure, diminished or absent point of maximal impulse, diminished heart sound, distended neckvein (CVP).
  - Respiratory:
    * Respirations: rate, depth, quality
    * Breach sounds
    * Chest tubes for patency and drainage
    * Autotransfuse chest tube drainage.
  - Neurological:
    * Level of consciousness
    * Pupillary size and reaction
    * Orientation
    * Movement and sensation of extremities.
  - Gastrointestinal—nausea, anorexia.
  - Urinary output (amount)-colour, pH and specific gravity.
  - Fluid and electrolytes balance:
    * Intake/output balance
    * Daily weight
    * Serum potassium and calcium levels
  - Presence of discomfort-pain, fatigue.
  - Ability to sleep
  - Behavior: Repression, fear, disorientation and hallucinations.
- Promoting oxygen/carbon dioxide exchange:
  - Preoxygenation and suction during intubation: suction as necessary after extubation.
  - Position with head only slightly elevated; turn side to side.
  - Encourage breathing exercises; incentive spirometry.
  - Encourage range of motion exercises and progressive activity.
- Promoting fluid and electrolytic balance:
  - Record accurate intake and output.
  - Maintain prescribed flow rates of parenteral fluid.
  - Give prescribed supplemental IV potassium chloride.

- Promoting comfort:
  - Give narcotic analgesia every 3 hours during first 24 hours then as needed.
  - Give frequent mouth care.
  - Control environment for comfort.
  - Change bedlinens when diaphoresis presents (assure patient it is common).
  - Plan activities to permit periods of sleep.
  - Provide backrubs for backache.
  - Splint incision during coughing.
  - Encourage patient to share feelings and experiences.
  - Support family visits.
- Promote activity:
  - Provide for passive than active range of motion exercises.
  - Encourage ambulation when permitted.
- Teaching:
  - Progressive return to physical activity as recommended by the physician.
  - Rehabilitation exercise programme.
  - Sexual activity usually permitted in 3 to 4 weeks.
  - Signs of overexertion include fatigue, dyspnea and pain.
  - Eat a balanced diet with prescribed modifications (Low Na^+, low fat).
  - Medications:
  - Name, dosage, schedule action and side effects of prescribed drugs use prescribed education as needed.
  - Signs that may persist: dyspnea, pain and night sweats.
  - Signs requiring medical attention fever, increasing dyspnea or chestpain with minimal exertion.
  - Need for ongoing medical care.

The nurse has to provide discharge instruction for the patient who undergoes cardiac surgery includes:
- Incision care:
  - Clean twice a day.
  - Care of sterile stips staples, sutures.
  - Incision massage with cocoa butter after 10 days.
- Showering:
  - Wash with soap that is unscented, gentle, bactericidal
  - No tube bath until incision is completely healed.
- Activity:
  - No lifting greater than 10 pounds.
  - No driving for 6 weeks.
  - No prolonged sitting.
  - Activity as tolerated, cardiac rehabilitation if ordered.
  - May resume sexual activity when comfort level allows.
- Nutrition:
  - Low sodium, low-fat and heart-healthy diet
  - Increase protein intake for 4 to 6 weeks.
- Medications:
  - Pain medications, do not drive or operate machine if taking narcotics.
- Miscellaneous
  - Women should wear a bra to help support chest TED stockings.
  - Daily weights - notify physician for gain of 6 pounds in 2 days.
  - Incentive spirometer three times a day.
  - Prevent constipation with fiber, fluids and stool softners.
  - Instruct any adverse symptoms should be reported to physician concerned.

ARTERIAL DISORDERS

Aneurysms

Aneurysms are outpouchings or dilation of the arterial wall and are a common problem involving aorta. Aneurysm is a Greek word meaning "widening". Aneurysms are points of weakness, dilation of outpouching of arteries to at least 1.5 times their normal size. Aneurysm occurs most commonly on the aorta but they can occur in any artery of the body. The other common sites include the femoral and popliteal artery.

Etiology

The exact cause of aneurysm is unknown. The several factors are associated with developments of aneurysm, including hypertension, smoking, atherosclerosis, trauma, syphilis, congenital abnormalities of the vessel infection, (TB) and connective tissue disorders that cause weakness on the wall of the vessel.

Pathophysiology

Most aneurysms are found in the abdominal aorta below the level of renal arteries. The aortic wall weakens and dilates with the turbulent blood flow. The growth rate of aneurysm is unpredictable, but the larger the aneurysm, the greater the risk of rupture. Thrombi are deposited on the aortic wall and can embolize. There are three types of aneurysm:
- A fusiform aneurysm involves a circumferential dilation of the vessel well and is relatively uniform in shape.
- A saccular aneurysm is pouch like with a narrow neck connecting the bulge to one side of the arterial wall.
- A dissecting aneurysm develops from a tear in the time of the artery that causes an accumulation of blood in the newly formed cavity between the intima and the media. They further classified according to type of tear and degree of hematoma.

A cause of aortic aneurysm is atherosclerosis with plaques composed of lipids, cholesterol, fibrin, and other debris deposited beneath the intima or lining of the artery. This plaque formation causes degenerative changes in the media (middle layer of arterial wall), leading to loss of elasticity, weakening and eventual dilation of aorta.

Clinical Manifestation

Patients with aneurysm are commonly asymptomatic. Abdominal aneurysm may be felt as a palpable mass and a systolic bruit may be heard. The patient may complain of abdominal or back pain. If the aneurysm leaks or ruptures, the patient will develop severe pain signs of shock, decreased RBCs count, and increased WBCs count.

Symptoms of thoracic aneurysm vary and depend on the size and placement of the aneurysm and its effect on the surrounding structures. Most patients may experience anterior chest wall, back, flank or abdominal pain or may develop signs of shock if the aneurysm leaks. Symptoms such as dyspnea, cough, wheezing may develop if the aneurysm puts pressure on the trachea or bronchi.

Management

Most aneurysms are found on routine physical or X-ray examinations (chest and abdomen), ECG, CT scan, and MRI may also be used to diagnose and assess the severity of aneurysms.

Examples

Aortography: Anatomic mapping of the aortic system by contrast imaging is not a reliable method, but it helps the surgeon with accurate information about the visceral, renal or distal vessels.

The goal of management is to prevent rupture of the aneurysm. Therefore, early detection and prompt treatment of the patient are imperative. Once an aneurysm is suspected, studies are performed to determine its exact size and location. A careful review of all body systems is necessary to identify and coexisting disorders, especially of the lungs, heart or kidney because they may influence the patient's risk of surgery.

The choice of treatment is surgery. The surgical technique involves:
- Incising the diseased segment of the aorta.
- Removing intraluminal thrombus or plaque;
- Inserting a synthetic arterial graft (Dacron or Polytetra fluoroethylene) which is sutured to the normal aorta proximal or distal to the aneurysm;
- Suturing the native aortic wall around the graft so that it will act as a protective cover.

Prior to surgery, every effort is made to bring the patient into best possible state of hydration and electrolyte balance. Any abnormalities in coagulation and blood cell count are corrected. The patients may receive antibiotics and baths with antiseptics before surgery. If aneurysm has ruptured immediate, surgical intervention is needed.

All aneurysm resections require cross-clamping of the aorta proximal or distal to aneurysm. When aneurysms are repaired electively, the patient is systematically anticoagulated with IV heparin before cross clamping aorta. This prevents clotting of pooled blood distal to the aneurysm. If surgery is emergent, no anticoagulative is indicated.

All patients undergoing aneurysmectomy should be placed in an intensive care unit with appropriate support services and equipment. The nursing role during the preoperative period should include teaching, providing support for the patient and family, and carefully assessing all body systems. It is imperative that problems be identified early and proper intervention instituted. In addition to maintaining adequate respiratory function, fluid and electrolyte balance, and pain control in the postoperative period, the nurse must monitor graft patency and renal perfusion. The nurse can also assist in preventing ventricular arrhythmias, infections and neurologic complications.

Aortic Dissection

Aortic dissection, occurring most commonly in the thoracic aorta, is a longitudinal splitting of the medial layer of the artery by a column of blood.

Etiology

Exact cause is unknown; but most people with aortic dissection problem have hypertension, or Marfan's syndrome.

Pathophysiology

Aortic dissection results from a small tear in the intimal lining of the artery, allowing blood to "track" between the intima and media and creating a false lumen of blood flow. As the heart contracts each systolic pulsation causes increased pressure on the damaged area, which further increases dissection. As it extends proximally, distally, it may occlude major branches of the aorta, cutting of blood supply to the areas such as the brain, abdominal organs, kidneys, spinal cord, and extremities. Occasionally a small tear develops distally and the blood flow reenters the true vested lumen. Aortic dissection differs from an aortic aneurysm. Aortic dissections are usually classified as:
- *Type I* involves the ascending aorta and descending thoracic aorta.
- *Type II* involves the ascending aorta only and
- *Type III* invovles the aorta distal to the subclavian artery.

Clinical Manifestation

The patient with acute aorta dissection usually has sudden severe pain in the back, chest, or abdomen. The pain is described as "tearing" or "ripping". The severe pain resembles MI. As the dissection progresses pain may be located both above and below the diaphragm. Dyspnea may also be present.

Management

The diagnostic studies used to assess dissection of aortas are history and physical examination, ECG, Chest X-Ray, CT Scan, transesophageal echocardiography, MRI, and aortography. The goal of therapy for aortic dissections without complications is to lower the BP and myocardial contractility to diminish the pulsatile forces within the aorta. The use of trimethapan and nitroprusside IV reduces BP and IV beta blockers may be used. Propranolol is used to decrease the force of myocardial contractility. Supportive treatment directed towards pain relief, blood transfusion and management of heart failure is indicated. Surgery is indicated when drug therapy is ineffective or when complications are present. Surgery invovles resection of the aortic segment containing intimal tear and replacement with synthetic graft material.

The nursing intervention includes:
- Bedrest—keep patient in semi Fowler's position and maintain quiet environment.
- Administrate narcotic or transquilizers as ordered to reduce anxiety.
- Continuous IV administration of anti-hypertensives.
- ECG monitoring.
- Monitoring of vital signs, level of consciousness (LOC).
- Preoperative care.
- Postoperative care.

ACUTE ARTERIAL OCCLUSIVE DISORDERS

The arteries are thick walled vessels that transport blood and oxygen from the heart to the tissues. Arterial disease can affect any artery of the body and can manifest itself as an acute or chronic condition. Disruption of the arterial blood flow can be caused by narrowing or complete obstruction of the wall of the vessels.

Acute arterial occlusion occurs suddenly without warning signs.

Etiology

Acute arterial occlusion caused by embolism, thrombosis of the already narrowed artery, or trauma, embolization of a thrombus from the heart or an atherosclerotic aneurysm is the most frequent cause of acute arterial occlusion. Heart condition in which thrombi are prone to develop include infective endocarditis, MI, mitral valve disease, chronic atrial fibrillation, cardiomyopathic and prosthetic heart valves.

Pathophysiology

The thrombi becomes dislodged and may travel to the lungs if they originate in the right side of the heart or to anywhere in the systematic circulation if they originate in the left side of the heart. Arterial emboli tend to lodge at sites of arterial branching or in areas of atherosclerotic narrowing. An acute arterial occlusion causes the blood supply distal to the embolus to decrease. The degree and extent of symptoms depend on the size and location of the obstruction, the occurrence of clots fragmentation with embolism to smaller vessels, and the degree of peripheral vascular disease already present. Sudden local thrombosis may occur at the location of an atherosclerotic plaque. Traumatic injury to the extremity itself may produce partial or total occlusion of a vessel from compression and shearing or laceration.

Clinical Manifestation

Signs and symptoms of an acute arterial occlusion usually have an abrupt onset. Clinical manifestation of it includes the six "Ps"—Pain, Pallor, Pulselessness, Paresthesia, Paralysis and Poikilotherma (adaptation of ischaemic limb to its environmental temperature, most often cool). Without immediate intervention, ischemia may progress to tissue necrosis and gangrene within hours. Paralysis is a late sign.

The nurse should note the symptoms that occur suddenly and are severe as follows:
- *Pain:* When the obstruction is complete, the pain is severe and constant and is not relieved by rest.
- *Pallor:* The limb typically appears pale and mottled.
- *Pulselessness:* Numbness, tingling and burning in the extremity are common when ischemia is severe.
- *Poikilotheremia:* The limb is typically cool, if not frankly cold to the touch.
- *Paralysis:* Mobility of the part in limited. The development of frank paralysis is an ominous sign because it may indicate the ischemic death of nerves in the extremity.

If perfusion is not rapidly restored, the limb will develop signs of necrosis and gangrene often is a matter of hours.

Management

Diagnosis of acute occlusion is primarily established through physical assessment of affected limb, Doppler Ultrasonic studies, ABI measurement, MRI and angiographing if indicated.

Drug therapy by immediate initiation of anticoagulant through continuous IV Hepatin. A few long term measures i.e. procedure used and treatment includes:
- Percutaneous balloon angioplasty.
- Intravascular ultrasound.
- Laser assisted balloon angioplasty (LABA).
- Peripheral atheroctomy.
- Intravascular stents.

The options for surgical repairs of acute arterial occlusions are:
- **Endarterectomy:** A direct opening is made into the artery to remove the obstruction.
- **Embolectomy:** Removal of embolus from artery.
- **Femoral:** Femoral bypass - A graft from one femoral artery to other.
- **Axilla femoral bypass:** A graft from axilla artery to femoral.
- **Femoral popliteal bypass.**
- **Aorta iliac bypsss.**

The patient may be undergoing varieties of emergency tests and procedures and will have extensive needs of teaching and support. Preoperative care focuses on the physical, emotional and psychosocial preparation of severely-stressed patient. The nurse is an important mediator between the patient and the rest of the treatment team and attempts to keep the channel of communication open while taking care of the person with acute arterial occlusion are as follows:

- Monitor the patient for any change in circulatory status to the affected limb. Monitor temperature, color, sensation and pain. A change in these parameters may indicate worsening occlusion.
- Monitor peripheral pulses bilaterally for presence, strength, quality and symmetry.
- Keeping the extremity warm, but do not apply direct heat or heat lamps.
- Avoid chilling.
- Maintain bedrest unless activity is specifically ordered.
- Keep the extremity flat or in a slightly dependent position to promote perfusion.
- Use an overbed cradle to protect a painful extremity from the pressure of linens.
- Use sheepskin and 4-inch forum mattress beneath the extremity.
- Do not use the knee gatch on the bed; instruct the patient not to cross the legs at the knee or ankle.
- Do not apply any restraint to the affected limb.
- Keep the head of the bed low to support circulation to the lower extremities.
- Monitor the effects of anticoagulant and thrombolytic therapy.
- Monitor prothrombin time, partial thromboplastin time, platelets and other studies.
- Assess for local and systematic bleeding.

The patient receives meticulous general surgical care. The complications of vascular surgery can affect virtually any organ system. The more invasion procedure, the greater the risk of complication. Potential complications include bleeding, infection at graft site, cardiac failure, myocardial injury to the adjacent organs and tissues (eg. ureters and nerves). The nurse is responsible for meticulous postoperative monitoring of all the body systems and supporting circulation and perfusion, preventing respiratory complication, supposing fluid balance, and promote wound healing and providing discharge instruction to the patient.

The discharge instructions after bypass graft surgery includes:
- Shower daily, clearing the incision gently with a mild or antibacterial soap without lotion of perfume added. Pat dry. Use a shower chair or stool to prevent falling if any instability. Avoid tube baths until healing is complete.
- Monitor the incision daily for signs of infections- redness, swelling, increased pain, discharge of suture or staple separation. Report any of these symptoms to surgeon promptly.
- Advance activity gradually as tolerated initiate a daily walking regime. Expect to feel fatigued and plan for rest periods throughout the day. Avoid lifting anything heavier than 10 pounds until approved by the surgeon.
- Resume a low fat, low cholesterol diet as tolerated. Use supplements as needed to ensure adequate calories, proteins and vitamin C during the healing period. Four to six small meals a day are often better tolerated than three large ones.
- Avoid constipation and straining at stool. Eat a high fiber diet with plenty of fluids to avoid constipation. Remain active. Take a stool softener daily plus a bulk-forming laxative if constipation cannot be managed through diets and fluids.
- Use prescribed pain medication as needed to ensure adequate rest and activity. Take oral medication with food to prevent gastric irritation.

CHRONIC ARTERIAL OCCLUSIVE DISEASE

Chronic peripheral arterial occlusive disease involves progressive narrowing and degeneration and eventual obstruction of the arteries to the extremities occurring predominantly in the legs. It may effect the aortoiliac, femoral, popliteal, tibial, peroneal vessels or any combinations of these areas. Arteriosclerosis obliterans is the most common form of chronic arterial occlusive disease.

Etiology

The leading cause of chronic arterial occlusion is the atherosclerosis a gradual thickening of the intima and media, which leads to narrowing of the vessel of lumen. Atherosclerosis primarily affects large arteries. The involvement is generally segmental with normal segments, interspersed between involved ones. The femoral popliteal area is the site most commonly affects in the non-diabetic persons. The patient with diabetes tend to develop disease in the arteries below the knee (specifically the anterior tibial, posterior tibial, and peroneal arteries). In advanced stages, multiple level of occlusions are seen.

The risk factors of peripheral vascular disease (PVD) include-increased age, smoking, hypertension, atherosclerosis, obesity, diabetes mellitus, stress, family history of PVD or atherosclerosis, sedantary lifestyle, hyperlipidemia.

Pathophysiology

Atherosclerosis, the build-up of cholesterol and triglyceride plaque within the arteries, combines with process of diffuse arteriosclerosis is calcification produced widespread, slowly progressive and narrowing of the arteries. Chronic arterial obstruction leads to progressively inadequate oxygenation of the tissues supplied by the obstructed arteries. The pain attributable to ischaemia is produced by end products of anaerobic cellular metabolism, such as lactic acid. This usually occurs in the larger muscle groups of the legs (buttocks, thighs and calves) during exercise. Once the patient stops exercising the metabolites are and pain subsides. As disease process becomes advanced, pain develops at rest. "Restpain" most often occurs in the feet or toes and indicates insufficient blood flow to the nerve supplying the distal extremity. The patient may notice rest pain more often at night and achieve partial relief by lowering the limb below heart level (eg. dangling the leg over the side of the bed). The clinical manifestations depend on the site and extent of the obstruction and the extent and the amount of collateral circulation.

Clinical Manifestation

- Intermittent claudication in:
  - Buttocks and upper thigh due to occlusion of aortoiline arteries.
  - Calves due to occlusion of femoral or popleteal artery.
  - If disease extends internal iliac artery results impotence and sexual dysfunction occurs in aortoiliac artery occlusion.
- Rest pain in advanced diseases precipitated by a predictable amount of exercise, relieved by resting and reproducible (Rest ischaemia).
- Diminished hair growth on affected extremities.
- Thick, brittle and slow growing nails.
- Shiny, thin, fragile, taut skin, dry and scaly.
- Cool temperature.
- Diminished or absent pulses.
- Palees blanched appearance with extremity elevation.
- Reddish discoloration: rubor with extremity in dependent position.
- Reactive hyperemia.
- Decreased motor function.
- Ulcer formation with advanced disease.
- ABI (Ankle-Bracheal Index) of 0.5–0.95.

The complication of chronic occlusion disorder is that ischemia leads to atrophy of the skin and underlying structure which in turn leads to decreased ability to heal, infection and necrosis and may result from even minor trauma (eg. diabetes). Ischaemic ulcer and gangrene are the most serious complications, may result in lower extremity amputation if blood flow is not restored.

Management

Various tests have been used to diagnose arterial occlusive disorder. Non-invasive tests include ultrasonography, segmental limb pressure, pulse volume recordings and exercise testing. In addition, Doppler ultrasound studies, duplex imaging, angiography, magnetic resonance angiography are also used.

The conservative therapy includes projecting the extremity from trauma, slowing the progression of atherosclerosis, decreasing vasospasm, preventing and controlling infection, and improving collateral circulation. The patient's risk factors should be assessed and proper intervention should be begun regarding cessation of smoking, weight reduction (if indicated) and control of lipid disorders. Hypertension should also be properly managed. The nurse should assist in teaching diet modification to reduce the intake of animal fat and refined sugars, proper care of the feet, and the avoidance of injury to the extremities. The patient with family history of cardiac, diabetes and vascular disease should be encouraged to obtain regular follow up case.

The common drugs used for arterial occlusive diseases include antiplatelets (aspirin, ticlopidine, dipyridamale) Xanthine derivative (Pentoxifylline) bihydrophridine (Nifedipine), israldipine, (Felodipine) and vasodilators (hydralazine, minoridil). The nurse should know the action of drugs and monitor the effects and side effects of the drugs and monitor the effect of claudication and exercise tolerace. Monitor BP and Pulse.

The patient with atherosclerosis should be taught and encouraged to do the following:

- Adjust calorie intake so that optimum weight can be achieved and maintained.
- Decrease dietary cholesterol to less than 200 mg/day.
- Substantially reduce saturated dietary fat.
- Restrict sodium to 2 g per day if edema is present.

The procedure/therapy used for acute care of the person with chronic arterial occlusive disease including:

- Percutaneous transluminal angioplasty with or without stent.
- Atherectomy.
- Arterial bypass.
- Patchgraft angioplasty, often in conjunction with bypass.
- Thrombolytic therapy/Anticoagulation.
- Endarterectomy (done rarely, with localized stenosis).
- Amputation required, if gangrene is extensive.

BUERGER'S DISEASE

Buerger's disease is an obstructive vascular disorder caused by segmental inflammation in the arteries and veins of the upper or lower extremities. It is also known as thromboanginitis obliterans (TAO).

Etiology

It typically occurs in men between the ages of 20 and 40 years but rare in women. The basic cause is unknown. But incidences are strongly associated with cigarette smoking—the disease does not occur in non-smokers.

Pathophysiology

Buerger's diseas causes an inflammatory response in the arteries, veins and nerves. There is infiltration of white cells and the area becomes fibroitic as healing occurs, which can result in vessel occlusion. Occlusion of the vessel occurs when development of collateral circulation around areas of obstruction. Necrotic lesions form at the tips of fingers and toes and recurrent superficial thrombophlebitis commonly occurs in both upper and lower extremities.

Clinical Manifestation

Symptoms include slowly developing claudication, cyanosis and coldness which can progress necrosis and gangrene. Rest pain is common. The risk of gangrene increases with the presence of collagen disease or atherosclerosis and in response to cold weather. The other symtoms may include color and temperature changes in the affected limb or limbs, parasthesia thrombophlebitis, and cold sensitivity, painful ulceration and gangrene.

Management

Buerger's disease is difficult to treat and management is focussed on assisting the patient to quit smoking and avoidance of trauma to the extremity. Patients are often told that they have choice between their cigarettes/Beedis and their legs. They cannot have both. In addition to cessation of smoking efforts, the patient has to avoid exposure to cold and protect the extremities from injury and trauma. Supportive psychotherapy and pharmacologic treatment of underlying anxiety disorders are sometimes helpful in assisting the patient to stop smoking. Although this disorder is difficult to treat, anticoagulants and vasodilator therapy have been used. A sympathectomy may help to eliminate vasospasm, but it must be performed early in the disease process. Amputation generally below the knee may be necessary in advanced cases.

RAYNAUD'S DISEASE

Raynaud's disease **(Fig. 5.3)** (arteriospastic disease is an episodic vasopastic disorder of the small cutaneous arteries, usually involving the fingers and toes. First described by Maurice Raynaud (1802).

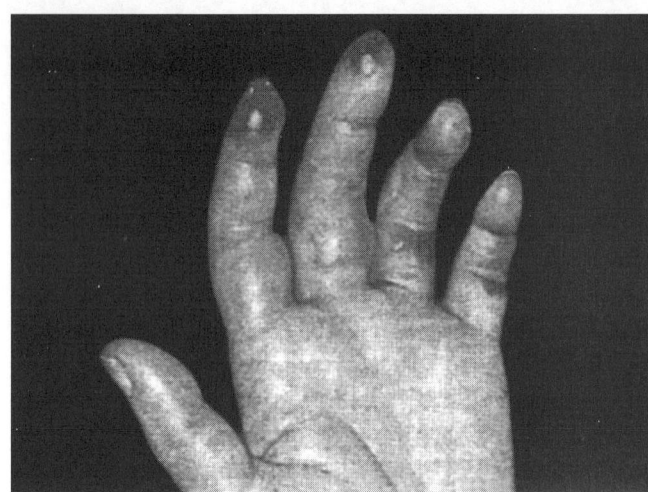

Fig. 5.3: Raynaud's phenomenon.

Etiology

The exact cause is not known. Associated disorder includes systemic sclerosis, systemic lupus erythematosus, rheumatid arthritis, hematological disorders, trauma, and arterial obstruction, other contributing factors include occupation-related trauma and pressure to the fingertips (e.g. typists, pianists and workers who use handheld vibrating equipments). Symptoms are commonly precipitated by exposure to cold, emotional upset, caffeine ingestion and tobacco use.

Pathophysiology

Vasoconstriction is regulated by alpha-2 receptors. Sympathetic stimulation or cold exposure causes the release of noradrenaline which activate the alpha-2 receptors and cause vasoconstriction and vasospasm. Persons with Raynaud's disease may have increased number of alpha-2 receptors. They may also have a decreased is betareceptors and calcitonin which are responsible for vasodilation. The pathological sequence is not completely understood.

Clinical Manifestation

The symptoms are symmetrical and bilateral. The vasospasm confined to the ditits and does not usually thumb. Only the tip of the finger distal to the metacarpophalangeal joint is typically affected. Toes may also be affected in same pattern. The disorder is characterized by three color changes (white, red and blue). Initially the vasoconstrictive effect produces pallor (white), followed by cyanosis (bluish purple). These changes are subsequently followed by rubor (Red) or hyperemia. The patient usually describes cold and numbness in the vasoconst rictive phase and throbbing aching pain; tingling and swelling in the hypermic phase. This type of episode usually lasts only for minutes but in severe cases, may persist for several hours. Complications include punctuate (small hole) lesions of the fingertips and superficial gangrenous ulcers in advanced cases. (See Figure 5.3 Raynaud's phenomenon.)

Management

Mild cases do not require any treatment. Patients are advised to have protection from cold by wearing loose, warm clothing or gloves when handling refrigerator, extreme should also be avoided and advised to stop smoking, avoid caffeine. Advise to immerse hands in warm water to decrease spasm. The drugs used are calcium channel blockers and beta-adrenergic blocking agents may help to some extent. Sympathectomy is considered only in advanced cases.

AMPUTATION AND ITS MANAGEMENT

Amputation is a surgical intervention commonly used in the treatment of peripheral vascular disease. It is the last resort of treatment when other medical and surgical measures have failed to save the limb. Amputation, although radical and traumatic for the patient, it can provide relief of chronic pain, the potential to walk against with the use of prosthesis and an improved quality of life.

The possible causes for indications or factors responsible for amputation are diabetes with pathology, peripheral vascular disease, birth defects, trauma and malignancy. Chronic tissue ischaemia that results in necrosis and then gangrene is the most common pathological sequence that results in amputation.

The goal of amputations is to preserve as much of the functional length of the extremity as possible while removing all infected of ischemic tissue. Lower extremity amputations are roughly classified as follows:
- Below the knee amputation (BKA).
- Above the knee amputation (AKA).
- Amputation of the foot and ankle (Symes).
- Amputation of the foot between metatarsus and tarsus (Hey's or Lisfracs).
- Hip diarticulation: Removal of the limb from the hip joint.
- Hemicorporectomy: Removal of half of the body from pelvis and lumbar areas.

Preoperative Care

The preoperative period focuses on the careful evaluation and preparation for surgery include carrying out routine diagnostic measure as indicated according to the underlying disease. Stabilization of patient from infection, diabetes and others. The nurse focuses on teaching and patient support in the preoperative period. Amputation can have tremendous psychological implication. This radical change in body image can evoke feelings of loss, anger, fear, shock and denial, so that psychological preparation of the patients in very essential preoperative teaching emphasizes care that will be provided in the postoperative period, pain management strategies, plans for prosthesis fitting, and a basic introduction to stump care routines. The patient should be told to anticipate the occurrence of phantom limb sensation, a sensation of aching, tingling or simple awareness of the amputated part. In addition, other routine for surgery performed by the nurses.

The nursing care of the person after amputation includes:
- Assess stump and monitor drainage for color and amount, report signs of increased drainage.
- Position of the patient with no flexion at hip or knee to avoid contractures and encourage prone position.
- Maintain patient in low-Fowler's or flat position after AK.
- Support stump with pillow for first 24-hours (according to physician or Surgeon's preference and avoiding flexion); place rolled bath blanket.
- Encourage exercises to prevent thromboembolism:
  - Active ROM of unaffected leg, ankle rotations and pumps.
  - Use of overhead trapeze when moving in bed.
  - Push-ups from sitting position in bed.
  - Quadriceps sets.
  - Lifting stump and buttocks off bed while lying flat on back to strengthen abdominal muscles.
- Teach care of stump:
  - Inspect for redness, blister and abrasions.
  - Wash stump with mild soap, rinse with water, and pat dry.
  - Avoid use of alcohol, oils and creams.
  - Remove stump bandage or stump sock and reapply as needed; use firm smooth figure of -8 Ace wrapping to reduce swelling and shape stump (if rigid dressing not used).
- Encourage patient to ambulate using correct crutch walking-techniques:
  - Keep elbows extended, limit elbow flexion to 30 degrees or less.
  - Avoid pressure on axilla.
  - Bear weight on palms of hands, not on axilla.
  - Maintaining upright posture (head up, chest up, abdomen in, pelvis in foot straight).
- Monitor patient's ability to use a prosthesis.

DISORDERS OF VEINS

Deep Vein Thrombosis/Thrombophlebitis (DVT)

The most common venous disorder, results from incompetent valves in the veins and obstruction of venous return to the heart usually results in a thrombus. The formation of thrombus (clot) in association with inflammation of the veins is called "Thrombophlebitis".

Etiology

Venous thrombosis typically results from at least one element of virchows traid: Venous stasis, damage to the endothelial lining of the vein, and hypercoagulopathy. The patients at risk for the development of thrombophlebotis usually has predisposing conditions to these three disorders. Risk factors for deep vein thrombosis are as follows:

- Advanced age - the elderly typically have a number of risk factors.
- Gender: DVT occurs more often in women.
- Positive history of thromboses.
- Immobility/stasis:
  - Surgery, bedrest, paralysis, fractured hip, spinal cord injury.
  - Prolonged sitting (automobile or air travel).
  - Obesity and pregnancy.
- Increased viscosity (Hypecoagulatable stumps)
  - Dehydration, fever and malneutrition.
  - Polycythemia vera and Severe anemias.
- Intimal damage:
  - Central and peripheral IV catheters, pacemaker wires, IV therapy.
  - IV drug abuse.
- Associated conditions/disorders:
  - Malignancy.
  - Varicose veins.
  - Inherited coagulation disorder.
  - Hemolytic anemia (Sickle cell anemia).
- Trauma:
  - Fractures especially involving the pelvis and long bones.
  - Burns.
- Use of oral contraceptives (risk primarily related to estrogen content).
- Chronic lung and heart disease (CHF, cerebrovascular disease).
- Cigarette smoking.
- Venous cannulation or catheterization).

Pathophysiology

Thrombi develop from platelets, fibrin and both red and white cells. They typically form in areas where the blood flow is slow or turbulent. The major elements of stasis increased coagulability, and intimal damage dramatically accelerate the process. Muscle spasm and changes in the intravascular pressure can cause the developing thrombus to dislodge and move towards the heart and lungs. The lungs are rich in heparin and plasmin activators and can effectively dissolve some thrombi. However, if the thrombus is not successfully dissolved, it can lodge in an artery and obstruct perfusion to the lung segment causing problems.

Clinical Manifestation

Clinical manifestation of the thrombophlebitis varies according to the size and location of the thrombus and the adequacy of collateral circulation. The patient with superficial thrombophlebitis may have a palpable firm, subcutaneous cord like vein. The area surrounding the vein may be tender to the touch, reddened, and warm. A mild systemic temperature elevation and leukocytoses may be present. Edema of the extremity may occur or may not occur.

The patient with deep thrombophlebitis may have no symptoms or have unilateral leg edema, pain, warm skin, and temperature greater than 38°C. If the calf is involved, tenderness may be present on palpation. Homan's sign, pain on dorsiflexon of the foot when the leg is raised is a classic but unreliable sign because it is not specific for DVT. If the inferior vena cava involved, the lower extremities may be edematous and cyanotic. If the superior vena cava is involved, the upper extremities, neck, back and face may be edematous and cyanotic.

The most serious complication of DVT are pulmonary embolism, chronic venous insufficiency and phlegmasia ceruleadolens.

Management

Various diagnostic studies are used to determine the site or location and extent of the thrombus or embolic which includes chest X-ray, APTT (activated partial thromboplastin time), PT (Prothrombin time) venous studies, venogram of the affected limb (Rarely), Lung scan and pulmonary angiogram.

The patients with DVT are treated with complete bedrest, because the patient on traditional heparian therapy will be on bedrest for 5 to 7 days. Patient on low molecular weight heparian can be out of bed after 24 hours if pain level permits. Patient can be treated with the use of local heat to extremity when inflammation is acute, fit the patient carefully for graduated compression stockings and teach correct use.

Patients are on anticoagulant therapy should be taught the action, dosage and side effects of medication, and they are advised to eat dark green and yellow leafy vegetables moderately because these are rich in vitamin K, which can counteract the effect of Coumadin (Warfran) and advise them to use alcohol only in moderation because it increases the anticoagulant effect.

In addition, patient should be taught the following:
- Risks and complications of DVT, signs and symptoms of complication.
- Risk, complications of heparin administration, signs and symptoms and complications.
- Bleeding precautions.
- Need for ongoing laboratory follow up of anti-coagulation levels after discharge.

The conservative treatment includes:
- Continuous IV heparin.
- Bedrest with bathroom privileges.
- Elevation of legs above the heart level.
- Anticoagulant therapy and heparin, warfarin.
- Elastic compression stockings.
- Measurement and charting of size of both thighs and calves every morning.
- Mild oral analgesics such as aspirin and codiene.
- NSAIDs
  Surgical procedure if indicated include.
- Intracaval filter insertion.
- Venous thrombectomy (rarely done).

The primary option is transvenous filteration device placed in the vena cava to trap embolie before they reach the heart and pulmonary vessels. Two types are currently in use the greenfield filter and bird's nest filter. Both filters are permanently implanted and rarely become dislodged or occluded. The nursing care of the patient with a vena caval filter includes:

- Assess venipuncture site for signs of bleeding or infection. Maintain an adhesive covering over the insertion site.
- Immobilize the extremity after the procedure per institution protocol or physician's order.
- Assess peripheral pulses, temperature, color and sensation in affected extremity per protocol. Assess for pain and presence of positive Homan's sign.
- Assess respiratory status and monitor pulse oximetry or blood gases as indicated. Position is partial or high Fowler's position.
- Implement bleeding precautions and associated safety measures if systemic anticoagulation is to be continued. Monitor appropriate laboratory test results (PTT, HB, HctINR).
- Teach the patient to monitor for signs of infection at insertion site. Signs of systemic bleeding (e.g. blood in stool, urine, gums, nosebleed easy bruises); bleeding precaution for home use, if anticoagulation is continued (e.g. use of soft toothbrush, electric razor, stool softener), symptoms to report to the health care provider (bleeding and infection) DVT. Pulmonary embolism-swelling and warmth in extremity, sudden chest pain, dyspnoea, tachypnoea, restlessness, filter occlusion.
- Localized pain, venous stasis, or swelling and unusual symptoms.

VARICOSE VEINS

Varicose veins or varcosites are prominent, abnormally dilated, tortous subcutaneous veins most frequently occur in saphenous system, most oftenly in the lower extremities because of the effects of gravity on venous presence.

Etiology

The aetiology of varicose veins is unknown. The increased venous pressure may result from congenital weakness of the vein structure, obesity, pregnancy, venous obstruction resulting from thrombosis or extrinsic pressure by tumors or occupations that require prolonged standing (eg. police constable, OT nurse, etc). It may be hereditary and effects chronic diseases such as cirrhosis or CHF.

Pathophysiology

As the veins enlarge, the valves are stretched and become incompetent allowing blood flow to be reversed. As back pressure increases and the calf muscle pump (muscle movement that squeezes venous blood back towards heart) fails. Further venous distention results. The increased venous pressure is transmitted to the capillary bed and oedema develops.

Clincial Manifestation

Discomfort from varicose veins varies dramatically among people and tends to be worsened by superficial thrombophlebitis. In addition, many patients voice concern about cosmetic disfigurement. The most common symptom of varicose veins is an ache or pain after prolonged standing, which is relieved by walking or by elevating the limb. Some patients feel pressure or a cramp like sensation. Swelling may accompany discomfort nocturnal leg cramps, especially in calf area occurs. The common complication is superficial thrombophlebitis. Ulceration may develop as a result of skin infections or trauma.

Management

A duplex ultrasound can detect obstruction and reflux in the vertease system with considerable accuracy. Treatment is not indicated if varicose veins are only a cosmetic problem. If incompetency of venous system develops, the care involves rest with the affected limb elevated, compression stocking and exercise such as walking. Sclerotherapy is a technique used in the treatment of unsightly superficial varicosites. Direct IV injection of a sclerosing agent such as sodium tetradecyl induces inflammation and results in eventual thrombosis of vein. After procedure leg is wrapped with an elastic bandage for 24 to 72 hours to maintain persons over the vein- local tenderness subsides within 2 to 3 weeks and eventually thrombosed vein disappears. After this patients are advised to wear compression stockings to prevent further varicosites.

The nurse should instruct patients to avoid sitting or standing for long time, maintain ideal body weight, take precautions against injury to the extremities and avoid wearing constrictive clothing. After vein ligation, the nurse should encourage deep breathing for promoting venous return. The extremities should be checked regularly for colour, movement, sensation, temperature presence of oedema and padal pulses. Postoperatively the extremities are elevated at a 15 degree angle to prevent development of verious stasis and oedema. Following measures are also to be taken.

VENOUS STASIS ULCER

Chronic venous insufficiency can lead to venous stasis ulceration, which may occur as a resultt of previous DVT.

Etiology

Leg ulcers can be caused by many conditions including venous hypertension, infection, diabetes mellitus, malignancy, connective tissue disorders, rheumatid arthritis and damage through DVT or VS, external injuries such as trauma, pressure, and insect bites.

Pathophysiology

The basic dysfunction is imcompetent valves of the deep veins. As capillaries rupture, RBCs breakdown and release haemosiderin causing a brownish discoloration of the skin due to the deposition of melanin, and hemosiderin. The venous stasis ulcers usually develop around the ankles, especially in the area of the medial malleoli. Loss of epidermis occurs, and portions of the dermis may also be involved, depending on the degree of venous stasis.

Clinical Manifestation

The skin of the lower leg is leathery, with a characteristic brownish or "brawny" appearance. Edema has usually been present for a prolonged period. The ulcer is concave lesion below the margin of skin surface. Pain may occur when the limb is in a dependent position or during ambulation. Pain is usually relieved by elevation of the foot. If the ulcer is not treated, infection may occur. Scar tissue is formed around the rim of the ulcer. Poor hygiene, debilitation, and inadequate nutritional status contribute to severity of ulcer.

Management

- Elevation of affected limb to reduce venous stasis and hypertension and edema.
- Extrinsic compression methods—Stocking's elastic bandages and hydrocolloid dressings.
- Routine prophylactic antibiotic therapy (Culture and Sensitivity if needed).
- Protein: Vitamin supplementation.
- Calorie limitation for weight reduction.
- Surgery: Excision of ulcer.

PULMONARY EMBOLISM

Pulmonary embolism is the most common complication in hospitalized patients.

Etiology

Thrombi in the deep veins can dislodge spontaneously. However, more common mechanism is jarring of the thrombus by mechanical forces, such as sudden standing, and changes in the rate of blood flow such as those that occur with Valsalvas manoeuvre. In addition, less common causes include fat emboli, (from fractured long bones), air emboli (from improper IV therapy) and amniotic fluids and tumours.

Pathophysiology

Most pulmonary embolies arise from thrombi in the deep veins of the legs. Other sites of origin include right side of the heart, upper extremities (rarely) and the pelvic veins (after surgery or childbirth). Lethal pulmonary embolie originate most commonly in the femoral or iliac veins. Emboli are mobile clots that generally do not stop moving until they lodge at a narrowed part of the circulatory system. The lungs are an ideal location for emboli to lodge because of their extensive arterial and capillary network. The lower lobes are more frequently affected because they have higher blood flow than the other lobes. Occasionally, the presence of deep vein thrombosis is unsuspected until pulmonary embolism occurs.

Clinical Manifestation

The severity of clinical manifestation depends on the size of the emboli and the size and number of blood vessels occluded. Most common are the sudden onset of unexplained dyspnoea, tachypnoea, or tachycardia. Other manifestations are cough, chest pain, hemoptysis, crackles, fever accentuation of the pulmonic heart sound, and sudden change in mental status as a result of hypoxaemia. Massive emboli may produce sudden collapse of the patient with shock, pallor, severe dyspnoea, and crushing chest pain. Some patients may have no pain. The complications of pulmonary embolism are pulmonary infarction and pulmonary hypertension.

Management

Diagnosis measures of pulmonary emboli include in addition to routin history need physical assent; venous studies, chest X-Ray, continuous ECG monitoring, ABGs, CBC, lung scan, and pulmonary angiography treatment measures includes:

- Oxygen by mask on Cannula.
- Establishment of IV route for drugs and fluids.
- Continuous IV heparin.
- Bedrest.
- Narcotics for pain relief.
- Thrombolytic agents in certain patients.
- Vena cava filter.
- Pulmonary embolectomy in life-threatening situation.

CHAPTER 6

Nursing Management of Hematological Disorders

INTRODUCTION

Hematology is the study of blood and blood forming tissues. This includes the blood cells, the bone marrow, the spleen and the lymph system. A basic knowledge of hematology is useful in clinical settings to evaluate the patient's ability to transport oxygen and carbon dioxide coagulate blood, and combat infection. Another important homeostatic function of the blood cells is removing old and dead cells. This functions is accompanied by the mononuclear phagocyte system (MPS). This is formerly known as the reticuloendothelial system (RES) is composed of monocytes and macrophages. Diseases associated with MPS are diverse in their underlying pathological manifestations disease course, and response to treatment. Most often the accompanying symptoms result from interference with normal development and function of the blood components; erythrocytes (RBCs) thrombocytes (platelets) leukocytes (WBCs) and altered hematopoiesis (blood cell production).

Normally, homeostasis is maintained through a balance between the rate of production of normal blood cells and the rate of destruction. Disorders of blood occurs when the balance is lost. Disturbances of the coagulation mechanism also result in blood disorder. Nurse has to play an important role in management of these conditions associated with hemotological disorders.

NURSES ASSESSMENT OF THE HEMATOLOGICAL SYSTEM

Most of the evaluation of the hematologic system is based on a thorough health history. In addition other key points to include are family history, drug history, exposure to chemicals and general nonspecific complaints offered by the patient.

Health History

A thorough history inccludes detailed information about the person's symptoms and through review system. The vagueness symptomatology of disorders of the hematological system makes a thorough assessment is essential, common symptoms include, shortness of breath, fatigue, bruising, tarry stools, constipation, lymphadenopathy, flue-like illness, and musculoskeletal pain. Unfortunately these symptoms occur in a vast number of other common disorders. The cause of any hematological abnormality must be assiduously pursued. The importance of accurate diagnosis, combined with the diverse and usually nonspecific signs and symptoms, makes it likely that the person will become involved in arduous diagnostic process. It is also important to learn whether the patient has had prior hematological problem (mononuculosis, malabsorption, liver disorders, thrombosis and spleen disorders and leukemia, etc.).

Family History

The existence of inherited hematological disorders such as sickle cell disease, and malignant tumors, requires detailed family history. Questions regarding disease or presence of symptoms among relatives should include reference to parents and siblings. Most specific disorders such as hemophilia may involve questions to grand fathers, uncles and nephews. For other disorders, female relatives need to be considered. Information regarding instances of severe or prolonged bleeding after trauma, dental extractions or surgery and occurrence of jaundice or anemia in relatives also should be obtained.

Drugs and Chemical

Drugs may induce or potentiate hematological disease. Most notable are the hematological effect of the cytotoxic drugs used in cancer therapy and the neutropenia associated with chloramphenical. Do not negate the importance of over the counter medication. Certain chemicals may exist a potentially harmful effect on hemopoietic system. To obtain a history of exposure to chemicals, an occupational history is useful. Some drugs affecting the hematologic function and laboratory values are as follows:

- Antituberculin (e.g. PAS) leads to leukocytes secondary to hypersensitivity and INH leads to neutropenia.
- Antifungal (e.g. amphotaracin B) leads to anemia.
- Antiseizure (e.g. carbomazepine) leads to anemia, leukopnea, thrombocytopenia.
- Antibiotic (e.g. chloromphenical)–anemia, neutrepenia, thrombocytoponea.
- Antihypertensin (e.g. Aldosterone) hemolytic anemia.
- Anti-inflammatory (e.g. phenylbutazone)–anemia, leukopenia, neutropenia, thrombocytopenia.

- Diuretics (chlorothiazic)-Thrombocytopenia (occasional).
- Antiarrhythmic (e.g. procainamide HCL)-Agranulocytosis.
- Antibacterial (e.g. bacterim, septran)-Anemia, leukopenia, neutropenia thrombocytopenia).
- Antineoplastics (immunosuppression)-Anemia leukopenia, neutropenia and thrombocytopenia).
- NSAIDs—Inhibition of platelet aggregation.
- Analgesia, antipyretics—Reduced platelet aggregation, prolonged bleeding time.

History of Fever, Fatigue and Malaise

Fever is common manifestation of many hematological disorders and information about history of fever should be obtained. In addition, information about fatigue and malaise are also obtained.

Physical Examination

A complete physical examination is necessary to accurately examine all systems that affect or are affected by the hematologic system. It is useful to recognize target organs and alteration that may reflect hematological disease. The nurse must be aware of signs and symptoms can be caused by hematological problems, even though these are not the obvious causes. The common assessment of abnormalities of hematologic systems and their causes include:

Skin

- Pallor of skin or nailbeds: Decrease in quantity of hemoglobin (anemia).
- Flushing: Increase in hemoglobin (polycythemia).
- Jaundice: Accumulation of bile pigments caused by rapid or excess hemolysis.
- Purpura, petachiae, ecchymois, hematoma: Hemostatic deficiency of platelets or clotting factors resulting hemorrhage into skin.
- Excoriation and pruritus: Scratching from intense pruritus secondary to disorders such as Hodgkin diseases; increased bilirubin.
- Leg ulcers: Common in sickle cell disease, especially prominent on the malleoli on the ankles.
- Brownish discoloration: Hemosiderin and melanin from the breakdown of erythrocytes, iron deposits, secondary to transfusional iron overload.
- Cyanosis: Reduced hemoglobin.
- Telengiectasis: Hyperemic spots caused by capillary or small artery dilation, small angioma with a tendency to hemorrhage.
- Angioma: Benign tumor consisting primarily of blood or lymph vessels.
- Spider nevus: Breached growth of dilated capillaries resembling a spider associated with liver disease and elevated estrogen levels as in pregnancy.

Nails

Rigid longitudinally, flattened concave—Chronic severe iron deficiency anemia.

Eyes

- Jaundiced sclera—Accumulation of bile pigments because of rapid or excessive hemolysis.
- Conjunctival pallor—Reduction in quantity of hemoglobin (anemia)
- Retinal hemorrhage—More frequent in concurrent states of thrombocytopenia and anemia than with thrombocytopenia alone.
- Dilation of veins—Polycythemia.

Mouth

- Pallor—Reduction in quantity of hemoglobin (anemia)
- Gingival and mucosole ulceration-Neutropenia, severe anemia.
- Gingival infiltration (swelling, reddening bleeding)—Leukemia caused by impeded movement of granulocytes and monocytes through gingivia tooth attachment into mucous membrane or by inability of impaired leucocytes to combat oral infections.
- Gingival or mucosal bleeding—Hemorrhagic disease, thrombocytopenia.
- Smooth tongue texture—Pernicious and iron deficiency anemia.

Lymph Nodes

Lymphadenopathy, tenderness—Normal response to infection in infants and children, cancerous invasion is causative factor in adult's enlargement caused by infection, foreign infiltrates, or metabolic disturbances especially with lipids.

Chest

- Widened mediastinum: Enlarged lymph nodes.
- Generalized sternal tenderness: Leukemia resulting from increased bone marrow cellularity causing increase in pressure and bone erosion.
- Localized sternal tenderness: Multiple myeloma as result of stretching periosteum
- Tachycardia: Compensatory mechanism in anemia to increase cardiac output.
- Murmurs: Usually systolic murmur in anemia caused by increased quantity and speed of low viscosity blood going through pulmonic valves.
- (Carotid bruits): Anemia caused by increased flow of ion viscosity blood swirling through blood vessels.
- Angina pectoris: Anemia.

Abdomen

- Hepatomegaly-leukemia, cirrhosis or fibrosis secondary to iron overload from sickle cell or thalassemia.

- Splenic bruits and rubs: Splenic infarction.
- Increasing abdominal girth: Hepatomegaly, splenomegaly, abdominal bleeding.

Nervous System

- Pain and touch, Position and vibratory sensation, tendon reflexes.
  - Impaired nervous system functions because of cobalamin deficiency or compression of nerve by masses.
- Decreasing level of consciousness: Intracranial hemorrhage needs thorough neurological examination.

Back and Extremities

- Back pain: Acute hemolytic reaction from flank pain because of renal involvement with hemolysis; multiple myeloma from enlarged tumors that stretch periosteum or weaken suppressive tissue causing ligament strain, muscle spasm, and sickle cell diseases.
- Arthralgia: Leukemia as a result of aching in bones that contain marrow, sickle cell disease from hemarthosis.
- Bone pain: Bone invasion by leukemia cells, bone demineralisation resulting from various hematoptotic and solid malignancies enhancing possibility of pathological fracture; sickle cell disease.

Diagnostic Studies of the Hemotological System

The nurse should recognise the need to thoroughly explain any diagnostic procedures to the patient. It is common for patient to be anxious when faced with illness. Therefore, instructions must be simple, clear and repeated when necessary to decrease anxiety and ensure the patient's compliance with preparatory protocol. Whether studies are performed on an outpatient or an inpatient basis. Written instruction regarding the procedure facilitates compliance. If a diverse ethnic population is served, it is helpful to have instructions translated into the patient's dominant language.

The repeated acquisition of blood specimen may be distressing for the patient. Some patients and staff members become concerned that amount of blood withdrawn for tests could lead adverse effects. Although multiple blood studies may be uncomfortable, it annoys in rate situation that diagnostic blood withdrawal predisposes the patient to significant volume loss. The nurse must capitalize on all appropriate opportunities to use independent nursing assessment and clinical judgement. For example, when there is suspicion of bleedings, it is important to perform guaiac test of the stool, nasogastric secretions or emesis and hematest of the urine.

The complete blood count studies and their purposes and normal values are as follows:

- RBC count
  - Hemoglobin (Hb) is a measurement of gas-carrying capacity of the red blood cells. Normal values male 13-18 g/100 ml, female 12-16 g/100 ml.
  - Hematocrit (Hct) is a measure of packed cell volume of RBCs expressed as a percentage of the total blood volume (Normal values male: 45-52 percent Female 37-48 percent).
  - Total RBC counts: Count of number of circulating RBCs (male 4.6-6.1 million/mm, female 4.0-5.4 million/mm).
  - Red cell indices: Mean corpuscular volume (MCV).
    - MCV is the determination of relative size of RBCs, low MCV reflection of microcytosis, high MCV reflection of macrocytosis (normal 80-95).
    - Mean corpuscular Hgb (MCH) is a measurement of average weight of Hb/RBC; low MCH indication of microcytosis or hypochromia, high MCH indication of macrocytosis (normal 27-33 Pg).
    - Mean corpuscular high concentrate (MCHC) is an evaluation of RBC saturation with Hb; Low MCHC indication of hypochromia high-MCHC evident in spherocytosis (normal 32-36 percent).
- WBC counts
  - WBC total count (TC) is the measurement of total number of leukocytes (normal 5000 to 10,000/mm).
  - WBC differential count (DC) is the determination of whether each kind of WBC is present in proper proposition, determination of absolute value by multiplying percentage of cell type to a total WBC count and dividing by 100 (neutrophil 55-70%, eosinophils 1-4%, basophils 0-1%, monocyte 2-6% and lymphocyte 25-40%) DC count totals 100%.
- Platelet counts is the measurement of number of platelets available to maintain platelet clotting functions (not measurements of quality of platelet function). Normal value of platelets is 150,000-400,000/mm.
- Erythrocytic sedimentation rate (ESR) measures the sedimentation or setting of RBCs and used as a nonspecific measure of many diseases, especially inflammatory condition. Increased ESR are common during acute and chronic inflammatory reactions when cell destruction is increased. The normal ESR in males: 1-15 mm in 1 hour; females:1-20 mm in 1 hour.
- Blood typing and Rh Factors ABO blood groups are named for the antigen found on the RBCs compatibility is based on the antibodies present in the serum.

Blood group	RBCs agglutinogen(s)	Serum agglutinogen(s)	Compatible donor blood groups	Incompatible donor blood groups
A	A	Anti-B	A and O	B and AB
B	B	Anti-A	B and O	A and AB
AB	A and B (universal recipient)	Neither	A, B, AB and O	None
O	Neither (universal donor)	Anti A and anti B	O	A, B and AB

Other Hematological Studies

Urine Studies

Bence Jones protein studies is an electrophoretic measurement used to detect the presence of Bence Jones protein, which is found in most cases of multiple myeloma. Negative findings indicate patient is normal. Nurses should acquire random urine specimen for urine study.

Radioisotope Studies

- Liver/spleen scan: Radioisotope is injected intravenously. Images from the radioactive emissions are used to evaluate the structure of the spleen and liver. Patient is not a source of radioactivity.
- Bone scan: Same procedure as spleen scan except used for the purpose of evaluating the structures of bone.
- Isotopic lymphangiography: Radionuclide study is used to assess lymph nodes and lymph system. Tecnitium 99 m is used. Technique is less invasive than radiographic lymphangiograph.

No specific nursing responsibilities for radioisotopic study.

Radiologic Studies

- *Lymphangiosgraphy:* The purpose is to evaluate deep lymph nodes. Radiopaque oil-based dye is infused slowly into the lymph vessels via small needles in the dorsum of each foot. Radiographs are taken immediately and on the next day.

The nursing responsibilities include:
- Inform the patient about what to anticipate.
- Obtain consent form.
- Assess for iodine sensitivity.
- Give preparatory sedation, if indicated.
- Instruct that patient's urine will be blue from the dye exretion for 1–2 days.
- Inform patient that transient fever-general malaise may be experienced for 12–24 hours.
- Watch for signs of oil embolus to lung (hacking cough, dyspnea, pleuritic pain and hemoptysis.
- Computed tomography (CT): A noninvasive radiologic examination using computer assisted X-ray evaluates the spleen, liver, or lymph nodes. No specific nursing responsibility required.
- MRI is the noninvasive procedure for sensitive images of soft tissue without using contrast dyes. No ionizing radiation is required. Technique used to evaluate spleen, liver and lymph nodes. Here nurse instructs patient to remove all metal objects and asks about any history of surgical insertion of staples, plates, or other metal appliances. Inform patient of need to lie still in small chamber.

Biopsies

- *Bone marrow:* Technique involves removal of bone marrow through a locally anaesthesized site to evaluate the status of the blood forming tissue. It is used to diagnose multiple myeloma, all types of leukemia, and some lymphomas and to stage of some tumors (e.g. breast cancer). It is also done to assess the efficacy of leukemic therapy.

  In these procedures, nurses have to explain the procedure to patient, obtain signed consent form, consider pre-procedure, analgesic administration to enhance patient's comfort and cooperation. Apply pressure while dressing after procedure. Assess biopsy site for bleeding.

- *Lymph node biopsy:* The purpose is to obtain lymph tissue for histologic examination to determine diagnosis and therapy. Open test is performed in operative room with direct visualization of the area and closed (needle) test is performed at bedside or in office. In this, the nurse must explain procedure to the patient. Obtain signed consent form. Use sterile technique in dressing changes after procedure. Carefully evaluate for wound for healing. Assess patient for complications, especially bleeding and edema.

Coagulation Studies

- Platelet count: Count of number of circulatory platelet (normal value) 1,50,000 to 4,00,000.
- Prothrombin test: Assessment of extrinsic coagulation by measurement of factors I, II, V, VII, X (PT: 12-25 seconds).
- International normalized ratio (INR): Standardised system or reporting PT based on reference calibration model and calculated by comparing the patient with PT with a central value. (The desired level of anticoagulation regimen 2.0-3.0).
- Activated partial thromboplastin time (APTT): Assessment of intrinsic coagulation by measuring factors I, II, V, VIII, IX, X, XI, XII, longer with use of heparin (30-45 seconds).
- Automated coagulation time (ACT): Evaluation of intrinsic coagulation status; more accurate than APTT, used during dialysis, coronary artery bypass procedure artenogram (Normal 150-180).
- Thromboplastin generation test (TGT): Reflection of generation of thromboplastin; if abnormal, second stage done to identify missing coagulation factor (Normal less than 12 seconds (100 percent).
- Bleeding time (BT) Is measurement of time small skin incision bleeds; reflection of ability of small blood vessels to constrict (Normal: 1-6 minutes).
- Thrombin time (TT): Reflection of adequacy of thrombin; prolonged thrombin time indication that coagulation is inadequate secondary to decreased thrombin activity (Normal 8-12-seconds).

- Fibrinogen: Reflection of level of fibronogen; increase in fibrinogen possible indication of enhancement of fibrin formation, making patient hypercoagulable; decrease in fibrinogen indicates that patient possibly predisposed to bleeding (normal 200–400 mg/dl).
- Fibrin split products: Reflection of degree of fibrinolysis; reflection of excessive fibrinolysis and predisposition to bleeding (if present); possible indication of disseminated intravascular coagulation (normal— less than 10 mg/L).
- Clot retraction: Reflection of clot shrinkage or retraction from sides of test tube after 24 hours; used to confirm platelet problem (normal 50–100% in 24 hours).
- Capillary fragility test (Tourniquet test, Leeds test): Reflection of capillary integrity when positive or negative pressure is applied to various areas of the body. Positive test indicates thrombocytopenia, toxic vascular reaction (normal: No petechia or negative).
- Protamine sulphate test: Reflection of presence of fibrin monomer (portion of fibrin remaining after elements that polymerize and stabilize detach); positive indication of predisposition to bleed and possible presence of dissemination intravascular coagulation (normally it is negative).

HEMATOLOGICAL DISORDERS

Management of persons with problems of the hematological system present challenges to the nurse because of the diversity and vagueness of the presenting symptomatology. Disease processes are as diverse as the components that make up the hematological system. For this reason, the nurse performs a complete and thorough ongoing assessment of the patient to determine the etiology of the patient's health concerns. Interventions should be focussed on supporting the patient's return to optimal function and resolution of hematological alterations. The nurse is responsible for assisting the patient to a better understanding of the hematological system and the complexities therein to obtain an optimal level of health.

DISORDERS OF ERYTHROCYTES

Common disorders of erythrocytes include underproduction (anemia) overproduction (erythrocytosis) and impaired hemoglobin synthesis (hemoglobinopathies).

Anemias

The term anemia refers to a deficiency in the number of circulating red blood cells available for oxygen transport. Anemia is a reduction below the normal in the number of erythrocytes, the quantity of hemoglobin, and the volume of packed red cells (Hct) caused by rapid blood loss, impaired production of RBCs, or increased destruction of erythrocytes. Because RBCs transport oxygen, erythrocytic disorder can lead to hypoxia. This hypoxia accounts for clinical manifestations of anemia. Anemia is not a specific disease, it is a manifestation of pathologic process.

Etiology

Anemia can result from primary hemotologic problems or can develop on a secondary consequence of defects in other body systems. The many kinds of anemia can be grouped according to either as a morphologic or an etiological classification. Morphologic classification is based on descriptive objective laboratory information about erythrocyte size and color. Aetiologic classification is related to the clinical condition causing the anemia such as decreased erythrocytic production, blood loss or increased erythrocytic production.

The etiologic classification of anemia are as follows:
- Decreased erythrocyte production:
  - Decreased hemoglobin synthesis
    * Iron deficiency (chronic blood loss and inadequate intake)
    * Thalassemias (decreased hemoglobin synthesis)
    * Sideroblastic anemia (decreased prophyrin)
  - Defective DNA synthesis
    * Cobalamin (vitamin B_{12}) deficiency of megaloblastic anemias.
    * Folic acid deficiency.
  - Decreased number of erythrocyte precursors (secondary to impaired production).
  - Aplastic anemia (drugs, chemicals, radiation, chemotherapy, virus congenital autoimmune mechanisms).
  - Anemia of leukemia and myelodysplasia.
    * Chronic disorders or diseases.
- Secondary to blood loss:
  - Acute
    * Trauma
    * Blood vessels rupture (hemorrhage).
  - Chronic
    * Gastritis, gastrointestinal bleeding, or other malignancy.
  - Bleeding ulcers, bleeding hemorrhoids.
  - Menorrhagia (menstrual flow).
- Increased erythrocytes destruction (Hemolysis):
  - Intrinsic
    * Abnormal hemoglobin (Hbs-sickle cell disease (anemia) genetic hemoglobinopathy).
    * Enzyme deficiency (G6PD) deficiencies or glucose-6 phosphate dehydrogenase.
    * Membrane abnormality (paraxysmal nocturnal hemoglobinuria).
    * Hereditary spherocytoses (inherited as autosomal dominant trait).
  - Extrinsic
    * Physical trauma (prosthetic heart valves and extracorporeal circulation).

- Antibodies (isoimmune and autoimmune-drug induced autoimmune response).
- Infectious agent and toxins (malaria).

Although the morphologic system is more accurate means of classifying anemias, it is easier to discuss patient care by focussing on the aetiologic problem. The relationship of morphological classification and etiologies of anemia are as given below:

- Normocytic, normochromic anemias may be due to acute blood loss, hemolysis, chronic renal disease, cancers, sideroblastic anemias, refractory anemia, diseases of the endocrine dysfunction, aplastic anemia pregnancy.
- Macrocytic, normochromic anemias may be due to cobalamin (vitamin B_{12}) deficiency, folic acid deficiency, liver disease (including effects of alcohol abuse) postsplenectomy.
- Microcytic, hypochromic anemia may be due to irondeficiency anemia, thalassemia lead poisoning.

Clinical Manifestations

The clinical manifestations of anemia are primarily caused by the body response to tissue hypoxia. The intensity of the manifestations varies depending on the severity of the anemia and presence of coexisting diseases. The severity of anemia can be determined by the Hb level:

- Mild states of anemia (Hb 10 to 14 g/dl) may exist without causing symptoms. If symptoms develop, they are usually caused by an underlying disease or a compensatory response to heavy exercise. These symptoms include palpitations, dyspnea and diaphoresis.
- Moderate states of anemia (Hb 6 to 10 g/dL) the cardiac pulmonary symptoms may be increased and may be associated with rest as well as activity.
- Severe anemia (Hb less than 6/dL) displays many clinical manifestation involving multiple body systems, which include:
  - Skin, pallor, jaundice, pruritus, (jaundice and pruritus due to hemolysis).
  - Eyes: Retinal hemorrhage, blurred vision, icteric conjunctiva and sclera (due to hemolysis).
  - Mouth: Glossitis and smooth tongue
  - Cardiovascular: Palpitations (mild and moderate), tachycardia, increased pulse pressure, systolic murmurs, intermittent claudication, angina, CHF and MI.
  - Pulmonary: Exertional dyspnea (mild), dyspnea (moderate), tachypnea, orthopnea and dyspnea at rest.
  - Neurologic: Headache, vertigo, irritability, depression, impaired thought process.
  - Gastrointestinal: Anorexia, hepatomegaly, splenomegaly, difficulty in swallowing and sore mouth.
  - Muscutoskeletal: Bone pain.
  - General: Sensitivity to cold, weight loss and lethargy.

Management

The numerous causes of anemia necessitate different nursing interventions specific to the needs of the patient. Nevertheless there are certain general components of care for all patients with anemia. The main problems are activity intolerance, alteration in nutrition, ineffective management of the respective regimen and hypoxemia. The plan of exercising care designed according to problems. However, dietary and lifestyle changes can reverse some anemias. Acute intervention for severe anemia include blood transfusion, drug therapy (e.g. erythropetin, vitamin supplements) and oxygen therapy and patient education regarding awareness care with therapy.

Iron Deficiency Anemia

Iron is present in all RBCs a heme in hemoglobin and is stored form. The heme in hemoglobin accounts for two-thirds of the body's iron. The other one-third of iron is stored as ferritin and hemosiderin in macrophages in the bone marrow, spleen and liver. Normally 1.5 mg of iron is lost daily through GI tract, sweat and urine. When the stored iron is not replaced, hemoglobin production is reduced, leads to iron-deficiency anemia.

Etiology

Iron deficiency may develop from inadequate dietary intake, malabsorptions, blood loss of hemolysis. The body loses approximately 1.5 mg iron daily; this loss is usually compensated for with daily dietary intake. This tenuous balance may be compromised by chronic blood loss, either physiological such as menstruation; or pathological form gastrointestinal or other bleeding. This compromise results in an iron deficiency anemia.

Common cause of gastrointestinal blood loss in adult are peptic ulcer, gastritis, esophagitis, diverticuli, hemorrhoids and neoplasia, genitouterine blood loss occurs primarily from menstrual bleeding. The average monthly menstrual blood loss is about 45 ml and causes the loss of about 22 mg of iron. Pregnancy contributes to iron deficiency because of the diversion of iron to the foetus for erythropoiesis, blood loss at delivery and lactation. In addition chronic renal failure, dialysis may induce anemia.

Clinical Manifestation

In the early course of iron deficiency, the patient may be free of symptoms. As the disease becomes chronic any of the general manifestations of anemia may develop. In some persons, in addition to pallor, specific symptoms may occur. Mild cases may develop fatigue and exertion dyspnea. Severe anemia causes the nails to become brittle and shaped (concave) and develop longitudinal ridges. Glossitis (Inflammation of tongue–the papillae of the tongue atrophy, and tongue has a smooth shiny, bright-red appearance and cheilosis (inflammation of lips–the corners of mouth may be cracked, reddened and painful). In addition, the patient may complain about headache, paresthesia, and burning sensation of the tongue, all of which are caused by the lack of iron in the tissues.

Management

The cells are characteristically hypochromic and microcytic and may be detected by observation of the peripheral blood smears or by blood cell indices (Ht, Hb. RBC). Diagnosis may be confirmed by a low serum iron levels and elevated serum iron binding capacity or by a low serum ferritin level or absent iron stores in the bone marrow endoscopy, colonoscopy may be used to detect GI bleeding.

The main goal of management is to treat the underlying disease that is causing reduced intake (malnutrition, alcoholism) or absorption of iron. In addition, efforts are directed towards replacing iron. This may be done through increasing the intake of iron. The patient should be taught which foods are good sources of iron. The role of nutrients is erythropoiesis and their sources are as follows:

- Cobalamin (vitamin B_{12}) has role in RBC maturation, found in red meats, especially liver.
- Folic acid also has role in RBC maturation found in green leaves, vegetables, liver, meat, fish, legumes and whole grains.
- Vitamin B_6 has role in hemoglobin synthesis, found in liver and muscle meat, eggs dried fruits, legumes, dark green leafy vegetable, whole grain and bread enriched with cereals, potatoes.
- Amino acids have role in synthesis of nucleoproteins, found in eggs, meat, milk and milk products (cheese, ice creams, poultry, fish, legumes and nuts).
- Vitamin C has role in conversion of folic acid to its active forms aids in absorption found in citrus fruits, leafy green vegetables, strawberries and cantaloupe.

The first step in medical therapy is to determine and correct the cause of anemia. Repletion of iron stores in the body may then be accomplished by the administration of iron. Oral iron supplements usually is given in the form of ferrous sulphate. Patient teaching is very essential for newly diagnosed patient, because ferrous sulphate may be irritating to GI tract. It should be taken after meals and with orange juice or vitamin C to increase the absorption. The person is told that the stools will be black or tarry and that symptoms of diarrhea or nausea should be reported to health care provider. Constipation is the major side effect of iron supplementation and a stool softener may be needed. When the patient cannot tolerate oral iron preparation or is unable to absorb iron properly, parenteral iron is administered by IM or IV administration of iron. Nutritional education is essential. Transfusion of packed RBCs in selected cases.

Megaloblastic or Macrocytic Anemia

Megaloblastic anemias refer to anemia with characteristics morphological changes caused by defective DNA synthesis and abnormal RBC maturated. The RBCs are large (macrocyte) and abnormal and are referred to as megaloblasts. Macrocytic RBCs are early destroyed because of their fragile membranes. Although the overwhelming majority of megaloblastic anemias result from cobalamin and folate deficiencies; their type of RBCs deformity can also occur from suppression of DNA synthesis by drugs from inborn errors of cobalamin and folic acid metabolism and from erythroleukemia (malignant disorder characterised by proliferation of erythropoietic cell in bone marrow). The common forms of megaloblastic anemia and their causes are as follows:

- Cobalamin (vitamin B_{12}) deficiency can result from dietary deficiency, deficiency of gastric intrinsic factor (due to gastrectomy, and pernicious anemia), intestinal malabsorption and increased requirement.

The deficiency results in impaired synthesis of DNA, resulting morphological changes in blood and bone marrow. General symptoms of anemia related to cobalamin deficiency develop because of tissue hypoxia (as stated earlier). Gastrointestinal manifestation includes a sore tongue, anorexia, nausea, vomiting and abdominal pain. Typical neuromuscular manifestation includes weakness, paresthesias of the feet and hands, reduced vibratory and position senses, ataxia, muscle weakness, and impaired thought process ranging from confusion to dementia. Because cobalamin deficiency related anemia has an insidious onset, it may take several months for these manifestations to develop.

Diagnosis of pernicious anemia is confirmed by an abnormal Schilling test result which demonstrates, the inability to absorb vitamin B_{12} unless intrinsic factor is also administered. Treatment consists of parenteral administration of vitamin B_{12}, usually once in a month by nurse in outpatient setting. The most common cause of relapse in person with pernicious anemia is that reluctance to continue therapy for life. Patient teaching is a focus of nursing care and discharge planning. In addition to general measures for anemia, the nurse should ensure that injuries are not sustained because of the diminished sensation to heat and pain resulting from the neurologic impairment. The patient must be protected from burns and trauma. If heat therapy is required, the patient's skin must be evaluated at frequent intervals to detect redness. Irritation from nasogastric tubes and restrictive clothing may not be procurred by the patient because of reduced pain sensations. A careful follow up is required.

- Folic acid deficiency also causes megaloblastic anemia. Folic acid required for DNA synthesis leading to RBC formation and maturation. Common causes of folic acid deficiency include the following:
  - Poor nutrition, especially a lack of green leafy vegetables, liver, citrous fruits, yeast, dried leaves, nuts and grains.
  - Malabsorption syndrome, particularly small-bowel disorders.
  - Drugs that impede the absorption and use of folic acid (e.g. methotrexate, oral contraceptives), as well as anti-seizure agents (e.g. phenobarbital, dephenylhydantine).
  - Alcohol abuse and anorexia (chronic alcoholism).
  - Hemodialysis patients, because folic acid is dialyzable.
  - Malnutrition.
  - Pregnancy causes increase in need for and use of folic acid. Deficiency during pregnancy may result in neural tube defects.
  - Increased requirement.

Clinical Manifestation

The clinical manifestation of folic acid deficiency is similar to those of cobalamin deficiency. This disease develops insidiously and the patient's symptoms may be attributed to other coexisting problems such as cirrhosis or esophageal varices. GI disturbances include dyspepsia and a smooth beefy red tongue. The absence of neurologic problem is an important diagnostic finding. This lack of neurologic involvement differentiate folic acid deficiency from vitamin B_{12} deficiency.

Laboratory findings include macrocytic anemia, megaloblastic changes in the bone marrow and a low serum folate level. Most persons respond promptly to oral folic acid and well balanced diet. Daily requirements for folic acid and 100 to 200 mg. The body is able to store approximately a 4-month supply of folic acid. Persons with anemia caused by a dietary deficiency can be treated with 1 mg of folic acid for 3-month period. Locate the cause and avoid or by corrective measures. Patients should be instructed in food rich in folic acid including organ meat, eggs, cabbage, broccoli, citrus fruits and brussels, sprouts. Boiling, steaming and canning for acid-rich foods reduces the amount of available vitamin persons who consume large amounts of are susceptible to folic acid deficiency. Advise patients to reduce or avoid alcohol.

Further, there are other forms of megaloblastic anemia which include:
- Drug-induced suppressions of DNA synthesis-resulting from folate antagonists. Metabolic inhibitions, alkylating agents, nitrous xoide.
- Inborn errors–heredity defective folate metabolisms Lesch-Nyham syndrome, defective of cobalamins.
- Erythroleukemia.

Thalassemia

Thalassemia is one of the common inherited single gene disorders in the world. As in iron-deficiency, it is a disease of inadequate production of normal hemoglobin. Hemolysis occurs in thalassemis, but insufficient production of hemoglobin is the predominant problem. In contrast to iron deficiency anemia, in which hemesynthesis is the problem, thalassemia involves problem with the globin protein.

Etiology

Thalassemias are a group of autosomal recessive genetic disorder commonly found in certain ethnic groups. An individual with thalassemia may have a heterozygous or homozygous form of the disease. A person who is heterozygous has one thalassemic gene and one normal gene and is said to have thalassemia minor or thalassemic trait, which is mild form of disease. A homozygous person has two thalassemia genes, causing severe condition known as thalassemia major.

Pathophysiology

Thalassemia is characterized by a decreased synthesis of one of the globin chains of hemoglobin. The beta chain is most often affected. As a result, there is decreased synthesis of hemoglobin and an accumulation of the alpha globin chain in the erythrocyte. These alterations result in decreased RBC production and a chronic hemolytic anemia.

Clinical Manifestation

The patient with thalassemia minor is frequently asymptomatic because the patient adjusts to the gradually acquired chronic state of anemia. Occasionally splenomegaly may develop in this patient, and mild jaundice may occur if malfored erythrocytes are rapidly hemolysed. The person who has thalassemia major is pale and displays general symptoms of anemia. In addition, the person has pronounced splenomegaly. Jaundice from RBC hemolysis is prominent. Chronic bone marrow hyperplasia leads to expansion of the marrow space. This may cause thickening of the cranium and maxillary cavity leading to an appearance resembling Down's syndrome. Thalassemia major is a life-threatening disease in which growth of both physical and mental are often retarded.

Management

Thalassemia minor requires no treatment because the body adapts to the reduction of normal hemoglobin. At present only treatment of thalassemia major is transfusion therapy and chelation therapy (therapy to reduce the iron overloading that sometime occurs with chronic transfusion therapy). No specific drug or diet therapies are effective in treating thalassemia. The nurse must be familiar with transfusion therapy and sensitive to the emotional needs of the patient who receive frequency transfusions. Avoid hopelessness and depression among population. Couple should be referred to genetic counseling.

Aplastic Anemia

One of the most severe forms of anemias related to reduced or impaired erythrocyte production is a group of disorders termed "aplastic" hypoplastic or pancytopenic "anemias". These anemias are life-threatening stem cell disorders, characterized by hypoplastic, fatty bone marrow and that result in pancytopenia.

Aplastic anemia is to an extent is a misnomer because in most cases, all marrow elements—erythrocyte, leukocytes and platelets are quantitatively decreased, although they are qualitatively normal.

Etiology

Aplastic anemia affects all age groups and both genders. The incidence is low, affecting approximately 4 persons per one million. There are various etiological types of aplastic anemia, but they can be divided into the major groups, i.e. congenital (idiopathic) or acquired are as:
- Congenital origin caused by chromosomal alterations. (approximately 30 percent of the aplastic anemia that appear in childhood). Fanconi syndrome, dyskertosis congenita, Shwachman-Diamond syndrome.
- Acquired as a result of exposure to:
  - Ionizing radiation, chemical agents (e.g. benzene, insecticide-DDT, arsenic, alcohol).
  - Viral and bacterial infections (e.g. hepatitis, parvovirus, miliary TB).
  - Prescribed medication (e.g. alkalating agents, antiseizure agents, antimetabolite, antimicrobial and gold).
  - Pregnancy.
  - Idiopathic.

Pathophysiology

Aplastic anemia usually is characterised by depression or cessation of activity of all blood-producing elements. There is a decrease in white blood cells (leukopenia) a decrease in platelets (thrombocytopenia) and decrease in the formation of RBC, which leads to an anemia. The process may be chronic or acute depending on the causative factor of the anemia.

Clinical Manifestation

Aplastic anemia usually develops insidiously. Clinically, the patient may have symptoms caused by suppression of any or all bone marrow elements general manifestations of anemia such as pallor, fatigue, and dyspnea as well as cardiovascular and cerebral responses may be seen. Pallor of skin and mucous membranes is characteristic in addition to fatigue, palpitation and exertional dyspnea. Infection of the skin and mucous membrane occur with severe granulocytopenia; hemorrhagic symptoms (bleeding into the skin and mucous membranes and spontaneous bleeding from the nose, gums, vagina and rectum) occur with severe thrombocytopenia.

Management

The diagnosis is confirmed by laboratory studies. Results of physical examination often are normal. The CBC characteristically reveals a pancytopenia (a marked decrease in the numbering of cell types). The reticulocyte count is low. Definitive diagnosis made by bone marrow examination and biopsy.

Management of aplastic anemia is based on identifying and removing the causative agent (when possible) and providing appropriate care until the pancytopenia reverses. In the past, treatment of aplastic anemia was aimed at mainly at stimulating hematopoiesis through and administration of steroids and androgens therapy. It has shown limited value and can produce toxic effects.

In recent years, bone marrow transplantation from a donor with identical human leukocyte antigen has emerged as the treatment of choice for the person younger than 40 years with severe aplastic anemia. The remainder of persons are treated with immunosuppressive therapy. The prognosis of persons depending on severity and method of treatment. Patients who are not successfully treated often die of complications associated with hemorrhage and infection.

Nursing care is based on careful assessment and management of complications of pancytopenia, primarily focused on preventing infection and monitoring signs of bleeding. To prevent infection in the hospitalised patient who is immunosuppressed, the following intervention should be included in the plan of care:
- Private room
- Protective isolation
- Provide and instruct the patient on meticulous hygiene
- Assessment and maintenance of oral care regimen
- Monitor invasive lines for signs of infection
- Avoid bladder catheterization.
- Instruct family and visitors on careful handwashing.

Nursing intervention aimed at the prevention of bleeding episodes include the following:
- Monitoring invasive line sites
- Testing urine and stools for blood
- Minimizing venipuncture and injections
- Avoiding rectal temperatures, medication and enema
- Instructing the patient on use of soft sponges for oral care.

Decreasing oxygen carrying capacity of the blood diseases, oxygen supply to the tissues, will lead to fatigue with activity. Measures to prevent fatigue include provide frequent rest periods, avoiding fatigue-producing activities, and monitoring the patient for signs of excessive fatigue or shortness of breath with activities. Patients are often hospitalised for several weeks depending on the type of treatment received. The nurse needs to assist the patient's developing coping strategies to deal with the anxiety and isolation of prolonged hospitalisation. Music and art therapies are helpful strategies to assist the patient in coping positively with the disease and treatment.

Education of the patient and family members is the cornerstone in the prevention of infection and avoidance of bleeding episodes. Teaching the person with aplastic anemia includes the following:

- Prevents infection:
  - Use good handwashing technique
  - Avoid sharing eating utensils and bath linens.
  - Take bath everyday (for every other day if skin is dry). Keep perineal area clean.
  - Use good oral hygiene
  - Eliminate intake of raw meat, fruits or vegetables
  - Report signs of infection immediately to health care provider.
- Prevent hemorrhage:
  - Observe for signs such as bloody urine, stool and patechae and report
  - Use a soft toothbrush or swab for mouth care and avoid the use of dental floss.
  - Keep mouth clean and free of debris
  - Avoid enemas or other rectal insertions
  - Avoid pricking or blosing the note forcefully
  - Avoid trauma, falls, bumps, and cuts, avoid contact with sports
  - Avoid use of aspirin preparations (anticoagulant effect)
  - Use an electric razor
  - Use lubrication and be gentle during sexual intercourse.
- Prevent fatigue:
  - Take frequent rest periods between ADL and activity
  - Avoid excessive work load or heavy lifting, and ask for assistance with sternum activity.
  - Increase time necessary for routine care.
  - Decrease activity if shortness of breath, dizziness or sensations of heaviness in extremities occurs.
  - Report signs of increased fatigue with activity to health care provider.

Hemolytic Anemias

Hemolytic anemia is defined as the premature destruction of erythrocyte occurring at such a rate that the bone marrow is unable to compensate for the loss of cells. Hemolysis can occur either extravascularly or intravascularly.

In cases of extravascular hemolysis, the spleen removes erythrocytes from circulation at a much more rapid rate, usually because of some perceived problems with the erythrocyte.

Examples are autoimmune anemias and hereditary spherocytosis. Extravascular hemolysis takes place in the macrophages of the spleen, liver and bone marrow.

Intravascular hemolysis is secondary to the erythrocyte lysing and spilling the cell contents into the plasma. This occurs as a result of an enzyme deficiency in the erythrocyte membranes or mechanical factors such as dialysis or prosthetic heart valves, which can prematurely weaken the erythrocyte. Hemolytic anemias can also develop as a result of abnormal hemoglobin synthesis as in the thalassemia and sickle cell disease. Intravascular hemolysis occurs within the circulation.

Etiology

The causes of hemolytic anemias may be acquired form or hereditary forms as briefed below.

- Acquired forms:
  - Immune system–mediated hemolysis is caused or associated with transfusion reactions, hemolytic disease of the newborn, and autoimmune hemolytic anemia. The mechanism of RBC destruction will be antibody mediated erythrocytes by enzymes of the complement system.
  - Traumatic hemolysis is caused by presence of prosthetic heart valves; structural abnormalities of the heart; hemolytic uremic syndrome; disseminated intravascular coagulation and hemodialysis. Here physical destruction of erythrocytic by "mechanical" means (trauma).
  - Infectious hemolysis are due to bacterial infection (clostridia, cholera, typhoid). Destruction occurs as a result of infection of erythrocytes.
  - Toxic (chemical) hemolysis occurs as a result of exposure to toxic chemical agents; hemodialysis or uremia; and venoms. Destruction due to chemical injury of erythrocytes. The chemical such as oxidative drugs, arsenic, lead, copper and snake venom.
  - Physical hemolysis are due to burns and radiation, destruction of erythrocyte by heat or radiation injury.
  - Hypophosphatemic hemolysis are due to hypophosphatemia (phosphate deficiency in plasma). Destruction, RBCs by diminished cellular production of substances required for erythrocyte life and function.
- Hereditary form:
  - Structural defects, i.e. plasma membrane defects, destruction due to fragility of the erythrocyte.
  - Enzyme deficiency, i.e. deficiency of glycolytic enzymes and deficiency of metabolic enzymes (i.e.

glucose-6-phosphate dehydrogenase). Destruction by diminished cellular function.
- Defects of globin synthesis or structure associated with:
    * Sickle cell anemias: There is increased membrane fragility and deformation during sickle cell crisis.
    * Thalassemia: There is defective hemoglobin structure and function.
    * Miscellaneous Hb defects: Defective Hb structure and function.

Pathophysiology and Clinical Manifestation

In warm-reacting anemias, antibodies (IgG) develop against an individual's own erythrocytes. These antibodies combine more readily at body temperature. Antibody coated RBCs are destroyed by the reticuloendothelial system, particularly the spleen symptoms depend on the onset. In episodes of severe hemolysis dyspnea, palpitations and congestive heart failure occurs. Jaundice, pallor and splenomegaly are common.

In cold reacting disease, IgM antibodies react, with antigens on the erythrocyte, optimally in cold temperature (less than 31°C) ischemia occurs when red cells clump in the capillary beds, causing cyanosis, pain and paresthesias. Hemoglobinuria also occurs.

Autoimmune reaction results when individuals develop antibodies against their own erythrocytes. Autoimmune hemolytic reactions may be idiopathic developing with no prior hemolytic history as a result of the immunoglobulin IgG covering of RBCs or secondary to other autoimmune disease (e.g. SLE), leukemia, lymphoma, or drugs (penicillin, indomethacin, phenylbutazone, phenacetin, quinidine, quninine and methyldopa).

Management

Diagnosis is confirmed by demonstrating the presence of the antibody or complement on the RBCs (direct Coomb's test) or in the serum 'indirect Coomb's test). Additional laboratory test findings will show a decreased Hct, increased reticulocytes, and an increased bilirubin.

Treatment depends on the cause of hemolysis. Mild cases require no treatment. Treatment and management of acquired hemolytic anemias involve general supportive care until the causative agent can be eliminated or at least rendered loss injurious to the erythrocytes. Supportive care includes administering corticosteroids and blood products or removing the spleen.

Nursing management consists of teaching the patient about the drug therapy, preparing the patient for surgery if indicated and helping the patient and family to cope with the illness. The patient and family need to be instructed regarding precipitating factors associated with autoimmune hemolytic anemias. Teaching should include preventive measures such as avoiding exposure to cold for persons with cold-reacting anemias.

Hereditary Spherocytosis

Hereditary spherocytosis (HS) is the most common problem of alteration in erythrocyte shape. It is inherited in an autosomal dominant trait it is characterized by a membrane abnormality that leads to osmotic swelling of the RBC and susceptibility to destruction by the spleen.

This anomaly occurs in 1 of every 5000 persons irrespective of their sex or race. It is usually detected in childhood; but, may appear initially in adulthood.

In this disease, there is deficit in the proteins that form the structure of the erythrocyte. This malformation of protein gives the cells a thick spherical appearance. This abnormal cell then becomes increasingly permeable to sodium, leading to increased energy demands by the cell. The circulating spherocytes become trapped in the spleen, where increased energy demands cannot be met and the cell dies.

Symptoms include those typically associated with anemia (pallor, fatigue, exceptional dyspnea), jaundice from the increased serum bilirubin level, and enlarged spleen from the increased RBCs destruction.

Diagnosis depends on observations of spherocytes in the peripheral blood smear and by laboratory demonstration of increased osmotic fragility of the RBCs. The reticulocytes count usually elevated, as is the serum bilirubin level.

The treatment for hereditary spherocytosis is splenectomy, which will correct the haemolytis, for the underlying sperocytosis will persist. The gallbladder is often also removed because of the increased incidence of gallstones in patients with HS.

Routine postoperative care is indicated for person who has undergone splenectomy or cholecystectomy. Nursing interventions include careful monitoring for infection and continuing monitoring for signs of anemia. Patient education should include wound management of surgery. Genetic counselling is indicated for couples considering childbirth. Energy conservation technique should be included in the teaching plan.

Enzyme Deficiency Anemia

Deficiency of enzymes in the pathways that metabolise glucose and generate adenosine triphosphate (ATP) commonly leads to premature RBC destruction, known as enzyme deficiency anemia. A most common clinically significant enzyme abnormality is that of "Glucose-6-phosphate dehydragenase" (G6PD)

Etiology

Hemolytic episodes in G6PD deficiency can be caused by viral and bacterial infection or oxidant drugs (antimalarial, antipyretics, sulfonamides, quinidine, vitamin K derivatives and phenacetin, chloramphenical.

Pathophysiology

The enzyme G6PD is responsible for the antioxidant reactions in the RBCs. The lack of this enzyme causes the cell to be susceptible to oxidizing agents. This exposure results in damage to the hemoglobin in RBC membrane and the subsequent release of hemoglobin into the circulation G6PD deficiency is a sex-linked disorder and directly affects the erythrocyte ability to resist oxidative damage consequently when G6PD is reduced there is a decrease in glucose used by the RBCs. If erythrocytes are exposed to oxidative foods and drugs the metabolic needs of RBC increases. However, G6PD deficiency interferes with glucose metabolism and leads to damage of older RBCs, which are then destroyed by hemolysis.

Clinical Manifestation

Hemolytic episodes persists for 7 to 10 days after exposure to oxidating agents. The patient may experience back pain, jaundice, and hemoglobinurin as evidence of hemolytic process.

Management

Diagnosis is established by assay for the enzyme. Managing the hemolysis seen in G6PD deficiency is realtively easy. Because, only older RBCs are destroyed by the oxidative agents, the younger cells survive. The cause of the hemolytic reaction must be removed. During the period of acute hemolyis, the patient will require rest, adequate hydration and assessing kidney function. Attention should be focussed on preventing hemolytic disorders by treating infections promptly and screening high risk individuals of G6PD deficiency before giving an oxidative drug.

Treatment is in the recognition of the disorder and cessation of the offending drugs. During a hemolytic episodes, hydration and blood transfusion may be necessary. Prompt treatment of infection is also important in managing patients. Nursing care includes management of episodes and educating patient and family on the precipitating factor of disorder, and its prevention. Teaching also focuses on the bacterial and viral illnesses and avoiding precipitating drugs.

Sickle Cell Disease (SCD)

Normal hemoglobin is composed of heme (red) and globin (protein component). The globin portion comprises of two pairs of polypeptide chains–alpha and beta. Each of the polypeptide chains has a specific amino acid sequence and number. Any deviation in the normal number of sequence of essential amino acids results in abnormal hemoglobin (Hgb) synthesis. Disorders of hemoglobin synthesis are categorised as "hemoglobinopathies". They result from abnormalities in one or both of the polypeptide chain or in any one of the more than 500 amino acids. One of the most common hemoglobinopathies is sickle cell disease (Hbs) or sickle cell anemia.

Etiology

Sickle cell disease (SCD) is a family of genetic disorder caused by abnormal properties conveyed to sickle cell RBC by mutant sickle cell hemoglobin (Hbs). It is an incurable disease that is often fatal by middle age.

Sickle cell anemia, one type of SCD is an autosomal recessive genetic disorder in which the person is homozygous for Hbs, characterized by a chronic hemolytic anemia, sickle cell anemia occurs predominantly in the black population, e.g. Afro-American.

Some persons may have sickle trait, a mild condition that may be asymptomatic. A person with sickle cell trait is heterozygous, with approximately 1/4 of the hemoglobin in the abnormal S from and 3/4 in the normal A form. If two parents have sickle cell trait, there is 25 percent chance with each pregnancy that the child will have sickle cell anemia.

Different terms are used with discussion of sickle cell anemia. Only the homozygous condition of HbS describes the classic form of the disease called Sickle Cell Anemia. The heterozygous state HbSA refers to the often asymptomatic condition called sickle cell trait. In addition, a category of sickling disorders called sickling syndrome is associated with presence of HbS. The phenotypes of sickle cell are:

Genetic relationship	Hb	SCD
Homozygous dominating	HbA, HbA	Sickle cell disease
Heterozygous	HbA, HbS	Sickle cell tract
Homozygous recessive	HbS HbS	Sickle cell anemia

Pathophysiology

The mutation that causes sickle cell hemoglobins (HbS) to develop, involves one amino acid. The basic abnormality lies within the hemoglobin fraction of the hemoglobin (Hb), where a single amino acid (valine) is substituted for another (glutamic acid) in the sixth position of the beta chain. This single amino acid substitution profoundly alters the properties of the Hgb molecule. This substitute leads to an abnormal linking reaction that causes development of deformed crescent shaped (sickle shape) cells when oxygen tension is lowered.

However, when the oxygen tention of RBCs decreases, HbS polymerizes causing the Hb of distort and realign the RBC into sickle shape. The sickle cell in circulation leads to increased blood viscosity, which prolongs circulation time. This decrease in circulation time causes an increase in the hypoxic time of the cell, promoting further sickling. The development of sickle cells leads to plugging, the small circulation further decreasing the cellular pH and oxygen tension. Anerobic metabolism occurs with resulting tissue ischemia in any organ.

When hypoxia occurs in a patient with sickle cell anemia, the RBCs containing HBs changes from a biconcave disk to an elongated, crescent or sickle cell. These sickling cell may clog the small capillaries. The resulting homeostasis promote a self-perpetuating cycle of local hypoxia, deoxygenation of more erythrocytes and more sickling. As blood vessels are occluded, thrombosis occurs. This can ultimately lead to ischemia and necrosis of the infarcted tissue from lack of oxygen. With repeated infarction there is gradual involvement of all body systems, especially the spleen, lungs, kidney and brain. The abnormal shape of the hemoglobin is recognised by the body and the cell is hemolysed. Sickle cells are also destroyed randomly. Initially sickling is reversible on reoxygenation but eventually becomes irreversible with cells being hemolysed and hemolytic anemia develops.

Clinical Manifestation

Infant with sickle cell anemia do not manifest symptoms until 10 to 12 weeks of age at which time most of the foetal hemoglobin (HbF) has been replaced by HbS. RBCs with high levels of HbF are resistant to sickling. Children with sickle cell disease manifest a general impairment of growth and development and a failure to thrive.

The effect of sickle cell disease varies greatly from person to person. Many of them with SCD possess reasonably good health. The typical patient is anaemic but asymptomatic except painful episodes. Anemia usually is severe, chronic and hemolytic.

Patients manifest the clinical manifestations of chronic anemia with pallor of mucous membranes, fatigue and decreased exercise tolerance. Because of the haemolyser jaundice is common patients are prone to gallstones (cholelithiasis). The painful vaso-occlusive episodes are the most common events in SCD. The pain is the manifestation of localised bone marrow necrosis affecting juxta articular areas of the long bones, spine, pelvis, ribs and sternum. The painful episodes occur once a year or twice a year; the duration of episode lasts from 1 to 10 days. Physical and probably emotional (stress) factors precipitate a painful episode. Physical factors include events that cause dehydration or change the oxygen tension in the body such as infection, overexertion, weather changes (cold), high Hgb levels, ingestion of alcohol and smoking.

Persons with SCD are particularly susceptible, primarily because most experience as anemia meningitis, sepsis, pneumonia and urinary tract infections. The sudden exacerbation of sickling can bring about a condition known as sickle cell crisis. Sickle cell crisis may be thrombotic, aplastic, megaloblastic or splenic sequestration. Shock is a possible development for sickle cell crisis. To sum up, clinical manifestation of SCD are:

Acute Episodes
- Pain usually in back, chest or extremities, may be localised migratory or generalised.
- Fever low grade, 1-2 days after onset of pain.
- Vaso-occlusive crisis occlusion of blood vessels by the sick cells may occur in area such as the brain (CVA), chest, liver or penis, leads to:
  - Acute chest syndrome: fever, chest pain, cough, dyspnea, pus infiltrate pulmonary infarction leads to pulmonary hypertension heart failure.
  - Priapism (condition of prolonged or constant erection of penis)
  - Jaundice caused by increased RBC destruction and release if bili rubin vaso-occlusive crisis are triggered by stress, cold water exposure, dehydration, hypoxia, and infection.

Chronic Problem
- Leg ulcers, usually of the medial malleolus.
- Renal problems is renal insufficiency from repeated infarction.
- Occular problem of microinfarctions of the peripheral retina, leading to retinal detachment and blindness.
- Musculoskeletal: The painful bone infarction of the hand foot syndrome (painful swelling and hands over foot), necrosis of femoral heads.

The major causes of mortality are renal and pulmonary failure.

Management

The diagnosis of sickle cell anemia should be considered with any black patient who has hemolytic anemia. In addition, routine CRC, Hct, Hb levels and others, the common screening test for sickle cell is peripheral blood smear, sickle cell preparation, sickle cell, hemoglobin electrophores have been useful in diagnosis.

There is no specific treatment for the disease. Patients with sickle cell disease should be advised to avoid high altitudes, adequate fluid intake, and treat infections promptly. Pneumovax and H-influenza vaccine should be administered. Therapy is usually directed towards alleviating the symptoms from complication of the disease. For example, chronic leg ulcers may be treated with bedrest, antibiotics, warm saline soaks, mechanical or enzyme debridements and grafting if necessary.

Patient should be assessed for infarction; and thrombosis resulting from anoxia may occur in brain, kidneys, bone marrow and spleen. He/she should be watched for complication such as:
- Increased intracranial pressure (Brain-CVA)
- Infections–lungs, urinary tract and bones
- Leg ulcers
- Bony complications–avascular necrosis in shoulder and hips
- Pulmonary complications
- Cardiovascular complication–arrhythmia and murmurs.
- Priapism (prolonged and painful erection)
- Hemorrhage and shock.

Take measures to correct them accordingly–Which includes taking nursing measures to promoting comfort and oxygenation; promoting hydration preventing infection; promoting tissue perfusion; promoting activity tolerance; facilitating family planning and genetic counselling; facilitate coping. In addition, teaching the person with sickle cell anemia includes:

- Knowledge of the disease
- Avoidance of situation that causes crisis (infection, high altitude, overexertion, emotional stress, alcohol, cigarette smoking and avoidance of trauma.
- Importance of adequate fluid intake.
- Availability of psychological support services and social resources.
- Need for medical checking.

ERYTHROCYTOSIS

Erythrocytosis refers to an abnormal increase in erythrocytes. The increase may be secondary to hypoxia (from high altitude or from pulmonary and cardiac disease) or certain erythroproteins producing tumors or primary disorder (polycythemia vera). With hypoxia, RBCs increase as a compensatory mechanism to carry additional oxygen.

Polycythemia Vera

Polycythemia vera is a myeloproliferative disorder of the pluripotent stem cell. Polycythemia is the production and presence of increased number of RBCs. The increase in erythrocytes can be so great that blood circulation is impaired as a result of the increased blood viscosity (hyperviscocity and volume (hypervolume).

Etiology

There are two types of polycythemia and includes primary polycythemia and secondary polycythemia. Although this etiology and pathogenism differ, clinical manifestation and complication are similar.

Polycythemia vera is considered a myeloproliferative disorder arising from a chromosomal mutation in a single pluripotent stem. Due to this there will be thrombocytosis and leukocytosis.

Secondary polycythemia is caused by hypoxia rather than increase in the development of the RBC. Hypoxia stimulates erythrocyte production. The need for oxygen may be due to high altitude, pulmonary disease, cardiac vascular disease, alveolar hypoventilation, defective oxygen transport, or tissue hypoxia.

Pathophysiology

Polycythemia vera is a bone marrow disorder characterised by erythrocytosis, usually with a simultaneous leukolytosis and thrombocytosis, hypervolemia, increased blood viscosity from the increased RBC mass and platelet dysfunction occur.

Clinical Manifestation

Symptoms usually are absent in early stage, circulatory manifestation of polycythemia vera occur because of the hypertension caused by hypervolemia and hyperviscosity. They are often the first symptoms and include subjective complaint of headache, vertigo, dizziness, tinnitus, and visual disturbances. In addition, patients may experience angina, CHF, intermittent claudication and thrombophlebitis, which may be complicated by embolisation. These manifestations are caused by blood vessel distension, impaired blood flow, circulatory studies, thrombosis and tissue hypoxia caused by the hypervolemia and hyperviscosity. The most serious complications is CVA secondary to thrombosis. Generalised pruritus may be striking symptoms and is related to histamine release from an increased number of vasophils and mast cells.

Hemorrhagic phenomena caused by either vessel rupture from overdistention or inadequate platelet function may result in petechae, ecchymosis, epistaxis or GI bleeding. Hemorrhage may be acute or catastrophic.

Hepatomegaly and splenomegaly from organ engorgements may contribute to patient complaints of satiety and fullness. The patient also experiences pain from peptic ulcer. Plethora (ruddy complexion) may also be present. Hyperuricaemia is caused by the increase in RBC destruction that accompanies excessive RBC products. Uric acid is one of the products of cell destruction. This may cause secondary form of gout (a form of arthritis).

Management

Polycythemia confirmed by lab test of blood where there is increase in Hgb, Hct, WBC (basophilia), platelets and platelet dysfunction, leucocyte alkaline phosphate, uric acid, cobalamin levels and histamine levels. Bone marrow examination in polycythemia vera shows hyper cellularity of RBCs, WBCs and platelets, splenomegaly also are found.

Once the diagnosis of polycythemia vera is made, treatment is directed towards reducing blood volume and viscosity and bone marrow activities. The goal of therapy is to decrease the red cell mass. Treatment options are phlebotomy (for diminished blood values) alkalating agents (busulfan, hydroxyurea, melphalan), radioactive phosphorous or interferon to inhibit bone marrow activity. Usual treatment is periodic phlebotomy aimed at maintaining the Hct and Hgb at normal level.

When acute exacerbations of polycythemia vera develop, the nurse has several responsibilities. Depending on the institutional policies, the nurse may either assist with or perform phlebotomy, fluid intake and output must be evaluated during hydration therapy to avoid overload (which further complicate the circulatory congestion) and underdehydration (which can cause the blood to become even more viscus). If myelosuppressive agents are used, the nurse must administer the drug as ordered, observe the patient and teach the patient above medication and side effects. Teach about importance of combined medical care, blood tests and phlebotomy. Repetitive phlobotomy may lead to iron deficiency and take measures accordingly. The complications are treated accordingly.

ANEMIA CAUSED BY BLOOD LOSS

Anemia resulting from blood loss may be caused by either acute or chronic.

Etiology/Pathophysiology

Acute blood loss occurs as a result of sudden hemorrhage causes of acute blood loss include trauma, complications of surgery and diseases that disrupt vascular integrity. There are two clinical concerns in such situation. First, there is sudden reduction in the total blood volume that can lead to hypovolemic shock. Second, if the acute loss is more gradual, the body maintains its blood volume by slowly increasing the plasma volume. Consequently, the circulating fluid volume is preserved. But the number of RBCs available to carry oxygen is significantly diminished.

The sources of chronic blood loss are similar to those of iron deficiency (e.g. bleeding ulcer, hemorrhoids, menstrual and postmenopausel blood loss).

Clinical Manifestation

The clinical manifestation of acute blood loss are caused by the body's attempt to maintain adequate blood volume and meet O2 requirements. Clinical manifestation of acute blood loss according to varying degrees of blood volume loss as follows:

Volume loss	Clinical manifestation
10%	None
20%	No detectable signs or symptoms at rest, tachycardia with exercise and slight postural hypertension
30%	Normal supine blood pressure and pulse at rest, postural hypertension and tachycardia with exercise
40%	Blood pressure, central venous pressure and cardiac output below normal at rest, rapid, threading pulse and cold and clammy skin
50%	Shock and potential death

Management

When blood volume loss is sudden, the body reacts by vasoconstriction. In this stage, erythrocyte, Hb, and Hct levels are usually low and reflect the blood loss. Care of these patients induce replacing blood volume to prevent shock and identify the sources of hermorrhage and stopping blood loss. IV fluid used in emergency includes dextran, hetastarch, albumin, or crystalloid electrolyte solution such as lactated ringers. Blood transfusion (Packed RBCs) may be needed of the blood loss is significant. The patient also needs supplemental iron because, the availability of iron affects the marrow production of erythrocytes. When anemia exists after acute blood loss, dietary sources of iron will probably not be adequate to maintain iron pools. For every 2 ml of blood lost, 1 mg iron is also lost. Therefore, oral or parenteral iron prepared are administered. Nursing intervention includes treating shock in acute blood loss and locating the cause and take measures everyday in both acute and chronic blood loss.

DISORDERS OF HEMOSTASIS

The hemostatic process involves the vascular endothelium, platelets, and coagulation factors, which normally function in concert to arrest hemorrhage and repair vascular injury. Disruption of any of these may result in bleeding or thrombolic disorders. The common disorders associated with platelet and coagulation are:
- Platelets
  - Thrombocytopenia: Decreased numbers of platelets
  - Thrombocytosis: Increased number of platelets.
  - Bleeding syndrome: Disorders of platelet functions.
- Coagulation
  - Congenital
    * Hemophilia A: Decrease of factor VIII
    * Hemophilia B: Decrease of factor IX
    * Von Willebrands: Decrease of factor VIII disease defective platelet aggregation
  - Acquired
    * Vitamin K: Decrease of factors II, VII, IX deficiency and X.
    * Disseminated intravascular: Stimulates first the clotting process then fibro-coagulation analytic process

THROMBOCYTOPENIA

Thrombocytopenia is defined as a lower than normal number of circulating platelets (ranges of 150,000 to 400,000).

Etiology

Platelet disorders can be inherited (e.g. Wiskott-Aldrich syndrome) but vast majority are acquired. Acquired disorders occur because of decreased platelet production, or increased platelet production and many abnormalities occur following ingestions of some foods and drugs:
- Decreased Platelet production.
  - Inherited
    * Fanconi's syndrome (Pancytopenia).
    * Hereditary thrombocytopenia.
  - Acquired
    * Aplastic anemia.
    * Hematologic malignant disorder.
    * Myelosuppressive drugs.

- Chronic alcoholism.
- Exposure to ionizing radiation.
- Viral infections.
- Deficiencies of cobalamin and folic acid.
• Increased Platelet Destruction
  – Nonimmune
    • Thrombotic thrombocytopenia purpura.
    • Pregnancy.
    • Infection.
    • Drug induced.
    • Severe burns.
  – Immune
    • Immune thrombocytopoenic purpura.
    • Human immunodeficiency virus infection.
    • Drug induced.
  – Splenomegaly.
• Drugs, spices and vitamin causing abnormalities in platelet function
  – Suppression of platelet production.
    • Thiazide diuretics, alcohol, estrogen and chemotherapeutic drugs.
  – Abnormal platelet aggregation.
    • NSAIDs: Ibuprofen, indomethacin naproxen
    • Antibiotics: Penicillin and cephalosporins
    • Analgesics: Aspirin and aspirin containing drugs
    • Spices: Ginger, cumin, turmeric, cloves and garlic.
    • Vitamins: Vitamin C and vitamin E
    • Heparin
    • Other drugs, chloroquine, digitoxin, methyldopa, oral hypoglycemic agents, phenobarbital, quinidone, quinine, refampin and sulphana.

Pathophysiology

The major signs of thrombocytopenia observable by physical examination are petechiae, ecchymosis, and purpura. Petechae occur only in platelet disorders. The person may give a history of menorrhagia, epistaxis and gingival bleeding. The patient is questioned about recent viral infections which may produce a transient thrombocytopenia; drugs in current use; and extent of alcohol ingestion.

Clinical Manifestations

In spite of different etiologies, clinical manifestation of thrombocytopenia, are similar. Thrombocytopenia most commonly manifested by the appearance of small, flat, pin point red or reddish brown microphages termed "Petechiae". When the platelet count is low, RBC may leak out of the blood vessels and into the skin to cause Petechiae, when petechiae are numerous, the resulting reddish skin bruise is termed "purpura". Larger purplish lesions caused by hemorrhage are termed ecchymoses. Ecchymoses may be flat or raised, pain and tenderness are sometimes present.

Prolonged bleeding often routine procedures such as venipuncture or IM injection may also indicate thrombocytopenia. Because this bleeding may be internal the nurse must also be aware of manifestations that reflect the type of blood loss including weakness, fainting, dizziness tachycardia, abdominal pain and hypertension.

The major complication of thrombocytopenia is hemorrhage. The hemorrhage may be insidious or acute and internal or external. It may occur in any areas of the body, including the joints, retina, and brain. Cerebral hemorrhage may be fatal.

Management

Diagnostic studies include complete laboratory studies to ascertain the status of all blood components. The most commonly used test for assessment of platelets are platelet count, peripheral blood smear and bleeding bone. In addition, bone marrow examination is performed to determine the presence of megakaryocyte (Precursor of platelets in the bone marrow), and other abnormalities such as neoplastic invasion, aplastic anemia or fibrosis.

The primary treatment modalities for immunothrombocytopenia purpura (ITP) are corticosteroid therapy and splenectomy. Steroids appear to decrease both antibody production and phagocytosis of the antibodycoated platelets. Splenectomy removes the principal organs involved in destruction of the antibody coated platelets. To sum up, the treatment modalities according to different etiologies are:

• Immune thrombocytopenic purpura (ITP):
  – Corticosteroids.
  – Platelet transfusions.
  – Intravenous immunoglobulin.
  – Danazol (an androgen).
  – Immunosuppressives (cyclophosphamide and azathioprine).
  – Splenectomy.
• Thrombotic, thrombocytopenic purpura (TTP):
  – Plasma infusion.
  – Plasmapheresis and plasma exchange.
  – High dose prednisone
  – Splenectomy.
• Decreased production problems:
  – Identification and treatment of cause.
  – Corticosteroids.
  – Platelet transfusion.
  – Thrombopoietin (investigational).

The goal during acute episodes of thrombocytopenia is to prevent or control hermorrhage. The nurse has to assess the bleeding sites and take measures accordingly as practised institutional policies and follow standard guidelines to prevent and control bleeding. In a woman with thrombocytopenia, menstrual blood may exceed the usual amount and duration. Counting sanitary napkins used during menses is another important intervention to detect blood loss. Fifty milliliters of blood will completely soak a sanitary napkin. Suppression of menses with hormonal agents may be indicated during predictable period of thrombocytopenia.

The proper administrations of platelet transfusion is an important nursing responsibility. Platelet concentrates, derived from fresh whole blood, can increase in the platelet level effectively. One unit of platelets, a yellow liquid that is usually 30 to 50 ml in volume can be derived by centrifuging 500 ml. of whole blood. Platelet concentrates from multiple units of blood (usually from 6 to 8 different donors) can be pooled together for a single administration. Platelet transfusion can also be prepared by pheresing single donors. This may be indicated when HLA matched platelets are needed, especially for patients requiring multiple platelet transfusions. Transfusion often must be administered twice weekly.

A primary concern in the nursing care of persons with a decreased number of platelets is the concomitant bleeding tendency. Bleeding associated with trauma is likely with a platelet count less than 60,000/mm. Spontaneous hemorrhage may be a life-threatening possibility when the platelet count is less than 20,000/mm. Ongoing nursing assessment of the patient is essential and includes alertness of increased ecchymoses, petehiae, bleeding from other sites and any change in mental status. The need for avoiding trauma is obvious. Person with platelets counts below 20,000/mm should have bleeding precautions instituted. These include the following:
- Test all urine and stools for blood (guaiac).
- Do not take temperature rectally.
- Do not administer intramuscular infections.
- Apply pressure to all venipunctures sites for 5 minutes and to all arterial puncture sites for 10 minutes.

In addition, the nurse has the responsibility of teaching the person with thrombocytopenia which includes the following:
- Nature fo the disorder.
- Signs of decreased platelets (Petechaie, ecchymosis, gingival bleeding, hematuria, menorrhagia).
- Name, dosage, frequency and side effects of prescribed medications (corticosteroids) and importance of not stopping corticosteroids abruptly.
- Measures to prevent injury:
  - Use a soft toothbrush or swab for mouth care.
  - Do not use dental floss.
  - Keep mouth clean and free of debris.
  - Avoid intrusion into rectum (e.g. rectal medication and enemas).
  - Use electric shaver.
  - Apply direct pressure for 5 to 10 minutes if any bleeding occurs.'
  - Avoid contact sports, electrice surgery and tooth extraction.
  - Avoid blood thinning drugs such as Aspirin, that decreases sticking ability of platelet.
  - Increase knowledge of contents of over the counter (OTC) medications and effects on platelets functioning. Read labels on OTC drugs.
- Need for follow up medical care.

THROMBOCYTOSIS

Thrombocytosis is defined as the presence of an abnormally high number of circulating platelets.

Etiology Pathophysiology

Mild bleeding syndrome may be caused by quantitatively normal but functionally defective platelets. The most common cause of platelet abnormality in drugs, particularly aspirin. Aspirin inhibits, the release of intrinsic platelet adenosine diphosphate (ADP) and produces a defect in platelet aggregation. The defect remains for the lifespan of the platelet.

Thrombocytosis can be categorised as reactive (hyperactive bone marrow) or essential (myeloproliferative syndrome). The associated conditions include polycythemic vera, myelofibrosis, splenectomy, iron deficiency anemia, chronic inflammatory diseases, hemorrhagic thrombocythermea, and advanced carcinoma. Clinical manifestation includes thrombosis, increased bleeding tendencies, platelet counts more than 1000,000/mL.

Management

The abnormality may be detected by a test of bleeding time or more sensitively, by platelet aggregation tests. Patients with disorders of platelet function have clinical manifestation and patient care needs similar to these of persons with thrombocytopenia. Treatment of thrombo cytosis include the control of underlying cause, myelosuppressive drug therapy, plasmapheresis to reduce circulating number of platelets; and antiplatelet agents (e.g. Aspirin, dipyridamole) **(Table 6.1)**.

DISORDERS OF COAGULATION

Hemophilia

Etiology/Pathophysiology

Hemophilia is a hereditary bleeding disorder caused by defective or deficient coagulation factors. The two major forms of hemophilia which can occur is mild to severe forms are hemophilia A (Classic hemophilia, factor VIII deficiency) and hemophilia B (Christmas disease, factor IX deficiency). The disorder termed "von Willebrand's disease" is a related disorder involving a congenitally acquired deficiency of von Willebrand compilation proteins. Factor VIII is synthesized in the liver and circulates complexed to von Willebrand's protein (VWP). And one more hemophilia C (Factor XI deficiency).

Table 6.1: Commonly used antiplatelet agents.

Drugs (dose)	Actions	Side effects
Aspirin (150–300 mg daily as single dose)	Irreversibly inactivates the enzyme cyclooxygenase and thereby inhibit platelet production of thromboxane A2	• It may cause allergic or asthmatic reactions • GI symptoms (e.g., nausea, vomiting, abdominal pain, diarrhoea) • Skin rashes • Neutropenia, GI hemorrhage • Headache, tinnitus • Neutropenia, hemorrhage, agranulocytosis
Clopidogrel	Inhibits ADP-induced platelet aggregation	

Hemophilias are inherited as sex-linked recessive disorders and are therefore almost exclusively limited to males. The incidence of hemophilia A (1:10,000) hemophilia B (1:100,000) of the male population. Hemophilia C is rare with incidence 2 to 3 percent.

The inherent pattern of these hemophilion are as follows:
- *Hemophilia A:* Recessive sex-linked (transmitted by female carriers, displayed almost exclusively in men).
- *Hemophilia B:* Recessive sex-linked (transmitted by female carriers, displayed almost exclusively in men).
- *von Willebrand disease:* (VWP dysfunction) Autosomal dominant, seen in both sexes, recessive (in severe form of the disease).

Clinical Manifestation

Clinical manifestation and complications related to hemophilia include:
- Slow, persistent, prolonged bleeding from minor trauma and small cuts.
- Delayed bleeding after minor injuries (the delay may be for several hours or days).
- Uncontrollable hemorrhage after dental extractions or irritation of gingiva with a hard-bristle tooth brush.
- Epistaxis, especially after blow to the face.
- GI bleeding from ulcers and gastritis.
- Hematuria from GU trauma and splenic rupture resulting from fall or abdominal trauma.
- Ecchymoses and subcutaneous hematomas (common).
- Neurologic signs, such as pain, anesthesia and paralysis which may develop from nerve compression caused by hematoma formation and
- Hemarthrosis (bleeding from joints) which may lead to joint deformity severe enough to cause unresolvable crippling (most commonly in knees, elbows, shoulders, hips and ankles).

Life-threatening bleeding involves retroperitoneal, intracranial soft tissue hemorrhages.

Management

A diagnosis of haemophila is made by specific assays for factors VIII, IX and XI. The partial thromboplastotime (PTT) which reflects the intrinsic pathway of coagulation, is prolonged in hemophilia A, hemophilia B and hemophilia C. The platelet count and prothrombic time is normal.

Treatment is replacement of the deficient coagulation factor. When bleeding episodes do not respond to local treatment, i.e., ice bags, manual pressure or dressings, immobilization, elevation, or topical coagulate such as fibrin foam and thrombin.

Fresh frozen plasma once commonly used for replacement therapy is rarely used now. Cryoprecipitate which primarily contains factor VIII and fibrinogen is prepared for plasma, frozen rapidly and kept frozen until used. Before administration, the cryoprecipitate is thawed slowly.

The standard therapeutic products, i.e. concentrate factor used in treating hemophilia today are:
- Factor VIII
  - Plasma derived products: Monoclate, Hemofil, Profilate, Huma
  - Recombination products: Recombinates, Kogenate,
- Factor IX
  - Plasma-derived products: Alpha-Nine, Mononine, Ronyne, Profilinine.
  - Recombination products: Bebulin, autoplex, FEIBA and Hyate.

Nursing interventions are related primarily to controlling bleeding and include the following.
- Stop the topical bleeding as quickly as possible by applying direct pressure or ice packing the area with Gelfoam or fibrin foam, and applying topical hemostatic agents such as thrombin.
- Administer the specific coagulation factor concentrate ordered to raise the patient's level of the deficient coagulation factor.
- When joint bleeding occurs it is important to totally rest the involved joint, in addition to administering antihemophilitic factors to help prevent crippling deformities from hemarthrosis. The joint may be packed in ice, analgesics are given to reduce joint pain. However, aspirin and aspirin containing compounds should never be used.
- As soon as bleeding ceases, it is important to ROM exercises and physical therapy. Actual weight bearing is avoided until all swellings has resolved and muscle strength has returned.
- Manage any life-threatening complication that may develop as a result of hemorrhage. Example includes nursing intervention to prevent or treat airway obstruction from hemorrhage into the neck and pharynic, as well as early assessment and treatment of intracranial bleeding.

In addition, the nurse must provide ongoing assessment of the patient's adaptation to the illness. Psychosocial support and assistance should be readily available as needed. Most of the long terms are related to patient education. The patients with hemophilia must be taught to recognize disease-related problems and to learn which problem can be resolved or borne and which require hospitalization. Immediate medical attention is required for severe pain or swelling of a muscle or joint that restricts movement or inhibits sleep and for a head injury, a swelling in the neck or mouth, abdominal pain, hematuria, melena and skin wound needed for suturing.

Daily oral hygiene must be performed without causing trauma. There are many potential sources of trauma. The patient can learn to prevent trauma by using gloves whenever needed to prevent cuts or abrasion from knives, hammer and other tools. The patient should wear a medic alert tag to ensure that health care providers know about the hemophilia in case of an accident. Since the hemophilia is hereditary, genetic counselling is necessary as preventive measures if needed.

Vitamin K Deficiency

Vitamin K, a fat soluble vitamin, is a cofactor in the synthesis of clotting factors II, VII, IX and X. Approximately 50 percent of required vitamin K is obtained from a normal diet and 50 percent is produced by intestinal bacteria.

Vitamin K deficiency can be anticipated in persons who have a decrease intake and who are given broad-spectrum antibiotics, (such as neomycin sulphate that decreases the growth of intestinal bacteria. Interference with vitamin K, absorption occurs with primarily intestinal disease (Ulcerative colitis, Crohn's disease) biliary disease and malabsorption syndrome drugs such as large doses of salicylates, quinine and barbiturates interfere with vitamin K function.

Symptoms are those of anemia superimposed on the underlying disorders that is bleeding of the mucous membrane and into the tissue. Postoperative hemorrhages may be observed. In severe cases, GI bleeding may be massive.

Management

Diagnostic features of vitamin K deficiency are prolonged PT and PTT. There is also a decrease in the levels of vitamin K dependent clotting factors.

Treatment consists of therepy for the underlying disorder and cessation of causative drugs. For mild disorders, a water soluble vitamin K preparation (menadione) is given orally or parenterally. In severe disorders, fat soluble vitamin K preparation (Phytonadione) may be given. Fresh frozen plasma will partially correct the disorder immediately whereas, vitamin K therepy takes 6 to 24 hours to be effective and does not have the complication of fresh frozen plasma.

Nursing management includes monitoring of vital signs and teaching regarding safety precautions to prevent bruising, eipsodes. The patient should be instructed to avoid tromatising brush, avoid intramuscular injections and apply direction immediately on any bleeding site.

DISSEMINATED INTRAVASCULAR COAGULATION (DIC)

Disseminated intravascular coagulation (DIC) is a serious bleeding disorder resulting from abnormally initiated and accelerated clotting.

Etiology

DIC is not a disease, it is an abnormal response of the normal clotting cascade stimulated by another disease process or disorders. The diseases and disorders are known to predispose in patient with DIC are as follows:
- Acute DIC
  - Shock: Hemorrhagic; cardiogenic; anaphylactic.
  - Septicemia.
  - Hemolytic process
    * Transfusion of mismatched blood.
    * Acute hemolysis from infection or immunologic disorders.
  - Obstetric conditions
    * Abruption placenta.
    * Amniotic fluid embolus.
    * Toxemia.
    * Septic abortion.
  - Tissue damage
    * Extensive burns and trauma.
    * Heat stroke.
    * Severe head injury.
    * Transplant rejections.
    * Postoperative damage, especially after extra-corporeal membrane oxygenation.
    * Fat and pulmonary emboli.
    * Snake bites.
    * Glomerulonephritis.
    * Acute anoxia (e.g. after cardiac arrest).
    * Prosthetic devices.
- Subacute DIC
  - *Neoplastic disease:* Adenocarcinoma, acute leukemias, metastatic cancer and pheochromocytoma
  - *Obstetric:* Retained dead fetus.
- Chronic DIC
  - Liver disease
  - SLE
  - Localized malignancy.

Others include vascular disease like aortic aneurysm and fat embolus, vasculitis and crush injuries, brain injury; burns ischemia.

Pathophysiology

The primary disease initiates the clotting process. The response is generalized and occurs throughout the vascular system, creating state of hypercoagulability. The fibrinolytic processes which normally operate to limit clot extension and dissolve clots are then stimulated. As clotting factors are depleted and fibrinolysis continue a state of hypocoagulability develops.

The most common sequela of DIC is hemorrhage. This paradox is caused by (1) decreased platelets (2) depletion of clotting factors, II, V, VIII and fibrinogen in the process and (3) the production of fibrin degradation products (FDP) through fibrinolysis. The FDP act as anticoagulants and increase the hemorrhagic tendency. As the disorder progresses, clinical manifestation may include bleeding of the mucous membranes and tissues (petechiae, ecchymosis); oral, gastrointestinal genitourinary and rectal bleeding and bleeding after injections and venipuncture may occur. Hypoxia, tachypnea, hemoptysis, hypotension, acidosis and fever may also be presented. The generalized clinical manipulation of DIC includes the following:

- Neurological
  - Confusion
  - Irritability
  - Headache
  - Dizziness
  - Seizures
  - Fevers
  - IICP
  - Vertigo
  - LOC.
- Sensory
  - Blurred vision
  - Intraocular hemorrhage
  - Inner ear-bleeding
  - Conjunctival hemorrhage
  - Epistaxis
- Cardiovascular
  - Tachycardia
  - Chest pain
  - Hypotension
  - Abscess and peripheral pulses
  - Abnormal or increased bleeding from venipuncture or IV insertion sites.
- Genitourinary
  - Progressive oliguria
  - Hematuria
  - Renal failure
  - Bleeding around-indwelling poley catheter
  - Severe bleeding during menstruation
  - Vaginal bleeding
  - Proteinuria.
- Gastrointestinal
  - Melena
  - High-pitched bowel sounds
  - Nausea
  - Vomiting
  - Abdominal distension
  - Hematemesis.
- Integumentary
  - Cool, moist skin
  - Cyanosis
  - Petechiae
  - Mottling
  - Ecchymosis
  - Purpura.
- General
  - Acidosis
  - Acral cyanosis.

Management

Diagnosis of DIC is confirmed by laboratory findings. Abnormal RBCs may be found on peripheral smear, fibrinolysis reflected in increased fibrin split products D-dimers and prolonged prothrombin time. Fibrinogen level plabectomy is decreased. PT, PTT and TT are prolonged. Assay shows decreased levels of factors V, VIII and LX.

The management of DIC always begins with treatment of primary disease. Once this has been inhaled, the goal is to control the bleeding and restore normal levels of clotting factors. Blood products such as fresh frozen plasma, platelet packs, cryoprecipitate, and fresh whole blood may be administered, to replace the depleted factors. Heparin has been used to inhibit the underlying thrombotic process; however, it too often promotes rather than decreases bleeding and its use is controversial.

Nursing managment of the patient with DIC is extremely challenging. The person who develops DIC is critically ill and commonly has numerous sites of bleeding. The amount and nature of drainage from chest and nasogastric tubes, oozing from surgical incisions and progressive discoloration for the skin should be noted and recorded. Continual observation for new bleeding site and for an increase or decrease in bleeding is an integral part of the nursing care plan, especially heparin therapy is being used. The susceptibility of these persons to bleeding present special problems. Medication should be given or ally or intravenously if at all possible; and small gauge needles should be used when other injections are necessary. All precautions to be taken to prevent hemorrhage as described earlier (Thrombocytopenia). Maintaining fluid balance is very essential. Person with DIC usually lose large quantities of blood and receive frequent transfusions and other fluid replacement. In addition to monitoring blood infusion rates carefully, the nurse must be alert to signs of fluid overload such a slow-bounding pulse, and increasing central venous pressure. Intake and output are to be maintained accurately.

Generally the patient is comatose and the presence of purpura, numerous intravenous lines, and drainage tube makes patient appear may upset the family members. Emotional support should be given by the nurse to family. And family to be educated accordingly regarding disease process and other treatment modality and precautionary guidelines.

DISORDERS OF WBCs

The white blood cells (WBC-Leukocyte) system is composed of neurophils, lymphocytes, monocytes, basophils and eosinophils. All but lymphocytes are derived from a common stem cell. The primary function of WBC is to provide humoral and cellular response to infections. Neutrophils are primarily responsible for phagocytosis and the destruction of bacteria and the infectious organism. Lymphocytes are the principal cells involved in immunity, which is responsible for the development of delayed hypersensitivity and the production of antibodies. Any compromise in the integrity of the WBC system renders a person susceptible to infection.

Leukopenia refers to a decrease in the total WBC counts (granulocytes, monocytes and lymphocytes). Granulocytopenia is a deficiency of granulocytes which incldue nutrophils, eosinophils and basophils.

Neutropenia

The neutrophilic granulocytes, which play a major role in phagocytizing pathogenic microbes are closely monitored in clinical practice as an indicator of patient's risk for infection. A reduction in neutrophils is termed "neutropenia" or granulocytopenia. Neutropenia is defined as a neutrophil count of less than 2000/mm.

Etiology

Neutropenia is not a disease, it is a syndrome that occurs with variety of conditions and can also be an expected effect, side effect, or unintentional effect of taking certain medication includes the following:
- Hematological disorders
  - Idiopathic neutropenia
  - Cyclic neutropenia
  - Aplastic anemia
  - Leukemia
- Autoimmune disorders
  - Systemic lupus erythematous
  - Felty's syndrome
  - Rheumatoid arthritis
- Infections
  - Viral (e.g. hepatitis, influenza; HIV, measles)
  - Fulminant bacterial infections (e.g. typhoid fever, military tuberculosis)
- Drug-induced causes
  - Antitumor antibiotics (daunorubicin, doxorubicin).
  - Alkylating agents (nitrogen mustard, busulfan and Chlorombucil).
  - Antimetabolites (methotreate, 60-mercaptepurine).
  - Anti-inflammatory drugs (phenylbutazone).
  - Antibacterial drug (chloromphenicol, trimetho-prime sulfamethoxazole penicillin).
  - Anticonvulsant drugs (phenytoin).
  - Antithyroids.
  - Hypoglycemia (tolbutamide).
  - Phenothiozines (chloropromazine).
  - Psychotropics (and antidepressants (clozapine, imipramine).
  - Miscellaneous (gold, penicillamine, mepacrine and amodiaquine).
  - Zidovudine (AZT).
- Miscellaneous
  - Severe sepsis.
  - Bone marrow infiltration (e.g. carcinoma, tuberculosis, lymphoma).
  - Hypersplenism (e.g. Portal hypertension, Fetty's syndrome, Storage diseases (Gaucher's disease).
  - Nutritional deficiency (Cobalamin and Folic Acid).

Pathophysiology

The patient with neutropenia is predisposed to infection with non-pathogenic organism that normally constitute normal body flora, as well as opportunistic pathogens. When the WBC count is depressed or immature WBCs are present, normal phagocytic mechanisms are impaired. Because of the diminished phagocytic response, the classic signs of inflammation—Redness, Heat, Swelling— May not occur. WBCs are the major components of pus; therefore, in the patient with neutropenia pus formation is also absent. Therefore, the presence of fever is of great significance in recognizing the presence of infection in a neutropenic patient.

Clinical Manifestation

When fever occurs in the neutropenic patient, it is generally assumed to be caused by infection and requires immediate attention because the immunocompromised, neutropenic condition can lead to a rapid, sometimes fatal progression of minor infections to sepsis. The mucous membranes of the throat and mouth, the skin, perineal area and pulmonary systems are common entry points for pathogenic organisms susceptible to hosts. Clinical manifestation related to these sites includes complaints of sore throat and dysphagia, appearance of the ulcerative lesions of the pharyngeal and buccal mucosa, diarrhea, rectal tenderness, vaginal itchings, or discharge, shortness of breath, and non-productive cough. These seemingly minor complaints can progress to fever, chills, sepsis, and systic shock if not recognized and treated in early stages.

Management

The primary diagnostic test for assessing neutropenia are the periheral WBC count and bone marrow aspiration and biopsy. A peripheral smear is used to assess for immature form of WBCs. The Hct level, reticulocyte count, and platelet count are done to evaluate general bone marrow function. Bone marrow aspiration or biopsy includes cultures of nose, throat sputum, urine, stool, blood as indicated and chest X-ray also is necessary to confirm concerned infection.

The factors involved in the nursing care and collaborative care of patients with neutropenia include:
- Determining the cause of the neutropenia.
- Identifying the offending organisms if an infection has developed.
- Instituting prophylactic, empiric or therapeutic antibiotic therapy.
- Administering hematopoietic growth factors (e.g. granulocyte colonystimulating factor (G-CSF).
- Instituting protection isolation practices such as strict handwashing, visitors' restrictions, private room, high efficiency particulate air (HEPA) infiltration, or laminar air flow (LAF) environment.
- Occasionally the cause of the neutropenia can be easily removed. (e.g. by termination of the medications by drug-induced condition).
- Patient teaching about precaution to prevent neutropenia.

NEUTROPHILIA

Neutrophilia is defined as a neutrophilia greater than 10,000/m. Such an increase is normal response to infections primarily bacterial infections. Prolonged elevation of neutrophil count, especially in the absence of an apparent cause, demands a diligent search for the underlying cause. Persistent elevated neutrophil counts are associated with polycythemia vera, myeloid metaplasia and various systemic and inflammatory disorders.

LEUKEMIAS

Leukemia is the general term used to describe a group of malignant disorder, affecting the blood and blood forming tissues of the bone marrow lymph system and spleen. Leukemia occurs in all age groups. It results in an accumulation of dysfunctional cells because of a loss of regulation in cell division. It follows a progressive course that is eventually fatal if untreated.

Etiology

The etiology of leukamia is unknown. Regardless of the specific type of leukemia, there is generally no single causative agent in the development of leukemia. Most results from combination of predisposing factors including genetic and environmental influences. Persons with specific chromosomal aberrations such as occurs with Down syndrome, Von Recklingh-ausens neurofibromatosis and Fanconi's anemia, have an increased incidence of acute leukemia. Chromic exposure to chemicals such as benzene, drugs that cause aplastic anemia, and radiation exposure have been associated with an increased incidence of disease. An increased risk for development of acute leukemia has been noted after cytotoxic therapy for Hodgkin's disease, non Hodgkin's lymphoma, multiple myeloma, polycythmia vera and breast, lung and testicular cancers.

Classification of Leukemia

The leukemias are classified as acute or chronic and are further divided according to cell type or maturity:
- Acute leukemia is characterized by the clonal proliferation of immature hematopoietic cells. The leukemia arises following malignant transformation of a single hematopoietic progenitore followed by cellular replication and expansion of the transformed clone. The most prominent characteristic of the neoplastic cell in acute leukemia is a defect if maturation beyond the myoloblast or promyelocyte level in AML and the lymphoblast level as ALL. Acute leukemias are subclassified as acute lymphoitic leukemia (ALL) or acute nonlymphoitic leukemia (ANLL) according to the specific morphology of the leukemia cell. ANLL further classified as acute myelogenous leukemia (AML) Promelocytic leukemia, monocytic leukemia and other varieties according to cell type.
- Chronic leukemia may be lymphocytic as in chronic lymphocytic leukemia (CLL) or granulocytic as in chronic granulocytic or myelogenous leukemia (CMD).

Acute Lymphocytic Leukemia (ALL)

Acute lymphocytic leukemia, usually occurs before 14 years of age, peak incidence is between 2–9 years of age and is older adults.

Pathophysiology

Acute lymphocytic leukemia is malignant disorder arising from a single lymphoid stem cell, with impaired maturation and accumulation of the malignant cells in the bone marrow. Diagnosis is confirmed by bone marrow aspirations or biopsy, which typically shows different stages of lymphoid development, from very immature to almost normal cells. The degree of immaturity is a guide to the prognosis, the greater the number of immature cells, the poorer will be the prognosis.

Clinical Manifestation

Signs and symptoms of ALL include anemia, bleeding, lymphadenopathy and a predisposition infection. Clinical manifestation include fever, pallor, bleeding, anorexia, fatigue and weakness; bone, joint and abdominal pain; generalized lymphadenopathy; infections of respiratory tract, anemia bleeding of mucous membrane, ecchymoses; weight loss; hepatomegaly; headache, mouth sores; neurologic manifestation including CNS involvement increased intracranial pressure, secondary to meningeal infiltration.

Management

Diagnostic findings reveals low RBC count, Hb, Hct, low platelet count low normal or high WBC count, transverse line of refraction at end of metaphysis of long bones on X-ray; hypercellular bone marrow with lymphoblasts. Lymphoblasts are also possible in CSF. A blood smear show immature lymph blasts.

Treatment of ALL include use of chemotherapeutic agents. Untreated patients have a median survival from MST of 4 to 6 months with current chemotherapeutic regimen MST is close to 5 years. Chemotherapic protocol for ALL involve three phases:

1. Induction: Often using vincristine and prednisone.
2. Consolidation: Using modified course of intensive therapy to eradicate any remaining disease, and
3. Maintenance: Usually combination of drugs including the antimetabolites 6-mercaptopurine and methotrexate.

The use of prophylactic treatment of the CNS (intrathecal administration of methotrexate with or without craniospinal radiation). Intrathecal administration and/or craniospinal radiation with eradicate leukemic cells.

The patients are advised to eat diet that contains high in protein, fiber and fluids; avoid infection (by handwashing, and avoiding crowds) and injury; take measure to decrease nausea and to promote appetite; maintain oral hygiene. Smoking and spicy and hot foods may alter taste or irritate buccal mucous membrane. These foods should be avoided and teach the patient about medication.

Acute Myelogenous Leukemia (AML)

Acute myelogenous leukemia (AML) is a disease of the pluripotent myeloid stem cell. The cause of AML is unknown. AML occurs at any age but occurs most often at adolescence and after the age of 55. There is increase in incidence with advancing age—peak incidence and is between 60-70 years of age.

Pathophysiology

AML arises from a single myeloid stem cell and is characterized by the development of immature myeloblasts in the bone marrow.

Clinical Manifestation

Clinical manifestations are similar to ALL, which includes fatigue, and weakness; headache, mouth sores, minimal hepatomegaly and lymphadenopathy anemia, bleeding, fever, infection and sternal tenderness.

Management

Diagnostic findings reveal low RC count, Hb, Hct low platelet count, low to high WBC count with myeloblasts greatly hypercellular bone marrow with myeloblasts.

Treatment includes the use of cytarabine, 6-thioquanine, and doxorubicin or daunomycin. Treated patients MST is in 2 to 3 years. In the untreated or patient unresponsive to therapy the MST is 2 to 3 months. Some studies show bone marrow transplantation may benefit the clients.

The patient and family should be instructed to avoid sources of potential infection. Signs of potential infection should be recognized and reported to health care provider. Precaution to minimize bleeding should be emphasized (soft bristled tooth brush and electric razor). The patient should be instructed to avoid possible injury or trauma (e.g. blow nose gently, avoid constipation). Dietary instruction should include the basics of nutritionally adequate diet, particularly high protein and high fiber foods. Adequate amounts of fluids (2000 to 3000 per day). Patients should be instructed about medication, effects, side effects and nursing measures.

Chronic Lymphocytic Leukemia (CLL)

The incidence of CLL increases with ages and is rare under the age of 35. It is common in men than women.

Pathophysiology

Chronic lymphocyte leukemia (CLL) is neoplasm of activated by lymphocytes. The CLL cells which morphologically resemble mature, small lymphocytes of the peripheral blood, accumulates in the bone marrow, blood lymph nodes and spleen in large number. CLL is characterized by proliferation of small, abnormal, mature B lymphocytes, often leading to decreased synthesis of immunoglobulin and depressed antibody response. The accumulation of abnormal lymphocytes begins in the lymph nodes then spreads to other lymphatic tissues and the spleen. The number of mature lymphocytes in peripheral blood smear and bone marrow are greatly increased.

Clinical Manifestation

Usually there is no symptom. Detection of disease is often during examination for unrelated conditions, chronic fatigue, anorexia, splenomegaly, lymphadenopathy and hepatomegaly. The onset is insidious with weakness, fatigue and lymphadenopathy. Symptoms include pruritic vesicular skin lesions, anemia, thrombocytopenia, and enlarged spleen. The WBC count is elevated to a level between 20,000 to 100,000. This increases blood viscosity, and a clotting episode may be the first manifestation of disease. Bone marrow briefly shows infiltration of lymphocyte.

Management

The MST of person with CLL is 4.5 to 5.5 years. As a general rule, persons are treated only when symptoms, particularly anemia, thrombocytopenia, or enlarged lymph nodes and spleen appear. Chemotherapeutic agents used in the treatment of CLL are most often one of the alkylating agents, such as chlorambucil and the glucocorticoids. Although no treatment is curative, remission may be induced by chemotherapeutics or radiation of the thymus, spleen or entire body. Patient and family education is that described for AML.

Chronic Myelogenous Leukemia (CML)

Chronic myelogenous leukemia (CML) occur between 25-60 years of age. Peak incidence is around at 45 years of age. Although the etiology of CML is unknown, benzene exposure and high doses of radiation have been associated with CML. Philadelphia Chromosome (translocation of chromosome 22 and 9) is identified in person diagnosed with CML.

Pathophysiology

The primary defect in CML is in abnormal cell leading to uncontrolled proliferation of the granulocytic cells. As a result, proliferation, the number of circulating granulocytes increases sharply.

Clinical Manifestation

There is no symptoms in disease. The classic symptoms of chronic types of leukemia also exist in CML. These include fatigue, weakness, fever, sternal tenderness, weight loss, joint pain, bone pain, massive splenomegaly and increase in sweating. CML commonly changes from a chronic indolent phase into a fulminant neoplastic process some time indistinguishable from acute leukemia. The accelerated phase of the disease (blostic phase) is characterized by increasing number of granulocytes in the peripheral blood. There is a corresponding anemia and thrombocytopenia. Fever and adenopathy also may develop.

Management

Diagnostic findings reveal low RBC count, Hb, Hct, high platelet count early, lower count later; increase in polymorphonuclear neutrophilis, normal number of lymphocytes, and normal or low number of monocytes in WBC differential; low leukocyte alkaline phosphate, presence of philadelphia-chromosomes.

The overall survival rate is poor. Only 30 percent patients will survive 5 years after diagnosis. After the onset of blast crisis the life expectancy decreased to 2 to 4 months and prognosis is grave.

The goal of therapy of CML is to control proliferation of WBC. The commonly used drugs are hydroxyurea and busulfan (monitor of WBC count needed with therapy).

Once CML is converted into blastphase of disease, anthracyclines and cytosine arabinocyde have been used. The only potential curative therapy of CML is the bone marrow transplant.

Nursing intervention of leukemia patients include taking measures to prevent infection, promoting safety, providing oral hygiene, preventing fatigue, promoting effective coping; and patient and family education regarding disease process, oral care, medications and follow up care.

Lymphedema

Lymphedema is an abnormal accumulation of lymph within the tissue caused by destruction in flow.

Lymphedema can be classified as primary or secondary:

- Primary lymphedema results from hypoplastic, aplastic or hyperplastic development of the lymphatic vessels. Symptoms may manifest at birth, during puberty or in middle age.
- Secondary or acquired lymphedema most often develops from trauma to the lymph nodes. Common causes include surgical removal of lymph node, radiation-induced fibrosis, inflammation, lymphomas and parasitic infection (filarial infection).

Pathophysiology

The lymphatic vessels carry lymph from the tissue back into venous circulation. This system is made up of small, thin, vessels that are found throughout the body in close proximity to the veins. The lymphatics begin as capillaries that drain the tissue of lymph (fluid similar to plasma) and tissue fluid that contains cells, cellular debris and proteins. The lymph flows through oval bodies called lymph nodes, which remove nucleus agents such as bacteria and toxin. The flow that drain into the thoracic duct and right lymphatic duct, which empty into the junction of the internal jugular vein and subclavian vein.

Pathophysiological changes may include (1) roughening of the surface of the symptomatic vessel, (2) dilation of some lymph channels with thickening and edema of the lymphatic tissue and (3) fibrosis and separation of elastic fibers that may present in inflammatory state. Recurrent episodes of lymphedema may cause fibrosis and hyperplasia of lymph vessels, leading to severe enlargement of the extremity called elephant basis.

Clinical Manifestation

Lymphedema of the lower extremities begin with mild swelling at the ankle, which gradually extend to the entire limb. Initially, the edema is soft and pitting, but it then progresses to firm, rubbery, non-pitting edema. Left leg swelling is more common than right leg swelling. This condition is aggravated by prolonged standing, pregnancy, obesity, warm weather and menstruation.

Management

Diagnostic test includes the use of lymphangiography. Radioisotope lymphography involves injections into the foot with subsequent scanning. A CT Scan may show a honey comb pattern in the subcutaneous compartment.

Treatment consists of elevating the foot of the best on blocks at a height of 8 inches, wearing compression support stockings, and using an intermittent pneumatic compression device. Monitoring the circumferences of the extremities can help in determining the effectiveness of treatment.

Diuretics can be prescribed to temporaily decrease the size of the limp. Long-term antibiotic therapy may be indicated to control recurrent cellulitis and infection. Surgery is restricted to severe cases of lymphedema that are unsuccessfully treated by medical management. Surgery also may be used to decrease the incidences of recurrent infection. Microsurgery involving vein grafting to small lymph vessels has been successful.

There is no special diet to treat lymphedema. However, the patient's receiving diuretic therapy required adequate potassium. Salty and spicy foods that predispose to fluid retention and edema should be avoided. Avoid standing still for long periods of times. If infection is present, advise bedrest with legs are elevated.

LYMPHOMAS

Lymphomas are malignant neoplasm originating in the bone marrow and lymphatic structures resulting in proliferation of lymphocytes. The cause for the currently rising incidence is not entirely understood. Two major types of lymphoma are—Hodgkin's disease and non-Hodgkin's disease.

Hodgkin's Disease

Hodgkin's disease is a malignant disorder of lymph nodes first described by Thomas Hodgkin in 1832. It is characterized by proliferation of abnormal giant, multinucleate cells called Reed-Sternberg cells which are located in lymph nodes.

Etiology

The etiology of the Hodgkin's disease is unknown, but there may be several factors that are thought to play a role in its development. The main interactive factors include infection with Epstein-Barr virus (EBV), genetic predisposition and exposure to occupational toxins. The first peak incidence in 30-40 years and second peak incidence occur at 55 to 77 years.

Pathophysiology

The presence of the Reed-Sternberg (RS) cell is the pathological hall mark of the disorder, but four histological substances of Hodgkin's disease have been recognized: Lymphocyte, predominant, nodular sclerosis, mixed cellularity and lymphocyte depletion.

Clinical Manifestation

The onset of symptoms in Hodgkin disease is usually insidious. The initial development is most often enlargement of cervical, axillary or inguinal lymph nodes. This lymphadenopathy affects discrete nodes that remain movable and nontender. The enlarged nodes are not painful unless pressure is exerted on adjacent nerves.

The patient may notice weight loss, fatigue, weakness, fever, chills tachycardia or night sweats. A group of initial findings include fever, night sweats and weight loss (termed B symptoms) correlate with a worse prognosis. After the ingestion of even small amounts of alcohol, individuals with Hodgkin disease may complain of a rapid onset of pain at the site of disease. The cause for the alcohol-induced pain is not known. Cough, dyspnea, strider, and dysphagea may all reflect mediastinal node involvement.

In more advanced disease, there is hepatomegaly, and splenomegaly. Anemia results from increased destruction and decreased production of erythrocytes. Other physical signs vary depending on where the disease has spread. For example, intrathoracic involvement leads to superior vena cava syndrome; enlarged retroperitoneal nodes may cause palpable abdominal masses or interfere with renal function; jaundice may occur from liver involvement and spinal cord compresses lead to paraplegia may occur with extradural involvement. Bone pain occurs as result of bone involvement.

Management

Peripheral blood analysis, lymph node biopsy, bone marrow examination and radiological evaluation are important means of evaluating Hodgkin's disease using all the information from the various diagnostic studies, a stage of disease is determined as given below:

- *Stage I:* Involvement of a single lymph node or a single extranodal site.
- *Stage II:* Involvement of two or more lymph node regions on the same site of the diaphragm or localized involvement of an extranodal site and one or more lymph node regions of the same side of the diaphragm.
- *Stage III:* Involvement of lymph node regions on both sides of the diaphragm may include a single extranodal site, the spleen, or other, now subdivided into lymphatic involvement of the upper abdomen in the spleen (ophiceliac and portal nodes). Stage III (1) and the lower abdomen nodes in the periaortic, mesenteric and iliac region (Stage III 2).
- *Stage IV:* Diffuse or disseminated disease of one or more extralymphatic organs or tissues with or without associated lymph node involvement; the extranodal

side is identified as H-hepatic, L-lung, P-pleura, M-marrow, D-dermal and O-osseous.

Treatment decisions made on the basis of stages of diseases as follows:

Stage	Recommended therapy
I, II (A or B)	Radiation
I, II (A or B with mediastinal mass 7-1/3 diameter of chest)	Combination chemotherapy followed by radiation to involved field
IIIA (minimal abdominal disease)	Combination of chemotherapy with radiation to involved sites
IIIB	Combination chemotherapy
IV (A or B)	Combination chemotherapy

The two chemotherapeutic regimens for Hodgkin's disease includes:

Drugs	Schedule
MOPP	
Nitrogen mustard	Days 1 and 8
Vincristine (oncorin)	Days 1 and 8
Procarbazine	Days 1 and 14
Predisone (circle 1 and 4 only)	Days 1 and 14
ABVD	
Dexorubiun (Adriamycin)	Days 1 and 15
Bleomycin	Days 1 and 15
Vinblastin	Days 1 and 15
Dacarbazine	Days 1 and 15

The nursing care of the Hodgkin's disease is largely based on managing pancytopenia and other side effects of the therapy. The patient undergoing radiotherapy will need special nursing intervention. Psychosocial considerations are just as important as they are with leukemia. The regimen of drug administration is a 2-week course each month or as ordered by the physician.

Non-Hodgkin's Lymphoma (NHL)

Non-Hodgkin's lymphoma (NHL) is a heterogenous group of malignant neoplasms of immune system affecting all ages.

Etiology

The cause of NHL is unknown, although viruses have been implicated. An association between the development of NHL and immunosuppressed status particularly with AIDS and organ transplant recipient has been reported. An increased incident has also been reported in persons with certain autoimmune disorders such as Sjögren's syndrome. Men once more are coming affected usually after 60 years. Burkitt's lymphoma, high grade tumor, is more common in children and persons with AIDS.

Pathophysiology

NHL's classified according to different cellular and lymph node characteristics. As more information about the cell types is discovered, evolving schemes have been used to describe different subtypes. A variety of clinical presentation and courses are recognized from indolent (slowly developing) to rapidly progressive disease. Common names for different types of NHLs include Burkitt's lymphoma, reticulum cell sarcoma, and lymphosarcoma.

Once classification separates the NHLs into lymphocytic, histiocytic and mixed cell types each of which may appear as nodular or diffuse on microscopic examination. These have been subdivided into "favorable" and "unfavorable" histology as follows:
- 'Favorable' histology
  - Nodular poorly differentiated lymphocytic lymphoma (NLPD).
  - Nodular mixed lymphocyte and histiocytic lymphoma (NML).
  - Well-differentiated lymphocytic lymphoma of the nodular (NLWD) or diffused type (DLWD).
- 'Unfavorable' histology
  - Nodular histiolytic (NHL).
  - Diffuse poorly differentiated lymphocytic (DPDL).
  - Diffused histiocytic lymphoma (DHL).
  - Diffused mixed lymphoma (DML).
  - Diffuse undifferentiated lymphoma (DUL).

In general, a nodular pattern of cell structure conveys more favorable prognosis than a diffuse pattern. All NHL involve lymphocytes arrested in various stages of development, but there is no hallmark feature in NHL that parallels the Reed-Sternberg cell of Hodgkin's disease.

Clinical Manifestation

NHL originate outside the lymphoid, the method of spread can be unpredictable, and the majority of patients have widely disseminated disease at the time of diagnosis. Primary manifestation is painless lymphoid enlargement. Patients most often have nonreader peripheral lymphadenopathy that may appear bulky. The liver and spleen may be moderately enlarged the symptoms that may occur include unexplained fever, night sweats, and weight loss plus symptoms of affected organs.

Management

The diagnosis of NHL is made by examination of pathological lymphoid tissue. Lymphoid biopsy establishes the cell type and pattern. Once the diagnosis is made, the extent of the disease (staging) must be determined. As with Hodgkin's disease, accurate staging is a staging work up similar to Hodgkin's disease.

Treatment of NHL involves radiotherapy and chemotherapy. Ironically, more aggressive lymphomas are more responsive to treatment and more likely to be cured.

In contrast, indolent lymphomas have naturally long course. But, are difficult to effectively treat. Radiotherapy alone may be effective treatment of stage I disease, but combination of radiation therapy and chemotherapy is used for other stages.

Initial chemotherapy uses allocating agents such as cyclophosphonormid and chlorambutil. However, numerous combinations have been used to try to overcome the resistance nature of the disease. The most common chemotherapeutic regimen is CDVP (Cyclophosphemide, doxoribicin, vincristine, prednisone). Other combination therapies include cyclophosphomide, (CVP) and cyclophoshamide vincristine (oncovin) procarbozine and prednison (CVPP). Furthermore, high dose therapy with peripheral blood stem cell or bone marrow transplantation is also commonly employed.

Biologic therapy such as interferon, interlukin-2 and tumor necrosis factor is also being investigated for treating NH. The nurse has a crucial role in assisting patients to develop a realistic approach to the illness and to meet successfully the demands and limitations imposed by illness and its treatment. The nurse has to provide some of the needed support and guidance as the person learns to incorporate the illness into daily life. For which patient teaching needs as points covered in Hodgkin's disease.

Infectious Mononucleosis

Infectious mononucleosis is an acute disease caused by a herpes-like virus, the Epstein-Barr virus (EBV). It occurs more often in young persons with the highest incidence occurring between 15 to 30 years of age.

It is a benign disease with favorable prognosis. The onset may be subtle, appearing almost as flu-like symptoms. Malaise is a common early complaint, and it is often accompanied by fever, lymphadenopathy, sore throat, headache, generalized aches, and pains resembling those of influenza and moderate enlargement of the liver and spleen. Pruritus, palatal petechias, jaundice and rash may be present. The mode of transmission is via intimate contact with the spread of virus through the saliva. Rupture of the spleen and encephalis are rare complications.

Management

Diagnosis of infection mononucleosis is established by the heterophil agglutination or monospot blood test. Other lab tests show there is an increase in atypical lymphocytes. At the height of the disease the WBC count may range between 10,000 to 20,000 cells/mm.

Infectious mononucleosis is self limiting and with rest. Affected persons usually recover spontaneously within 2 to 3 weeks. Effectiveness of antiviral therapy has not been established. The use of corticosteroid may be indicated in severe cases with tonsillar enlargement and potential airway obstruction. Acetaminophen is effective in relieving fever, sore throat, and myalgias. Most persons can return to activities that do not require heavy exertion in 1 to 2 weeks and to normal activities in 4 to 6 weeks. Some persons have persistent fatigue for several months. Nursing management is supportive and focusses on the relief of symptoms and promotion rest.

The patient is instructed to avoid heavy lifting or contact sports at least one month until splenomegaly resolves. An enlarged spleen is susceptible to rupture. Additional teaching includes the need for increasing fluids and to use appropriate handwashing to prevent the spread of disease. Person with this disease is to be cautioned against donating blood and avoid events that oral secretions of the infective person should not spread to others.

Multiple Myeloma

Multiple myeloma or plasma cell myeloma is a condition in which neoplastic plasma cells infiltrate the bone marrow and destroy bone.

Etiology

There are many predictions regarding the etiology of this condition, including chronic inflammation, chronic hypersensitivity reactions, and viral influences, but no actual cause has been found.

Pathophysiology

The disease process involves excessive production of plasma cells. Plasma cells are activated B cells, which produce immunoglobulins (antibodies) that normally serve to protect the body. However, in multiple myeloma malignance plasm cells infiltrate the bone marrow and produce abnormal and excessive amount of immunoglobulin (usually IgG, IgA, IgD, IgE). This abnormal immunoglobulin formed as myeloma protein. Furthermore, plasma cell production of excessive and abnormal amounts of cytokins (IL-4, IL-5, IL-6) also plays an important role in pathological process of bone destruction. As myeloma protein increases normal plasma cells are reduced which further compromises the body's normal immune response. Ultimately the plasma cell destroys bone and invades the lymph nodes, spleen and kidneys.

Clinical Manifestations

The condition develops slowly and insidiously. The patient often does not manifest symptom until the disease advanced at which time, skeletal pain is the major manifestation. Pain in the pelvis, spine and ribs is particularly common. Diffuse osteoporosis develops as the myeloma protein destroys more bone. Osteolytic lesions are seen in the skull, vertebrae and ribs. Vertebral destruction can lead to collapse of vertebrae with ensuing compression of the spinal cord, requiring emergency measures to prevent paraplegia (radiation, surgery, chemotherapy). Loss of bone integrity can lead to pathological fractures. Bony degeneration also causes calcium to be lost from bones, eventually causes hypercalcemia.

Hypercalemia may cause, renal, GI, or neurologic changes such as polyuria, anorexia and confusion. Later hyperuricemia and renal failure may occur. There may be symptom of anemia, thrombocytopenia, and granulocytopenia, all of which are related to the replacement of normal bone marrow elements with plasma cells.

Management

Diagnosis conformed by required laboratory, radiologic and bone marrow examination.

Treatment includes administering pamidronate (for skeletal pain) and maintaining an adequate hydration are primary nursing considerations to minimize hypercalemia. In addition, weight bearing helps bones reabsorb some of the circulation. Calcium and corticosteroids may augment the excretion of calcium. Once chemotherapy is initiated, the uric acid levels rise because of the increased cell destruction. Hyperuricemia must be resolved by ensuring adequate hydration and using allapurinol.

Suitable analgesics may be used to reduce pain. There may be potential for pathological fracture, the nurse must be careful when moving and ambulating the patient. Braces, especially for spine may also help to control pain. The patient's psychosocial needs require skilled management sometime.

Disorders of Spleen

The spleen performs many functions and is affected by many illnesses. The term "hypersplenism" refers to the occurrence of splenomegaly and peripheral cytopenia (Anemia, leukopenia, thrombocytopenia).

There are many different causes of splenomegaly which includes:
- Hereditary hemolytic anemias: Sickle cell disease, Thalassemia.
- Autoimmune cytopenia: Acquire hymolytic anemia.

Immune Thrombocytopenia

- Infections and inflammation: Bacterial endocarditis, Infectious mononucleosis, SLE, sarcoidosis, HIV infection and viral hepatitis.
- Infiltrative diseases: Acute and chronic leukemia, lymphemias, polycythemia cera.
- Congestion: Cirrhosis of liver, congestive heart failure.

When the spleen enlarges, its normal filtering and sequestering capacity increases. Consequently, there is often a reduction in the number of circulating blood cells. A slight to moderate enlargement of the spleen usually asymptomatic and found during a routine examination of the abdomen. Even massive splenomegaly can be well tolerated, but the patient may complain of abdominal discomfort and early satiety. Other techniques to assess the size of the spleen includes TC colloid liver-spleen scan, CT scan and ultrasound scan.

Occasionally laparotomy and splenectomy are indicated in the disorder or treatment of splenomegaly. Splenectomy can have a dramatic effect in increasing peripheral RBCs, WBC and platelet count. Another major indication of splenectomy is splenic rupture. The spleen may rupture from trauma, inadvertent tearing during other surgical procedure and diseases such as mononucleosis.

Nursing responsibilities for the patient with spleen disorders vary depending on the nature of the problems.

BLOOD TRANSFUSION

Traditionally the term Blood Transfusion meant the administration of whole blood. Blood transfusion now has broader meaning because of the ability to administer specific components of blood, such as platelets, RBCs, or plasma. Blood component therapy is frequently used in managing hemotologic diseases. Many therapeutic and surgical procedures depend on blood product support. However, blood component therapy only temporarily supports the patient until the underlying problem is resolved. Because transfusions are not free from hazards, they should be used only if necessary. Nurses must be careful to avoid developing a complacent attitude abouit this common but potential dangerous therapy.

Type of Blood Components

The type of blood components and their indications for use are as given below:

Red Blood Cells

- *Packed RBCs (PRBCs):* RBCs separated from plasma and platelets. Packed RBCs are prepared from whole blood by sedimentation or centri–fugation. One unit contains 250-350 ml. PRBCs indicated for severe or symptomatic anemia, and acute or moderate blood loss. Use of RBCs for treatment allows remaining components of blood (e.g. platelets, albumin and plasma) to be used for other purposes. There is less danger of fluid overload as compared with whole blood. PRBCs are preferred RBC source because they are more components or specific.
- *Autologous PRBCs:* Used in elective surgery for which blood replacement is expected. These units may be stored for upto 35 days.
- *Washed RBCs:* RBCs are washed with sterile isotonic saline before transfusion. These are used when previous allergic reactions to transfusion. These are used when previous allergic reactions to transfuson. There is increased removal of immunoglobulins and proteins.

- *Frozen RBCs:* Frozen RBCs prepared from RBCs using glycerol for protection and frozen. They can be stored for 3 years at –188.6°F (–87°C). Frozen RBCs are indicated when autotransfusion is needed, or patient with previous febrile reactions to transfusion. There are infrequently because filters remove WBCs, i.e. they relatively free from leukocytes and microemboli, but they are expensive.

    Since RBCs are frozen in a glycerol solution, cells are washed after thawing to remove glycerol. They must be used within 24 hours of thawing. Successive washing with saline removes majority of WBCs and plasma proteins.
- *Leukocyte-poor RBCs:* RBCs from which most leukocytes have been removed. It is used when client has previous sensitivity to leukocyte antigens from prior transfusions or from pregnancy. In this, fewer RBCs than packed RBCs washed leukocyte poor RBCs units have more RBCs than nonwashed.
- *Neocytes:* RBC units with high number or reticulocytes (young RBCs). They are used in transfusion-dependent anemias. There will be fewer problems with iron overload, but expensive.

Other Cellular Component

- *Platelets*
    - Random donor packs: Platelets are prepared from fresh whole blood within 4 hours after collections. One unit contains 30-60 ml of platelet concentrate. In this, platelets are separated from RBCs by centrifuges: given in 50 ml of plasma. Platelets are used when bleeding caused by thrombocytopenia, Thrombocytopenia, and disseminated intravascular coagulation (DIC). In this, plasma base is rich in coagulation factors. Platelets preparation can also be packed, washed or made leukocyte poor.
    - Pheresis packs: Multiple units of platelets can be obtained from one donor by platelet pheresis. Platelets from an HLA-matched donor are separated by apheresis. They can be kept at room temperature for 1-5 days depending on type of collection and storage bag used. It is used for allosensitized persons with thrombocytopenia. The bag should be agitated periodically. Expected increase is 10,000/mkl/u. Failures to have rise may be due to fever, sepsis, splenomegaly or DIC.
- *Granulocytes:* Granular leukocytes separated by apheresis. It is used for granulocytopenia from malignancy or chemotherapy. Allergen sensitiza-tion may occur with chills and fever.

Plasma Components

- *Fresh frozen plasma (FFP):* Freezing of plasma within 4 hours of collection. Here, liquid portion of whole blood separates from cells and frozen. One unit contains 200–250 mL. Plasma is rich in clotting factors but contains no platelets. It may be stored for one year. It must be used within 2 hours after thawing. It may be indicated when bleeding is caused by deficiency in clotting factors (e.g. DIC clotting deficiencies, hemorrhage, massive transfusion, liver disease, hemophilia, defibrination. It should be administered through a filter. Use of plasma in treating hypovolemic shock is being replaced by pure preparations such as albumin plasma expanders.
- *Factor concentrate VIII and IX:* Prepared from large donor pools. Heated to inactivate HIV. It is used in VIII; hemophilia A and IX hemophilia B. There is increased risk of hepatitis (VIII, IX) and thromboembolism (IX). It can be given in small volumes.
- *Cryoprecipitate:* Precipitated material obtained from FFP when thawed. It is used for hemophilia A. Infection of burns, hypofibrinogenaemia, uremic bleeding. It contains factor VIII, XIII and fibrinogen.
- *Serum albumen:* (Normal serum albumin, plasma proteinfraction). In this albumin is chemically processed from pooled plasma. Albumin is prepared from plasma. It can be stored for 5 years. It is available in 5 percent or 25 percent solution. Albumin 25 g/100 ml is osmotically equal to 500 ml of plasma. Hyperosmolar solution acts by moving water from extravascular to intravascular space. Serum albumin is used in hypovolemic shock, hypoalbuminemia, burns and hemorrhagic shock. Its use has no risk of the hepatitis, does not require ABO compatibility, but lack of clotting factors, hypotension may occur if PFF is given faster than 10 ml/min.
- *Immunoserum globulin:* Obtained from plasma of preselected donors with specific antibodies. It is used in hypogammaglobinemia and used as prophylaxis for hepatitis A and tetanus. It is given intramuscularly.

Administrative Procedure of Blood Components

Blood components can be administered safely through a 19-gauge or larger needle into a free-flowing IV line. Larger size needles (e.g. 19 gauge) may be preferred if rapid transfusions are given. Smaller size needles can be used for platelets, albumin and cryoprecipitates. Peripherally inserted central catheters (PICCs) are not recommended because of increased incidence of clogged lines due to slow blood flow. The blood administration tubing with a filter should have a stop cock or other means to develop a closed system, with blood open to one part and isotonic saline solution infusing through the other. Dextrose solutions or lacted ringers should not be used because they induce RBCs hemolysis. No other additives (including medications) should be given via the same tubing unless the tubing is cleaned with saline solution.

When the blood or blood components have been obtained from the blood bank, positive identification of the donor blood and recipient must be made. Improper product to patient identification causes transfusion reactions, thus placing a great responsibility on nursing personnel to carry out the identification procedure appropriately. The nurse should follow the policy and procedure at the place of employment (hospital or institution or nursing home). The blood bank is responsible for typing and crossmatching the donors' blood with the recipients blood.

The blood should be administered as soon as it is brought to the patient. It should not be refrigerated on the nursing unit. If the blood is not used in right way, it should be returned to the blood bank.

During the first 15 minutes or 50 ml of blood infusion, the nurse should stay with the patient. If there are any untoward reactions, they are most likely to occur at this time. The rate of infusion during this period should be not more than 2 ml/minute. Blood should not be infused quickly unless an emergency exists. Rapid infusion of cold blood may cause the patient to become chilled. If rapid replacement of large amounts of blood is necessary, a blood warming device may be used.

After the first 15 minutes, the rate of infusion is governed by the clinical conditions of the patient and the product being infused. Most patients not in danger of fluid overload can tolerate the infusion of 1 unit of packed RBCs over 2 hours. The transfusion should not take more than 4 hours to administer. Blood remaining after 4 hours should not be infused because of the length of time it has been removed from refrigeration.

If a blood transfusion reactions occur, the following steps should be taken:
- Stop the blood transfusion.
- Maintain a patent IV line with saline solution.
- Notify the blood bank and the physician immediately.
- Recheck identifying tags and numbers.
- Monitor vital signs and urine output.
- Treat symptoms as per physician's order.
- Use the blood bag and tubing and send them to blood bank for examination.
- Complete transfusion reaction reports.
- Collect required blood and urine specimens at intervals stipulated by hospital policy to evaluate for hemolysis.
- Document on transfusion reaction form and patient chart.

The blood bank and laboratory are responsible for identifying the types of reaction.

The major non-immunological transfusion reaction include the following:
- *Circulatory overload:* Can occur when blood is given too rapidly or in large quantities. The elderly are particularly vulnerable. Patient develops signs of fluid overload and pulmonary congestion. The transfusion is stopped and oxygen and diuretic may be administered. The signs and symptoms of circulatory overload includes:
  - Dyspnea
  - Peripheral edema
  - Chest tightness
  - Jugular vein distention
  - Headache
  - Rales
  - Hypertension
  - Abnormal heart sounds
  - Cough
  - Hypertension
  - Cyanosis
- *Sepsis:* Bacterial contamination may occur at any time during the collection or handling of blood. Signs of sepsis begin almost immediately. The transfusion is stopped and the patient receives antibiotics and treatment for shock if it occurs. The signs of sepsis include:
  - Fever greater than 40°C.
  - Abdominal Cramps.
  - Nausea.
  - Vomiting.
  - Diarrhea.
  - Septic shock.
- *Disease transmission:* Hepatitis, CMV, and HIV are the most common diseases transmitted by blood transfusion. Hepatitis A and B are effectively identified with current screening capabilities but hepatitis C is still readily transmissible.

The following points are to be kept in mind when patient is receiving a blood transfusion.
- Carefully check all of the following:
  * Identity of patient to receive transfusion.
  * The label of the unit of blood for the name of the person for whom it is intended; make certain that if matches the patient's wrist band before administering the blood.
  * Expiration date of the blood.
  * Color and consistency of blood (if bag appears to have clots, gas or a dark purple color, it could be contaminated and should not be infused).
- Obtain base line vital signs and check again at frequent intervals throughout the procedure.
- Administer all blood products through micron mesh filters.
- Assess patient for any unusual sensation felt throughout the transfusion (This information helps with early identification of any reaction that occurs).
- Infuse blood within 4 hours after it is taken from the blood bank (to prevent bacterial growth).

- If blood cannot be infused within 4 hours, return it to the blood bank for proper refrigeration.
- Follow facility guidelines for proper disposal of empty blood bag and tubing.
- Record patient's response to the infusion.
- Report any adverse effect to the primary care provider immediately.
- Return the blood bag and tubing to the laboratory for testing if a reaction occurs.

Complication of Blood Transfusion

The complications of transfusion therapy may be significant and necessitate judicious evaluation of the patient. The common immunological reaction to blood transfusion and identification, management are as follows:

- Acute hemolytic reactions caused by transfusion of ABO-incompatible blood. This is an example of a type II Cytotoxic hypersensitivity reaction. When infusion of ABO-incompatible whole blood, RBCs or components containing 10 ml or more RBCs antibodies in the recipient's plasma attach to antigens on transfused RBCs causing RBC destruction. The chemical manifestations include chills, fever, low-backpain, tachycardia, tachypnoea, hypotension, vascular collapse, hemoglobinuria, haemoglobinemia, bleeding, acute renal failure, shock, cardiac arrest and death.

  When it occurs following measures to be taken immediately.
  - Treat shock if present.
  - Draw blood samples for serological testing slowly. To avoid hemolysis from the procedure, use a new venipuncture (not an existing central line and avoid small gauge needles. Send urine specimen to the laboratory.
  - Maintain BP with IV colloid solution. Give diuretics as prescribed to maintain urine flow.
  - Insert indwelling catheter or measures voided amounts to monitor hourly urine output. Dialysis may be required if renal failure occurs.
  - Do not transfuse additional RBC containing components until the transfusion service/blood bank has provided newly cross-matched unit.

  Acute hemolytic reactions can be prevented by meticulously verify and document patient identification from sample collections to component infusion and transfuse blood slowly for first 15-20 minutes with nurse is at patient's side.

- Febrile, nonhemolytic reaction: reactions are most common. It may be due to sensitization to donor WBCs, platelets or plasma proteins. There will be sudden chills and fever (Rise in temperature of greater than 1°C), headache, flushing, anxiety, muscle pain. When it occurs measures to be taken immediately include:
  - Give antipyretics as prescribed—Do not give aspirin to thrombocytopenia patients.
  - Do not restart transfusion unless physician orders.
  - This reaction can be prevented by considering and administering leucocyte poor blood products (filtered, washed, or frozen) for patients with a history of two or more such reactions.

- Mild allergic reactions may be due to sensitivity to foreign plasma proteins. There will be flush in, itching, urticaria (hives). The nursing intervention included here are:
  - Administering antihistamine as directed.
  - If symptoms are mild and transient, transfusion may be restarted slowly.
  - Do not restart transfusion if fever or pulmonary symptoms develop.

  This reaction can be prevented by prophylactic treatment with glucocorticosteroids or antihistamines. (Decadron, Benydryl) given 30–60 minutes before blood transfusion.

- Anaphylactic and severe allergic reaction are due to sensitivity to donor plasma proteins and/or infusion of IgA proteins to IgA deficient recipient who has developed IgA antibody. In this, there is anxiety, urticaria, wheezing, tightness and pain in chest, difficulty in swallowing, progressing to cyanosis, shock and possible cardiac arrest. This can be managed with following measures:
  - Initiate CPR if indicated.
  - Have epinephrine ready for injection (0.4 mL of a 1:1000 solution SC or 0.1 mk of 1:1000 solution diluted to 10 mL with saline for IV use).
  - Do not restart transfusions.

  This reaction can be prevented by transfusing extensively washed RBC products from which all plasma has been removed. Alternatively use blood from IgA deficient donor. Use autologous components.

- *Delayed hemolytic reactions:* In this there is fever, chills, backpain, jaundice, anemia, hemoglobinurea. Nursing intervention includes: monitor adequately urinary output and degree of anemia, treat fever with tybenol (PML). May need further blood transfusions. This will be prevented by doing more specific type and crossmatch when giving patient blood.

- Post transfusion graft versus host disease: There will be anorexia, nausea, diarrhea, high fever, rash, stomatitis, liver dysfunction. For which there is no effective treatment. Administer steroids. This can be prevented by giving irradiated blood products.

- *Noncardiac pulmonary edema:* There will be fever, chills, hypotension cough, orthopnoea, cyanosis, shock. Here, stop transfusion; continue IV saline; administer steroids as directed; give furosemide (Lasix) and epinephrine as ordered.

- *Cardiac overload:* Occurs when fluid administered faster than the circulation can accommodate. Due to this, cough, dyspnea, pulmonary congestion, headache, hypertension, tachycardia and distended neck vein occurs. When it occurs, nursing measures include:
  - Place patient upright with feet in dependent position.
  - Administer prescribed diuretics, oxygen and morphine
  - Phlebotomy may be indicated.
  - Cardiac overload can be prevented by
  - Adjusting transfusion volume and flow rate based on patient size and clinical status.
  - Have blood bank divide unit into smaller aliquots for better spacing of fluid input.
- *Sepsis:* Occurs when transfusion of bacterially-infected blood components. There will be a rapid onset of chills, high fever, vomiting, diarrhea, marked hypotension or shock. Nursing interventions here include:
  - Obtain culture of patient's blood and send bag with remaining blood and tubing to blood bank for further study.
  - Treat septicaemia as directed antibiotics, IV fluids and vasopressors.

Sepsis can be prevented by collection, process storing and transfusion of blood products according to blood banking standards and infusion within 4 hours of starting time.

Prevention is the key to management of transfusion. Accurate prescreening of potential donors, meticulous laboratory testing, and close patient monitoring are all essential components of care. The common screening guidelines for blood donors includes that persons with any of following are not permitted to donate blood.

- History of infectious diseases such as hepatitis HIV infection and AIDS tuberculosis, syphilis or malaria.
- Malignant diseases.
- Allergies or asthma.
- Polycythemia vera.
- Abnormal bleeding tendencies.
- Hypotension (current).
- Anemia (current).
- Recent pregnancy or major surgery.
- Men with at least one homosexual or bisexual contact since 1975 (concern for AIDS).
- International travel to malarial areas or high risk countries (concern for AIDS).
- Blood transfusion during last 6 months.
- History of jaundice.
- Diseases of the heart, lung or liver.
- Immunizations or vaccinations with attenuated viral vaccine rubella or rabies vaccine.
- Hemoglobin level below 13.5 g/dl for men, or 12.4 g/dl for women.
- Abnormalities in vital signs particularly fever.

CHAPTER 7

Nursing Management of Genitourinary Disorders

INTRODUCTION

Urology is the study of urinary tract and renal is related to kidneys. Urological and renal nursing (renourological nursing) is the study of the urinary tract and kidneys and nursing management of disorders of urinary tract as well as kidneys. Nursing professional have played an vital role in this area and needs to have an understanding of terminology assessment, pathophysiology and treatment for disorders of urinary system to enhance the delivery of adequate and appropriate care to respective patient.

NURSING ASSESSMENT OF GENITOURINARY SYSTEM

Subjective renal assessment begins with an assurance begins with an assessment of the patient's overall state of health and perceptions of what constitutes good health, rather than merely listening of documented health problems and concerns. The interview that explores any patient concerns or health problems especially any urinary tract symptoms which includes:

- *Dysuria:* Pain/burning with voiding.
- *Frequency:* Voids multiple times during the day either in large or small amounts.
- *Nocturia:* Awakens to void; abnormal when it occurs multiple times during the sleep cycle.
- *Hematuria:* Red blood cells in the urine may be gross (visible to eye) or microscopic (detectable with urine screen and microscope).
- *Hesitancy:* Difficulty initiating voiding.
- *Polyuria:* Urine output greater than 3000 mL/24 hours.
- *Oliguria:* Urine output less than 400 mL/24 hours.
- *Anuria:* Urine output less than 100 mL/24 hours.
- *Urgency:* The need to void immediately.
- *Urine odour:* Foul smell associated with urine.
- *Frothing:* Excessive foaming of urine.
- *Myoglobinuria:* Red-brown at times black, pigment in the urine.

When a kidney problem is suspected, the nurse asks the patient directly about the symptoms, moderate or severe renal disease can cause significant observable pathological changes. The clinical significance of urinary tract symptoms are as follows:

- *Dysuria:* Found in urinary tract infection (UTI).
- *Frequency:* Urinary tract infection, retention, hyperglycemia with increased fluid intake, prostatic hypertrophy.
- *Urgency:* UTI, bladder irritation, trauma, and tumor.
- *Nocturia:* Diuretics, prostatic hypertrophy, renal failure/insufficiency, increase fluid intake and congestive heart failure.
- *Hesitancy:* Partial urethral obstruction, posturinary catheter removal, CNS or spinal cord disease, postprostatectomy and laxity of perineal muscles in older women.
- *Frothing:* Presence of protein in the urine.
- *Foul odor:* Urinary tract infections.
- *Polyuria:* Diabetes mellitus, hormonal abnormality, diabetes inspidus high output renal failure.
- *Oliguria:* Renal failure, urinary retention/obstruction.
- *Anuria:* Renal failure, total obstructions (trauma, mass).
- *Myoglobinuria:* Muscle tissue breakdown following extreme physical exertion or massive trauma (myoglobin in muscle Hb) can result in renal failure.
- *Hematuria:* Renal calculi, urinary tract infection, inflammation of the kidney or bladder, trauma to the kidney or urinary tract. Posturinary catheter removal and menses.

The patient should be questioned about the presence or history of disease that are known to be related to the renal or other urologic problems, which includes hypertension, diabetes mellitus, gout or other metabolic disorders, connective tissue disorders, skin or upper respiratory tract infections of streptococcal origin, tuberculosis, viral hepatitis, congenital disorders, neurologic condition and specific urinary problems such as cancer, infections, BPH, calculosis, etc.

Diagnostic Studies of Genitourinary System

Diagnostic studies are important in locating and understanding the problems of the urinary system. The nursing responsibilities related to diagnostic studies include providing the patient with an adequate information of the procedure. The period during a diagnostic work up is typically a time of anxiety for most patients for which patient should be explained regarding the diagnostic procedure and also should be instructed on personal responsibility during particular study according to procedures. Diagnostic studies of the urinary system often cause embarrassment and emotional stress. Examination of the urinary system may be perceived as intrusion on a personal body area. The nurse should alleviate anxiety by providing privacy and protecting the patient's modesty.

Here are the usual diagnostic studies and the routine responsibilities of nurses.

URINE STUDIES

Urinalysis

This is a general examination of urine to establish baseline information or provide data to establish tentative diagnosis and determine whether further studies are to order. Here, the nursing responsibilities are:
- Try to obtain first urinated morning specimen.
- Ensure that specimen is examined within 1 hour of urinating.
- Wash perineal area if soiled with menses or faecal material.

Creatinine Clearance

Creatinine is a waste product of protein-breakdown (primary body muscle mass). Clearance of creatinine by the kidneys approximates the GFR. Normal finding is 85–135 ml/min.

Nursing responsibilities in this test are to:
- Collect 24-hours urine specimen.
- Discard first urination when test is started.
- Save urine from all subsequent urination for 24 hours and add specimen to collections container.
- Ensure urine collection container used.

Urine Culture (Clean Catch "Midstream")

This study is done to compress suspected urinary tract infection and identify causative organisms. Normally bladder is sterile, but urethra contains bacteria, and a few WBCs. If properly collected, stored and handled: < 10,000 organisms/ml usually indicate no infections. But > 100,000/mL indicates infection.

When collecting a mid stream urine specimen, the nurse has to collect needed equipments which include:
- Sterile container for the urine.
- Three sponges (cotton or gauze) saturated with cleansing solution and follow general direction.
- Touch only the outside of the collecting container.
- Collect the urine in container well after urinary stream is started and follow special directions as given below.

For Female
- Keep labia separated throughout the procedure.
- Cleanse the meatus with one front to back motion with each of the three cleansing sponges.

For Males
- Retract the foreskin of man in uncircumcised.
- Cleanse the glans with each of the three cleansing sponges.

The collected specimen are ideally transported to the laboratory within 30 minutes or promptly refrigerated.

Concentration Test (Fishberg)

This study evaluates renal concentration ability. The test is used to determine ability of kidney to conserve fluid and to establish differential diagnosis for diabetes insipidus and psychogenic polydypsia. The normal readings are:
- Urine volume 300 ml/12 hours.
- Specific gravity 1.020 to 1.035.
- Urine osmolality of 850 mOsm/kg or greater.

In this test, instruct patient to fast after given time in evening (in usual procedure). No fluid can be taken during test period. For period 8–12 hours usually during night. First morning void ensures maximal concentration. Three-hourly urine specimen are collected for volume, specific gravity, and osmolality after test period. Patient should be observed for signs of vascular collapse.

Urine Cytology

This study is to identify charges in cellular structure indicative of malignancy, especially bladder cancer. Here obtain urine and send immediately to laboratory. The first morning specimen should not be used.

Timed Urine Collection

A timed urine collection involves pooling of all the urine patient excretes over specific period of time. The test is often required for urological diagnosis. The duration of urine collection may vary from 2 to 4 hours, with 24 hours collection being the most common. The pooled urine specimen is examined for sugar, proteins, sediment (blood cells and casts). 17 ketosteroids, electrolytes, catecholamines, and breakdown products of protein metabolism. These tests provide information on:
- The ability of kidneys to excrete and conserve various salts.
- The production of various hormones that are excreted in urine.
- Changes in the body regulation of glucose metabolism.
- Identification of organisms difficult to recognize through routine urine culture and
- The presence of abnormal cells and debris in the urine. While collecting a timed urine specimen, the nurse
- Instructs the patient to empty the bladder and discard the urine at the appointed time to start the test.
- Save the urine from all subsequent voidings.
- Provide specific directions for storing the urine. Some specimen need to be kept cold during the collection period, and some need preservatives and some need no special care.
- Instruct the patient to void into a separate receptacle before defecating to avoid contaminating the specimen.

- Instruct the patient to empty the bladder and add the urine to the collection at the appointed time to end the test.
- Send the designated amount (properly labeled) to the laboratory.

Timed urine test also may involve collecting urine from more than one source (e.g. through the nephrostomy tube) follow instructions accordingly.

Blood Chemistries

- *Blood urea nitrogen (BUN)*: This study is most commonly used to identify presence of renal problems. Concentration of urea, in blood is regulated by rate at which kidney excretes urea. The normal finding is 5.20 mg/100 ml. Test indicates ability of kidneys to excrete nitrogenous wastes. BUN can be affected by high protein diet, blood in GI tract and catabolic state (injury, infection, fever and poor nutrition). Be aware that when interpreting BUN, nonrenal factors may cause increase (e.g. rapid cell destructions from infection, GI bleeding, trauma, athletic activity with excessive muscle breakdown and corticosteroid therapy).
- *Serum creatinine*: This is more reliable than BUN as a determinant of renal function. Creatinine is end product of muscle and protein metabolism and is liberated at a constant rate. Normal finding in men: 0.85–1.5 mg/100 ml and in women 0.7–1.25 mg/100 ml. Test indicates ability of kidneys to excrete creatinine. Serum creatinine gives a rough estimate of GFR. No specific preparation needed for test. Diet and metabolic rate have little effect on creatinine values.
- *Uric acid*: This study is used as a screening test primarily for disorders of purine metabolism but can indicate kidney disease as well. Values depend on renal function and rate of purine metabolism and dietary intake of food rich in purines. Normal values is 2.5–5.5 ml/dl in women and 4.5–6.5 ml/dl in men.
- *Sodium (Na+)*: It is main extracellular electrolyte determining blood volume. Usually values stay within normal range until late stages of renal failure. Normal findings are 135-145 m Eq/litre.
- *Potassium (K+)*: Kidneys are responsible for excreting majority of body's potassium. Potassium determinations are critical because potassium is one of the first electrolytes to become abnormal. Elevated K+ levels of > m Eq/L can lead to muscle weakness and cardiac arrhythmias. Normal findings is 3.5–5.5 m Eq/L.
- *Calcium (Ca+)*: Calcium is main mineral in bone and helps in muscle contraction, neurotransmission, and clotting. In renal disease, decreased absorption of calcium leads to renal osteodystrophy. Normal findings is 9–11 mg/dL (4.5–5.5 mEq/L).
- *Phosphorous*: Phosphorous balance is inversely related to a calcium balance. In renal disease, phosphorous levels are elevated because the kidney is the primary excretary organ. Soft tissue calcification may occur in both phosphorous in Ca- are elevated. Normal findings is 2.8–4.5 mg/dl.
- *Bicarbonate* (HCO_3^-): Most patients in renal failure have metabolic acidosis and low serum HCO_3 levels. Normal finding is 20–30 m Eq/L.

Radiological Studies

- *KUB (Kidney, Ureter, Bladder) X-ray films:* This study involves flat-plate X-ray examination of abdomen, and pelvis and delineates size, shape and position of kidneys. In this gross visualization of KUB location of calcifications and stones are possible. For this test bowel cleansing sometimes is ordered.
- *IVP (Intravenous Pyelography):* X-ray examination visualizes urinary tract after IV injection of contrast material (dye).

  The purposes of IVP are:
  - Determination of size and location of kidneys.
  - Demonstrations of presence of cysts or tumors.
  - Outline of filling of renal pelvis.
  - Outline of ureters and bladder.

  In this procedure:
  - X-ray film of abdomen (KUB) taken to identify size and position of kidneys.
  - Radiopaque dye given intravenously.
  - X-ray films of kidneys taken at 3-, 5-, 10 and 20-minutes interval.

  For this procedure, preparation includes:
  - Evening before procedure, give cathartic or enema to empty colon of feces and gas.
  - Keep patient on NPO status 8 hours prior to the procedure.
  - Before the procedure, assess the patient for any history of allergy to iodine, shelfish, or dyes to avoid anaphylactic reactions.
  - Inform patient that a feeling of warmth, flustering of the face, and salty taste in the mouth may occur as the dye is injected.
  - Inform the procedure involved, lying on table and heavy serial X-rays taken.
  - Inform patient that numerous X-ray and films are taken during the procedure. This does not indicate a problem.
  - During the procedure, patient should be carefully monitored for signs and symptoms of a reaction to dye, including respiratory distress, diaphoresis, urticaria, instability of viral signs or unusual sensations. Emergency equipment should be available.
- After the procedure, fluids are forced to help excrete or flush out the contrast material and prevent renal failure.

- *Nephrotomogram:* X-ray is taken with rotating tubes. Multiple exposures are taken to visualize specific sections of the kidney after IV injection of contrast material (dye). Explain procedure and prepare patient as for IVP.
- *Retrograde Pyelography:* This is performed for visualization of urinary tract. X-ray of urinary tract is taken after the injection of contrast material into kidneys, cystoscope is inserted and urethral catheters are inserted through it into renal pelvis. Contrast material (Radiopaque matter is injected through the catheters. X-ray films are taken of renal collecting structure. Here also prepare patient as for IVP and
    - Inform patient that pain may be experienced from distension of pelvis and discomfort from cystoscope.
    - Inform patient that general anesthesia may be given for procedure.
- *Cystogram:* In this, contrast material is instilled into bladder via cystoscope or catheter. Its purpose is to visualize bladder and evaluate vesicoureteral reflux. Nursing responsibility is as in cystoscope.
- *Renal Angiography:* The purpose of this test is to visualization of renal circulation. Particularly, useful in evaluating renal contrast material (dye) often injected directly into femoral artery by passing a catheter through artery to level of renal arteries.
  Nursing implications are the same as for IVP.
    - Patient must be observed for dye-induced acute renal failure and bleeding at arterial puncture site especially in the first 4 hours.
    - The pressure dressing should be checked for fresh bleeding.
    - The puncture site should be checked for tenderness or swelling.
    - Vital signs and distal pulses must be assessed frequently for every 15 minutes and 4 hours.
    - Bed rest should be maintained for 8 hours after the procedure.
- *Ultrasound:* In this, small external ultrasound probe is placed on patient's skin. Conductive gel is applied to the skin. Noninvasive procedure involves passing sound waves into body structure and recording images as they are reflected back. Computer interprets tissue density based on sound waves and displays it in picture form. Study is most valuable in detection of renal or perirenal masses. Differential diagnosis of renal cysts, solid masses and identification of obstruction It can be used safely in patients with renal failure. Since this procedure is painless and noninvasive. A full bladder is required to delineate the abdominal structure.
- *CT Scan:* This study provides excellent visualization of kidneys and renal circulation using an X-ray beam rotated around body. A kidney size can be evaluated, tumors, abscesses, suprarenal masses (e.g. adrenal tumors, pheochromocytomas) and obstruction can be detected.

  Advantage of CT over ultrasound is its ability to distinguish subtle difference in density. Use of IV administered contrast material during CT accentuates density of renal tissue and helps differentiate masses. Whole body CT scanner segments kidneys. If dye is used, the same nursing implications apply as listed in IVP.
- *MRI:* Computer generated films rely on radio waves and alteration in magnetic field. It is useful for visualization of kidneys. It has not been not proven useful for detecting urinary calculi or calcified tumors. In this, there is need to explain procedure to the patient. Have patient removed all metal objects. Patient with a history of claustrophobia needs to be sedated.
- *Renal radionuclide imaging (RRI):* In renal scan, radioactive isotopes are injected. IV radiation detector probes are placed over kidney and scintillation counter monitors radioactive material in kidneys. Purpose is to show blood flow, glomerular filtration, tubular function and excretion. Radioisotope distribution in kidney is scanned and mapped. Test is usual in showing location, size and shape of kidney and in general assessing blood perfusion and its ability to secrete urine. Abscesses, cysts and tumors may appear or coast spots because of presence of non-functioning tissue.

  This procedure requires no dietary or activity restriction. Inform patient that no pain or discomfort should be felt during test.

Endoscopy

Endoscopy: i.e., cystoscopy study involves use of tubular lighted scope to inspect bladder. Lithotomy position is used. It may be done using local or general anesthesia. The nursing responsibilities include:
- Before the procedure, force fluids or give IV fluids if general anesthesia is to be used.
- Ensure that consent form is signed.
- Explain procedure to the patient.
- Give preoperative medication.
- After procedure, explain that burning on urination, pink tinged urine and urination frequency are expected effects after cystoscopy.
- Do not let patient walk alone immediately after the procedure because orthostatic hypotension may occur.
- Offer warm sitz bath, heat and mild analgesics to relieve discomfort.

Urodynamics

Urodynamics: i.e., cystometrogram. This study involves insertion of catheter and instillation of water or saline solution into bladder. Measurement of pressure exerted against bladder wall is recorded. Purpose is to evaluate bladder tone, sensations of filling, and bladder (detrusor) stability. This test needs explain procedure to the patient and observe patient for manifestation of urinary tract infections after the procedure.

Invasive Procedure

Invasive procedure: i.e., renal biopsy is the technique usually done as a skin (percutaneous) biopsy through needle insertion into lower lobe of kidney. Purpose is to obtain renal tissue examination to determine type of renal disease or to follow progress of renal disease. Before the procedure, ascertain coagulation status through patient history, medications, history, CBC, hematocrit, prothrombin time and bleeding and clotting time, type and crossmatch for patient's blood. Ensure that consent form is signed. Be aware that IVP or ultrasound study is done before biopsy. After procedure, apply pressure dressing to biopsy site and check frequently for bleeding.

- Bedrest must be maintained with the patient flat, in a supine position and motionless for 4 hours after renal biopsy.
- Coughing is avoided for first 4 hours after biopsy.
- Blood pressure and pulse should be taken on the following schedule.
  - Every 15 minutes for 1 hour, every 30 minutes for 1 hour, every hour for 2 hours until it becomes stable.
- Bedrest should be maintained for 24 hours.
- Urine is observed for hematuria for first 24 hours and biopsy.
- Patient should avoid heavy lifting for 10 days after biopsy.
- Assess patient for flank pain. Monitor hematocrit levels.

INFLAMMATORY DISORDERS OF URINARY SYSTEM

Urinary Tract Infections (UTI)

Infections of the urinary tract may appear as a variety of disorders. Infections may be broadly classified as upper and lower UTI, based on the patient's symptoms. Terminology may specifically delineate the site of inflammations or infection. Examples of terms are 'pyeloenephritis' (involvement of kidneys and kidney pelvis) and cystitis (involvement of bladder). Lower UTIs involve the urinary bladder (cystitis), urethra (urethritis) and prostatitis. Upper UTI may involve kidney and renal pelvis (pyelonephritis).

Etiology

The urinary tract above the urethra is normally sterile. Several physiologic and mechanical defense mechanisms assist in maintaining sterility and preventing UTIs. These defenses include normal voiding with complete emptying of the bladder. Normal antibacterial ability of bladder mucosa and urine, ureterovesical junction competence, and peristaltic activity that propels urine towards bladder. An alteration in any of these defence mechanisms increases the risk of contracting a UTI.

Common microorganisms causing urinary tract infections are:
- *Escherichia coli*
- *Proteus*
- Enterococci
- *Pseudomonas*
- *Klebsiella*
- Staphylococci
- Enterobacter
- *Candida*
- Serratia

The risk factors associated with development of urinary tract infections are:
- Female due to:
  - Short urethra, close proximity to vagina and anus.
  - Postmenopausal decrease in estrogen and loss of vaginal lactobacilli, which prevent infection.
  - Diminished ureteral peristalsis (e.g., pregnancy).
  - Use of diaphragm.
- Structural abnormality:
  - Stricture urethra.
  - Incompetent ureterovesical function anomalies.
- Obstruction:
  - Compression of growing uterus against ureter, compression of growing uterus against ureters. (e.g., tumor, fibroids).
  - Presence of tumors, calculi, prostatic hypertrophy.
  - Iatrogenic causes.
- Impaired bladder innervation:
  - Congenital spinal cord malformation.
  - Spinal cord injury.
  - Multiple sclerosis.
  - Urinary stasis.
  - Neurogenic bladder.
- Chronic diseases:
  - Gout, diabetes mellitus, hypertension, sickle cell disease.
  - Polycystic kidney disease, multiple myeloma.
  - Glomerulonephritis.
  - Immunosuppression.
- Instrumentation:
  - Catheterization.
  - Diagnostic procedures.
  - Incomplete-bladder emptying.
- Age:
  - Decreased acidity of urine.
  - Anemia and malnutrition.
- Renal scarring from previous UTIs.

The mode of entry of bacteria into the genitourinary tract can always be traced with certainty. There are four major pathways exist:

1. *Ascending infection:* From the urethra it is the most common cause of genitourinary tract infection in men and women. As the female urethra is short and rectal bacteria tend to colonize the perineum and

vaginal vestibule, females are especially susceptible to ascending urinary tract infections. A common factor contributes ascending infection is urologic instrumentation (catheterization cystoscopy). Sexual intercourse has been shown to be a major precipitating factor of UTI in women. Sexual intercourse promotes milking of bacteria from vagina and perineum and may cause minor urethral trauma that predisposes women to UTIs. UTIs associated with sexual intercourse can develop as quickly as 12 hours after intercourse.

2. *Hematogenous spread:* Occurs infrequently. With the exception of tuberculosis, renal abscesses are perinephric abscesses. Bacteremia is more likely to complicate UT when structural and functional abnormalities exist and when the urinary tract is normal.
3. *Lymphogenous spread is rare:* Bacterial pathogens travel through the rectal and colonic lymphatics to the prostate and bladder through the preuterine lymphatic in the female genitourinary tract.
4. Direct extension from another organ occurs with extra peritoneal abscesses, especially those associated with inflammation, bowel disease, fulminant, pelvic inflammatory disease in women, paravesical abscesses and genitourinary tract fistula and pyelonephritis.

Pathophysiology

Normally urine produced in kidneys flows unobstructed through urinary tract. Urine is sterile unit which reaches urethra. Most UTIs result from gram-negative organisms, such as *E. coli, Klebsiella, Proteus* or *Pseudomonas*, that originate in the persons own intestinal tract and ascend through the urethra to the bladder. During micturition urine may flow back the ureters (vesicoureteral reflux) and carry bacteria from the bladder up through the ureters to the kidney pelvis. Whenever urinary stasis occurs, such as with incomplete emptying of the bladder, renal calculi, or genitourinary obstructions, the bacteria have a greater opportunity to grow. Urinary stasis also promotes a more alkaline urine which facilitates bacterial growth. UTI occurs primarily when host resistance is impaired due to above stated causes.

Clinical Manifestation

The symptoms that bring the person with UTI seek medical attention typically include frequency, urgency, dysuria, (burning on urination) cloudy or foul-smelling urine, suprapubic discomfort, and hematuria, bacteriuria, upper UTIs and pyelonephritis are associated with fever, flank pain, costovertebral angle tenderness, nausea, and vomiting. Most persons, however, are asymptomatic or minimally symptomatic. In these persons, UTI is identified only on routine examination of the urine. Bacteriuria and positive urine cultures serve as basis for diagnosing lower UTIs.

Management

Diagnostic test includes urinanalysis, culture and sensitivity test before starting medication. If necessitated, advance test like IVP cystogram.

Medication typically used is the treatment of urinary tract infections include anti-infectives, analgesics and anticholenergies.

- *Trimethoprimsulfamethoxazole* (Bactrim, Septran) is folate antoganist, enzymatic inhibition of bacterial synthesis, when patient is on the medication:
    - Increase fluid intake to 1500 ml/day.
    - Monitor intake and output.
    - Observe for adverse reactions (rash, hives, etc.).
- *Nitrofurantoin* interferes with bacterial enzyme systems. When patient is on this medication.
    - Administer with food or milk.
    - Avoid exposure of the drug to light.
    - Space dose equally around the clock.
- *Ciprofloxacin* inhibits DNA-gyrase, preventing bacterial DNA replication. During this treatment, nurse:
    - Instructs the patient to avoid antacids.
    - Encouirage intake of at least 1500 ml/day.
    - Monitor intake and output.
    - Assess nausea, vomiting and diarrhea.
- *Amoxicillin* inhibits mucoprotein synthesis in the cell wall of rapidly dividing bacteria. During this treatment, the nurse, should:
    - Observe for urticaria or rash.
    - Assess renal, hepatic, and hematological function.
    - Administer round the clock without skipping doses.

Analgesics such as penozopyridine (pyridin, urogenic), local anesthetic action on urinary mucosa. Administer after meals. Instruct patient that urine may turn orange and will stain fabrics. Avoid use more than 5 days.

Anticholinergic such as propantheline bromide (probanthin). Potent antimuscarinic activity, decreases bladder spasm. Administer one hour before meals do not crush medications, assess bowel sounds, and postural hypertension.

Additional treatment includes increasing fluid intake to 3 to 4 liters per day unless it is contraindicated. Increased fluid intake helps to dilute the urine, lessens irritation and burning, and provides a continued flow of urine to minimize stasis and multiplication of bacteria in the urinary tract. Sitz bath may provide comfort for individual with urethritis. And regular intake of vitamin C in sufficient dose to be excreted in the urine can reduce bacterial growth due to ascorbic acid. Lemon juice may be provided to increase ascorbic acidity to prevent growth of bacteria.

Health education to be given to the public to reduce urinary tract infections in the community are regarding:
- Symptoms of urinary tract infections.
- Need for prompt medical attention when symptoms of UTI occurs.

- Need to continue drug therapy even though symptoms abate.
- Importance of following care and repeat urine culture.
- Maintenance of fluid intake of 3 to 4 L/day if patient's health permits as increased fluid intake helps flush bacteria out of the urinary system.
- Avoidance of bubble bath, powders, and harsh soaps in the perineal area.
- Wearing of cotton underpants as nylon and synthetic fabrics do not allow ventilation and may facilitate bacterial growth.
- Avoidance of tight-fitting pants that may irritate the urethra.
- For women, importance of wiping perineal area from front to back to prevent introducing bacteria into the urethra.
- Need to shower instead of tubbath for persons with recurrent urinary tract infections.
- Need to increase fluid intake before and after sexual intercourse and empty the bladder immediately after intercourse.
- Avoidance of urinary stasis by voiding approximately every 2 to 4 hours.
- Need for regular intake of vitamin C or cranberry juice or lemon juice to help prevent urinary tract infections.

Cystitis

Cystitis is the inflammation of the urinary bladder.

Etiology

The incidence of cystitis is very high in women followed by older men and young children especially in girls. These age and sex variation in the frequency of cystitis are related to anatomic differences or pathologic changes in the groups at risk. The adult female urethra is short and the proximity to rectum and vagina predisposes women to the risk of bladder contamination. Bacterial contamination of the bladder can be the result of poor personal hygienic practices and sexual intercourse.

In children, vesicoureteral reflux is usually the pre-existing abnormality. In men, the longer urethra (of which the proximal two-thirds is normally sterile) and the antibacterial property of prostatic secretions provide protection from bacterial infections, unless there are predisposing causes such as BPH.

Pathophysiology

Once cystitis has occurred, it may remain localized in the urinary bladder for years without ascension to the kidneys or may be completely resolved after initial treatment. Although the bacterial infection may be self-limiting, the urinary tract should be evaluated if there is recurrence, even in the patients who have no symptoms. The risk of recurrent symptomatic infection is increased when there are urinary tract abnormalities. Asymptomatic bacteriuria can occur and is no synonymous with UTI. It indicates that bacteria can be present in the urine. Tissue invasion must occur for an infection to exist. Pyuria (the presence of WBCs in the urine) usually signals this occurrence and is the characteristic laboratory findings in symptomatic UTI.

Clinical Manifestation

The manifestation of cystitis are frequency and urgency of urination, suprapubic pain, dysuria, foul-smelling urine and pyuria. Hematuria may or may not occur in symptomatic UTI. The presence of fever, nausea, vomiting, and flank tenderness usually indicates pyelonephritis. About half of all persons with significant bactesiuria have no symptoms or may reflect nonspecific signs such as increased fatigue, anorexia, or changes in cognitive ability. The incidence of asymptomatic bacteriuria increases greatly with age. Asymptomatic bacteriuria is more likely to occur in women over 65 years of age.

Diagnostic Studies

- Urinalysis for presence of WBC.
- Urine for gram stain.
- Urine for culture and sensitivity with clean-catch urine.
- IVP, cystoscopy if indicated.

The nurse should be aware that noninfectious agents also cause irritative bladder symptoms similar to UTI and intravesical chemotherapy or pelvic radiation.

Management

Uncomplicated cystitis are treated with antimicrobial therapy which includes, bactrim, septra, nitrofurantoin and cephalexin, of which single time therapy or 1 to 3 days or therapy. Prophylactic antibiotic therapy is given to prevent recurrence of after treatment of UTI. Acute intervention for a patient with cystitis includes an adequate fluid intake if this is not contraindicated which helps increase feelings or urgency and frequency and also dilute the urine to reduce irritation in the bladder. Potential bladder irritants like coffee, alcohol, citrus juices, chocolate and highly-spiced food or beverages should be avoided. The patient should be instructed to take complete course of treatment as prescribed and periodical urine examination should be done, i.e. gross or microscopic hematuria. Presence of WBCs, malodor and sediment and follow health education as in UTI. Acute intervention for a patient with cystitis includes an adequate fluid intake if this is not contraindicated which helps increased feeling of urgency and frequency and also dilutes the urine to reduce irritation and the bladder.

Glomerulonephritis

Glomerulonephritis is a disease, that affects the glomeruli of both kidneys, i.e. inflammation of the glomeruli. Although the glomerulus is the primary site of inflammation, tubular, interstitial, and vascular changes also occur.

Etiological factors are many and varied; they include:
- Immunological reactions (systematic lupus erythematosus and streptococcal infection).
- Vascular injury (hypertension).
- Metabolic disease (diabetes mellitus) and
- Disseminated intravascular coagulation.

Glomerulonephritis is divided into a number of classifications which may describe:
- The extent of damage (diffuse or focal).
- The initial cause of the disorder (systematic lupus erythematosa, streptococcal infection, scleroderma
- The extent of change (minimal or widespread).

Glomerulonephritis exists in acute, latent and chronic form.

Acute Glomerulonephritis

Acute poststreptococcal glomerulonephritis (APSGN) is most common in children and young adults, but all age groups can be affected.

Etiology

APSGN develops 5 to 21 days after an infection of the pharynx or skin (e.g., streptococcal sore throat, impetigo) by certain nephrotoxic strains of group A beta hemolytic streptococci. The person produces antibodies to the strepotcoccal antigen. The antigen-antibody complexes are deposited in the glomeruli and activated compliment. Compliment activated causes an inflammatory reaction to the injury. This response to the injury is also a decrease in the filtration of metabolic waste products from the blood and an increased permeability of the glomerulus to larger protein molecules.

Pathophysiology

APSGN is a result of an antigen-antibody reaction with glomerular tissue that produces swelling and death of capillary cells. The antigen-antibody reaction activates the complement pathway, resulting in chemotaxis of polymorphonuclear leukocytes with release of lysosomal enzymes that attack the glomerular basement membrane. The responses in the membrane is an increase in all three types of glomerular cells (i.e. endothelial, mesangial, and epithelial) causing an increase in membrane porosity with resultant proteinuria and hematuria. Renal function is depressed by scarring and obstruction of the circulation through the glomerulus. Signs and symptoms reflect damage to the glomeruli with leaking of proteins and RBCs into the urine and varying degrees of decreased glomeruli filtrations, with retention of metabolic wastes products, sodium and water.

Clinical Manifestations

Typical patient complaints include shortness of breath, mild headache, weakness, anorexia, flank pain. The early clinical manifestation of APSGN includes hematuria, proteinuria, azotemia, increased urine-specific gravity, elevated ESR, oliguria, elevated antistreptolysine *'O titerited*. Later chemical manifestations include circulatory congestion, hypertension, edema and end-stage renal failure. Signs and symptoms which may include generalized body edema, hypertension, oliguria, hematuria with a smoky or rusty appearance, and proteinuria. Fluid retention occurs as a result of decreased glomerular filtration. The edema appears initially in low pressure tissue such as around the eyes (Periorbital edema), but later, progresses to involve total body as ascitis or peripheral edema in the legs. Smoky urine is indicative of bleeding in the upper urinary tract. The degree of proteinuria varies with severity of glomerulonephropathy. Hypertension primarily results from increased ECF.

Management

The diagnosis of APSGN is based on a complete history and physical examination and laboratory studies to determine the presence or history of a group. A extrahemolytic streptococci in a throat or skin lesion. Urinalysis provides important data such as presence of proteinuria, hematuria and cell debris.

Serum BUN and urine creatinine clearance test indicates renal function status. Test to determine infection includes ESR and anistreptolysis 'O'titter, and *renal* biopsy is indicated.

The management of APSGN focuses on lymptomatic relief. Rest is recommended until the signs of glomerular inflammation (Proteinuria, hematuria) and hypertension subside. Edema is treated by restricting sodium and fluid intake and by administering diuretics. Severe hypertension is treated with antihypertensive drugs. Dietary protein intake may be restricted if there is evidence of an increase in nitrogenous wastes (e.g., elevated BUN value). The restriction varies with proteinuria.

Persistent infection is treated promptly to help prevent an increase in antigen-antibody complex formation. Patients with poststreptococcal glomerulonephritis are given a course of prophylactic antibiotics, the drug of choice is penicillin. Prophylactic therapy may be continued for months after the acute phase of illness. Diuretic therapy is implemented when severe overload develops. Elevated blood pressure is controlled by antihypertensive drugs only after fluid control has proved to be unsuccessful.

There is no specific treatment for APSGN. General management focussed on prevention, i.e. early defection and prompt treatment of URTI. Fluid retention is often managed by dietary sodium restrictions and nurse should be constantly alert for signs and symptoms of fluid overload and bedrest is prescribed during the acute phase of illness.

The recovery period for acute glomerulonephritis may be as long as 2 years; therefore, patient teaching is important. Proteinuria, hematuria and cellular debris may exist microscopically even when other symptoms subside. Although fatigue may be present, these persons usually feel well. They often need to be convinced of the importance of follow-up care.

Teaching includes:
- Nature of illness and effect of diet and fluids on fluid balance and sodium retention.
- Diet teaching regarding prescribed sodium and fluid restrictions.
- Medication regimen: dose, frequency, side effects, need to continue regimen as prescribed.
- Need to balance activities with rest of fatigue present.
- Avoidance of infection which may exacerbate illness.
- Signs and symptoms indicating need for medical attention (hematuria, headache, edema, or hypertension).
- Importance of follow-up care.

Chronic Glomerulonephritis (CGN)

Chronic glomerulonephritis is a syndrome that reflects the end stage of glomerular inflammatory disease.

Etiology

Most types of glomerulonephritis and nephrotic syndrome can eventually lead to chronic glomerulonephritis (CGN). Although CGN may follow the acute disease, most of the persons have no history of the disease or source of predisposing infection. Some persons with minimal impairment in renal function continue to feel well and show little progression of disease. The progression of renal deterioration may be insidious or rapid, resulting in end stage of renal disease.

Pathophysiology

Chronic glomerulonephritis is characterized by progressive destruction (sclerosis) of glomeruli and gradual loss of renal function. The glomeruli having varying degrees of hypercellularity and become sclerosed (hardened). The kidney decreases in size. Eventually there is tubular atrophy, chronic interstitial inflammation, and arteriosclerosis.

Clinical Manifestation

Various symptoms of renal dysfunction may lead the person to seek health care, including headache, especially in the morning; dyspnea on exertion, blurred vision, lassitude, weakness or fatigue. Other signs of CGN include edema, nocturia, and weight loss. Early in the disease process, urinalysis may reveal albumin, casts and blood despite normal renal function tests. The ability of kidneys to regulate internal environment will begin to decrease as more glomeruli become scarred resulting in fewer functional nephrons. The syndrome is characterized by proteinuria, hematuria and the slow development of uremic syndrome as a result of decreasing renal function.

Management

CGN is often found coincidentally when an abnormality on urinalysis or elevated blood pressure is detected. It is common to find that the patient has no recollection or history of acute nephritis or any renal problems. A renal biopsy is performed to determine the exact cause and nature of the glomerulonephritis. However, now some of them use ultrasound and CT scan as diagnostic measure.

No specific therapy exists to arrest or reverse this disease process. Treatment is supportive and symptomatic. Hypertension and urinary tract infections should be treated vigorously. With any exacerbation of hematuria, hypertension and edema, the patient is returned to bedrest, and treatment is similar to that of acute glomerulonephritis is instituted. Signs of pulmonary edema and congestive cardiac failure are closely monitored. Women with CGN who become pregnant appear to be susceptible to toxemia and to spontaneous abortion, needs close observation by obstetrician. Protein and phosphate restrictions may slow the rate of progression of renal failure.

For prevention or to reduce risk, known infection should be treated promptly. Care involves teaching the patient to live healthfully to avoid infections (as in AGN), to eat balanced diet within the prescribed limit, to take prescribed medications appropriately to maintain follow-up health care, and to report to concerned physician about any exacerbation and signs and symptoms.

Nephrotic Syndrome

The term nephrotic syndrome describes a clinical course that can be associated with a number of disease conditions. Nephrotic syndrome or nephrosis is not a single disease entirely but a constellation of symptoms including albuminuria, hypoalbuminuria, edema, hyperlipidemia, and lipiduria. This syndrome causes damage to the glomeruli with resultant proteinuria. It is most often seen in children.

Etiology

Some of the more common causes of nephrotic syndrome are:
- *Primary glomerular disease:*
  - Membranous proliferative glomerulonephritis.
  - Primary nephrotic syndrome.
  - Focal glomerulonephritis.
  - Inherited nephrotic disease.
- *External causes:*
  - Multisystem disease
    - Systemic lupus erythematous.
    - Diabetes mellitus.
    - Sickle cell disease.
    - Amyloidosis.
  - *Infections:*
    - Bacterial (streptococcal, syphylis).
    - Viral (herpes zoster, HIV and hepatitis).
    - Protozoal (malaria).

- Neoplasms:
  - Hodgkin's disease.
  - Solid tumors of lungs, colon, stomach and breast.
  - Leukemia.
- Circulatory problems:
  - Severe congestive heart failure.
  - Chronic constrictive pericarditis.
- Allergic reaction:
  - Insect bites, bee sting and pollen.
  - Drugs (penicillamine, NSAIDs, captopril and heroin).

Pathophysiology

The initial physiological change is nephrotic syndrome is a derangement of cells in the glomerular basement membrane (GBM) resulting in increased membrane porosity and significant proteinuria. As protein continues to be excreted, serum albumin is decreased (hypoalbuminemia), thus decreasing the serum osmotic pressure. The capillary hydrostatic fluid pressure in all body tissues becomes greater than the capillary osmotic pressure in all body tissues becomes greater then the capillary osmotic pressure and generalized edema results. As fluid is lost into the tissues, the plasma volume decreases stimulating secretion of aldosterone to retain more sodium and water, which decreases the glomerular filtration rate to retain water. This additional fluid also passes out of the capillaries into the tissue leading to even greater edema.

Clinical Manifestations

The characteristic manifestation includes peripheral edema, massive proteinuria, hyperlipidemia, and hypoalbuminiemia. Characteristic blood chemistries include decreased serum albumin, decreased serum protein, and elevated serum cholestrol. The increased glomerular membrane permeability found in nephrotic syndrome is responsible for the massive excretion of protein in the urine. There is the decreased serum protein and subsequent edema formation. Ascitis and anasarca (severe generalized edema) develop if there is a severe hypoalbuminemia.

The diminished plasma oncotic pressure from the decreased serum proteins stimulates hepatic lipoprotein synthesis which results in hyperlipidemia. Initially cholesterol and low-density lipoproteins are elevated. Later fat bodies (fatty casts) commonly appear in the urine. Alterations of the humoral and cellular immunoresponse results in infection. Calcium and skeletal abnormalities may occur; results in hypocalcemia, blunted calcemic response to parathyroid hormone, hypoparathyroidism and osteomalacia. With nephrotic proteinuria loss of clotting factors can result in relative hypercoagulable state, i.e. hypercoagulability with thromboembolism is most serious complication.

Management

Treatment of nephrotic syndrome is symptomatic, that is focused on reduction of albuminuria, controlling edema, and promoting general health. Management of edema includes the cautious use of angiotensin converting enzyme (ACE) inhibitors, NSAIDs and a low-sodium (2 to 3 g per day), low to moderate-protein diet (0.5 to 0.6 kg per day). Dietary salt restrictions are a key to managing edema. In some individuals, thiazide or loop diuretics may be needed. If the urine protein loss exceeds 10 g/24 per hour, additional dietary protein may be needed. Corticosteroids and cyclophosphamide may be used for the treatment of severe cases of nephrotic syndrome.

A major nursing intervention for a patient with nephrotic syndrome is related to edema. It is important to assess edema by weighing the patient daily, accurately recording intake and output, and measuring abdominal girth or extremity size. Comparing this information daily provides the nurse with a tool for assessing the effectiveness of treatment. The edematous skin needs careful cleaning. Trauma should be avoided and the effectiveness of diuretic therapy must be monitored. Measures should be taken to avoid exposure to person with known infections. The nurse should handle the patient properly with their altered body image due to edema. A sodium-restricted diet is usually prescribed.

The patient and family should be educated regarding:
- The effects of nephrotic syndrome on the kidneys and the possibility of the need for dialysis or renal transplant in the future.
- Medication regimen, name, dose, actions, side effects and the need to complete prescribed antibiotics.
- Nutrition: increased calories, adequate protein and decreased sodium.
- Self assessment of fluid status, including signs and symptoms of hypovolemia and hypervolemia.
- Signs and symptoms requiring medical attention: Increased edema, dyspnea, fatigue, headache and infection.
- Promotion of good health habits to prevent infection, including nutritionally adequate diet, exercise, adequate rest, and sleep and avoidance of source of infection.
- Need for follow up care to monitor renal function.

Goodpasture's Syndrome

Goodpasture's syndrome is an example of cytotoxic (type II) autoimmune disease, is characterized by the presence of circulating antibodies against GBM and alveolar basement membrane (ABM).

Etiology and Pathophysiology

It is a rare disease that is seen mostly in young male smokers. Although the primary target organ is the kidney, the lungs are also involved. The pathologic nature of the syndrome results when binding of the antibody causes an inflammatory reaction mediated by complement fixation and activation. The causative factors for development of autoantibody production are unknown, although type A influenza viruses, hydrocarbon, penicillamine, and unknown genetic factors may be involved.

Clinical Manifestations

The clinical manifestations include hemoptysis, pulmonary insufficiency, crackles, rhonchi, renal involvement with hematuria and renal failure, weakness, pallor, and anemia. Pulmonary hemorrhage usually occurs and may precede glomerular abnormality by weeks or months. Abnormal diagnostic findings include low hematocrit and hemoglobin levels, elevated BUN and serum creatinine levels, hematuria and proteinuria, circulating serum anti-GBM antibodies parallel to the activity of the renal disease.

Management

Management consists of corticosteroids, immunosuppressive drugs (e.g., cyclophosphamide), plasmapheresis and dialysis. Plasmapheresis removes circulating anti-GBM antibody and immunosuppressive therapy inhibits further antibody production. Renal transplantation can be attempted once the circulating anti-GBM antibody titer decreases.

Nursing management appropriate for critically-ill patient who is experiencing symptoms of acute renal failure and respiratory distress. The patient and family need instructions cocnerning current therapy, medications and complications of disease processes. The complication of Goodpasture's syndrome is rapidly progressive glomerulonephritis. (This also occurs as complication of APSGN, SLE and illustrative disease).

Renal Artery Stenosis

Renal artery stenosis is a partial occlusion of one or both renal arteries and their major branches.

Etiology

Renal artery stenosis can be due to the atherosclerotic narrowing or fibromuscular hyperplasia. It is the cause of approximately 5 percent of all cases of hypertension. The end result is a narrowing of the lumen of the arteries supplying the kidneys. Obstruction of the renal arteries can be caused by aneurysm, thrombosis and emboli.

Pathophysiology

Renal artery stenosis results in a major reduction in blood flow to the kidneys. This change in renal perfusion causes increased secretion of renin and activation of renin-angiotensin-aldosterone system. The end result is acceleration of hypertension, which, if untreated, leads to further pathological changes in the kidneys.

Clinical Manifestation

The clinical manifestation of renal artery stenosis includes:
- Abdominal bruits.
- Hypertension.
- Disparity in kidney size.
- Disparity in kidney shape.
- Delayed appearance of contrast medium in renal anteriogram.
- Hyperconcentration of contrast media in kidneys, calyceal system on intravenous pyelogram.
- Lesion evidenced on renal arteriogram.
- Increased serum creatinine level with captopril challenge.
- Changes in blood flow on duplex doppler ultrasonography.
- Detection of change in blood flow within vessels on MRI.

Management

A renal arteriogram is the best diagnostic tool for identifying renal artery stenosis. The goals of therapy are control of blood pressure, and restoration of perfusion to the kidney. Beta-blocker or angiotension converting enzyme inhibitors are used to manage hypertension. Analgesics are used to manage pain associated with vascular occlusion. Preventing pulmonary embolism is critical in persons with renal vein thrombosis. Anticoagulants are indicated for patients with renal artery occlusion or renal vein thrombosis.

Surgical revascularization of the kidney is indicated when blood flow is decreased enough to cause renal ischemia or when evidence indicates that renovascular hypertension is present and surgical intervention may result in the patient becoming normotensive. The surgical procedure normally involves anastomosis between the kidney and another major artery, usually spleenic artery or aorta. Percutaneous transluminal angioplasty may be used as an alternative to surgery, especially in older patients who are poor surgical risks. Person with renal artery stenosis and hypertension that does not respond to medication may need a nephrectomy.

Patient should be educated regarding the lower cholestrol including maintaining a diet low in animal fat and increasing aerobic exercises. Patients should be instructed to monitor their blood pressure at home and report any abnormalities to health care provider. If anticoagulant therapy is prescribed, the patient and family should understand precautions to take to avoid injury and signs and excessive bleeding. And patient should be taught to recognize signs and symptoms and report immediately to the concerned healthcare provider.

Renal Vein Thrombosis

Renal vein thrombosis may occur unilaterally or bilaterally trauma, extrinsic compression (e.g. tumor, aortic aneurysm), renal cell carcinoma, pregnancy, contraceptive use, and nephrotic syndrome are associated with renal vein thrombosis.

The patient has symptoms of flank pain, hematuria or fever or has nephrotic syndrome. Anticoagulation is an important treatment because there is a high incidence of pulmonary emboli. Corticosteroids may be used in the patient with nephrosis. Surgical thrombectomy may be performed instead of or along with anticoagulation.

Nephrosclerosis

Nephrosclerosis consists of sclerosis of the small arteries and arterioles of the kidneys. There is a decreased blood flow, which results in patchy necrosis of the renal parenchyma. Ischemic necrosis and destruction of glomeruli with subsequent fibrosis also occurs.

Etiology

Whereas renal artery stenosis results in hypertension, hypertension causes nephrosclerosis or damage to the renal arteries, arterioles and glomeruli. Hypertension is the major cause of end-stage renal disease.

Pathophysiology

In benign nephrosclerosis, the renal arterial vessels show thickening and narrowing of their lumina, and some glomerular capillaries are sclerosed and collapsed. Renal blood flow can be reduced as the result of these vascular changes. The renal tubules can also be affected, resulting in tubular atrophy signs and symptoms are mild, i.e. mild proteinuria from glomerular damage. Nocturia may occur due to tubular concentrating ability and urinary casts may be present due to tubular injury. Later mild renal insufficiency leads to risk for acute failure.

In malignant nephrosclerosis, the major changes are necrosis and thickening of the arterioles and glomerular capillaries and diffuse tubular loss and atrophy. Gross hamaturia occurs with RBC casts, heavy proteinuria and elevated plasma creatinine. Malignant nephrosclerosis is a medical emergency, and high blood pressure must be lowered to prevent permanent renal damage as well as damage to other vital organs.

Clinical Manifestations

The signs and symptoms of nephrosclerosis are the same as those of chronic renal failure. By the time the signs and symptoms develop, the disease has progressed to an extreme point. Deterioration in renal function progresses gradually. Accelerated or malignant nephrosclerosis is associated with malignant hypertension or complication of hypertension characterized by a sharp increase in blood pressure with a diastolic pressure greater than 130 mm Hg. The patient is usually an young adult, with a male to female ratio 2:1. Renal insufficiency progresses rapidly.

Management

Treatment of nephrosclerosis is focussed on early detection and treatment of hypertension. Causative factors are sought and treatment to lower blood pressure is initiated. When significant renal damage exists, stabilizing the person's current level of function or slowing deterioration of the kidney tissue is the goal. Control of hypertension is continued. For hypertensive emergencies, potent vasodilator such as diazoxide and sodium nitroprusside are used. IV medications usually act rapidly to lower blood pressure. Sodium nitroprusside is given as a continuous IV drip. Monitor the patient continuously for headache, hypotension, muscle twitching, tachycardia, restlessness and retrosternal or abdominal pain. Nursing care of the patient with nephrosclerosis is same as in chronic renal failure. During drug therapy, monitor the patient closely for tachycardia, hypotension, hyperglycemia, and marked sodium and water retention.

Obstructive Uropathies

Obstruction of the urinary system occurs in any portion of the urinary tract from the urinary calyces in kidney to the urethral meatus. Patients with obstructions have characteristic signs and symptoms, depending on the location and extent of the obstruction. Uncorrected urinary obstruction can lead to renal failure.

Obstruction may be congenital or acquired and due to intrinsic and extrinsic which include:
- *Intrinsic* causes such as anamolies, diverticuli, tumors or benign growth within the urinary tract, e.g. narrowing of ureteropelvic junction, bladder neck hyperplasia, urethral stricture, BPH and meatal stenosis.
- *Extrinsic* causes such as tumors, adhesions, retroperitoneal fibrosis, or prolapsed adjacent organs or functional causes as a result of neurologic or psychogenic factors, e.g. are pelvic and abdominal tumors or prolapsed uterus. Functional causes are vesicosphincter dyssynergia after spinal cord injury and neurogenic bladder secondary to diabetes.

The major causes of urinary tract obstructions according to location are as follows:
- Lower urinary tract:
  - Bladder neoplasms
  - Urethral strictures
  - Calculi
  - Tumors
  - Benign prostatic hypertrophy (BPH).
- Ureteral obstruction
  - Calculi
  - Trauma
  - Nephroptosis (floating or dropped kidney)
  - Enlarged lymph nodes (lymposarcoma reticuli-cell carcinoma, Hodgkin's disease.
  - Congenital anamoly.

- Kidney
  - Calculi
  - Ptosis
  - Polycystic kidney disease
  - Pregnancy (usually right-sided).

The common condition of obstructive uropathies discussed are as follows:

Hydronephrosis

Hydronephrosis is the dilation of the renal pelvis and calyces with urine. It may occur either unilaterally or bilaterally. It is due to causes of obstruction of urinary tract.

Pathophysiology

Obstruction of any part of the urinary system from the kidney to the urethra will generate pressure that may cause functional and anatomic damage to the renal parenchyma. When any part of the urinary tract is obstructed, urine collects behind the obstruction, producing dilation of the urine collecting structures. Muscles of the affected area contract in an effort to push the urine around the obstruction. Partial obstruction may produce slow dilation of structures above the obstruction without functional impairment. As the obstruction increases, pressure builds up in the tubular system behind the obstruction causing a backflow of urine and dilation of the ureter (hydroureter). The urine back-up eventually reaches the kidney causing dilation of the kidney pelvis (hydronephrosis). Pressure build up in the renal pelvis leads to destruction of kidney tissue and eventually renal failure.

Due to obstruction, urine flow is decreased, even to the point of stagnation. This stagnant urine provides a culture medium for bacterial growth and rarely is obstruction seen without some infection. The specific effects that occur with obstruction depend on the location extent (partial or complete) and duration of the obstruction. Obstruction in the lower urinary tract causes bladder distension. If this is prolonged, muscle fibres become hypertrophied and diverticuli (herniated sacs of bladder mucosa) develop between the hypertophied muscle bands. Since the diverticulum holds stagnant urine, infection often occurs and bladder stones may form.

The obstruction of the upper urinary tract can progress rapidly to hydronephrosis because of the small size of the ureters and kidney pelvis. Increased pressure causes partial ischemia between the renal cortex and medulla and the dilation of the renal tubules leading to tubular damage. Urinary stasis in the dilated pelvis leads to infection and calculi, which add to the renal damage. Some urine flow back up the renal tubules into the veins and lymphatics as a compensatory mechanism. The unaffected kidney then takes on increased elimination of waste products. With prolonged obstruction, the unaffected kidney hypertrophies may function almost (80 percent) as effectively alone as both kidneys did before the obstruction. Obstruction of both kidneys leads to renal failure.

Clinical Manifestation

Hydronephrosis occurs without any symptoms as long as kidney function is adequate, and urine can drain. An acute upper urinary tract obstruction will cause pain, nausea, vomiting, local tenderness, spasm of the abdominal muscle, and a mass in the kidney region. The pain is caused by stretching of the tissue and by hyperperistalisis. Because of the amount of pain is proportional to the rate of stretching a slowly developing hydronephrosis may cause only a dull flank pain, whereas a sudden blockage of the ureter, e.g. form a stone, causes a severe stabbing (colicky) pain in the flank or abdomen. The pain may radiate to the genitalia and thighs and is caused by the increased peristaltic action of the smooth muscles of the ureter in an effort to dislodge the obstruction and force urine past it. Reflex reaction to the pain causes nausea and vomiting. An extremely dilated kidney may press on the stomach, causing continued gastrointestinal symptoms. This may indicate uremia.

When the bladder is distended from the lower urinary tract obstruction, the person will experience abdominal discomfort and feel the need to void although voiding will not be possible. The bladder may be palpated above the symphysis pubis. There may be urge to void usually 250 to 500 ml nocturia, hematuria and pyuria may also be present.

Management

The diagnosis can be made on complete examination and routine renourogical tests. The medical management is in specific to the cause of the urinary tract obstruction. Treatment centers around re-establishing adequate drainage from the urinary system, such as placing a ureteral catheter above the point of obstruction. Strictures may be successfully dilated.

Surgery is indicated to relieve the obstruction and preserve kidney function. Procedures include pyeloplasty and catheter or stent insertion into the kidney or bladder (nephrostomy, ureterostomy or suprapubic cystotomy). Severe kidney damage may necessitate nephrectomy.

The person with acute obstruction has severe colic, can be treated with narcotics (morphine, meperidine) in combination with antispasmodic drugs (Probanthin, balladona prep). General nursing management of urinary obstruction includes pain management, fluid balance assessment, prevention of urinary complications and patient teaching. The patient should be monitored for signs and symptoms of infection. Patients and families should be taught postoperative care of incisions and care and management of indwelling catheters if applicable. Information about medications, diet, fluid restrictions and signs and symptoms of infection and recurrent obstruction should be included in the teaching plan.

Renal Calculi (Stones)

Urinary stones (urolithiasis) may develop at any level in the urinary system but are most frequently found within the kidney (nephrolithiasis). Renal calculi are crystallization of minerals around an organic matrix such as pus, blood, or devitalized tissue. Most stones consist of calcium salts or magnesium-ammonium phosphate, the remainder are cystine or uric acid stones.

Etiology

Many factors are involved in the incidence and type of stone formation, including metabolic, dietary, genetic, climatic and occupational influence are as follows:
- *Metabolic:* Abnormalities that result in increased urine levels of calcium, oxaluric acid, uric acid or citric acid.
- *Climate:* Warm climates that cause increased fluid loss. Low urine volume and increased solute concentration in urine.
- *Diet:*
  - Large intake of dietary proteins that increases uric acid excretion.
  - Excessive amounts of tea or fruit juices that elevate urinary oxalate level.
  - Large intake of calcium and oxalate.
  - Low fluid intake that increases urinary concentration.
- *Genetic factors:* Family history of stones formation, cystinuria, gout or renal acidosis.
- *Lifestyle:* Sedentary occupation and immobility.

No demonstrable cause can be found for more than half of the renal stones that occur (idiopathic). However, a major predisposing factor is the presence of UTI. Infection increases the presence of organic matter around which minerals can precipitate and increases the alkalinity of the urine by the production of ammonia. This results in precipitation of calcium phosphate and magnesium-ammonium phosphate. Stasis of urine also permits precipitation of organic matter and minerals. Other factors associated with the development of stones include long-term use of antacids, vitamin D, large doses of vitamin C and calcium carbonate.

Pathophysiology

Most stones are *calcium* (oxalate and phosphate) anything that leads to hypercalciuria is a predisposing factors for renal stones. Factors that contribute to calcium stone formation will include hypercalcemia and/or hypercalciuria resulting from hyperparathyroidism vitamin D intoxication, multiple myeloma, immobilization, severe bone disease, cancer, renal tubular acidosis, prolonged intake of steroids and increased intake of calcium.

The contributing factors of *uric acid* stone formation are high purine diet, gout renal failure, blood dyscrasiasis, use of thiazide diuretics and alkalysing agents. The factors contributing to *cystine* stone formation are cystinuria resulting from genetic disorder of amino acid metabolism.

The other important factors in the development of stones include obstruction with urinary stasis and urinary *infection*. With urea spitting bacteria (e.g. *Proteus, Klebsiella, Pseudomonas,* and some species of *Staphylococci*). These bacteria cause the urine to become alkaline and contribute to the formation of calcium-ammonium phosphate stones (struvite or triple phosphate stones). Infected stones when they are entrapped in the kidney may assume a staghorn configuration as they enlarge. Infected stones are frequent in the patient with an external urinary diversion and long term indwelling catheter. Neurogenic bladder or retention of urine.

Clinical Manifestations

Urinary stones cause clinical manifestation when they cause obstruction to urinary flow, common sites (**Fig. 7.1**) of obstruction are at the ureteropelvic junction (UPJ), in the ureter at the point it crosses the iliac vessels and at the ureterovesical junction (UVJ). Symptoms include abdominal or flank pain (usually severe), hematuria and renal colic. The pain may be associated with nausea and vomiting. If the stone is nonobstructing, pain may be absent. If it produces obstruction in a calyx or at UPJ, the patient may experience dull costovertebral flank pain or even colic. Pain resulting from the passage of a calculus down the ureter is intense and collicky. The patient may be in mild shock with cool, moist skin. As a stone nears the UVJ, pain will be felt in the lateral flank and sometimes down into the testicles, labia, or groin. Other clinical

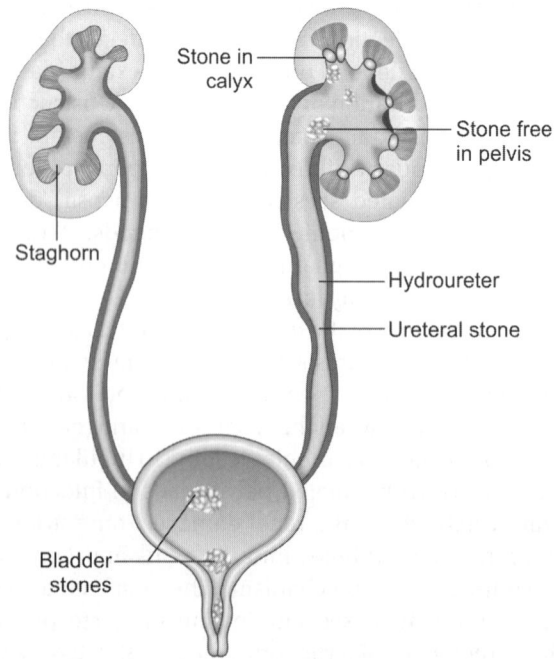

Fig. 7.1: Location of calculi in the urinary tract.

manifestations include the presence of urinary infections accompanied by fever, vomiting, nausea, and chills.

Management

The diagnostic studies performed to determine the presence of renal stones include kidney, ureters and bladder (KUB) X-rays IV or retrograde pyelography; ultrasound; CT; and cystoscopy. Additional studies include urinalysis and serum calcium and serum uric acid levels.

Evaluation and management of patient with renal calculi consists two current approaches. The first approach is directed towards management of acute attack. This involves treating the symptoms of pain, infection or obstruction as indicated for the individual patient. At frequent intervals, narcotics are typically required for relief of renal colic pain. Many stones pass spontaneously. However, stones larger than 4 mm are unlikely to pass through the ureter. The second approach is directed toward evaluation of the etiology of the stone formation and the prevention of further development of stones. Information to be obtained from the patient includes family history of stone formation, geographic residence, nutritional assessment including intake of vitamins A and D, activity pattern (active or sedentary), history of periods of prolonged illness with immobilization or dehydration and any history of disease or surgery of the GI or GU tract.

Therapeutic measures according to urinary stone are as follows:
- *Calcium oxalate:*
    - Increase hydration.
    - Reduce dietary oxalate.
    - Give thiazide diuretics.
    - Give cellulose phosphate to cholate calcium and prevent GI absorption.
    - Give potassium citrate to maintain alkaline urine.
    - Give cholestyramine to bind oxalate.
    - Give calcium lactate to precipitate oxalate in GI tract.
- *Calcium phosphate:* Treat underlying causes and other stones.
- Struvite or tripla phosphate stones ($MgNH_4PO_4$)
    - Administer antimicrobial agents, acetohydroxamic acid and antibiotics.
    - Use surgical intervention to remove stone.
    - Take measure to acidify urine.
- *Uric acid stones.*
    - Reduce urinary concentration of uric acid.
    - Alkalinize urine with potassium citrate.
    - Administer allopurinol.
    - Reduce dietary purines.
- *Cystine*
    - Increase hydration.
    - Give alpha-penicillamine and tiopronin to prevent cystin crystallization.
    - Give potassium citrate to maintain alkaline urine.

And adequate hydration, dietary sodium restrictions, dietary changes, and the use of above-stated medication minimize stone formation. High fluid intake at least 3000 ml per day is recommended. Dietary intervention may be important in the management of urolithiasis. Recent research suggests that a high dietary calcium intake, which was previously thought to contribute to kidney stones, may actually lower the risk by reducing the urinary excretion of oxalate, a common factor in many stones. Initial nutritional management should include limiting oxalate-rich foods and thereby reducing oxalate excretion. Foods high in purine, calcium or oxalate contents are as follows:
- *Purine:* High sardines, herring, mussels, liver, kidney, goose, venison, meat soups and sweetbread.
  Moderate: Chickens, almond, crab, veal, mutton, bacon, pork, beef, ham.
- *Calcium:* Milk, cheese, ice cream, yogurt, sauces containing milk, all beans (except green beans) lentils, fish with fine bones (e.g., sardines, kippers, herring, salmon) dried fruits, nuts chocolate, cocoa and ovaltine.
- *Oxalate:* Spinach, rhubarb, asparagus, cabbage, tomatoes, beets, nuts, celery, parsley, runner beans, chocolate, cocoa, instant coffee ovaltine, tea and worcestestrone sauce.

Indication for endourologic, lithotripsy or open surgical removal of stones include the following:
- Stones too large for spontaneous passage.
- Stones associated with bacteriuria or symptomatic infection.
- Stones causing impaired renal function.
- Stones causing persistent pain, nausea and vomiting.
- Inability of patient to be treated medically.
- Patient with one kidney.

Stones in the lower ureter may be removed by endourologic procedure, i.e. cystoscopic manipulation. General anesthesia may be required, and care is similar to that after cystoscopy.

The percutaneous lithotripsy, extracorporeal shock wave lithotripsy are used to remove stones and the cancel a laser therapy is used to remove stone in the lower ureters. It is pulsed dye laser system designed to break up calculi that have migrated to the lower ureters. The laser probe is inserted through:
- Ureterolithotomy
- Pyelolithotomy
- Nephrolithotomy.

Nursing intervention includes proper assessment and take suitable measure to reduce pain, risk for infection, correcting altered urinary eliminate and reduce anxiety. If any procedure to be performed on the patient, take actions accordingly including health education to patients and family.

Strictures

A stricture is a narrowing of the lumen and is sometimes congenital but is usually acquired. Strictures may occur in the bladder neck, urethra, or ureters.

Etiology

Strictures of the bladder neck may be congenital or may result from chronic prostatitis in men or cystitis in women. The causes of urethral strictures include trauma from accidents (e.g. those resulting in fractured pelvis), gonorrheal infections, and urethral instrumentation. The membranous urethra is a common site of stricture caused by instrumentation, because of its location (the urethral curve just below the prostatic urethra) and because of the surrounding rhabdospincter muscle prevents easy distension. Meatal stenosis, a narrowing of the urethral opening are common. Ureteral strictures may be caused by severe or chronic infection, radiation therapy, and retroperitoneal abscess formation from inflammatory bowel disease and perforation. Urethral strictures occur more often in men than women because of the length of the urethra.

Pathophysiology

Narrowing of the urethra can result from chronic infection that leads to inflammation of the lining. The inflammation causes a hyperplasia of the lining, and the strictures develop. The truama may completely severe the urethra. When the urethra is anastomosed, stricture frequently occurs at the surgical site. One of the leading causes of urethral stricture is a tumor that puts pressure against exterior of the urethra, resulting in stricture of the lumen.

Clinical Manifestation

The first symptom of urethral stricture is usually a decrease in the urinary stream and difficulty in initiating the stream. Other symptoms are those of UTI and urinary retention. Severe urethral strictures result in a complete urinary obstruction, leading to the signs and symptoms of hydronephrosis.

Management

Strictures can sometimes be avoided by the proper management of inflammatory process or traumatic injuries. Treatment of existing strictures includes dilation, use of a catheter for temporary or permanent drainage, for ureteral or urethral strictures, and surgery. Some patients are taught to dilate urethra themselves between office visits to keep strictural areas open. Nursing intervention includes informing the patient about the procedure, preparing the patient for the procedure, and assessing the patient's need for management, education and follow-up care. Education for the patient and family centers on recognition of early signs and symptoms of a decrease in urine stream and urine retention. Education should be focussed on high risk groups.

Renal Tumor

Renal tumor arises from the cortex or pelvis and calyces.

Tumor arising from both areas may be benign or malignant.

Etiology

Exact causes of renal tumor is not known, but certain risk factors have been linked to the disease. The most common risk factor for all concerns of urinary system is cigarette smoking. Occupational exposure to textile dyes, rubber metallurgy, paint, and leather has been implicated in the development of renal cell carcinoma. Other risk factors are the use of phenacetin-containing analgesies and exposure to asbestos, cadmium and gasoline.

Pathophysiology

Renal carcinoma usually develops unilaterally but may occur bilaterlly. In *Stage I*, the margins are well-defined (encapsulated) and compress the kidney parenchyma during growth rather than infiltrating the tissue. The upper pole of the kidney is usually involved and the tumor is usually large at the time of diagnosis. In *Stage II*, the tumor invades the fat surrounding the kidney. *Stage III* consists of local metastasis either through direct extension or through the renal vein or lymphatic (lymph node involvement). Distant metastasis during *Stage IV* are primarily in the lungs or bone; but other areas, such as the liver, spleen, bone, opposite kidney, or brain may also be involved. Prognosis is based on the stage and advancement of the disease at diagnosis.

Clinical Manifestation

There are no characteristic early symptoms. Generalized symptoms of unexplained weight loss, fever, weakness and anemia are the earlier manifestation. The classic manifestation of gross hematurial, flank pain, and flank palpable mass are those of advanced disease. Painless hematuria is the most frequent sign of renal cell carcinoma.

Management

Several studies are used to diagnose adenocarcinoma of the kidney which include IVP, CT scan MRI. Angiography, radionuclide isotope scanning and biopsy.

Unless the person is a poor surgical risk or has extensive metastasis, the diseased kidney is removed (nephrectomy), through a transabdominal, flank, lumbar or thoracoabdominal approach. Radical or partial nephrectomy may be performed accordingly. Radiation is used postoperatively for residual or recurrent tumors and is also beneficial for symptomatic bone metastasis. The use of chemotherapeutic agents in combination with immunomodulating agent has shown some benefits. Interleukin-2 has shown some promise for the treatment of renal cell carcinoma. The side effects of interleukin-2 can be severe and include severe hypotension rigors and anaphylaxis. Hormonal therapy with progesterone, testosterone and antiestrogen is useful in some patients.

If surgery is the treatment chosen, patient and family teaching will focus on peroperative instructions. Preoperative instructions may include a discussion of the type and length of surgery, type of anesthesia, and the need for IV Line, catheter, or other drains. Instruction in the use of an incentive spirometer are crucial because inadequate ventilation is frequent problem postoperatively. The patient is informed of the pain medication routine, e.g. management of the patient after nephrectomy is similar to the patients undergoing abdominal surgery and urinary diversion surgery.

Wilm's Tumor

Wilm's tumor is a common renal tumor of infants and children. It is mostly hereditary. The most common manifestation is abdominal swelling, or distension. This distention is often noticed by parents or is found routine examination. Other symptoms include pain, fever, hematuria and hypertension.

These tumors respond well to multimodality therapy which includes surgical and radiation therapy.

Bladder Cancer

The most frequent malignant tumor of the urinary tract is transitional cell carcinoma of the bladder. Most bladder tumors are papillomatous growth within the bladder.

Etiology

The primary etiology of bladder cancer is exposure to aniline dyes used in the textile industry. Cigarette smoking is associated with an increase in bladder tumors. Cancer of the bladder is most common between the ages of 60 to 70 years and more in men than women. Risk factors include cigarette smoking, exposure to dyes used in the rubber and cable indsutries, and chronic abuse of phenacitin containing analgesics. Women treated with radiation of cervical cancer and patient who has received cyclophosphomide also have increased risk, but reasons are not known yet.

Pathophysiology

Tumors of the bladder range from small benign papilloma to large invasive carcinomas. Most neoplasms are of the transitional cell type because the urinary tract is covered with transitional epithelium. These neoplasms begin as papillomas. Therefore, all papillomas of the bladder are considered premalignant and are removed when identified. Carcinoma of the bladder graded and staged as follows:

Grades	Differentiation
Grade I	Well differentiated
Grade II	Medially differentiated
Grade III	Poorly differentiated
Grade IV	Anaplastic

Stage	Tissue involvement
Stage O	Mucosa
Stage A	Submucosa
Stage B	Muscle
Stage C	Perivesicle fat
Stage D	Lymph node

Clinical Manifestations

Gross painless hematuria is the first sign of bladder tumor in most patients. It is usually intermittent, lessening the person's concern and delaying medical care. Hematuria may be accompanied by urgency and dysuria. Some patients are asymptomatic until obstruction occurs. Painless hematuria is seen in renal tumor; so it should be investigated. Cystitis may be first symptom of the bladder tumor, since the tumor acts as a foreign body into the bladder causing inflammation. Symptoms of renal failure result from obstruction of the ureters. Sometime, it causes one to seek medical care. Vesicovaginal fistula (VVF) may occur before symptoms develop. The presence of renal failure or VVF indicates a poor prognosis because they usually occur after the tumor has infiltrated widely.

Management

When cancer is suspected, urine specimen for cytology can be obtained to determine the presence of cancer cells. Bladder cancers can be detected using IVP, ultrasound, CT or MRI. However, the presence of cancer is confirmed by cystoscopy and biopsy.

Chemotherapy is primarily palliative or used before radiation therapy. CMV (Cisplatin, methotrexate, and vinblantine) with or without doxorubicin hcl is most frequently used therapy. Thiotepa may be instilled into the bladder as a topical treatment for noninvasive bladder cancer. Before instillation of thiotepa, the patient receives 8 to 12 hours of IV hydration. The dwell time for thiotepa is 12 hours after which the drug is drained.

External cobalt radiations of large invasive tumours may be recommended before surgery to retard tumour growth. Super voltage irradiation can be given when the patient physically cannot tolerate include a variety of procedures. Transurethral resection (TUR), with fulguration (electrocautery) is used for the diagnosis and treatment of superficial lesions with low recurrent rate. This is also used to control bleeding in advanced tumors. Laser photo coagulation, and open loop resection (snaring of polytypes of lesion) with fulguration are also used. Postoperative management as in any surgical procedure is with avoidance of alcoholic beverages, analgesics and stool softener.

Renal Trauma/Trauma of Urinary Tract

Assessing the integrity of the urinary tract must be part of the evaluation of any person with traumatic injury to the lower trunk. A continual increase in the incidence of traumatic renal injuries is related to an increase in the mechanization and speed of transportation and to the increase in violent crimes and injuries. Injuries particularly related to the urinary tract damage include fractures of the pelvis, penetrating blows to the body and blunt trauma.

Etiology

The majority of incidence occur in men younger than 30 years of age. Blunt trauma is the most frequent cause. Injury to the kidney should be considered in multiple or sports injuries, traffic accidents and falls. It is especially likely when the patient injures the abdomen flank or back. Penetrating injuries may result from violent encounters (e.g. gunshot, or stabbing incidents) or from surgical procedure errors. Pelvic fracture may result in bladder perforation and urethral tearing. A sharp blow to the body particularly to the lower back, may result in contusion, tearing or rupture of a kidney.

Pathophysiology

If trauma of the urinary tract occurs for any reason, urine output may be scant or absent after trauma, urine if present, may be bloody and symptoms of peritonitis may appear. The first symptoms of trauma to the kidney usually are hematuria and pain or tenderness of the upper abdominal quadrant and flank on the involved side. Signs of shock may be present if hemorrhage is extensive.

Management

Clinical findings include a history of trauma to the area of the kidneys. Diagnostic test used to facilitate diagnosis of trauma to urinary tract incldues KUB, cystogram, IVP, renal angiography and CT scan. Laboratory test includes serial urinalysis and hemoglobin, BUN and creatinine levels.

The severity of renal trauma depends on the extent of the injury treatment, range from bedrest, fluids and analgesics to surgical exploration and repair of nephrectomy. Initial treatment includes controlling bleeding, preventing shock and promoting urinary drainage. A cystotomy may be performed to provide urinary drainage when injuries involve the bladder and urethra. Vital signs, fluid balance records, and hematocrit levels are monitored to assess bleeding.

Complaints of pain may indicate ureteral colic, signifying obstruction of the ureter by a clot. Surgery is required to control severe haemorrhages; otherwise the kidney is allowed to heal spontaneously. Bedrest is maintained until gross hematuria resolves; thereafter, activity progress according to tolerance and absence of haematuria. When urethral injuries are suspected, great care must be taken when inserting urinary catheters to prevent further urethral injury.

A kidney may become loosened and 'float' or become displaced (nephroptosis). If symptoms of obstruction occurs, the kidney may be sutured to its anatomical site (nephropexy). Postoperatively the patient's hips are elevated to prevent tension on the suture line. Nephrectomy may be indicated depending on the severity of the trauma.

Nursing interventions vary with type and extent of associated injuries. Specific intervention related to renal trauma include ensuring increased fluid intake, providing comfort, measures, monitoring intake and output, observing for haematuria, determining the presence of myoglobinuria, assessing the cardiovascular status, and monitoring potentially nephrotoxic antibiotics. Care of the person is similar to nephrectomy or urinary diversion procedures.

Teaching should include preventive strategies such as wearing a seat belt when on automobile, following safety rules, when riding bicycle or walking, and wearing protective equipment when participating in contact sports. Person with one kidney should be cautioned regarding participation in contact sports.

Urinary Retention

Urinary retention is the inability to empty the bladder. The kidneys are producing sufficient urine, but the person is unable to expel the urine from the bladder.

Etiology

The causes of urinary retention are either mechanical or functional. *Mechanical causes* may be congenital or acquired and include anatomic blockage of urine flow in the lower urinary tract.

- Congenital:
  - Urethral stricture
  - Urinary tract malformation
  - Spinal cord malformation
- Acquired:
  - Calculus
  - Inflammation
  - Trauma
  - Tumor
  - Hyperplasia
  - Pregnancy

Functional causes include impairment of urine flow in the absence of mechanical obstruction which includes:
- Neurogenic bladder dysfunction.
- Ureterovesical reflux.
- Decreased peristaltic activity of the ureter.
- Detrusor muscle atrophy.
- Anxiety, i.e. fear of pain after surgery.
- Medications, i.e., anesthetics, narcotics, sedative, antihistamines, antihypertensives, antiparkinsonism, anticholinergics and antispasmodics.

Pathophysiology

An inability to void results from blockage of the urethra. The end result and primary feature of urinary retention is inability to void. The bladder becomes distended with urine and is sometimes displaced to either side of the midline. Percussion over full bladder produce a "Kettle drum" sound. Discomfort occurs from pressure of the bladder on other organs, and the person has an urge to urinate. Restlessness and diaphoresis also may occur with a full bladder. Voiding 25 to 50 ml of urine at frequent intervals often indicates retention with overflow. The intravesicular pressure increases as the bladder continues to fill with urine.

As the bladder overfills, the restoring capacity of the spincter is taxed. A small amount of urine flows out of the bladder to reduce the intravesicular pressure to the level where the spincter can control the flow of urine once again. The patient may state that the bladder continues to feel full. As the bladder fills again, the cycle is repeated. The urine-specific gravity is normal or high in the presence of retention with overflow because the kidney's ability to produce urine is not impaired.

Management

Urinary retention is urological emergency and if untreated can lead to kidney damage. Intervention for urinary retention is aimed at re-establishing the urine flow. The diagnosis of urinary retention is based on determining the amount of residual urine after voiding attempts. Urine yield of 250 to 300 ml after catheterization is indicative of retention. Routine studies of urorenal systems including a complete history and physical examination with particular attention to GU systems are helpful in identifying retention.

Medications used in urinary retention is determined by the etiology. Retention due to sensory/neurological problems may be treated with cholenergic drugs. The drugs which stimulate bladder contraction should not be used if obstruction is suspected. Obstruction occurs below the bladder, continuous drainage must be provided to prevent damage to the kidney. One means of providing drainage is by the use of 'cystostomy' tube (usually Foleys, Malicot, or Pezzor Catheter) which is placed directly into the bladder through a suprapubic incision. If surgery like nephrostomy or pyelostomy indicated can be performed with proper preparation followed by post procedure care appropriately.

Urinary Incontinence

Urinary incontinence is voluntary unpredictable expulsion of urine from the bladder is encountered in several temporary or permanent conditions, due to cerebral clouding, infection, disturbance of CNS pathways cerebral lesions), disturbance of urethrobladder reflex (upper or lower motor neuron) and tissue damage.

Etiology

Anything that interferes with bladder or urethral spincter control can result in urinary incontinence. Causes may be transient (e.g. caused by confusion or depression, infection, medications, restricted mobility or stool impaction); congenital disorders that produce incontinence include exstrophy of the bladder, epispadias, spina bifida with myelomenigocele, and ectopic ureteral orifice; *acquired* disorder includes functional incontinence, stress incontinence, urge incontinence, overflow incontinence, reflex incontinence, incontinence after trauma or surgery:

- Functional incontinence is loss of urine due to problems of patient mobility or environmental factors. It may result from variety of factors including urinary tract dysfunction, environmental causes (no toilet facilities) and locomotor and cognitive factor, causes include pathological, anatomical, or physiological factors affecting the urinary tract, as well as external factors. Many of these factors reversible such as infection, atrophic vaginitis, acute fecal impaction, confusion, restriction, immobility, medical conditions that cause polyuria and drug side effects. Inability to control urination is a problem that frequency leads to emotional distress and can seriously impair a person's social activities.

- Stress incontinence is a sudden increase in intra-abdominal pressure causes involuntary passage of urine. It occurs as a result of incompetence of the bladder outlet or urethral closure. Any activity leading to an increase intra-abdominal pressure on the bladder can result in urinary incontinence. Activities leading to stress incontinence, including lifting, exercising, coughing and sneezing or laughing.

- Urge incontinence is the involuntary loss of urine associated with an abrupt and strong desire to void (urgency). It is a condition which occurs randomly when involuntary urination is preceded by warning of few seconds to a few minutes. Leakage is periodic but frequent. Nocturnal frequency and incontinence are common conditions; it may appear with varying severity during psychological stress. *Motor urge* incontinence caused by detrusor muscle instability; Sensory urge incontinence caused by hypersensitivity of bladder. The incontinence occurs as a result of uninhibited detrusor contractions. When active detrusor contraction over come urethral resistance, urine leakage occurs. This type of incontinence is seen in patients with multiple sclerosis or after CVA (stroke), Ca, bladder, and other cerebrovascular disorders.

- Overflow (Paradoxic) incontinence. Involuntary loss of urine associated with overdistension of the bladder is called overflow incontinence. It is a condition when the pressure of urine is overfull, bladder overcomes spincter control. Leakage of small amounts of urine is frequent throughout the day and night. Urination may also occur frequently in small amounts. Bladder is remaining distended and usually palpable. This disorder caused by outlet obstruction (Prostate hyperplasia, bladder neck obstructs in urethral stricture) or by underactive destrusor muscle caused by myogenic or neurogenic factors (e.g. herniated disc, diabetic neuropathy). It may also occur after anesthesia surgery (hemorroidectomy, herniorraphy, cystoscopy) and neurogenic bladders and after radical pelvic surgery.

- Reflex incontinence is a condition which occurs when no warning or stress precedes periodic involuntary urination. Urination is frequent, moderate in volume and occurs equally during the day and night. It is caused when spinal cord lesion about S2 interfers with CNS inhibition disorders result in detrusor hyperreflexion and interferes with pathways coordinating detrusor contraction and spincter relaxation.
- Incontinence after trauma or surgery. Vesicovaginal or urethrovaginal fistula may occur in women. Alteration incontinence control in men involves proximal urethral sphincter (bladder neck and prostatic urethra) and distral sphincter (external straited muscle). Fistula may during pregnancy, after delivery of a baby, as a result of hysterectomy or invasive cancer of cervix; or after radiation therapy. Incontinence is found as postoperative complication after transurethral, perineal or retropubic prostatectomy.

Pathophysiology

Bladder sphincter control is necessary for urinary continence. Such control requires normal voluntary and involuntary muscle action coordinated by a normal urethrobladder reflex. As the bladder fills the pressure within the bladder gradually increases. The detrusor muscle within the bladder wall responds by relaxing to accommodate the greater volume. When the bladder has filled to capacity, usually between 400 and 500 ml of urine; the parasympathetic stretch receptors located within the bladder will be stimulated. The stimuli are transmitted through afferent fibres of the reflex once for micturition. Impulses are then carried through the efferent fibers of the reflex are to the bladder, causing contraction of the detrusor muscle. The internal sphincter, which is normally closed, reciprocally opens and urine enters the posterior urethra. Relaxation of the external sphincter and perineal muscles follows, and urine is released. Completion of this reflex can be interrupted and voiding postponed through release of inhibitory impulses from the cortical center, which results involuntary contraction of the external sphincter. If any part of this complex control system is interrupted, urinary incontinence will result. As stated earlier, the causes of urinary incontinence are disturbances of cerebral control, disturbances of urethrobladder reflex, bladder disturbance, relaxed muscullation, psychogenic disturbances, etc.

Management

Urinary incontinence can be diagnosed by a variety of urodynamic examinations. A cystomyogram and electromyogram are done to evaluate the detrusor muscle of the bladder as well as sphincter and perineal activity. An ultrasound of the bladder, cystoscopy and IVP are also done to assess the structures and functioning of urinary tract.

Treatments of urinary incontinence can be categorized as behavioral, pharmacological and surgical. A combination of therapies is often used. Behavioral techniques include bladder training, timed voiding, prompted voiding, and pelvic muscle exercises. Behavioral therapies help people to regain control of their bladder. Bladder training teaches people to resist the urge to void and gradually expand the intervals between voiding. *Pelvic floor* electrical stimulation uses mild electrical impulses to stimulate muscle contractions.

The common medication for urinary incontinence are as follows:

- Estrogens (Premarim, Estratab, Estrace) binds the protein responsible for estrogen effects; relieves atrophic vaginitis and restores urethral suppleness. Here the nurse has to explain risk of blood clots, review signs of thrombophlebitis and encourage smoking cessation. Examples of estrogen are quinstrediol and estraiol.
- Anticholinergic agents such as Pro-Bantine, Oxybutynine, Dicyclomin decrerase the spasticity of bladder, are direct smooth muscle relaxation of bladder. This may cause postural hypertension, for which instruct the patient to change position slowly and assess bowel sounds. These drugs should not be used in patients with glaucoma.
- Cholinergic agents such as bethanecol, neostigmines, treat flaccid bladder by stimulating contractions of the bladder. If used, administer medication on empty stomach, monitor vital signs and intake and output and instruct patients to ambulate with caution.
- Alpha-adrenergic blocks such as prazosin, phenoxybenzamine, phenylpropanolamine, reduce spasticity of the bladder neck. When administering these drugs, monitor orthostatic vital signs; monitor intake and output and daily weight the patient and instruct patient to avoid OTC medication unless instructed by physician.
- Sympathomimetics such as ephedrine, phenylephrine, increase in bladder neck and urethral tone. During its administration monitor for dysrhythmias, assess vital signs and instruct patient on potential side effects of dizziness, headache or dyspnea.

- Alpha-adrenergic blockers such as phenylpropanolamine. Imipramine increases urethral resistance. This should be administered several hours before bedtime. Instruct patient to avoid caffeine containing beverages.
- Calcium channel blockers such as nifedipine, diltiazine, verapamil, reduce detrusor contractions. When it is used, monitor blood pressure and heart rate and assess for orthostatic hypertension and monitor intake and output.

Surgical approaches vary, depending on the underlying problem. For example, a transurethral resection of the prostate is used to treat BPH. Several surgical procedures help correct anatomic malposition of the bladder neck and urethra that causes female stress incontinence, e.g. Vesicourethroplexy. Pre and postoperative measures are taken accordingly.

The nurse must recognize both the physical and the emotional problems that accompany incontinence. The patient's dignity, privacy, and feeling of selfworth must be maintained or enhanced. Most persons suffering from incontinence can be helped with proper diagnosis and modern therapeutic approaches.

A person with stress incontinence can be taught to do pelvic floor (perineal) muscle exercises (Kegel exercises). The patient should contract the pelvic muscles as though trying to stop the flow of urine, while relaxing the abdomen, thighs and buttocks. Each contraction is held for a few seconds and followed by relaxation for the same period of time. Contraction and relaxation times are gradually increased. These exercises should be repeated in sets of 10 or more contractions and done four to five times each day over several weeks. Consistency and persistence are necessary for success and exercise regimens have to be individualized. Vaginal weights (cones) or biofeedback may help patient gain awareness and control of their pelvic muscles. Vaginal weight training involves holding small weight within the vagina by tightening the vaginal muscles. These exercises should be performed for 15 minutes twice daily for 4 to 6 weeks.

The nurse has a major responsibility to help the patient with incontinence problems in a variety of settings. In the hospital, nursing measures aimed at maintaining urinary continence include: identifying transient causes and assessing patient for signs of bladder infections, fecal impaction, or bladder distention. The nurse should offer the urinal or bedpan or help the patient going to the bathroom every 2 hours or at scheduled intervals. Assuming the usual position for urination (standing for the man and sitting and leaning forward for the woman) or using relaxation techniques often help a patient urinate successfully, particularly in unfamiliar settings. Applying pressure over the bladder area (credes maneuver) may be helpful when bladder outlet distruction is not a problem. The nurse should ensure that the patient has privacy and is not rushed when trying to urinate. Technique to stimulate urination includes running water in the sink, placing hands in water, and pouring warm water over the perinium. Fluid intake patterns monitored and fluids encouraged.

If bladder retaining cannot be achieved, external appliances or intermittent self catheterization may be indicated. Several external appliances that prevent soiling, decreasing odor, and improved body images are available for men. External appliances for womens are not useful in most situations. However, newly developed inserts, patches, pessaries and bladder neck support devices are useful for some women with stress incontinency. Keeping the skin clean and dry is essential to prevent skin irritation and breakdown.

The nursing responsibilities are often measured for different types of incontinency as follows:

- Stress incontinence:
  - Perineal muscle exercises (e.g. Kegel exercises) i.e.,
    * Tighten the perineal muscle as if to prevent voiding hold for 3 seconds, then relax.
    * Inhale through pursed lips while tightening perineal muscles.
    * Bear down as if to have a bowel movement. Relax and then tighten perineal muscles.
    * Hold a pencil in the fold between the buttock and thigh.
    * Sit in the toilet with knees held wide apart. Start and stop the urinary stream.
  - Weight loss if patient is obese.
  - Insertion of vaginal pessary, estrogen vaginal cream.
  - Insertion of condom catheters, or penile clamp, surgery.
  - Urethral inserts, patches or bladder necks support devices to correct underlying problem.
- Urge incontinence:
  - Treatment of underlying cause.
  - Instructions to have patient urinate more frequently or on time schedule.
  - Anticholinergic drugs, propantheline or imopramine at bed time.
  - Calcium channel blockers, condom catheters, vaginal estrogen creams.
- Overflow incontinence:
  - Urinary catheterization to decompress bladder.
  - Implementation of cre's Valsalva's maneuver.
  - Alpha-adrenergic blockers, i.e. Prazosin to decrease outlet resistance.
  - Bethanechol to enhance bladder contractions.
  - Intermittent catheterization.
  - Surgery to correct underlying problem.
- Reflex incontinence:
  - Treatment of underlying cause.
  - Decompression to prevent ureteral reflux and hydronephrosis.

- Intermittent self-catheterization.
- Alpha-adrenergic blockers (Prazosin) to relax internal spincter.
- Diazepam or baclofen to relax external sphincter.
- Prophylactic antibiotics.
- Surgical sphincterectomy.
- Incontinence after trauma or surgery:
  - Surgery to correct fistula.
  - Urinary diversion surgery to bypass urethra and bladder.
  - External condom catheter.
  - Penile clamp.
  - Placement of artificial implantable sphincter.
- Functional incontinence: Modification of environment or careplan that facilitates regular easy access to toilet and promote patient safety (better lighting ambulatory assistant equipment, clothing, alteration, timed voiding, different toileting equipment).

Reno-Ureteral Surgery

The most comon indication for nephrectomy are: renal tumor, polycystic kidneys that are bleeding or severely infected, massive traumatic injury to the kidney and the elective removal of a kidney from a donor. Surgery involving the ureters and kidneys is most commonly performed to remove calculi that becomes obstructive, correct congenital anomalies, and divert urine when necessary. Now laparoscopic nephrectomy is also performed to obtain a kidney from a living, related donor to be transplanted into a person with end stage renal disease.

Preoperative Care

The basic needs/routines of the patient undergoing renal and ureteral surgery are similar to those of any patient who experiences surgery. In addition, it is especially important preoperatively to ensure adequate fluid intake and a normal electrolyte balance. The patient should be told that there will be probably a flank incision on affected side and surgery will require a hyperextended, side-lying position. This position frequently causes the patient to experience muscle aches after surgery. If nephrectomy is planned, the patient must be assured that one working kidney is sufficient to maintain normal renal function.

Postoperative Care

The specific postoperative needs of a patient are related to urine output, respiratory status and abdominal distension.

In the immediate postoperative period, urine output should be determined at least every one to two hours. Drainage from various catheters should be recorded separately. The catheter or tube should not be clamped or irrigated without a specific order. The total urine output should be at least 30 to 50 ml per hour. It is also important to assess for urine drainage on dressing and to estimate the amount. Daily weighing of the patches is important. The same scale, dress should be weighed.

Postoperatively it is important to ensure adequate ventilation. The patient is often reluctant to turn, cough and take deep breath because of the incisional pain. Adequate pain medication should be given to ensure the patient comfort and ability to perform coughing and deep breathing exercises. Frequently additional respiratory devices such as an incentive spirometer are used every two hours while the patient is awake. In addition, early and frequent ambulation assists in maintaining adequate respiratory function.

Abdominal distention is common in these surgery; may be due to paralytic ileas caused by manipulation and compression of the bowel during surgery. For which, oral intake is restricted until bowel sounds return to normal until IV fluids are recommended.

Urinary Diversion

Urinary diversion may be performed with and without cystectomy. Urinary diversion procedures are performed to treat cancer of the bladder, neurogenic bladder, congenital anomalies, strictures, trauma to the bladder, and chronic infection with deterioration of renal function. Numerous urinary diversion techniques and bladder substitutes are possible including an incontinent urinary diversion, continent urinary diversion catheterized by patient, or an orthotopic bladder so that patient voids urethrally.

- Incontinent urinary diversion is diversion to the skin requiring an appliance. The simplest form is the cutaneous ureterostomy, but scarring and strictures led to the use of ileal or colonic conduits, preferably ileal conduit.

  In ileal conduit ureters are implanted into part of ileum or colon that has been resected from intestinal tract. Abdominal stoma is created. It helps relatively good urine flow with few physiological alteration. External appliances need to continually collect urine. This procedure is more complex. Postoperative complication may be increased. Reabsorption of urea by ileum occurs. Meticulous attention is needed to care for stoma and collecting device.

- A continent urinary diversion is an intra-abdominal urinary reservoir that is catheterizable or with an outlet controlled by the anal sphincter. Continent diversions are internal pouches created similarly to the ileal conduit. Reservoirs have been constructed from the ileum, ileocecal segment or colon. Here, ureters are excised from bladders and brought through abdominal wall and stoma is created. External appliance is necessary because of continuous urine drainage; possibility of stricture or stenosis of small stoma.

Periodic catheterization may be required to dilate stomas to maintaining patency. Nephrostomy may be performed and catheter is inserted into pelvis of kidney. Procedure may be done to one or both kidneys and may be temporary or permanent. It is most frequently done in advanced disease as palliative procedure. There is high risk of renal infection predisposed to calcious formation from catheter. Nephrostomy tube may have to be changed every month. Catheter must never be clamped.
- Orthotopic bladder substitutes can be derived from various segments of the intestine. An isolated segment of the distal ileum is often preferred. Various procedures include the hemiKock pouch, studer pouch, and the ilear W-neobladder. In these procedures, the bowel is surgically reshaped to become a neobladder. The ureters and urethra are sutured into the neobladder. Orthotopic bladder substitute allows for natural micturation. Incontinence may be possible problem needing intermittent catheterization.

Preoperative Care

The patient is awaiting cystectomy and urinary diversion must be given a great deal of informations. The nurse must assess ability and readiness to learn and teach the details about the procedure to the patient. The patient's anxiety and fear may be decreased by giving proper information. A discussion of social aspects of living with a stoma (including clothing, changes in body image, and sexuality, exercises and odor) provides the pattern with facts that may lay some fears. The patient who will have continent diversion must be taught to catheterize and irrigate the pouch and be able to adhere to a strict catheterization schedule. Like this; every information should be provided to the patient undergoing surgery.

The basic needs of the patient requiring urological surgery are the same as those of any other surgical patient. Special emphasis must be placed on promotion of ventilation and adequate urine output, prevention of distention and hemorrhage and attention to drainage tubes and dressings.

The care of the person after urological surgery needs emphasis on the following:
- Promote ventilation:
  - Encourage breathing exercises.
  - Encourage self-turning in bed frequently.
  - Encourage ambulation.
- Monitor patency and output of urinary catheter.
- Prevent complications:
  - Change wet dressings to protect skin.
  - Restrict food and oral fluids if bowel sounds are absent.
  - Encourage fluids to 3000 ml/day when permitted.
  - Monitor for bright red blood on dressing or in urine.
- Administer analgesics to control pain.

The following guidelines should be used for changing a urinary pouch:
- Explain procedure to patient, being sure to include sensory information.
- Assemble all supplies.
- Empty the pouch and gently remove the pouch from the skin.
- Cleanse the peristomal skin with mild soap and water. Rinse and pat dry.
- Wash mucus secretions off the stoma gently.
- Measure the diameter of the stoma and cut a corresponding opening in the skin barrier and the pouch or select the corresponding size of percute pouch.
- Apply skin seal around the stoma is desired. Allow the area to dry completely.
- Attach the pouch to the skin barrier. The pouch and skin barrier may be applied to the skin separately or together. In the early postoperative period, it is easier to attach the pouch to the skin barrier and then apply the system in one piece to the skin.
- Apply the pouch and skin barrier around the stoma, keeping the adhesive area free of wrinkles or creases. Press gently and firmly into place. The value at the bottom of the pouch must be closed or attached to drain tubing and collecting bag.

Renal Failure

Renal failure is severe impairment or total lack of kidney function, in which there is an inability to excrete metabolic waste products and water, as well as functional disturbance of all body systems. Renal failure may be acute in onset (developing in hours to days) or chronic (developing slowly and progressively over a course of several years). Renal failure refers to a significant loss of renal function, when only 10 percent of renal function remains, the person is considered to have end stage renal disease.

Acute Renal Failure (ARF)

Acute renal failure is a clinical syndrome characterized by a rapid decline in renal function with progressive azotemia (an accumulation of nitrogenous waste products such as BUN) and increasing levels of serum creatinine. Urine output is generally less than 40 ml/hr (Oliguria) but may be normal or even increased. ARF can be further divided into prerenal, intrarenal or intrinsic and postrenal etiologies.

Etiology

- *Prerenal*: Causes consist of outside the kidneys than reduce renal blood flow and lead to decreased glomerular perfusion and filtration. This is caused by intravascular volume depletion, decreased cardiac output, or vascular failure secondary to vasodilation or obstruction.

- Hypovolemia can lead to decreased renal perfusion, which can be due to:
    - Hemorrhage
    - Dehydration
    - Vomiting
    - Gastric suction
    - Diabetes insipidus
    - Diabetes mellitus
    - Wound drainage
    - Cirrhosis
    - Inappropriate use of diuretics
    - Diaphoresis
    - Burns
    - Peritonitis.
  - Decreased cardiac output:
    - Congestive heart failure
    - Myocardial infarction
    - Precardial temponade
    - Cardiac arrhythmias/dysrythmias
    - Open heart surgery
    - Cardiogenic shock.
  - Systemic vasodilation/decreased peripheral resistance:
    - Sepsis (Septic shock)
    - Acidosis
    - Anaphylaxis
    - Neurologic injury.
  - Hypotension/hypoperfusion:
    - Cardiac failure
    - Shock
  - Renal vascular obstruction:
    - Thrombosis of renal arteries
    - Bilateral renal vein thrombosis
    - Embolism.
  - Drugs that may complicate prerenal azosimin include NSAIDS, which block synthesis of vasodilating prostaglandins and angiotensin converting enzyme (ACE) inhibition which blocks synthesis of angiotensin.
- *Intrarenal causes*: Prerenal disease can lead to intrarenal disease (tubular necrosis) if renal ischemia is prolonged. Intrarenal failure is caused by damage to kidney tissues and structures and include tubular necrosis, nephrotoxicity and alteration in renal blood flow.
  - Tubule/Nephron damage.
    - Acute tubular necrosis (most common cause)
    - Acute glomerulonephritis
    - Acute pyelonephritis
    - Rhabdomyolysis.
  - Vascular changes
    - Coagulopathies
    - Malignant hypertension
    - Taxemia of pregnancy
    - Systemic lupus erythematous
    - Sclerosis
    - Stenosis.
  - Nephrotoxin/Nephrotoxic injury
    - Allergic-antibiotic (sulfonamide, rifampin) NSAIDs, ACE inhibitor.
    - Antibiotics: Gentamicin, tobramycin, amphotericin B, Polymyxin B, neomycin, kanamycin, vancomycin.
    - Chemical: Carbon tetrachloride and lead
    - Heavy metals: Arsenic, mercury
    - Iodinated radiographic contrast media (IVP dye)
    - Drug-induced interstitial nephritis—NSAIDs, tetracycline furosemide, thiazide, phenytoin, penicillin, sulphonamide and cephalosporins.
- *Postrenal causes*: Involve mechanical obstruction of urinary outflow, between the kidney and the urethral meatus, which includes ureteral and bladder neck obstruction due to:
  - Calculi formation
  - Benign prostatis hyperplasia
  - Prostate cancer
  - Bladder cancer
  - Trauma (to back, pelvis or perineum)
  - Strictures
  - Spinal cord disease.

Pathophysiology

The kidneys receive approximately one fourth of the cardiac output; therefore, they are very sensitive to alteration in perfusion. Most cases of ARF are caused by ischemic episode. Ischemia causes nephron damage, although maintaining of fluid and electrolyte balance is possible 25% of nephron functioning. A urinary output of at least 400 ml/day is necessary for adequate excretion of wastes. The decreased GFR that occurs in ARF is responsible for the increased BUN and serum creatinin levels. The kidneys respond to hypoperfusion in the release of renin and adaptive response to maintain perfusion to the glomerular bed. ARF developes when these adaptive responses are ineffective in maintaining normal kidney function.

The pathophysiology of ARF is not completely understood. Nephrotoxic factors and ischemia produce acute renal failure (ARF). The possible pathologic process involved in ARF include the following.

- *Renal vasoconstriction:* Hypovolemia and decreased renal blood flow stimulate renin release, which activates the angiotensin-aldosterone system and results in constriction of the peripheral arteries and the renal afferent arterioles. With decreased renal blood flow, there are decreased glomerular capillary pressure and glomerular filtration rate (GFR) as well as tubular dysfunction and ultimately oliguria.
- *Cellular edema:* Ischemia causes an anoxia, which leads to endothelial celloedema. Cellular edema

raises tissue pressure above capillary flow pressure; consequently blood flow through the arterioles may still be altered after treatment of the underlying conditions. Inadequate renal blood flow further depresses the GFR.

- *Decreased glomerular capillary permeability:* Ischemia alters glomerular capillary permeability. This in turn reduces the GFR, which significantly reduces blood flow and leads to tubular dysfunction.
- *Intratubular obstruction:* When tubules are damaged, interstitial edema occurs, and necrotic epithelial cells accumulate in the tubules. This accumulated debris also lowers the GFR by obstructing the tubules and increasing intratubular pressure.
- *Leakage of glomerular filtrate:* Glomerular filtrate leaks back into plasma through holes in damaged tubular membranes, which decreases intratubular fluid flow.

Clinical Manifestation

Clinically ARF may progress through phases of onset oliguria, diuresis and recovery. In some situations, the patient does not recover from ARF, and chronic renal failure results.

- The onset is the initial phase of injury to the kidney. Reversal or prevention of kidney dysfunction is possible at this stage by early intervention. In this phase, there is hypotension, ischemia, hypovolemia are seen. Symptoms are subtle, which last for hours to days.
- Oliguria phase follows within one day of the onset. Major problems of the phase include inability to excrete fluid loads, regulate electrolysis and excrete metabolic waste products.

    When urine output is less than 400 ml/24 hours, there is inability to excrete metabolic wastes; increased serum urea nitrogen and creatinine. BUN may increase 20 mg/dl/day. The symptoms include nausea, vomiting, drowsiness, confusion, coma, gastrointestinal bleeding, asterixis, pericarditis. These last for 1-3-weeks, may extend to several weeks in older patients.

    When urine output is less than 30 ml/24 hours, there is inability to regulate electrolytes (hyperkalemia, hyponatremia, acidosis, hypocalcemia, hyperphosphatemia); inability to excrete fluid overload, (fluid overload, hypervolemia); hematological dysfunction (anemia, platelet dysfunction, leukopenia) cases may require dialysis. The symptoms are nausea, vomiting, cardiac dysrhythmias, ECG changes, Kussmaul's breathing (rapid, deep respirations) drowsiness, confusion, coma, edema, CCF pulmonary edema, neck vein distention, hypertension, fatigue, bleeding, infection. The duration also is dependent upon type of toxic injury and duration of ischemia.
- *Diuretic phase:* The diuretic phase begins gradual increase in daily urine output of 1 to 3 liter per day, but may reach 3 to 5 liters or more per day. There is increased production of urine (deficit in concentrating ability of tubule and osmotic diuretic effect of high BUN), slowly increasing excretion of metabolic wastes, hypovolemia, loss of sodium, loss of potassium, high BUN initially; BUN gradually returns to baseline. Symptoms include, urine output up to 4-5 liters per day, postural hypertension, tachycardia, improving mental alertness and activity, weight loss, thirst, dry mucus membranes and decreased skin turgor. These last for 2-6 weeks after onset of oliguria, but duration may vary accordingly.
- *Recovery phase:* The recovery phase begins when the GFR increases so that BUN and serum creatinine levels are starting to stabilize and then decrease. Kidneys are returning to normal functioning, some residual renal insufficiency. Thirty percent of patients do not attain full recovery of GFR. There is decreased energy levels which last for 3-12-months.

The clinical manifestations of acute renal failure according to body system are:

- Urinary
    - Decreased urinary output
    - Proteinuria
    - Casts
    - Decreased specific gravity
    - Decreased osmolality
    - Increased urinary sodium.
- Cardiovascular
    - Volume overload
    - Congestive heart failure
    - Hypotension (early)
    - Hypertension (after development of fluid overload)
    - Pericarditis
    - Pericardial effusion
    - Arrhythmias.
- Respiratory
    - Pulmonary edema
    - Kussmaul's respiration
    - Pleural effusion.
- Gastrointestinal nausea and vomiting
    - Anorexia
    - Stomatitis
    - Bleeding
    - Diarrhea
    - Constipation.
- Hematologic anemia (development within 48 hours)
    - Leukocytosis
    - Defect in plaslet functioning.
- Neurologic
    - Lethargy
    - Convulsions
    - Asterixis
    - Memory impairment.

- Others
  - Increased susceptibility to infection
  - Increased BUN
  - Increased creatinine
  - Increased potassium
  - Decreased pH
  - Decreased bicarbonate
  - Decreased calcium
  - Increased phosphate.

Management

The most important tool for distinguishing prerenal, intrarenal and postrenal causes the history, including a thorough review of recent clinical events and drug therapy. Urinalysis is an important diagnostic test. Urine sediment containing abundant cells, casts or protein suggests intrarenal ATN is associated with abundant urinary casts. Normal urine sediment is possible in both prerenal and postrenal causes. Hematuria, Pyuria and crystals may be associated with postrenal causes. If needed, further tests may be necessary such as CT, MRI, renal ultrasound, retrograde pyelogram and renal scan.

The use of medications in the treatment of ARF is determined by the underlying cause and the presenting symptoms. Hypovolemia is treated with hypotonic solutions such as OUSI saline. If hypovolemia is due to blood or plasma loss, packed red blood cells and isotonic saline are administered. Volume replacement's rates must match volume losses on a 1:1 basis. Loop diuretics are used to manage potassium levels. Doses of up to 320 mg/day of fusomide may be required to produce adequate diuretics. Renal failure from nephrotoxin or ischemia is treated with agents that increase renal blood flow. These include renal-dose dopamine, mannitol and loop diuretics.

Inflammatory states as in acute glomerulonephritis are treated with glucocorticosteroids. Patients with impaired renal functions may have altered responses to therapeutic doses of many medications. Uremia alters the protein binding sites, absorption, distribution and metabolism of many drugs. NSAIDs and ACE inhibitors are contraindicated in patients with acute renal failure.

When conservative management is not effective, dialysis is required. Dialysis, the process by which waste products in the blood are filtered through a semi-permeable membrane, is indicated. When the patient with ARF is fluid overloaded, and/or has rapidly progressive azotemia, hyperkalemia, and metabolic acidosis are used. Three methods are used. Hemodialysis, peritoneal dialysis and continuous renal replacement therapy.

While taking care of the person with acute renal failure following points to be kept in mind which include maintaining fluid and electrolytic balance:

- Maintain fluid restrictions.
  - Monitor intravenous fluid carefully.
  - Keep accurate records of intake and output.
  - Weigh patient daily.
  - Monitor vital signs frequently, including postural signs.
  - Assess fluid status of patient frequently.
  - Administer phosphate binding medications as prescribed.
  - During diuretic phase.
  - Assess for changes in mental status indicative of low serum levels.
  - Assess for presence of irregular apical pulses indicative of hypokalemia.
- Maintaining nutrition:
  - Provide fluid in small amounts during oliguric phase; gingerable and other effective scent soft drinks may be tolerated better than other fluids.
  - Provide diet:
    - Restricted in protein as prescribed.
    - High in carbohydrates and fat during protein restrictions.
    - Low in potassium during hyperkalemia, high in potassium during hypokalemia.
  - Take measures to relieve nausea (antiemetic and comfort measure).
- Maintaining rest/activity balance:
  - Maintain bedrest in the acute phase.
  - Assist patient with activities of daily living to conserve energy.
  - Promote early ambulation when renal status permits.
  - Provide for planned rest periods.
- Prevent injury:
  - Assess orientation, reorient confused patient.
  - During bedrest, keep side rails raised and use padded rails as necessary.
  - When patient is ambulatory, assess motor skills and monitor ambulation and assist patient as necessary.
  - Assess patient for signs of bleeding.
  - Protect patient from bleeding: instruct patient to use soft tooth brush, perform guaiac test on stool, emesis and nasogastric returns.
- Preventing infection:
  - Avoid source of infection: limit visitors to well adults.
  - Assess for signs and symptoms of infection.
  - Maintain asepsis for indwelling lines or catheters.
  - Perform pulmonary hygiene.
  - Turn weak or immobile patients every 2 hours and as needed.
  - Provide meticulous skin care.
  - Bathe patient with superfat soap.
  - Administer prescribed antipruritic agents.
- Facilitate coping:
  - Encourage development of nurse-patient relationship to assist patient to express feelings as desired.

- Promote patient independence (autonomy).
- Assist patient to explore alternative way of coping.

In addition, patient and family education to be given to take care of the person with acute renal failure as follows:
- Causes of renal failure and problems with recurrent failures.
- Identification of preventable environmental or health factors contributing to the illness such as hypertension and nephrotoxic drugs.
- Prescribed medication regimen, including name of medication, dosage, reason for taking, desired and adverse effects.
- Prescribed dietary regimen.
- Explanation of risk of hypokalemia, and reportable symptoms (muscle weakness, anorexia, nausea, vomiting and lethargy).
- Signs and symptoms of returning renal failure (decreased urine output, without decreased fluid intake, signs of fluid retention and increased weight).
- Signs and symptoms of infection, methods to avoid infection.
- Need for ongoing follow-up care.
- Option for the future, explanation of transplantation and dialysis there is a possibility.

Chronic Renal Failure (CRF)

Chronic renal failure involves progressive, irreversible destruction of the nephrons in both kidneys. The disease process progresses until most nephrons are destroyed and replaced by non-functional scar tissue.

Etiology

Although there are many different causes of chronic renal failure, the end result is a systemic disease involving every body organ. The causes of chronic renal failure includes the following:
- Glomerular dysfunction
  - Glomerulonephritis.
  - Diabetic nephropathy.
  - Hypertensive nephrosclerosis.
- Systemic disease
  - Sickle cell anemia.
  - Scleroderma.
  - Polyarteritis nodosa.
  - Systemic lupus erythematosus.
  - HIV-associated nephropathy.
  - Vasculitis.
- Urinary tract obstruction
  - Prostatic and bladder tumors.
  - Lymphadenopathy.
  - Ureteral obstruction.
  - Calculi.
- Others
  - Chronic pyelonephritis.
  - Nephrotic syndrome.
  - Polycystic kidney disease.
  - Renal infarction.
  - Cyclosporin nephrotoxicity.
  - Multiple meloma.

Pathophysiology

Chronic renal failure differs from acute renal failure in which the damage to the kidneys is progressive and irreversible. Progression of CRF is through four stages, decreased renal reserve, renal insufficiency, renal failure and end-stage renal disease (ESRD):
- *Decreased renal reserve (renal impairment):* This stage is characterized by normal BUN and serum creatinine levels and an absence of symptoms. 45-75 percent loss of nephron function and GFR 40-50 percent of normal.
- *Renal insufficiency:* In this there is 75-80 percent loss of nephronfunction and 20-40 per cent GFR normal. BUN and serum creatinine levels begin to rise. Easy fatigue, weakness, mild anemia, mild azotemia, (which worsen physiological stress), nocturia, polyuria are seen.
- *Renal failure:* In this there are 10-20 percent GFR normal, increase in BUN and serum creatinine levels, anemia, Azotemia, metabolic acidosis. Low urine specific gravity, polyuria, nocturia and symptoms of renal failure are present.
- *End-stage renal disease (ESRD) or uremia:* In this stage there are more than 85% of loss of nephron, less than 10 percent of normal GFR, BUN and serum creatinine at high levels. Anemia, azotemia, metabolic acidosis and urine specific gravity are fixed at 1.010 oliguria and symptoms of renal failure appear. It is at this stage where most of the patients face much difficulty in carrying out basic activities of daily living because of the cumulative effect and extent of the symptoms.

Clinical Manifestations

As renal function progressively deteriorates every body system becomes involved. The clinical manifestations are a result of retained resistances, including urea, creatinine, uremia, is a syndrome that incorporates all the disturbances seen in the various systems throughout the body in chronic renal failure. The body system manifestation in chronic renal failure causes signs, symptoms and assessment parameters as follows:
- Hematopoietic system affected may be due to decreased erythroproteins by the kidney; decreased survival time of RBCs, bleeding, blood loss during dialysis, mild thrombocytopenia and decreased activity of platelets. The signs and symptoms are anemia, fatigue, defects in platelet function, thrombocytopenia, ecchymosis and bleeding. Assessment parameters include hematocrit, hemoglobin, platelet count and observing for bruising, haematemesis or melena.
- Cardiovascular system affected may be due to fluid overload, renin-angiotensin mechanism; overload

anemia, chronic hypertension, calcification of soft tissues, uremic toxins of pericardial fluid and fibrin formation on epicardium. These lead to hypervolemia, hypertension, tachycardia, dysrhythmias, CCF, pericarditis for which monitoring of vital signs, body weight, ECG, heartsounds, electrolytes pain is needed.

- Respiratory system affected due to compensatory mechanisms for metabolic acidosis, uremic toxins, uremic lung and fluid overload. These lead to tachypnea. Kussmaul's respirations, uremic fetor (or uremic halitosis), tenacious sputum, pain with coughing elevated temperature, hilar pneumonitis, pleural friction rub, and pulmonary edema, which needs respiratory assessment, arterial blood gas results readings, inspection of oral mucosa, monitoring vital signs and pulse oximetry.
- Gastrointestinal systems affected may be due to change in platelet activity, serum uremic toxins, electrolyte imbalances and urea converted to ammonia by saliva. This leads to anorexia, nausea and vomiting, gastrointestinal bleeding, abdominal distention, diarrhea, and constipation, which need monitoring of intake and output, hematocrit, hemoglobin, guaic test for all stools, assessment for quality of stools, assess for abdominal pain.
- Neurological system affected due to uremic toxins, electrolyte imbalance, cerebral swelling, resulting from fluid shifting, which leads to lethargy, confusion, stupor, coma, sleep disturbances, unusual behavior, asterixis and muscle irritability. This requires monitoring level of consciousness, level of orientation, reflexes, EEG and electrolyte levels.
- Skeletal system may be affected due to decreased calcium absorption and decreased phosphate excretion. These give rise to renal osteodystrophy, renal rickets, joint pains, retarded growth, it needs assessment of levels of serum phosphorus, serum calcium, and for joint pain.
- Skin may be affected due to anemia, retained pigment, decreased size of sweat glands, decreased activity of oil glands, dry skin, phosphate deposits and excretion of metabolic waste products through the skin. These give rise to pallor, pigmentation, pruritis, ecchymosis, excoriation and uremic frost, which needs observation for bruising, assessment of color and integrity of skin and observe for scratching.
- Genitourinary system affected due to damaged nephron. This gives rise to decreased urine output, decreased urine specific gravity, proteinuria, casts and cells present in the urine, and decreased urine sodium, which requires monitoring of intake and output, serum creatinine, BUN, serum electrolytes, urine-specific gravity and urine electrolytes.
- Reproductive system may be affected due to hormonal abnormalities, anemia, hypertension, malnutritions and medication. This leads to infertility, decreased libido, erectile dysfunction, amenorrhea, and delayed puberty which require monitoring intake and output, vital signs, hematocrit and hemoglobin.

In addition, Psychological changes including personality and behavioral changes, emotional liability, withdrawal and depression are commonly observed. Fatigue and lethargy contribute to the patient's feeling of sickness. The changes and body image caused by edema, integumentory disturbances, and access devices (fistulas, catheters) lead to further anxiety and depression.

Management

When a patient is diagnosed as having chronic renal insufficiency, conservative therapy is attempted before maintenance of dialysis begins. Because of the multisystemic effects, chronic renal failure may have serious abnormalities in laboratory values and which are characteristics of person with CRF. Diagnostic measures include identification of reversible renal disease by renal ultrasound, renal scan (if indicated), CT scan (if indicated), hematocrit and hemoglobin levels, BUN, serum creatinine and creatinin clearance level, serum electrolyte, urinalyses and urine culture.

Initial management of patient with chronic renal failure is focussed on controlling symptoms, preventing complications and delaying the progression of renal failure. The treatment goals for the person whose CRF are:

- Stabilization of the internal environment as demonstrated by:
  - Mental altertness, attention span, and appropriate interactions.
  - Absence or control of peripheral and pulmonary edema.
  - Control of electrolyte balance within the following limits:
    * Sodium: 125 to 145 mEq/L
    * Potassium: 3-6 mEq/L
    * Bicarbonate: > 15 mEq/L
    * Calcium: 9-11 mg/dl
    * Phosphate: 3-5 mg/dl.
  - Serum albumin: > 2g/dl.
  - Control of protein catabolism and protein metabolic wastes as indicated by following parameters.
    * Urea nitrogen: < 100 mg/dl
    * Creatinine: < 10 mg/dl
    * Uric acid: < 12 mg/dl.
  - Absence of joint inflammation and pain.
  - Control of anemia
    * Hematocrit: ≥ 33 percent
    * Ferritin: > 50-100 mg/ml
    * Iron saturation: > 20 percent.
- Absence of infection.
- Absence of bleeding.

- Blood pressure controlled at:
  - < 140/90 mm Hg sitting and
  - < 10 mm Hg postural change in standing.
- Control of coexisting disease including heart failure, anemia, dehydration.
- Absence of toxicity from inadequately excreted medications.
- Nutrient intake sufficient to maintain positive nitrogen balance.
- Anorexia and nausea are controlled.
- Pruritis controlled.

Medications are used to control blood pressure, regulate electrolytes and control intravascular fluid volume accordingly as prescribed. For example, therapies to lower serum potassium levels are regular insulin administration intravenously, sodium bicarbonate IV, calcium gluconate, dialysis, kayexalate (Sodium polystyrene sulfonate) and dietary restriction of potassium (40–50 mEq/L and treatment of concurrent disorders like anemia, GI disturbances, etc.

While taking care of person with chronic renal failure following points are to be kept in mind:
- Maintain fluid and electrolyte blance.
  - Monitor for fluid and electrolyte excess.
    - Assess intake and output every 8 hours.
    - Weigh patient every day.
    - Assess presence of and extent of edema.
    - Auscultate breach sounds.
    - Monitor cardiac rhythm and blood pressure every 8 hours.
    - Assess level of consciousness with the interval of every 8 hours.
  - Encourage patient to remain within prescribed fluid restriction.
  - Provide small quantities of fluid spaced over the day to stay within fluid restrictions.
  - Encourage a diet high in carbohydrate and within the prescribed sodium, potassium, phosphorus and protein limits.
  - Administer phosphate-binding agents with meals as prescribed.
- Prevent infection or injury.
  - Promote meticulous skin care.
  - Encourage activity within prescribed limits but avoid fatigue.
  - Protect confused person from injury.
  - Protect person from exposure to infectious agents.
  - Maintain good medical/surgical asepsis during treatment and procedures.
  - Avoid aspirin products.
  - Encourage use of soft tooth brush.
- Promote comfort.
  - Medicate patient as needed for pain.
  - Medicate with prescribed antipruritic use of emollient bath, keep skin moist, and control environmental temperature to modify pruritis.
  - Encourage use of damp cloth to keep lips moist, give good oral hygiene.
  - Encourage rest for fatigue, however, encourage self-care as tolerated.
  - Provide calm and supportive atmosphere.
- Assist with coping in lifestyle and self concept
  - Promote hope.
  - Provide opportunity for patient to express feelings about self.
  - Identify available community resources.

In addition, patient and family teaching is needed while taking care of the person with chronic renal failure.
- Relationship between symptoms and their causes.
- Relationships among diet, fluid restriction, medication and blood chemistry values.
- Preventive health care measures: oral hygiene, prevention of infection and avoidance of bleeding.
- Dietary regimen, including fluid restrictions, i.e.
  - Prescribed sodium, potassium, phosphorus and protein restrictions.
  - Label reading and identifying nutritional content of foods.
  - Use of small frequent feedings to maintain nutrient intake when anorexia or nauseated.
  - Fluid prescription and sources of fluid in diet.
  - Avoidance of salt substitute containing potassium.
- Monitoring of fluid excess:
  - Accurate measurements and recording of intake and outputs.
  - Monitoring weight gain and edema.
- Medication:
  - Action, doses, purpose and side effects of prescribed medications.
  - Avoidance of over-the-counter (OTC) drugs, especially aspirin, cold medication and NSAIDs.
- Planning for gradual increase in physical activity including rest periods to conserve energy.
- Measures to control pruritis.
- Planning for following health care:
  - Symptoms requiring immediate medical attention: changes in urine output, edema, weight gain, dyspnea, infection, increased symptoms of uremia.
  - Need for continual medical follow up.
  Add dialysis and kidney transplantation.

Dialysis Therapy

If complications of ARF become marked (e.g., fluid volume overload with congestive heart failure, hyperkalemia [> 6.0 mEq/liter], and severe metabolic acidemia [pH < 7.20]), aggressive therapy with dialysis may be necessary.

Continuous Arteriovenous Hemofiltration for Acute Renal Failure

An alternative to peritoneal and hemodialysis in the treatment of critically ill patients with renal failure and/or fluid overload is continuous arteriovenous hemofiltration (CAVH). This technique uses a hemofilter that facilitates removal of water, electrolytes, and small to medium molecular weight molecules from the vascular space, while conserving the cellular and protein contents of circulating blood. The blood enters the extracorporeal circuit by an arterial access, flows through the hemofilter, and returns to the patient by way of a venous access. Blood flow is driven by the hydrostatic blood pressure; no pump is used.

The mechanism underlying hemofiltration involves the use of a transmembrane pressure gradient. This pressure gradient is achieved by the net difference between hydrostatic and osmotic pressures. The hydrostatic pressure consists of two components. These include the arterial blood pressure, which drives fluid across the semipermeable membrane into the ultrafiltrate compartment, and the pressure exerted by the fluid within the ultrafiltrate system, which drives fluid from the fibers into the ultrafiltrate. The pressure opposing the hydrostatic pressure is the colloidal osmotic pressure exerted by the plasma proteins, which do not pass through the semipermeable membrane.

The filter replacement fluid used is determined by the patient's electrolyte values, and the ultrafiltration flow rate is geared to the patient's needs. If the objective is to remove extracellular fluid only, ultrafiltration is regulated at a low rate (approximately 100–300 ml/hour) without subsequent intravenous replacement; if the objective is to clear both extracellular fluid and toxic substances (e.g., urea, potassium), then high ultrafiltration rates and filter replacement fluid are used. The final composition of the ultrafiltrate might include the following: sodium 150 mEq/liter, chloride 114 mEq/liter, potassium 0, bicarbonate 37 mEq/liter, magnesium 1.6 mEq/liter, calcium 2.5 mEq/liter. Clotting of the extracorporeal circuit is prevented by the administration of flow dose heparin. The dose is titrated depending on the patient's coagulation status.

Nursing care of patients undergoing continuous arteriovenous hemofiltration involves patient and equipment preparation, attachment, monitoring of patient and the hemofilter, and termination of hemofiltration. A baseline assessment, including the clinical history, physical examination, and hemodynamic profile, is essential. The hemodynamic profile includes vital signs and measurement of hemodynamic pressures (e.g., central venous, pulmonary artery, pulmonary capillary wedge pressure, and arterial pressures). The patient's weight is ascertained, and baseline laboratory data (e.g., hematology, coagulation, and chemistry profiles) are established.

An access site is established. The most commonly used sites are the femoral artery and vein; the saphenous or subclavian veins may also be used as the venous access. Scribner-type wrist shunts involving the radial or ulnar arteries and median cubital or basilic vein may also be cannulated. The hemofilter is primed, heparinized, and attached to the patient. The hemofilter must be secured carefully to the patient to prevent accidental disconnection.

Continuous monitoring of the patient's hemodynamic status is recommended and best achieved using an arterial line. Ideally, use of the pulmonary artery catheter more closely reflects the patient's fluid status. The nurse observes the flow rate every 15 minutes; outputs are recorded hourly. The goal is to remove a large amount of fluid each hour and to replace part of this volume. This results in a net loss of fluid and selected solutes (e.g., urea). The desired hourly fluid balance is specified by the physician. Laboratory values are followed closely to identify trends. It is essential to avoid fluctuations outside the normal range. Aseptic shunt care is imperative; monitoring of pulses distal to the access site is essential.

Patient/family educatiaon should include information about the function, purpose, and standard care of patients receiving continuous arteriovenous hemofiltration. Areas of greatest concern include the frequency of patient monitoring and the special equipment involved. The nurse should emphasize that the frequency of care is standard practice for patients receiving this form of therapy.

CHAPTER 8

Nursing Management of Disorders of Reproductive System

INTRODUCTION

The reproductive system is inter-related with other systems including the neurologic, endocrine and urinary system and also with general physiologic function. For example, estrogen (produced primarily in woman's ovaries) influence on bone density and testosterone (produced primarily in a man's testes) influence muscle mass. The reproductive system is also directly related to sexual function and is therefore, intricately interwoven into the complex, sensitive and frequently stress-laden area of psychosocial mores and cultural values regarding sex.

Conditions affecting healthful functioning of the reproductive system of men and women take a high toll in loss of life and acute and chronic physical and emotional stress. Reproductive nursing refers to nursing the disorders of the reproductive system both in men and women. The nurse has a responsibility to assist in general health education to refer patients for appropriate health care, and to understand the treatment available as the nursing care needed when disease develops.

The male reproductive system consists of the external structure—the penis and the scrotum—and the internal structures including prostate gland, the seminal vesicles and several ducts. The female reproductive system consists of the breasts, the uterus, the ovaries, the fallopian tubes and the vagina and the external genitalia (the vulva) as well as ligaments at pelvic bones. A sound knowledge of reproductive system is essential.

NURSING ASSESSMENT OF THE MALE AND FEMALE REPRODUCTIVE SYSTEM

As stated before, reproductive system is inter related with other systems. Therefore, problems in other systems are often interrelated with problems and stresses within the reproductive system. The nurse must elicit general information as well as information especifically relating to the reproductive system.

Reproduction and sexual issues are often considered extremely personal and private. The nurse must develop trust to elicit such information. A professional demeanour is important while taking a reproductive or sexual history which include genitourinary assessment of female and male.

Female Genitourinary Assessment

Every woman who enters the health care system should have a complete gentitourinary health histories which include the urinary system, menstruation, sexual activity, contraceptive use, pregnancies and gynecological problems or surgeries. In addition, breast health, physical abuse and sexual assault should be screened. The following outline summarises the interview items, symptoms, and health promotion activities to be included in assessment:
- Current breast health.
- Problem with breasts:
  - Breast pain/tenderness.
  - Lumps.
  - Skin dimpling.
  - Lesions or changes in the skin.
  - Discharge from nipples.
- Current genitourinary health.
- Urinary symptoms including infections and voiding dysfunction:
  - Dysuria
  - Frequency
  - Urgency
  - Hematuria
  - Nocturia
  - True incontinence (loss of urine without warning)
  - Stress incontinence (loss of urine with cough or sneeze).
- Menstrual history:
  - Age at menarchy (first menses).
  - Last menstrual period.
  - Interval of frequency; regular or irregular.
  - Duration.
  - Menstrual flow: light, medium or heavy (number of pads or tampoons used in a specified time period).
  - Menorrhagia (increased amount or duration of flow).
  - Dysmenorrhea (pain with menstruation) frequency or severity.
  - Bleeding between periods.
  - Postcoital bleeding (bleeding after intercourse).
  - Postmenopausal bleeding: essential to assess for any bleeding since menopause to screen for endometrial cancer).
  - Postmenstrual syndrome symptoms: irritability, depression, weight-gain, headaches, breast tenderness and breast swelling.

- Obstetrical history:
  - Number of pregnancies (gravida).
  - Pregnancy outcomes:
    - Term: Number of births between 37 and 42 weeks of pregnancy.
    - Premature: Number of births before 37 weeks of pregnancy.
    - Living: Number of children living.
    - Abortions: Spontaneous or elective.
  - Types of deliveries: Vaginal, forceps or caesarian.
- Perimenopausal symptoms:
  - Hot flashes/flushes.
  - Headaches.
  - Night sweats.
  - Vaginal dryness.
  - Mood swings.
  - Numbness and tingling.
- Vulvovaginal problems:
  - Discharge, color, amount and odor.
  - Vaginal itching.
  - Lesions or lumps.
  - Dyspareunia (pain with intercourse).
  - Vaginisms (spasms of muscles around vagina)
  - History of STDs.
- Sexual health:
  - Sexually active; monogamous versus multiple partners; male/female/both.
  - Satisfaction or problems related to sexual activity.
  - Changes in ability to engage in sex; vaginal dryness, female sexual disorders, inhibited orgasm or pain with intercourse.
- Health promotion practices:
  - Contraceptive choice, proper use of method, satisfaction and side effects.
  - Pelvic examination: last pap smear and results.
  - Condom use.
  - Breast, self examination.
  - Vulvo self examination.
  - Mammogram.
  - Personal hygiene; douche, bubble baths, use of tampoon, and feminine sprays.
- Family history:
  - Breast cancer.
  - Cervical, ovarian or endometrial cancer.
  - Diethystilbestrol (DES) use, (Previously used to prevent spontaneous abortion; since it has been associated with cervical adenoses and cervical and vaginal carcinoma and congenital anomalies GU tract. It was banned in 1971).

In addition any history of medication taken in surgeries include dilation and currettage, hysterectomy, oophorectomy, repair of cystocele, repair of rectocele, salpingectomy, tubal sterilization.

Male Genitourinary Assessment

A male genitourinary history includes current health status as well as past medical history, which includes bladder, kidney function, the penis and testes, possible hernias, sexual health and health promotion activities. The following outline summarizes symptoms and health promotion behavior to be included in the assessment.

- Current genitourinary health status.
- Screen for urinary symptoms including infections, voiding, dysfunction or prostate problem:
  - Dysuria (pain with urination).
  - Frequency.
  - Urgency.
  - Hematuria.
  - Nocturia.
  - Urinary retention.
  - Straining.
  - Hesitancy.
  - Change in force/caliber of stream.
  - Dribbling.
  - History of prostate problems.
  - History of urinary infections.
- Screen for incontinence:
  - True (loss of urine without warning).
  - Stress (loss of urine with cough/sneeze).
- Screen for problem with penis such as skin lesions, cancer or STDs:
  - Pain.
  - Lesion or sores.
  - Discharge.
  - History of STDs.
- Screen for problems with testes such as torsion, cancer or infections and problems with the scrotum such as hydrocele, hernia or varicocele:
  - Lump or swelling in testes.
  - Bulge or swelling in scrotum.
  - Change in size of scrotum.
  - History of hernia.
- Assess sexual health:
  - Sexually active: monogamous versus multiple partners male/female/both.
  - Satisfaction with or problem related to sexual activity.

Physical Examination

The examination of the external genitalis uses inspection and palpation.

Male Genitalia

An examination should be performed with the patient lying or standing. The standing position is generally preferred. The examiner should be seated in front of the standing patient. Gloves should be used during examination of male genitalia.

- *Pubis:* The nurse observes the diamond-shaped pattern of hair distribution. The absence of hair is not normal. The skin is also evaluated. The pubic hair should be inspected for nits, lice or scabies.
- *Penis:* The nurse notes the size and skin texture of the penis and any lesions, scars or swelling. The lesion caused by chancres, genital warts, herpes or penile cancer. The location of the urethral meatus, as well as the presence of absence of a foreskin should be noted. If present, foreskin should be retracted to note cleanliness and replaced over the gland after observation. The glands are compressed to note any discharge and its amount, color and odor are present. The nurse also palpates the penile shaft for tenderness, masses and observes the ventral and dorsal aspects.
- *Scrotum and Testes:* The nurse performs a complete skin examination by lifting each testes to inspect all sides of the scrotal sac. The scrotum is inspected for size, symmetry, swelling, inflammation and/or lesions. Palpation of scrotum is done to note changes in consistency or the presence of masses. It is important to note if the testes are distended. The left testes usually hangs lower than the right. Undescended testes is a major risk factor for testicular cancer, as well as a potential cause of male infertility. The patient also be taught TSE (Testes Self examination).
- *Inguinal region and spermatic cord:* The examiner insepcts the inguinal region for rashes, lesions, or lymphadenopathy, which may suggest pelvic organ infections. The nurse has to make the patient cough or bear down and notes any conspicuous bulging in the inguinal canals. The nurse also palpates the area for any bulging as the patient again coughs or bears down. The nurse palpates the inguinal and femoral pulses and the local lymph nodes.

    The spermatic cord is located posteriorly in the scrotal sac. The nurse follows the cord on each side. The inguinal region is gently palpated using the forefinger or small finger and by pushing up through the loose scrotal skin to the abdominal wall along the inguinal region. At this point, the patient again bears down and coughs. The nurse determines whether the strain produces bulging of the intestine through the ring, indicating the presence of hernia a condition which requires follow up.
- *Anus and prostate:* The anal sphincter and perineal regions are inspected for lesions, masses and hemorrhoids; A digital examination is required for all patients who have symptoms of prostate trouble such as difficulty in initiating the flow and urge to void frequently.

    The prostate gland is palpated by means of rectal examination with the patient standing with the hips flexed over an examination table or in a side lying position. Before the examination, advise the man that he may feel as though he needs to have a bowel movement. The patient is asked to bear down while a lubricated index finger is gently inserted into the canal and then the rectum. The prostrate and seminal vesicles are palpated. The size, shape and consistency of the lobes and the median sulcus of prostrate are noted. The normal prostate is 2.5 by 4 cm, smooth, heart-shaped, rubbery and non-tender. Rectal examination is most important step in the diagnosis of prostate disease.
- *Male breasts:* The male breast can be easily and quickly examined during routine physical examination. Barring some rare cases, breast cancer does not occur in males, mostly it occurs frequently in the areolar area. The inspection of skin and areolae for the presence of any swelling, retractions or lesions are noted. The breast, areola, and axillae are then palpated for mass.

Female Breasts and External Genitalia

Physical examination of women often begins with inspection and palpation of the breasts and then proceeds to the abdomen. Examination of the abdomen provides an opportunity to detect pain or any masses that may involve the genitourinary system.

- *Breasts:* In a menstruating women, the ideal time to examine the breast is several days after menstruation, when they are less tender and nodular. Breasts are examined first by visual inspection. The nurse, with the patient being seated, observes the breasts for symmetry, size, shape, skin color and texture. Vascular patterns and the presence of unusual lesions. The patient is asked to put her arms at her sides, arms over head, lean forward and press hands on hips. The nurse observes for any abnormalities during these maneuvers. The axillae and the clavicle also be examined for any abnormalities.

    When the patient assumes a supine position, a pillow is placed under the back on the side to be examined. The patient is asked to put the arm above and behind the head. These maneuvers flatten the breast tissue and make palpation easier. The breast is then palpated in a systemic fashion using a vertical line, a clockwise or a spoke approach. The nurse should use the distal fingers pads for palpation. The tail of Spence should be included in the examination because this area and the upper outer quadrant are the areas where most breast malignancies develop. Finally, the nurse should palpate the area around the areolae for masses. The nipple should be compressed to determine the presence of discharge or any masses. The color, consistency and odor of any discharge should be documented.

- *External genitalia:* The nurse uses gloves for examination of the external genitalia. The monspubis, the labia majora, the labia minora, the perinium and the anal region are inspected for characteristics of skin hair distribution and contour. Lesions, swellings and discharges are noted.

    The nurse separates the labia to the maximum to inspect the clitoris, the urethral meatus, the vaginal orifice, the hymen, the preineum, and the anal region. Any inflammation or cysts on Bartholin's gland or Skene's glands are noted.

Internal Pelvic Examination

Women who are scheduled for pelvic examination should be advised to avoid douching, sexual intercourse and applying any vaginal preparations (medicinal or deodorant) for at least 24 hours before examination. The most common position for the pelvic examination is the lithotomy position. Sim's (lateral position) and knee chest position also are used sometimes.

During the speculum examination, the nurse observes the walls of the vagina and cervix for inflammation, discharge, polyps and suspicious growths. During this examination, it is possible to take a pap smear and collect secretions for culture and study under the microscope (i.e. wet smears).

After the speculum examination, a bimanual examination is performed to allow assessment of the size, shape and consistency of the uterus, ovaries and tubes. The tubes are not normally palpable. Abdominal palpation is performed to rule out or discover abnormalities. Enlargement of the uterus is detected by palpating in the midline of the lower abdomen. Enlargement of the fallopian tubes and ovaries may be detected by the palpation of the right and left quadrant.

DIAGNOSTIC STUDIES OF REPRODUCTIVE SYSTEM

Many diagnostic tests that are performed to assess problems occurring in other body systems also provide valuable data on the condition of the reproductive system. The following are the most commonly used diagnostic studies in the assessment of the reproductive system and the nurses' responsibility regarding these diagnostic tests. To understand many of the diagnostic studies of the reproductive system, it is important to understand the concepts of sensitivity and specificity. Sensitivity addresses the issue of how well a test identifies people with a particular disease (screening test), specificity testing answers the question of how well a test eliminates those individuals without disease. The goal of sensitivity testing is to avoid false-positive results. It is the nurse's responsibility to ensure that the patient understands the purposes of any test being performed.

Urine Studies

- *Pregnancy testing:* Occurrence of pregnancy is generally validated by measuring outputs of human chorionic gonadotropin (hCG) in the urine by means of an immunologic test. hCG is detected in urine to ascertain whether a woman is pregnant. Hydatidiform mole and chorioepithelioma 'in men and women) may also be detected.

    Nursing responsibility is to obtain through menstrual history from patient, including birth control methods, determine presence or absence of presumptive signs of pregnancy (e.g. breast changes or increased whitish vaginal discharge).
- *Hormone testing:*
    - Testosterone level: In the tumors, developmental anomalies of the testes can be detected. For which the nurse instructs patient to collect 24 hours urine specimen. Keep it refrigerated.
    - Follicle stimulating hormone (FSH) assay: This test indicates gonadal failure because of pituitary dysfunction.

        Female: Follicular phase : 2–5 i.u/24 hr.
        Mid cycle : 8–40 i.u./24 hrs.
        Leutal phase : 2–10 i.u./24 hrs.
        Menopause : 35–100 i.u./24 hrs.
        Male : 2–15 i.u./24 hrs.

For FSH assay, patient is instructed to collect 24 hours urine specimen indicates phase of menstrual cycle if menopausal and if an oral contraceptives or hormones.

Blood Studies

- *Prolactin assay:* This test detects pituitary dysfunction that can cause amenorrhea. In this, nurse observes venipuncture site for bleeding or hematoma formation.
- *Serum hcG assay:* hcg is detected in serum to ascertain whether a woman is pregnant. Here nurse instructs the patient to have blood drawn in laboratory. Elicite where she is in her menstrual cycle, whether she has missed menses and if so how late she is.
- *Serum androgen and testosterone levels:* These tests ascertain whether elevated androgens are due to adrenal or ovarian dysfunction. Serum testosterone is also drawn to assess cause of amenorrhea.
- The nurse collects health history to eliminate potential sources of interference with accuracy of results (e.g. use of steroids or barbiturates or presence of hypothyroidism or hyperthyroidism).
- *Serum progesterone:* This test is frequently used to detect functioning corpusluteum cyst. Here nurse observes venipuncture site for bleeding or hematoma formation. Includes last menstrual period and trimester of pregnancy since progesterone level varies with gestation

- *Serum estradiol:* This test measures ovarian function. It is particularly useful in assessing estrogen-secreting tumors and states of precocious female puberty. Normal values depend on laboratory that performs test and should be obtained from that laboratory. It may be used to confirm premenopausal time. Increased serum estradiol levels in men may be indicative of testicular tumor. Here the nurse observes venipuncture site for bleeding or hematoma formation.
- *Serum FSH:* This test indicates gonadal failure due to pituitary dysfunction; it is used to validate menopause. In females; follicular phase: 4-30 ml u/ml; Mid cycle: 10-90 ml u/ml; Luteal phase: 4-30 ml u/ml: Menopause 40-250 ml u/ml. In males: 4-25 ml/ml. In this test no food or fluid restrictions are required. State phase of menstrual cycle; if menopausal or if oral contraceptive or hormones.

Syphilis Studies

- *Nontreponimal serologic tests include:* Wasserman (complement fixation), Venereal disease research laboratory (VDRL), (flocculation), Rapid plasma reagin (RPR) (agglutination). These tests are non-specific antibody test used to screen for syphilis. Positive reading can be made within 1-2 weeks after appearance of primary lesion (chancre) or 4-15 weeks after initial infection.

  Here the nurse tells the patient that fasting is unnecessary,
- Informs the patient that blood sample will be drawn. Observe venipuncture site for bleeding or hematoma formation. Obtain data to determine presence or absence of problems such as hepatitis, pregnancy and autoimmune diseases that may interfere with the accuracy of results.
- *Treponemal:* Test fluorescent treponemal antibody absorption (FTAAbs). This test detects syphilis antibodies. It also detects early syphilis with great accuracy. It is usually performed if results of nontrepenoma testing are questionable. In this, the nurse tells the same as in venipuncture care.
- *Miscellaneous studies*
- Dark field microscopy is a direct examination of the specimen obtained from potential syphilitic lesion (chancre) performed to detect treponoema. The Nurse has to avoid direct skin contact with open lesion.
- Wet mounts is a direct microscopic examination of specimens of vaginal discharge which is performed immediately after collection. This determines presence or absence and number of trichomonas organisms, bacteria, white and red blood cells, and candidal buds or hyphae. Other clues or causes of inflammation or infection may be determined.

  In this, the nurse explains the procedure and purpose to patient. Instructs the patient not to douche before examination. Prepare collection of specimens (glass slide, 10-20 percent potassium hydroxide (KOH) solution, sodium chloride (NaCl) solution, and cotton tipped applicators).
- *Cultures:* Culture specimens of vaginal, urethral or cervical discharge are taken and used to assess presence of gonorrhea or chlamydia. Rectal and throat cultures may also be taken depending upon data obtained from sexual history. Here, nurse has to obtain specific contact and sexual history inclusive of oral and rectal intercourse. Instruct against douching before examination. Obtain urethral specimen from men before void. Instruct women who are sexually active with multiple partners to have at least a yearly culture for gonorrhea and chlamydia. Instruct sexually active men to have any discharge evaluated immediately rule out gonorrhea strains that do not cause classic symptoms of dysuria.
- *Gram's stain:* This presumptive test is used for rapid detection of gonorrhea. Presence of gram-negative intracellular diplococci generally warrants initiation of treatment. Not highly accurate for women. The nursing responsibility is as in culture.

Cytologic Studies

- *Pap smear:* Microscopic study of exfoliated cells via special staining and fixation technique detects abnormal cells, cells most commonly studied are those obtained directly from endocervix; vaginal pool and endometrial lining of uterine activity.

  In this procedure, instruct women who are sexually active, and who are over age of 18 to have pap smears according to cancer society guidelines. Arrange for smear at mid cycle time. Instruct patient not to douche for at least 24 hours before examination. Collect careful menstrual and gynecologic history.
- *Nipple discharge test:* Cytologic study of nipple discharge is performed here indicates whether hormonal preparation or other drugs are being taken, breastfeeding or history of amenorrhea. Instruct patient demonstration of breast self examination or examination of breasts that nipple discharge should always be evaluated.

Radiological Studies

- *Soft tissue mammography:* Low dose X-ray image of breast tissue on photographic film is used to assess breast masses, recent breast enlargement, and nipple discharge to detect malignancy. It is usually an outpatient procedure. For which instruct patient about risks (radiation) and advantages of the examination. Instruct regarding cancer society recommendation.
- *Contrast mammography:* This test is used to evaluate abnormal nipple discharge. It is particularly effective

in detecting non-palpable intraductal papillomas. Test consists of injection of radiopaque dye in breast duct. Here determine actual or possible allergy to contrast medium.
- *Ultrasound:* This test measures and records high frequency sound waves as they pass through tissues of variable density. It is very useful in detecting masses greater than 3 cm such as ectopic pregnancies, IUDs, ovarian cysts and hydatidiform moles.

Invasive Procedures

- *Breast biopsy:* Histologic examination of excised breast tissue is performed, either by needle-aspiration or excisional biopsy. Here, prior to surgery, instruct patient about operative procedure, and sedation. After surgery, perform wound care and instruct patient about breast-self-examination.
- *Hysterosalpingogram:* This test instillation of radioscopic dye through cervix into uterine cavity and subsequently through and out of fallopian tubes. Spot X-ray images are taken to detect abnormalities of uterus and its adnexa (ovaries and tubes) as dye progresses through them. Test may be most useful in diagnostic assessment of fertility (e.g. to detect adhesions near ovary, an abnormal uterine shape or blockage of tubal pathways).

  Here inform patient about procedure and that it may be fairly uncomfortable, especially shoulder pain. Determine possibility of dye allergy.
- *Colposcopy:* Direct visualization of cervix with binocular microscope that allows magnification and study of cellular dysplasia and vascular and tissue abnormalities of cervix. This test is used as a follow-up study for abnormal pap smear and for examination of women exposed to DES in utero. Biopsy of cervix may be taken during colposcopic examination. This test is valuable in decreasing number of false-negative cervical biopsies. The nurse has to instruct patient about the outpatient procedure. Inform patient that this examination is similar to speculum examination. Explain purpose of procedure and prepare patient for it.
- *Conization:* Cone shaped sample of squamocolumnar tissue of cervix removed for direct study. In this, the nurse explains purposes and method of procedure and that it requires use of surgical facilities and anesthesia. Instruct patient to rest for at least 3 days after procedure. Also discuss necessity for 3 week follow up check.
- *Loop electrosurgical excision of transformation zone (LEETZ):* It is excision of cervical tissue via an electrosurgical instrument. Here the nurse explains purpose and method of procedure and that it may be done in the physician's office for further diagnostic testing.
- *Loop electrosurgical excision procedure (LEEP):* Same as LEETZ.
- *Culdotomy, culdoscopy and culdocentesis:* Culdotomy is an incision made through posterior forni of cul-de-sac and allows visualization of peritoneal cavity (i.e. uterus, tubes, and ovaries).
- Culdoscope can then be used to study these structures closely. This technique is valuable in fertility evaluations. Withdrawal of fluid (Culdocentesis) allows examination of fluid characteristics.
- *Laparoscopy (Peritoneoscopy):* This method of entry into the abdomen allows visualization of pelvic structures via fiberotopic scopes inserted through small abdominal incisions. Instillation of carbon dioxide into cavity improves visualization. This technique is used in diagnostic assessment of uterus, tubes, and ovaries. It can be used in conjunction with tubal sterilization.

  In this, the nurse explains purpose and method of procedure. Before surgeon instructs patient about procedure, prepare abdomen, and reassure patient about sedation. Tell patient to rest for 1-3 days after surgery. Inform patient of probability of shoulder pain because of air in the abdomen.
- *Dilation and currettage:* The operative procedure dilates cervix and allows curretting of endometrial lining. This test is used in assessment of abnormal bleeding patterns and cytologic evaluation of lining. In this, instruct the patient before surgery, about the procedure and sedation. Tell patient that overnight hospitalizations is occasionally required. Perform postoperative assessment of degree of bleeding (frequent pad checking first 24 hours).

Fertility Studies

- *Semen analysis:* Semen is assessed for volume (2-5 ml), viscosity, sperm count (Greater than 20 million/ml), sperm motility (60 percent motil) and percent of abnormal sperm (60 percent with normal structures). Here, instruct patient to bring in fresh specimen within 2 hours after ejaculation (may be by masturbation).
- *Basal body temperature assessment:* This measurement indicates indirectly whether ovulation has occurred (temperature rises at ovulation and remains elevated during secretory phase of normal menstrual cycle). In this, the nurse instructs woman to take her temperature using special basal temperature thermometer. (Calebrated in tenths of degrees) every morning before getting out of bed. Tell the woman to record temperature on graph.
- *Huhner test or Sim's-Huhner:* Mucus sample of cervix is examined 2-8 hours after intercourse. Total number of sperm is assessed to number of live sperms. This test is performed to determine cervical mucus is "hostile"

to passage of sperm from vagina to utera. Here nurse must instruct couple to have an inter-course an estimated time of ovulation and be present for test within 2-8 hours after intercourse.
- *Endometrial biopsy:* In this outpatient procedure, small currette is used to obtain piece of endometrial lining to assess endometrial changes common to progesterone secretion after ovulation. Here advise patient that test must be performed postovulation. Explain that procedure should cause only short period of uterine cramping.
- *Hysterosalpinogram:* Same as invasive procedure.
- *Serum progesteron:* Same as blood studies.

REPRODUCTIVE PROBLEMS OF FEMALES/WOMEN

Disease and disorders of the female reproductive system threatens the physical and emotional health of many women, infection process and disorders of menstruation are common and pervasive problem. Malignant neoplasm destroys child-bearing potential and numerous lives.

Vaginitis

Infection and inflammation of the vagina, cervix and vulva tend to occur when the natural defenses of the acidic vaginal secretions (maintained by sufficient estrogen level) and the presence of Lactobacillus are disrupted. The woman's resistance may also be decreased as a result of aging, poor nutrition and the use of the drugs that alter the mucosa organism gain entrance to the areas through contaminated hands, clothing, douche nozzles and during intercourse, surgery and childbirth.

Etiology

The cause of following infections of vagina are as follows:
- Monilial vaginitis caused by candida albicans (fungus).
- Trichomoniasis caused by *Trichomonas vaginalis* (Protozoa).
- Bacterial vaginosis caused by *Gardnerella vaginalis* and *Corynebacterium vaginale*.
- Severe recurrent vaginitis caused by candida albicans.
- Foreign body.
- Allergens or irritants.

Most lower genital tract infections are related to the sexual intercourse. Intercourse can transport organisms, injure tissues, and alter the acid-base balance of the vagina. All of these increase risk for inflammation or infections of the vagina. The risk factor associated with infections of the vulva and vagina include the following:
- Pregnancy.
- Age—Premenarche and postmenopause.
- Low estrogen levels.
- Dermatological allergies.
- Diabetes mellitus—alteration in carbohydrate metabolism.
- Oral contraceptive use.
- Inadequate hygiene.
- Douching.
- Treatment with broad spectrum antibiotics and use of steroids.
- Use of vaginal contraceptives—foams and inserts.
- Intercourse with infected partner.
- Frequent intercourse with multiple partners.
- Tight, nonabsorbent and heat-retaining clothing.

Pathophysiology

The vagina is normally protected from infection by its acid pH and the presence of normal flora such as Döderlein's bacilus. Any factor that alters the normal vaginal physiology may dispose to infection. If the pH or vaginal mucosa is altered or the woman resistance is decreased by aging-related changes, stress, or diseases and her risk to infection increase. The use of antibiotics which destroys the normal protective flora of the vagina also increases the risk of infection. The risk factors listed in etiology causes vaginitis.

Clinical Manifestations

The clinical manifestation of vaginitis varies according to its causes which include:
- *Monilial vaginitis:* Commonly found in mouth, gastrointestinal tract and vagina. There is white, curd-like, cheesy discharge, characteristic patches on vaginal walls and cervix and foul odor, severe burning, itching, and dyspareunia.
- *Gardnerella associated bacterial vaginosis:* Grayish-white, hormonous watery discharge with fishy or foul odor; scant amount and may or may not have other symptoms.
- *Foreign body:* Blood tinged serosanguineous or purulent disease usually with foul odor discharge may be thick or thin.
- *Allergens or irritants:* Increase in usual type and amount of secretions, itching and burning rash.

Management

Genital problems are evaluated by performing a history including sexual history and physical examination and obtaining the appropriate laboratory and diagnostic studies. The diagnosis of vaginitis is made by microscope analysis of vaginal secretions (e.g. KOH analysis, wet smear, or Gram's stain) and culture of the discharge. Serological testing and urine culture may also be used. The management of vaginitis is primarily pharmacological which includes accordingly as follows:
- *Monilial vaginitis:* Diagnosed by KOH microscopic examination—pseudohyphase pH 4.0-4.7 and treated by antifungal agents which includes:

- Clotrimazole (Mycelax, lotriman) applicator intravaginally HS for 7 days.
  - Micronazole (Monistat) Cream intravaginally HS for 7 days.
  - Tioconazole 6.5 percent (Vagistat-l) intravaginally HS for 1 dose.
  - Fluconazole (Diflucan) one tablet orally stat.
  - Nystatin (Mycostatin) suppositories daily or bid for 14 days.
- *Trichomoniasis:* Metronidazole (Flagyl) orally for 7 days or 2 g stat. For both partners symptomatic therapy is suggested.
- *Bacterial vaginosis.* If sexually transmitted; metronidazole (Flagyl) for 7 days and ampicillim 500 mg orally or clindamycin (Cleoun) 300 mg orally for 5 days bid for 7 days: Examine and treat both partners. Intravaginal treatment with metro-Gell applicator bid for 5 days; Clindamycin phosphate 2 percent vaginal cream) applicator HS for 7 days.
- *Foreign body:* Removal of objects, antibiotic specific to secondary infection.
- *Allergens or irritants:* Removal of possible allergens or irritant; topical steroid ointment as needed.

Nursing management focusses primarily on the appropriate use of prescribed therapy and measures to prevent reinfection. The nurse instructs the woman to clean the genital area thoroughly with soap and water and dry well before applying any medication. The hands should be washed properly before and after treatment. The nurse advises the woman to remain recumbent for 30 minutes after insertion of suppository or cream to facilitate absorption and prevent loss from vagina. Tampons should be avoided during treatment. If vaginal drainage is present, the woman is encouraged to wear minipad. Sitz bath can be comforting. The woman is instructed to refrain from intercourse while the infection is being treated and the male partner should use a condom until all symptoms of inflammation have been resolved.

Prevention of infection is an important consideration. The following measures reduces the incidence of vaginal infections which include:
- Cleanse the general areas thoroughly with mild soap and water daily:
  - Wipe genital area from front to back after bowel movements.
  - Avoid use of vaginal irritants (e.g. harsh deodarants and perfumed soap, deodarant sprays, douches).
  - Do vaginal irrigation as ordered.
  - Avoid routine douching, which can alter the vaginal pH.
- Use underwear with cotton crotch and change panties daily; avoid using any clothing that is tight in the crotch or thighs. Avoid wearing underpant while sleeping.
- Assess sexual partners for any sign of infection (e.g. discharge, lesions, reddened areas on genitalias):
  - Use a barrier method of contraception.
  - Avoid any sexual practice that is painful or abrasive.
  - Avoid anal genital intercourse.
  - Cleanse genital area of self and partner and void before and after intercourse.
- Change tampons or napkins frequently during menstruation.
- Treat athletes foot and "jook itch" with over-the-counter-antifungals.
- Consider using Vitamin C 500 mg per orally (PO) bid to increase the acidity of vaginal secretions.
- Recognize the signs of infection and respond promptly.

CERVICITIS

The term 'Cervicitis' includes number of conditions characterized by inflammation and infection of the cervix. Cervicitis has been linked with cervical cancer.

Etiology

Chlamydia trachomitis, Neisseria gonorrhea, Staphylococus aureas and herpes virus all can cause cervicitis, chlamydia is the most common cause of infection. It is sexually transmitted.

Pathophysiology and Clinical Manifestation

Leukorrhea may be the only sign and the amount may not be significant. On examination, the cervix is grossly erythematous and edematous, and there is usually a mucoid purulent discharge. But the amount may be so small that patient does not notice it. There may be the mucopurulent discharge with postcoital spotting from cervical inflammation. The woman commonly has no subjective signs but may report pruritis, burning, lower abdominal pain, or dyspareunia. Symptoms of a urinary tract infection may also be present. Cervical stenosis, salpingitis and infertility are possible sequelae of chronic disease.

Management

Diagnosis is confirmed by the existing signs and symptoms. Vaginitis if present is treated first, the cervix is cultured and appropriate pharmacological therapy is initiated. Gonococcal cervitis is treated with one dose of cephlox IM plus oral doxycycline for 7 days and one dose of oral azithromycin to treat concurrent chlamydial infection. Other organism may be treated as mentioned in the vaginitis. If the woman cervitis does not respond to antibiotics, cryosurgery or laser therapy may be necessary. Treat partners with same drugs.

Cryosurgery is a safe outpatient procedure. Women are told that a watery discharge is common after treatment but it resolves in several weeks. Healing is usually complete within 6 weeks. Women are also told that they may experience mild to moderate cramping during procedure. Take preventive measure of cervicitis as mentioned in vaginitis.

BARTHOLINITIS (BARTHOLIN'S CYSTS)

Bartholin's cysts are one of the most common disorders of the vulva. They result from obstruction of a duct, which may become infected. Thickened mucous, stenosis or mechanical trauma may initiate the process.

Pathophysiology and Clinical Manifestation

The infection is usually unilateral but can be bilateral. Neisseria gonorrheae is the most common infecting organism. The secretary function of gland continues and the duct fills up with fluid, producing severe inflammation, enlargement of the gland and tissue edema. The area becomes tender, and even walking may be difficult. The pain is constant, and dyspareunia can be severe. The abscess may rupture, resulting in temporary symptom relief, but usually reforms. Occasionally, the acute inflammation resolves leaving scar tissue that can form a cyst. The cyst usually is nontender but may interfere with ambulation and intercourse.

Management

Cultures are taken and woman is treated for any underlying infection process. If the cysts are symptomatic, incision and drainage may be performed. The cysts tend to recur and a permanent opening for drainage of the gland may need to be constructed by placing a tiny WORD catheter through a stab wound into the cyst cavity. The catheter remains in the cyst for 3 to 4 weeks until healing has occurred and a new duct is formed. This procedure is also useful when infection is present. Laser can also be used to remove the cyst. Total gland excision may be performed in older women who have suffered repeated abscesses or when cancer is suspected.

Nursing intervention focusses on comfort. Mild analgesics and sitz baths help relieve pain, yes the most procedures are performed on an outpatient basis, the nurse instructs the woman on the safe use of these interventions at home and reinforces the need to report any signs of infection.

PELVIC INFLAMMATORY DISEASE (PID)

Pelvic inflammatory disease (PID) is a general term that refers to acute subacute, recurrent or chronic infection of the reproductive organs—pelvic peritoneum, veins, or connective tissues. PID is an infectious condition of the pelvic cavity that may involve infection of the fallopian tubes (Salpingitis), ovaries (oophoritis) and pelvic peritoneum (peritonitis). The infection may be confined to just one structure or be widespread.

Etiology

PID is rare during pregnancy and occurs at the time of premenarchal, postmenopausal and is found among celibate women. It occurs in women using IUDs more often than in women using other forms of contraception. Women are at increased risk for Chlamydial infection (i.e. those women younger than 24 years of age and having multiple sex partners or a new sex partner) should be routinely tested, for Chlamidia. In addition, known risk factors include low socio-economic status, early onset of sexual activity, multiple sex partners, frequent douching (three or more times per month), cigarette smoking and a prior history of STDs. Surgery on the reproductive organs, child bearing and abortion all lower the women's resistance to infection and provide portal of entry for pathogens.

Pathophysiology

PID is often the result of untreated cervicitis. The organism infecting the cervix ascends higher into the uterus, fallopian tubes, ovaries and personal cavity. Pathogenic organisms usually are introduced from outside the body and pass up the cervical canal into the uterus. Common causative organism include gonococci, Chlamydia, hemopilus. These organisms as well as mycoplasma streptococci and anaerobes may gain entrance during sexual intercourse or after pregnancy termination, pelvic surgery or childbirth.

There is a growing evidence that the presence of bacterial vaginosis also increases the risk of acquiring a pelvic infection. The causative organism invades the pelvis by way of the fallopian tubes or through the uterus veins or lymphatics. Many of the pathogen lodge in the fallopian tubes and create an acute or chronic inflammatory reaction. Purulent material collects in the tubes, adhesions and strictures form and sterility which is one of the most serious consequences of PID is occuring. Partial obstruction of the tubes may predispose a woman to ectopic pregnancy because of the fertilized ovum cannot reach the uterus. Inflammatory adhesions become so severe that surgical removal of the uterus, tubes and ovaries may be necessary. The infection usually remains localized in the lower abdomen and pelvis, although abcesses may form.

Clinical Manifestation

Women with PID usually go to a health care provider when they experience lower abdominal pain. So the clinical manifestation of acute PID includes severe abdominal pain, lower abdominal cramping, intermenstrual bleeding, dyspareunia, fever and chills, malaise, nausea and vomiting. The pain typically starts gradually and is constant. The intensity may vary from mild to severe, and movements such as walking can increase the pain. Pain increases during intercourse. Spotting after intercourse and abnormal vaginal discharge is common. A sensation of pelvic pressure and back pain may also be present, as well as foul-smelling purulent vaginal discharge. Symptoms often appear after the onset or cessation of menses. Abdominal palpation reveals pain and tendency to the lower quadrants of the abdomen, which is confirmed on pelvic examination. Masses may be felt indicating enlargement of the fallopian tubes or ovaries or the presence of an abscess.

Management

PID is a chemical diagnosis based on the patient's signs and symptoms. The diagnosis is based on the data obtained during bimanual portion of the pelvic examination. Diagnostic studies include WBC count and culture of any purulent secretions. A laparoscopy may be done to visualize pelvic structures and accomplish drainage of abscess and lysis of obstructing adhesions. Ultrasonography may be used to evaluate masses.

Treatment is aimed at eradicating the infection and preventing complications. Immediate complication of PID includes septic shock and Fitz-Hugh-Curtis syndrome, which occurs when PID spreads to the liver and causes acute prehepatitis. Long term complication includes ectopic pregnancy, infertility and chronic pelvic pain PID is usually treated on an outpatient basis. The patient is given a combination of antibiotics such as Cefoxitin and doxycycline to provide broad coverage against the causative organism. The patient must have no intercourse for 3 weeks. Her partner must be examined and treated. Physical rest and oral fluids are encouraged. Hospitalization may be necessary if the woman is acutely ill. Broad spectrum antibiotics are used until drug sensitivities are determined. Salpingectomy may be necessary if an abscess is found and more radical surgery is needed when all the reproductive organs have been compromised by the infection. If the woman has an IUD, it is removed.

Nursing interventions are largely supportive. Bedrest is a semi-Fowler's position and is recommended to assist pelvic drainage. Heat applied to the abdomen may be comforting, but tube or sitz baths should be avoided during the period of active infection. The vaginal discharge is copious and commonly purulent and may cause pruritis and excoriation. Other nursing measures include managing fever, monitoring vital signs, monitoring intake and output and providing emotional support.

The nurse instructs the woman to cleanse the perineal region every 3 to 4 hours and maintain scrupulous hygiene after urination and defecation. Tampoons should not be used and drainage pads should be changed frequently. A minimum of 3000 ml of fluid is daily recommended. Women treated as outpatients are remained for the seeking of appropriate follow-up because PID can have serious life-long consequence for fertility. The woman's sexual partner may be treated with antibiotics at the same time. The importance of using condoms to prevent reinfection or future infection is stressed.

Problems of Menstruation

Menstrual cycles are influenced by hormones from the hypothalamus gonadotropin-releasing hormone and anterior pituitary (FSH and LH). These hormones influence the development of a dominant follicle and egg within one ovary and resulting production of estrogen during the follicular phase of the cycle. The estrogen from the ovary causes the growth of the endometrial lining of the uterus. Following ovulation, the corpus luteum (site of ovulation) produces progesterone that further develops and stabilizes the endometrial lining, building a suitable lining to receive a fertilized egg. The progesterone dominant part of the menstrual cycle is called the luteal phase because of the essential part of the corpus luteum plays. When a fertilized egg does not implant in the endometrial lining, the corpus luteum is not maintained and production of progesterone falls. In response to decreasing level of progesterone, the endometrial lining is shed. This shedding is referred to as "menstruation" or woman's menses or her period. The first day of menses is considered the start of day 1 of the menstrual cycle. Menses may be irregular during first few years after menarche and the years preceding menopause. Once established, a woman's menstrual cycle usually has a predictable pattern. However, considerable normal variation exists among women in cycle length as well as in duration, amount characteristic and menstrual flow.

Almost all women experience problems with their menstrual cycle at some point in their reproductive years. Problems produce a variety of symptoms that may be directly or indirectly related to pelvic organs. Most problems are self manageable and are rarely brought to the health care provider's attention unless they become severe or persistent.

PREMENSTRUAL SYNDROME

Premenstrual syndrome (PMS) is defined as a cluster of distressing physical and behavioral symptoms that occur as the second half of the menstrual cycle and are followed by a symptom-free period. PMS constitutes a group of somatic, behavioral, cognitive and mood symptoms distressing enough to impair interpersonal relationships or interfere with urinal activities.

Etiology and Pathophysiology

The etiology and pathophysiology of PMS are not well understood. But these may the result of a wide variety of hormonal, psychological and nutritional factors. Women with PMS have genetically determined sensitivity to one or more of the neurotransmitter systems such as serotonin. This sensitivity results in heightened response to the normal cyclic fluctuation of the ovarian hormone. Other proposed causes include estrogen and progesterone imbalances and nutritional deficiency of pyridoxine (Vit B_6) or magnesium.

Clinical Manifestation

PMS is extremely variable in its clinical manifestation. Variations are common between women and for an individual woman, from one cycle to another. Commonly occurring physical symptoms include, breast discomfort, peripherial edema, abdominal bloating, episodes of binge, eating and headache. Abdominal bloating and breast-swelling are apparently caused by local fluids' shifts because total body weight does not generally change symptoms of autonomic nervous systems arousal such as heart palpitation and dizziness have been reported. Women may experience anxiety, depression, irritability and mood swings. The symptoms can be grouped on the basis of possible etiology:

- *Anxiety:* (Nervousness, mood swings, irritability) may be due to high serum estrogen, low serum progesterone, elevated adrenal androgen and possible disturbance of thyroid axis.
- Water-related symptoms (weight gain, swelling of extremities, breast tanderness, abdominal bloating) may be due to high serum aldosterone, retention of sodium and water, decreased colloid osmotic pressure in abdomen.
- *Cravings:* (Craving for sweets, increased appetite) may be due to increased carbohydrate tolerance and low red cell magnesium levels.
- Depression (forgetfulness, crying, confusion, insomnia) due to causes mentioned in the anxiety.

In addition, headache, heart pounding, fatigue, dizziness or faintness may be present.

Management

There is no objective means of diagnosing PMS existance and the diagnosis is primarily established by exclusion. A woman is considered to have PMS if her symptoms interfere with activities of daily living. Symptoms that occur in three consecutive menstrual cycles confirm the diagnosis.

Numerous treatments have been suggested, including both pharmacological and nonpharmocological strategies. But no treatment has been proved to be effective in all cases. The use of oral contraceptive produces symptoms similar to PMS in some women but also relieves symptoms in some women, diagnosed with the disorder. Treatment attempted to reduce number and severity of symptoms and restore the women's psychological health. Treatment strategies for PMS include:

- Pharmalogical Strategies:
  - *Combination oral contraceptives:* Used for women with no contraindication.
  - *Selective serotonin reuptake inhibitions (SSRI):* Antidepressants—Good relief for mood symptoms.
  - *Prostaglandin inhibitors:* Administration 2-4 times daily at onset of symptoms.
  - *Diuretics:* Administration during luteal phase.
  - Tranquilizers, Gonadotrophic inhibitor (Denazol).
  - Evening primrose oil (natural therapy).
- Non-pharmacological Strategies:
  - *Diet:* Well-balanced, avoid caffeine, alcohol. Reduce refined carbohydrates and adequate intake of vitamin B6.
  - *Stress management:* Relaxation techniques-Abdominal breathing, mental imagery and progressive muscle relaxation.
  - *Exercise*: Aerobics, walking and swimming.
  - *Education and counseling:* Knowledge of possible causes and treatment daily dairy maintaining family understanding, support groups, assertiveness training.
  - Sex and marital therapy.

The nurse helps the woman and her family by teaching following points:

- Teach possible causes of conditions and treatment.
- Teach relaxation techniques.
- Teach patient to do the following:
  - Avoid stressful activities during premenstrual period. Fatigue exaggerate symptoms.
  - Take medication as prescribed.
  - Reduce or eliminate smoking and alcohol consumption.
  - Reduce or eliminate consumption and caffeine.
  - Follow a regular exercise program.
  - Eat well-balanced diet with adequate protein and reduced intake of salts and refined sugars.
  - Incorporate stress-reducing strategies into daily lifestyle.
  - Increase intake of food high in vitamin B and magnesium (green leafy vegetable, legumes and whole grain cereals).

DYSMENORRHEA

Dysmenorrhea is defined as abdominal cramping or discomfort associated with menstrual flow. It involves uterine pain with menstruation and is commonly called menstrual cramps.

Etiology

The two types of dysmenorrhea are primary (when no pathology exists) and secondary (when a pelvic disease or condition in the underlying cause). Primary dysmenorrhea is not associated with pelvic pathology and occurs in the absence of any organic disease. Its severity usually declines after pregnancy by the age of 30. Secondary dysmenorrhea occurs in response to organic disease such as PID endometriosis, leiomyomas (uterine fistoids) and IUD use.

Pathophysiology

Primary dysmenorrhea is not a disease. It is caused by either an excess of prostaglandin F2Alpha (PGF2Alpha) and/or an increased sensitivity to its neuptors. The sequential stimulation of the endometrium by estrogen followed by progesterone results in a dramatic increase in prostaglandin production by the endometrium. With the onset of menses, degeneration of the endometrium releases prostaglandin. Locally prostaglandin increases myometrial contractions and construction of small endometrial blood vessels with consequent tissue ischemia and increased sensitization of the pain receptor resulting in menstrual pain. Prostaglandin absorbed into the circulating systems may be responsible for symptoms of headache, diarrhea and vomiting.

Secondly dysmenorrhea is usually acquired after adolescence, occurring most commonly in the 30's and 40's. Common pelvic conditions that cause secondary dysmenorrhea include endometriosis, chronic PID, uterine fibroids and adenomyosis.

Clinical Manifestation

Primary dysmenorrhea starts 12 to 24 hours before the onset of menses. The pain is most severe. The first day of menses and rarely lasts more than 2 days. Characteristic manifestation include lower abdominal pain that is colicky in nature, frequently radiating to the lower back and upper thighs. The abdominal pain is often accompanied by nausea, diarrhea, fatigue, headache and light headedness.

Secondly dysmenorrhea usually occurs after the woman has experienced problem-free periods for some time. The pain which may be unilateral is generally more constant in nature; usually continues longer than primary dysmenorrhea. Depending on the cause of symptom such as dyspareunia (Painful intercourse) painful defecation, or irregular bleeding may occur at times other than menstruation.

Management

Primary dysmenorrhea is treated with prostaglandin inhibition which blocks prostaglandin synthesis and metabolism. NSAIDs are effective for many women because these drugs inhibit prostaglandin synthesis. The drugs used commonly are NSAIDS (Ibuprofen, Mefenamic acid (Ponstel), Naproxen, Ketoprofen. Nursing intervention during drug therapy includes: Teach the patient to:
- Take drug on an empty stomach unless GI irritation develops.
- Report the occurrence of any unexplained bleeding (of menorrhagia epistasis).
- Mefenamic acid should be taken with meals, or antacids to decrease GI irritation. It should not be taken for more than 7 days. Treatment of secondary dysmenorrhea is aimed at the underlying organic cause. Options include both pharmacological and surgical interventions.

Women rarely seek professional help for mild primary dysmenorrhea. However, women who are consistently unable to engage in normal activities because of menstrual pain should be encouraged to seek medical care. Women often ask nurses what can be done for minor discomfort associated menstrual cycles. They should be advised that during acute pain, relief may be obtained by lying down for short periods, drinking hot beverages, applying heat to the abdomen or back, and taking an anti-inflammatory drug or mild analgeisa. The nurse can suggest noninvasive pain-relieving practices such as distraction and guided imagery.

The nurse instructs the patient that NSAIDs are most effective when taken at the onset of the menses before pain becomes severe, and can be buffered with food or antacid if GI irritation occurs. Other health care measures can reduce the discomfort of dysmenorrhea. These include regular exercise, maintenance of proper nutritional habits, avoidance of constipation, maintenance of good body mechanics, and avoidance of stress and fatigue, particularly during the time preceding menstrual periods. Staying active and interested in activities may also help. Women should be taught when dysmenorrhea occurs as well as how to treat it. Education and supportive therapy can provide women with a foundation for coping with this common occurrence and increase feelings of control and self-reliance. Constipation should be avoided. If pain occurs, the nurse can suggest that the woman—use local heat, which helps dilate blood vessels and relieve ischemia and use of progressive relaxation strategies.

AMENORRHEA

Amenorrhea refers to the absence of menstruation.
- *Primary amenorrhea* exists if the first menses had not occurred by the age of 16. It usually results from a genetic, endocrine or congenital developmental defect and is often associated with disorders of pubertal development.
- *Secondary amenorrhea* exists when a previously menstruating woman ceases to menstruate for more than 3 to 6 months (3 months in a woman with a history of regular menstrual cycle). Skipping an occasional single period is normal. Pregnancy is the most common causes of secondary amenorrhea.

Etiology

Anovulation is the most common cause. For missing menses, once pregnancy has been ruled out. Additional causes of secondary amenorrhea is usually a response to environmental variable, such as altered function of the hypothalamus, pituitary gland, ovaries, thyroid, or adrenal gland. Second amenorrhea also is a side effects of some medication, and women who take oral contraceptive may experience amenorrhea for upto

6 months after discontinuing the pill. To sum up, the causes of amenorrhea are as follows:

- Hypothalamic—Pituitary axis
  - Reversible CNS—mediated insults (e.g. emotional stress-anorexia nervosa or severe dieting, strenuous exercise, post-pill syndrome and chronic or acute illness).
  - Prolactinoma and other causes of hyperprolactinemia (e.g. drugs).
  - Cramopharyngioma and other brainstem or parasellar tumors.
  - Congenital conditions (e.g. isolated gonadotropin deficiency).
  - Trauma (e.g. head injury with hypothalamic contusion).
  - Infiltration process (e.g. Sarcoidosis).
  - Vascular disease (e.g. hypothalamic vasculitis).
  - Pituitary tumors.
  - Sheehan's syndrome.
- Ovaries
  - Autoimmune disease (often involving thyroid, adrenal, islet cells).
  - Premature menopause (idiopathic) or resistant-ovary syndrome.
  - Polycystic ovary disease.
  - Congenital or genetic condition (e.g. Turner's Syndrome).
  - Infection (e.g. Mumps, oophoritis).
  - Toxins (especially alkylating chemotherapeutic agents).
  - Radiation.
  - Trauma, torsion (rare).
- Uterovaginal Outflow Tract
  - Asherman's syndrome (Postcurrettage loss of endo-metrium).
  - Mulleriah dysgenesis.
- Hormonal Synthesis and Action
  - Male pseudohermaphroditism (e.g.testicular feminization).
  - 17-Hydroxylase deficiency.

Pathophysiology

Pathophysiology of amenorrhea is based on the causes. Prolonged secondary amenorrhea is common among certain groups of conditioned athletes such as gymnasts and long distance runners, because normal menarche is believed to be required approximately 17 percent of body weight. Weight loss may result in amenorrhea. The consequences of prolonged amenorrhea are not fully known.

Clinical Manifestation

Absence of menses and signs and symptoms of underlying causes and effects.

Management

The diagnostic work up for amenorrhea includes a detailed history and careful examination of the reproductive system. Pregnancy should be ruled out as a possible cause. The treatment depends on the cause. An organic problem is corrected if possible. Hormone therapy may be required.

The nurse teaches the woman about the problem, its causes and the diagnostic studies are planned. Teaching may include information about weight gain, stress reduction, and reducing the energy drain of strenuous exercise. Women may need counseling and support to deal with feelings of threat to their self concept and concern overfertility that may be caused by the amenorrhea.

DYSFUNCTIONAL UTERINE BLEEDING (DUB)

Dysfunctional uterine bleeding (DUB) is defined as excessive or irregular uterine bleeding with no demonstrable cause. It can take many forms including excessive flow, prolonged duration of menses and intermenstrual bleeding.

Etiology

Irregular vaginal bleeding is a common gynecologic concern. Frequently occurring irregularities include oligomenorrhea (long intervals between menses), secondary amenorrhea (cessation of menses for at least 6 months) menorrhagia (excessive menstrual bleeding) and metrorrhagia (irregular bleeding or bleeding between menses).

The causes of DUB during childbearing and postmenopausal years are as follows:

- Menorrhagia (Prolonged profuse menstrual flow during regular periods) is caused by submucous myomas, pregnancy complications, adenomyosis, endometrial hyperplasia, malignant tumors and hypothyroidism.
- Metrorrhagia (bleeding between periods) is caused by endometrial polyps, endometrial and cervical cancer, exogenous estrogen administration.
- Polymenorrhea (increased frequency of menstruations) is caused by anovulation; shortened luteal phase.
- Cryptomenorrhea (usually light menstrual flow)—caused by hymenal or cervical stenosis, Asherman's syndrome (uterine synechiae), oral contraceptives.
- Menometrorrhagia (Bleeding at irregular intervals occurs as a result of any conditions causing intermenstrual bleeding; sudden onset is indication of malignant tumors or complications of pregnancy.
- Oligomenorrhea (menstrual periods more than 35 days apart) may be caused by anovulation from endocrin causes (Pregnancy, menopause) or systemic (excessive weight loss); estrogen-secretory tumors.

- Dysfunctional uterine bleeding (An abnormal bleeding without known organic cause).
The cause is unknown.

Irregular bleeding may be caused by dysfunction of the hypothalmic-pituitary-ovarian axis such as pituitary adenoma. Changes in lifestyles such as marriage, recent moves, a death in the family, financial stress, and other emotional crises can cause such dysfunctions. (Psychologic factors can influence endocrine function).

Pathophysiology

Dysfunctional uterine bleeding may occur between or during their menstrual periods. When menorrhagia is present, the woman may soak a tampoon or pad every 1 to 2 hours or a week or more. The exact cause of the anovulatory episode is not understood; but it may represent a dysfunction of the hypothalmic-pituitary-ovarian axis that results in continuing estrogen stimulation of the endometrium. The endometrium outgrows its blood supply, partially breaks down and is sloughed in an irregular manner. Anovulation may also result from thyroid or adrenal abnormalities.

Management

The diagnostic work of DUB starts with a thorough history of the frequency, amount and duration of bleeding. Laboratory test may include blood counts to estimate blood loss, pregnancy tests, thyroid studies, ovulation tests and coagulation studies. Papanicolaou (Pap) smears, pelvic examinations, ultrasonography, endometrial biopsy, and sonohysterography may be employed to assess for structural problems and cancer.

Treatment depends on the nature of the problem (menorrhagia or amenorrhea), degree of threat to the patient's health and whether children are desired in the future. The cause of bleeding guides medical care. In the absence of an organic cause, the preferred treatment is usually conservative. There are pharmacological options to stop heavy bleeding or reduce it. Further blood loss in subsequent menstrual cycles include the use of estrogens, progestrins, NSAIDS, antifibrinolytic agents, and gonadotroph in releasing hormona agonists such as danazol. All patients with menorrhagia shouild be assessed for anemia and treated as indicated.

Surgery may be indicated depending on the underlying cause of the irregular vaginal bleeding. Dilation and Curettage (D and C) was once a common therapy for excessive bleeding or for spotting in perimenopausal woman. Now D and C is used only is extreme cases of bleeding or for older women when endometrial biopsy and ultrasonography provide diagnostic information. Endometrial ablations done by laser or electrosurgical technique has been successful with many 80 percent cases with uncontrolled menorrhagia. If menorrhagia is caused by uterine fibroids, a hysterectomy may be performed or a myomectomy removal of fibroids without removal of the uterus may be performed if the patient wants to preserve her uterus. Hysterectomy may be necessary for those women whose bleeding cannot be controlled with hormones, who are symptomatically anemic and whose lifestyle is compromised by persistent bleeding.

Mostly care of the DUB cases are provided in the outpatient setting, the nursing role is largely educational. Educating the women about characteristics of the menstrual cycle assists them to identify normal variations. This knowledge can help dispel apprehensions and misconceptions. If the patient's menstrual cycle pattern does not fall within the range of normalcy, the nurse should urge her to visit her health care provider. Myths concerning activities allowed during menstruation are common. The nurse should be prepared to clarify the facts. The patient should be assured that bathing and hairwashing are safe. A daily warm tub bath may actually relieve some of the associated pelvic discomfort. Women can swim, exercise, have intercourse and basically continue that usual daily activities.

The nurse teaches the woman to accurately assess the amount of bleeding in terms of number of pads or tampons, type of pad or tampon and degree of saturation. The nurse helps the woman set up and maintain an accurate record of the bleeding in the form of diary. Frequent changing of tampons or pads meet comfort and hygienic needs during menstruation. The selections of internal or external sanitary protection is a matter of personal preference. Tampons are convenient and make menstruation hygiene easier, whereas pads may provide better protection. Using a combination of tampons and pads and avoiding superabsorbant tampons may decrease the risk of toxic shock syndrome (TSS). TSS is an acute condition caused by toxins of *Staphylococcus aureus*. TSS causes high fever, vomiting, diarrhea weakness, myalgia, and sunburn like rash.

The nurse also encourages the woman to express her concerns and fears. Anxiety related to infertility or fear of cancer can be intense but remain unexpressed.

ENDOMETRIOSIS

Endometriosis is the presence of normal endometrial tissue in sites outside the endometrial cavity. The most frequent sites are in or near the ovaries, the uterosacral ligaments, and the uterovesical peritoneum. However, endometrial tissues can be found in many other locations such as the stomach, lungs, intestines and spleen. The tissue responds to the hormons of the ovarian cycle and undergoes mini menstrual cycle similar to the uterine endometrium.

Etiology

The etiology of endometriosis remains unknown. But there are multiple theories and lines of research. The condition may be hereditary because it occurs more often in women whose mothers had the disorder. Theories include the congenital presence of endometrial cells out of their normal locations, the transfer of endometrial cells by means of the blood or lymph system, and menstrual fluid containing endometrial cells up the fallopian tubes and into the pelvic cavity. A more recent theory suggests a possible immune mechanism in the etiology of endometriosis.

Pathophysiology

With each menstrual period, the seeded endometrial cells are stimulated by ovarian hormones and bleed into the surrounding tissues, causing inflammatory response. Encased blood may lead to palpable masses known as chocolate cysts. Occasionally the cystes rupture and spread endometrial cells deeper into the pelvis. Repeated inflammation and healing may create adhesions severe enough to fuse pelvic organs or cause bleed of bladder strictures. The ovaries are the most common site of involvement, and the process is usually bilateral. The pelvic peritoneum; the anterior and posterior culdesac; and the uterosacral, round, and broad ligaments are other common sites. Endometriasis progresses gradually and usually does not produce symptoms until the woman is 30 to 40 years of age.

Clinical Manifestation

The classic feature is menstrual pain and discomfort that becomes progressively worse. Other possible symptoms include abdominal pain, dyspareunia, irregular menses, bowel problems and urinary dysfunction. The most common symptoms are secondary dysnaemorrhea, infertility, pelvic pain and dyspareunia and irregular bleeding. Less common symptoms include backache, painful bowel movements and dysuria. Pelvic examination reveals a fixed, retroverted uterus that is enlarged, tender and nodular.

When the ectopic endometrial implants "menstruate" the blood collects in cyst like nodules that have a characteristic bluish black look. Nodules in the ovaries are sometimes called chocolate cysts, because of the thick chocolate colored material they contain. When a cyst ruptures, the pain may be acute and the resulting irritation promotes the formation of adhesions, which fix the affected area to another pelvic structures. The adhesions may become severe enough to cause a bowel obstruction, or painful micturition. Adhesion involving the uterus, tubes, or ovaries may result in infertility.

Management

Diagnosis of endometriosis is confirmed by the laparoscopy. The endoscopy is used to carefully map out and describe the extent of disease involvement and biopsy of suspicious tissue can be obtained during procedure. Ultrasound and MRI may also be used for differentiation of cystic lesion and detecting stage of the disease. Treatment of endometriosis is influenced by the patient's age, desire to get pregnant, symptom of severity, and the extent and location of disease. When symptoms are not disruptive, a watch and wait approach is used. When endometriosis is identified as a possible cause of infertility, therapy will proceed more rapidly.

Drug therapy is used to reduce symptoms. Drugs are selected to inhibit estrogen production by the ovary so that the endometrial tissue shrinks. The various drugs are used to imitate a state of pregnancy or menopause, since both natural conditions relieve symptoms, continuous use of (for 9 months) combined progestin and oestrogen causes regression of endometrial tissue. Oral contraceptive with minimal estrogen and high levels of progestins may be used to produce endometrial strophy. Disadvantages to this approach include irregular bleeding and symptoms such as nausea, fatigue and depression.

Drugs with antigonatropic action such as danazol may be used to suppress ovarian activity. Danazol stops endometrial proliferation, prevents ovulation, and produces atrophy of ectopic endometrial tissue. The newest and most expensive therapy is injectable gonadotropin-releasing hormone analog (Leuprolids lupron). It causes a hypestrogenic state resulting amenorrhea. The side effects include hot flushes, vaginal dryness or emotional lability as in menopause.

Surgical intervention may be necessary if the disorder does not respond to drug therapy. For women wishing to get pregnant, conservative surgical therapy is used to remove implants that may block the fallopian tube. Also, adhesions are removed from the tubes, ovaries and pelvic structures. Efforts are made to conserve all tissues necessary to maintain fertility. Definitive surgery involves removal of the uterus, tubes, ovaries and as many endometrial implants as possible.

Nurses should educate women about endometriosis with special attention to the common symptoms. The nurse reassures the woman that endometriosis can be treated. The nurse teaches about the prescribed drugs all the management of side effects. Strategies to manage chronic pain are particularly important. The importance of ongoing care and follow up is reinforced. If surgery is the treatment the nursing care is similar to that of the general preoperative and postoperative care of patient undergoing laparotomy.

UTERINE PROLAPSE

The most commonly occurring problems with pelvic support are uterine prolapse, cytocele and rectocele. The uterus may undergo minor displacement in ways that are considered to be normal variations with little or no clinical effects. Uterine prolapse represents a severe uterine problem in which the uterus protrudes through the pelvic floor apertuor genital hiatus. It is usually associated with a cystocele or rectocele.

Etiology

Usually vaginal childbirth increases the risk of these problems, i.e. uterine prolapse, cystocele, or rectocele. Uterine prolapse occurs most often in multiparous caucasian women as a resposne to injuries to the muscle and fascia of the pelvis incurred during childbirth.

Women without any children may also have these problems which include the following:
- Systemic conditions such as obesity and chronic pulmonary disease, and local conditions such as ascites and uterine or ovarian tumor are other causes for these problems.
- Chronic coughing, constipation, genetic predisposition and estrogen deprivation after menopause can also contribute to prolapse. The decrease in estrogen that normally accompanies the perimenopause also reduces some connective tissue support.

Prolapse usually develops gradually, suggesting that the effects of aging play a major role. As the uterus begins to drop, the vaginal walls become relaxed and the bladder may herniate into vagina (cystocele) or the rectal wall may herniate into the vagina (Rectocele).

Pathophysiology

Variations in the normal position of the uterus or prolapse can result from congenital or acquired abnormalities of the pelvic support structures. Acquired weakness occurs after birth, surgery, and closely spaced pregnancies and in response to obesity and the loss of tissue elasticity with aging. The severity of the prolapse is designated by degree. In first degree prolapse, the cervix still rests within the lower part of the vagina. In second degree prolapse the cervix is at the vaginal opening, i.e. cervix protrudes through the introitus, the entire uterus suspended by its stretched ligaments, hangs below the vaginal orifice. Before menopause the uterus hypertrophie's end is engorged and become flabby. The vaginal mucosa thickens and stasis ulcers may develop. Anterior and posterior vaginal wall relaxation often accompany prolapse, allowing for the development of cystocele or rectocele. Older women may have these conditions for years before seeking medical attention.

Clinical Manifestation

Patient with first degree prolapse experiences few symptoms but may report sensations or heaviness or fullness and a feeling that something is falling out or something coming down" of the vagina. In more severe prolapse, when the cervix protrudes at the introitus, the patient may complain of feeling like she is sitting on a ball. With severe prolapse, the woman is clearly aware of the mass. Vaginal bleeding, discharge and infection may be present. Leukorrhea or menometrorrhagia may develop in premenopausal women with prolapse as a result of uterine engorgement. After menopause discharge and bleeding with prolapse usually results from injection and ulceration.

Women may have dyspareunia, a dragging or heavy feeling in the pelvis backache and bowel or bladder problems if cystocele or rectocele also present. The woman with a cystocele may complain of urinary incontinence (stress incontinence) accompanying any activity that increases the intra abdominal pressure, such as coughing, laughing or lifting. The patient with rectocele may complain of chronic constipation and develop hemorrhoids. When third-degree uterine prolapse occurs the protruding cervix and vaginal walls are subjected to constant irritation and tissue charge may occur.

Management

Uterine prolapse can be readily identified in pelvic examination. If a cystocele is present, the vaginal outlet is relaxed with a thin walled smooth bulging mass present in the anterior vaginal wall below the cervix. The mass descends when the patient is asked to bear down. If retrocele is present, palpitation of the vaginal area reveals, a thin walled rectovaginal septum projecting into the vagina. Many women are found to have both a cystocele and rectocele.

Treatment depends on the degree of prolapse and how much the woman's daily activities have been affected. Pelvic muscle strengthening exercises (Kegel exercises) may be effective for some women. Postmenopausal woman with first degree prolapse are treated with estrogen therapy to maintain the tone and integrity of the pelvic floor muscle. Exercise therapy is suggested for all women. If pain or bleeding occurs, the uterus may be manually repositioned and supported by the insertion of vaginal pessaries. Pessary is a device that is placed in the vagina to help a support the uterus. A wide variety of shapes exists including rings, arches and balls. They are made of hard rubber or plastic that maintain the uterus in a forward position by exerting pressure on the ligaments attached to the posterior wall of the cervix. When a woman first received a pessary, she also needs instruction for its cleaning follow up. Pessaries that are left in place for long periods are associated with erosion, fistulas and increased incidence of carcinoma. Conservative treatment with estrogen, exercise and a pessary may also be employed for cystocele or rectocele if the woman experiences mild symptoms.

If more conservative measures are not successful, surgery is indicated, surgery to repair cystocele, rectocele and more advanced prolapses is undertaken when symptoms significantly interfere with patient's lifestyle. The procedures designed to tighten the vaginal wall termed 'anterior and posterior colporrhaphy'. They are frequently combined with hysterectomy. Cystocele repair may be done abdominally and combined with a uterovesical suspension's procedure called a Marshall-Marchatti-Krantz procedure to correct stress incontinence.

Nurse can assist women to avoid or decrease problem with pelvic support by teaching them how to do exercises to strengthen their pelvic floor muscles. Exercise teaching is an important nursing intervention for any patient with uterine prolapse. The woman is instructed to tighten the muscles of the perineum as if to stop the flow of urine maintain the tension for 5 seconds at a time and repeat the exercise in sets of 10. The exercise is repeated 10 to 12 times daily. Knee-chest exercises are used less often but may be orderered to stretch or strengthen the pelvic ligament. Corrective exercises for poor posture may also be prescribed.

The nurse encourages obese patients to lose weight to reduce intra-abdominal pressure. Chronic cough and chronic constipation are also corrected, because these conditions contribute to weakness of the muscle wall. Women fitted with a pessary needs to be taught how to insert it and withdraw it if the device becomes displaced or uncomfortable. Pessaries are removed and cleaned once every few weeks or months as recommended.

If vaginal surgery is necessary, the preoperative preparation usually includes a cleansing doucher in the morning of surgery. A cathartic and cleansing enema are usually given when a rectocele repair is scheduled. A perineal shave is done. The below-mentioned guidelines may be followed when the woman undergoing vaginal surgery:
- Provide perineal care after each voiding or defecation:
  - Poor sterile normal saline over vulva and perineum.
  - Cleanse perineum as needed with sterile cotton balls; cleanse away from vagina towards rectum.
  - Dry perineum as needed with sterile cotton balls.
- Encourage sitz baths after sutures are removed.
- If douches are ordered during immediate postoperative period:
  - Use sterile equipment and sterile solution.
  - Insert douche nozzle very gently and rotate carefully.
- Avoid pressure on suture line:
  - Prevent a full bladder; keep urinary catheter patent.
  - Use measures to prevent constipation.
  - Teach patient to avoid the Valsalva's maneuver.
  - Keep patient flat or in low Fowler's position in bed.
- Provide an icepack for perineal discomfort (severel seal plastic bags or glove make an acceptable pack).
- Encourage leg exercises.
- Encourage deep breathing.
- Monitor intake and output.
- Note characteristics of urine and stool. The discharge preparation after vaginal surgery, if the patient and family need, following should be advised by the nurses:
  - Perform daily douches and tub baths as prescribed.
  - Avoid staining at stool.
  - Use stool softener and laxative as prescribed.
  - Avoid lifting for 6 weeks.
  - Avoid sexual intercourse until physician gives permission (usually about 6 weeks).
  - Avoid jarring activities.
  - Avoid prolonged standing, walking or sitting, continue leg exercises for 6 weeks.
  - Vaginal sensation may be lost for several months postoperatively but sensation will return.
  - Eat high-fiber diet and drink 300 ml of fluids daily.

FISTULAS

A fistula is an abnormal tunnel-like opening between hollow internal organs or between an organ and the exterior of the body.

Etiology

Fistulas can develop from a variety of causes but usually the result of surgery, childbirth, trauma, carcinoma, radiation therapy. Gynecologic procedures cause urinary tract fistulas. The name of the fistula indicates the connecting structures. Fistulas can develop between the vagina and the rectum (rectovaginal), bladder (vesicovaginal) or urethra (urethrovaginal), vescicovaginal fistulas are the most common followed by rectovaginal.

Pathophysiology

Conditions that cause fistulas to form typically compromise the blood supply and cause tissue damage. Tissue sloughs and a channel gradually develop between the affected tissue and the vagina. The result is a constant leak of urine or escape of flatus or fecal material through the vagina. This is highly distressing to the patient and creates an offensive odor. The drainage excoriates and irritates the vaginal and vulvular tissue.

Clinical Manifestation

When vesicovaginal fistulas (between the bladder and vagina develops some urine leaks into the vagina, whereas with rectovaginal (between rectum and vagina) flatus and feces escape into the vagina. In both instances, excoriation and irrigation of vaginal and vulvular tissue occur and may lead to severe infections. In addition, wetness and offensive odors may develop causing embarrassment and severely limiting socialization.

Management

Fistulas are diagnosed primarily through pelvic examination. A fistulagram, which involves the inejction of dye into the vagina, may be used to assess the exact location and severity of the fistula.

Small fistulas may heal spontaneously if the tissue is allowed to rest. Surgery is otherwise necessary to close fistula tract. Tissue inflammation and edema must be treated first, and this can take months. Either anterior or posterior colporrhaphy may be used. It may be necessary to temporarily divert the urinary or fecal stream in complex situation. A folley, ureteral or nephrostomy catheter is used to keep the area well drained and is left in place for weeks in some patients. With urinary diversion many urinary fistulas are able to heal spontaneously. Bowel rest contributes to healing rectovaginal fistulas and the patient may be placed on total parenteral nutrition (TPN). A diverting colostomy may also be performed if surgical intervention becomes necessary.

If fistulas are being conservatively managed, nursing interventions focus on comfort and prevention of infection. The nurses teaches woman that a chlorine solution makes an effective deodorizing douche and this solution is also excellent for perineal irrigation. A solution of 5 ml of household bleach to 1 liter of water is appropriate. Douching should be performed at low pressure to prevent forcing the solution through the fistula tract. Sitz baths and careful cleaning with mild soap and water is also helpful.

Postoperative care focuses on tissue healing. A small amount of serosanguineous drainage is expected but the patient is carefully monitored for evidence of continued fecal or urinary drainage. Douches may be ordered, and the nurse administers gently and at low pressure to protect healing tissue. Bedrest is often enforced for several days, perineal hygiene is great importance. But preoperatively and postoperatively the perineum should be cleansed every 4 hours. Warm sitz baths should be changed frequently. The patient is encouraged to maintain an adequate fluid intake. Encouragement and reassurance are needed in helping the patient to cope with her problems.

Postoperatively nursing care emphasises on avoidance of stress on the repaired areas and prevention of infections.

Postoperative care should be taken on catheters than the indwelling cataheter, usually in place for 7 to 10 days, in drainage at all times oral fluids should be urged to provide for internal catheter irrigation. Minimal pressure and strict asepsis used if catheter irrigation becomes necessary. The first stool after bowel surgery may be purposely delayed or prevent contamination of wound. Later stool softeners or laxatives may be given.

Surgical repair of fistulas is not always effective, even in the best conditions. Therefore, supportive nursing care for patients and her significant others is specifically important.

NEOPLASMS OF THE FEMALE REPRODUCTIVE TRACT

Cervical Polyps

Cervical polyps are benign pedunculated lesion that generally arises from the endocervical mucosi and are seen protruding through the cervicle or during speculum examination. The two main types of cervical polyps are:
1. Endocervical from the canal in the opening of the cervix
2. Ectocervical from the lower portion that protrudes into the vagina. Endocervical polyps tend to occur in middle-aged women. Ectocervical polypse are found most often in postmenopausal woman.

Pathophysiology

Most polyps are asymptomatic and discovered on routine pelvic examination. Endocervical polyps are usually reddish purple to cherry red, smooth soft growth that may vary in size from a few millimeters to 2 or 3 cm in diameter and length. They are usually attached to the mucosa by a narrow pedicle and may be single or multiple in number. Ectocervical Polyps are pale or flesh-colored, round and elongated and often attach with a broad pedicle. Most polypoidal structures are vascular, and both types of polyps may become infected and necrotic at the tip.

Clinical Manifestation

The classic symptoms is intermenstrual bleeding, particularly after intercourse or douching. Leukorrhea may be present. The chronic irritation and bleeding can lead to cervicitis, endometritis, or even salphingitis.

Management

Cervical polyps are usually diagnosed direct inspections and can be removed safely in clinic. The procedure causes minimal bleeding, but if bleeding should occur, it can be controlled by electrical or chemical cautery. All the excised tissues are sent for pathological examination. Antibiotics may be given prophylactically particularly if there is any evidence of tissues necrosis or cervicits. Simple removal of polyps is usually curable. The nurse encourages the woman to rest and avoid strenous activities after polyps removal. A prineal pad can be provided to absorb drainage. The nurse instructs the woman to report any significant bleeding or infection. And instruct her to avoid tampon use, douches and sexual intercourse for about a week while healing takes place.

Cervical Cancer

Cervical cancer is the seventh most common type of cancer in women following breast, colorectal, lung, endometrial and ovarian cancers and lymphoma.

Etiology

Exact cause is unknown, but has a close association existing between early and frequent sexual contact with multiple partners and cervical viral infections, particularly the human papilloma virus (HPV). The HPV has been isolated in the vast majority of precancerous and cancerous changes of the cervix. It is spread predominantly through sexual contact. Studies have found a high incidence of cancer cervix in prostitutes. The rest factors of cervical cancer include the following:

- Actual risk factors:
  - Low socioeconomic status.
  - Early age at first coitus.
  - Multiple sexual partners.
  - History of STD.
  - High risk male partner.
  - Compromised immunity (HIV, HPV infections).
  - Early age at first pregnancy.
  - Prostitution.
  - Multiparity.
- Potential risk factors:
  - Heavy use of talc.
  - Cigarette smoking.
  - Use of oral contraceptives.
  - Vitamin A and C-deficiency.
  - Derangement of folic acid metabolism.
  - Intrauterine exposure to DES.
  - Diabetes.
  - Nulliparity.
  - Frequent douching.

Pathophysiology

Majority of cervical concerns are squamous cell, arising from the epidermal layer of the cervix, cell dysplasia indicates the presence of a precursor lesion, typically called "Cervical intraepithelial neoplasia" (CIN) which has been divided into the following three stages:

CIN I : Mild to moderate dysplasia.
CIN II : Moderate to severe dysplasia.
CIN III : Severe dysplasia to carcinoma in situ.

Women diagnosed with dysplasia may experience disease regression, persistence or a progression to carcinoma. There are usually no signs or symptoms of dysplasia and the diagnosis is based on cytologic findings. Cervical can spread through the blood, by direct extension, a lymph invasion. As the lymph node grows larger, venous blood flow is obstructed and leg edema, ureteral obstruction or hydronephrosis may occur. Hematogenous spread can occur to the lungs, mediastinum, liver and bone, prognosis based on the stage of the disease, depth of invasion and vascular involvement of the tumor.

Clinical Manifestation

Cervical cancer is asymptomatic in the early stages. As the disease progresses, the woman may experience thin, watery vaginal discharge, and occasional bloody spotting, especially after sexual intercourse or douching. In addition, metrorrhagia, postmenopausal bleeding, polymenorrhea occurs as early symptoms. With advanced disease, a foul smelling discharge may develop from sloughing of the epithelial tissue. Pain is usually a late sign and can involve pelvic, flank, lower back and abdomen. The growing tumor may place pressure on the rectum and bladder causing irritation and discharge. Hemorrhage is possible with advanced infiltrative tumors, which may also erode the walls of adjacent organs and create fistula. In addition with loss, anorexia, anemia, dysuria and rectal bleeding also may be present.

Management

Early detection is important to ensure positive outcomes. Routine pap smear screening begins once a woman engages a regular intercourse or turns 18 years old. The pap smear is a screening test but not a diagnostic tool. The diagnosis of cervical cancer can be confirmed only by biopsy. Two most common methods for obtaining cervical biopsy are conization or punch biopsy. Colposcopy allows for microscopic examination of the cervix and improves the accuracy of the biopsy process. In addition to CT scans, IVP, cystoscopy, progesto-sigmoidoscopy, and barium meal studies of the lower GI tract are based on diagnostic adjuncts.

Chemotherapy has not played a significant role in the management of cervical cancer. Squamous cell cancers tend to be relatively unresponsive to drug treatment. Cervical cancer is treated according to the stage of disease as briefed below:

- *Stage 0:* Carcinoma in situ, intraepithelian carcinoma. Treatment options are cryosurgery, conization, laser surgery, hysterectomy, 5-year survival rate is 95-100 percent.
- *Stage 1:* Carcinoma is strictly confined to the cervix (extension to the corpus should be disregarded).
- *Stage Ia:* Preclinical carcinoma of the cervix that is those diagnosed by microscopy. Treatment options are simple hysterectomy or radiation (Cesium implant).
- *Stage Ia1:* Minimal microscopically evident stomal invasion.
- *Stage Ia2:* Lesions detected microscopically that can be measured. The upper limit of the measurement should not show a depth of invasion of more than 5 mm taken from the basis of the epithelium, either surface or glandular from which it originates and a second dimension, the horizontal spread must not exceed 7 mm. Larger lesions should be staged as Ib.
- *Stage Ib:* Lesions of greater dimensions than 1a2, whether seen clinically or not, performed space involvement should not alter the staging but should be specifically recorded so as to determine whether it should affect treatment decisions in future. Treatment options are radiation, and or radical (Werthem's)

hysterectomy. Survival rate is 75 to 85 percent radiotherapy (external or implant).
- *Stage II:* Involement of the vagina but not the lower third or infiltration of the parametric but not out of the sidewall. Treatment of radical hysterectomy of nodes or radiotherapy.
- *Stage IIa:* Involvement of the vagina but no evidence of parametrial involvement.
- *Stage IIb:* Infiltration of the parametrial but not out of the side wall.
- *Stage III:* Involvement of lower third of the vagina or exteretion to the pelvic side wall. All cases with hydronephrosis or nonfunctioning kidney should be included unless they are known to be attributable to other cause treatment in radiation.
- *Stage IIIa:* Involvement of the lower third of the vagina but not out of the pelvic side wall of parametrics are involved.
- *Stage IIIb:* Extension on to the pelvic side wall or hydronephrosis or nonfunctional kidney.
- *Stage IV:* Extension ouitside the reproductive tract, i.e., extensions beyond true pelvic or clinical involvement of the mucosa of the bladder or rectum, no state classification with bullous edema is alone. Treatment options are radiation, surgery (e.g. exenteration) and chemotherapy survival rate is 5-15 years.
- *Stage IVa:* Involvement of the mucosa of the bladder or rectum.
- *Stage IVb:* Involvement of the distant metastasis or disease outside the true pelvis.

Surgical management deals in later part of this chapter.

The guidelines for care of the woman undergoing internal radiotherapy are as follows:
- *Preimplantation:* Nursing care before the insertion of the radioactive implant usually includes the following:
  - Provide cleansing enema to empty the bowel.
  - Insert Folley catheter to keep the bladder empty and small during treatment.
  - Provide betadine douche and shake pubic area if ordered.
- *Implantation period:* Nursing care during the 24 to 72 hours treatment includes the following:
  - Insert gauze packing into the vagina to separate the rectum and bladder from the irradiated area. One or two stitches may be placed in the labia to support the holder in position.
  - Maintain strict bedrest.
    * Elevate head of bed no more than 20 degrees. Keep the patients as flat as possible.
    * Assist the patient to turn from side to side as needed for comfort.
  - Provide low residue diet and possibly antimotility agents to prevent bowel distension.
  - Administer analgesic as needed for uterine cramping, which can be severe.
  - Perform routine perineal cleansing if drainage is present, provide room deodarizer if discharge is foulsmelling.
  - Ensure a minimum fluid intake of 2500 ml daily.
  - Visit patient frequently from room door way for emotional support.
  - Provide diversional activities appropriate to activity restrictions.
  - Monitor implant for proper placement; keep long-hand-led forceps, and lead-lined container in the room in case of dislodgement.
  - Monitor complications:
    * *Infection:* Increased vaginal redness or swelling; increasingly dark, foul-smelling drainage; cloudy urine and fever.
    * *Thrombophlebitis:* Painful leg swelling, positive Horman's sign.

Staff who are involved in internal radiotherapy should follow the following radiation precautions:
- Time at the bedside limited—each contact should last not more than 30 minutes.
- Children and pregnant women/staff should not visit during treatment.
- Staff members should wear a dosimeter during every patient contact to monitor radiation exposure.
- Lead shield may be installed at the side and foot of the bed.
- Staff should use the principles of distance, time, and shielding in all contacts with the patients.
- Implant is always handled by means of long-handled forceps, never with hands. A lead-lined container should be present in the room for use if the implant dislodges.
- A sign that clearly identifies the radiation hazard is pasted on the room door including contact number of radiation safety officer.

The hospitalization period for intracavitary radiotherapy is short, and the patient is discharged soon after the removal of the implant. The woman must learn several self-care skills for home management and should be aware of the sign and symptoms of potential complication. Radiotherapy causes fatigue, vaginal stenosis, loss of vaginal lubrication and induced menopause. The nurse should teach the woman regarding careful vaginal douches, techniques and local application of estrogen cream (to prevent bleeding) and regular vaginal dilation (to prevent vaginal narrowing and fibrosis). If a woman has spouse or sexual partner, regular sexual intercourse usually at least three times per week is one method of minimizing stenosis. Manual oturator can be used to dilate vagina after lubrication. Sexual intercourse may be resumed about 3 weeks after discharge by using proper lubricants. Other self-care measures include gradually increasing activity, maintaining a liberal fluid intake to prevent urological problems and adjusting the diet to prevent bowel problems (e.g. constipation or diarrhea). The nurse teaches about signs and symptoms that indicate complications. The woman should promptly report unusually heavy discharge, foul-smelling urine, low-grade fever, persistent bowel problems or pain. Radiotherapy can cause fistula in the pelvis. The importance of follow-up care and monitoring is emphasized while teaching.

UTERINE LEIOMYOMA (FIBROIDS)

Leiomyomas (fibroids, myomas fibromas) are the most common benign tumors of the female genital tract. Leiomyomas are benign tumors of muscle cells origin that contain varying amounts of fibrous tissue.

Etiology

The exact etiology is not completely understood. The stimulus for growth is unclear but it is thought to be related to estrogen, because leiomyomas are rare before menarche and often decrease in size after menopause. The tumors often enlarge during pregnancy, and with the use of contraceptives. Women who smoke tend to be relatively estrogen deficient and have been found to have a lower incidence of leiomyomas. Tumors can react enormous proportions weighing as much as 50 pounds.

Pathophysiology

Leiomyomas originate in the myometrium are classified by the anatomical locations. Submucous myomas lie just beneath the endometrium and compress it as they grow. They can develop a pedicle and protrude into the uterine cavity or even through the cervical canal. Intramural myomas lie within the uterine muscle, and subserous tumors lie at the serosal surface of the uterus or may bulge outward from the myometrium. The external tumors also tend to become pedunculated.

Clinical Manifestation

The majority of women with leiomyomas are asymptomatic and may go undetected even when large in size, particularly if the woman is obese. The development of the symptoms depends on the location, size and condition of the tumor. Menorrhagia is the most common symptom. Bleeding can result from distortion and congestion of surrounding vessels or ulceration of the overlying endometrium. Bleeding usually takes the form of premenstrual spotting or prolonged light bleeding, after the menses. Metrorrhagia is associated with venous thrombosis or necrosis in the surface of the tumor, particularly if it extrudes through the cervix. The blood loss may be significant enough to create an iron-deficiency anemia that does not respond to iron therapy.

Pain is not a characteristic symptom although it can result from tumor degeneration or with myometrial contractions that attempt to expel myoma from the uterus. If the pedicle stalk becomes twisted it can cause sudden, severe pain. Women often report sensation of heaviness in the pelvis or "a bearing down" feeling especially with large tumors. The tumor may cause pelvic circulated congestions and create backache, constipation or dysmenorrhea. The woman even notices and increases in abdominal girth.

Management

Chemical diagnosis is based on the characteristic pelvic findings of an enlarged uterus destorted by nodular masses. Diagnosis confirmed through the use of MRI and CT scan, pelvic sonography, and hysterography or hysteroscopy.

Treatment depends on the symptoms, the age of the patient, her desire to bear children and the location and size of the tumor or tumors. Persistent heavy menstrual bleeding causing anemia and large or rapidly growing fibroids are indications of surgery. Drug therapy does not play a major role in management of leiomyomas. However, GnRH agonists may be used to reduce the level of circulating estrogens and shrink the tumor. Leiomyomas are the most common indication for hysterectomy. No diet or activity restricts for leiomyomas.

ENDOMETRIAL CANCER

Cancer of the endometrium (Uteri corpus) is the most common form of gynecological cancer and it primarily affects the woman over 50 years of age.

Etiology

The major risk factor for endometrial cancer is estrogen in particular unposed estrogen. Additional risk factors include increasing of age, obesity, diabetes-mellitus, nulliparity, late menopause (after the age of 52) and hypertensions. Obesity is a risk factor because adipose (fat) cells store estrogen which increases endogenous estrogen and increases its availability. Pregnancy and birth control pills are protective factors. In addition, the use of estrogen replacement therapy (ERT) and the use of tamoxifen for breast cancer and other causes of endometrial cancer.

Pathophysiology

Cancer arises from the lining of the endometrium; most tumors are pure adenocarcinomas. The precursor may be a hyperplasic state that progresses to invasive carcinoma. Hyperplasia occurs when estrogen is not counteracted by progesterone. Direct extension develops into the cervix and through the uterine serosa. An invasion of the myometrium occurs in regional lymph nodes including the paravaginal and para-aortic, become involved. Hematogenous metastases develops concurrently.

The usual sites of metastases are lung, bone, liver and eventually the brain. Malignant cells found in the peritoneal cavity, presumably by tubal transport, and their presence is included in staging prognostic factors include histologic differentiation, uterine size at time of diagnosis; myometrial invasion, peritoneal cytology, lymph nodes and adnexal metastasis and tumor size. Endometrial cancer grows slowly, metastasizes late and is amenable to therapy if diagnosed early.

Clinical Manifestation

The first sign of endometrial cancer is abnormal uterine bleeding usually in postmenopausal women. Occasionally women have a purulent, blood-tinged discharge. Pain is late symptom and usually occurs with metastatic disease.

Management

Endometrial biopsy may be taken and examined for high risk women to detect early. The other methods for detection of endometrial cancer includes—endometrial aspiration, endometrial washing, dilation and currettage, pap smear, and combination of methods.

Endometrial cancer is treated according to its stages:

Stage I : Confined to corpus.
Stage II : Involves corpus and cervix.
Stage III : Extends outside the corpus but not outside the pelvis (vaginal wall).
Stage IV : Involves bladder rectum or outside pelvis.

The most common treatment is total abdominal hysterectomy with bilateral salpingo-oophorectomy (TAH-BSO). Radiation and surgery are often combined to treat in early state of the disease. Hormonal therapy (Progestin) and chemotherapy (doxorubicin, cyclopholpomide, cisplatin are often added for stage III and IV diseases).

Nursing care associated with hystrectomy and radiotherapy followed. Nurses play a major role in health teaching about the importance of the careful assessment of all dysfunctions, uterine bleeding in postmenopausal population. Endometrial cancer is treatable disease.

Gestational Trophoblastic Neoplasia (GTN)

Gestational trophoblastic neoplasia (GTN) is the term used to describe choriocarcinoma and related diseases such as hydatid form mole and invasive mole.

The etiology of GTN is not thoroughly understood. The hydatid form mole often precedes malignant diseases. GTN is an abnormal pregnancy characterized by a degeneration or abnormal growth of the tropho-blastic tissue of the placenta, usually in the absence of an intact fetus. It produces a serum marker, human chorionic gonadotropin (hCG) whose levels are directly related to the number of tumor cells.

Early stage of GTN may be similar to normal pregnancy. As the disease progresses, most of the women experience uterine bleeding. Rapid uterine growth occurs. Often accompanied with nausea and vomiting.

Management

The diagnosis of GTN usually accomplished by ultrasonography, aminography, and analysis of HCG levels. Other diagnostic measures may be employed to rule out the presence of metastasis.

Suction currettage is the most common method used for evacuation of molar pregnancy, although hysterectomy may be selected if the woman does not desire future pregnancies.

Intravenous ocytocin may be used to assist in expulsion of the tissue, which is then sent for extensive HPE.

OVARIAN CYSTS

Benign tumors of the ovary are many and varied. The cause of most of them is unknown. For purpose of clarity, they are divided into cysts and neoplasms. Cysts are usually soft, surrounded by thin capsules, and are seen mainly during the reproduction years. Follicle and corpus luteum cysts are common ovarian cysts. Epithelial ovarian neoplasms are extremely varied. They may be cystric or solid, small or extremely large. Cystric teratomas or dermoids originate from germ cells containing bits of any type of body tissues, such as hair or teeth.

Pathophysiology

Benign cysts and tumors develop from a variety of physiological imbalance. Elevated levels of luteinizing hormone may cause hyperstimulation of the ovaries. Follicular cysts depend on gonadotropins for growth and generally occur during the menstrual years and resolve spontaneously simple cysts occur commonly during menopause.

The characteristics of various type of benign ovarian cysts and tumors are as follows:
- Cysts
  - Follicular cysts:
    * Most common form of cysts.
    * Frequently multiple, range in size from a few mm to as large as 15 cm in diameters.
    * Depend on gonadotropin for growth.
    * Occur during menstrual years and usually resolve spontaneously.
    * May cause menstrual irregularities if blood estrogen is elevated.
  - Corpus luteum cysts:
    * Less common variety.
    * Associated with normal ovarian function or elevated progesterone.
    * Average diameter 4 cm.
    * May appear purplish red from bleeding within corpus luteum.

- May cause delayed menstrual bleeding from progesterone secretions.
- Menorrhagia common.
  - Theca Lutein cysts:
    - Least common variety.
    - Usually bilateral and produce significant ovarian enlargement upto 30 cm in diameter.
    - Develop from prolonged and excessive stimulation by gonadotropins.
    - Associated with hydatide form mole 50 percent of the time and choriocarcinoma 10 percent of the time.
- Epithelial tumors
  - Serous tumors
    - Found in all age groups.
    - Can be extremely large filling pelvis or abdomen.
  - Mucinous Tumors
    - Occur in second to third decade of life.
    - May be bilateral.
    - Can reach spectacular size and largest form.
  - Endometroid tumors
    - Small lesions, purplish-blue in color.
    - Large tumors called "chocolate cysts" because they contain chocolate color clots.
    - Very low malignancy potential.
  - Mesonephroid Tumors
    - Usually multifocal.
    - Involve peritoneal surfaces and may cause interestinal or urinary tract complications.
    - Characterized by papillary proliferation without mitotic activity.

Clinical Manifestation

Ovarian masses are often asymptomatic until they are large enough to cause pressure in the pelvis, constipation, menstrual irregularities, urinary frequency, a full feeling in the abdomen, anorexia and peripheral edema may occur depending on the size and locations of the tumor. Here there may be an increase in abdominal girth. Pelvic pain may be present if the tumor is growing rapidly, severe pain results when cyst twists in its pedicle (twisted ovarian cyst).

Management

Palpation of the reproductive organs during pelvic examination commonly reveals the presence of any mass or enlargement of the ovary. Any mass palpated in a postmenopausal women requires further investigation which includes ultrasonography and CT scan, etc. and confirm diagnosis.

Many ovarian cysts resolve spontaneously. If the cyst does not decrease in size, oral contraceptive may be prescribed to shrink it. Surgery is usually recommended only when the cyst is larger than 8 cm or occurs after menopause or before puberty. A cystectomy rather than oophorectomy will be performed if possible.

Woman should be educated regarding disease, importance of follow up care; nurse should reassure the patient who has undergone surgery. If woman goes surgical menopause, estrogen replacement therapy is initiated.

OVARIAN CANCER

Malignant neoplasms of the ovaries occur at all ages including infancy and childhood. It occurs most frequently in women between 55 to 65 years of age.

Etiology

The etiology of ovarian cancer is not understood but several factors appear to be associated with it like hereditary, endocrine, environment of the ovarian cancer. Women who have mutation of the BRCA-1 gene have increased susceptibility of ovarian cancer. Incidence rates are high in industrialized areas, which point to environmental influences. Exposure to talc and asbestos, diets high in meat and animal fats and high milk consumption all appear to be linked with the cancer.

Breastfeeding, multiple pregnancies, oral contraceptives use (more than 5 years) and early age at first birth seem to reduce risk of ovarian cancer. It is thought these factors have a protective effect because they reduce the number of ovulatory cycles the women experience. Women who are not exposed to these factors may have risk of getting ovarian cancer.

Pathophysiology

Ovarian cancer is a broad term that can be divided into many categories depending on the cell type of origin. The four main types of ovarian neoplasms are as follows:
- Epithelium: Serous, mucinous and edometroid.
- Germ cell: Teratomas (mature and immature) dysgerminoma (occurs less than 20 years)
- Gonadal stroma: Granulosa (theca, serotils, leydig cells)
- Mesenchyma: Fibroma, lymphoma, sarcoma.

Ovarian cancer has two pattern of metastasis: Lymphatic and direct. Primary lymphatic drainage of the ovary is through the retroperitoneal nodes surrounding the renalilium. Secondary drainage is through the inguinal lymphatics. Ovarian cancer also metastasizes directly to the abdominal cavity.

Clinical Manifestation

In its early stages ovarian cancer is usually asymptomatic. As malignancy grows a variety of symptoms, develops which includes pelvic discomfort, lowback pain, weight change, abdominal pain, nausea, and vomiting, constipation and urinary frequency. Further increase in abdominal girth, bowel and bladder dysfunction, menstrual irregularities, and ascitis can occur. An ovarian malignancy should be considered when abnormal uterine bleeding occurs.

The stages of the ovarian cancer includes the following:
- Stage I   : Limited to ovaries.
- Stage II   : Involving one or both ovaries with pelvic extentions.
- Stage III   : Involving one or both ovaries with intraperitoneal metastasis outside pelvis or positive lymph nodes.
- Stage IV   : Involving one or both ovaries with distant metastasis (e.g. liver, lungs).

Management

The early diagnosis of an ovarian cancer usually occurs by chance rather than successful screening. Although no screening test exists today still routine tests like MRI, CT scan and ultrasonography are used. Laparotomy is the primary tool for both diagnosis and staging.

Surgery is the primary therapeutic approach and usually involves TAH-BSO. Ascitic fluids or washings are submitted for cytology. All the tissues of the pelvis are carefully assessed, and biopsies of any suspicious tissues are sent for analysis.

Adjuvant therapy is often employed based on the stage of the diseased as follows:

Stage I   : Chemotherapy.
Stage II   : Instillation of radioactive phosphorous into the peritoneum or combined chemotherapy.
Stage III and IV   : Surgical removal of tumor.

The patient receives the standard postoperative teaching appropriate for any major abdominal surgery. Patient teaching concerning the diagnosis, surgery, and adjuvant therapy for ovarian cancer is an integral aspect of nursing care apart from routine surgical nursing measures. Ongoing supportive measures are initiated because of poor prognosis.

VULVAR CANCER

Vulvar cancer is rare and invasive disease; it accounts for the just 5 percent of malignance of the female genital tract. Similar to cervical cancer, preinvasive lesions are referred to as vulvar intraepithelial neoplasia (VIN) precede invasive vulvar cancer.

Etiology

Preinvasive disease (vulvar carcinoma in situ) is occurring more commonly in younger women possibly because of factors such as exposure to papilloma virus and HIV. The exact etiology of this cancer is still unknown. Etiological factors are believed to include STDs involving the vulva and the use of tight-fitting apparel or nylon under-garments, perineal deodorants, and trauma. Herpes, syphilis and other lesions have all been associated with development of carcinoma. Immunosuppression, diabetes, smoking and hypertension also have been linked. But cause and effect of relationship have not been established.

Pathophysiology

Most of the cancers of the vulva are squamous in 'origin'. The initial lesion often arises, from an area of intraepithelial neoplasia, which can eventually form a firm nodule and ulcerate. The lesion can develop anywhere in the vulva, but 70 percent of the lesions arise on the labia. The lesions usually are localized and well demarcated.

Clinical Manifestation

Patient with vulvar neoplasia may have symptoms of vulvar itching or burning, pain, bleeding or discharge.

Management

Diagnosis of vulvar cancer is based on pathology report on the biopsy of the suspicious lesion. VIN managed by eradicatory lesion is medically with 5-fluorouracil (S-Fu) or surgical excision. The standard treatment for invasive carcinoma is radical vulvectomy. It involves excision of the mons pubis, terminal portion of urethra and vagina, excision of portions of the round ligaments in saphenous veins and selected lymph node dissection.

Nursing care of the woman undergoing radical vulvectomy are as follows:
- Preoperative care:
  - Explain treatment and plan of care.
  - Administer enemas and douches as prescribed.
  - Provide emotional support.
  - Teach deep-breathing exercises and leg exercises.
- Postoperative care:
  - Maintain bedrest for 72 hours in semi-Fowler's position.
    * Support legs with pillows.
    * Turn every 2 hours.
    * Encourage frequent deep-breathing and use of incentive spirometer.
    * Encourage leg exercises.
    * Avoid stress on suture lines.
    * Assess for signs of complications—atelectasis and deep vein thrombosis.
  - Assess discomfort level and ensure, adequate analgesive.
    * Use PCA pump if possible to allow patient to control dosage.
  - Monitor wound healing
    * Provide perineal hygiene and give sitz baths when ordered; keep perineum dry.
    * Cleanse wound bid and after defecation.
    * Maintain patency of Foley catheter.

- Provide low residue diet.
- Provide diversional activities.
- Encourage expression of feelings.
- Discharge teaching
  - Use support host for 6 months, elevate legs frequently.
  - Can resume sexual activity in 4 to 6 weeks.
  - Discuss possible need for lubrication and positive changes with coitus and genital numbness may be present.
  - Avoid staining with defecation.
  - Discuss signs and symptoms of complications to report to physician.
  - Note the possible altered directional flow of urine.

SURGERIES OF THE FEMALE REPRODUCTIVE SYSTEM

A varieties of surgical procedures are performed when benign or malignant tumors of the genital tract are found. A hysterectomy may be done either vaginally or abdominally. A vaginal route is often used when vaginal repair is to be done in addition to removal of the uterus. The abdominal route is used when large tumors are present and the pelvic cavity is to be explored or when the tubes and ovaries are to be removed at the same time. The abdominal route can present more postoperative problem because it involves incisions and the opening of the abdominal cavity. The common surgical procedure on the female reproductive tract are as follows:

- Oophorectomy—Removal of an ovary.
- Salpingectomy—Removal of fallopian tube.
- Bilateral salpinge—Oophorectomy (Bil S and O); Removal of both ovaries and fallopian tubes.
- Total hysterectomy—Removal of the entire uterus, including the cervix may be referred to as a TAH (total abdominal hysterectomy). Procedure can be done vaginally or abdominally.
- Subtotal hysterectomy—Removal of the uterus without cervix (Rare).
- Panhysterectomy—(Total abdominal hyperectomy and bilateral salpingo-oophorectomy; Removal of the entire uterus and both fallopean tubes, and ovaries also called TAH-BSO).
- Hystero-oophorectomy—Removal of the uterus and an ovary.
- Hystero-salpingectomy—Removal of the uterus and fallopian tube.
- Radical hysterectomy (Wertheim procedure)—TAH-BSO, partial vaginectomy and dissection of the lymph nodes in the pelvis.
- Vaginectomy—Removal of vagina.
- Pelvic exenteration—Radical hysterectomy, total vaginectomy, removal of the bladder with diversion of urinary systems and resection of bowel with colostomy.
- Anterior pelvic exenteration—Above operation without bowel resection.
- Posterior pelvic exenteration—Above operation without bladder removal.

Nursing care of the woman undergoing hysterectomy are as follows: (in addition to routine nursing intervention for any surgery).

Preoperative Care

- Verify patient understanding of the procedure and anticipated care.
- Administer prescribed enemas, laxatives and douches.
- Verify completion of prescribed skin preparation.
- Promote circulation and oxygenation:
  - Apply antiembolic hose.
  - Teach deep breathing, effective coughing, use of incentive spirometer, how to splint abdomen, and how to change position.
  - Teach leg and feet exercises.
  - Teach how to use PCA for pain control.
  - Encourage expression of feelings and concerns.

Postoperative Care

- Promote comfort:
  - Administer analgesics and encourage PCA use.
  - Administer antiemetics as needed.
- Promote circulation and oxygenation:
  - Encourage, turning, deep-breathing, coughing and use of intensive spirometer.
  - Encourage leg and feet exercise every hour while in bed.
  - Maintain use of antiembolic hose as ordered.
  - Encourage frequent ambulation.
  - Assess signs and symptoms of thromboembolisms.
- Maintain fluid and electrolytic balance:
  - Accurately record all output and drainage.
- Promote elimination:
  - Monitor effectiveness of bladder emptying after catheter removal. Catheterize for residual if ordered.
  - Monitor signs and symptoms of returning peristalism.
  - Encourage frequent ambulation and a liberal fluid intake.
  - Teach diet modifications to prevent constipation.
- Provide discharge teach in:
  - Teach signs of urinary tract infection.
  - Provide teaching regarding incision care.
  - Instruct patient to avoid heavy lifting, prolonged sitting and long car drive.
  - Tell the patient to refrain from coitus for about 6 weeks and not to douche unless prescribed by her physician. Vaginal bleeding or discharge may persist for upto 6 weeks.
  - Help patient to anticipate the occurrence of mood swings and emotional lability during healing.

INFERTILITY

Infertility is the inability to achieve pregnancy after at least one year of regular sexual intercourse without contraception. The problems may be considered primay if the couple has never conceived or secondary if conception was successfully achieved in the past.

Etiology

Infertility may be caused by either female factors or male factors. The common causes of infertility in men and women are as follows:
- Female
  - Developmental: Uterine abnormalities.
  - Endocrine: Pituitary, thyroid, and adrenal dysfunction, ovarian dysfunction (inhibit maturation and release of ovum).
  - Diseases: PID (especially gonococcus), fallopian tube obstructions. Diseases of cervix and uterus that inhibit passage of active sperm.
  - Other: Malnutrition, severe anemia and anxiety.
- Male
  - Developmental: Undescended testes, other congenital abnormalities (inhibit development of sperm).
  - Endocrine: Hormonal deficiency (pituitary, thyroid, adrenal), inhibit the development of sperm.
  - Diseases: Testicular destruction from disease, orchitis from mumps, and prostatitis.
  - Others: Excessive smoking, fatigue, alcohol, excessive heat (hot baths) use of marijuana.
- Both Male and Female
  - *Diseases:* STDs, cancer-causing obstructions (inhibit transport of ovum or sperm).
  - *Others:* Immunological incompatibility (inhibit sperm penetration of ovum) and marital problems.
  - *Diethylstilbestrol (DES),* exposure in utero (suggested but not proved as a cause of male infertility).

Pathophysiology

Three basic categories of infertility account for 95 percent of reproductive dysfunction: Anovulation, anatomical defect of the female genital tract and abnormal sperm production. The common cause in male and female explained in etiology.

The most frequent female causes of infertility include ovulation factor, such as anovulation or inadequate corpus luteum, tubal obstruction, or dysfunction such as endometriosis or damage from pelvic infections, and uterine or cervical factors such as leiomyoma or structural anomalies. Risk factors for infertility include increasing age, tobacco and illicit use of drugs, excessive exercises, severe dietary restriction and specific occupational and environmental exposure.

Clinical Manifestation

In addition to clinical manifestation of the causes of infertility, infertility itself can produce profound psychological effects. When couple find themselves unable to have children, the trauma can affect every aspect of their lives and marriage. The experience of diagnosis and treatment can be an emotional roller coaster of raised expectations and dashed hopes.

Management

A detailed history and general physical examination of the woman and her partner provide the basis for selecting diagnostic studies. The possibility of medical or gynecologic diseases is explored before tests are performed to evaluate whether the cause is female infertility. These tests include ovulatory studies, tubal patency studies and postcoital studies.

The purposes of an infertility evaluation are to establish the cause of infertility and provide a basis for determining medical or surgical treatment options. The process can be physically painful as well as emotionally and economically stressful. The common diagnostic testing for infertility includes the following:
- Male
  - Semen analysis to determine presence, number and motility of sperms.
  - Testicular biopsy if sperm count is low or absent, the presence of sperm indicates obstruction of vas deferens.
- Female
  - Basal body temperature chart to determine that ovulation is occurring.
  - Postcoital test of cervical secretion, measure the ability of sperm to penetrate cervical mucosa and remain active and determine quality of mucous.
  - *Endometrial biopsy:* Determine whether ovulation is occurring (if in endometrium).
  - *Laparoscopy:* Examine the pelvis and determine patency of fallopian tubes.
  - *Hysterosalpingography:* Determine patency of uterus and fallopian tubes.
- Male/female
  - Hormonal tests to determine whether problem is hormonal.

Treatment

Artificial insemination is simple, safe, inexpensive and highly successful infertility treatment when male infertility is the cause. Semen may be deposited by a cervical-vaginal route, intracervically, or intrauterine. A few drops of semen are injected as close to the time of ovulation as possible. Treatment may use the partner's semen (homologous) or donor (heterologous). The fertility donor is carefully determined and the sperms are screened for HIV. This can be an emotional topic for some couples and may induce strong reactions.

Alternative approach to infertility management includes the following:

- *In vitro Fertilization (IVF) and Embryo Transfer:* One or more ova are recovered from the ovarian follicles and fertilized with the partners sperm in a Petri dish.

  Oocyte retrieval is performed by means of ultrasound-guided needle aspiration. The cleaved ova are placed in the patient's uterus through a small catheter about 48 hours after retrieval. Pregnancy rates are related to the number of embryos placed and vary from 18 to 30 percent.

- *Gamete Intrafallopian Transfer (GIFT):* Oocytes aspirated from follicles are mixed with washed sperm and placed in the uterine tube via laparoscopy. This approach appears to achieve a higher pregnancy rate than IVF. The proembryo travels towards the uterus, following the natural time table for implantation in 4 days.

- *Zygote Intrafallopian Transfer (ZIFT) and Tubal Embryo Transfer (TET):* These procedures are similar to GIFT except transfer to the fallopian tubes occurs at the zygote stage, about 16 to 18 hours after oocyte insemination. TET involves transfer of embryos into the fallopian tube around 40 to 48 hours after oocyte insemination.

- *Surrogate Mothers:* Surrogate mothers are women who contract to conceive by artificial insemination and give the baby to the semen donor after delivery. Many social and legal implications with the process have received recent attention through some extremely public law suits over custody of the child.

- *Ovum Transfer:* A donor provides the ovum, which is fertilized with the partner's sperm. The embryo is transferred to the infertile woman's uterus after about 5 days via a small catheter. Pregnancy rates have been as high as 25 to 50 percent.

The management of infertility problem depends on the cause of infertility is secondary to an alteration in ovarian function, supplemental hormone therapy to restore and maintain ovulation may be attempted. Drugs used to induce ovulation include clomiphene citrate (clomid), human menopausal gonadotropin (Pergonal) and bromocriptine (Parlodel).

When a tubal blockage exists, the woman should be referred to a specialist to discuss whether surgical correction (Transcervical balloon tuboplasty-TBT) or IVF is more appropriate. Chronic cervicitis and inadequate estrogenic stimulation are cervical factors causing infertility. Antibiotic therapy is indicated for cervicitis. Inadequate estrogen stimulation is treated by administration of estrogen.

When a couple has not succeeded in conceiving while under infertility management, an option is intrauterine insemination with the husband's or donor's sperm. IVF may be used. Assisted reproductive technologies (ART continue to develop rapidly since the first IVF baby was born in 1978. ARTs include IVF, GIFT, ZIFT, donor gametes, and embryocryo preservation. With the increasing embryocryo preservation assisted hatching, and intracytoplasmic sperm injection, couples have an increased potential for pregnancy. The use of ART poses many ethical, legal, social and financial concerns.

Nurses can assist women experiencing infertility by providing information about the reproductive process and infertility evaluation and addressing the psychologic and social distress that can accompany infertility. Removing or reducing psychologic stress can improve the emotional climate, making it more conducive to achieving a pregnancy.

The nurse has a major responsibility for teaching and providing emotional support throughout the infertility testing and treatment period. Feelings of anger, frustration, grief and helplessness may heighten as more and more diagnostic tests are performed. Infertility can generate great tension in a marriage as the couple exhaust their financial and emotional resources. Recognizing and taking steps to deal with the psychologic factors that surface can assist the couple to cope up in better way with the situation. The nurses also play a role in promoting fertility which includes teaching of prevention of infections, responsibility for infertility, early diagnosis and treatment.

PROBLEMS OF THE BREAST

Breast problems are significant health concerns to women. In a woman's lifetime, there is a one in eighth chance that she will be diagnosed with breast cancer (Few breast cancers are found in men). Whether benign or malignant, intense feeling of shock, fear and denial often accompany the initial discovery of a lump or change in the breast. These feelings are associated both with the fear of survival and with the possible loss of a breast. Throughout history, the female breast has been regarded as a symbol of beauty, sexuality and motherhood. The potential loss of a breast or part of a breast may be devastating for many women because of the significant psychologic, social, sexual and body image implications associated with it.

BENIGN BREAST PROBLEMS

Benign breast disease is common and accounts for about 90 percent of all breast problems. Because there is no universally-accepted classification system for benign disorders.

Cystic Breast Disease

Fibrocystic changes in the breast constitute a benign condition characterized by changes in the breast tissue.

The change includes the development of excess fibrous tissue hyperplasia of the epithelial lining of the mammary ducts, proliferation of mammary ducts and cystic formations. The changes produce pain by nerve irritation from connector tissue, edema and by fibrosis from nerve pinching.

Etiology

The underlying cause of cystic breast disease is not fully understood. Changes in the breast are cyclic and thought to be caused by hormonal imbalance or the exaggerated response of breast tissue to ovarian hormone. Breast tenderness is more pronounced during or before the menstruation. Cystic breast disease is most common in nulliparous women between the ages of 40 and 50 years but can occur at any age. Occurrence is least frequent after menopause.

Pathophysiology

Fibrocystic changes do not increase the risk of breast cancer for majority of patients. Masses or nodularities can appear in both breasts and are often found in the upper, outer quadrant, and usually occur bilaterally. Changes once thought be abnormal such as microcysts, apocrine change, adenosis, fibrosis, and varying degrees of hyperplasia are now reorganized as part of the involutional process of breast. These changes include the presence of lumps, of varying size, nipple discharge, and breastpain (mastodynia or mastalgia). Cystic lesions are soft, well demarcated, and freely movable. The process is almost always bilateral with most lesions located in the left breast. The cyst may contain clear, milky, straw colored or yellow to dark brown fluid. Occasionally the contents may be blood tinged.

Clinical Manifestation

Manifestation of fibrocytic changes include one or more palpable lumps that are usually round, lobular, well delienated and freely-movable within the breast. Some lumps are fibrous and do not contain cysts. There may be accompanying discomfort ranging from tenderness to pain. The lump is usually observed to increase in size and perhaps in tenderness before menstruation. Cysts may enlarge or shrink rapidly. Nipple discharges associated with fibrocystic breasts is often milky, watery milky, yellow or green.

Management

The woman who discovers a mass or masses in her breast should seek the advice of the health care provider. A needle aspiration generally comprise the presence of cyst. Biopsies in women with fibrocystic disease may be indicated for women with increased risk for breast cancer.

The woman with cystic changes should be encouraged to return regularity for follow-up examination throughout life. She should also be taught breast self-examination (BSE) to self-monitor the problem. Severe fibrocystic changes may make palpation of the breast more difficult. Any new lumps or changes in the breasts should be evaluated and changes in symptoms should be reported and investigated.

Many type of treatment have been suggested for a fibrocystic condition. These include the use of a good support bra, dietary therapy (low-salt diet, restriction of methylxanthioses such as coffee, tea, cola, chocolate), vitamin E therapy, analgesics, Danazol (Danocrine), diuretics, hormone therapy, antiestrogen therapy, and surgical therapy (Subcutaneous mastectomy).

The role of the nurse in the care of the patients with benign breast disorders is primarily that of educator and facilitator. The nurse should be knowledgeable about benign conditions, understand their medical management, be able to provide and clarify information and support the patient emotionally and physically through diagnosis and treatment.

A woman with fibrocystic breast, should be told that she may expect recurrence of the cyst in one or both breasts until menopause and that cysts may enlarge or become painful just before menstruation. Additionally she should be reassured that cysts do not "turn into cancer". Any new lump that does not respond in a cyclic manner over 1 to 2 weeks should be examined promptly. The nurse teaches BSE to those women who are not familiar with it and stresses its use every month. Teaching breast models can also be helpful. Women should be taught to recognize through touch their normal breast tissue and the location and size if any lesion is present. They should report significant changes, that differ from the normal cyclic fluctuations or that appear at a different time in the menstrual cycle.

The use of mild analgesics and wearing a firm supportive brassiere may provide comfort and reduce pain. The use of warm and moist heat may be beneficial to relieve aching pain, eliminating caffeine consumption and decreasing salt content before menstruation to relieve bloating and weight gain can be recommended.

FIBROADENOMA OF BREAST

Fibroadenoma is a common cause of discrete benign breast lumps in young women (less than 25 years).

Etiology/Pathophysiology

The possible cause of fibroadenoma may be increased estrogen sensitivity in localized area of the breast. Fibroadenoma are tumors of fibroblastic and epithelial origin thought to be caused by hyperestrinisms. They are estrogen-dependent and associated with menstrual irregularities. Tumors are slow growing and often are stimulated by pregnancy and lactations.

Regressions may occur after delivery. Fibroadenomas tend to regress at menopause and become hyalinized. "Giant" fibroadenomas grow very rapidly to 10 to 12 cms in diameter but are not prone to malignant change than smaller lesions. Dimpling or nipple retraction is not associated with fibroadenoma.

Clinical Manifestation

Fibroadenomas are usually small, painless, round, well-delineated and very mobile. They may be soft but are usually solid, firm and rubbery in consistency. There is no accompanying retraction or nipple discharge. The lump is often painless. The fibroadenoma may appear as a single unilateral mass, although multiple bilateral fibrodenomas are reported. Growth is slow and often ceases when size reaches 2 to 3 cm. Size is not affected by menstruation. However, pregnancy can stimulate dramatic growth. Fibroadenomas are rarely associated with cancer.

Management

Fibroadenomas are easily detected by physical examination and are often visible on mammographs. Definitive diagnosis, however requires biopsy and tissue examination.

Surgical removal is the standard treatment of fibroadenoma. Many can be removed under local anesthesia in a OPD setting. Surgery is not urgent in women under 25 years of age. In women over 35, all new lesions should be examined using an excisional biopsy. Fibroadenoma is not reduced by radiation or are not affected by hormone therapy. The nurse frequently has the opportunity to counsel a young woman with fibroadenoma. During the contact, the benign nature of the lesions should be stressed and follow-up examination and BSE should be encouraged.

BREAST INFECTIONS

Mammary Duct Ectasia

Ductal ectasia is a benign breast disease of perimenopausal and postmenopausal women involving the ducts in the subareolar area. It usually involves several bilateral ducts.

Etiology

Mammary duct ectasia, also referred to as plasma cell mastitis, is a benign condition of unknown etiology. Some believe an anaerobic bacteria may be implicated. Another causative factor may be bacterial infections that result from stasis of fluid in the large ducts of the breasts. The primary risk factor is the age between 45 to 55.

Pathophysiology

Mammary duct ectasia involves inflammation of the ducts behind the nipple, duct enlargement, and a collection of cellular debris and fluid in the involved ducts. As the inflammatory response resolves, the ducts become fibrotic and dilated. Nipple discharge usually is bilateral and ranges from serous to thick, sticky or pastelike. Drainage may be green, greenish brown or blood stained. Nipple itching, suggestive of Paget's disease, may accompany transient pain in the subareolar and inner quadrants of the breast. On palpation the areolar area may feel warm like, the nipple may be red and swollen or flat and retracted. The condition is not associated with breastfeeding.

Clinical Manifestation

Nipple discharge is the primary symptom. This discharge is multicolored and sticky. Ductal ectasia is initially painless but may progress to burning, itching and pain around the nipple, as well as swelling in the areolar area. Inflammatory signs often are present. The nipple may retract and the discharge may become bloody in more advanced disease. Ductal ectasia is not associated with malignancy.

Management

Treatment varies depending on the severity of the problem. Because of the chronic nature of the problem, most women are monitored with routine physical examination of the breast. The symptoms of mammary duct ectasia may engender the fear of malignant disease in the patient. Once the benign nature of the chronic condition is affirmed, fears generally are dispelled, and most women are able to deal with their symptoms. Although there is no cure for mammary duct ectasia, antibiotics are prescribed for acute inflammatory episodes, such as the development of an abscess. If the chronic discharge can no longer be tolerated, surgical excision of the retroareolar ducts is performed.

The nurse must be cognizant of the chronic yet benign nature of this condition and offer support and understanding care. The woman is taught how to cleanse the breast to minimize the risk of infection. Good handwashing and personal hygiene measures are stressed. Wearing a supportive yet nonconfining brassiere padded with sterile guaze and changing the bra daily or as necessary helps prevent abscess formation. The nurse teaches the woman signs and symptoms indicative of abscess should be reported immediately.

Acute Mastitis and Abscess

Mastitis is an inflammatory condition that occurs most frequently in lactating women. There are two types of mastitis, i.e. acute or chronic. The acute form is a rare condition, almost always found in breastfeeding mothers during the first 4 months of lactation. It occurs most frequently from "*Staphylococcus aureas* or *staphylococcus epidermides* infection that spreads from a crack in the skin surface of the nipple (cracked nipple) to underlying breast tissue. It may be confined to only one quadrant of the breast.

Symptoms include a fissured nipple, fever, chill, localized tenderness and erythema. Purulent discharge from the nipple is usually not observed.

The chronic form of mastitis can follow acute mastitis or have a slow and insidious onset. Both acute and chronic mastitis are caused by the same bacterial agents. The chronic form occurs more in older women, and the symptoms can be microinflammatory breast cancer. The infection usually arises in the sweat or sebacous glands and spreads in the breast. Symptoms of chronic mastitis include a painful breast mass that involves the nipple and areola and a low grade fever.

Pathophysiology

In both acute and chronic mastitis there is edema and congestion of the periodical and interlobular stromata. The ducts are distended from the accumulation of neutrophils and retained secretions. If an abscess forms its central core may be necrotic and contain creamy, yellow exudate. Fibrosis of the involved tissue can develop after treatment. Both acute and chronic mastitis can mimic breast cancer, but recent lactation usually excludes the acute forms the need for further assessment.

Clinical Manifestation are explained above in acute and chronic mastitis.

Management

Acute mastitis is easy to diagnose in a nursing mother. Treatment with antibiotics resolves infectious process. In older women, because the conditions have similarities to inflammatory breast carcinoma, surgical incision and drainage of the inflammatory exudate are performed to determine the cause. Antibiotics can then be prescribed.

When acute mastitis is the result of an infection during lactation, most women immediately stop breastfeeding. Breastfeeding should continue unless an abscess in forming or purulent drainage is noted. The infant is not affected by sucking on the involved breast, and antibiotic therapy is not required. Continued breastfeeding is believed to reduce the pain and lessen the volume of milk that can be a source of bacterial growth. If breastfeeding is discontinued, the woman is instructed to keep her breasts as empty as possible by pumping. If the breast is not emptied, it will become engorged and pain will increase. The woman is instructed to complete the entire course of antibiotics and not discontinue them when symptoms are relieved. The older women are more anxious about their diagnosis of cancer. Emotional support and frank discussion are made until biopsy results. Both mastitis require antibiotic theory, rest analgesics, application of local heat.

Breast Cancer

Breast cancer is the most common malignancy, it is second only to lung cancer. It is the leading cause of death from cancer among women.

Etiology

The underlying cause of breast cancer is still unknown but number of risk factors have been identified, which includes the following:
- *Age and Gender:* The incidence of breast cancer is increased with age. Nearly two-thirds of breast cancers are found in postmenopausal women usually after 50 years. The reason for the age-related increase is thought to be the increased probability of mutagenic changes occurring over a longer lifespan rather than any instability inherent aging cells. Breast cancer may be inherited (BRCA-I gene) or noninherited.
- *Menstrual and Reproductive History:* The risk of breast cancer is increased when menstruation begins at an early age (11-12 years) and extends to a late menopause (about age 55). Nulliparity (childless women) and women who bear their first child near or after the age of 30 years and also family history of mother or sister or both had breast cancer may increase risk.
- *Hormones and Oral Contraceptives:* Hormonal replacement therapy at menopause has created a great deal of cancer and controversy, because of the increased incidence of breast cancer associated with it. There is no evidence yet to suggest a causal relationship between oral contraceptives and incidence of and survival from breast cancer.
- *Diet and Body Weight:* Animal data and description of epidemiology of breast cancer incidences strongly suggest an association of dietary factors specifically a high-fat diet. With an increased risk of breast cancer. This claim is largely unproved. Body weight, height, obesity and increased body mass have been reported to be associated with an increased risk of breast cancer but still is controversial. In obesity, fat cells store estrogen.
- *Benign Breast Disease:* Fibrocystic condition of the breast is not associated with breast cancer. However, biopsy proven atypical hyperplasia is associated with increased risk.
- *Radiation Hazard:* Three groups of women who received low level radiation exposure demonstrated an increased breast cancer risk, which was perticularly notable if the exposure occurred in the early years (less than 30 years), radiation damages DNA.
- *Alcohol:* A suggested small increase in risk with moderate alcohol consumption has been reported, although limitation in methodology have been cited, and results require confirmation.

Pathophysiology

Tumors of the breast arise in the epithelial cells either ductal or lobular tissues and are referred to carcinomas. A number of histological subtypes also have been identified, but are not commonly seen nor are they invasive as ductal and lobular carcinomas when the tumor is confined within a duct or a lobule and has not invaded surrounding tissue it is considered localized or in situ carcinoma of the breast. Infiltrative ductal or lobular carcinomas are tumors that have spread directly into surrounding tissues and may have distant metastases if they have penetrated the axillary internal mammary nodes of the systemic circulation.

The breast is divided into four quadrants, upper inner, upper outer lower inner and lower outer. Most breast tumors are located in the upper outer quadrant, but they can occur in any area of the breast of the invasive breast tumors, infiltrative ductal carcinoma is the most prevalant histological cell type followed by infiltrating lobular carcinoma. Brief review of selected histological types of breast cancer their incidence, characteristics and prognosis are as follows:

- Infiltrating ductal carcinoma (Incidence 70 percent) Characterized by stony hard mass, gritty texture; may appear bilaterally and prognosis is poor, common involvements are in axillary nodes.
- Medullary carcinoma (5-7 percent) characterized by soft mass, often reaches large size, may be circumscribed and prognosis is favorable.
- Mucinous or colloid carcinoma (5 percent): Slow growing; can reach large size may occur with other tumor type. Prognosis is good if tumor is predominantly mucinous.
- Invasive lobular carcinoma (4 percent): Multicentricity is common and may involve both breasts. Prognosis is similar to ductal type.
- Paget's disease (3 percent): Scaly, eczematoid nipple with burning, itching, discharge, two-thirds have palpable underlying mass. Prognosis is related to histological type of underlying tumor.
- Inflammatory breast cancer (lesser than 1 percent): Skin red, warm, indurated with obstructive lymphangitis (Pequ d'orange) appearance). Prognosis is poor. Often presents with palpable nodes and evidence of metastasis.
- Lobular carcinoma in situ (2.5 percent): Usually found in incidental finding in benign breast specimens (high risk for development of invasive cancer). Prognosis is good.

Clinical Manifestation

Breast cancer is detected in a single lump or mammographic abnormality in the breast and is difficult to differentiate from benign tumors. With more advanced tumors a variety of signs and symptoms are helped in differentiating a benign tumor from malignant tumor. Benign tumors usually have well defined edges, are encapsulated and are freely movable. The shape of a malignant tumor is more difficult to define and is less mobile on palpation. Usually the result of the tumor becoming 'fixed' and adhering to the chest wall. If palpable, breast cancer is characteristically hard, irregularly shaped, poorly delineated, nonmobile and nontender. As the tumor infiltrates into surrounding tissues, it can cause retraction of the overlying skin and create what is referred to as dimpling. A small percentage of breast cancers cause nipple discharge. The discharge is usually unilateral and may be clear or bloody. Nipple retraction may occur. Plugging of the dermal lymphatics can cause skin thickening and exaggeration of the usual skin markings, giving the skin the appearance of an orange peel (Pseudo-orange) a pseudo-orange breast sign indicates lymphatic obstructive tissue tumor growth with resulting edema. The breast resembles an orange peel with large prominent pores. These signs are ominous and usually reflect advanced disease. To sum up, clinical manufacture of breast cancers are:

- Lump that is
  - Irregular, star-shaped.
  - Firm to hard in consistency.
  - Fixed, not mobile.
  - Poorly defined or demarcated.
  - Usually not tender, but can occasionally cause discomfort.
  - Single.
- Presence of skin or nipple retraction.
- Nipple discharge.
- Pseudo-orange appearance (dimpling) of the skin.

Management

The management of breast cancer is both complex and controversial. Treatment options are ever changing and influenced by new and better surgical techniques, new cytotoxic drug combinations and more accurate knowledge of breast cancer growth and dissemination.

Diagnosis is confirmed on the basis of history including risk factors physical examination of breast and lymphatics. Mammography, ultrasound biopsy, estrogen progesterone receptor assays, and other molecular studies (DNA ploidy, sphase, P53, HER-2/ncu). And staging work-up made on the basis of CBC, platelet count, calcium and phosphate levels, LFT sentinel node biopsy, chest X-ray, bone scan, CT scan of chest, abdomen, pelvis and MRI.

At present, there is wide range of treatment options available to both patient and the care providers attempting to make critical decisions about what treatment to select. Many prognostic factors are considered when treatment decisions are made about a specific breast cancer. These factors include lymphnode status, tumor size, histologic classification and the identification of histologic subtypes. All of these enter into the staging of breast cancer. The most widely accepted staging method is AJCC (American Joint Committee on Cancer).

TNM System as given below:

Primary Tumor (T)

T	0	No evidence of primary tumor
T	is	Carcinoma in skin
T	1	Tunmour less than or equal to 2 cm
T	2	Tumor greater than 2 cm but less than or equal to 5 cm
T	3	Tumor greater than 5 cm
T	4	Extension to chest wall and inflammation

Regional Lymph Node (N)

N	0	No tumor in regional lymph nodes.
N	1	Metastasis to movable ipsilateral nodes.
N	2	Metastasis to matted or fixed iphilateral nodes.
N	3	Metastasis to ipsilateral internal mammary nodes.

Distant Metastasis (M)

M	0	No distant metastasis.
M	1	Distant metastasis (include spread to ipsilateral supraclavicular node)

Stage Grouping

Stage 0	Tis	N_0	M_0
Stage I	T_1	N_0	M_0
Stage II A	T_0	N_1	M_0
	T_1	N_1	M_0
	T_2	N_0	M_0
Stage II B	T_2	N_1	M_0
	T_3	N_0	M_0
Stage III A	T_0	N_2	M_0
	T_1	N_2	M_0
	T_2	N_2	M_0
	T_3	$N_1 N_2$	M_0
Stage III B	T_4	Ang N	M_0
	Ang T	N_3	M_0
Stage IV	Ang T	Ang N	M_1

The role of systemic drug therapy is the treatment of breast cancer (chemotherapy and endocrine therapy) is either eradicate or impede the growth of micrometastatic disease.

Chemotherapy refers to the use of cytotoxic drugs to destroy cancer cells. The chemotherapy agents and protocol effective for treating breast cancer include the following:

- *Single agents:* Cyclophosphamide, melphalan, thiotepa, doxorubicin and epirubicin.
- Protocols using various agents
  - CMF – Cycle phosphamide, methotrexate 5-Fluoracil (5 Flu)
  - CPF – Cyclophosphamide, prednisone, 5-Flu
  - CMF/VA – CMF/Vincristine, doxorubicin (A).
  - CMF/VP – CMF/V. prednisone.
  - AC – Doxorubicin cyclophosphamide.
  - FAC – 5 Flu
  - FEC – 5 Flu Epirubicine cyclophosphonamide.
  - LMF – Melphalan-methotrexate, 5-Flu

Hormonal therapy has been a useful treatment modality for breast cancer. Tamoxifen citrate (Nolvadex) is the usual first choice of treatment in postmenopausal estrogen receptor positive women with or without nodal involvement. Tamoxifen, an antiestrogen drug, blocks the estrogen receptors sites of malignant cells and that inhibits the growth-stimulating effect of estrogen. Side effects are minimal including hot flashes, nausea, vomiting, dry skin, vaginal bleeding, menstrual irregularity and other commonly associated with estrogen.

Radiation therapy used in three situations of breast cancer which:

1. As the primary treatment to destroy the tumor or as a companion to surgery to prevent local occurence.
2. To shrink a large tumor to operable size and
3. As the palliative treatment for pain caused by local recurrence and metastasis. Lumpectomy is always followed by radiation.

Surgery is the main way of breast cancer treatment, especially when the disease is localized without distant metastasis. When primary, localized breast cancer (less than 2 to 4 cm and no metastasis) is disgnosed and two surgical options may be offered: modified radical mastectomy with or without breast reconstruction or breast sparing (lumpectomy procedures). The goal of both surgical procedures is to control local regional disease, to accurately stage the disease, so that patients at high risks for recurrence are identified and to provide the best chance for long-term survival in addition to achieving the best cosmetic results. The ovarian long-term survival rates for these two surgical methods are approximately the same. Modified radical mastectomy is now considered the standard form of mastectomy surgery.

- Modified radical mastectomy involves the removal of the whole breast, some fatty tissues and dissection of the axillary lymph nodes. The pectoral muscles and surrounding nerves are left intact. The cosmetic results avoid the chest devastating chest wall defects, shoulder and arm limitations and skin graft requirements that accompanied the more radical procedure.
- Breast sparing procedure known as partial mastectomy, wedge resection or lumpectomy involve the least removal of breast tissue and therefore have the best cosmesis. The contraindication for use of breast-sparing procedures include the following:
  - Pregnancy, first and second timesters preclude the use of radiation therapy.
  - Locally-advanced or inflammatory breast cancer.

- Multiple lesions located in separate quadrants of the breast or diffuse malignant or indeterminate—Appearing micro calcifications.
- Prior irradiation of the breast.
- History of callagens—vascular disease, which is recognized as having poor tolerance to the effect of radiation therapy.
- *Tumor size:* large tumor in a small breast, which will not allow adequate resection of tumor.
- *Breast size:* large pendulous breasts which are difficult to irradiate; small breasts which may result in an unacceptable cosmetic outcome.
- *Location of tumor:* Tumors that are located beneath the nipple necessitate removal of the nipple-areola complex, which has questionable value compared with mastectomy.

NURSING MANAGEMENT OF THE PATIENT UNDERGOING MASTECTOMY

The period between the diagnosis of breast cancer and the selection of the treatment plan is difficult period for the woman and her family. During this period, the woman may be very self focussed, verbalizing her conflict and indecisions frequently. Appropriate nursing interventions during this period include exploring the women's usual decision-making pattern, helping the woman accurately evaluate the advantages and disadvantages of the options, providing information relevant to the decision and supporting the patient once the decision is made. During this period, the woman may exhibit signs of distress or tension, such as tachycardia, increased muscle tension and restlessness, whenever she focuses on the decision to be made. The nurse should assess the woman's body language motor activity, and affect during periods of high stress and indecision so that appropriate intervention can be carried out.

Irrespective of the surgery planned, the patient must be provided with sufficient information to ensure informed consent. Some patients need extensive and detailed information. For others this only increases anxiety. Sensitivity to individual needs is essential. Preoperative diagnostic studies must be completed. Teaching is the preoperative phase includes instruction in turning, coughing deep breathing, a review of postoperative exercises, and explanation of the recovery period from the time of surgery until discharge.

The woman who has had a modified radical mastectomy needs specific nursing intervention. Restoration of the functioning of the arms in the affected side after mastectomy and axillary lymph node dissection is one of the important goals of the nursing activities. The woman should be placed in a semi Fowler's position with the arm on the affected side elevated on a pillow. Flexing and extending the fingers should begin in the recovery room with progressive increase in activity is encouraged.

Postoperative mastectomy exercises are isntituted gradually at the surgeon's direction. These exercises are designed to prevent contractures and muscle shortening, maintaining muscle tone, and improve lymph and blood circulation. The difficulty and pain encountered by the woman in performing the previously simple tasks include in the exercise program may cause frustration and depression. The goal of all exercises is return to full range of motion gradually within 4 to 6 weeks.

Postoperative discomfort can be minimized and administering analgesic about 30 minutes before initiating exercises. When showering is appropriate, the flow of warm water over the involved shoulder often has a soothing effect and reduces joint stiffness. Whenever possible, the same nurse should work with the woman so that progress can be monitored and problem can be identified.

Measure to prevent or reduce lymphedema must be used by the nurse and taught the woman. The affected arm should never be dependent even while the person is sleeping. Blood pressure readings, venipunctures, and injection should not be done on the affected arm. Elastic bandages should not be used postoperatively. The woman must be instructed to protect the arm on the operative side from even minor trauma such as pinprick or sunburn. If trauma occurs to the arm, the area should be washed thoroughly with soap and water. A topical antibiotic ointment and a bandage or other sterile dressing should be applied. When lymphedema is acute, an intermittent pneumatic compression sleeve may be prescribed. This device applies mechanical massage to the arm. Manual massage is also effective in mobilizing subcutaneous accumulation of fluid. Elevate the arm, so that it is level with the heart, diuretics, and isometric exercises may be recommended to reduce fluid volume in the arm.

Psychological Management

Throughout interaction with a woman with breast cancer, the nurse must keep in mind the extensive psychologic impact of the disease. All aspects of care must include sensitivity to the woman's efforts to cope with a life-threatening disease. An open relationship in which the woman can express her fears and feelings is essential. The nurse can help meet the woman's psychologic needs by doing the following:

- Assist her to develop a positive but realistic attitude.
- Helping her to identify sources of support and strength to her, such as her partner, family and spiritual practices.
- Encouraging her to verbalize her anger and fears about her diagnosis and impact it will have on her life.
- Promoting open communication of thoughts and feelings between the patient and her family.
- Providing accurate and complete answers to question about her disease treatment options, and reproductive and lactation tissue (if appropriate).

- Offering information about community resources which can help.

Before the discharge, the patient is instructed about wound care management, exercise guideline and sensory change precaution, assessment and management of lymphedema, and prevention of trauma and infection. The following precautions should be taken with the patient after mastectomy:

- Ensure that affected arm is never used for blood pressure, injections or venipunctures.
- Wear no constricting clothing or jewellery, including wrist watch on affected arm.
- Do not carry heavy objects (pocket book, packages) in affected arm.
- Wear rubber gloves when washing dishes.
- Use unaffected arm when removing items from hot oven or protect by wearing a padded glove pot holder.
- Use a thumb when sewing wash needle pricks and cover as necessary.
- Take care when trimming finger nails and cuticles; avoid using scissors for this task.
- Use softening lotion or creams to keep skin in soft and nipple conditions.
- Outdoor activities:
  - Wear gloves when gardening.
  - Avoid sunburn-wear protective clothing or use sunscreen liberally.
  - Use insect repellent in an area where biting or stinging insects may be located.
  - Tend to cuts and scratches immediately by washing and applying protective covering.

Postmastectomy arm exercises includes the following:
- Ball squeezing
- Pulley motion
- Handball climbing
- Elbow pull-in
- Crossed arm
- Scissors
- Sword of hope.

MALE BREAST PROBLEMS

Gynecomastia

Gynecomastia, a transient enlargement of one or both breasts is the most common breast problem in men. It usually occurs in pubertal boys during the time of rapid testicular growth between the ages of 1 to 15 years. This condition is seen in men aged 45 years and older, and also it is seen in obese men because obesity increases the rate of conversion of androgens to estrogen in patient with cirrhosis of liver, because of the incomplete hepatic clearance of estrogen. Gynecomastia may develop in men who are receiving drugs such as estrogen, cimitedine, certain antibiotics (isonized) antihypertensive agents (reserpine and methyldopa) calcium channel blockers and digoxin.

Pathophysiology

Gynecomastia is caused by hormonal imbalance. As a result of the large estrogen secretion, hyperplasia (overdevelopment) of the stromata, and ducts in the mammary gland occurs. The primary cause of gynemastic in the older man is the aging process may be due to increase of plasma testesterone. Symptoms of gynecomastia include a firm, circular, disk-like circumscribed, tender mass beneath the areola, it is usually bilateral at onset. In adolescent boys the condition is transient and last for approximately 12 to 24 months.

Gynecomastia may also be a symptom of other problems. It is seen accompanying developmental abnormalities of the male reproductive organ. It may also accompany organic diseases including testicular tumors, cancer of the adrenal cortex, pituitary adenomas, hyperthyroidism and liver disease.

Management

In suspected clients with gynecomastia, a human chorionic gonadotropin-beta subunit (hcG-B level should be obtained). This finding assists in ruling out malignant testicular germ cell condition, which can manifest with gynecomastia and an elevated hcG-B level. Chest and mediastinal roentgenogram may be used. In older men biopsy of breast is taken and examined.

Surgery is used for cosmesis only when the gynecomastia persists over a long period of time and is not associated with an underlying disease process.

The nurse who cares for men with gynecomastia must offer sympathetic understanding. Most men are intensely embarrassed about the condition because breast constitutes a serious assault on male self-image. The condition is visible whenever the man removes his shirt for work or recreation and frequently results in taunts and jokes. Similar problem exists when the person undergoes mastectomy for looking asymmetrical chest. The patients who are treated with hormonal therapy for prostatic cancer should be warned that gynecomastia is one of the side effects of treatment. The nurse should convince the person by using all his or her skill to cope up with problem associated with gynecomastia in men.

Male Breast Cancer

Generally, breast cancer has bean found in 1 percent of men. The presentation, diagnosis, and treatment are similar as those for women with the breast cancer. The family history places men at increased risk for breast cancer.

The symptoms are commonly seen at the time of diagnosis include a firm mass directly beneath the nipple in the subareolar area, most frequently in the left breast. A lesion in the upper outer quadrant is the next most frequent location for tumor growth. Bloody nipple discharge with nipple inversion is common. Evidence of Paget's disease of the nipple (eczema), itching, ulceration and local tenderness also may be present. Metastasis may occur to bone, the lungs and the liver.

Management

Treatment for a primary localized tumor is modified radical mastectomy with node dissection. Breast-sparing procedure is usually not used in men. When axillary nodes are involved in the disease process, systemic adjuvant therapy (chemotherapy and hormonal) is advised. CMF and FAC are prescribed.

A man for whom breast cancer is diagnosed faces unique psychosocial stressors that the nurse needs to address on an individual basis. The use of tamoxifen has reduced the need for palliative surgeries such as orchidectomy. The male patient is treated for breast cancer in an uncommon occurrence; however, the nurse will need to be sensitive to his unique needs and tailor the standard surgical care routines to the individual situation.

Male Reproductive Problems

Men's reproductive health care is one dimension of an emerging speciality area in nursing practice. Traditionally, problem of the male reproductive system have been viewed only as problem of urination or fertility. As with women, men have unique biological and social health care need. Often the complexity of the male reproductive system and the multiple psychosocial needs of the patient have been minimized in today's health care system. Consequently, myths and knowledge deficits related to the specifics of sexual function are common in the male population. It is important to provide health care that is sensitive to the unique problems of the male. Problems of the male reproductive system can involve a variety of structures (penis, urethra, bladder, ejaculatory duct, prostate, prepuce, testis, scrotum, epidymis, vas deferens, rectum), and create anxiety for both the patient and nurse providing care. Anxiety and fear may also cause the patient to delay seeking help for a problem or practising health-promoting behaviors. Our society often does not encourage men to admit or seek help for problems related to their sex organs. The nurse should be particularly sensitive to the possible embarrassment with the male reproductive problems.

Problems of Scrotum and its Contents

The skin of the scrotum is susceptible to number of common skin diseases. The most common condition of the scrotal skin are fungal infection, dermatitis (neurodermatitis, contact dermatitis and seborrhea dermatitis) and parasitic infection (scabies and lice), are dealt in integumentary nursing or dermatological nursing.

The scrotal sac contains the testes, epididymis, and part of the spermatic cord. Other associated structures include nerve, lymphatic, and vascular networks. These structures are responsible for the production and storage of sperm and provide the pathway for ejaculation. The testes are also involved in hormonal production primarily of testosterone. Consequently, any disorder related to these structures have the potential to affect male fertility adversely as well as interfere with testosteron production. Pathologies of these structures include problems with swelling, twisting cords, trauma, and carcinoma. The testes are particularly sensitive to changes in scrotal environment, such as fluctuation in temperatures and blood flow. Infection is also a common problem.

EPIDIDYMITIS

Epididymitis is an inflammatory process of epididymis and is the most common intrascrotal inflammation in adult males.

Etiology

Epididymitis usually secondary to an infectual process (sexually or non-sexually transmitted), with trauma or urinary reflux down the vas deferens. It is most often caused by an ascending infection via the ejaculatory duct through the vas deferens into the epididymis. There are three means of introduction of the infection into the duct system:
1. Infection may be introduced when surgical or diagnostic procedure are performed. The most common organism for contamination is "*Escherichia coli*".
2. Structural malformation or developmental of structural insufficiencies in the child may contribute to problem of urinary reflux. Reflux of sterile or infected urine causes chemical irritation in the epididymis and cause of inflammation.
3. Adult male between the age 19-35 years, sexual transmission is the most common means of infection. *Chlamydia trichomatis* and *Neisseria gonorrhea* are caused in heterosexual male, *E coli* and *H. influenzene* are the causes in homosexual males.

Pathophysiology

Epididymitis results from inflammation of the epididymis and scrotal sac. Fluid accumulation in the scrotal sac is an inflammatory response to the infection process. Excess fluid loss into the interstitial space of the scrotal sac leads to diminished blood flow, nerve damage and resultant pain and swelling. Inflammatory fluids also can form pockets of pus called abscesses. Heat generated from the inflammatory process can negatively affect the testicular function of the spermatogenesis. Consequently, complication of epididymitis include testicular infarction, chronic pain from nerve damage, abscess formation and infertility.

Clinical Manifestation

The most common clinical manifestations are severe tenderness, pain in the scrotal area, and noticeable swelling of one or both the sides of the scrotum. The onset of pain may be insidious, gradually increasing over hours or days, the scrotal swelling can cause pain on ambulation and discomfort that is exacerbated by wearing restrictive clothing. Men with epididymitis often walk with type of "waddle" to help spare the scrotum from rubbing up against the thighs or clothing. Elevation of the scrotum will reduce the pain (Prehns signs). Other symptoms include an increase in temperature of the scrotum and symptoms include an increase in temperature. A urethral discharge may also be present, with color and consistency varying according to the types of causative organism. Urethritis is often associated with epididymitis and associated symptoms include burning on urination, frequency, urgency and general malaise.

Management

Assessment of the patient with symptoms of epididymitis should include a sexual history. For young children, it should include question to determine possible sexual abuse and any history of recent urinary examination or instrumentation. In elderly male, question focuses on history or symptoms of urinary obstruction or recent urinary examination. Urinanalysis, urine and urethral cultures are needed to determine the specific organism and its sensitivity to various antibiotics as well as to provide information for needed medications. Further scrotal ultrasound and radionuclide scanning is performed when diagnosis is questionable.

The nature of the patient's pain is assessed, whether the pain is bilateral or unilateral, and if the pain is of sudden onset or has developed over hours or days. The nurse also notes if pain is relieved by elevating the scrotum. Any symptoms of dysuria are documented such as burning, frequency, urgency, fever and general malaise. A recent history of urethral discharge or change in the discharge is important to help determine the possible type of causative organism. The color, consistency and amount of any discharge are documented.

The patient is also observed for the classic "Waddle" or a somewhat rolling gait, indicating that the patient is attempting to protect his scrotum. Swelling of the scrotum is documented, as well as whether it is on one or both the sides. Palpation of the scrotum at this time is generally differed to avoid causing severe pain. For patients with chronic recurrent epididymitis, aspiration fluid for the epididymis can be performed.

Treatment of epididymitis usually consists of pain management, medication to treat the infection and supportive care. NSAIDs such as ibuprofen may be used to decrease the inflammation and relieve the discomfort and swelling. If severe pain, narcotics may be used. Stool softeners are given to prevent constipation and reduce straining on defecation, which may cause severe pain in the inflamed scrotum. Eradication of infection generally is accomplished by giving oral antibiotics (broad spectrum).

In younger men, less than 35 years of age, the most common cause is through sexual transmission of either gonorrhea or Chlamydia. The use of antibiotics is important for both partners if the transmission through sexual contact. Patients should be encouraged to refrain from sexual intercourse during the acute phase. If they do engage in intercourse, condoms should be used. Bedrest with the scrotum elevated in towel, application of ice packs, and the use of scrotal supports when the swelling is less severe and it will also help decrease the discomfort caused by the heavy sensation resulting from enlarged scrotum. Bedrest is maintained until the patient is painfree, then a scrotal support is worn for approximately 6 weeks. The patient is instructed to avoid work that would strain the lower abdomen and scrotal area.

ORCHITIS

Inflammation or infection of the testicle is known as "Orchitis". In this, testes are inflamed, painful, tender and swollen.

Etiology

Orchitis may be caused by pyogenic bacteria, gonococci, tubercle bacilli or viruses. It generally occurs after an episode of bacterial or viral infections such as mumps, pneumonia, tuberculosis or syphilis. It can also be a side effect of epididymitis, prostatectomy, trauma, infections mononucleosis, influenza, catheterization or complicated urinary tract infection.

Pathophysiology (Clinical Manifestation)

Inflammatory fluid seeks from the testicle into the serus membrane lining the epididymis and the testicle to create unilateral or bilateral swelling. Hydrocele (a collection of fluid within the tunica vaginalis testis) is frequently associated with orchitis. The signs and symptoms of orchitis are the same as those of epididymitis. However, because orchitis is caused by a systemic infectious process rather than a localized infection, more systemic symptoms are present. Consequently the patient may also have clinical manifestation of nausia, vomiting, and pain radiating to the inguinal canal. As a result of inflammation and fibrosis, some degree of atrophy occurs, which may lead to sterility. Unless both testes are severely involved, infertility is rare. Mumps orchitis is condition contributing to infertility.

Management

Treatment involves the use of antibiotics (if the organism is known) pain medication on bedrest with the scrotum elevated on an ice pack. Any pubertal boy or man who is exposed to mumps usually is given gamma globulin immediately unless he has already had mumps or been vaccinated for the disease. Mumps orchitis could easily be decreased by childhood vaccination against mumps. Broad spectrum antibiotics are given for common bacterial causes. If hydrocele is present, the fluid may be aspirated to reduce pressure on the testes. If the hydrocele is surgically trapped within the first 2 days the potential for testicular atrophy is decreased; however, a tap should only be done when edema is persistent because a chance exists that surgical decompression may exacerbate the inflammation.

Patient education focuses on measures to reduce discomfort from gonodal swelling and alleviate systemic symptoms. During the acute phase of gonadal swelling, the scrotum may be supported with the same method used for the patient with epididymitis. Warm or cold compression may be applied to help reduce swelling and increase comfort. Antibiotics are administered for bacterial causes. Rest and an increased fluid intake are encouraged for all patients. Anti-inflammatory medication is given to help reduce pain and swelling.

TESTICULAR TORSION

Testicular torsion is a condition which involves a twisting of the spermatic cord that supplies blood to the testes and epididymitis in which testicular circulation is acutely impaired.

Etiology

Testicular torsion is most commonly seen in young males under the age of 20. Torsion may follow activities that put sudden pull on the cremasteric muscle, such as jumping into cold water, blunt trauma, or bicycle riding. It may also occur at night when there is less gravitational pull from the testes on the cord allowing more movement and consequent twisting.

Pathophysiology

Torsion interrupts the blood supply to the testes leading to ischemia and severe unrelieved pain that may be aggravated by manual elevation of the affected side. The scrotum is swollen, tender, and red. The affected side is usually elevated because the twisting and shortening of the cord pulls up the testicle. The cremasteric reflex, elicited by stroking the inner aspect of the thigh to cause reflex refraction of the testicle is usually absent on the side of the suspected torsion. Although the scrotum appears infected because of the swelling and redness, both urinalysis and blood tests are typically normal. Fever is rarely present. Absence of pain after a time may indicate infarction and necrosis. Gangrene may be a serious sequelae.

Clinical Manifestation

The patient experiences severe scrotal pain, tenderness, swelling, nausea, and vomiting. Urinary complaints, fever and WBCs bacteria in the urine are absent. The pain does not usually subside with rest or elevation of the scrotum. Pain is localized to testis and radiates to groin and lower abdomen, severe in nature; similar episodes of self-limiting pains are not unusual. Vomiting is common. Fever, dysuria are rare. On examination, testis may be in elevated position with abnormal lie, testes will be swollen and tender, epididymis also may be tender. Cremasteric reflex is usually negative. Pain is constant (Prehn's sign).

Management

Diagnostic studies may include an orchiogram or testicular scan, which qualitatively measures the blood flow to the testis. Doppler studies also help to diagnose torsion.

Detorsion (a process of untwisting the spermatic cord) can be attempted manually. Torsion constitutes a surgical emergency. If manual detorsion is unsuccessful. Unless it resolves spontaneously, surgery to unturn the cord and restore the blood supply must be performed quickly. The torsion causes ischemia to the testis, leading to necrosis and possible need for removal (orchidectomy). If orchidectomy is performed, a testicular prosthesis is usually inserted. Orchioplexy performs in nongangrenous testicles. As for the nursing care, often orchioplexy and orchiectomy are similar. Ice bags and scrotal elevation may be ordered to reduce swelling. The nurse continues to monitor the patient for signs of testicular necrosis and fever in the case of orchioplexy. A small pentose drain may be placed in the scrotum which will necessitate dressing change.

After surgery the patient should be instructed to limit stair climbing to two flights and not to lift or carry heavy objects for 4 weeks and is instructed to refrain from sexual intercourse/activities for 6 weeks. The use of scrotal support for at least 3 weeks is recommended to control edema. Sitz baths may help relieve any discomfort.

Body image disturbance may include fears of castration (orchiectomy), loss of masculinity, sterility and impotence. The nurse provides specific information about the physiological changes resulting from testicular atrophy or surgical removal of testicles. The patient is still able to have an erection after trauma or surgery to the testicles. Fertility may or may not be affected if there is still a remaining healthy testicle. Counseling on alternative means of conception may be suggested. The patient is reminded that the appearance of the scrotum will not be altered if a testicular prosthesis is inserted after orchiectomy.

Other Benign Problems on Testis

The other problems include congenital problem, i.e. crypto-orchidism, acquired problem such as hydrocele, spermatocele and varicocele.

- Crypto-orchidism (undescended testes) is failure of the testes to descend into the scrotal sac before birth, which needs surgery to locate and suture the testes to the scrotum.
- Hydrocelo is a nontender, fluid-filled mass that results from interference with lymphatic drainage of the scrotum and swelling of the tunica vaginalis that surround the testes, diagnosis is done by transillumination. No treatment is indicated unless the swelling becomes very large and uncomfortable in which an aspiration or surgical drainage of the mass is performed.
- Spermatocele is a firm, sperm-containing, painless cyst of the epididymis that may be visible with transillumination. The cause is unknown, and surgical removal is the treatment.
- Varicocele is a dilation of the veins that drain the testes. The scrotum feels worm-like when palpated. The cause is unknown. The varicocele is usually located on the left side of the scrotum as a consequence of retrograde blood flow from the left renal vein. Surgery is indicated if the patient is infertile. Repair of the varicocele may be performed through injection of a sclerosing agent or by surgical ligation of the spermatic vein.

TESTICULAR CANCER

Etiology

The etiology of testicular cancer is still unknown. Testicular tumor occurs primarily in men between 20 to 40 years of age. Testicular tumors are more common in males who have had undescended testes (cryptorohidism) or a family history of testicular cancer or anomalies. Other predisposing factors include a history of mumps, orchitis, inguinal hernia, in childhood, maternal exposure to DES, and testicular cancer in the contralateral testis.

Pathophysiology

Testicular tumors may develop from the cellular components of the testis or from the embryonal precursors (germ cell tumor). Testicular tumors are divided into germinal or nongerminal. Germ cell tumors are further divided into two groups; seminomatous and nonseminomatus. The tumors of mixed cell types can also occur. Testicular germ cell tumors are almost malignant. Nongerm cell tumors are rare, usually benign and can occur at any age.

Clinical Manifestation

Clinical manifestations of testicular cancer are often subtle and go unnoticed by the male until he notices a feeling of heaviness or dragging in the lower abdomen and groin areas. The patient may notice a lump in his scrotum as well as scrotal swelling and a feeling of heaviness. The scrotal mass usually is nontender, painless, very firm and cannot be transilluminated. Other symptoms are nonspecific such as back pain, weight loss and fatigue. Manifestation associated with metastasis to other system include back pain, cough, dyspnea, hemoptysis, dysphagia (difficulty in swallowing), alteration in vision, mental status, papilledema and seizures.

Management

Palpation of the scrotal contents is the first step in diagnosing testicular cancer. Additional tests that aid in diagnosis include a testicular sonogram and MRI. If testicular tumor is suspected, blood may be drawn to look for the tumor markers of the glycoprotiens, alpha-fetoprotein (AFP) and human chorionic gonadotropin (hCG). Biopsy of the testis is contraindicated because of the highly metastatic character of testicular carcinoma. Testicular cancer is histologically classified as germ cell tumor, i.e. seminos and nonseminomas.

As with many forms of cancer, the survival of the patient is closely associated with early recognition of the tumor. In any suspected case of testicular cancer, the testis is usually removed immediately. Orchidectomy consists of enbloc excision of the spermatic cord, the contents of the inguinal canal and the testes with the tunical attached. The adjacent area is explored for metastases. The specimen are then examined to determine the cancer cell type. Staging of the disease as well as pathological findings determine the course of treatment. The staging of the testicular neoplasia is as follows:

Stage I : No metastasis, confined to testis.
Stage II : Metastasis to retroperitonal lymph nodes or other subdiaphragmatic area.
Stage III : Metastasis to mediastinal and supraclavicular nodes or other areas above diaphragm.

Treatment of testicular cancer based on tumor type is as follows:

Stage 0 : Benign form needs surveillance.
Stage I : Seminomatous orchiectomy and radiation therapy.
Nonseminomatous orchiectomy, modified retroperitoneal lymph node dissection and radiotherapy.

Stage II : Seminomatous/nonseminomatous orchiectomy, radiation therapy/modified full retroperitoneal lymphnode dissection.

Stage III : Seminomatous/nonseminomatous.

Combination of chemotherapy and full retroperitoneal lymph nodes dissection.

Nongerminal testicular tumors treatment consists of four modes of treatment (orchiectomy, radiation, lymphodenectomy and chemotherapy).

The nurse explains the effects of orchiectomy and fertility and nurse gives patient teaching, which includes focuses on the planned treatment in its expected effects of surgery, chemotherapy and radiation therapy.

In addition, every male between puberty and 40 years of age should be taught and encouraged to perform monthly testicular self examination (TSE) for the purpose of detecting testicular tumors or other scrotal abnormalities such as varicoceles and the nurse should teach the patient how to do a self examination with particular emphasis in males with a history of an undescended testis or a previous testicular tumor. The guidelines for self examination of the scrotum are as follows:

- During a shower or bath is the easiest time to examine the testes, warm temperature makes the testes hang lower in the scrotum.
- Use both hands to feel each testis. Roll the testes between the thumb and first three fingers until the entire surface has been covered. Palpate each one separately.
- Identify structures. The testis should feel round and smooth like a hard-boiled egg. Differentiate the testis from epididymis. The epididymis is not as smooth as the egg-shaped testis. One testis may be larger than the other. Size is not as important as texture. Check for lumps, irregularities, pain in the testes or a dragging sensation. Locate the spermatic cord, which is usually firm and smooth and goes up towards groin.
- Choose a consistent day of the month such as birth date, that will make it easy to remember for examination of testes. The examination can be performed more frequently if desired.
- Notify the doctor at once if any abnormalities are found.

PROBLEMS OF PROSTATE

Prostatitis

Infections of the prostate occurs infrequently, but it can result in chronic problems that are difficult to eradicate. Prostatitis cause long term discomfort and problems with fertility.

Etiology

A number of inflammatory conditions can affect the prostate gland after a male reaches puberty. The four most common forms of prostatitis are acute bacterial prostatis, chronic bacterial prostatitis, nonbacterial prostatitis, and prostatodynia. Bacterial prostatitis is frequently associated with an indwelling urethral catheter, urethral instrumentation or trauma. Common causative organisms are *Escherichia coli, Psudemonos, Enterobacter, Proteus, Chlamydial trachomatis, Neisseria gonorrhea* and group D *Streptococci*. Chronic bacterial prostatitis should be considered in men with a history of recurrent bacteriuria. Nonbacterial prostatitis may occur after a viral illness or it may be associated with other STDs particularly in a younger adult. The etiology is not known and a culture reveals no causative organism. Prostadodynia has the same symptoms as prostatitis (irritation, and pelvic pain on urination), but no evidence of inflammation. The condition is limited to younger men.

Pathophysiology

Bacterial prostatitis generally results from an organism reaching the prostate gland by one of the following routes; ascending from the urethra descending from the bladder, and invasion via the bloodstream or the lymphatic channels. The prostate gland becomes swollen, inflammed and painful because of either a bacterial infection or other inflammatory process. The prostate surrounds the urethra and when it becomes swollen it can compress the urethra and cause urinary obstruction. Men with prostatitis typically complain of changes in voiding patterns, such as difficulty starting the stream or the need to strain on urination. Low back pain, pelvic pain and perinial pain are other common symptoms. Pain during or after ejaculation may be experienced. In addition, the patients with bacterial prostatitis frequently complain of symptom of UTIs, that can include urgency, frequency, painful urination and hematuria. Bacterial infections cause fever, chills and general fatigue.

Clinical Manifestation

Acute bacterial prostatitis results in manifestation of fever, chills, dysuria, urethral discharge, increased urinary frequency and urgency, low back, rectal, pelvic and perineal pain, and acute cystitis with cloudy and smelly urine. The prostate is extremely swollen, tender, firm and warm to touch. The complication of prostatitis are epidymitis and cystitis. Sexual functioning may be affected as manifested by postejaculatory pain libido problems and erectile dysfunction. Prostatic abscess is a rare complication.

The symptoms of chronic prostatitis may be absent or rare generally milder than that of acute prostatitis. These include backache, perineal pain, ejaculatory pain, mild dysuria, and increased frequency of urination. Factors that may contribute to chronic prostatitis include urethral obstruction, persistent infection above the urethra, and prostatic pathological condition such as congestions, hyperplasia and prostatic calculi. It predisposes the patient to recurrent UTI. The prostate feels irregularly enlarged firm and slightly tender on palpation.

Management

Urine cultures are usually obtained to determine the organisms causing bacterial prostatitis. Culture of prostatic secretion can verify a diagnosis of bacterial infection. Patients with nonbacterial prostatitis usually have negative urine culture, but prostatic secretions can show an increased number of leukocytes and fat-containing macrophages.

Treatment is conservative and consists of antibiotics for 30 days to prevent chronic infection, forced fluids, physical rest, stool softeners to decrease irritation of the prostate from hard feces and local application of heat by sitz baths. Prompt treatment of prostatitis may prevent edema and resultant urinary obstruction. The specific antibiotics for acute bacterial prostatitis are ciproflaxacin (cipro) and trimethoprim sulfamethoxazole (Bactrim). Antispasmodics, analgesics and stool softeners are often prescribed to provide relief from painful symptoms. The non-bacterial prostatitis and prostatodynia are difficult to treat because no bacteria are found in urine or prostatic fluid. Treatment usually consists of anti-inflammatory agents, hot sitz baths and sexual activities that result in ejaculation. Antibiotics are ineffective against calculi and surgical excision is required. Prostatectomy may be necessary to eradicate infection.

The patient with acute bacterial prostatitis experiences prostate pain when standing, when urinating and during ejeculation. Nursing interventions are aimed at relief of pain and fever, bed rest and maintenance of adequate hydration. The patient with chronic prostatitis should be instructed regarding the long-term nature of the problem. Because the prostate can serve as a source of bacteria, fluid intake should be kept at a high level. Antibiotics may have to be taken for number of months. Activities that drain the prostate, such as intercourse (use a condom to protect the partner from infection), masturbation and prostatic massage are often helpful in the long-term management of this problem. Chronic prostatitis may eventually lead to erectile dysfunction for which the patient may need to seek treatment.

The patient is taught how to take warm sitz bath. Use anti-inflammatory medication and avoid allergy producing foods that may be excerbating the inflammation. The patient should refrain from sexual activity until the antibiotic has started to work, approximately 2 weeks into therapy. After 2 weeks regular ejaculation is encouraged to promote "flushing" of the prostate gland. Complete course of antibiotic should be taken. Abstaining from alcohol and OTC drugs (of decongestants) help exacerbation of the symptom of urinary obstruction. The continued stool softeners can decrease irritation to the inflamed prostate infection.

BENIGN PROSTATIC HYPERPLASIA (BPH)

The prostate gland, located below the bladder, surrounding the urethra and is responsible for contributing to ejaculatory fluid. During puberty the prostate grows rapidly. After puberty, growth tapers off by the age of 30 years. Changes in the size of the gland next occurs after the age of 50, when the gland begins to atrophy and becomes nodular.

Benign prostatic hypertrophy (hyperplasia, BPH) is an enlargement of portions of this gland that eventually cause problems with urination. Parts of the gland may be atrophy, whereas other parts become large and nodular.

Etiology

BPH is common problem in men over the age of 50. The changes in the size and shape of the prostate are associated with increased androgen levels. Although the cause is not completely understood, it is thought that the primary cause is an increased number of cells resulting from endocrine changes associated with aging process. Excessive accumulation of dihydroxy-testosterons (the principal intraprostatic androgen), stimulation of estrogen and local growth hormone action are proposed causes.

Pathophysiology

The changes that occur in the prostate gland of older men can create a number of problems with the associated urinary system. When the enlarged nodular tissue of the prostate impinges on the urethra, the urethra elongates and compresses causing obstruction of urinary flow. This can result in a compensatory hypertrophy of the bands of bladder muscle. This in turn increases the trabeculation (contouring) of the bladder wall providing pockets of urinary retention. These trebeculated areas show up on ultrasound. Because of the muscular thickening, the bladder has less capacity. Muscle tone can diminish over time. Consequently, bladder cannot empty completely at each voiding (residual urine); the urine becomes alkaline from stasis and is a fertile medium for bacterial growth.

Clinical Manifestation

In BPH urethral and bladder changes can result in symptoms of urinary obstruction and irritation. Often the symptoms of obstruction are gradual and not noticed by the male until acute urinary retention occurs. Symptoms of gradual obstruction include a decrease in the urinary stream with less force on urination and often dribbling at the end of voiding. Other related symptoms include hesitancy, a difficulty in starting the stream, intermittency and inability to maintain a constant stream. The patient may also complain of a sense of incomplete emptying of the bladder. Straining and urinary retention are the symptoms that often convince the patient to seek medical help.

Symptom of irritation often accompany the obstructive problems. Nocturia from incomplete emptying is common. Dysuria, urgency, and urge incontinence are symptoms associated with loss of muscle tone in the bladder and changes in the angle of the bladder neck. The patient also has symptoms of UTIs because of incomplete emptying and the increased risk of infection. As the prostate enlarges, so does the vasculature and when straining takes place, these vessels may break and cause hematuria.

To brief the clinical manifestation of BPH, includes prostate gland enlarges, becomes more nodular; straining on urination, hesitancy in starting urine flow; decreased urine stream; postvoid dribbling; nocturia; dysuria, hematuria and urgency.

Other problems that can arise from BPH are kidney disorders caused by backflow of urine. Hydronephritis and pyelonephritis are possible sequelas to urinary obstruction. Anemia may also occur if blood loss is severe, or as a result of secondary insufficiency. Calculi may develop because of the alkalinization of the residual urine.

Management

Diagnostic test for BPH includes the following.
- Primary screening.
  - History including symptoms of voiding problems.
  - Physical examination, including digital rectal examination (DRE).
  - Urine analysis with culture.
  - Serum creatinine and blood urea nitrogen.
  - Prostate-specific antigen (PSA)—A blood test to estimate the volume of prostate.
- Secondary screening.
  - Urodynamic flow studies—Cystourethroscopy, uroflowmetry, IVP.
  - Transrectal ultrasound.
  - Cystoscopy (for surgical candidates).

To primary treatment for BPH is now referred to as "watchful waiting". When there are not symptoms or only mild ones, a conservative noninvasive wait-and-see approach is taken. If the patient begins to have signs or symptoms that indicate an increase in urethral obstruction, further treatment is indicated. The numerous treatment options for BPH can be categorized as pharmocologic, nonsurgical invasive and surgical invasive options.
- Pharmocologic hormone manipulation can be used to cause regression of hyperplasic tissue through suppression of androgens. The drugs used for BPH include antibiotics. Finasteride (Proscar), Alpha-adrenergic receptor blocks such as Prazosin (Minipress), Tetrazosin (Hytrin), Tamsulosin (Flomax) Doxazosin (cardura) and Herbal medicine extracted from plant (phytotherapy), i.e., can palmetto have been used.
- Nonsurgical invasive can include intermittent catheterization or indwelling catheter can be temporarily used to reduce symptoms and bypass the obstruction. The other non-surgical invasive procedure includes stents and coilsm balloon dilation and heat [Transurethral microwave antenna (TUMA)].
- Surgery is indicated when there is a decrease in urine flow sufficient to cause discomfort, persistent residual urine, acute urinary retention because of obstruction with no reversible precipitatory cause, or hydronephrosis. Treatment of symptomatic BPH primary involves resection of the prostate. The selection of a surgical approach to remove the tissue depends on the size and position of the prostatic enlargement. The usual surgical procedure for BPH are as follows:
  - Laser ablation
    * Transurethral, ultrasound guided and laser-induced prostatectomy (TULIP)
    * Visual laser ablation of the prostate (VLAP).
  - Transurethral resection of the prostate (TURP)-by using resectoscope.
  - Transurethral incision of the prostate (TUIP).
  - Suprabubic prostate resection.
  - Retropubic prostate resection.
  - Perineal prostate resection.

Nursing Management

Nurse is most directly involved with the care of prostate having surgical intervention, the focus on nursing management will be on preoperative and postoperative care.

Preoperative care includes all routine of the person undergoing any surgery. In addition, urinary drainage must be restored before surgery. A urethral catheter such as coude (curved-tip) catheter may be needed to restore drainage-septic technique is important at all times to avoid introducing bacteria into the bladder. Antibiotics are usually administered before any invasive surgical procedures. Any infection of the urinary tract must be treated before surgery. Restoring urine drainage and encouraging high fluid intake (2 to 3 L/day unless contraindicated) are also helpful in managing the infection. The patient is often concerned about the impact of the impending surgery on his sexual functioning. The nurse should provide an opportunity for the patient and the partner to express that concerns and proper counseling given by the nurse appropriately.

Postoperative care includes the management of complication of surgery. The main complications of prostatectomy are hemorrhage, bladder spasms, urinary incontinence and infection. Nursing management of the patient following traditional resectoscope and surgery include:

- Promoting adequate urine elimination—maintain patency of catheter.
- Controlling discomfort from bladder spasms and straining by using narcotics, belladona and opium suppositories and stool softener.
- Preventing infection by using antibiotics—IV or oral.
- Relieving anxiety.

Postoperative nursing care for the person undergoing prostate surgery are as follows:
- Maintain patency of catheter system.
- Monitor appearance of urine, red to light pink (24 hrs) to amber (3 days).
- Monitor patient for signs of water intoxication after TURP (confusion, agitation, warm moist skin, anorexia, nausea, vomiting).
- Instruct patient not to try to void around catheter, explain feeling of needing to void from pressure of catheter.
- Avoid use of enemas and rectal thermometers.
- Give prescribed medication (analgesics, antispasmodics) as needed; tell patients spasm will decrease in intensity and severity within 24 to hours.
- After catheter removal
  - Monitor signs of urinary retention.
  - Monitor for continence, teach perineal exercises if dribbling occurs.
  - Encourage increased fluids and frequent voiding.
- Change dressings, frequently around suprapubic wounds after suprapubic prostatectomy to prevent skin maceration.
- Give patient opportunities to discuss feelings about sexuality and possible incontinence.
- Teach patient to:
  - Avoid vigorous exercises, heavy lifting (over 20 pounds) and sexual intercourse for at least 3 weeks.
  - Avoid driving for 2 weeks.
  - Avoid straining with defecation using stool softeners or mild laxatives if needed.
  - Drink at least 2500 ml of fluids per day to prevent urinary stasis and infection and to keep stools soft.
  - Diet high in fiber facilitates the passage of stool.
  - Notify doctor if urinary stream diminishes or if bleeding occurs.

CANCER OF THE PROSTATE

Cancer of the prostate is the most common cancer in men.

Etiology

The cause of prostatic cancer is basically unknown. Prostatic cancer is an androgen-dependent adenocarcinoma. Factors such as sexual activity socioeconomic class, alcohol use have not been shown significant factors. Factors that may affect the development of prostate cancer include hormonal changes and viral infections. Hormonal changes during aging are the reason that prostate cancer is seen almost exclusively in men over age of 40. Positive antibody titers to herpes simplex and cytomagalovirus have been found in men with prostate cancer. Other risk factors include a history of multiple sexual partners, episodes of STDs, the presence of cervical cancers in sexual partners and industrial exposure to cadmium.

Pathophysiology

Cancer of the prostate often starts as a discrete localized hazard nodule in an area of senile atrophy. It is often caused by an adenocarcinoma that arises in peripheral regions of the gland. The growth is generally on the outer portion of the gland, compression of the urethra and subsequent voiding symptoms are not common until late in the disease. The tumor is slow-growing and usually being in the posterior or lateral portions of the prostate. It can spread by three routes. Direct extension is by continuity to the seminal vescicles, urethral mucosa, bladder wall and external sphincter. The cancer later spreads through the prineural lymphatic system to the regional lymphnodes. The vein from the prostate seem to be the mode of spread to the pelvic bones, head of femur, lower lumbar spine, liver and lungs.

Clinical Manifestations

Prostate cancer is asymptomatic in the early stages. Eventually, the patient may have symptoms similar to those of BPH, including dysuria hesitancy, dribbling, frequency, urgency, hematuria, nocturia and retention. The prostate feels hard, enlarged and fixed on rectal examination. The enlargement is usually unilateral, pain in the lumbosacral area, which radiates down to the hips or legs. When coupled with urinary symptoms may indicate metastases. To sum up, clinical manifestation of prostate cancer include:
- Often no symptoms if cancer is confined to the gland.
- Symptoms of urinary obstruction and symptoms of urinary tract infection.
- Low back pain, malaise, aching in legs, a hip pain if cancer has metastatized.

Management

Early recognition and treatment is required to control growth. Primary screening for prostate cancer consists of palpation of the gland during DRE, a blood test for PSA (a glycoprotein that is detected in the epithelial cells of the prostate) and TRUS (transrectal ultrasound). Biopsy, needle aspiration, open biopsy, bone screening, grading and staging.

A symptom of staging prostate cancer has been developed to classify the location, size and spread of the tumor and guide treatment decision. DUKES system of staging the prostatic neoplasia are as follows:

Stage A : Microscopic lesions found in prostate gland removed because of benign hypertrophy.
Stage B : Nodules confined to prostate gland, no capsular adherence, or urethral involvement: normal serum acid phosphatase level.
Stage C : Carcinoma involving prostatic capsule, seminal vesicles, urethra, bladder and pelvic lymph nodes or a malignant tumor of lesser extent with elevated serum acid phosphatase levels.
Stage D : Findings as in Stage C plus evidence of extrapelvic lesions or osseous involvement.

Treatment included according to stages as follows:

Stage A : Continue medical follow-up, observation, TURP or total prostatectomy and radiation therapy.
Stage B : TURP, total prostatectomy with or without lymphodectotomy as radiation therapy.
Stage C : Hormone manipulation: e.g. 2H—releasing hormone analogues. Orchiectomy, radical resection of prostate and radiation therapy.

The types of surgical procedures performed in prostate are:
- Transurethral resection done when enlargement of the medial lobe surrounding urethra-BPH. No incision, removal by way of urethroscopy.
- Suprapubic resection performed when extremely large mass of obstructive tissue and prostatic cancer. Low midline abdominal incision through bladder or prostate gland.
- Retropubic resection-performed when large mass is located high in pelvic area—Prostate cancer, low midline abdominal incision into prostate gland (bladder is not incised).
- Perineal resection, performed when large mass is located low in pelvic area—Prostate cancer. Here incision is made between scrotum and rectum.
- Radical perineal resection is done when mass extends beyond the capsule, includes lymph node dissection—Prostate cancer. Here there is large perineal incision between scrotum and rectum.

For all procedures, three-way Foley catheter with 30 ml by urethra is used as drainage tube. The complication of surgical procedures include hemorrhage, water intoxication, incontinence, obstruction, infections, wound infection, impotence and sterility may occur.

Preoperative and postoperative phases of therapy are the same as for BPH. Nursing intervention for patient who undergoes radiation therapy and chemotherapy as in other malignancies (Oncological nursing). If the patient is to have a perineal approach in surgery, he is given a bowel preparation which may include enemas, cathartics and sulfasalazine (Azulfidine) or neomycin preoperatively and only clear fluids the day before surgery to prevent fecal contamination of the operative side.

Additional postoperative care includes:
- Caring for the perineal wound.
- Restoring urinary and bowel continence.
- Promoting sexual function and psychological counseling.
- Dealing with grief.

PROBLEMS OF THE PENIS

Health problems of the penis are rare if sexually transmitted infectious diseases are excluded. Structural problem of the penis is typically related to the head of the penis and the foreskin. The head of the penis is susceptible to diseases caused by irritation, cancer and trauma. Foreskin also is a source of structural difficulties that can affect urinations, cause pain and interfere with blood flow to the penis. Functional problems of the penis primarily involves disorders of erection. Problems of the penis may be classified as congenital, problems of the prepuce, problems with the erectile mechanism and cancer.

Congenital Problem of Penis

Hypospadias is a urologic abnormality in which the urethral meatus is located on the ventral surface of the penis anywhere from the corona to the perineum. Hormonal influences in utero, environmental factors and genetic factors are possible causes. Surgical repair of hypospadias may be necessary if it is associated with chordee or if it prevents intercourse or normal urination. Surgery may also be done for cosmetic reasons or emotional well-being.

Epispadias and opening of the urethra on the dorsal surface of the penis, is a complex birth defect that is usually associated with other genitourinary tract defects. Corrective surgery to place the urethra in a normal position in the penis is usually done in childhood.

Phimosis and Paraphimosis

Etiology

Phimosis is a condition in which the opening of the prepuce or foreskin is unable to be retracted behind the glans. The condition may be congenital or acquired as a result of inflammation or infection. It is caused by edema or inflammation of the foreskin of an uncircumcised male. This results in the foreskin constricting around the head of the penis making retraction difficult. It is generally caused by poor hygiene techniques that allow bacterial and yeast organisms to become trod under the foreskin.

Paraphimosis conversely, is a condition in which the prepuce is retracted over the glans and forms a constriction at the base of the glans. This is usually as a result of manipulation of the foreskin over the glans to infection. Chronic irritation may cause senile carcinoma. Healing of the irritation or infection causes scar tissue formation, which can worsen the acquired phimosis and if the constriction of the foreskin at the head of the penis is severe enough, it causes urinary obstructions and painful urination.

Constriction is also a major problem with paraphimosis. The constriction at the base of the glans usually results in swelling of the glans. If the swelling is not reduced, blood vessels to the glans are compressed, reducing flow. Inadequate blood flow can result in the necrosis of the glands.

Management

Treatment for severe cases of phimosis may consist of incisions in the foreskin to reduce the contracture and widen the opening. Congenital phimosis may be successfully treated by gentle repeated stretching of the foreskin over the glans.

Circumcision may be performed if the prepuce cannot be satisfactorily retracted. Circumcision, the surgical removal of the foreskin of the penis may be done for religious, cultural or hygienic reasons. Parents are encouraged to make the final decisions after considering all the advantages and disadvantages.

Circumcision is done to prevent recurrence of paraphimosis. When the penis is circumcised, the wound is covered with gauze generously impregnated with petrolatum. Bleeding usually is controlled by applying pressure on dressing that may be bulky and must be removed before the patient can void. It is removed cautiously and replaced after voiding with a fresh petroleum dressing.

Patient education focuses on strategies to reduce the inflammation. Hot soaks and oral antibiotics are often used to treat the swelling and infection that can result from phimosis. Cool compresses are used for paraphimosis. The cool compress is applied to the penis and the penis is elevated for a short period before a gentle attempt is made to reduce the prepuce. Antibiotics, warm soaks and sometimes circumcision or dorsal slit of the prepuce may be required. Careful cleaning followed by replacement of the foreskin generally prevents these problems.

If circumcision has been necessary, the nurse teaches the patient how to change the petrolatum dressing and observe for signs of infection. The nurse also instructs the patient to be alert for signs of bleeding. If severe bleeding occurs, a firm dressing should be applied to the penis and the patient should be taken to medical aid. For the emergency treatment room, an estrogen preparation may be prescribed for the adult patient for several days after surgery to prevent painful erections.

Cancer of the Penis

Cancer of the penis is rare apart from cancer associated with the STD, human papilloma virus (HPV) and in men who were not circumcised as infants.

Etiology

The incidence of penile cancer depends greatly on hygienic standards and cultural and religious practices. It almost never occurs in a male who was circumcised at birth. Circumcision after puberty does not decrease the risk of cancer when compared with the incidence among uncircumcised males. Circumcision removes the prepuce or foreskin, which provides a haven for bacteria. The bacteria act on disquamated cells, producing smegma, which is irritating to the tissue of the glans penis and the prepuce. The chronic irritation is considered to be the carcinogenic. Trauma and STDs are thought to be considered as penile cancer rather than causative.

Pathophysiology

Penile cancer starts as a small lesion usually on or under the prepuce and extends until the entire glans and shaft are involved. The initial lesion may assume a variety of forms. It may appear as a small bump, resemble a pimple or wart or occur as a non-healing ulcer with the edges rolled inward. The latter associated with earlier metastases and a poorer 5-year survival. The most common type of malignancy is squamous cell carcinoma. Phimosis is present in patient with penile cancer, may obscure the lesion. The lesion may then cause erosion through the prepuce, resulting in a foul odor and discharge. Bleeding may or may not be present. Urethral and bladder involvements are rare. Eventually the disease can become autoamputative. If left untreated, death occurs in 2 to 3 years.

Clinical Manifestation

Clinical manifestation of penile cancer includes weakness, fatigue, malaise and weight loss. Men may complain of itching and burning under the prepuce and an occasional foul discharge. A 1-year delay before seeking treatment occurs in 15-50 percent cases. Biopsy is performed to establish diagnosis. However, benign penile lesions occurs infrequently. Metastasis occurs at the regional femeral and iliac nodes and is associated with significantly worse prognosis. The stages of penile cancer includes the following.

Stage A : Lesions confined to glans or foreskin.
Stage B : Shaft or corpora cavernosa invaded by tumor.
Stage C : Shaft involvement, lymph nodes involved but operable.

Stage D : Shaft involvement, lymph nodes inoperable and metastases to distant sites.

Management

Treatment is usually surgical. Treatment in the early stages is laser removal of the growth. A radical resection of the penis may be done if the cancer has been spread. Surgery, radiation, or chemotherapy may be tried depending on the extent of the disease, lymph node involvement or metastasis.

Stage 0 : Circumcision.
Stage A : Partial penectomy or amputation of the penis.
Stage B : Total amputation of the penis.
Stage C : Total amputation and perineal urethrostomy.
Stage D : Hemipelvectomy or hemicorporectormy if scrotum and anus.

The nurse teaches the patient about the potential side effects of radiation in the perineal area. Radiation in this location can cause the skin to become dry, itchy and sensitive. Special gels that are safe to use during radiation may be applied to the affected area. Urethral strictures may develop several months to years after radiation therapy. The nurse informs the patient of symptoms of urethral structure, which includes difficulty starting or stopping the urine flows. Frequent UTI and nocturia and bowel pattern may change during radiation therapy.

The emotional devastation of a diagnosis of penile cancer is difficult to assess. The proposed surgery may be unthinkable to the patient, who is frequently in a state of shock. The scope of support and sexual counseling needed by the patient is beyond the expertise of most nurses. The patient is referred for sexual counseling with experts who can clearly explain the options.

ERECTILE DYSFUNCTION/IMPOTENCE

Erectile dysfunctions is the inability to attain or maintain an erect penis that allows satisfactory sexual performance. Impotence is the inability of a man to have an erection firm enough or sustain an erection long enough for sexual intercourse.

The term satisfactory is defined by the couple involved and may vary from couple to couple. The ability to have an erection depends not only on healthy psychological state, but also on adequately functioning neuorological, vascular and hormonal system. The brain is the controlling organ for sexual arousal. The brain perceives sexual stimuli and controls the psychological changes that occur during arousal.

Etiology

The two fundamental causes of impotence are physical and psychological. Physical cause includes changes in bloodflow to the penis and neurogenic dysfunctions. Diseases such as diabetes, lupus and rheumatoid arthritis can damage blood vessels and cause obstruction of blood flow in the penis. Anemia and dehydration can cause insufficient blood volumes to maintain an erection. Cardiac diseases and antihypersensitive drugs can interfere with the capillar blood pressure. The risk factors of impotence are as follows:
- Stress.
- Fatigue.
- Drug effects, e.g. antihypertensive agents, beta blockers, or alcohol.
- Diabetes mellitus.
- Vascular diseases, e.g. hypertension or peripheral vascular disease.
- Neurological disorder, e.g. if multiple sclerosis, or spinal cord injury and Parkinson's disease.
- Effects of colorectal, cystectomy or selected prostatectomy procedures.
- Trauma to the perineal area.
- Psychological factors of fear, anxiety, anger, frustrations, performance:
  – Anxiety, i.e. fear of not performing well during sexual intercourse and fatigue.

Pathophysiology

Inability of the brain to respond to sexual stimuli can interrupt the signals to the parasympathetic nervous system, that release a transmitter substance causing the small arteries in the penis to dilate. The result is insufficient blood flow to fill the network of sinusoids inside the corpora cavernosa (erectile chamber) that cause the penis to enlarge and become firm. When the blood volume in the erectile chamber is inadequate, they cannot create enough pressure to block blood return. Blood drains from the penis and erection cannot be maintained.

The sympathetic nervous system controls both orgasm and ejaculation. The two functions there form can occur without an erection.

After ejaculation or when sexual stimulation diminishes the arteries on the penis constrict, reducing blood flow and the veins expand to allow disengorgement.

Clinical Manifestation

The clinical manifestation of impotence includes the following:
- Inability to have an erection.
- Inability to sustain an erection.
- Inability to have an erection firm enough for penetration (incomplete erection).

Management of Impotence

Diagnostic tests for impotence include CBC, urinalysis, BUN, creatinine and fasting blood sugar, cholesterol level, hormonal studies and nocturnal monitoring of penile tumescence. Invasive studies include arteriogram (dye injection to sudy blood flow) and cavernosometry and psychological test is also performed.

Several new medications for impotence are under development. Sildenafil (Viagra) has been released for use and attracted by many persons. Viagra can cause lowering of blood pressure and cardiac arrest. Other side effects are headache and GI disturbances. Topical agents are occasionally used to enhance venous congestion of the penis, e.g. nitroglycerin ointments—topical vasodilator. Topical and oral agents are often combined with other therapies to treat impotence. Hormonal therapy (Testosterone) increases libido. Vasodilators can induce penile erections by means of increased blood flow, sinusoidal relaxations and increased venous resistance. These generally used drugs are Papaverine and Pentolamine combination injected by a patient into the corpus cavernosum of the penis or inserted into the tip of the penis via suppository. The drug combination may include prostaglandin E (PGE). Many medications have side effects that inhibit erectile function. Modify the dosage or change of drug when needed.

External vacuum devices are sometimes used to achieve an erection for a short time. These devices are cylinders that fit over the penis and use a suction pump to pull blood into the penis. A band is applied to the proximal aspect of the penis when the erection is achieved to impede the venous return. The erection may be maintained for approximately 30 minutes. These devices contraindicated for patients with bleeding disorders, sickle cell anemia and severe circulatory compromise.

Counseling and sexual therapy classes may be suggested for patients who have identified psychological impotence. Surgical treatment of impotence include vascular reconstructive surgery, inflatable prosthesis, self contained inflatable prosthesis and semirigid/malleable prosthesis.

The man experiencing erectile dysfunction requires a great deal of emotional support, for both himself and his partner. The patient needs reassurance and then confidentiality will be maintained. Nurses are in a unique position of conducting routine health assessments on men seeking any form of medical treatment.

Priapism

Priapism is a painful condition, characterized by prolonged erection greater than 4 to 6 hours. Penile ischemia can result causing permanent impotence or necrosis of the penis.

Etiology

- Caused by either prolonged venous occlusion or arterial blood engorgement.
- Possible side effects of some impotence therapies.

Treatment

- Treatment is directed as the specific cause.
- Options include administration of alpha antogonists directly into the corpora cavernosa, and IV therapy to re-establish acid-base balance.
- Pain management is a high priority (infertility, vasectomy, male sterilization).

SEXUALLY TRANSMITTED DISEASES

Sexually transmitted diseases (STDs) are diseases that usually can be transmitted from one person to another with heterosexual or homosexual intercourse or intimate contact with the genitalia, mouth or rectum. Historically they have been referred to as veneral diseases. Although diseases are sexually transmitted there are some notable exceptions to sexual transmission. During pregnancy, the fetus may become infected in utero by placental transmission, and the neonate may acquire congenital syphilis or be stillborn. Infants of mothers with gonorrhea may contract an infection of the eyes (ophthalmic neonoatarum) during birth, and unless treated it can lead to permanent blindness.

Until the 1980, only five veneral diseases (Syphilis, gonorrhea, chancroid, lymphogranuloma venerium and granuloma inguinale) were regularly monitored. In 1960s, several diseases were added to the list of STDs. These include "*Chlamydia trachomatis*, genital herpes, human papilloma virus (HPV), genital myeoplasmas, cytomegalovirus, hepatitis B, vaginitis, enteric infections and ectoparasitic disease. Early in the 1980s the human immunodeficiency syndrome emerged as major STD. We shall discuss some of the important STDs.

Gonorrhea

Etiology

Gonorrhea is caused by *Neisseria gonorrhea*, a gram-negative diplococcus. Mucosa with columnar epithelium is susceptible to gonococcal infection. This tissue is present in the genitalia (the urethra in men, the cervix in women), the rectum and the oropharynx. The disease is spread by direct physical contact with an infected host, usually during sexual activity. Neonates can develop a gonococcal infection after passage through an infected birth canal. The delicate gonococcus is easily killed by drying, heating or washing with an antiseptic solution. Consequently, indirect transmission of instruments or linen are rare. The incubation period is 3 to 4 days. The disease confers no immunity subsequent to reinfection.

Pathophysiology

In men the gonococcus is introduced into the anterior urethra during sexual activity. Because most men are diagnosed and treated early complications and residual effects of gonorrhea are uncommon among men. Sterility from orchitis or epididymitis can occur as a residual effect. But this is rare.

The incidence of asymptomatic gonorrhea in men is believed to be low. However, there is an increasing awareness of the importance of men with asymptomatic infection in the transmission of gonorrhea.

Gonorrhea in women, most often begins as asymptomatic cervicitis and the infection can be present for extended periods without causing noticeable signs. Hence there are a high number of infected asymptomatic women. These women do not receive treatment unless gonorrhea is diagnosed through screening or unless women is identified by a sexual partner and presents herself for treatment. In cases of untreated gonorrhea, women, the residual effects of chronic PID, infertility and ectopic pregnancies are well known. Other complication of untreated gonorrhea in both men and women include dermatitis, carditis, meningitis and arthritis.

Clinical Manifestation

The most common signs and symptoms of gonorrhea are as follows:

A. 1. In Heterosexual men there is:
   - Urethritis—Often first symptoms.
   - Severe dysuria—Especially with first voiding in morning.
   - Purulent discharge from urethra
   - Swelling of the penis and balantitis—rare symptom.
   2. In homosexual and bisexual men, there is
   - Rectal gonorrhea is common—usually asymptomatic and discovered by rectal culture.
   - Pharyngeal gonorrhea—usually asymptomatic.
B. *In women:* Women rarely have early distressing symptoms such as men have. When symptoms are present they include the following:
   - Slight purulent vaginal discharge.
   - Vague feeling of fullness in pelvis.
   - Discomfort or aching in abdomen.
   - If bladder is involved—burning frequency and urgency usually causes the person to seek medical attention.

The symptoms are so light that they may be ignored.

Management

The most reliable way to confirm gonococcal infection is to isolate the organism in culture. Prevention of gonorrhea and its complications can be achieved in three stages. The first and most crucial stage is primary prevention that is prevention of the disease. The second stage or secondary prevention involves prevention of complication of the disease such as PID. The third stage or tertiary prevention is reversal of the damage caused by the disease, such as by tubal reconstruction.

Early treatment of infected person is the most effective method of prevention of new infections of sexual partners. Education to acquaint people with the symptoms of gonorrheas is efficacy of condoms, and availability of diagnosis and treatment sources. The treatment which necessarily include the following.

- *Uncomplicated gonorrhea:* Cefixine (Suprax) 400 mg orally in single dose or Ceftrinaxacin 500 mg orally single dose plus Azithromycin—1 gm orally in single dose or doxyecycline 100 mg orally tid 7 days.
- Follow up cultures after completion of treatment (usually 7 days).
- Case finding.
- Treatment of contacts.
- Instruction on abstinence from sexual intercourse and alcohol.
- Re-examination if symptoms persist or recur after completion of treatment.
- Repeat serological test for syphilis at one month.

Syphilis

Syphilis is caused by a spirochete, *Treponema pallidum* that gains entry into the body through either the mucus membrane or skin during intercourse. The organism is readily destroyed by physical and chemical agents including heat, draining and mild disinfectants such as soap and water. The incubation period is usually 3 weeks. However, symptoms can appear as early as 9 days or as long as 3 months after exposure which in case of rectal infection in homosexuals.

Pathophysiology

The signs and symptoms of syphilis developed in four stages as follows:

1. *Primary stage:* The duration of stage is 2-8 weeks. There will be a hard sore or pimple on vulva or penis that breaks and forms painless, draining chancre; may be a simple chancre or groups of more than one, may be present also on lips, tongue, hands, rectum or nipples, chancre heals leaving almost invisible scar.
   Exudate from lesions and chancre are highly contagious.
   Duration of stage is 3-8 weeks.
2. *Secondary stage:* Appears 2-4 weeks after chancre appears, extends over 2-4 years. Signs and symptoms depends on site, low-grade fever, headache, anorexia, weight loss, anemia, sore throat, hoarseness, reddened and sore eyes, jaundice with or without heptatitis, aching of joint muscles, long bones; sores on body or generalized fine rash (cutaneous eruptions) condylomatoa auminate (veneral warts) in rectum or genitalia.
   Exudates from lesions highly contagious, blood contains organisms. Duration of state is 1-2 years.

3. *Latent stage:* No clinical signs—Absence of signs and symptoms. Duration will be 5-20 years. Contagious for about 2 years; not contagious to others after that. Blood contains organism and may be transmitted placentally to fetus. Duration of stage is throughout life or progresses to late stage.
4. *Late stage:* Appearance 3-20 years after initial infection. Non-infectious Chronic (without treatment) is possibly fatal. The characteristic finding includes the following.
    - *Benign:* Tumor-like mass (Gummas) on any area of the body. They are chronic destructive lesions affecting any organ of the body especially skin, bone, liver and mucus membrane.
    - *Cardiovascular:* There will be damage to heart valves and blood vessels aortic valve insufficiency or occular aneurysm of thoracic aorta and aortitis.
    - *Neurosyphilis:* Spinal fluid possible contains organism. There will be meningitis, general paresis (Personality changes for minor to psychotic tremors. Physical and mental deterioration). Paralysis, and Taber dorsales (ataxia, areflexia, paresthesias, lightening pains, damaged joints-charcots joints) paresis, insomnia, confusion, delirium, impaired judgement and slurred speech.

Management

Management of syphilis is aimed at eradication of all syphilitic organisms. [Early syphilis (primary, secondary, or early latent)] treated with a single dose of Benzathin Penocillin-G (IM) at single visit. Other antibiotics used are Doxycycline, Tetracycline or Erythromycin. Syphilis lasting below 1 year is treated with three weekly injections of Benzathin Penicillin (G) (IM). The symptomatic neurosyphilis is treated by aqueous crystalline penicillin (IV) daily for 14 days followed by penicillin or Benzathin weekly for 3 doses. The other antibiotics such as Doxycyclin, Tetracyclin and Erythromycin are used.

Appropriate antibiotic treatment of maternal syphilis before 10th week of pregnancy prevents infection of the fetus. All patients with neurosyphilis may be carefully monitored with periodic serologic testing, clinical evaluation for 6-month interval and repeat CSF examination for at least 3 years. Specific management is based on the presenting symptoms. Take preventive measures as in gonorrhea.

Herpes Genitalis

Herpes genitalis (Genital herpes-HSV-2) is caused by infections with herpes virus hormonis type 2 (HSV-2) HSV-2 can be transmitted from genitalis to mouth through oral-genital contact. Once acquired, herpes genitalis is a 'life-long' disease and carries with it not only intense and recurrent discomfort, but also anxieties about future childbearing malignancy, and sexual and marital function. In early pregnancy, women infected with herpes have an increased change of miscarriage. It endangers the fetus during delivery, caesarian delivery is often necessary. It is also associated with cervical cancer.

Pathophysiology

The incubation period is 3 to 7 days. The primary lesions appear as a vesicle on the external genitalia in men; often on the rectum in homosexual men and on the vagina, cervix or external genitalia of women. These lesions often ulcerate, especially when located on moist surfaces. Following primary herpes, the virus persists in a latent or unrecognized form in most patients. It is believed that latent infections are localized in the ganglia of sensory nerves to the genitalia. When the host factors favor it, the latent infection becomes clinically apparent as recurrent herpes.

Clinical Manifestation

A patient with primary HIV-2 infection may initially complain of burning or tingling at the side of inoculation. Vesicular lesions, which may occur on the penis, scrotum, vulva, perineum, perianal region, vagina, cervix, contain large quantities of infectious viral particles. The lesion scrupture and form shallow, moist ulcerations. Finally, crusting and epitheliazation of the erosions occur. Primary infections tend to be associated with local inflammation and pain, accompanied by systemic manifestations of fever, headache, malaise, myalgia and regional lymphadenopathy.

Urination may be painful from urine touching active lesions. Retention may occur as a result of HSV urethritis or cytitis. A purulent vaginal discharge may develop with HSV cervicitis. The duration of the symptoms is longer and the frequency of complications is greater in women. Transmission of genital herpes, therefore, can occur by sexual contact with an excreter of virus who is free from symptoms. Primary lesions are generally present 17 to 20 days, but new lesions sometimes continue to develop for 6 weeks.

Management

Diagnosis of genital herpes is usually based on the patient's symptoms and history. Other diagnostic measures include viral isolation by tissue culture and cytologic examination of vesicular exudate for multinucleated giant cells.
- Primary infection:
    - Acyclovir (Zovirax) 400 mg orally tid and 7-10 days
    - Acyclovir 200 mg orally five times a day and 7-10p days
    - Famiclovir (Famvir) 250 mg orally tid and 7-10 days
    - Vallyclovir (Valtrex) 1 gm orally twice a day for 7-5 or 10 days.

- Recurrent infection
  - Acyclovir 400 mg orally three times a day and 5 days or.
  - Acyclovir 200 mg orally five times a day x 5 days or.
  - Famciclovir 125 mg orally twice a day x 5 days.
  - Valcyclovir 500 mg orally twice a day x 5 days.
  - Attempt to identify trigger mechanisms).
  - Yearly pap smear.
  - Abstinence from sexual contact while lesions are present. However, it may shed virus without lesions.
  - Provision of symptomatic intervention.
  - Confidential counseling and testing of HIV.

Above drugs are used as daily suppressive therapy for frequent recurrence and severe infection as directed by doctor.

CHLAMYDIAL INFECTIONS

Chlamydia trachomatis, a gram-negative bacterium, is recognized as a genital pathogen that is responsible for an increasing variety of clinical illnesses.

Etiology

Chlamydia trachomatis is caused by *C. trachomatis*, chlamydial infection is recognised as the most prevalent of the STDs. Age, number of sex partners, socio-economic status and sexual orientation are predictors of infection with *C. trachomatis*.

- *Age:* Infection is rather one, two to three times higher, in sexually active, women under the age of 20 years. The rates of urethral infection are higher teenage males than for adult men.
- *Number of sex partners:* Persons with several sex partners are at higher risk of infection.
- *Socioeconomic status:* Persons at lower socio-economic stratum are at increased risk for infection with *C. trachomatis*.
- *Sexual preference:* The prevalence of urethral chlamydial infection among homosexual men is one-third then among heterosexual men. Chlamydial infections can be transmitted to infants during delivery, causing conjunctivities and pneumonia in many. The incidence of chlamydial is highest in young, promiscuous, indigent, unmarried women who live in the inner city and in those who have had a prior history of STDs.

Pathophysiology

Chlamydia trachomatis is an intracellular parasite that has specific requirements for adenosine triphosphate (ATP) and amino acids. There are two stages in the life cycle of the organism. In stage I, the infective stage, the elementary body attaches to the host cell and the ingested by phagocytosis. In stage II, the elementary body undergoes metamorphosis to become a reticulate or initial body. This is the metabolic phase of the life cycle. The initial body duplicates by binary fission and changes into elementary body. The host cell, which contains the elementary body, undergoes lysis, liberating infectious organisms that are capable of reinfecting new cells.

The chlamydial infection in males include urethritis, post-genocal urethritis, prostitis, conjunctivitis, pharyngitis and subclicinal LGV. In addition, female cervicitis includes chlamydial infection transmitted to infants by mothers causing conjunctivitis, pneumonia, asymptomatic pharyngeal carriage and gastrointestinal carriage.

The complication in men includes epididymitis, prostratitis Reiter's syndrome, sterility and rectal strictures, and in women, salpingitis, endometritis, perihepatitis, ectopic pregnancy, infertility vulvar/rectal carcinoma and rectal strictures are the complications.

Management

Chlamydial infections respond to treatment with doxycycline (vibramycin) azithomycin (zithromax) or ofloxacin (floxin). It is important that the patient encourages sexual partner(s) to seek care as soon as possible to avoid reinfection of the patient and complications in the partner. Patients who are sexually active should be advised to wear condoms or use of spermicides to prevent reinfection. Social and emotional support of these pati-ents is important as it is with any person with STD.

Lymphogranuloma Venereum

Lymphogranuloma venereum (LGV) is a chronic STD caused by specific strains of *C. trachomatis* are, i.e. serotype L1, L2 and L3 of *C trachomatis*.

The disease is contracted by vaginal, anal or oral intercourses, primary inoculation with the organism may occur at any site involved in closed contact. The incubation period is 3 to 30 days. Lymphadens it is of regional lymph node drainage the site of primary infection occurs and the disease spreads by way of the lymphatic system.

Pathophysiology

The three clinical phases of infection in LGV are:
1. Inoculation and appearance of the primary lesion.
2. Lymphatic spread and generalized symptoms and
3. Late complication.

In individual case, any one of the phases may be absent or unnoticed. The primary lesions which is transient appears as papula, small erosion or vesicle. These are present in the prepuce and glans penis in male and vagina and cervix in females. They are painless. Local edema may be present. If the rectum is infected, a bloody discharge followed by mucopurulent discharge, diarrhea and cramping.

Involvement of the lympatic occurs 1 to 4 weeks after the appearance of primary lesion. Penile, vulvar and anal infection can lead to inguinal or femoral lymphadenopathy. Marked inflammation occurs resulting in necrosis, buboes, absesses and inguinal lymph nodes, and infection of surrounding tissue. Healing occurs by fibrosis after several weeks or months and which damages lymph nodes and disrupt nodal function.

Constitutional symptoms that occur during the stage of regional lymphadenopathy include fever, chills, headache, meningitis, anorexia, myalgia, and arthalgia. Complication of untreated anorectal infection include perirectal absess, fisutala, in ano, and rectovaginal, rector vesical and ishiorectal fistulas.

Management

LGV is treated with 2-week course of tetracycline, sex partners should also be treated. The patient may require much counseling and teaching as they deal with their disease. Because the fluctuant lymph nodes may be disturbing to the patient self-image, social and emotional support is very much important.

Chancroid

Chancroid is an STD caused by a gram-negative bacillus. *Haemophilus ducreyi:* Chancroid has been established as a cofactor for HIV transmission and high rate of HIV infection among patients with chancroid.

Pathophysiology

The initial lesions are acutely tender genital ulcers, lymphadenopathy, and tender buboes. The buboes which are fluctuant, inguinal node masses may suppurate and lead to abscesses. Exudate from the ulcers or aspirate from the buboes is stained and a "shool-of-fish" pattern may be noted on microscopic examination by some one experienced in interpretation. In women, the lesions of the chancroid are most often found in the labia, anus, clitoris, vagina and cervix. Some women do not have lesions but may have mild vaginitis. In men, the lesions appear on the prepuce, glans or shaft of the penis.

Clinical Manifestation

The ulcers found in chancroid are typically ragged and irregular. They are highly infectious and autoimmunity occurs resulting in multiple lesions. The ulcer appears excavated, have a granulating purulent surface and are painful. Often edema of the surrounding tissue is persistent. The buboes which are most often unilateral, painful and spheric in shape. The skin over the buboes is inflamed. These buboes tend to become softer in abscess form. These abscesses in turn may suppurate and rupture, further spreading infection usually appear when inguinal abscess is formed.

Management

Follow-up is essential, because, treatment failure may occur. The individual is taught to report any sign or symptom that persists or worsen during treatment and abstain from sexual activity until lesions are healed. Proper use of condom should be stressed.

Granuloma Inguinale (Donovanoses)

Granuloma inguinale or granuloma venereum is believed to be most often transmitted by sexual contact, although nonsexual transmission has been reported.

Etiology

Granuloma inguinale caused by a gram-negative bacillus "Calymmatobacterium (Donovania) granulomatis" is widely referred to as Donovan Bacillus. The disease is mildly contagious and probably requires repeated exposure for spread of infection. Predisposing factors are poorly understood. The disease is most common in men than women and is particularly common in homosexual men. The incubation period varies from several days to several months.

Pathophysiology

Lesions appear on the genitalia and in the perianal areas. The most common sites of lesions are the prepuce and glans in men and the vagina and the labia in women. The infection first appears with development of subcutaneous nodules. These elevated areas eventually ulcerate, producing sharply defined painless lesions. The ulcers enlarge slowly and bleed on contact. With ulceration, the infection tends to spread along the pubic region. Involvement of the lymph nodes is uncommon but can occur and produce occlusions of the lymphatics resulting in elephantasis.

Management

Treatment with suitable antibiotics and clinician follow-up of anyone diagnosed with granuloma inguinale is extremely important due to the possibility of the treatment failure. All persons should be advised to abstain from sexual activity until all sexual partners complete a course of treatment.

Condylomata Acuminata (Genital Warts)

Condylomota acuminata (Genital Warts) is caused by human papillomavirus (HPV) and highly contagious STD is seen frequently in young, sexually active adults.

Etiology

Genital warts are sexually transmitted and are the most commonly recognized clinical signs of genital HPV infections. They are important because of their possible role in the development of cervical cancer. The incubation period of the virus is generally 1 to 6 months, but may be longer. The disease is most common in adolescent girls and young women. HPV can remain dormant for decades before recurrences occur.

Pathophysiology

Minor trauma during the sexual intercourse can cause abrasions that allow HPV to enter the body. The epithelial cells infected with HPV undergo transformation, proliferate and form a warty growth. Immunosuppressed persons, pregnant women and diabetics are most susceptible to HPV. Genital warts occur in or around the vulva, vagina, cervix perineum, anal canal, urethra and glans penis. They enlarge during pregnancy and may cause haermorrhage or obstruction during delivery.

Clinical Manifestation

Condylomata acuminatal lesions are discrete single or multiple papillary growths that are white to gray. The warts may grow and coalese to form large cauliflower-like masses. In men, the warts may occur on the penis and scrotum, around the anus and or in the urethra. In women, the warts may be located on the vulva, vagina and the cervix and in preanal area. During pregnancy, genital warts tend to grow rapidly. An infected mother transmits the conditions to her newborn. Bleeding on defecation may occur with anal warts. The genitalis and anorectal region as well as urethra, bladder and oral mucosa may be affected. Research has linked HPV infection with cervical and vulvalar cancer in women and with anorectal and squamous cell carcinoma of the penis in men.

Management

Warts may be confused with condylomata, secondary syphilis, carcinoma or benign tumors. Serologic and cytologic testing should be done. If dysplasia confirmed by pap smear, colposcopic examination and biopsies should be performed. Virapap a test that uses DNA hybridization techniques can be used.

The primary goal, when treating visible genital warts, is the removal of the symptomatic warts. The removal may or may not decrease infectivity. One common treatment is the use of 80 percent and 90 percent trichloroacetic acid (TCA) applied directly to the wart surface. Petroleum jelly is applied to the surrounding normal skin to minimize irritation before a small amount of TCA is applied to the wart with a cotton swab. A sharp stinging pain is often felt with initial acid contact, but this quickly subsides. TCA is not washed off after treatment. It can be used in pregnant women.

Podophyllin (10-25%) a cytotoxic agent is recommended therapy for small external genital warts when it is used, it is applied carefully to each wart with normal tissue being avoided, and is then thoroughly washed off in 1 to 4 hours. The substance encourages the sloughing off of skin containing viral particles. Podophyllin has local (e.g. pain, burning) and sestemic (e.g. nausea, dizziness, leukopoenia respiratory distress), toxic symptoms. It is contraindicated in pregnant women.

Patient managed treatment is also an option. Podofilox liquid and gel are available (condylox and condylox gel). Patient applies solution or gel for 3 successive days followed by 4 days if no treatment can be repeated upto 4 weeks.

If the wart does not regress with any of these therapies, treatment such as cryotherapy with liquid nitrogen, electrocautery, laser therapy 5-Fluoracid, and surgical excision may be indicated.

Prevention of HPV should be stressed. It includes:
Avoiding sexual relationship with persons in known high-risk groups.
- Using latex condoms if having sexual intercourse
- Avoiding anal intercourse.
  Cesarean delviery may be indicated for warts obstructing the pelvic outlet or if a vaginal birth would cause excessive bleeding of the warts.

Trichomoniasis

Trichomoniasis is caused by the protozoan, "*Trichomonas vaginalis*". Evidence suggests that the incubation period range between 4 to 28 days. It is most often sexually transmitted by such as towels, toilet seats, and so on. The parasite commonly exists in vaginal or cervical secretions and in seminal fluid. It is estimated that one of five females will have a trichomonal infection during one's life time.

Pathophysiology (Clinical Manifestations)

Trichomoniasis is commonly viewed as an innoculous infection. Yet there are serious implications for health. During the postpartum period in women who have trichomoniasis, the rate of persistent fever, prolonged vaginal discharge and endometritis is twice as high as in women who do not harbour the organism. Majority of patients with trichomoniasis have cervical rosions and leukorrhea and has been suggested that chronic irritation may predispose to cervical cancer.

Management

The CDC recommends that both partners be treated simultaneously with metronidazole to prevent reinfection by the untreated partner at a later date. Vaginal inserts of metronidazole in the woman alone are less effective. The drug is known to cross the placental barrier. For this reason it is not given to pregnant women until after the first trimester.

Bacterial Vaginosis

Bacterial vaginosis is the most common vaginal infection among women of childbearing age. Studies have linked it with preterm labor, infections of amniotic fluids, postpartum uterine infections, and PID. It is characterized by an overgrowth of normal flora resulting from introduction of other flora and altered vaginal pH related to sexual activity or poor hygienic practices.

Pathophysiology

Bacterial vaginosis infection characterized by a small amount of homogenous gray or grayish, white discharge. The discharge usually has a disagreeable odor and because it is less irritating than discharge caused by other organism, pruritis is mild or absent. On inspection, the vaginal walls are slightly reddened and the discharge appears to adhere to the mucosal lining.

Management

Self-care measures should be emphasized. These include use of condoms for 4 to 6 weeks after diagnosis, limiting hygienic douching to vinegar and water and wiping from front to back after voiding.

Hepatitis B Virus

Hepatitis B virus (HBV) is a DNA virus that causes acute or chronic hepatitis, cirrhosis, and hepatocellular carcinoma. There are more than 300 million persons infected world over. The risk of developing HBV infection is greatest in infants at birth and declines with age.

Etiology

Transmission from mother to neonates if mother is positive for hepatitis B antigen (HBcAg). HSV transmitted sexually and risk factors include multiple sexual partners, a history of STD and homosexuality especially with receptive anal intercourse. It is also transmitted by drug abusers who share needles and by needle sticks by health care workers. It is not transmitted through blood transfusion. Other risk factors include patients on hemodialysis and those who are hospitalized.

Pathophysiology

The hepatitis caused by HBV results in the same symptoms seen in other types of hepatitis. The liver is inflamed and the patient may have jaundice, anorexia, slight fever and gastrointestinal upset, etc.

Management

The centre of disease control of prevent (CDC) recommends vaccination for persons identified as being at high risk, including residents of correctional or long-term care facilities, persons seeking treatment for STD, prostitutes, homosexuals and promiscuous heterosexuals. The CDC also recommends that all children regardless of their exposure to risk stated against HBV. The vaccine is given at birth, 1 month and 6 months. If serum HBs Ag is not detected after 5 to 7 years, a booster dose of the vaccine should be considered. Vaccination also is recommended for all health care providers/workers possibly by needle sticks. Postexposure prophylactive treatment with hepatitis B immune globules (HBIG) given to the person who had sexual contact with HBV positive partner of HBV carriers.

In addition to those diseases already discussed, pediculosis pubis molluscum conagiosum and scabies are considered to be STDs.

Role of Nurses in Prevention of Control of STDs

The nurses' first responsibility in STD control is to educate person who have sexually transmitted infection or may develop one. Nurses must be knowledgeable about the most prevalent diseases and the signs and symptoms, methods used in diagnosis, treatments and where individual can obtain help and information. Many approaches to curtailing the spread of STDs have been advocated and have met with varying degrees of success. Nurses should be prepared to discuss practices with all patients, not only those who are perceived to be at risk. These 'safe' set practices include abstinence, monogamy, with an uninfected partners, avoidance of certain high risk sexual practices, and use of condoms and other barriers to limit contact with potentially-infectious body fluids or lesions. Sexual abstinence is a certain method of avoiding all STDs, but few adults consider this as feasible alternative to sexual expression. Limiting sexual intimacies, outside of a well-established monogamous relationship can reduce the risk of contracting a STD.

Nurses can exert influence on the community by taking an active role in education programs. Patient teaching should include the following:

- Explain the importance of taking all antibiotics as prescribed. Symptoms will improve after 1-2 days of therapy, but organism may still be present.
- Teach patient about the need for treatment of sexual partners with antibiotics to prevent transmission of disease.
- Instruct patient to abstain from sexual intercourse during treatment and to use of condoms when sexual activity is resumed to prevent spread of infection and prevent reinfection.
- Explain the importance of follow up examination and reculture at least once after treatment if appropriate to confirm complete cure and prevent relapse.
- Allow patient and partner to verbalize concerns to clarify areas that need explanation.

- Instruct patient about symptoms of complications and need to report problems to ensure proper follow up and early treatment of reinfection.

    Explain precautions to take, such as being monogamous, asking potential partners about sexual history, avoiding sex with partners, who has IV drugs or who have visible oral, inguinal, genital, perineal or anal lesions, using condoms; voiding and washing genitalia after intercourse (coitus) to reduce the occurrence of reinfection.

- Inform patient regarding state of ineffectivity to prevent a false sense of security, which might result in careless sexual practices and poor personal hygiene.

    All sexually active women should be screened for cervical cancer.

HIV INFECTION AND AIDS

HIV infection is one of the most dreadful diseases. Individuals infected with HIV has thus far eventually developed 'Acquired Immunodeficiency Syndrome (AIDS)'. AIDS severally compromises the body's ability to fight various infections and some forms of cancer. The incidence of HIV infections and AIDS continues to increase steadily worldwide. Therefore, nurses must understand the critical concepts related to this problem. AIDS was considered to be universally fatal until quite recently.

Advances in drug treatment, however, are delaying the onset of AIDS for selected persons infected with HIV and are giving new hopes to infected persons.

Etiology

AIDS is an acquired viral disease. The virus integrates itself into CD4 (T4 helper) cells, causing immune dysfunction and rendering the infected person unusually susceptible to life-threatening infections and malignancies. The causative agent of AIDS is infection with HIV, a human retrovirus that belongs to the Lentivirus subfamily. Several human retroviruses have been identified. Two of them, HIV-1 and HIV-2 have been associated with T4 helper cell depletion, resulting in loss of cellular immunity characterized by AIDS.

The routes for transmission of HIV are well-documented, which includes:
- Directly from person to person by sexual contact.
- Direct inoculation with contaminated blood products, needles, or syringes and
- From infected mothers to her fetus or newborn.

HIV is a fragile virus that can only be transmitted under specific conditions that allow contact with infected body fluids, including blood, semen, vaginal secretions, cerebrospinal fluid, saliva, tears and breast milk. However, blood, semen and vaginal' secretions are the primary routes of infection. Epidemiological studies indicate that transmission through body fluids such as saliva, tears and breast milk is inefficient and unlikely to produce infection.

HIV is not transmitted by casual contacts, including sneezing, coughing, spitting, handshakes, contact with potential secretions on toilet seats, bath tubs, showers, swimming pools, utensils, dishes or lime used by infected persons. Mosquito bites are not a source of infection.

HIV is a blood born STD. During any form of sexual intercourse, (anal, vaginal or oral), the risk of infection is considerably greater for the partner who received the semen, although infection can also be transmitted to an inserted partner. The increased risk occurs because the receiver has prolonged contact with the semen; this helps to explain why women are more easily infected than men during heterosexual intercourse. The risk factors for HIV infection are summarised as follows:

- Sexual practices:
    - Unprotected sex (without condom use).
    - Multiple sexual partners.
    - Anal or oral sexual activity.
    - Improper condom use or condom breakage.
    - Open sore, lesions or irritations in the genital area.
- Contaminated blood.
- Contaminated needle (For SC or 1M or IV, etc).
- Occupational exposure:
    - All health care workers-acute care long-term care, and home care (Doctors, Nurses and others).
    - Dental workers.
    - Correction officers and law enforcement personnel (Police and others).
- Perinatal exposure (during pregnancy, birth or breastfeeding).

Approximately 25 percent children of HIV-positive mothers are infected with HIV.

Pathophysiology

The natural history of HIV infection is associated with unpredictable course of disease progression. Many patients undergo a prolonged period of clinically-silent infection, often lasting for more than 10 years. Although the virus is consistently detectable throughout this time, patients typically have only soluble immunological alterations. Once the patient becomes symptomatic, however, decreases in the number of T4 helper cells can be detected and viral replication increases.

The life cycle of HIV is similar to that of the other retroviruses, mature visions interact with specific host receptors and then use the host cell for viral replication. HIV interacts with the CD4 glycoprotein, which occurs on the membrane of the specific cells, primarily the CD4+(T4) helper lymphocytes. The CD4 protein may also be found on the surface of several other cells as well, including some monocytes, macrophages, glial cells and gastrointestinal cells (GI). Presence of the CD4 and glycoprotein allow the virus fuse to the host cell. The viral core is subsequently injected into the cell cytoplasm, where the viral ribonucleic acid (RNA) genome is translated into dioxyribonucleic acid (DNA) by a retroviral enzyme called reverse transcription. Infection and subsequent viral replication eventually depletes the hosts T4 helper cells, resulting in a dramatics loss of the protective immune response against invading microorganism.

Many potential cofactors may be associated with HIV disease progression. These cofactors which may be viral, host, or environmental are thought to directly influence the replication of HIV or the severity of its pathogenic effects. Viral co-factors that may influence the progression of the disease include herpes simplex virus (HSV) cytomegalovirus) (CMV) Epstein-Barr and (EBV).

Host Co-factors may include variety of cytokines and intracellular mediators. Environmental co-factors may induce hyperactivation of the immune system, resulting in an expansion of the pool of HIV, and replicating cells. As viral replication increases and depletes the body of T4 lympocytes, the body's defense mechanism is progressively weakened. Infections that were once disarmed by the healthy immune system are eventually able to cause serious and potentially life-threatening disease. The spectrum of HIV infection ranges from a symptomatic to potentially life threatening opportunistic infection.

Clinical Manifestation

The early phases of infection with HIV varies from person to person. Some individuals experience symptoms similar to flu or mononucleosis, consisting of fever, fatigue, nausea, vomiting, headache, rash or lymphadenopathy. Symptoms may be mild or serious enough to warrant hospitalization. It is during this time that the viral load (amount of HIV present) is very high, CD and helper cells drop dramatically and the person converts to seropositive HIV status. The initial phase of infection may be followed by a period of latency that may last from several months to 10 years or more. During this time, the person may be completely asymptomatic or experience only mild symptoms such as fatigue. As the immune system becomes further compromised, the symptoms of AIDS develop. Clinical manifestations associated with AIDS are primarily those of opportunistic infections. The common symptoms include the following:

- Chills and fever
- Night sweats
- Dry productive cough
- Dyspnea
- Lethargy
- Confusion
- Stiff neck
- Seizures
- Headache
- Malaise
- Fatigue
- Oral lesions
- Skin rash
- Abdominal discomfort
- Diarrhea
- Weight loss
- Lymphadenopathy
- Progressive generalized edema

The complications of HIV disease present a complex picture of opportunistic infections, neoplasms or condition related to immunodeficiency. If not treated in time, symptoms of opportunistic infection also develop. The common AIDS—Related opportunistic infection includes the following:

- *Bacterial infections:* Mycobacterium avium complex (MAC), *Mycobacterium tuberculosis* causes fever, diarrhoea and profound wasting.
- *Fungal infections:* Candidiasis (Thrush or vaginal infection), Cryptococcosis (causes meningitis), histoplasmosis (Associated with fever and weight loss).
- *Protozoal infection:* Cryptosporidium (causes fulminant diarrhea) *Pneumocytis*, Carinu (Ac. Resp. failure), *Toxoplasma gondii* (causes encephalitis).
- Viral infections HSV, CMV, (cause Retinitis, blindness).
- *HIV related cancer:* Kaposis sarcoma, non-Hodgkin's lymphomas, cervical cancer.

HIV can cross the blood-brain barrier, attach to microglial cells and cause encephalopathy or more dysfunction.

Management

HIV infection or AIDS is diagnosed when an individual with HIV has at least one of these additional conditions:

- CD4+T cell count drops below 200/ml
- Development of one of the following opportunistic infections (OIs):
  - *Fungal:* Candidiasis of bronchi, trachea, lungs or esophgus pneumocystis carinii pneumonia (PCP), disseminated or extrapulmonary hissopharmosis.
  - *Viral:* Cytomegalovirus (CMV) disease other than liver, spleen or nodes CMV retinitis (with loss of vision); herpes simple with chronic ulcer or bronchitis, pneumonitis, or esophagitis, progressive multifocal leucoencephalopathy (PML), extrapulmonary cryptococcosis.
  - *Protozoal:* Disseminant or extrapulmonary coccidiomycosis, toxoplasmosis of the brain; chronic intestinal isosporiasis; chronic intestinal cryptosporidiasis.
  - *Bacteria:* Mycobacterium tuberculosis (any site); any disseminated or extrapulmonary mycobacterium including MAC or *M. Kansasii*, recurrent pneumonia; recurrent salmonella septicemia.
- Development of one of the following opportunistic cancers: Invasive cervical cancer and Kaposi Sarcoma (KS). Burkitts lymphoma, immunoblastic lymphoma, or primary lymphoma of the brain.
- *Wasting syndrome occurs:* Wasting syndrome defined as a loss of 10 percent or more of ideal body mass.
- *Dementia develops:* The most useful screening test for HIV are those that detect HIV-specific antibodies.

The most commonly used test is the enzyme-linked-immunosorbent assay (ELISA). A positive ELISA must be confirmed by the western blot technique. Both depend on antibody formation. The following steps are used in the process of testing blood for antibodies to HIV:
- A highly sensitive enzyme immunoassay (EIA, ELISA) is done to detect serum antibodies that bind to HIV antigens on test plates; blood samples that are negative on this test are reported as negative.
- If the blood is LIA reactive, the test is repeated.
- If the blood is repeatedly EIA reactive, a more specific confirmatory test, such as the western blot (WB) or Immunoflurescence assay (IFA) is done.
    * Western blot (WB) testing used purified HIV antigens electrophoresed on gels. These are incubated with serum samples of antibody in the serum, it is present it can be detected.
    * IFA is used to identify HIV in injected cells. Blood is located with a fluorescent antibody against pH or p24 antigen and then examined using a fluorescent microscope.
- Blood that is reactive in all of the first three steps is reported as HIV antibody positive.
- If the results are indeterminant, testing should be repeated within 6 months. Consistently in determinant test results require the use of polymerase chain reaction (PCR), viral culture, and other diagnostic measures;
    * PCR analysis DNA extracted from lymphocytes and/or HIV from serum using an invitro amplification procedure.
    * A cell culture system can be used to grow viruses from infected lymphocytes.

Since these tests are expensive and difficult to do, they are usually not used for screening purposes, but may be done in situations where the index of suspicion is high and antibodies are negative. HIV can be classified as laboratory categories as follows: (CDC 1993).

Category I : Greater than or equal to 500 CD 4 + Cells.
Category II : 200 to 499 CD4 + Cells.
Category III : Less than 200 CD4+ Cells.

HIV classification for adolescents and adults according to revised centers for Disease Control and Prevention (CDC 1993) as Clinical Categories are as follows:

Category A: One or more of the following conditions are occurring in a adolescent or adult with documented HIV infection. Conditions listed in categories B and C must not have occurred.
- Asymptomatic HIV infection.
- Persistent generalized lymphadenopathy.
- Acute (Primary) HIV infection with accompanying illness or history of acute HIV infection.

Category B: Symptomatic conditions occurring in an HIV infected adolescents or adult that are not included among conditions listed in category C and that meet at least one of the following criteria:
- The conditions are attributed to HIV infection or are indicative of a defect in cell-mediated immunity.
- The conditions are considered by physicians to have a clinical course or management that is complicated by HIV infection.

Examples of conditions in clinical category B include but are not limited to:
- Bacterial endocarditis, meningitis, pneumonia, or sepsis.
- Candidiasis and oropharyngeal (thrush).
- Cervical dysplasia, severe, or carcinoma.
- Constitutional symptoms such as fever (greater than 38.5°C) or diarrhea lasting for more than a month.
- Hairy leukoplakia, oral.
- Herpes zoster (Shingles), involving at least two distinct episodes or more than one dermatome.
- Idiopathic thrombocytopoenic purpura.
- Listeriosis.
- *Mycobacterium tuberculosis* infection and pulmonary.
- Nocardiosis.
- Pelvic inflammatory disease.
- Peripheral neuropathy.

Category C: Any condition that has occurred, the person will remain in Category C, i.e:
- The conditions clinical category C are strongly associated with severe immunodeficiency, occur frequently in HIV- infected patients and cause serious morbidity or mortality.
- According to proposed classification system, HIV-infected patient would be classified on the basis of both:
    - The lowest accurate (not necessarily the most recent) CD4+ lymphocyte determination and
    - The most severe clinical condition diagnosed regardless of the patients current clinical condition.

Treatment

There are no specific treatment in the early stages of HIV infections. Respiratory treatment may become necessary as the patient's disease progresses. Standard precautions are necessary when the patient is hospitalized or being treated at home. Treatment associated with maintenance and improvement of nutritional status also usually become necessary. Specific treatment related to opportunistic infections are briefly discussed as given below:

Respiratory System
- *Pneumocystis carinii pneumonea (PCP):* There will be nonproductive cough, hypoxemia, progressive shortness of breath, fever, night sweat and fatigue.

This is diagnosed by chest X-ray, induced sputum culture and bronchoalveolar lavage. It can be treated by Bactrim, Cleocin Mepron and Crosicosteroids.
- *Histoplasma capsulatum:* In this, there will be pneumonia, fever, cough weight loss, disseminated disease. Diagnosis made by sputum culture, serum or urine antigen assay. This is treated by using amphotericin, B, itoconazole (Sporanax) and fluconazole (Diflucon).
- *Coccidioides immitis:* There will be fever, weight loss, cough, test includes sputum culture, serology, treatment as in histoplasma capsulature.
- *Mycobacteria TB:* There will be a productive cough, fever, night sweats, weight loss, diagnosis by chest X-ray, sputum for AFB and culture. Treated by antituberculosis drugs, INH, Streptomycin, Reampicin.
- *Kaposi sarcoma:* There is dyspnea, respiratory failure, chest X-ray and biopsy all helps to diagnose. Cancer chemotherapy and radiation are the treatments.

Integumentary System

- *HSV1 and HSV2:* Orolabial mucocutaneous ulcerative lesions (Type 1) genital and perineal mucocutaneous ulcerative lesion (Type 2) Do viral culture and treat with acyclovir, famiclovir valacyclovir (valtrex).
- *Varicell Zoster vira (VZV):* Shingles, erythematous maculopapular rash along dermatromal planes, pain, pruritus are seen. Do viral culture and treat with acyclovir famuclovir (famvir) valtrax and foscarret (foscavir).
- *Kaposis Sarcoma:* Firm, flat, raised nodular, hyperpigmented, multice lesions found in skin, Do biopsy lesions. Treat with cancer chemotherapy, alpha interferon, radiation of lesions.
- *Bacillary angiomatosis:* Erythematus vascular papules, subcutaneous nodules are seen on skin. Do Biopsy and treatment with erythromycin, doxycycline.

Eye

- CMV retinitis: Lesions on the retina, blurred vision, loss of vision. Do ophthalmoscopic exam and treat with canciclovir (cytovene) foscarret or cidofovir (vistide).
- HSVI: Blurred vision: corneal lesions, acute retinal necrosis, or ophthalmoscopy examination. Treat with acyclovir, famciclovir, etc.
- VZV: Ocular lesions, acute retinal necrosis. Do ophthalmoscopy and treat with antiviral drugs.

GI System

- *Cryptosporidium muris:* Watery diarrhea, abdominal pain, weight loss, and nausea are seen. Do stool examination, small bowel or colon biopsy. Treat with anti-diarrheals, flaramomycine, azithromycin, asovaquone and sandostatin (octreotide).
- *CMV:* Stomatitis, esophagitis, gastritis, colitis, diarrhea, bloody diarrhea, pain, weight loss. Do endoscopic visualization, culture, biopsy for ruling out the causes and treat with ganciclovir and antiviral drugs.
- *HSV:* Vescicular eruption on tongue, buccal, pharyngeal or perioral esophage 1 mucose seen. Do viral culture, administer antiviral drugs.
- *Candida-Albicans:* There will be whitish-yellow patches in mouth, esophagus, GI tract. Do microscopic examination for scraping from lesion, culture. Administration of flucanozole, nystatin, clotrimazol (lotrimin), itroconazole and amphotericin B are helpful.
- *Mycrobacterium avium Complex (MAC):* There will be watery diarrhea, weight loss. Do small bowel biopsy with AFB stain and culture. Administer clarithromycin (Biaxin) rifampin, ciproflaxacin, azithromycin according to culture.
- *Isospora belli:* Diarrhea, weight loss, nausea, abdominal pain are seen. Do stool examination. Small bowel colon biopsy. Treat with trimethoprim sulfamethoxazole, pyrimethamine + folinic acid.
- *Salmonella:* Gastroenteritis, fever and diarrhea. Do stool and blood culture. Administer ciprofloxacin, ampicillin, amoxicillin-Sep.
- *Kaposi sarcoma:* There will be diarrhea, hyperpigmented lesions in mouth and GI tract. Do GI series and biopsy. Treat cancer with chemotherapy, alpha-interferon and radiation.
- *Non-Hodgkin's lymphoma:* There will be abdominal pain, fever, night sweats, weight loss, Do lymph node biopsy and treatment with chemotherapy.

Neurologic System

- *Toxoplasma gondii:* There is cognitive dysfunction, motor impairment, fever, altered mental status, headache, seizures, sensory abnormalities, diagnosis by MRI, CT scan toxoplasma serology and brain biopsy, Treat with pyrimethamine + folinic acid + sulfadiazine, clindamycin azithromycin clarithromycin.
- *JC Papovirus:* Progressive multifocal leuko-encephalopathy (PML), Mental and motor declines; diagnosis by MRI, CT scan and brain biopsy; effective antiretroviral therapy may help.
- *Cryptococcal meningitis:* There is cognitive impairment, motor dysfunction, fever, seizures, headache, CT scan, serum, antigen test, CSF analysis and will help to diagnosis. Treatment with amphaterrcin B, flucystosine, flucanozole, helps.
- *CNS lymphomas:* Cognitive dysfunction, motor impairment, aphasia, seizures, personality charges, headache, Do MRI, CT scan. Treat with radiation and chemotherapy.

- *AIDS dementia complex (ADC):* There is insidious onset of progressive diementia. Do CT scan. Effective antiretroviral therapy may help.

Nursing Management

Health assessment of all patients should include an appraisal of potential risk factors for HIV infection. For obtaining complete, accurate sexual history including past and present sexual activities, skilful interviewing techniques and professional relationship based on trust are required. Nurses need to be able to explain the need for information on intimate sexual activities and phrase questions in appropriate but comprehensive terms.

A major goal of health promotions is to prevent disease. HIV infection is preventable until a vaccine is available; education and behavioral changes are the only effective tools. Educational messages should be specific to the patients' need, culturally sensitive, language appropriate and age-specific. Nurses are excellent resources for this type of education, but nurses must be comfortable with and knowledgeable about sensitive topics such as sexuality and drug use. Risk-reducing sexual activities decrease the risk of contact with HIV through the use of barriers. Barrier should be used when engaging in insertive sexual activity (oral, vaginal or anal) with partner who is known to HIV infected or with partner whose HIV status is not known. The most commonly used barrier is the male condom. The major points for correct use of male condom are as follows:

- Use only condoms (rubber) that are made out of latex or polyurethane.
  - Natural skin. Condoms have pores that are large enough for HIV to penetrate.
- Store condom: in a cool, dry place and protect them from trauma. The friction caused by carrying them in back pocket, for instance can wear down the latex.
- Do not use condom if the expiration date has been over or if the package looks worn or punctured.
- Lubricants used in conjunction with condoms must be water soluble.
  - Oil based lubricants can weaken latex and increase the risk of tearing or breaking.
  - Nonlubricated, flavoured condom can provide protection during oral intercourse.
- The condom must be placed on the erect penis before any contact is made with the partner's mouth, vagina or rectum to prevent exposure to pre-ejaculatory secretions that may contain HIV.
- Remove the penis and condom from the partner's body immediately after ejaculation and before the erection is lost.
  - Hold the condom at the base of the penis and remove both at the same time.
- This keeps semen from leaking around the condom as the penis becomes flaccid.
- Remove the condom after use. Wrap in tissue and discard. Do not flush down the toilet as this can cause plumbing problem.
- Condoms are not reusable. A new condom must be used for every act of intercourse.

Now female condoms are also available. Use can be complicated. So careful instructions and practice are required as given below.

- Female condoms consists of a polyurethane sheath with two springs from rings:
  1. The small ring is inserted into the vagina and holds the condom in place internally. This ring can be removed if the condom is to be used in anal intercourse. It should not be removed by the condom to be used for vaginal intercourse.
  2. The larger ring surrounds the opening to the condom. It functions to keep the condom in place externally while protecting the external genitalia.
- Use only water soluble lubricants with female condoms:
  - Female condoms come prelubricated and with a tube of additional lubricant.
  - Lubrication is needed to protect the condom from tearing during sexual intercourse and can also decrease the noise that results from friction of the penis against the condom.
- Some men feel that female condom is better than the male condom. Some others like male condoms better. The only way to find out which type of condom works better is to try the both.
- Practice inserting the female condom. The steps shown in figure. Lubrication makes the condom slippery, but do not get discouraged. Just keep trying.
- During sexual intercourse, ensure that the penis is inserted into the female condom through the outer ring. There is a chance that penis will miss the opening, thus making contact with the vagina and defeating the purpose of the condom.
- Do not use a male condom at the time when a female condom is used.
- After intercourse, remove the condom before standing up.
  - Twist the outer ring to keep the semen inside. Gently pull the condom out of the vagina and discard.
  - Do not flush down the toilet, as this can cause plumbing problem.
- Do not reuse female condom.

Cleansing the equipment before use is a risk reducing activity. It decreases the risk for those who share equipment.

The patient should be taught to recognize clinical manifestation that may indicate progression of the disease so that prompt medical care can be initiated. An overview

of the symptoms the patient should report includes the following:
- Report the following signs and symptoms immediately:
  - Any change in level of consciousness, lethargy, hard to arouse, unable to arouse, unresponsive and unconscious.
  - Headache accompanied by nausea and vomiting, changes in vision, changes in ability to perform coordinated activities, or after any head trauma.
  - Vision changes; blurry or black areas in vison field, new floaters.
  - Persistent shortness of breath related to activity and not relieved by a short rest period.
  - Nausea and vomiting accompanied by abdominal pain.
  - Dehydration, unable to eat or drink, because of nausea, diarrhea, or mouth lesions; severe diarrhea or vomiting, and dizziness when standing.
  - Yellow discoloration of the skin.
  - Any bleeding from the rectum that is not related to hemorrhoids.
  - Pain in the flank with fever and unable to urinate for more than 6 hours.
  - New onset of weakness in any part of the body, new onset of numbness that is not obviously related to pressure, new onset of difficulty in speaking.
  - Chest pain not obviously related to cough.
  - Seizures.
  - New rash accompanied by fever.
  - New oral lesions accompanied by fever.
  - Severe depression, anxiety, hallucinations, delusions or possible danger to self or others.
- Report the following signs and symptoms within 24 hours:
  - New or different headache, constant headache not relieved by aspiring or acetominop.
  - Headache accompanied by fever, nasal congestion or cough.
  - Burning, itching or discharge from the eyes.
  - New or productive cough.
  - Vomiting 2-3 times a day.
  - Vomiting accompanied by fever.
  - New, significant or watery diarrhea (more than 6 times a day).
  - Painful urination, bloody urine and urethral discharge.
  - New significant rash (widespread, painful, itchy, or following a path down the leg or arm, around the chest or on the face).
  - Difficulty in eating because of lesions.
  - Vaginal discharge, pain or itching.

Nursing Diagnosis commonly used in HIV infections include the following:
- Altered family processes.
- Altered nutrition: less than body requirement.
- Altered oral mucus membrane.
- Altered sexuality problems.
- Altered thought processes.
- Anticipatory grieving.
- Anxiety.
- Body image disturbance.
- Caregiver role strain.
- Chronic low self-esteem.
- Decisional conflict.
- Diarrhea.
- Fatigue.
- Fear.
- Hyperthermia.
- Ineffective denial.
- Ineffective individual coping.
- Noncompliance.
- Pain.
- Powerlessness.
- Relocation stress syndrome.
- Self-care deficit.
- Situational low esteem.
- Sleep pattern disturbance.
- Social isolation.
- Spiritual distress.

CHAPTER 9

Nursing Management of Endocrine Disorders

INTRODUCTION

The endocrine system is an integrated chemical communication and coordination system that enables reproduction, growth and development with the nervous and immune systems, the endocrine system maintains the internal homeostasis of the body and coordinates response to external and internal environment changes. The endocrine system is composed of glands and glandular tissues that synthesize, store and secret chemical messengers (hormones) that travel through the blood to specific target cells throughout the body. The specificity of the system is determined by the affinity of reception on the target organs and tissues for a particular hormone, the 'lock and key' mechanism.

The endocrine system consists of the hypothalamus, anterior and posterior pituitary, thyroid, parathyroid, adrenal cortex, adrenal medulla pancreas, gonads, peneal body and thymus glands. Specialized endocrine cells are also located along the gastrointestinal tract. The hormones from these glands are vital to this important life transactions of the organism, including differentiation, reproduction, growth and development, metabolism adaptatation and sexual function.

NURSING ASSESSMENT OF THE ENDOCRINE SYSTEM

Normal function of all the hormones influence four broad domains which include maintenance of a normal internal environment, energy production, storage and utilization; growth and development; and reproductive and sexual functions. Hormones affect every body tissue and system causing great diversity in the signs and symptoms of endocrine dysfunction. Therefore, assessment of the endocrine system is often difficult and requires keen clinical skills to detect mainfestations because of disruption in maintenance of normal internal enviornment, inadequate energy production, storage and utilization, abnormal growth and development and abnormal reproductive and sexual function.

Systemic assessment of multiparameters is necessary to define the healthiness of a person's endocrine system or needs. The anatomical location of endocrine glands preludes their direct assessment. Endocrine dysfunction may result rom deficient or excessive hormone secretion, transport abnormalities, and inability of the target tissue to respond to a hormone or inappropriate stimulation of the target tissue to respond to a hormone, or inappropriate stimulation of the target tissue receptor. A thorough history from the patient or significant others is absolutely necessary. Special attention should be paid to the patient history, regarding fluid and nutritional intake, elemination pattern, energy level, perceptions of changes in body characteristics, reproductive and sexual function and tolerance to stressors.

Fluid/Nutritious intake: May be increased or decreased intake may not be associated with weight loss or weight gain, and also cover quantity and quality of food and fluids including alcohol and tolerance of foods.

Elimination patterns: Includes frequency, approximate amount, and color of urinary eliminations the presence of nocturia or dysuria the frequency of the color of bowel movements, constipation, diarrhea, etc.

Energy level: Performing proper activity of daily living, etc. Perception of changes in body includes changes in hair distribution, body proportions, voice, skin pigmentation, etc.

Reproduction and sexual related problems: Fragility, menstruation and pregnancy in females and impotence in males.

Tolerance to stressors: Physical and psychological stressors such as intolerance to heat and cold infection, irritation, euphoria, depression, crying and anger.

The collection of objective data about endocrine system requires a complete physical examination which includes inspection, palpation and other assessment skills.

The nurse should observe the patient's general appearance and appropriateness of dress for ambient temperature. Assessment should include the following:

- *Body size:* Height and weight compared to the table of standards or estimation of normality, size of the hand and extremities, proportionality and posture and facial features.
- *Skin:* Skin color, pigmentation, texture, coarseness, leathery texture excessive thinness, size of the sweat glands, diaphoresis, acne, strial, echymoses and vitiligo.

- *Hair:* Texture, distribution, brittleness and alopecia.
- *Face:* Color, erythema, especially on cheeks (Plethora), pained, anxious expression.
- *Eyes:* Eyebrows, hair distribution, visusl scuity, lens opacity, shape, position, movement of eyelids, lid lag, visual fields, extraocular movements, edema.
- *Nose:* Mucosa, noisy breathing.
- *Mouth:* Buccal mucosa, condition of teeth, malocclusion and mottling, tongue size and fasciculations (localized, uncoordinated uncontrollable twitching of single muscle groups) shape and size of jaw.
- *Voice:* Huskiness or hoarseness, volume, pitch and slurring.
- *Neck:* Symmetry; alignment; forceful carotid pulsation, unusual bulging of thyroid lobes behind the sternocleidomastoid muscles; trachia in midline, dullness, thickening, flabbiness of vocal cords, polyps, gray-brain hyperpigmentation on posterior neck and axillae (acanthosis nigricans); when inspecting the thyroid gland observations should be made first in the normal position, preferably with side lighting, then slight extentions and then as the patient swallows some water.
- *Extremities:* Size, shape, symmetry, proportionately (distance from symphysis pubis to foot; approximately half of total height) edema.
  - *Hands:* Tremors (a piece of paper is placed on outstretched fingers, palmdown, to assess fine tremor), muscle strength grip, thenar (ball of the thumb, westing, dupuytrens, constracture, clubbing muscle wasting.
  - *Legs:* Muscle weakness (assessed by having the seated patient extend one leg to a horizontal position; ability to hold this position for 2 minutes usually indicates normal muscle strength) bowing, color and amount of hairs, size of feet, corns, celluses and pedal pulses.
  - *Toes:* Masceration, fissures, deformities, toenails with fungal infection
  - *Reflexes:* Particularly deep tenden reflexes, relaxation time
  - *Pulses:* Rate and rhythm.
  - *Thorax:* Gynecomastia in men.
  - *Abdomen:* Increased pigmentation of scars, purplish pain on light palpation.
  - *Genitalia:* Decreased hair distribution (diamond pattern in women may indicate virilizing adrenal tumor) size of the testes, clitoral enlargement.

Inspection and palpation are used to check skin turgor, mucous membrane moisture, and jugular vein distention and to check for the presence of edema. These data will give information about the fluid and electrolyte status of the person which can be charged with almost any endocrine problem routine palpation required for thyroid, parathyroid gland and routine palpation required for thyroid, parathyroid gland and pancreas to determine the size, shape and symmetry. In addition, assessment of vital signs (TPR, BP, heart sound) routine done.

Diagnostic Studies of the Endocrine System

Accurately performed laboratory tests aid and confirm diagnosis of problems of the endocrine system. The commonly used tests are as follows:

Pituitary Studies

- *Serum studies:* Include test of growth hormone, somatomedin (insulin-like growth factor 1); GH release after exercise; insulin-induced hypoglycemia, prolactin level; FSH an LH; water deprivation tests.
- *Radiological studies:* Still X-ray, CT scan, MRI.

Thyroid Studies

- *Serum studies:* Include test for T4, T3, T3 resin uptake, Free T4, Free T3, radioactive iodine uptake TSH and calcitonin.
- *Radiological studies:* Thyroid scan.

Parathyroid

- *Serum studies:* Parathyroid hormones (PTH), total serum calcium phosphorous, 125-Dihydroxy vitamin D3 tests
- *T Radiological:* Skeletal X-ray, CT scan.

Adrenal Studies

- *Serum studies:* Cortisol, aldosterone, ACTH stimulation, dexamthosone suppression (overnight), metyrapone suppression tests.
- *Urine studies:* 17-Ketosteroid, aldosteron, free cortisol vanillylmandelic acid.

Pancreatic Studies

- *Serum studies:* FBS, oral glucose tolerance, capillary glucose monitoring and glycosylates Hb.
- *Urine studies:* Glucose (Sugar), ketone, glucose and acetone tests.

DISORDERS OF PITUITARY GLAND

Hyperfunction of the Anterior Pituitary Gland (Hyperpituitarism)

The hypothalamus and pituitary gland form a unit that controls the function of several endocrine glands—Thyroid, adrenals, and gonad as well as a wide range of physiological activities.

Etiology

Hyperfunction of the anterior portion of the pituitary gland may involve one or more hormones. A cause from the pituitary gland itself is deemed primary. If the cause is from interference with the pituitary pathway (i.e. if cause of stems from the hypothalamus) the problem is considered secondary.

Tumors of the pituitary gland are common cause of hyperfunction. Pituitry hyperfunction also can result from pituitary hyperplasia.

The cause of hyperplasia is not always known, but may be due to altered feedback signals cause the hypersecretions.

Diminished feedback from target organ secretions can result in hyperplasia and hypersecretion.

The cause of pituitary tumors or adenomas are unknown pituitary adenomas and functioning or nonfunctioning, depending on whether or not they secrete a homone. Most adenomas are benign, but can be come quite aggressive and grown to large sizes. They are classified according to the hormone being secreted. For examples, prolactinomas and growth hormons secreting tumor adenomas also are classified according to tumor size as given below:

- *Enclosed:* No invasion into the floor of the sella turcica.
- *Invasive:* Destruction of part or all of the sella turcica.
- *Microadenoma:* Enclosed tumor less than 10 mm in diameter.
- *Macroadenoma:* Enclosed tumors greater than 10 mm diameter; these tumor may show suprasellar extension.

Pathophysiology

Pituitary adenomas may depend on intrasellar adenomas, less than 1 cm in diameter that present with manifestations of hormonal excess without sellar enlargement or extraseller extension. Panhypopituitarism does not occur. Macroadenomas are the tumors larger than 11 cm in diameter and caused generalized sellar enlargement. Tumor 1 to 2 cm in diameter and confined to the sell turcica. These tumor can usually be sucessfully treated. Larger tumors especially those with suprasellar, sphenoid sinus or lateral extension are much difficult to manage and treat. Panhypopituitarism (insufficiency of pituitary hormone caused by damage or deficiency of pituitary gland), and visual loss increase in frequency with tumor size and suprasellar segment. Alteration is physiological functioning that occurs with pituitary tumors result from the presence of space occupying mass in the cranium and from the effects of the excessive secretions of hormones by functional neoplasm. In contrast, another alteration may result from the compression of glandular tissues by the tumor mass, that can cause a decrease in the secretion of one or more anterior pituitary hormones and is caused by a nonfunctional adenoma. Alteration may be neurological and endocrine alteration.

Neurological alteration occurs because the growing tumor presses on the dura, diaphragm sellae, or adjacent structure, including optic chiasm, caranial nerve II, III, IV and VI may be involved causing visual defects. Tumor may involve the neighboring bony structure and lobes further may compress or infilltrate hypothalamus. Sudden increase in size with rapid onset of neurological signs may lead to pituitary apoplexy hemorrhage into the tumor.

Endocrine alterations are depending on which hormone the adenoma is secreting a variety of effects may be seen.

Clinical Manifestation

The clinical manifestation of pituitary hormone secreting tumors include the following:

Neurological Manifestation

- Visual defects often is first seen as losses in superior temporal quadrants with progression to a hemianopia or scotomas and finally to total blindness.
- Headache
- Somnolence
- Rarely signs of increased intracranial pressure (hydrocephalus and papilledema)
- With very large tumors, disturbance in appetite, sleep, temperature regulation, and emotional balance because of hypothalamic involvement.
- Behavioral changes and seizures with expansion causing compression of the temporal or frontal lobe (very rare).

Endocrinal Manifestations

- Prolactin hypersecretion
  In females
  - Menstrual disturbances, such as irregular menses, anovulatory periods, oligomenorrhea or amenorrhea.
  - Infertility.
  - Galactorrhea.
  - Manifestations of ovarian steroid deficit; such as dyspareunia, vaginal mucusal atrophy, decreased vaginal lubrication and decreased libido.

  In males
  - Decreased libido and possible erectile dysfunction.
  - Reduced sperm count and infertility.
  - Gynecomastia
  - Galactorrhea.

  And both males and females have depressed levels of gonadal steroids.
- Growth hormone hypersecretion (acromegaly)
  - Macroadenoma with resultant headache and visual changes.
  - Changes in facial features (coarsening of features) increased size of nose, lips and skin folds; prominence of supraorbital ridges; growth of mandible resulting in prognathism and widely-

- spaced teeth; soft tissue growth resulting in facial puffiness.
- Increased size of the hands and feet and weight gain.
- Deepening of voice from thickening of vocal cords.
- Increased vertebral bodies resulting in thoracic kyphosis.
- Enlarged tongue, salivary glands, spleen, liver, heart, kidney and other organs; cardiomegaly results in increased blood pressure and signs and symptoms of congestive cardiac failure.
- Elevated blood pressure even without cardiac failure.
- Snoring, sleep apnea and respiratory failure.
- Dermatological changes; acne, increased sweating, oiliness, development of skin tags.
- Hypertrophy progressing to atrophy of skeletal muscles.
- Backache, arthralgia, or arthritis from point damage and bony overgrowth.
- Peripheral nerve damage, such as carpal tunnel syndrome or neuropathies, from bony overgrowth and change in nerve size.
- Impaired glucose tolerance progressing to diabetes mellitus.
- Changes in fat metabolism resulting in hyperlipidemia.
- General changes in mobility; presence of lethargy and fatigue
- Osteoporosis.
- Radiographic findings indicative of bony proliferation in hands, feet, skull, ribs and vertebrae.
- Electolyte change, increased urinary excretions of calcium; elevated blood phosphate level.

Gonadotrophic hypersecretion: The incidence of gonadotrophic hypersecretion occurs more in male than female, highest incidence is in middle age, in which follicle-stimulating hormone (FSH) is more common and also luteinizing hormone (LH) secretion. The clinical mainfestation, the ptient will have history of normal pubertal development and fertility, but there will be hypersecretions of only FSH result in secondary to hypogonadism.

Management

In addition to history and physical examination, diagnosis is confirmed by routine pituitary studies.

Pituitary adenomas are treated with surgery, radiation or drugs to suppess hypersecretion by adenoma. Pituitary surgery is initial therapy of choice by many surgeons, and the transphenoidal microsurgical approach to the sella turcica in the procedure of choice. Transfrontal craniotomy is required only in the occasional patient with massive suprasellar extension of the adenoma.

Pituitary radiation is usually reserved for patients with larger tumors who have had an incomplete resectin of large pituitary adenomas. Both surgery and radiation have its own advantages and complications. The common complication in hypopituitarism, damage to optic nerve mechanism, seizures, radionecroses of brain tissue.

Medical management of pituitary adenoma became feasiblity with the availability of bromcriptive, a dopamine agonist, bromocriptine a dopamine agonist. The drug is most sucessful in the treatrment of hyperprolactinemia and is also useful in selected patients with acromegaly or Cushing's disease. Octreotide acetate, a analogy is used in the therapy of acromegaly and TSH secreting adenomas.

The patient with pituitary adenoma will need teaching and support to deal with a variety of issues including body image, changes, anxiety, sexual functioning, active tolerance and homegoing medications.

The patients who have undergone surgery with transphenoidal resection are advised to avoid activities causing incrased intracranial pressure. Bending over at the waist, blowing to the nose forcefully, coughing and straining with defecation can increased intracranial pressure. Teaching should be inclusive of strategies to prevent constipation and its avoidance of such activity. Assistance may be needed with activities of daily living.

PROLACTIN HYPERSECRETION

Prolactin (PRL) hypersecretion is the most common endocrine abnormality caused by hypothalamic-pituitary disorders and PRL is the hormone most commonly secreted in excess by pituitary adenoma.

Etiology

The causes of prolactinemia are physiological, pathological and pharmacological and include the following:
- *Physiological:* Prolactinoma, primary hyperthyroidism chronic renal failure, polycystic ovarian syndrome; Cushing's disease; hypothyroidism, acromegaly, chest wall trauma; spinal cord injury and idiopathic.
- *Pharmacological*
    - Psychotrophic agent: Neuroleptics (phenothiazone, chlorpromozon and haloperidol.
    - Antidepressants: Trycyclics, impiramine, monoamino oxidase inhibitors.
    - Anxiolytics: Benzodiazepines.
    - Antiemetics: Metoclopramide, sulpiride.
    - Opiates: Methodone, morphine.
    - Gastrointestinal agents: Metodopramide, cisapride, dompiridone
    - Bet blockers: Ranitidine, cemetidine, femotidine
- Antihypertensive: Resrpin, methyldopa.
- Calcium Channel Blocker: Verapamil
- Hormones: Estrogens, Thyrotrophin-releasing hormone (TRH).

Pathophysiology and Clinical Manifestation

Normal serum prolactin levels are usually less than 20 mg/ml. Prolactin is a natural contraceptive (inhibits gonadotropin-releasing hormone (GRH) and is necessary for lactation).

The clinical manifestations of PRL excess are the same regardless of cause. The classic features are galactorrhea and amenorrhea in women and galactorrhea, decreased libido or erectile dysfunction in men.

Pathophysiological mechnism of prolactin hypersecretion include dopamine disorder, hypersecretion of pituitary tumors, hypothalamic thropin, releasing hormones stimulation, neugenic secretions triggered by chest irritation (rib fracture) anorectomy, or herpes zoster and decreased clearance of prolactin as seen in chronic renal failure.

Management

The assessment of patient with galactorrhea or unexplained gonodal dysfunction with normal or low plasma gonadotrophin levels should include a history regarding menstrual status, pregnancy, fertility, sexual function and symptoms of hypothyroidism or hypopituitarism. Current and previous use of medication shall be documented.

All patients with PRL-secretioning macroadenomas should be treated, because of the risks of further tumor expansion. Hypopituitarism and visual impairment. Treatment for patient with microadenoma is also recommended to prevent early osteoporosis.

Surgical treatment of choice is resection of the adenoma with the transsphenoidal approach. Medical treatment consists mainly of brocogrippine, a potent domain against the stimulate, dopamine and affects hypothalemia and pituitary levels. The dosage 2.5 to mg/dl orally in divided doses. Side effects such as dizziness postural hypertension, nausea, that can be minimized by gradually increasing the dose. Another drug used is pergolide mesylate (dose 25 to 300 mg/dl).

The teaching needs of the hyperprolactinemia are similar to those of person with hyperpituitarism.

GROWTH HORMONE HYPERSECRETION

Growth hormone (GH), an anabolic hormone promotes protein synthesis and mobilizes glucose and free fatty acids. Overproduction of GH which is usually caused by a benign pituitary adenoma (tumor) causes gigantism or acromegaly chracterized by soft tissue and bony overgrowth.

Pathophysiology

In acromegaly, chronic GH hypersecretion is usually related to a pituitary adenoma. The secretion remains episodic, although the number, amplitude, and duration of secretory episodes increased and occur randomly. The characteristic nocturnal surge is absent, and there are abnormal responses to suppression and stimulation. Therefore, glucose suppressibility is lost and GH stimulation by hypoglycemia, is usually absent. Most of the deterious effects of chromic GH hypersecretion are caused by its stimulation of excessive amount of insulin like growth factor-1 (IGF-1 a protein secreted by the liver) and palsma levels of this are increased in acromegaly. The growth promoting effects of IGF-1 lead to the characteristic proliferation of bone, cartilage and soft tissues and increase in size of other organs to produce the classic clinical manifestation of acromegaly. The insulin resistance and carbohydrate intolerance seen in acromegaly appear to be direct effect of GH and not due to IGF-1 excess.

Clinical Manifestation

Symptoms of acromegaly begin insidiously in the third and fourth decades of life and both genders are affected equally. When the problem develops after epiphyseal closure bones increase in thickness and width. Physical features include enlargement of the hands, feet and paranasal and frontal sinuses include enlargement of the hands, feet and paranasal and frontal sinuses and deformities of the mandible and spine. In addtion, enlargement of the soft tissue (e.g. tongue, skin, abdominal organs causes manifestation such as speech difficulties and hoarseness, coarsening of facial features, abdominal distention and sleep apnea. The sleep apnea may be related to upper airway narrowing or may be central in origin. Persons with acromegaly may have hypertension, cardiomegaly, left ventricular hypertrophy, diaphoresis, oily skin, peripheral neuropathy, proximal muscle weakness, and joint pain, women exhibit menstrual disturbances.

The enlarged pituitary gland can exert pressure on surrounding structures, leading to visual disturbances and headaches. HG mobilizes stored fat for energies; it increases free fatty acids levels in the blood and predisposes patients to atherosclerosis. Prolonged secretion of GH is diabetogenic which leads to hyperglycemia.

Management

Diagnostic measures include evaluation of plasma GH and IGF 1 levels, IGF binding protein 3 (IGF BP-3), oral glucose tolerance tests. MRI, CT scan for locating tumor and ophthalmologic examination.

The therapeutic goal in acromegaly and gigantism is to return GH levels to normal. This is accomplished by surgery, radiation, drug therapy, or combination of the three.

Surgery is most commonly accomplished with transsphenoidal approach, in which an incision is made in the inner aspects of the upper lip and gingiva. The sella turcica is entered through the floor of the nose and sphenoid sinuses.

The goal of transphenoidal microsurgery removes only the GH - secreting adenoma. Sometimes pituitary gland may be destroyed and removed, which result in deficiency of hormone of anterior pituitary which requires parental administration of the essential hormones produced by target organs (glucocorticoids, thyroid hormone and certain sex homones).

Conventional radiotherapy is also successful, although a much longer period is required to reduce GH levels to normal streotactic radiosurgery (gamma surgery) may be applied to small, surgically inaccessible pituitary tumors.

Drug therapy may include the use of bromocriptine (parlodel), a dopamine agonist or octreotide (Sandostatin), a somastatin analog that reduce GH levels to within the normal range in many patients. The GH lowering effects of these drugs are seldom complete or permanent and they are often used adjuvant to other therapies or to reduce tumor size before surgery.

Nursing interventions include assessment of signs and symptoms of abnormal tissue growth and evaluates physical size of each patient from time to time, and physical application, symptom of diabetes mellitus and cardiovascular disease.

The individual treated surgically needs skilled neurosurgical nursing care and must be prepared before surgery for postoperative care. Nursing intervention includes preoperative instillation of bacteracin nose drops, discussion of mouth breathing, mouth care, ambulation, pain control, activity and hormone replacement. The patient should be instructed to avoid vigorous coughing, sneezing and straining at stool (valsalva maneuver) to prevent CSF leakage from the point at which sella turcica was entered, and skilled postoperative neurosurgical care should be procide. The complication of surgical intervention includes transient diabetes insipidus, meningitis, infection, CSF rhinorrhea and hypopituitarism. Dieting and activities recommended according to problem rised, e.g. DM, CHF, etc.

HYPOPITUITARISM

Hypopituitarism is a rare disorder that involves a decrease in one or more of the anterior pituitary hormones, i.e. Growth hormones (GH) Adrenocorticotropic hormone (ACTH), Gonadotropic hormone (GTH), Protactin (PRL), Thyroid stimulation hormone (TSH) and non-functioning pituitary adenomas. Any combination of deficit of the six major harmones may occur in hypopituitarism.

Etiology

Hypopituitarism may be classified in number of ways, isolated, partial or panhypopituitary transient or permanent idiopathic or organic, and primary (Pituitary) or secondary (affecting hypothalamic releasing factors). Several disorders can interfere with the function of interior pituitary gland and cause hyposecretion of one or more hormones or hypopituitarism which includes the following:

- *Tumors:* Craniopharyngioma; primary CNS tumors; nonsecreting pituitary tumor.
- *Ischemic changes:* Sheehan's syndrome Ischemic changes following postpartum hemorrhage or infections resulting shock
- *Developmental abnormalities.*
- *Infections:* Viral encephalities, bacteremia and tuberculosis.
- *Autoimmune disorders*
- *Radiation:* Damage, particularly after treatment of secreting adenomas of pituitary gland
- *Trauma:* Including surgery.

Pathophysiology

In hypopituitarism, the symptoms vary widely depending on the cause and the endocrine dysfunction present. If tumor is the cause, symptoms resulting from growth of a space-occupying lesion in the cranium, effects resulting from pressure on the optic chiasm and potential disturbances of the cranial nerves III, IV, and VI. If the tumor arises from regions surrounding the pituitary such as Rathke's pouch (craniopharyngiomas), the hypothalamus, or the third ventricle, the neurological signs and symptoms will be more severe and include manifestation of increased intracranial pressure.

The endocrine dysfunction may be the result of hypothalamic damage of primary pituitary disease. The most frequent pathophysiological alteration results from lack of synthesis and secretion of ganodotropin. The patients with hypopituitarism exhibit all or only selected aspects of these hormonal deficiency. Usually the pathological alteration progresses slowly.

Clinical Manifestations

Clinical findings associated with pituitary hypofunction vary with the degree and speed of onset of pituitary dysfunction and are related to hyposecretion of the target glands. The symptoms are often and commonly included weakness, fatigue, headache, sexual dysfunction fasting hypoglycemia, dry and skin, diminished tolerance stress, and poor resistance to infection. In the adults, premature wrinkling around the eyes and mouth is common. Psychiatric symptoms include apathy, mental slowness, delusions, orthostatic hypertension. The common clinical manifestation of hypopituitarism include the following:

- Manifestation based on causes, such as bacteremia, viral hepatis, autoimmune disorders and trauma.
- Manifestation such as vision changes, papilledema or hydrocephalus if cause is tumor
- Manifestation of gonadotropin deficiencies.

- Decreased Serum levels of FSH, LH and gonadal steroids.
- Children- delayed puberty.
- Adults.
  - Women—Oligomenorrhea, or amenorrhea, uterine and vaginal atrophy, potential atrophy of breast tissue, loss of libido, decrease in body hair and decreased breast size.
  - Man—loss of libido, decreased sperm count, possible erectile dysfunction, decreased testicular size, decreased total body hair, impotence.
- Manifestations of growth hormone deficiency.
  - Children
    - Stunted growth (below third percentile) with normal body proportions, excessive subcutaneous fat, poor muscle development.
    - Immature facial features and immature voice.
    - Slow growth of nails and thin hair.
    - Delayed puberty but eventual normal sexual development.
    - Decreased level of GH.
  - Adults
    - Severe, short stature
    - Immature faces
    - Moderate obesity
    - Decreased muscle mass and weakness
    - Lassitude
    - Emotional liability
    - Decreased basal levels of GH or decreased response to provocative testing.
    - Some person may have normal GH level with low level somatomeding (IGF-1).
- Manifestations of prolectin deficiency.
  - Failure to lactate in the postpartum women (Sheehan's syndrome).
  - Decreased serum levels of prolactin.
- Manifestations of Thyroid stimulating hormone (TSH) deficiency. Signs and symptoms of secondary hypothyroidism-anorexia, bulimia.
  - Decreased serum levels of TSH and thyroid hormone.
- Manifestation of ACTH deficiency
  - Signs and symptoms of secondary ACTH insufficiency; no hyperpigmentation
  - Decreased levels of ACTH, glucocorticoids and adrenal and organs (aldosterone levels may be normal).

Management

The decision to treat a patient is based on symptoms of a mass lesion including headache, impaired vision, and cranial nerve palsy and other factors include concerned hormonal deficiency. Treatment of hypopituitarism consists of surgery, or radiation for tumor removal, permanent target gland hormone replacement and nutrition dietary plan. Replacement therapy is carried out with corticosteroids, thyroid hormone, and sex hormones. Gonadotropin can some time restore fertility.

A primary nursing role in anterior pituitary insufficiency is assessment and recognition of subtle signs and symptoms. Nursing care focusses on assisting the patient to effectively cope with change in the body image and teaching about treatment protocol. Some symptoms are reversible once the treatment is initiated. Treatment with sex steroids helps to initiate the development of sexual characteristics and adolescent entering puberty. Treatment with sex steroids restores secondary sexual characteristics in adults, and treatment with gonadotropins restores fertility in the women with normal menstrual cycles. Helping patients identify their strength, coping strategies may help them to deal with body image disturbances and decreased self-esteem that may result from their illness.

Patient education is another focus of nursing care. The patient must be prepared for various diagnostic tests including blood tests and roentgenograms, CT scans, or MRI of the head. If a tumor is a cause of the deficiency, the tumor is removed. Hormonal replacement of therapy with gonadal steroids and gonadotropin in adolescents and in adults are individualized. The patient needs to be taught about prescribed dedication GHs are given subcutaneously. Gonadal steroids are given orally to restore sexual characteristics and gonadotropin or clomiphene is used in women to induce ovulation if pregnancy is desired. Patients should be taught that steroids are effective in preventing premature bone demineralization. Patient who declines hormone therapy, particularly women, need to be monitored periodically for accelerated bone loss and must take adequate calcium.

HYPERFUNCTION OF POSTERIOR PITUITARY

The hormone secreted by the posterior pituitary are antidiuretic hormones (ADH), is also called arginine vasopressin (AVP) and oxytocin. These hormones are formed in the hypothalamus and stored in the posterior pituitary. ADH contributes to fluid balance by controlling renal reabsorption of free water. It also has potent vasoconstriction properties. Oxytocin controls lactation and uterine contraction. Oxytocin excess is not recognized as a clinical problem. This hormone is administered pharmacologically in the management of labor.

SYNDROME OF INAPPROPRIATE ANTI-DIURETIC HORMONE

Syndrome of inappropriate anti-diuretic hormone (SIADH) is also called Schwartz-Bartter syndrome occurs as a result of the excessive release of ADH (vasopressin), resulting in fluid and electrolyte imbalance of those indicated by the plasma osmotic pressure.

SIADH is characterized by fluid retention, serum hypo-osmality, dilutional hyponatremia, hypochloremia, concentrated urine in the presence of normal or increased intravascular volume and normal renal function.

Etiology

SIADH has various causes which include the following:
- *Pulmonary disorders:* Malignant neoplasms (e.g. oat cell adenocarcinoma of lung), tuberculosis, ventilator patients receiving positive pressure and lung abscesses pneumonia, COPD.
- *Other malignancies:* Duodenum, pancreas, prostatic lymphoma, sarcoma, leukemia, Hodgkin's lymphoma, non-Hodgkin lymphoma and thymonia.
- *CNS disorders:* Tumors infection (meningitis), trauma (subarachnoid hemorrhage), cerebrovascular accident, surgery GBS, SLE, encephalitis and skull fracture.
- *Endocrine disorders:* That result in hypovolemia and impair free water excretion, particularly if associated with fluid replacement (adrenal insufficiency and anterior pituitary insufficiency).
- *Drugs:* Such as clofibrate, chlorpropamide, thiazides, vineristine, cyclophosphomide, morphine, general anesthetic agents, opiods, trycyclic antidepressants and carbamazopine, oxytocin and narcotics.
- *Stressors:* Fear, acute infections, pain, anxiety, trauma and surgery.

Pathophysiology

In patients with SIADH total body water increases because of water retention and hypo-osmolar state results from hyponatremia. ADH release follows one of four patterns.
- ADH release is erratic and unrelated to plasma osmolality.
- ADH release varies with plasma osmolality, but osmostat has been reset, and ADH release occurs at lower plasma osmolality.
- ADH release is normal, but the patient is more sensitive to the released ADH or some unmeasured factor, that increases water retention is released. ADH or some unmeasured factor, that increases water retention is released.
- The abnormally-released ADH or the increased sensitivity of cells to ADH increases the permeability of the distal renal tubules and collecting ducts to water, and water reabsorption by the kidney increases. Intravascular volume increases but edema does not occur due to natriuresis (urinary sodium excretion). Natriuresis is a result of enhanced glomerular filtration and decreased proximal tubular sodium reabsorption, even with hyponatremia. Hyponatremia results in hypo-osmolality and creates an osmolar gradient across the blood brain barrier and other cellular membrane. This osmolar gradient results in water movement into the brain and other cells and cellular hydration.

Clinical Manifestation of SIADH

- *Early symptoms:* Anorexia, nausea, vomiting, weight gain, muscle weakness, irritability, mild disorientation, malaise, hostility, anxiety unco-operativeness.
- Late symptoms: Lethargy, headache, decreased deep tendon reflexes coma and seizures.
- Fluid and electrolyte changes:
  - Decreased plasma sodium and plasma osmolality.
  - Increased urinary sodium and urinary osmolality.
  - Decreased urinary volume.
  - Absence of edema.

Management

The treatment goal is to restore normal fluid volume and osmolality medical management of acute SIADH focuses on treating the etiologic factor (e.g. carcinoma or infection) and correcting or at least restoring toward normal, the plasma sodium level and plasma osmolality. Water restriction is the first priority. Water may be restricted to as little as 500 ml/day oral salt intake is increased if the patient is able to take oral nutrients.

In chronic SIADH, water restriction of 800 to 1000 ml/day is recommended. Regardless of etiology, demeclocyclin (Occlimycin) a tetracyclin that causes nephrogenic diabetes insipidius is useful. This drug blocks the action of ADH source, severe hyponatremia is treated with hypertonic saline and loop diuretic such as lasix.

Nursing care of the person with SIADH includes the following:

Perform Careful Nursing Assessment

- Identify patients at high risk.
- For high-risk patient, monitor daily weights, daily intake and output accurately, daily serum and urinary sodium levels and osmolality, vital signs and neurological states every 4 hours. Report any decrease below normal and serum sodium (1-1.25 m Eq/L) any signs of fluid retention (increased weight and decreased output) and any neurological changes (headache, or nausea or decreased responsiveness or LOC).
- For patients with diagnosed SIADH being treated aggressively with hypertonic sodium or loop diuretics, the frequency of monitoring is increased to every 1 to 2 hours. Any deterioration in neurological status is reported immediately.
- For patients with chronic SIADH, monitor weight daily to weekly and report any increase not attributed to

dietary changes or any complaint of nausea, headache or lethargy. Monitoring by the nurse in OPD is the same as for the hight risk person.

Provide Supportive Care

- Restrict fluids as prescribed until normalization of serum sodium (if appropriate).
- Control discomfort from thirst:
  - Space fluid intake throughout the 24 hours period.
  - Use inches, which allow more frequent relief of thirst with less fluid intake.
  - Provides frequent mouth care.
- Administer drugs and fluids as ordered.
- Positioning head of bed. Flat or with no more than 10 degrees of elevation to enhance venous return to heart and increase left atria filling pressure and reducing antidiuretic hormone release.
- Positioning side rails up because of potential alteration in mental status.
- Turning of patient every 2 hours, proper positioning, range of motion exercise, massage (if patient is bedridden.)
- Use of seizure precautions such as padded side rails and dimlighting.
- Assistance with ambulating.
- Provision from frequent oral hygiene.
- Patient and family teaching should include the information about the following:
- Review the purpose and management of fluid restriction.
- Review self-monitoring required on a long-term basis (intake and output measurement, weight change).
- Discuss drug therapy as appropriate.

DIABETES INSIPIDUS (DI)

Pituitary Diabetes Insipidus (DI) results from lack of sufficient ADH either from inadequate levels of circulating ADH, insufficient pituitary release of ADH or accelerated degradation of circulating ADH. Central DI occurs where any organic lesion of the hypothermia. In fundibular, stem or posterior pituitary interferes with ADH synthesis, transport, or release.

Etiology

The cause of pituitary DI may be central brain or pituitary tumors, head trauma, encephalitis, meningitis, hypophysectomy or cranial surgery. The cause is often idiopathic. Nephrogenic DI is a second form of the disorder and results from failure of the renal tubules to respond to ADH. The cause of nephrogenic DI may be chronic renal failure, sickle cell anemia, and Sjögren's syndrome. Diabetes insipidus may be transient or permanent. Postsurgical DI is permanent, transient DI associated with pregnancy is caused by an excessive amount placental secreted vasopressinase that neutralizes ADH activity.

Pathophysiology

The lack of adequate ADH or an ineffective kidney response to ADH results in insufficient water reabsorption by the kidney. The loss of excessive water from the body (polyuria) stimulates the perception of thirst (polydipsia). If the problem stimulates the perception of thirst (polydipsia). If the problem is long standing, diabetes insipidus can result in an increased bladder capacity and hydronephrosis. When inadequate water replacement occurs, CNS and vascular changes from hyperosmolality and volume depletion can occur.

Clinical Manifestation of DI

Polyuria: Increased urination, as much as 20, frequencies of urine per day may be excreted; urine is dilute with specific gravity of 1.005 or less osmolality of 200 or less.

Polydipsia: Increased thirst, patient favors cold or ice drinks.

- Only slightly elevated serum osmolality because of water intake usually is maintained. (Most patients compensate for fluid loss by drinking large amount of water).
- Abnormal results of tests for urine concentration:
  - Water deprivation test; No increase in urine concentration with either pituitary or nephrogenic DI.
  - ADH replacement; Increase in urine osmolality with pituitary
  - DI, but no response with nephrogenic DI.
- Sleep disturbance from polyuria.
- Inadequate water replacement results in:
  - Hyperosmolality; irritability, mental dullness, coma, hyperthermia
  - Hypovolemia; hypertension, tachycardia, dry mucus membrane, poor skin turger. Weight loss, shock and constipation.

Management

The therapeutic goal is maintained of fluid and electrolyte balance. This goal may be accomplished by IV administration of fluid (saline and glucose) and by hormone replacement with ADH (vasopressin) administer either SC, IM or IV. In acute DI, fluids should be administered at rate that decreases the serum sodium by about 1 mEq/2 every 2 hours. Clofibrate Atromid), Carbamazepine (Tegretol) and thiazide may also be prescribed for symptomatic DI. For long-term therapy, desopress in acetates. An analog of ADH that is administered as a nasal preparation and does not have the vasoconstrictive effects, is the preferred therapy.

Nursing care of the patient with DI is based in the clinical symptoms. Fluid volume deficit manifested by hypertension, tachycardia and rapid, shallow respiration can be detached early by frequent assessment. Polyuria and nocturia can cause disturbances in rest and sleep pattern.

Nursing intervention for the person with diabetes insipidus focus on the following:
- Maintain fluid and electrolyte balance: Monitor intake and output, daily weight, urine specific gravity, vital signs (orthostic), skin turgor, and neurological status every 1 to 2 hours during the acute phase, then every 4 to 8 hours until discharge and again return to physician or OPD clinics.
- Provide fluids be sure patient can reach them.
- Administer drugs as ordered, which includes
  - Arginine vasopressin 0.25-0.5 mg SC or IM
  - Lysin vasopressin (Dypressin) 3-8 dose/24 hr-nasal spray.
  - Pitressin tannate in oil, 10-40 mg /1-3 doses/week IM.
  - Desmopressin (DDAVP) s-10 mg/dose/1-2-doses/24 hr. Nasal inhalation.

Except desmopressin, other preparations mentioned here interact with V1 and V2 receptors. This pressor side effects can occur including abdominal cramping, hypertension and angina.

In addition, patient and family teaching should include inform about diagnostic test, drug therapy and side effects and instruction regarding self management.

DISORDERS OF THE THYROID GLAND

Thyroid hormone, thyroxine (T4) and triiodothyronine (T3) which is the more active form, regulate energy metabolism and growth and development. Alterations in the thyroid gland may be associated with hypersecretion, hyposecretion of normal secretion of thyroid hormone. Thyroid disorders are manifested as hyperfunction (thyrotoxicosis), hypofunction, inflammation or enlargement (goiter may interfere with surrounding structures and can be associated with increased, normal or decreased hormone production.

HYPERTHYROIDISM

Hyperthyroidism is defined as sustained, increased synthesis and release of thyroid hormone by the thyroid gland. Thyrotoxicosis is hypermetabolism that results from excess circulating levels of T4 T3 or both. Hyperthyroidism and thyrotoxicosis usually are together as in Graves' disease. However, in some forms of thyroiditis, thyrotoxicosis may occur without hyperthyroidism.

Etiology

The incidence of hyperthyroidism is 4 to 10 times greater in women and the highest frequency is in the 30-50 years age group. The cause and definitions of different hyperthyroidism includes the following:
- *Toxic diffuse goiter* (Graves' disease) is an autoimmune disorder characterized one or more of the following diffuse goiter, hyperthyroidism, infiltrate ophthalmopathy and infiltration dexmopathy. The etiology is unknown. The patient who is genetically susceptible becomes sensitized to and develops antibodies (TSABs) against various antigens within the thyroid gland and often other tissue as well. TSABs (thyroid stimulating antibodies) stimulate the TSH receptor on the thyroid hormone. Precipitating factors such as insufficient iodine supply, infection and stressful life events may interact with genetic factors that control immunology and metabolic abnormalities to cause Graves' disease.
- *Toxic multinodular goiter* (Plummer's disease) is a disorder characterized by the presence of many thyroid nodules and a milder form of hyperthyroidism is seen with Graves' disease. Plummer's disease frequency is highest in women and it is more common in iodine deficient areas.
- *Toxic adenoma* Single or occasionally multiple adenomas of follicular cells that secrets and function independent of TSH.
- *Thyroiditis* is an inflammatory process in the thyroid and can have several causes such as subacute granulomatus (de Quervains) thyroiditis which is due to bacterial or fungal infection. There is increased amount of T4 and T3 released during acute inflammatory process; transient hyperthyroid states followed by return to state, and eventually to hyperthyroid state chronic immune thyroid. (Mashimotos thyroiditis) as a gland is destroyed by the recurring inflammatory exacerbations; hyperthyroid state usually requires no treatment.
- *T3 thyrotoxicism* T3 level elvated but cause is unknown. T4 but have signs and symptoms of thyrotoxicosis.
- *Hyperthyroidism caused by metastatic thyroid cancer* Rare because thyroid cancer cells do not concentrate iodine efficiently may occur and may large follicular carcinoma.
- *Pituitary hyperthyroidism* Rare pituitary adenomas may secrete excesses TSH; treatment involves removal of pituitary tumor.
- *Chronic hyperthyroidism* Chronic gonadotropin has weak thyrotropin activity; tumors such as choriocarcinoma, embryonal cell carcinoma and hydatixform mole have high concentrations of chorionic gonadotropins that can stimute T4 and T3 secretions; hyperthyroidism disappear with treatment of tumor.
- *Struma ovarii* Ovarion dermoid tumor made up of thyroid tissue that secretes thyroid hormone.
- *Factitious hyperthyroidism* Results from ingestion of exogenous thyroid extraction.
- *Iodine induced hyperthyroid* Over production of thyroid hormone resulting from administration of supplemental iodine to a person with endemic goiter.

Pathophysiology

In hyperthyroidism from any cause, the normal regulating control of thyroid function is lost, resulting in an increased concentration of thyroid hormone and increased peripheral manifestations of thyroid hormone excess. Thyroid hormone increases metabolic rate and calorigenises alters protein, fat and carbohydrate metabolism, directly stimulate some body systems such as bone and bone marrow and increase sympathetic (adrenergic) activity. The underlying pathophysiology of all manifestations is not known. However, the effects of hyperthyroidism on body system are well known and occur in large part because of the interaction of the hypermetabolic static, increased circulation and adrenergic stimulation.

In Graves' disease, ophthalmopathy, may precede, coincide with are following hyperthyroidism. The changes may be infiltrative or noninfiltrative or both. In infiltrative, the eyeballs protrude from the orbits (exophthalmos proptosis). This is due to impaired venous drainage from the orbits which causes increased fat deposits and fluid (edema) in retroorbital tissues. Because, if increased pressure, the eyeballs are forced to outward and protrude. In noninfiltrative, the upper lids are usually retracted and elevated with sclera above the iris visible. When the eyelids do not close completely, the exposed corneal surfaces become dry and irritated. Serious consequences such as corneal ulcer and eventual loss of vision occur.

Clinical Manifestation

The manifestation of thyroid hyper functions are systemwise and include the following:

Cardiovascular systolic hypertension; increased rate and force of cardiac contractions; bound and rapid pulse; increased cardiac output; cardiac hypertrophy; systolic murmurs; arrhythmias; palpitations; atrial fibrillation (in order adult); angina.

Respiratory increased respiratory rate; dyspnea on mild exertion.

Gastrointestinal increased appetite, thirst; weight loss; increased peristalsis; diarrhea, frequent defecation; increased bowel sound; splenomegaly and hepatomegaly.

Integumentary warm, smooth, moist skin; thin, brittle nails detached from nail bed (nydrolysis); hair loss (may be patchy); acropachy (clubbing), palmer erythema; fine silky hair premature graving (in mendioaphoresis; vitiligo).

Musculoskeletal fatigue, muscle weakness especially proximal, proximal muscle wasting; pretibial myxedema; dependant edemas osteoporosis.

Nervous system Difficulty in focussing eyes. Nervousness; fine tremor (of fingers and tongue); insomnia; liability of mood, delirium; restlessness; personality changes of irritability, agitation; exhaustion; hyper reflexion of tendon reflexes; depression, fatigue, apathy (in older adult); Lack of ability to concentrate; stupor; and coma.

Reproductive Menstrual irregularities; amenorrhea; decreased libido.

Others Intolerance to heat; increased sensitivity to stimulant drugs; elevated basal temperature, lid lag, stare, eyelid retraction, exophthalmos, goiter, raid speech.

Ophthalmopathy in Graves' Disease

Signs

Bright eyes stare: Results from retraction of the upper eyelid.

- Lid lag: on downward gaze, upper lidlag, behind the globe movement and sclera seen between lid and limbus.
- Globe lag: Globe lag behind lid with upward gaze.
- Lid movement; Jerky and spasmodic.
- Eyes partly open when sleeping.
- Periorbital edema.

Symptoms

- Sense of irritation and excessive tearing.
- Feeling of pressure behind eyes.
- Complaints of blurred or double vision, easy tiring of eyes.

Complication

- Corneal ulceration.
- Optic nerve involvement (optic neuropathy).
- Myopathy of extraocular muscles.

Management

When hyperthyroidism is suspected, various diagnostic tests are necessary to confirm diagnosis in addition to history and physical examination and ophthalmologic examination, which includes ECG and laboratory tests such as serum T3 Ru, T4, free T3, TSH levels, and TRH stimulation test, and thyroid scan also is useful.

Three classes of medications are used in the treatment of hyperthyroidism, which include the following:

1. *Antithyroids* of thioamide, which inhibit the synthesis of thyroid hormone and propylthiouracil (PTU) and methimazole (Tapezole)
2. *Iodides* Which primarily inhibits the release of thyroid hormone, e.g., Radioactive iodine (RAI). RAI therapy are being increasingly used because:
   - It can be given on outpatient basis.
   - It is safer for wider range of patients including elderly persons who are poorer surgical runs.
   - It can result in faster improvement in thyroid function than antithyroid drug therapy and
   - Although still controversial, can be used in women of childbearing age.

It is administered orally in one dose, average dose 80 to 90 per/g of thyroid tissue. Treatment can be repeated after six months.

3. Beta-adrenergic blockers such as propranolol (Inderal) calcium antagonists the effect; thyroid hormone on body cells.

Surgery is no longer the treatment of choice with Graves' diseases, if indicated, surgical techniques include the removal of one lobe (subtotal thyroidectomy) or removal of the gland (total thyroidectomy).

Nursing Management

A restful, calm, quick room should be provided because of increased metabolism causes sleep disturbances. Provision of adequate rest may be a challenge because of the patient's irritability and restlessness. Nursing intervention may include:

- Placing the patient in a cool room, away from very ill patients and noisy high traffic areas.
- Using light bed coverings and changing the linen frequently if the patient is diaphoretic.
- Encouraging and assisting with exercise involving large muscle groups (tumors can interfere with small muscle coordination) to allow the release of nervous tension and restlessness.
- Restricting visitors who upset the patient and
- Establishing a supportive, trusting relationship to help the patient to cope with aggravating events and lessen anxiety.

If exophthalmos is present, there is potential for corneal injury related to irritation and dryness. The patient may have orbital pain. Nursing intervention to relieve eye discomfort and prevent corneal ulceration include applying artificial tears to soothe and moisten conjunctival membrane, salt restriction may help to reduce preorbital edema. Elevation of the patient's head promotes fluid drainage from the preorbital area; the patient should sit upright as much as possible. Dark glass reduces glare and prevent irritation from smoke, air currents, dust and dirt. If the eyes cannot be closed, they should be lightly taped for sleep. To maintain flexibility, the patient should be taught to exercise the intraocular muscles several times a day, by turning eyes in the complete range of motion. Good grooming can be helpful in reducing the loss of self-esteem that can result from an altered body image. If the exophthalmos is severe, treatment may include suturing the eyelids together, administering corticosteroids, radiation of retro-orbital tissues, orbital decompression, or corrective lid or muscle surgery.

If surgery is scheduled, the patient must be adequately prepared to avoid postoperative complications, routine nursing intervention followed according to surgical procedure.

The person receiving radiation therapy of the thyroid gland should be taught the following:

- Flush the toilet two or three times after each use.
- Increase intake of fluids to aid in RAI's excretion.
- Use separate eating utensils and separate towels and wash clothes. Wash these and underclothes and bedlinen separately.
- Rinse bathroom sinks and tube thoroughly after use, and wash hands carefully after using the bathroom.
- Sleep alone for few days and avoid kissing and intercourse (although amount of radiation in the patient's body is minimal).
- Avoid prolonged physical contact with anyone.
- Do not breastfeed.
- Delay pregnancy for 6 months after therapy.
- RAI should not be used in pregnant women because of the teratogenic effects on fetus, and the placenta transports iodine early.

The following measures to be taken when the person with thyroid crisis or storm by the nurses include:

- Monitor the patients temperature, intake output, neurological status and cardiovascular status every hour.
- Initiate an IV Line for medication and fluids.
- Administer increasing doses of oral propylthiouracil as ordered (200 to 300 mg every 6 hours may be given) after a loading dose of 800 to 1200 mg orally.
- Administer iodine preparation as ordered. Sodium iodine given IV twice daily or an oral preparation may be ordered.
- Administer propranolol 1 to 20 to 80 mg per oral or 2 to 10 mg IV as ordered. Propranolol can worsen asthma or CHF because it constricts bronchial smooth muscles and causes a decrease in cardiac output.
- Initiate measures to lower body temperature, including external cooling devices, cold baths and acetaminophen. Salicylates are contraindicate because they inhibit thyroid hormone binding to protein carries and thus increase free thyroid hormone levels.
- Initiate other supportive therapy as ordered, including oxygen, cardiac glycosides, and treatment measures for the precipitating event.
- Maintain quiet, calm, cool, private environment until crisis is over.
- Maintain continuity of care.
- Decrease stressers by use of patient education, comfort measures or family support.

As recovery ensures, the nurse must continue to provide intervention that addresses the outcomes related to hyperthyroidism. These include but or not limited to:

- Initiate other supportive therapy as ordered, including oxygen, cardiac glycosides, and treatment measures for the precipitating event.
- Maintain quiet, calm, cool, private environment until crisis is over.

- Maintain continuity of care.
- Decrease stressers by use of patient education, comfort measures of family support.

As recovery ensures, the nurse must continue to provide intervention that addresses the outcome related to hyperthyroidism. These include but or not limited to:
- Promote adequate rest:
  - Provide a quite, comfortable enviornment.
  - Provide back rubs.
  - Use home remedies such as hot milk to assist in promoting sleep.
  - Encourage quiet periods even if the patient does not sleep.
- Maintain increase activity tolerance:
  - Encourage short walks if cardiac output is stable.
  - Space activity between rest periods.
- Maintain adequate nutrition intake:
  - Monitor intake and output every 8 hours
  - Weight daily
  - Monitor nutritional intake
  - Provide frequent high-protein and high caloric meals.
- Promote good eye care:
  - Perform visual assessment every shift.
  - Initiate appropriate measures such as using dark glasses, or elevating head of bed; using artificial tears and tapping the eyelids closed at various intervals.
  - Report any new complaints immediately.
- Facilitate improved coping. Offer patient's intervention to help them relax, such as music, backrubs, and distraction.
- Enhance patient knowledge–Regarding diseases signs and symptoms, explain medication use, purpose, dosage, schedule and side effects; precaution during RAIT, self monitoring.

HYPOTHYROIDISM

Hypothyroidism is a metabolic state resulting from a deficiency of thyroid hormone that my occur at any age. Congenital hypothyroidism results in a condition called cretinism.

Etiology

Hypothyroidism may result from the following:
- *Loss or atrophy of thyroid tissue* Autoimmune thyroiditis, ablative therapy for hyperthyroidism, thyrotoxic drugs, congenital agenesis, maldevelopment, or radiation for head and neck malignancy.
- *Loss of trophic stimulation* Pituitary dysfunction (pituitary or secondary hypothyroidism) or hypothalamus dysfunction.
- *Miscellaneous alterations* Deficit in hormone biosynthesis; peripheral resistance to thyroid hormone, idiopathic factors or environment factor (iodine deficiencies).

The most frequent causes and their brief description are as follows:
- *Goiter* Any enlargement of the thyroid gland is not associated with hyperthyroidism, hypothyroidism, cancer or inflammation is referred to as simple goiter; endemic goiter due to iodine deficiency. Sporadic goiter occurs sporadically in regions that are not the locus of the endemic goiter. Mostly seen in females and family history of goiter.
- *Thyroiditis*
  - Acute thyroiditis (acute pyogenic thyroiditis) results from infection of thyroid by pyogenic organisms: symptoms include pain, and tenderness in thyroid, dysphasia, fever, malaise, treatment, symptomatic.
  - Subacute nonsuppurative thyroiditis (Dequavain thyroiditis and Granulomatous thyroditis) results from vital infections of thyroid gland, may follow an upper respiratory infection, most often seen in 4th and 5th decades of life, symptoms include pain in the thyroid, fever, hoarseness, dysphasia, pallitations, nervousness; lassitude, thyroid moderately enlarged, subsides in few months, treatment usually symptomatic, aspirin for mild cases, glucocorticoids when disease is unresponsive to other measures.
  - Subacute lymphocytic thyroiditis (Painless thyroiditis, lymphocytic thyroiditis). It is a form of thyroiditis increasing in frequency; etiological factor unknown but possible autoimmune symptoms include self-limiting form of hyperthyroidism and nontender enlarged thyroid gland, which may be followed by hypothyroidism treatment symptomatic during hyperthyroidism phase may include beta-adrenergic blockers but not *propylthiouracil* (not effective) monitor annually for hypothyroidism.
  - Chronic thyroiditis (Hashimoto's thyroiditis, Riedel's thyroiditis) is a rare form of thyroiditis, cause is unknown. Extensive fibrosis gland occurs; symptoms include insidious onset, symptoms form compression of traches, esophagus, and recurrent laryngeal nerve, gland enlarged hard; hypothyroidism can occur, treatment is symptomatic with surgery for symptoms of compression, and thyroid replacement for hypothyroidism.
- *Ablative therapy:* Total thyroidectomy, hypophysectomy, and radiation therapy of pituitary or thyroid gland cause is iatrogenic hypothyroidism. Patients undergoing these treatments must take thyroid hormone replacement for life.

Pathophysiology

The patients with hypothyroidism may or may not have a goiter. An enlarged thyroid gland is seen when the disease results from thyroiditis. Defective hormone biosynthesis, peripheral resistance to thyroid hormone, and environment factors. All these conditions reduce thyroid hormone production and as a result, TSH secretions is increased because of lack of negative feedback. Increased thyroid mass then results from the increased stimulation. In contrast, hypothyroidism results from lack of TSH, (secondary hypothyodism) growth of the thyroid gland are not stimulated. The three types of thyroiditis are acute, subacute, chronic occur (already briefed in etiology). And regardless of the cause, lack of thyroid hormone results in a general depression of basal metabolic rate and slows the development of functioning of the every system of the body. Alteration in the integumentary cardiovascular, nervous, musculoskeletal, alimentary and reproductive system are seen one of the major changes in accumulation of hyaluronic acids and alterations of the ground substances producing mucinous–edema Myocoedema and third space fluid effusions. Myocodedema coma represents the most severe form of hypothyroidism and ultimately can occur in any patient with untreated prolonged hypothyroidism. Precipitating factors include, sedatives narcotics, exposure to cold, surgery, infection and trauma.

Clinical Manifestations

The major manifestations of cretinism are defective physical development and mental retardation in infants/children. Affected infants may exhibit a large posterior fontanels, squinting, excessive sleeping, thickened skin and lips, enlarged tongue, abdominal distention, vomiting and a hoarse cry. Dull facial expression, feeding and respiratory difficulty, peripheral cyanoses, and supraclavicular and periorbital edemas umbilical hernias and hypothermia. Hypothyroids in childhood is due to autoimmune thyroiditis (Symptom explained in earlier pages).

Hypothyroidism in the adult is characterized by an insidious and non-specific slowing of body process. The system-wise clinical manifestation of hypothyroidism are as follows:

- *Cardiovascular:* Increased capillary fragility, decreased pulse rate, varied changes in blood pressure; cardiac hypertrophy, weak contractility, distant heart sounds, anemia, tending to develop CHF, angina and MI.
- *Respiratory:* Dyspnea; decreased breathing capacity.
- *Gastrointestinal:* Decreased appetite, nausea and vomiting; weight gain, constipation, distended abdomen and enlarged scaly tongue.
- *Integumentary:* Dry, thick inelastic, cold skin; brittle nails; dry, spares, coarse hair, poor turgor of mucosa; generalized interstitial edema; puffy face and decreased sweating; pallor.
- *Musculoskeletal:* Fatigue; weakness; muscular aches and pains; slow movement; arthralgia.
- *Nervous:* Apathy; lethargy; forgetfulness; slowed mental processes; hoarseness; slow, slurred speech; prolonged relaxation of deep tendon muscles; stupor, coma, parenthesis; anxiety, depression; polyneuropathy.
- *Reproductive:* Prolonged menstrual periods or amenorrhea; decreased libido and infertility
- *Others:* Increased susceptibility to infection; increased sensitivity to narcotics, barbiturates, and asthenia, intolerance to cold, decreased hearing; sleepiness and goiter.

Management

Studies of thyroid function useful for diagnosing hypothyroidism include serum T3 RU, T3, T4 serum cholesterol, ECG. Serum cholesterol, ECG, Serum TSH, and TSH stimulation tests. Other tests may be needed to determine the true hormonal status.

The therapeutic objective in hypothyroidism is restoration of a euthyroid state as safely and rapidly as possible with hormone replacement in the adult, a low-caloric diet is indicated to promote weight loss. Synthetic oral thyroxine synthroid, levothyroid is the drug of (sodium-levothyroxine) choice to treatment of hypothyroidism. In the young, otherwise, healthy patient, maintenance of replacement dose can be started at once. In the older adults, patients, and person with compromised cardiac status, a small initial dose (12.5 to 25 mg/L) is recommended because the usual dose may increase myocardial angine and cardiac arrhythmias. Any chest pain experienced by a patient starting thyroid replacement should be reported immediately and ECG and cardiac enzyme tests are performed.

Treatment consists of pharmacological therapy described. Surgery may be performed for large goiter, particularly those compressing adjacent tissues and organs.

Nursing Management

Assessment of the patient who is suspected of having hypothyroiditis based on clinical manifestations that usually occur. If the patient has any edema, coma, mechanical respiratory support will be necessary as well as cardiac monitoring. The nurse will be administering all medications IV since the paralytic ileus associated with myxedema causes unreliable absorption of oral medications. If the patient is hyponatremic, hypersonic saline may be infused. The nurse should monitor hypothermia. For the assessment of the patient progress vital signs, body weight, fluid intake and output visible edemas should be monitored. Cardiovascular assessments also follow, and take measures accordingly as in acute interventions.

The nursing interventions required by the patients with hypothyroidism vary greatly depending on the severity of disease. Because the hypothyrodic state is reversed slowly, the patient will not return to the premorbid health state for 2 to 3 months. Potential nursing intervention include the following:

- Promote activity to the level of patient tolerance. At first the patient will have a very limited tolerance and only be able to move around in the room. Activities should be increased gradually:
  - Monitor the cardiovascular response to new activities. If the patient complains of chest pain or develops an unacceptable heart rate, stop the activity and then resume at a slower rate.
  - Monitor blood pressure, pulse and respirations before, during and after each activity.
- Promote positive body image:
  - Provide information that helps the patient and significant others understand the relationship of body changes to hypothyroidism.
  - Educate about reversible body changes.
  - Stress the positive changes that have occurred.
- Promote normal bowel elimination:
  - Monitor bowel elimination.
  - Maintain adequate fluid intake
  - Increase bulk in the diet.
- Treat hypothermia:
  - Monitor temperature every 2 to 4 hours.
  - Maintain environment temperature that is comfortable for the patient
  - Use blankets to increase body temperature if necessary.
- *Facilitates* Intake of a nutritional diet that is low in calories and includes food from all food groups.
- Promote comfort:
  - Use nonmedicinal comfort measures such as massage, cool or warm heart and distraction to pain control.
  - If medications are used, monitor carefully. Patient will have a lower tolerance for sedatives and depressant medications.
- Provide for self care needs. At first the patient may require complete care for hygiene, toileting and dietary needs.
- *Facilitate* patients understandings of the relationship between the sexual problems and the hypothyroidism.
- Maintain skin integrity:
  - Monitor skin condition each shift.
  - Institute preventive care measures such as sheepskin pads and soft sheets.
  - If patient is unable to or does not turn be on his/her own, assist in turning in every hour.
- Facilitate safe environment and orientation to environment:
  - Monitor neurological status every shift.
  - Reorient that patient frequently uses resources such as current events, clocks and newspapers.
  - Maintain a safe environment; remove any clutter, keep bed low, and keep bed rails up.
  - Check on patient frequently, especially at night, and use night-lights to prevent confusion.
  - Inform significant others of relationship between mental status and hypothyroidism.
  - Involve patient as much as possible in decision about care.

In addition, the nurse helps the patient and family caregivers learn how to continue the plan of care after discharge. The importance of compliance with medications and follow up care should be stressed.

CANCER OF THE THYROID GLAND

Cancer of the thyroid gland less prevalent than other forms of cancer and only very small percentage of thyroid neoplasm are malignant. Two general types of malignant neoplasm are found which include:

1. Those arising from follicular epithelium (Papillary, follicular, medullar and anaphasic).
2. Those arising from parafollicular tissue. Thyroid-lymphoma. The characteristics of the five forms of primary malignant neoplasms of the thyroid include the following:
   - *Papillary* The incidence of this cancer is 65% usually occurs in young persons, more in females than males. The prognosis is good. Rarely causes death in young person if occult or intrathyroidal. Metastasis is intra-glandular lympathics, slows growing tumor.

     It is asymptotic. Occult (Less than 1.5 cm in diameter) Intrathyroidal (greater than 1.5 diameter, but does not extend through surface and extrathyroidal extends through thyroid surface. It is well differentiated psammoma body found in 40% of tumors and virtually diagnostic of malignant nature. Tumors appear as a cold sport on thyroid scan. Growth partially depends on TSH.
   - *Follicular* The incidence of this cancer is 20%. Usually occurs after 40 years; more in female. Metastasis occurs early by blood vessels in sites bones, lung, liver. Prognosis is good if minimally invasive lesion; symptom of goiter may have been present for years; Tumor is well differentiated to poorly differentiated, cyst formation and calcification; tremors may appears as "hot" areas on thyroid scan. Suppressive thyroid therapy can cause regression of metastatic lesion.
3. *Anaplastic:* The incidence of this cancer is 5% usually occurs after 60 years more in females than males; Metastasis by direct invasion to adjacent structures;

highly malignant prognosis varies with cell type (giant cell-6 months, and small cells-5 years symptoms include hoarseness, inspiratory strider, pain dysphasia signs of invasion adjacent areas. Two cell forms of tumour, giant cell and small cell.

4. *Thyroid lymphoma:* The incidence of this cancer is 5%. Occurs usually after 40 years, more in women than men. Metastasis by lymphatic system; gland fixed to other structures. Prognosis is good. Patient may have long history of previous goiter, rapid enlargement of goiter, hoarseness, dysphasia, pressure sensation dyspnea and some pain: Tumor usually is in nodular histocytic form. It is strongly associated with Hashimotos thyroiditis.

5. *Medullary:* The incidence of this type of cancer is 5% usually occurs after 50 years, both in male and female equally. Metastasis is by interglanular lymphatic and blood vessels. Prognosis is moderate (10 years survival estimated). Because of tumor produces hormone, possible survival is estimated). Because of tumor produces hormone, possible, paraendocrine manifestation such as carcinoid syndrome, watery diarrhea, Cushing's syndrome, tumor of C-cells of thyroid, not accelerated, some appear as 'cold' spots on the thyroid scan; may produce ACTH, prostaglandin for carcinoembryonic antigen. It occurs as a familial form as apart of multiple endocrine neoplasia (MEN).

Management

Diagnosis of the thyroid cancer has been simplified by the acceptance of the fine needle biopsy and obtaining tissue samples from solid tumors or fluid cysts. Radionuclide imagery, ultrasound tests and thyroid suppression tests are helpful in thyroid cancer.

Medical management of person with thyroid cancer includes use of all modalities of cancer treatment: surgery, radiation, hormoneal suppression, and chemotherapy.

Care of the patient with thyroid nodule first focuses on helping patient through the diagnostic process. Thyroid nodule occurs frequently, and most are not to be concerned. No one diagnostic test is completely reliable. Depending on the patient characteristics, various tests may be performed. The nurse prepares the patient for each test, focusing particularly on education.

When surgery is indicated, nurse has to prepare the patient for surgery by performing required routine measures preoperatively and postoperatively, which includes patient teaching regarding general preoperative and postoperative care. Particularly in thyroid surgery, patient needs to, learn how to cough, and move the head and neck postoperatively without placing strain on the suture line. Thus, the patient is taught preoperatively to support the neck by placing both hands behind the neck when moving the head or when coughing.

The nursing intervention during postoperative care of the person after thyroid surgery includes the following:
- Monitor for and report signs of complications.
  - Laryngeal nerve damage; hoarseness and weak voice.
  - Hemorrhage of tissue swelling:
    * Bleeding on dressing; check back of dressing by slipping hand gently under the neck and shoulders.
    * Choking sensation.
    * Difficulty in coughing or swallowing.
    * Sensation of dressing being too tight even after it loosened.
  - Calcium deficiency (tetany):
    * Early signs: tingling around mouth or of toes and fingers, decreasing serum calcium levels.
    * Later signs: positive Chvostek's and Trousseau's signs and grand malseizures.
  - Respiratory distress associated with any signs just listed.
- Provide emergency care:
  - Keep emergency supplies readily available.
    * Tracheotomy set for laryngeal nerve damage. Oxygen and suction equipment suture removal set for respiratory obstruction hemorrhage.
    * IV calcium gluconate or calcium chloride (for tetany)
  - For acute respiratory diseases:
    * Call for immediate medical help.
    * Raise head of bed.
    * Loosen dressing over incision.
    * Give calcium as ordered, if signs and symptoms of tetany present.
    * If loosening dress does not relieve symptoms of respiratory distress and if medical help is not readily available, remove clips or sutures as instructed.
  - Provide comfort
    * Avoid tension on suture lines: encourage patient to support head when turning by placing both hands behind neck.
    * Give prescribed analgesics as necessary.
  - Maintain nutritional status
    * Start soft foods as soon as tolerated only fluids may be tolerated initially.
    * Encourage a high carbohydrate and high-protein diets.
  - Teach patient
    * ROM exercises to neck when suture line healed to prevent permanent limitations.
    * Need for life-long thyroid hormone replacement therapy after a total thyroidectomy.
    * Any special care measures related to the underlying disease.
    * Need for follow up care.

DISORDERS OF PARATHYROID GLAND

Hyperparathyroidism

Hyperparathyroidism is a condition involving increased secretion of parathyroid hormone (PTH). PTH has following functions:
- Maintenance of normal serum calcium.
- Regulate bone resorption of calcium.
- Regulates reabsorption of calcium from glomerular filtrate.
- Regulates phosphate and bicarbonate excretion in kidney tubule.
- Regulates calcium absorption in intestine; influenced by estrogen, drestrogen in women and activated vitamin D (1,25-dihydroxycholecalciferol calcitriol).
- Calcium regulates pores of cell membranes, movement of sodium, and thus depolarization and resultant action potential in nerves and muscles.

In short, PTH helps regulates calcium, and phosphate levels by stimulating bone resorption, renal tubular reabsorption of calcium and activation of vitamin D.

Etiology

Hyperparathyroidism is classified as primary, secondary, or tertiary.
- Primary parathyroidism is due to an increased secretion of PTH leading to disorders of calcium, phosphate, and bone metabolism. The excessive concentration of circulating PTH usually leads to hypocalcemia and hypophosphatemia. The most common cause is a benign neoplasm or a single adenoma in the parathyroid gland. It is most common in women and usually occurs between 30 and 70 years.
- Secondary hyperparathyroidism appears to be compensatory response to states that induce or cause hypocalcemia, the main stimulus of PTH secretion. Disease condition associated with secondary hyperparathyroidism include vitamin D deficiencies, malabsorption, chronic renal failure and hyperphosphatemia.
- Tertiary hyperparathyroidism occurs when there is hyperplasia of parathyroid glands and the loss of feedback from circulating calcium levels. Thus, there is autonomous secretion of PTH, even with normal calcium levels. It is observed in the patient who has had a kidney transplant after a long period of dialysis treatment of chronic renal failure.

Pathophysiology

Primary hyperparathyroidism is result of one or two major problems. The exaggeration of the normal effects of PTH on skeletal, renal and gastrointestinal system and the associated hypercalcemia. Hypersecretion of PTH results in continued stimulation of target organs and elevates serum calcium. The normal negative feedback of serum calcium on PTH and secretion is lost or ineffective. Increased PTH, increased bone resorption enhances the reabsorption of calcium from the glomerular filtrate, and increases calcium absorption through the gastrointestinal tract.

In the skeletal system: There are increased PTH, increased bone resorption resulting in osteopenia and in very severe cases, cysts and fractures. From osteitis fibrosa cystica. Joint changes also occur. In the renal system, increased PTH enhances the reabsorption of calcium from the glomerular filtrate, reabsorption of phosphate and alteration in the excretion of bicarbonate. Production of activated vitamin D increases elevated PTH effects the GI tract are indirect and occur through the action of vitamin D. The activated vitamin D results in increased agent of vitamin D. The activated vitamin D. The activated vitamin D results in increased calcium absorption through GI tract. These processes result in elevated serum calcium which in itself leads to neurological, musculoskeletal, cardia, GI and renal alteration.

In both secondary and tertiary hyperparathyroids, the calcium level is chronically low. In chronic renal failure the low calcium results from hyperphosphatemia, a decreased production of activated vitamin D and a decrease in calcium absorption. There also may be a decreased sensitivity of bone to the action of PTH. This process results in hyperplasia and excessive production of PTH are usually able to keep the calcium level close to normal, but at the expense of bone destruction The bone lesions are characterized by osteomalacia, osteosclerosis and osteitis fibrosa cystica.

Clinical Manifestation

Hyperparathyroidism has varying symptoms. The sytemwise clinical manifestations are as follows.
- *Cardiovascular:* Arrhythmias, shortened QT interval on ECG, and hypertension.
- *Gastrointestinal:* Vague abdominal pain, anorexia, nausea and vomiting, constipation, pancreatitis, peptic ulcer disease, cholelithiasis, weight loss and appetite.
- *Integumentary:* Skin necrosis and moist skin.
- *Musculoskeletal:* Skeletal pain, backache, weakness, fatigue, pain on weight bearing; osteoporosis, pathologic fracture of long bones; compressed fractures spine and decreased muscle tone.
- *Neurologic:* Personality disturbances, emotional irritability, memory impairment, psychosis, delirium confusion, coma; incoordinations; hyperactive deep tendon reflexes; abnormalities of gait; psychomotor retardation and headache.
- *Renal:* Hypercalciuria, kidney stones (nephrolithiasis), urinary tract infection and polyuria.

- *Others:* Corneal calcification on slit-lamp examination, serious complications are renal failure, pancreatitis, collapse of vertebral bodies, cardiac changes and long bone and rib fractures.

Management

An increased serum PTH levels and persistent hypercalcemia are criteria for establishing diagnosis of PHPT and other causes of hypercalcemia and increased serum ruled out. PTH measured by radioimmunoassay. Serum calcium level will exceed 10 mg/dl Elevation in other lab test include urine calcium, serum chloride, uric acid, creatinin amylase bone changes are detected by radiological studies-Ray, MRI, CT scan ultrasound for location and adenoma.

The treatment objectives are to relieve symptoms and prevent complication caused by excess PTH. The choice of therapy complications causes excess PTH. The choice of therapy depends on the urgency of clinical situation, the degree of hypercalcemia, the underlying disorder, the status of renal, renal and hepatic function, the clinical presentation of patient.

Plicamycin mithracin and antihypercalcemic agent, lowers the serum calcium in 48 hours, used for metastatic parathyroid carcinoma and severe bone diseases. It has many side effects. Biophosphonate such as pamidronate (Aredia) used to inhibit osteoclastic bone resorption. Destrogon progesterone can reduce calcium levels in postmenopausal woman. Oral phosphate can be used to inhibit calcium absorption effects of vitamin D in intestine. Diuretic may be given to increase the urinary excretion of calcium. In several cases to correct fluid volume deficit and promote calcium excretion by administration of saline, lasix and drugs as ordered.

Parathyroid tumors should be removed surgically. The goal is to restore normal parathyroid function and hypercalcemia or hypocalcemia. The amount of parathyroid tissue removed depends upon the appearance of each gland.

Nursing care of the patient depends upon the treatment. During the acute preoperative period, patients are treated medically which consists continuing hydration, administration of loop diuretics, replacement of electrocytes and administration of sodium chloride and other prescribed medication.

Postoperatively, the care requirements are very similar to these required after thyroidectomy. Potential physiological complication includes hemorrhage, hypocalcemia and airway obstruction. The patients respiratory, cardiovascular, neurological and fluid volume state are monitored routinely.

The nursing intervention includes:
- Have a tracheotomy set and IV calcium preparation readily available.
- Report any signs of hemorrhage, hypocalcemia, or airway obstruction.
- Assess mental status and motor strength.
- Perform complete respiratory assessments. Keep head of bed elevated 30 degrees to facilitate respiration. Encourage deep breathing, coughing and tuning 2-4th hourly.
- Increased ambulations at patient's tolerance take into account mental status and weakness.
- Maintain fluid intake at prescribed levels or enough to achieve 1000 ml or more if serum calcium levels are normal or 2000 ml or more if they are higher.
- Teach patient and significant others about:
  - Prescribed drug
  - Prescribed diet if any
  - Electrolyte replacement if any
  - Fluid intake requirements
  - Wound care
  - Symptoms to report: those indicating infection, hypercalcemia, or hypercalcemia.
  - Follow-up care requirements.

HYPOPARATHYROIDISM

Hypoparthyroidism or inadequate circulatory PTH, is characterized by hypocalcemia resulting from lack of PTH to maintain serum calcium levels. It may be pseudohypoparathyroidism (idiopathic) or true hypoparathyroidism (iatrogenic).

Etiology

The causative factors of true hypoparathyroidism may be classified into three major categories surgically induced, idiopathic and functional:
- The most common cause of hypoparathyroidism is iatrogenic that is accidental removal of parathyroids or damage to the vascular supply of the glands during neck-surgery (e.g. thyroidectomy, radical neck surgery).
- Idiopathic hypoparathyroidism resulting from the absence, fatty replacement or atrophy of the glands as a rate disease that usually occurs early in life and may be associated with other endocrine disorders because many of these persons have abnormal antibodies directed against parathyroid gland. The cause is unknown.
- Functional hypoparathyroidism is the result of chronic hypomagnesemia, which may be seen in malabsorption or alcoholism, and appear to impair PTH release.
- In pseudohypoparathyroidism, the excretion and release of PTH are normal. But there is target tissue resistance to PTH. The cause is unknown may cause by genetic defect resulting in hypocalcemia in spite of normal or high PTH levels is often associated with hypothyroidism and hypogonadism.

Pathophysiology

A deficiency of tissue resistance to PTH results in decreased bone resorption, decreased activation of vitamin D and thus decreased intestinal absorption of calcium, increased renal excretion of calcium and decreased renal phosphorus. The result is hypocalcemia and hyperphosphatemia. The major physiological alterations result from the effect of low calcium levels on neuromuscular irritability, nerves show decreased threshold of excitation, repeated responses to a single stimuli and in severe cases continuous activity of muscular spasms (tetany). Cardiac activity is altered. Calcification of basal ganglia and lens of the eye may occur. The severity of the hypocalcemia and chronicity of the problem indicate the sign and symptoms seen with true hypoparathyroidism. In mild cases which results in any slightly decreased serum calcium levels, the patient may be asymptomatic.

The patient with pseudohypoparathyroidism may have the same signs and symptoms as seen with true hypoparathyroidism. In addition, such patients may have skeletal and developmental abnormalities including short stature, round face, short neck, stocky body, and discrete bone lesions. The most common bone lesion is unilateral or bilateral shortenings of the fourth of fifth metacorpal or metatarsal bone. Mental retardation may also be present. The patient has low serum calcium and high serum phosphorus levels with normal to PTH level on radioimmunoassay.

Clinical Manifestation

The clinical features of acute hypoparathyroids are due to slow serum calcium levels. Sudden decrease in calcium concentration gives rise to syndrome called tetany. This is characterized by tingling of the lips, fingertips, and occasionally feet and increased muscle tension leading to paresthenias and stiffness. Painful tone spasms of smooth and skeletal muscles particularly of the extremities and face dysphagia, a constricted feeling of throat and laryngospasm. Chvostek's sign (facial muscle spasm when the face is tapped below the temple) and Trousseau's sign (carpopeda spasm when arterial circulation is interrupted by applying BP Cuff).

To sum up, the true hypoparathyroidism and clinical manifestation includes the following:

- *Neuromuscular manifestation:* Changes in nerve activity affect peripheral motor and sensory nerves.
  - Numbness and tingling paresthesia around mouth, tips of fingers and some times in the feet.
  - Tetany with positive Chvostek's and Trousseau's signs, spasms of wrists, fingers, forearm feet and toes.
  - Fatigue, weakness, painful cramps, osteosclerosis, soft tissue calcification and difficulty in walking
  - Convulsions that may consist of tonic spasms of the total body or the more typical tonic clonic activity.
  - Laryngeal stridor and dyspnea.
  - *Other neurological signs:* headache, painful edema, elevated CSF pressure, local signs and symptoms, including gait changes, tremors, rigidity, and spasms; possible signs of parkinsonism, hyperactivity, deeptendon reflexes paresthesia of perioral area, hands and feet.
- *Emotional:* Mental manifestation—irritability, depression, anxiety, emotional liability, memory impairment, confusion, frank psychoses, personality changes, disorientation, etc.
- *Cardiovascular manifestation*
  - Decreased contractility of heart muscle.
  - Decreased cardiac output from congestive heart failure.
  - Prolonged QT and ST intervals and occasional dysrhythmias (ECG)
  - Resistance to effect of digitalis preparations.
- *Eye manifestation:* Eye changes including lenticular opacities, cataracts, papill edema. Eventualy there will be loss of total sight.
- *Dental manifestation:*
  - Enamel defects seen on the tooth crown.
  - Delayed or absent tooth eruption.
  - Defective dental root formation.
- *Integumentary:* Dry, scaly skin, hair loss on scalp and body, thin patchy hair, brittle nails, fragile nails, vitiligo, skin infection (Candidiasia).
- *GI and Renal Manifestation:* Abdominal cramps and urinary and fecal incontinence, urinary frequency, malabsorption, and steatorrhea.

Management

The main objectives of treatment are to treat tetany when present and prevent long-term complication by maintaining normal serum calcium level (eucalcaemia). The first priority of trachea in correcting calcium levels to prevent tetany. This is achieved by giving IV calcium gluconate or calcium chloride. Airway pathway must be maintained.

Tetany is treated with IV infusion or slow push of calcium salts (calcium salts can cause hypotension and cardiac arrest—thin slow push) long-term therapy consists of the administration of vitamin D and possibly supplemental calcium and oral phosphate binders.

The cause of hypoparathyroid is the identified and long term therapy is started as soon as possible. Normal serum calcium levels are maintained by supplemental dietary and elemental calcium by dietary phosphate restriction and phosphate-binding agents such as aluminium hydroxide and by vitamin D therapy to increase GI absorption of calcium. Vitamin D preparation includes ergocalciferol, or calcitriol, or calderol.

Nursing care of the patient with hypoparathyroidism requires close assessment for signs of tetany. The patient may experience anxiety and in effective breathing pattern as a result of the signs and symptoms of the disease. The nurse should be readily available to answer the patient questions. The patient should be kept in a room from where the nurses' station can be visible. The patient's call light should be answered promptly. The nurse needs to keep attending on any patient complaint. Hyperventilation which can accompany anxiety worsens the hypocalcemia because hyperventilation causes respiratory alkalosis, which in turn causes more of the ionized calcium to bind to serum protein. The decrease in ionized calcium exacerbates symptoms of hypocalcemia. Thus, a patient should be supported to prevent hyperventilation. Keeping patient informed of their serum calcium levels will also help them feel in control and lesser anxiety. The patients are assessed for following by the nurse:

- Chvostek's and Trousseau's signs.
- Airway patency.
- Mental status orientation.
- Emotional status; anxiety and irritability
- *Vital sign:* Pulse rate and rhythms.

Any abnormal changes should be reported immediately so that treatment can be instituted and prevent seizure. Safety precaution to prevent nature of disease; need for long-term therapy, medication, administration, monitoring signs of:

- *Infective treatment:* recurrence of tetany.
- *Signs of hypercalcemia:* thirst, poluria, lethargy, muscle tone, constipation.
- *Complication:* Renal stones (flank pain i.e. pain radiating down into groin) and need for continual follow-up care and dietary changes.

DISORDERS OF ADRENAL GLAND

The adrenal gland is essential to life. Without the hormone cortisol and aldesterone produced in the adrenal cortex, the body's metabolic processes responds inadequately to even minimal physical and emotional stressors such as changes in the temperature, exercises or excitement. More severe is stressors such as serious infections, surgery, or extreme anxiety would possibly result in shock and death. The adrenal medulla secretes hormones are also produced by sympathetic nervous system although more slowly.

There are three main classifications of adrenal steroid hormones.

- *Glucocorticosteroids:* Regulate metabolism, increased blood glucose level and are critical in the physiologic stress response. In humans, the primary glucocorticoids is cortisol.
- *Mineralocorticosteroid:* Regulate sodium and potassium balance. The primary in mineralocorticoid is aldosterone.
- *Androgens:* Contribute to growth and development of both genders and to sexual activity in adult women.

The term corticosteroids refers to any one of these three types of hormones produced by the adrenal cortex. Dysfunction of the adrenal gland can be manifested as increased or decreased function of the cortex or increased function of the medulla.

CUSHING'S SYNDROME

Hyperfunction of the adrenal cortex, cortisol excess leads to Cushing's syndrome. Cushing's syndrome is spectrum of clinical abnormalities caused by excess corticosteroids particularly glucocorticoids.

Etiology

The causes of Cushing's syndrome may be divided into three major groups:

1. *Primary Cushing's syndrome:* Excessive cortisol production resulting from adrenal adenoma or carcinoma also called adrenal Cushing's syndrome.
2. *Secondary Cushing's syndrome:* Excessive cortisol production resulting from adrenal hyperplasia, because of excessive ACTH production. These excessive ACTH production results from either.

   Increased release of ACTH from the pituitary gland because of pituitary of hypothalamic problem also called Cushing's disease or pituitary Cushing's syndrome.
3. *Iatrogenic Cushing's syndrome:* Excessive cortisol levels resulting from chronic glucocorticoid therapy.

Pathophysiology

The major result of Cushing's syndrome is excessive production of cortisol early in the noniatrogenic disorders, the most prominent alteration is loss of the normal diurenal secretory pattern. With loss of diurenal pattern, the morning level of cortisol production may not be abnormally elevated, but levels during the day do not show the normal decrease below the morning peak, at later stages cortisol elevated at all times.

The pathophysiological factors associated with cortisol excess primary result from exaggeration of all the known actions of glucocorticoids and includes alteration in the:

- Protein, fat and carbohydrates metabolism.
- Inflammatory and immune responses.
- Water and mineral metabolism.
- Emotional stability.
- RBCs and platelets levels.

Excessive cortisol may disturb secretion of other anterior pituitary hormones (Prolactin, thyrotropin, LH and GH) and cause alteration in sleep patterns. Some of these alterations may contribute to the clinical picture. In many instances, cortisol excess is also associated with excessive production of androgen, this results in virilization in females. Adrenal tumors may secrete cortisol, androgens and aldosterone in various proportion depending on the hormone-produced excess clinical manifestation occurs.

Clinical Manifestation

The clinical manifestation of Cushing's syndrome can be body systems and are related to excess levels of corticosteroids. Although manifestation of glucocorticoids excesses usually predominated symptom of minor corticoids and regan excess may also be seen. They are as follows:

- Glucocorticoids (cortisol)
  - *General appearance:* Truncal centripedal obesity, thin extremities, rounding of face (moon face) fat deposits, on back neck and shoulder (Buffalo hump).
  - *Integumentary:* Thin fragile skin, purplish-red striae, Potential hemorrhages; bruises; cheeks plethora, acne, poor wound healing.
  - *Cardiovascular:* Hypervolemia, hypertension, edema of lower extremities.
  - *Gastrointestinal:* Increase in secretion of pepsin and hydrochloric acid and anorexia.
  - *Urinary:* Glycosuria, hypercalciuria and kidney stones
  - *Musculoskeletal:* Muscle waisting in extremities, and proximal muscle weakness; fatigue, osteoporosis, awkward gait, back and first pain weakness and growth retardation in children.
  - *Immune:* Inhibition of immune response
  - *Hematologic* leukocytosis, lymphopenia, polycythemia and increased coagubility.
  - *Fluid Electrolyte:* Sodium and water retention, edema, hypokalemia
  - *Metabolic:* Hyperglycemia, negative nitrogen balance, dyslipidemia.
  - *Emotional:* Psychic stimulation, euphoria, irritability, hypomania, to depression, emotional liability, moodswings.
2. Mineral corticoid (Aldosterone)
   - *Fluid Electrolyte:* Marked sodium and water retention, tendency toward edema marked hypokalemia.
   - *Cardiovascular:* Hypertension, hypervolemia, dysrhythmia and CHF.
3. Androgens
   - *Integumentary:* Hirsutism acne, loss of scalp hair and coat hair on face and total body.
   - *Reproductive:* Menstrual irregularities oligomenorrhea enlargement of clitoris in females, gynecomastia and testicular atrophy in males and changes in libido.
   - *Musculoskeletal:* Increase in muscle development.

Management

Medical management is focussed on identifying the cause of the problem and removing the cause of cortisol excess if possible. Various diagnostic procedures are preformed to confirm the diagnosis and differentiation among the various causes of cortisol excess. Abnormal signs include granulocytosis, lymphocytopoenia, eosinopenia, hyperglycemia signs include granulocytosis, lymphocytopenia, eosinopenia, hyperglycemia, glycosuria, hypercalciuria, and osteoporosis, hypokalemia, alkalosis, etc.

The treatment of choice for Cushing's disease is transsphenoidal surgical removal of the pituitary ademosis hyperphysectomy. Adrenolectomy is indicated for adrenal tumor or hyperplasia. Currently transperitoneal or retroperitoneal laparoscopic surgery is performed to remove adrenal tumor less than 5 cm in size.

Those who do not cope with surgery, are treated with mitotane (Lysodren). This drug suppresses cortisol production, alters peripheral metabolism of cortisol and decreases plasma and urine corticosteroid level. This action results as "medical adrenality" Metyrapone, ketoconazole and cytadren may be used to inhibit cortisol synthesis. And long corticosteroid therapy lead in the cause of the problem. Gradually it should reduce to complete the side effects of anticortisol should be monitered, which includes anorexia, nausea, vomiting, GI bleeding, depression, vertigo, skin rashes and diplopia.

If surgery is anticipated the patient should be brought to optimal physical condition. Hypoglycemia and hypertension must be controlled and hypokalemia is corrected with diet and potassium supplements. A higher protein diet meal plan helps correct the protein depletion. Vitamin A supplementation may be given to counteract the problem of delayed healings.

Nursing Management

The patient with excessive cortisol secretion needs skilled nursing care. The patient can be crtically ill. During the acute period, the primary focus of care is on high priority needs of supporting coping, restoring fluid balance, and preventing infections and injuries. While providing physical care of the patients, the nurse has to take following measures:

- Decrease controllable stressors
  - Provide continuity care.
  - Explain all procedures slowly and carefully.
  - Spend time with patient and listen carefully.
  - Avoid sudden noises, temperature changes, drafts and unnecessary invasion of privacy.
- Monitor physiological coping
  - Ensure blood pressure and pulse remain stable.
  - Take vital signs at least every 2 to 4 hours.

- Control fluid volume excess.
  - Restrict fluids as prescribed; distribute fluid throughout the 24 hours; use ice chips to prevent thirst.
  - Provide a diet low in sodium as necessary.
  - Provide potassium replacement as ordered oral-intake foods high in potassium.
  - Monitor daily weight, intake and output for every 4 to 8 hours and laboratory values of sodium, potassium, chloride, bicarbonate and pH.
- Prevent infection and falls
  - Monitor temperature every 4 hours.
  - Assess mouth, lungs and skin every shift for early signs of infection and report signs immediately.
  - Limit staff and visitors with signs and symptoms of upper respiratory infection.
  - Institute preventive care; sterile technique for invasive procedures routine turning, coughing and deep breathing every 2 hours; oral hygiene. Before breakfast, after meals, and at bed time.

If person undergoing adrenal surgery following intervention to be followed during preoperative and postoperative period:

- Preoperative
  - Provide supportive care.
  - Assist patient with usual preoperative care.
  - Maintain nutritional status with a high protein, prescribed calorie diet with adequate minerals and vitamins.
  - Assist with correction of fluid and electrolyte imbalance.
  - Assist with hormonal therapy as prescribed.
  - Assist with measures used to prevent or treat crisis of adrenal hormonal excess of deficit.
  - Administer prescribed IV fluids and glucocorticoids before surgery
- Postoperative
  - Establish monitoring schedule, detect complications of surgery and adrenal crisis, blood pressure alterations, blood glucose alterations fluid and electrolyte imbalances.
  - Because the patient may have unusual activity intolerance, pace postoperative activities with alternate periods of rest and a gradual increase in self care.
  - Provide measures to minimize effects of postural hypertension:
    * Supply ACE bandages or elastic stockings.
    * Assess effects of posture on blood pressure.
    * Assist or accompany the patient during ambulation while blood pressure remains labile.
  - Provide measures to decrease risk of infection in the immunosuppressed patient (e.g. strict surgical asepsis, deep breathing and avoiding contact with person with infections).
  - Administer cortisol replacement as typically prescribed:
    * IV route for first 24 to 48 hours.
    * Oral route when patient is able to tolerate food by mouth.
  - Administer mineralocorticosteroid (fludocortisone) replacement, if prescribed, this is typically prescribed when cortisol replacement is less than 40 to 50 mg/24 hours in the patient with bilateral adrenalectomy.
  - Assist patient and family in learning about required hormonal replacement:
    * Bilateral adrenalectomy: Maintenance dose of cortisol and mineralocorticoids.
    * Untilateral adrenalectomy doses of cortisol dependent on degree of suppression of HPA axis.

IATROGENIC CUSHING'S SYNDROME

Iatrogenic Cushing's syndrome occurs when a patient takes large doses of exogenous glucocorticoids for their therapeutic anti-inflammatory effects. The clinical situation in which glucocorticoids might be used for their anti-inflammatory and immunosuppressive effects include the following:

- *Eyes surgery or trauma:* Usually given as drops, ointment, or intraorbital systemic effects minimal.
- *Dermatologic disorders:* Used as ointments; can have systematic effects if used over large parts of the body or used daily.
- *Autoimmune diseases:* Rheumatoid arthritis, systemic lupus erythematosus and scleroderma.
- Rheumatoid arthritis, systemic lupus erythematosus scleroderma.
- *Hematological disorders:* Hemolytic anemias, thrombocytopenia, lymphomas leukemias.
- *Allergic reaction:* Anaphylaxis, contact dermatitis, transfusion reaction.
- *GI disorders:* Ulcerative colitis, Crohn's diseases, hepatitis
- *Nephrological disorders:* Nephrotic syndrome.
- *Neurological diseases:* Head trauma and surgery to prevent cerebral edema and increased intracranial pressure.
- *Cardiopulmonary diseases:* Asthma, COPDs myocarditis.
- *Transplantation:* Renal, liver, heart, beta-cell transplantation.
- *Others:* Part of many protocols for various malignancies.

Pathophysiology

Long-term therapeutic doses of glucocorticoids can result in the full clinical picture of Cushing's syndrome. Bone changes are great in Iatrogenic Cushing's syndrome. Syndrome often develops vascular necrosis. There are mild fluid and electrolyte imbalance. Severe myopathy may occur. Peptic ulcer occurs more often. Patients who receive glucocorticoids are very susceptible to cataract formation and are susceptible to all types of infections.

Management

A different type of problem, cortisol deficit can occur when glucocorticoids are given for a prolonged period. They must be withdrawn slowly to remove adrenal insufficiency. Blood glucose levels may be monitored frequently if there is a history of diabetes mellitus. For hyperglycemia the experience of most of the people can increase in appetite. If the weight gain is a problem, a calories restricted diet may be necessary. To prevent GI problem steroids should be taken with food or antacids. Stools should be guiactested regularly to monitor early signs of GI irritation. If fluid retention problem, sodium restriction diet is prescribed. Take measures to prevent fluid and electrolyte problem accordingly. In addition, monitor signs of infection and assessment of psychological and emotional status, anxiety, depression and mood swings.

Patient receiving prolonged therapeutic glucocorticoid therapy need considerable teaching to be able to manage therapy and to identify signs and symptoms of complication which include the following:

- Take drug as prescribed.
  - Do not miss a dose or stop medication suddenly.
  - Drug must be withdrawn slowly under physician's supervision.
  - If nausea and vomiting occur and drug cannot be taken, notify physician immediately.
  - Keep sufficient tablets always to avoid missing a dose.
  - Take drug with food or antacids
  - With every other day, therapy, take twice the normal dose every other day at 8 hours.
  - If traveling, carry medication with one does not keep (do not ship them).
- Monitor self and report side effects of weightgain, edema, behavior changes, GI bleeding, increased urination, or thirst or signs of infections.
- Check blood glucose levels if directed.
- Prevent infection:
  - Avoid persons, especially children, with infections.
  - Avoid crowded, poorly ventilated places.
  - Care of wounds carefully.
  - Report any signs which may include feelings of increased weakness, feeling poorly and having less energy.
- Maintain a nutritious diet, including foods from all groups, follow direction for any prescribed diet (low calorie, high potassium, low sodium).
- *Carry out a regular exercise program:* walking helps to strengthen muscles and decrease bone problem.
- Have yearly eye examination.
- Consult physician regularly as instructed.

ALDOSTERONISM

Aldosteronism or aldosterone excess can be either primary (Conn's syndrome) or secondary. Primry aldosteronism results from bilateral nodular hyperplasia or from a single aldosterone, producing adenoma. Secondary aldosteronism occurs frequently and results from the presence of exogenous conditions, that stimulate the renin angiostenism-aldosterone system which includes:

- Cardiac failure
- Liver disease
- Nephrosis
- Renal artery stenosis
- Bartter's syndrome
- Idiopathic cyclic edema
- Pregnancy
- Hypovolemic states
- Estrogen therapy.

Pathophysiology

In primary aldosteronism, excessive aldosterone is secreted and stimulate the reabsorption of sodium in kidney in exchange for potassium and hydrogen, which results water retention, further volume expansion and hypertension. Further and hydrogen, which results water retention, further volume expansion and hypertension. Further, retinopathy develops headache in clinical findings. The loss of intracellular and extracellular potassium changes the excitability of muscle membrane, resulting in muscular weakness, intermittent parenthesis and sometimes diminished deep tendon reflexes. Paralysis may occur. Severely low levels of potassium leads to loss of concentrating ability of the kidney tubules leading to increased water loss, polyurea, nocturia, and polydipsia. Further, it leads to hypernatremia excessive loss of hydrogen results in hypokalemia alkalosis, producing signs and symptoms of tetany.

Secondary aldosteronism results when increased renin secretion is stimulated by the various pathological factors, which leads to hypokalemia and alkalosis and hypertension depending on the severity of the exogenous cause.

Management

Blood test and urine tests reveal alteration in serum electrolytes. Hypertension and hyperkalemia are key factors; these should be treated accordingly as described concerned chapters.

- If primary aldosteronism results from an aldosterone secreting adenoma treatment of choice in surgical resection, i.e. untilateral adrenalectomy.
- In blatant hyperplasia medical treatment with sodium restriction potassium replacement therapy and spironolactone the choice of treatment.

- In secondary aldosteronism, medical treatment for the abnormal secretion and water retention is sodium restriction. K2 replacement and diuretics provide nursing care accordingly.

ADRENOCORTICAL INSUFFICIENCY

Addison's Disease

Adrenocortical insufficiency (hypofunction of the adrenal cortex) may be primary (Addison's disease) or secondary from a lack of pituitary ACTH.

Etiology

Inadequate secretion of cortisol may occur as a result of:
- Insufficient secretion of ACTH resulting from hypothalamic pituitary disease (secondary).
- Insufficient secretion of ACTH and adrenal atrophy resulting from suppression of hypothalamic-pituitary function by long-term exogenous glycocorticoids given in therapeutic doses (iatrogenic) or
- Destruction of the adrenal cortex itself (primary).

Primary insufficiency also called Addison's diseases can result from several causes which include:
- Idiopathic atrophy, probably caused by autoimmune abnormality.
- Infiltration of adrenal glands with cancer.
- Impairment of blood flow from vasculitis or thrombosis.
- Hemorrhage and infarction secondary to septicemia (Waterhouse-Friderichsen syndrome).
- Destruction of adrenal glands by chemical such as mitotane.
- Congenital hypoplasia.
- Surgical removal of adrenal glands.
- Metastases to adrenal glands.

Pathophysiology

Primary adrenocortical insufficiency deprives the body of both minerlocorticosteroids and glucococorticoids. These hormonal losses decreases body's ability to retain sodium and secrets potassium. The loss of sodium decreases extracelluler electrolytes and fluid volume. The decreased volume along with decreased vascular tone, diminished cardiac output, and decreased renal perfusion. Excretion of waste products is inhibited. The loss of glucocorticoids in Addison's disease decrease hepatic gluconeogeneses and increases tissue glucose uptake. Muscle strength is lost. Various GI disorders may occur and mental and emotional functioning and stability are impaired. The loss of negative feedback of glucocorticoids with pituitary secretion of ACTH results uncontrolled ACTH release along with lipoprotein. Various changes in sexual characteristics may result from a decrease in adrenal androgen or from the general debility associated with insufficiency.

Secondary adrenal insufficiency results in similar pathophysiological disturbance except that the fluid and electrolytic imbalance because of aldosterone in response to the renin–angiotensin system. Adrenal crisis (Addisonian crisis) is a severe exacerbation of adrenal insufficiency, occurring in any person with chronic insufficiency regardless of the cause.

Mental and emotional changes are some of the symptoms and may include lethargies, loss of vigor, depression, irritability and loss of ability to concentrate. Patient can become increasingly apathetic and be unable to participate in and ADL.

The clinical manifestations of adrenal insufficiency also can be seen in most body systems and related to deficit levels of corticosteroids, which also include symptoms of aldosterone and androgen.

- Glucocorticoids
  - *General appearance:* Weight loss.
  - *Integumentary:* Bronzed or smoky hyperpigmentation of face, neck, hands, especially creases, buccal membranes, nipples, genitalia and scars (if pituitary function normal), vitiligo, alopecia.
  - *Cardiovascular:* Hypotension, tendency to develop refractory shock; vasodilators.
  - *Gastrointestinal:* Anorexia, nausea, vomiting, cramping, abdominal pain diarrhea or constipation.
  - *Urinary:* No glycosuria
  - *Musculoskeletal:* Fatigability.
  - *Immune:* Propensity toward autoimmune diseases.
  - *Hematologic:* Anemia, lymphocytosis.
  - *Fluid and electrolyte:* Hyponatremia, hypovolemia, and dehydration, hyperkalemia.
  - *Metabolic:* Hypoglycemia, insulin sensitivity and fever.
  - *Emotional:* Neurasthenia, depression, exhaustion or irritability confusion, and delusions.
- Aldosterone:
  - *Fluid and electrolyte:* Sodium loss, decreased volume of extracellular fluid, hyperkalemia and salt craving.
  - *Cardiovascular:* Hypovolemia, tendency toward shock, decreased cardiac output and decreased heart size.
- Androgens:
  - *Integumentary:* Decreased axillary and pubic hair (women).
  - *Reproductive:* No effect in men. Decreased libido in women.
  - *Musculoskeltal:* Decrease in muscle size and tone.

Management

In addition to clinical feature, a diagnosis of Addison's disease can be made when cortisol levels are subnormal and fail to raise over basal levels with ACTH stimulation tests. Tests under plasma cortisol serum electrolyte, Tuberculin test, CT scan are MRI also used.

Pharmacological treatments of adrenal crisis include the following:
- Administration of glucocorticoids and mineral corticoids, e.g. Decadran, hydrocortisone, fluid cortisone.
- Initiation of volume replacement, e.g. IV normal saline.
- Administration of glucose, e.g. IV dextrose.
- Administration of vasopressors.

Treatment includes identification of precipitating factors and initiate treatment accordingly. Nursing care that is related to nursing diagnosis includes promoting activity, facilitates coping, promoting comfort, balance, preventing injury, promoting good nutrition, promoting comfort, improving self exteem, and patient teaching regarding disease and treatment and follow-up.

DISORDERS OF PANCREAS

The pancreas is along, tapered, labular, soft gland that between 60 and 90 g. It lies behind the stomach and anterior to the first and second vertebrae, The pancreas perform exocrine and endocrine function.The islets of Langerhans are the areas of endocrine activity and they release their secretions into the portal circulation. However, the secretions are also pancrine. Pancrine diffuse to neighboring cells to exert their action, rather than traveling to their target tissues through the blood like endocrine secretions. The islets account for less than 2% of the gland and alpha, beta, and delta cells. Glucon is synthesized by the alpha cells, insulin, by the beta cells gastrin and somatostatin by the delta cells. Any deficiency in the endocrine function of the pancreas insulin leads diabetes mellitus.

DIABETES MELLITUS (DM)

Diabetes mellitus is a group of metabolic diseases characterized by hyperglycemia resulting from defect in insulin secretion, insulin action or both. The basis of the abnormalities in carbohydrate, protein and fat matabolism in diabetes is the deficient action of insulin on the target tissue of skeletal muscle, adipose tissue, and liver. Uncontrollable DM may result in long-term damage, dysfunction, and failure of various organs, especially the heart, kidneys, and eyes.

Etiology and Classification of DM

The diagnosis label of diabetes mellitus (DM) carries many physiologic and socio-economic ramification and therapeutic requirement. Therefore, accurate classification of the degree of glucose tolerance and type of diabetes are important. In July 1997, a new diagnostic and classification system for diabetes was published by an expert committee on the diagnosis and classification of diabetes mellitus of the American Diabetes Association. The new system reflects the etiology and pathophysiology of diabetes with two major categories being type 1 diabetes mellitus, (previously termed insulin-dependent DM or Juvenile onset DM) and type 2 diabetes mellitus (previously termed "noninsulin dependent DM or maturity-onset DM).

The classification of diabetes and other disorders of glucose tolerance with the defining characteristics are as follows:

Type 1 Diabetes Mellitus

Type 1 diabetes mellitus is characterized by autoimmune beta-cell destruction, which is attributed to a genetic predisposition coupled with one or more viral agents and possible chemical agents. It is immune mediate. The characteristics include:
- Insulinopence (insulin deficit) and dependent on exogenous insulin sustain life.
- Onset generally before age 30, but may occur at any age, including old age.
- Person's body built is generally lean, rarely obese.
- Variable rate of beta-cell destructions.
- Clinical presentation is usually rapid (polyuria, polydipsia, polyphagia weight loss).
- Majority of persons (85-90%) have one or more of the following autoantibodies present at the time when fasting hyperglycemia is initially detected.
- Islet cells autoantibodies (ICA).
- Insulin autoantibodies (IAA).
- Glutamic acid decarboxylase autoantibodies (GAD).
- Tyrosine phosphatase IA-2 or IA-2B autoantibodies.
- Strong human leukocyte antigen (HLA) associations.
  - Linkage of DQA and B genes
  - Influenced by DRB genes.

Idiopathic diabetes has some defined characteristics; which include the following:
- No immunological evidence for beta cell destruction.
- No HLA association.
- Strongly inherited.
- Most individuals effected are of African or Asian origin.
- Episodic ketoacidosis with varying degrees of insulin deficiency below episodes.

Type 2 Diabetes Mellitus

Majority of 90% of people with diabetes mellitus have type 2 has strong genetic influences but has no correlation with HLA type has been found. The defining characteristics will include:
- The absolute requirement of exogenous insulin is episodic.

- No requirement for exogenous insulin to sustain life at least initially.
- Ranges form a picture of predominantly insulin resistance with mild relative insulin deficiency to a picture of more severe insulin secretory defects with insulin resistance.
- Persons usually are obese; those who are not obese by traditional criteria, usually have abdominal adiposity.
- Onset usually after 40, but may occur at any age.
- No autoimmune HLA association.

Other Disorders of Glucose Tolerance

- *Genetic defects of beta cell function:* Previously termed maturity onset diabetes of youth (MODY) impaired insulin secretion without defects in insulin action. Autosomal dominant inheritance is present. Abnormalities in the three genetic loci have been determined to date.
- *Genetical defects in insulin action:* Not available.
- *Diseases of the exocrine pancreas:* Pancreatitis, trauma and infection, pancreatectomy, pancreatic carcinoma, cystic fibrosis and hemochromatosis.
- *Endocrinopathies:* Acromegaly, Cushing's syndrome, glucagonoma, pheochromocytoma.
- Drug induced
  - Permanent destruction of beta cells (vacorcrat poison) IV Pentamidine.
  - Impairment of insulin action (nicotinic acid, glucocorticoids) thiazidediuretics.
  - Impairment of insulin secretion, thready precipitating DM in an individual with insulin resistance (e.g. drug-induced hypokalemia).
- *Infections:* Congenital rubella and cytomegalovirus.
- *Uncommon forms:* immune mediatal: stiffman syndrome, anti-insulin receptor antibodies.
- *Genetic syndromes associated with DM:* Turner's syndrome, Down syndrome, and Klinefelter's syndrome.
- *Gestation DM:* Pregnancy related.
- *Impaired glucose tolerance (IGT):* Glucose levels are higher than normal but do not meet diagnostic criteria for DM. Generally obese person will have insulin resistant and are at increased cardiovascular risk.
- *Impaired fasting glucose:* Fasting glucose levels are higher than normal but lower than those in IGT or DM.

Pathophysiology

The hallmark of diabetes is insulin deficiency, either absolute or relative. In absolute insulin deficiency, the pancreas produces either no insulin or very little insulin, as seen in type 1 DM. In relative insulin deficiency the pancreas produces either normal or excessive amounts of insulin, but the body is unable to use it effectively, such that glucose levels remain elevated. This latter deficit is called "Insulin" that glucose levels remain elevated. Resistance and is seen in type 2 DM. Basically it is failure of the pancreas to produce enough insulin to overcome this insulin resistance that participates clinical type 2 DM.

Basically it is failure of the pancreas to produce enough insulin to overcome this insulin resistance that participates clinical type 2 DM in predisposed individuals.

This absolute or relative insulin deficiency results in significant abnormalities in the metabolism of the body fuels. The body needs fuel for all its functions. For building new tissue, and for repairing tissue. The fuel comes from the food that is ingested which is composed of carbohydrates, protein and fats. It is important to understand and emphasize to patient that diabetes is not a disease of glucose alone although the patient that diabetes is not a disease of glucose alone, although the diagnostic criteria that have been devised use the serum glucose level as the marker of diagnosis and control of the diseases. It is important that nurse helps patients understand that diabetes is a disease that effects how the body utilizes all foods carbohydrates, fats and protein.

The insulin requiring organs are the liver skeletal muscles and adipose tissue. The consequences of either absolute or relative insulin deficiency at the levels of these organs are as follows:

- *Liver:* Hyperglycemia, hypertriglyceridemia, and ketone production
- *Skeletal muscle:* Failure of glycost uptake and amino acid uptake
- *Adipose tissue:* Lipolysis resulting in elevated free fatty acids level in the circulation.

This situation is worsened by the consumption if dietary carbohydrates which are metabolized into glucose and fail to be utilized by the liver and skeletal muscles, with resultant progressive hyperglycemia and glycost when the blood glucose level reaches the renal threshold (approximately 180 mg/dl) in normal kidney, the kidneys cannot keep up with reabsorbing the glucose from the glomerular filtrate and glycosuria results. Glucose attracts water and an osmotic diuresis occurs, resulting in polyuria (increased urination). This polyuria results in the loss of water and electrolysis, particularly sodium chloride, potassium and phosphate. The loss of water and sodium results in thirst and increases fluid intake (polydipsia) are triggered as the cell becomes starved of their fuel. This glycosuria leads to rapid weight loss in Type 1 DM and pathological metosia in Type 2 DM in both types, dehydration and electrolyte disturbances lead to fatigue and listlessness. Serum lipid abnormalities (TGs) very low density lipoprotein (VLDLS) and some time cholesterol may be elevated. This leads to depletion in all electrolytes K, Na, CI) if is not treated, complications will develop. Actually, the patient can develop nausea, and vomiting, and conditions can advance to hyperglycemic coma or diabetic ketoacidosis (DKA). Chronically, the patient can develop microvascular and macrovascular complication or neuropathy.

Clinical Manifestation

Early symptoms include polyuria, polydipsia, polyphagia, visual blurring, fatigue, weight loss and late signs and symptoms include coma and chronic complications. Normally insulin and its counter regulatory hormones maintain blood glucose within range of 70 to 110 mg/dl. Elevated blood glucose level produce symptoms related to the degree of actual or relative insulin deficiency. When absolute insulin deficiency of decreased insulin activity occurs, glucose is not used properly. Glucose remains in the blood stream and produces an osmotic effect on intracellular and interstitial fluid. This shift in fluid balance results in clinical manifestation of frequent urination (polyuria) and thirst (polydipsia). Without sufficient insulin, the patient may experience hunger (polyphagia) as the body turns to other energy resources besides glucose; first fat and then protein. Acute and chronic complications from hyperglycemia are closely associated with the type of diabetes mellitus and circumstances in which it occurs.

Management

Management of diabetes mellitus is primarily aimed at achieving a balanced diet, activity, and medication together with appropriate monitoring, patient, and family education. These components are equally necessary for effective control of diabetes.

Diagnosis of diabetes mellitus can be made on the basis of the following:
- Complete history and physical examination.
- Blood tests, including fasting blood glucose, post-prandial blood glucose, glycocylated, hemoglobin, cholesterol and triglyceride levels, blood urea nitrogen and serum creatinine, electrolysis.
- Urine for complete urinalysis, microalbuminuria, culture and sensitivity glucose and acetone.
- Funduscopic examination—delayed eye examination.
- Neurologic examination.
- Blood pressure.
- Monitoring of weight
- Doppler scan.

Treatment of Type 1 DM

Treatment of Type 1 DM involves an insulin, diet and exercise. The discovery of insulin by Banting and Best in 1921 occupies as major place in medical history. Today common insulin used for DM are as follows:
- Quick-acting insulin lipro, regular (bufferal).
- Intermediate acting insulin: NPH, Lente.
- Combination insulin 70% NPH and 30% regular.

Insulin differs in speed of effect onset time of greater action (peak) and how they act duration. Insulins are classified as quick, intermediate, and long-acting. Dietary carbohydrate and activity must be coordinated with insulin action so that:
1. Insulin is available for optimal metabolism when the food that was eaten is absorbed and
2. Food is available while insulin is acting to prevent hypoglycemic reactions.

Two principles are useful in coordinating food and insulin.
1. The carbohydrate intake must be coordinated with insulin actions.
2. Regular or quick-acting insulin requires that a supplemantal snack of 15 gram of carbohydrate be given to match the peak action of the insulin. For example, (1) 10 AM injection of regular insulin in plan.

The nurse must clarify the insulin prescription in terms of the type strength and species. Any change in any one of the properties may lead to difference in action. When the insulin prescription is changed, careful patient monitoring is necessary to identify clinical effect. The steps of administration of insulin are as given below.
- Wash hands thoroughly.
- Roll intermediate or long-acting insulin between palms of hands to mix insulin. Note: Always, insulin bottle before using for first time. Make sure that it is proper type and concentration, expiration date not over and top of the bottle is in perfect condition.
- Prepare insulin injection is same manner as for any injection.
- Select proper injection sites and inject following procedure for any subcutaneous (SC) injection. In site where SC tissue is adequate, inject commercial insulin needles at 90-degree angle. For sites with minimal SC tissues pinches up skin and insert needle at 45-degree angle.
- If blood appears in syringe after needle insertion, select new site for injection. Aspiration is not necessary.
- After injecting insulin, apply some pressure, with dry cotton ball (or 2X2) at site when withdrawing needle.
- Hold cotton ball in place for a few seconds but do not massage.
- Destroy and dispose or single-use syringe safely.
  Note: When instructing patient to self-inject insulin, use the following guidelines (if appropriate).
- Aspiration does not need to be done before injection.
- Disposable syringe can be used for several injections.

Problems with insulin therapy are hypoglycaemia, allergic reactions, lipodystrophy and the Somogyi effect.

Treatment of Type 2 DM

Currently four classes of medication are available to improve diabetes control for patient with type 2 DM.

The common oral medication type 2 DM includes the following:

- *First-generation sulfonylureas:* Which stimulate release of insulin from pancreatic islets; decrease glycogenolysis and gluconeogenesis and enhance cellular sensitivity to insulin. They are tolbutamide (Orinse) acetohexamide (Dymelar), tolazamide (Tolanase), chlorpropamide (Diabenase).
- *Second-generation sulfonylurea:* Which stimulate release of insulin from pancreatic islets, decreased glycogenolysis and gluconeogenic, enhance cellular sensitivity to insulin. They are glipizide (Glucotrol) glybunde.
- *Meningitis* stimulate a rapid and short lived release of insulin from pancreas, e.g. Repoglunide (Prandin).
- *Biguanide* Decrease the rate of hepatic glucose production and augments glucose uptake by tissues, e.g. Metformin (glucophage).
- *Alpha-glucosidase* Intubitory works on the brush border of the small intestine to slow the breakdown of disaccharides and polysaccharides into monosaccarides; delays subsequent ansorption of glucose. Examples acarbone (Precose), miglitol (Glyset).
- *Thiazolidinediones* Decreases peripheral insulin resistance in skeletal muscle without stimulating insulin secretion, e.g. Troglitazone (Rezulin).

Oral agents are not oral insulin or substitute for insulin. The patient must have some functional endogenous insulin or for oral agents to be effective. They may be combination of oral agencies or with insulin to achieve goal-ranged control. Dietary control should be provided before starting oral agents. The hypoglycemic action of oral medications can be enhanced are prolonged by means of the concurrent administration of drug such as anticoagulants, salicylates, alcohol and propranolol. Drugs that can suppose oral agent action include thyroid preparation, corticosteroids, and thiazide diuretics.

Therapy is the cornerstone of care of person with diabetes mellitus. The recommended diet can only be defined as a dietary prescription bases on nutritional assessment and goal. Nutritional assessment is used to determine what the individual with diabetes is able and willing to do. Sensitivity to cultural, ethnic and financial consideration is important when developing meal planning approaches. The overall goal is to assist persons with diabetes in making changes in nutrition and exercise habits leading to improved metabolic control. The specific goals of nutritional therapy include:

- Maintenance of normal blood glucose level as possible by balancing food intake and insulin or glucose lowering medication and activity.
- Achievement of optimum serum lipid level.
- Provision of adequate calories for maintaining or attaining reasonable weight for adults, normal growth and development rate in children, and adolescents, increased metabolic needs during pregnancy, and lactation, or recovery from catabolic illness.
- Prevention and treatment of acute complications, such as hypoglycemia, and long-term complication such as renal disease, neuropathy, hypertension and cardiovascular disease.
- Improvement of overall health though optimal nutrition.

Principles that the nurse should teach the patient and reinforce, including the following:

- *Eat according to the prescribed meal plan:* A dietary need related to the specific patient's body weight, occupational age activities and type of diabetes individual response to a dietary prescription should be monitored and appropriate adjustment should be made when necessary.
- *Never skip meals* This is particularly important for patient taking insulin or oral agents. The body requires food at regularly-spaced intervals throughout the day. Insulin and oral agents prescribed to fit the schedule. Omissions or delay of meals can result hypoglycemia.
- Learn to recognize, appropriate, food portions; can result in accurate portion allotments.

Exercise

Regular, consistent exercise is considered an essential part of diabetic management. Exercise contributes to weight loss, reduces tryglycerides and cholesterol, increases muscle tone, and improves circulation. Exercise plans for persons with diabetes should keep in minerals both benefit and risks of exercise as follows:

- Benefits of exercise for the person with diabetes include:
  - Improves insulin sensitivity.
  - Lowers blood glucose during and after exercise.
  - Improves lipid profile.
  - May improve some hypertension.
  - Increased energy expenditure; Assists with weight loss, preserve lean body mass.
  - Promotes cardiovascular fitness.
  - Increases strength and flexibility.
  - Improves sense of well-being.
- Risks of exercises for the person with diabetes:
  - Precipitation or exacerbation of cardiovascular disease, angina, dysrhythmias and sudden death.
  - Hypoglycemia if taking insulin or oral-agents.
    * Exercise related hypoglycemia.
    * Late onset postexercises hypoglycemia.
  - Hyperglycemia after every strenuous exercise.
  - Worsening of long-term complication
    * Proliferative retinopathy
    * Peripheral neuropathy
    * Autonomous neuropathy.

Before entering titany type of exercise program, all patient should have a complete history in physical examination, with particular attention to the cardiovascular system and any existing long-term complications. An exercise stress ECG is recommended for all persons over 30 years of age. The general guidelines for exercise program for the person with diabetes includes the following:

- *Exercise type:* Aerobic (low impact for type 2 DM) start with light level.
- *Exercise session:* Each session should eventually include:
  - 5 to 10 minutes of warm-up stretching and limbering exercises.
  - 20-30 minutes of aerobic exercises and heart rate in target zone (as defined by the physician) or perceived exercise rating.
  - 15-20 minutes of light exercise and stretching to cool down.
- *Exercise frequency:* 3 to 5 times per week.
- *Special precautions:*
  - Consider the insulin/oral agent regimen (may need to decrease insulin).
  - Consider the plan for food intake—Discuss with healthcare provider. May need to take extracarbohydrates before exercise.
  - Check blood glucose before, during, afterward (for baseline).
  - If glucose is over 250 mg/dl, check urine ketones; if negative, okay to exercise; if positive, take insulin; do not exercise until ketones are negative.
  - Exercise should not cause shortness of breath and should be stopped with any onset of chest pain or dyspnea.
  - Carry diabetic ID card and bracelet.
  - Carry source easily absorbed carbohydrates (three glucose tablets or hard candies).
  - Do not exercise in extreme heat or cold.
  - Inspect feet daily and after exercise.
- Precautions for selected persons:
  - Person with insensitive feet should choose good shoes for walking and avoid running and jogging. Swimming and cycling may also be included.
  - Persons with proliferate retinopathy should avoid exercises associated with valsalva maneuvers or that cause jarring and jointing of head or exercises with head in low position.
  - Persons with hypertension should avoid exercises associated with valsalva maneuvers and exercise involving intense exercises of tarso and arms (Exercises involving the lower extremities preferred).

Exercise does not have to be vigorous to be effective. The blood glucose-reducing effects of exercise can be attained with mild exercise such as brisk walking. The exercise selected should be enjoyable to foster regularity. Exercise is best done after meals, when the blood glucose level is rising.

COMPLICATIONS OF DIABETES MELLITUS

The complications of DM are classified as acute and chronic. Acute complications include hypoglycemia, diabetes ketoacidism (DKA), and hyperglycemic hyperosmalor nonketonic coma (HHNC).

Diabetic Ketoacidosis

Diabetic ketoacidosis (DKA) are referred to as diabetic acidosis and diabetic coma may develop quickly or over several days or weeks. It can be caused by too little insulin accompanied by increased calorie intake, physical or emotional stress or undiagnosed diabetes, may be due to indequate treatment of existing DM; insulin is not taken as precribed; infection; change in diet; insulin or exercise regimen. DKA mostly likely to occur in Type 1 DM and also seen in Type 2 DM.

In DKA, an assessment finding includes the following needs immediate intervention:
- Dry mouth
- Thirst
- Abdominal pain
- Nausea and vomiting
- Gradually increasing restlessness, confusion, lethargy
- Flushed dry skin
- Serum glucose greater than 300 mg/dl
- Eyes appear sunken
- Breath orders of ketones
- Rapid, weak pulse
- Labored breathing (Kussmaul's respiration)
- Fever
- Urinary frequencies
- Glycosuria and Ketonuria

Diagnostic measures include blood work (immediate blood glucose, CBC, Keton pH, electrolytes) BUN, ABG, urinalysis including Sp. Gr. PH sugar assessment.

The preferred treatment for DKA is the low dose insulin. IV infusion method. In this method 5 to 10 units of insulin per hour is normal saline solution is administered until ketodosis is reversed. This insulin therapy is continued until a blood glucose level of 250 mg/dl is reached. When the glucose level is reached in level, a solution contains 5% dextrose in saline is given to prevent hypoglycemia along with IV or SC insulin as needed to maintain in blood glucose level fluid and electrolyte therapy aimed at replacing extracellular and intracellular water and deficits of sodium, chloride, bicarbonate, potassium, phosphate magnesium and nitrogen. Ongoing monitoring includes monitoring vital signs, level of consciousness cardiac rhythm, oxygen saturation, and urine output. And assess breath sound for fluid overload, monitor serum glucose and serum potassium, and anticipated posssible administration of sodium bicarbonate with severe acidosis (pH lesser than 7-0).

HYPERGLYCEMIC HYPEROSMOLAR NON-KETONIC COMA (HHNC)

HHNC in the acute complication of Type 2 DM. It occurs in the patient with diabetes, who is able to produce enough insulin to prevent DKA but not enough to prevent severe hyperglycaemeia, Osmotic diuresis and extracellular fluid depletion. Increasing hyperglycemia causes intracellular dehydration because of a shift of the fluid from the intracellular to the extracellular space. This causes neurologic abnormalities such as somnolence, coma, seizures, hemiparesis, and aphasia. There is usually a history if inedequate fluid intake, increasing mental depression and polyuria.

HHNC constitutes a medical energy. The management of both DKA and HHNC is similar except that HHNC requires greater fluid replacement. Diagnostic measures followed as in DKA. The primary management of HHNC involve intravenous rehydration with hypertonic solution (OUS Normal saline). Hypertonic solutions are indicated, because patient is hyperosmolar. As the patient is rehydrated, the hyperglycemia resolves. Intravenous insulin is generally not needed. Once the patient is stabilized, attempts to detect and correct the underlying precipitating cause should be initiated.

When hospitalized, the patient (DKA or HHNC) is closely monitored with appropriate blood and urine tests. The nurse is responsible for monitoring blood glucose and urine output and ketones as well as using laboratory data to direct care. Areas that need monitoring are administration of IV fluids to correct dehydration, administration of insulin therapy to reduce blood glucose and serum acetone, administration of electrolytes to correct electrolyte imbalance, assessment of renal status, assessment of cardiopulmonary status related to hydration and electrolyte levels, and monitoring the level of consciousness. And vital signs should be assessed often to determine the presence of fever, hypovolemic shock, tachycardia and Kussmaul's breathing.

According to assessment, proper reporting and recording are maintained to take measures of any deviation accordingly. Hyperglycemia may be caused by intake of too much food; too little or no diabetic medication; inactive and emotional physical stress; and poor absorption of insulin.

The clinical manifestation of hyperglycemia, include the following:
- Elevated blood glucose
- Increase in urination
- Increase in appetite followed by lack of appetite
- Weakness, fatigue
- Progression of DKA or HHNC.
- Blurred vision
- Headache
- Glucosuria
- Nausea and vomiting
- Abdominal cramps

Treatment of hyperglycemia includes:
- Physician attention
- Continuation of diabetic medication as ordered.
- Frequent checking of blood and urine specimen and recording results.
- Hourly drinking of fluids.

Preventive measures for hyperglycemia include:
- Taking of prescribed dose of medications at proper time.
- Accurate administration of insulin or oral agents
- Maintenance of diet.
- Maintenance of personal hygiene
- Adherence to sick-day rules when ill.
- Checking of blood for glucose as ordered.
- Contacting physician regarding ketonuria
- Wearing diabetic identification.

CHRONIC COMPLICATIONS OF DM

The chronic complication of diabetes mellitus are classified microvascular (small blood vessels) and macrovascular (large blood vessels).

These are consequences of the duration and degree of hyperglycemia. These changes of:
- *Microvascular:* Diabetic retinopathy, diabetic nephropathy, neuropathy systemetrical sensory peripheral polyneuropathy, painful peripheral neuropathy, mononeuropathy, radioculopathy and amyotrophy.
- *Macrovascular:* Dyslipidemia, hypertension (coronary artery diseases). The signs and symptom of different diabetic neuropathy as follows:
  - Peripheral sensory polyneuropathy
    * Classic symmetrical glove-and stocking distributions.
    * Paresthesia, hyperesthesias.
    * Pain (characteristics vary; may be sharp, stabbing lancinating, aching, etc.)
    * Loss of sensation to pinprick, vibration and temperature.
    * Loss of deep tendon reflexes.
    * Muscle wasting and weakness.
  - Autonomic
    * Orthostatic hypertension.
    * Cardiac denervation.
    * Anhidrosis.
    * Gustatory sweating.
    * Gastroparesis, with delayed gastric emptying, nausea, emesis.

- Diarrhea.
- Bladder atony/annoyance.
- Erectile dysfunction.
  - Mononeuropathy
    - Cranial nerve palsy (III, IV, VI, and VII).
    - Ulnar nerve palsy.
    - Carpal tunnel syndrome.
  - Amyotrophy
    - Acute anterior thigh pain or numbness.
    - Weakness to hip flexion on examination.
    - Quadriceps wasting.
  - Radioculopathy
    - Follows dermatomal distribution on trunk
    - Paresthesis.
    - Hyperesthesia.
    - Pain.
    - Numbness.

Treatment of diabetic neuropathy by medication, particular as painful diabetic neuropathy, includes.

	Min	Max
Prepoxyphene with Darvon	1tab QID	2 tab 4th hrly (Darvocet N-100)-Min
Amitryptyline HCl (Elavil)		
Carbemazepine (Tegreso)	25 mg tid	100 mg tid
Phenotoin (Dilantin)	100 mg hrs	100 mg gid
Gabapentin (neurontin)	300 mg h	600 mg QID
Capsaican (zostrex)	Apply topically	

HYPOGLYCEMIA IN DM

Hypoglycemia or low blood glucose occurs when proportionately too much insulin is in the blood for the available glucose. This causes the blood glucose to drop to less than 50 mg/dl.

The cause of hypoglycemia include the following:
- Alcohol intake with food.
- Too little food delayed omitted, inadequate intake.
- Too much exercise without compensation.
- Diabetes medication or food taken at wrong time.
- Loss of weight with change in medication.
- Use of beta blockers interfering with recognition of symptoms.
- A decrease in available blood glucose can result sypathetic nervous system activation and the release of epinephrine. This results in manifestations of cold sweats, weakness, trembling, nervousness, irritability pallor. And increased heart rate. The clinical manifestation of hypoglycemia varies with each patient. The brain depends on a constant supply of glucose because it is unable to stone glucose or glycogen. If that supply is indequated, the patient will experience confusion, fatigue, and abnormal behavior that can resemble alcohol intoxication.

The clinical manifestation of hypoglycemia includes the following:
- Blood glucose less than 50 mg/dl
- Cold, clammy skin
- Numbness of fingers, toes, mouth
- Rapid heart beat
- Emotional changes
- Headache
- Nervousness
- Faintness, dizziness
- Unsteady gait, slurred speech
- Hunger
- Changes in vision
- Seizures, coma.

Treatment of hypoglycemia needs:
- Immediate ingestion of 5-20 gm of simple carbohydrates.
- Ingestion of another 5-20 gm of simple carbohydrates in 15 minutes if no response or relief.
- Contacting of physician if no relief is obtained.
- Discussion with physician with medication dosage.

Preventive measure of hypoglycemia includes:
- Taking of prescribed medications at proper time.
- Accurate administration of insulin or oral agents.
- Ingestion of all ordered diet foods at proper time.
- Provision of compensation for exercise.
- Ability to recognize and know symptoms and treat them immediately.
- Carrying of simple carbohydrate (Sugar).
- Education of friends, family employees about symptoms and treatment.
- Checking blood glucose as ordered.

HYPOGLYCEMIA IN NON-DM

Hypoglycemia in the nondiabetic person is characterised by subnormal plasma glucose, generally less than 50 mg/dl. It may be asymptotic, may cause adrenergic symptoms (anxiety, irritability, palpitation, diaphoresis, and pallor) or may cause neurologlycopenic symptoms with more severe hypoglycemia. Neurologlycopenic symptoms include mental confusion, seizures, and coma may be associated with severe trauma (e.g. motor vehicle accidents). A firm diagnosis rests with the documents of Whipple's triad.
- Appropriate signs and symptoms.
- Appropriate abnormal blood glucose and
- Responses to normalized blood glucose with carbohydrate ingestion.

Classification

Hypoglycemia in nondiabetics may be broadly classified as either fasting or nonfasting (reaction) hypoglycemia. Fasting hypoglycemia generally results in neuroglycopoenic symptoms whereas ready hypoglycemia generally results in neuroglycopenic symptoms, whereas ready hypoglycemia is usually associated with mere adrenergic symptoms.

The cause fasting hypoglycemia includes the following:
- Insulin Excess
    - Exogenous insulin surreptitiously.
    - Sulfonylurea ingestion (accidental in individual without DM, surreptitious use and pharmacy dispensation error).
    - Insulin producing islets cell tumor insulinomo- benign or malignant.
    - Islets hyperplasia.
    - Nesidioblastosis.
- Increased hepatic glucose production
    - Advanced renal disease.
    - Advanced liver disease.
    - Ethnol use, especially in the setting of poor nutrition.
    - Severe sepsis.
    - Secure malnutrition.
- Counter regulatory hormone deficiency.
    - Hypopituitarism
    - ACTH deficiency.
    - GH deficiency.
- Hypothyroidism C.
- Nonislets cell tumors; mesenchymal tumor.
- Autoimmune disease, Antibodies that stimulate the insulin receptor (rare).

Reactive hypoglycemia generally occurs 3 to 5 hours after meals, related to either primary delay in insulin secretion (idiopathic) or rapidly rising postprandial glucose related to rapid gastric emptying postgastric surgery. Failure of the pancreas to keep pace with this rapidly rising postprandial glucose results in later insulin hypersecretion and hypoglycemia. Reactive hypoglycemia person have an increased of type 2 DM.

Management of these hypoglycemia detects the cause and correct the hypoglycemia. Fasting hypoglycemia person using insulin or sulfonylureas surreptitiously should be educated regarding deleterious effects and referred for counseling. Reactive hypoglycemic persons need focus on a prevention or hypoglycemia episodes by:
- Delaying the postprandial glucose rise through increased dietary fiber and the use of complex carbohydrates
- Enhancing insulin sensitivity through exercise and weight reduction towards desirable body weight.

THE DIABETIC FOOT

One of the complications of DM is diabetic foot. Three major factors play a role in the diabetic foot: neuropathy, ischemia, and sepsis. Amputation commonly results.

Sensory impairment leads to painless trauma and potention for ulceration. Motor impairment contributes to wasting of intrinsic muscles in the feet, resulting in foot deformity. Foot deformities alter the normal gait and pressure distribution. Friction and resultant callosities may develop and result in fractures in the ankle or forefoot and ultimately there is a significant deformity called a Charcot foot. Anhidrosis as manifestation of autonomic neuropathy can result in excessive dryness and cracking of the skin, which also contributes to infection. A macrovascular and microvascular alteration produces tissue ischemia and may lead to sepsis. The triad of neuropathy, ischemia, and sepsis result in gangrene and ultimately leads to amputation.

Gangrene may be classified as dry or wet. Dry gangrene occurs when tissue death is not associated with inflammatory changes. Aggressive glycemic control and hospitalization for IV antibodies to limit spread of infection are necessary. Amputation of effected toes is often necessary. The area must be kept dry to prevent wet gangrene. Wet gangrene is gangrene coupled with inflammation, septicemia, and shock may occur. Pediatric care is critical to attain and maintain a health proper toe nail trimming and use of orthotic extra depth. Extra-width of custom-molded shoes can prevent ongoing trauma and ultimately the amputation associated with the diabetic foot.

Prevention of microvascular disease, neuropathy, and macrovascular disease should be major focus of the diabetic care. Thorough interim histories, interim physical examination, and measurements of laboratory parts meters will allow for early diagnosis. Therefore, allowing for early intervention and risk factor modifications and prevention of end-stage diseases.

Proper care of the feet is crucial for the patient with peripheral vascular disease. The guidelines for patient teaching regarding foot care includes the following:
- Wash feet daily with a mild soap and warm water. Test water temperature with hand first.
- Pat feet dry gently especially between toes.
- Examine feet daily for cuts, blister, swelling and red, tender areas. Do not depend on feeling sores. If eye sight is poor have lanolin
- Use on feet to prevent skin from drying and craking. Do not apply between toes.
- Use mild foot powder on sweaty foot. Powder feet only, not shoes.
- Do not use commercial remedies to remove calluses or corns.
- Cleanse cuts with warm water and mild soap, covering with clean dressing. Do not use iodine, rubbing alcohol, or strong adhesives.

- Report skin infections or non healing sores to health care provider immediately.
- Cut toenails even with rounded contour of toes. Do not cut down corners. Soak nails before cutting.
- Separate overlapping toes with cotton or lamp's wool.
- Break in new shoes slowly. Avoid open toe, open-heal, and high healed shoes. Leather shoes are preferred to plastic ones. Wear slippers with soles. Do not go barefoot. Shake out shoes before use.
- Wear clean, absorbent (cotton or wool) socks or stockings that have not been mended. Colored socks must be colorfast.
- Do not wear clothing that leaves impressions, hindering circulation.
- Do not use hot water bottles or heating pads to warm feet. Wear socks for warmth.
- Guard against frostbite.
- Exercise feet daily either by walking or by flexing and extending feet in suspended position. Avoid prolonged sitting, standing, or crossing of legs.
  In addition, consider the following:
- Assess for signs and symptoms of SIADH:
  - Specific symptomatology reflects alterations in cerebral function.
  - Assess for confusion, disorientation, irritability, restlessness, lethargy; tremors, seizure activity, hyper reflexia.
  - Hemodynamic status: Vital signs—Arterial blood pressure, peripheral pulses, heart rate and rhythm; respiratory rate and patter; body temperature.
    * Body weight.
    * Signs of fluid overload.
  - Laboratory parameters:
    * Serum osmolality: <280 mOsm/kg.
    * Serum sodium: <130 Eq/liter.
  - Urine osmolality: to serum osmolality.
  - Urine sodium: >180 mEq/liter.
    * Urine specific gravity: 1.030.
    * Other serum electrolytes.
    * Potassium and chloride
- Assess thought/behavioral process.
- Specific neuralgic parameters:
  - General cerebral functions: Consciousness and mentation.
  - Immediate memory—Ask patient to repeat another series of numbers backwards; ability to calculate; abstractum reasoning.
  - Thought content: Spontaneous, logical; flight of ideas, inappropriate recurrent thoughts, or excessive repetition of thoughts.
- Inquire of family/significant others us to recent change in behavior or personality. Have such changes occurred suddenly or gradually
- Are the changes in behavior response associated with some event?
- Implement measure to foster optimal thinking and expression of thoughts:
- Specific considerations:
  - Provide quiet environment with minimal distractions.
  - Allow adequate time for communication; be accessible to patient/family
  - Provide explanations in clear, concise terms; repeat questions or directions to the patients understanding
- Involve patient and family/significant others in decision making regarding care and activities.
- Collaborate with patient and family/significant others to develop/implement prescribed therapeutic regimen:
- Fluid restrictions:
  - Discuss reasons for strict fluid intake, balanced with output.
  - Encourage patient/family to ask questions and express concerns.
  - Assist patient/family to develop plan as to when and how much fluid will be gested per 24-hour schedule.
  - Teach patient/family how to record intake and output accurately.
- Implement therapeutic regimen:
- Fluid intake:
  - Initial intake limited to urine output/24 hr.
  - As serum sodium level moralize and CNS symptoms additional fluid is given equal to that estimated insensible losses (i.e. fluid lost via skin, lungs).
  - Aggressive fluid therapy:
  - Administration (IV) of 3% hypertonic saline.
  - Administer/monitor diuretic therapy.
  - Furosemide therapy in conjunction with prescribed fluid replacement therapy.
  - Hypertonic peritoneal dialysis may be considered to relieve fluid excess.
  - Close ongoing monitoring of the following is necessary to evaluate effectiveness of therapy
  - CNS function
  - Intake/output and body weight
  - Cardiac status, cardiopulmonary function: Syspnea, tachypnea, productive cough with pink-tinged sputum, presence of adventitious breath sounds-crakles, wheezes.
  - Laboratory parameters
- Emphasize importance of daily weight
  - Identify fluids especially enjoyed by patient.
- Offer praise for accomplishments in implementing fluid restricion.

- Remain accessible to patient/family.
- Lend a listening and concerned ear.
- Consult nutritionist to perform comprehensive nutritional assessment
- Implement fluid restriction on nutritional regimen as prescribed.
- Explain therapeutic regimen to patient/family.
- Encourage fluids/foods with high sodium content
- Perform assessment of patient's immediate environment for potentially injurious equipment or materials.
- Minimize neurologic/neuromuscular stimulation.
- Institute seizure precautions: Bed in low position, side rails padded; pharyngeal airway and suction equipment at beside.

CHAPTER 10

Nursing Management of Integumentary Disorders and Burns

INTRODUCTION

Derm or dermis derived from Greek words means "Skin" Dermis in the thick layer of living tissue below the epidermis containing blood capillaries, nerve endings, sweat glands, hair follicles and other structures.

Integument or skin is the largest organ exposed to the external environment and provides the first line of defense of the body yet at the same time it is affected by changes in the internal environment. Problems of the skin are often present in difficult management challenges. Clothing and cosmetics can disguise or cover some skin problem, but many a problem cannot be hidden so easily. The emotional impact of skin problem often is more serious than skin problem itself. Dermatology is the study of the skin and its problem. Dermatological nursing is that which deals with all the nursing aspects of dermatological conditions.

Nursing Assessment of the Integument System

Assessment of the integument provides data about how the person is affected by and is coping with both external and internal environment. Data obtained in the assessment provide the basis for identification of actual or potential nursing problems related to the skin, infection, fluid and electrolyte balances, nutritional imbalances, or inadequate oxygenation of tissues. Baseline observations are useful for identifying changes that may occur.

Assessment of the skin begins at the initial contact with the patient and continues throughout the examination. Specific areas of the skin are examined during examination of other areas of the body unless the chief complaint is that of a dermatological nature.

Patient's History

The patient's history is an important part of the health assessment and is included with the physical examination. If during a general history, the patient describes a skin problem or skin discomfort, itching or superficial pain. Then further data are obtained. The informations will be as follows:

- *Usual skin conditions:* Appearance, color, moisture, texture, or integrity.
- *Onset of the problem:* Initial sites where changes were first noticed; skin appearance at onset; any other symptoms noted at the time of onset such as pain or itching.
- *Changes since onset:* Changes in location of lesions, changes in appearance, increase in size and new symptoms such as pain or itching.
- *Specific known cause:* For example contact with poisoning, exposure to known allergen or stress.
- If cause is unknown:
  - Recent exposure to sensitizing substances, such as metals, chemicals, detergents or poisonous plants.
  - Description for a new drug such as penicillin.
  - Occupations that may cause contact with potential skin irritants or hands constantly in water.
  - Recreational activities, for example, painting, camping or gardening.
  - Exposure to sun burn, photosensitivity, or skin cancer or cold frost bite.
- *Alleviating factors:* Physician prescribed or self-prescribed things.
- Psychological reaction to skin changes; withdrawal from social activities, cosmetics for cover-up; feelings about the problem, i.e. body image.
- Previous trauma, surgery or prior disease that involves the skin.

Physical Examination

The skin is an organ that can be examined by direct inspection and observation with no tools but a good light. Palpation is also used in gathering data about certain type of lesions. General principles when conducting an assessment of the skin are as follows:

- Be prepared:
  - Have a private examination room of moderate temperature with good lighting and a room with exposure to daylight preferred.
  - If the lighting is inadequate, lesions may be missed or described inaccurately. If the room temperature is not well-controlled, vasoconstriction, vasodilation and papillary erections occur, giving false data.
  - Ensure that the patient is comfortable and in a dressing gown that allows easy access to all skin areas.
- Be systemic:
  - Proceed from head to toe.
  - If only some parts of the skin are inspected, an improved parameter may be omitted or a lesion missed.

- Be thorough:
  - Look at all areas carefully. If the person is lying down, ensure to examine the back especially the sacral area.
  - Lift folds of tissue, such as under the breasts or gluteal folds.
  - The examiner's embarrassment of the examine may result in inadequate data.
  - Do not forget to assess the mucus membrane as well.
- Be specific:
  - Perform a general inspection and then a lesion-specific examination.
  - When lesions are identified, describe the lesions using metric system and established parameters color, size and shape.
- Compare symmetrical parts:
  - Compare the right side with left side.
  - When observing changes in skin color, or tissue shape, always compare one side of the body with other to differentiate structural from pathological changes as well as symmetry of manifestation.
- Record the data:
  - Unrecorded data are lost data.
  - Baseline observations indicating normality of abnormality are needed for comparison with subsequent finding.
  - Changes need to be recorded to determine progress toward achieving desired outcomes.
  - Use appropriate terminology and nomenclature when reporting or documenting.
- Use appropriate technique:
  - Palpation is used during physical assessment of the skin.
  - Lesions are palpated for density, induration and tenderness.
  - Standard precautions need to be observed during palpation, and the examiner should determine whether it is appropriate to use gloves.

The objective data to be collected when examining the skin for general health status include skin color, temperature, moisture, elasticity, turgor, texture, thickness and odor. Brief description of these are as follows:

Color

Changes in color are best obtained in the lips, mucous membranes of the mouth, earlobes, finger nails and toe nails and the extremities. The lip shows rapid color changes. Color of the skin varies with the amount of melanin in the cells, and with the blood supply. Skin colour may be masked by cosmetics curtaining. Inaccurate assessment of skin color may be attributed to factors such as conducted in a poorly lit room, room temperature excessive, the presence of edema, poor hygiene or positioning. The possible color changes in certain conditions are as follows:

- Redness (Erythema) is due to vasodilations more rapid blood flow and more oxygenated blood. It can be seen in conditions like blushing, heat, inflammation, fever, alcohol ingestion, extreme cold below 15°C hot flushes, and polycethemia.
- Whiteness (Pallor) due to:
  - Vasoconstriction, slower blood flow, less blood in capillaries, seen in cold, fear and shock.
  - Partially obstructed blood flow, less blood in capillaries seen in vasospasm, thrombus, narrowed vessels and arterial insufficiency.
  - Fluid between blood vessels and skin surgeries seen in edema.
  - Descreased oxygenation of blood from decreased hemoglobin seen in anemia.
  - Loss of melanin seen in vitiligo.
- Bluish (cyanosis) is due to deoxygenated hemoglobin, noticed in earlobes, lips, mucous, membranes of mouth, nail beds, seen in heart or lung diseases, inadequate respiration, peripheral blood vessal obstruction, venous disease, cold and anxiety.
- Yellow (Jaundice) due to increased bile pigment in blood eventually distributed to skin and mucous membrances and to sclera of eye. This is usually seen in liver disease, obstruction of bile ducts, chronic uraemia and rapid hemolysis.
- Brown due to increased melanin deposits; normal in brown black races. This is found in aging, sunburn, anterior pituitary, adrenal cortex, or liver diseases.
- Dullness due to:
  - Vasoconstriction in dark skin found in cold, fear, shock.
  - Partially obstructed blood flow in dark skin, found in vasospasm thrombus, narrowed vessels and arterial insufficiency.
  - Fluid between blood vessels and skin surface of dark skin found in edema.

The color of the skin indicates degree of blood supplied to and temperature of the skin and oxygen supply and fluid supply to the skin.

Skin is assessed as being dry, moist and oily. Dry skin is usually seen in elderly ones because of diseased activity of sebaceous glands. Dry skin is also seen in dehydration: persons with hypothyroidium have thick, dry and leathery skin. Moist is caused by the presence of water or sweat in the surfaces. Overheating produces sweating. Hyperthyroidism cases have moist smooth skin. Stressors, shock or any situation stimulate sympathetic nervous system and increase fluid loss through shock gland diaphoresis. In as much as vasoconstriction occurs imulation causes cold, clammy skin. Oily skin is seen in adolescence due to excess sebum formation.

The skin is highly elastic and moves freely over most areas. It loses mobility, when it becomes stretched, this occurs with edema, when the interstitial space becomes filled with fluid, skin becomes rigid in the person with scleroderma. Turgor is a tissue tension and is measured by the speed of the skin's return to normal position of fullness after it has been stretched. Decreased turgor may be due to aging or dehydration. The elasticity and turgor tested at the portion of skin over the sternum. Texture and roughness may occur normally on exposed areas, especially elbows and soles of the feet. The skin of an infant is usually soft and smooth, whereas elderly person may roughen and lack underlying tissue substance atrophy. Roughness is seen in hypothyroidism, hypertrophic scarring.

Normal skin is uniformly thin over the body except over the palms and soles. A callus or painless overgrowth of epidermis may develop over these areas as a result of pressure or friction. And normally clean skin is usually free from odour except for areas that contain apocrine sweat glands. Odor occurs because of bacterial composition of protein matter and some draining skin lesions.

In addition to skin assessment, assessment of accessory structures of skin, i.e. hair and nails also is very essential.

Hair growth pattern and distribution are indications of the persons' general state of health. Excessive hair growth is hypertrichosis, usually related to heredity or hormonal changes. Hair loss alopecia is normally with age. Abnormal hair loss may be because of hormonal imbalance, general ill health, infections of the scalp, typhoid fever, chronic liver disease, stressor and some medication antimetabolite or heparin. Hair should be free from lice and nits. Hair loss on the dorsum of the toes may indicate decreased arterial circulation.

The appearance of the nails' changes with age and with ill health. Changes in hardness, brittleness, roughness or shape may indicate some metabolic diseases, nutritional imbalances include vitamin deficiency or digestive disturbances. Pale nail beds indicate hypoxia, clubbing of finger is associated with chronic hypoxia. Paronychic an infection of the tissue surrounding the nail characterized by red shiny skin and painful swelling, it may result in psoriasis dermatitis.

Lesions of Skin

When lesions are observed, the following parameters are used for description, type, color, size, shape and configuration, texture, effect of pressure, arrangement, distribution and variety. The following skin changes are observed in skin lesions.

- Changes in color or texture
  - Spot: It is circumscribed; flat; color change, termed as macule, e.g. Freckle, Pimple, Blemish.
  - Discoloration reddish-purple: It is bleeding beneath the surface; injury to tissue, termed as "Contusion, e.g. bruise.
  - Soft whitening caused by repeated wetting of skin termed as "maceration", e.g. occurs between toes after soaking.
  - Flake: Dry cells of surface termed as "scale", e.g. dandruff, psoriasis..
  - Roughness from dried fluid: i.e. Dry exudate over lesion termed as "crust" scab. e.g. eczema, impetigo.
  - Roughness from cells: It is a leathery thickening of outer skin layer is termed as "lichenification" e.g. callus on foot.
- Changes in shape
  - Fluid-filled lesions:
    * Less than 1 cm: clear fluid vesicle, e.g. blister, chickenpox
    * Greater than 1 cm: clear fluid bulla, e.g. larger blister, pemphigus.
    * Small, thick yellowish fluid pustule, e.g. Acne.
  - Solid mass-cellular growth.
    * Less than 1 cm papule, e.g. small mole, raised rash.
    * 1 to 2 cm nodule, e.g. enlarged lymph node.
    * Greater than 2 cm tumor, e.g. Benign or malignant tumor.
    * Excessive connective tissue over scar keloid, e.g. overgrown scar.
  - Swelling of tissue
    * Generalized swelling: fluid between cells edema, e.g. inflammation swelling and itching.
    * Circumscribed surface edema, transient; some itching, e.g. allergic reaction.
- Breaks in skin surface
  - Oozing, scraped surface: Loss of superficial structure of the skin abrasion, e.g. "Floor burn scrape".
  - Scooped out depression: Loss of deeper layer skin ulcer, e.g. pressure or stasis ulcer.
  - Superficial linear skin breaks: Scratch marks, frequency of finger nails excoriations, e.g. scratching.
  - Linear Cracks or Cleft: Slit or splitting of skin layer, Fissure, e.g. Athlete's foot.
  - Jagged cut: Tearing of skin surface laceration. e.g. accidents, cut by blunt edge.
  - Linear cut, edges approximation: cutting by sharp instrument incision, e.g. knife cut.
- Vascular lesions
  - Small, flat, round, purplish and red spot are due to intradermal or submucous hemorrhage petechia. e.g. bleeding tendency, decreased platelets and vitamin C deficiency.
  - Spider-like: red, small, due to dilation of capillaries, arterioles or venules, telengiectasias, e.g. liver disease and vitamin B deficiency.
  - Discoloration, reddish purple: escape of blood into fissures ecchymosis, e.g. trauma to blood vessels.

The following terminology is used for lesion configuration and lesion distribution:

- Lesion configuration
  - Annular—Ring shaped.
  - Gyrate Ring—Spiral shaped.
  - Iris lesion—Concentric rings or bull's eye.
  - Linear—In a line.
  - Nummular-discoid-coinlike.
  - Polymorptious—Occurring in several forms.
  - Punctuats—Marked by points or dots.
  - Serpiginous—Snake-like.
- Lesion distribution
  - Asymmetric—Unilateral.
  - Confluent Merging together.
  - Diffuse—Wide distribution.
  - Discrete—Separate from other lesion.
  - Generalized—Diffuse distribution.
  - Grouped—Cluster of lesions.
  - Localized—Limited area of involvement that is clearly identified.
  - Statellite—Single lesion and close proximity to a large grouping
  - Solitary—A single lesion.
  - Symmetric—Bilateral distribution.
  - Zosteriform—Band like distributional song a dermatome area.

Common assessment abnormalities of the integumentary system are as follows:

- Alopecia is loss of hair localized or generalized. It may be due to hereditary, friction, rubbing, traction, trauma, stress, infection, inflammation, chemotherapy, pregnancy, emotional shock, tinea cupitis and immunological factors.
- Angioma is a tumor consisting of blood or lymph vessels. It is due to normal increase with aging, liver disease, pregnancy and varicose veins.
- Carotenaemia Carotenosis: Yellowish discoloration of skin, no yellowing of sclerac, most noticeable on palms and soles. It is due to vegetable containing carotene, e.g. carrots, squash and hypothyroidism.
- Comedo black heads and white heads: Keratin, sebum micro-organisms and epithelial debris within a dilated follicular opening. It is due to acne vulgaris.
- Cyanosis: Slightly bluish-gray or purple discoloration of the skin problems, vasoconstrictions, asphyxiation, anemia, leukemia and malignancies.
- Cyst: Sac containing fluid or semisolid material. It is due to obstruction of a duct or gland and parasitic infections.
- Depigmentation (vitiligo): Congenital or acquired loss of melanin resulting in white, depigmented areas. It may be due to genetic chemical and pharmacologic agents, nutritional and endocrine factors, burns and trauma inflammation and infection.
- Ecchymosis: Large, bruise-like lesion caused by collection, collection of extravascular blood in dermis and subcutaneous tissue. It may be due to trauma, and bleeding disorders.
- Erythems: Redness occurring in patches of variable size and shapes. It may be due to heat, certain drugs, alcohol, ultraviolet rays, any problem that causes dilation of blood vessels to the skin.
- Excoriation: Superficial excavations of epidermis. It may be due to pruritis and trauma.
- Hematoma: Extravasation of blood of sufficient size to cause visible swelling. It is due to trauma and bleeding disorders.
- Hirsutism is male distribution of hair in women. It is due to abnormality of gonads or adrenal glands, decrease in estrogen levels and familial trait.
- Intertrigo: Dermatis of overlying surfaces of the skin. It may be due to moisture, obesity monitor infections.
- Jaundice: Yellow or yellowish-brown discoloration of skin best observed in the sclera secondary to increased bilirubin in blood. It is found in liver disease, REC hemolysis, pancreatic cancer, and common bile duct obstruction.
- Keloid: Hypertrophied scar beyond margin of incision or trauma.
- Lichenification: Thickening of the skin with accentuated skin making. It may be due to repeated scratching, rubbing and irritation.
- Mole melanocytic nevus: Benign overgrowth of melanocytes. It is due to defects of development, excessive numbers and large irregular moles and often familial.
- Petechae: Pinpoint, discreate deposit of blood less than 1 mm to 2mm in the extravalcular tissues and visible through the skin or mucous membrane. It is due to inflammation, marked dilation, blood vessel trauma, blood dycrasia that results in bleeding tendencies, e.g. thrombocytopenia.
- Telangiectasia: Visibly dilated, superficial, cutaneous small blood vessels commonly found on face and thighs. It may be due to aging, acne, sun exposure, alcohol, liver failure, corticosteroid medication, radiation, certain systemic diseases, skin tumors and normal variant.
- Tending: Failure of skin to return immediately to normal position after gentle pinching. It is due to aging, dehydration, cachexia.
- Vericosity: Increased prominence of superficial veins. It may be due to interruption of venous return, e.g. from tumor, incompetent values and inflammation.

Diagnostic Studies of Integumentary System

Diagnostic studies provide information to the nurse in monitoring the patient conditions and planning appropriate interventions. The common diagnostic studies of the integumentary system are as follows:

- *Biopsy:* It is one of the most common diagnostic test used in the assessment of skin lesions. Techniques of biopsy include punch, incisional, excisional and shave subsection.

- Punch: Here, special punch biopsy instrument of appropriate size is used. Instrument rotated to appropriate level to include dermis and some fat, suturing may or may not be done.
- Excisional: Is useful where good cosmetic results and entire removal desired. Skin is closed with subcutaneous and skin sutures.
- Incisional: Elliptical incision made in lesion is too large to excise. Adequate specimen obtained without causing an extensive cosmetic defect.
- Shave subsection: Single edged razor blade used to shave off lesions performed on superficial lesions. Provides full thickness specimen of stratum corneum.

Nursing responsibilities during biopsy include verify that consent form is signed if needed. Assist with preparation of site anesthesia, procedure and hemostasis. Apply dressing and give postprocedure instruction to patient. Properly identify specimen.

- *Microscopic Test:*
  - Potassium Hydroxide: Hair, scales or nails examined for hyphae of fungal infection. Specimen is put on a glass slide and 10 to 40 percent concentration of potassium hydroxide added. In this instruct the patient regarding the purpose of test. Prepare slide.
  - Tzank test (Wrights and Giemsas Stain): Fluid and cells from vesicles or bullae examined. Used to diagnose herpes virus. Specimen put on slide, stained, and examined microscopically. Nurse instructs the patients regarding purpose and use. Use sterile technique for collection of fluid.
  - Culture: The test identifies fungal, bacterial, and viral organisms.
    - For fungi, scraping performed if the fungus is systematic involving skin.
    - For bacteria, material obtained from intact pustules, bullae, or abscesses.
    - For viruses, bullae scraped and exudate taken from center of lesion.

    In culture, nurse instructs patient regarding purpose and specific procedure. Properly identify specimen. Follow instruction for storage of specimens if not sent the same to laboratory.
  - *Mineral slides:* To check for infestation, scrapings are taken place in slide with mineral oil. Here, nurse instructs patient of purposes of test, prepare slide.
  - *Immunofluorescent studies:* Some cutaneous diseases have specific abnormal antibody proteins that can be idealized by fluorescent studies. Both skin and serum can be examined. Here, nurse informs patients of purpose of test and assists in obtaining specimens.
- *Other Test:*
  - *Woods light:* Examination of skin with long wave ultraviolet light causes specific substance to fluorescence, e.g. Pseudomonal organism, fungal infection, vitiligo. Explain the purpose of examination and inform patient it is not painful.
  - *Diascopy:* Examination of the skin using gentle pressure with a transparent object to check lesion vascularity. Explain the procedure to patient.
  - *Patch Test:* Used to determine whether patient is allergic to any testing material. Small amount of potentially allergenic matter applied under the occlusion, usually skin on back.
  - In this, nurse explains purpose and procedure to the patient. Instructs patient to return 48 hours for removal of allergens and evaluation. Inform patient of revaluation is needed at 96th hour.

COMMON SKIN PROBLEMS

Skin problems may result from various causes, such as parasitic infection, fungal, bacterial and viral infections, reaction to substances encountered externally or internally taken new growth.

PARASITIC INFECTIONS

Pediculosis (Lice Manifestation)

Occurs mostly among children. People on crowded buses. Pediculis Lice are most often found among people who live in overcrowded dwellings with inadequate hygienic facilities.

Pathophysiology

Lice obtain their nutrition by sucking blood from the skin. They leave their eggs or nits on the skin surface attached to the hair shaft and this results in the transfer from one person to another. Three types of lice infest humans; the headlouse, the body louse and pubic louse.
- The head louse pediculus humanus capitis attaches itself to the hair shaft, laying about eight eggs a day. The eggs are firmly attached to the hair or threads of clothing, ova hatch in one week. They may be viewed with a hand lens or flash light and appear as grayish; glistening oval bodies. The head louse usually is confined to scalp and beard. Transmission occurs through use of infected persons' hats, brushes or combs.
- The body louse pediculus humanus corporis resides mainly in the seams of clothing around the neck, waist and thighs. The bite causes minute hemorrhagic points and severe itching. Transmission by direct contact or by way of clothing, bedding and towels.
- The pubic louse phthirus pubis differs slightly from the head and body louse. It resembles a tiny crab, having claw-like pincers that attach firmly to the pubic hair. Nits are visible in the pubic hair. It is transmitted by sexual contact, bed clothing, towels and occasionally toilet seats.

Clinical Manifestation

Minute, red, noninflammatory, point flush with skin; progression to popular wheat-like lesions. i.e., pinpoint erythema, raised macules and pruritis. The bite of the insect with contamination from saliva, head parts and feces-causing intense itching. Scratching may lead to further trauma with the possibilities of secondary infection and enlarged cervical lymph nodes. Secondary excoriations in intracapular region; firmly attached to hair shaft in head and body lice.

Management

Diagnosis is made by physical examination of the appropriate body part. A magnifying glass may be helpful in spotting symptoms and treatment of pediculosis consists of topical application of the pediculicide such as lindane, permethrin, pyrethrin and malathion. When pyrethrin or lindanes are used, a second application of the 7 to 10 days may be necessary. Directions for application differ according to the product and body location. So it should be applied accordingly as per manufacturers' instructions. Contact screening with bed partners. Playmates showed head gear and contacts treated if necessary. Persons with head lice should be instructed to soak comb, brushes and hair utensils in hot water and pediculicide shampoo for 15 minutes. Clothing and bedding should be laundered in hot water and dried on light heat or dry-cleaned.

Scabies

Scabies is caused by the female itchmite (Sarcoptes Scabiei). It is prevalent during periods of overcrowding and occurs in all age groups and socioeconomic levels.

Pathophysiology

The female itchmite penetrates the stratum corneum and burrows into the skin. Within several hours of the skin penetration, the itchmite lay a large number of eggs and deposits fecal pellets. The larva mature in 10 to 14 days and move to the skin surface, where the females are impregnated; the cycle then repeats itself. The incubation period varies; but often a long period elapses before symptoms are noted. Delayed hypersensitivity is thought to be a major factor in the lapse between infestation and symptoms. The incubation period in persons with no previous exposure is 4 to 6 weeks.

Clinical Manifestation

The classic symptoms of scabies are intense itching and lesions that resemble wavy brownish, thread-like lines occurring most commonly on the hands especially the interdigital webs., flexer surface of the wrist posterior inner surface of the elbows, anterior axillary folds, nipples in the females, belt line, gluted creasos and male genitalia. The head and neck are rarely involved. Pruritis may be severe, especially at night pruritis thought to be a result of a hypersensitivity reaction. Secondary infection with excoriations and pustule may result from scratching. Scratching destroys burrows. Vesicles are filled with serus fluid may contain mite.

Management

Diagnosis is made on the basis of sign and symptoms and identifying the itchmite under microscope. The goal of therapy is elimination of the itchmite and treatment of complications.

- Scabies treatment: Patient and all family members.
    - Lindane Kwell, Scabies for with the follow:
        * Apply at bed time in a thin layer over the entire body from neck down.
        * Wash off in 8 to 12 hours.
        * Give a second treatment in 24 hours if prescribed.
    - Crotamiton 10% (Eurax.)
        * It is less effective than lindane.
        * Bathe before initial application and after each treatment.
        * Repeat treatment as prescribed.
    - Benzyl Benzoate Emulsion
        * Give two overnight treatments one week apart as prescribed.
        * Not widely available. Apply as directed by the physician.
- Treatment for complication from scabies.
    - Postscabies dermatitis with pruritis: topical or oral corticosteroids.
    - Secondary infection with systemic antibiotics.
    - Postscabies papules or nodules treated with coal tar gels.

And teaching the patient with scabies include the following.

- All family members should be treated simultaneously whether or not symptoms present.
- Be sure that all external body areas below the neck covered by the prescribed scabiecide.
- Wash underclothing and bed and bath linen in hot water on the day of treatment; dry in dryer or iron after dry; clothing and bedding that cannot be laundered should be placed in plastic bags for at least one week. Parasite cannot survive longer than 4 days off the human skin.
- Signs and symptoms may not disappear until 1 or 2 weeks after treatment; pruritis of hands and feet may persist for upto 3 months.

FUNGAL INFECTIONS

Fungi are larger and move complex than bacteria. They may be unicellular, such as yeasts, or multicellular such as molds. Many types are pathogenic to humans causing common skin disorders or serious systemic diseases such as blastomycosis. Certain types of fungi cause few symptoms, whereas other produce inflammation or hypersensitivity reaction.

Candidiasis

Candidiasis is caused by candida albicans, a yeast-like fungus, normally inhabits in the GI tract, mouth and vagina, but not usually on the skin. Candidiasis, moniliasis, the inflammation associated with the organism overgrowth on the skin is caused by the toxins that are released. Other predisposing factors are pregnancy, use of birth control pills, poor nutrition, antibiotic therapy, diabetes mellitus and other endocrinal disorder, inhalational corticosteroids and immunosuppressed conditions. Overgrowth of C. albicans causes candidiasis.

Pathophysiology

Candidiasis of the mucous membrane is thrush, the lesions are white spots that look like milk curd on the buccal mucosa and may extend down the esophagus. Vaginal thrush causes intense itching with a thick, white vaginal discharge. Candidiasis of the skin appears as pruritic, eroded, moist-inflammed areas with vesicles and pastules, and it occurs mostly in body folds such as beneath the breasts, in the inter-gluteal fold or in the groin.

Clinical Manifestation

The classic clinical manifestation of candidiasis is the presence of satellite lesions on the periphery of the general inflammation. The symptoms and signs of mouth, vagina and skin are as follows:
- Mouth: White cheese like patches leaving erosions when removed.
- Vagina: Vaginitis with red, edemations, painful vaginal wall, white patches, vaginal discharge, pruritus, pain on urination and intercourse.
- Skin: Diffuse papular erythematous rash with pin-point satel-lite lesion around edges of affected area.

Management

Diagnosis of candidiasis at any site made by clinical appearance and microscopic examination and culture.

Treatment aimed at elimination of the precipitating factors. Other measures including keeping the skin dry to avoid maceration; wearing loose absorbent clothing; and using topical medications such as powders, this helps the skin dry. Nystatin myostatis is an antifungal available in tablets, powder or vaginal suppositories and lozenges, amphotericin; cloterimazole, ciclopirox and ketconazol are effective against yeast infections. The sum up measure to prevent candidiasis are:
- Eradication of infection with appropriate medication.
- Skin hygiene to keep it clean and dry.
- Avoidance of lubricants.

Dermatophytoses

There are several different types of dermatophytosa tinea or superficial fungal infection of the skin and its appendages. The most common types are tinea capitis, tinea corporis, tinea cruris and tinea pedis.

Tinea Capitis

Tinea capitis is appropriately called ringworm of the scalp; can be caused either by species of "Microsporum or by Trichophyton fungi". The infection is transmitted readily, especially in crowded condition where poor hygiene exists although many children show a high resistance. Minor scalp trauma facilitates implantation of the spores; therefore, the infection can spread by contaminated barbers' instruments, combs or sharp brushes. It has worldwide distribution, primarily among pre pubertal children.

The characteristic lesion is round with erythema, a slight scaling, and some postules appearing at the edge of the lesion. Hair loss occurs with the hair shaft broken off at skin level. The hair loss is only temporary because the lesions usually heal without scarring. Usually tinea capitis is noninflammatory, a painful inflammation condition is called "Keroin".

Management

Griseofulvin is an antifungal agent effective in the treatment of all the dermatophytosis. The adult dose of tinea cupitis is 500 mg orally, and absorption enhanced when the drug is administered after a high fat meal. Infection usually resolves within 4 to 6 weeks. A mild antifungal agent, such as tolnaftate or haloprogin may be applied twice daily as ordered. The patients should be advised for shampooing head twice a week, cutting hair short facilitates shampooing. It may cause psychological trauma in children. Therefore, the hair is best left at an acceptable length. Daily shampooing avoids infection.

Tinea Corporis

Tinea corporis is dermatophytic infection commonly referred to as ringworm. It occurs in children living in hot and humid climates.

The lesions of tinea corporis occur on non and hairy parts of the body and are flat with an erythmatous scaling border and clearing center. They are typical annular appearance, well-deepened margins with fine cigarette paper scale and erythmatis.

Because of the dermatophytoses thrive in moist warm environment, the affected area should be kept clean and dry and overbathing to be avoided. A bland dusting powder can be used to promote dryness. Loose underclothing should be worn.

Mild infections are treated with cold compress; topical antifungals for isolated patches, creams or solution of miconazole Monistat and clotrimazole, Lotrimain. other than topical fungicide. Oral griseofulvin for severe infections.

Tinea Cruris

Tinea cruris is dematophytes commonly referred to as 'Jock itch' which occurs most commonly in men, especially who have tinea pedis and those who frequently wear athletic suppress or right shorts. It also occurs in women who wear tight pantyhose or slacks.

Tinea cruris the lesion of. the warm, moist, inter triginous areas of the groin. The lesions are bilateral and extend outward from groin along the inner thigh. The color ranges from brown to red, scaling is absent and pruritus is unusually present.

Lesions are well defined border in groin area.

Treatment includes topical antifungal cream or solution.

Tinea Pedis

Tinea pedis is most common dermatophytosis commonly referred to as "athletes foot". There are several forms of tinea pedis. It is rarely seen in children or women, but is widespread among young men especially those wearing shoes in hot climates. Walking barefoot in gymnasiums or ground swimming pool are susceptible to acquire infection.

The most common form of tinea pedis is intertriginous form. The fungal involvement usually begins in the toe webs, especially in the fourth interspace and may extend to the under-surface of the toe or on the plantar surface.

The person may be asymptomatic or may experience itching and burning in the affected area. The nails may become discolored, thickened or distorted onychomycosis. There will be interdigital scaling and maceration, erythema and blistering, pruritus and painful.

Treatment includes topical antifungal cream or solution.

The person with tinea pedis needs to be taught meticulous foot hygiene after the toes are dried thoroughly a light dusting of antifungal powder is applied to promote dryness. Caking the powder should be avoided. Socks should be of an absorbant material such as cotton, and may need to be changed more than once daily to promote dryness. A major focus of nursing is to initiate activities that lessen infection, such as wearing sandals, going barefoot, to decrease tissue moisture and using good foot hygiene, which includes washing the feet frequently and drying well between the toes.

Tinea Unguium

Tinea unguium is a dermatophytes. In this only few nails on one hand is affected; nails on toes are possibly affected. Fungal scale close to outer margin or lesion, brittle, thickened, broken nails with white or yellow discoloration.

Treatment modalities include:
- Tropical antifungal cream or solution.
- Griseofulvin moderately successful in fingernails.
- Poor response on toe nails.
- Debridement of toe nails to normal contour if problematic.

BACTERIAL INFECTIONS

The skin is covered with numerous micro-organisms especially bacteria. Most bacteria that normally inhabit in the skin are nonpathogenic. The skin provides an ideal environment for bacterial growth with abundant supplies of warmth, nutrients and water. Bacterial infections occur when the balance between the host and the micro-organisms is altered. This can occur on primary infection following a break in the skin. It can also occur as a secondary infection to already damaged skin or as a sign of a systemic disease. The common bacterial infections of the skin are as follows:

Impetigo

Impetigo is a common skin infection caused by staphylococci or beta-hemolytic streptococci or combination of both. It can occur at any age group but mostly in children. It occurs during summer or early fall. Factors that promote development of impetigo include tropical climates, uncleanliness, poor hygiene, poor nutrition and poor health.

Impetigo begins as a small thorn-walled vesicle that ruptures, easily and leaves a weeping denuded spot. It becomes pustular and dries to form a honey colored crust that appears stuck in the skin. The process, which is superficial may extend below the crust. Usually it is confirmed to face but may occur elsewhere. Clinical management includes vesiculopustular lesions that develop thick, honey-colored crust surrounded by erythema, pruritic most common in face.

Treatment consists of maintaining cleanliness and applying topical antibiotics. The crusts must be removed and the lesions washed gently two or three times daily to prevent further crust formation. Warm soaks or saline compress may be necessary to soften crusts that adhere firmly. Topical antibiotics are applied thrice a day. Systemic antibiotics such as oral penicillin, benzeathine pencillin I M erythromycin are prescribed.

Folliculitis

Folliculitis is usually caused by staphylococcis aureas, but occasionally caused by other bacteria. It may be caused by drainage from other infection. Predisposing factors include uncleanliness, maceration, infection, chemical irritation and injury.

Bacterial infections of the hair follicle may be superficial in the epidermis around the hairfollicle or deep in the tissue surrounding both the lower and upper portions of the hair follicle. Small pustules at hair follicle opening with minimal erythema, development of crusting most common on scalp; beard, extermities in men, tender to touch. Deep folliculitis produces a more severe inflammatory response. Sycoses barbae, barber's itch is deep folliculitis of the beard, in which hair do not fall out or break such as occurs with tinea barbae. Hordeolom Stye is deep folliculitis of the cilia of eyelids. There is usually swelling of the surrounding eyelid, with cursing along the edge of the eyelid.

Treatment of superficial folliculitis includes cleansing with soap and water and supplying topical antibiotics. Warm compresses are applied to encourage resolution of deep folliculities. Topical antibiotics such as neosporin, hasten healing. Healing is usually without scarring and loss of involved hair follicles.

Nursing management focuses on teaching patients about the prescribed therapy and about avoiding predisposing factors.

Furuncles and Carbuncles

Furuncles or boils are deep folliculitis that originate either superficial folliculates or as a deep nodule around hair follicle.

Furunculosis is the appearance of several furuncles. An infection that involves several surrounding hair follicles is termed as carbuncles.

Etiology

The causative organism is usually *Staphylococcus*, but occasionally furuncles can be caused by other bacteria. Both furuncles and carbuncles occur most often in obese poorly-nourished, fatigued, or otherwise susceptible persons whose hygiene may be poor, in debilitated elderly people and in persons with poorly controlled diabetes mellitus.

Pathophysiology

Local swelling and redness occur together with severe local pain which is decreased by moving the involved part as little as possible. Within 3 to 5 days, the lesion becomes elevated or "points up" the surrounding skin becomes shiny and the center or 'core' turns yellow. A carbuncle has several cores. The boil will usually rupture spontaneously but it may be surgically incised and drained. A drainage occurs, the pain is immediately relieved. The drainage soon changes from a yellow purulent material to a serosanguineous discharge. All drainage usually subsides within a few hours in a few days, the redness and swelling subside gradually.

Clinical Manifestations

In furuncles, there will be tender erythematous area around hair follicle; draining of pus and core of necrotic debris on rupture; they are most likely to occur on face, back of the neck, axillae, breasts, buttocks, perineum, thighs whereas carbuncles are usually limited to the nape of the neck and back. In addition to lesion, malaise, regional adenopathy, and elevated temperature are seen in furunculosis.

Management

For furuncles: Incision and drainage, occasionally antibiotics, meticulous care, of involved skin, frequent application of warm and moist compresses.

For funculosis: Warm compresses; systemic antibiotic after culture and sensitivity study of drainage usually semi synthetic penicillanase-resistant, oral penicillin such as oxacillin. Measures to reduce surface stphylococci include antimicrobial cream to nares, armpits, and groin and antiseptic to entire skin; often recurrent with scarring; incision and drainage of life lesions; prevention or correction of predisposing factors; meticulous hygiene.

For carbuncles: Treatment as in furuncles; often recurrent despite production of antibodies healing slow with scar formation.

Nursing care focuses on preventing this spread of infection. Patients are cautioned to keep their hands away from the discharge to prevent spread of infection.

Erysipelas

Erysipelas is a type of cellulitis usually caused by a hemolytic Streptococci and *S. aureus*. Elderly people with poor resistance are most often affected. Erysipelas may follow a puncture wound, ulcer or chronic dermatis.

Erysipelas is characterized by localized inflammation and swelling of the skin and subcutaneous tissues, usually of the face, scalp, hands, and genitalia. A bright, sharp line separates the diseased skin from the normal skin. The lesions are hot and red. The infection spreads via the lymphatic system and bloodstream.

Gramstain culture and sensitivity will determine the appropriate antibiotic therapy. Local lesions should be immobilized and elevated to decrease local edema. Wet to dry dressings may decrease pain and dry-up bullous lesions. Moist heat may also be used. If abscess formation occurs, incision and drainage are indicated. Nursing intervention focuses on helping patients assume responsibility for treatment and completing the treatment. It is imperative that the patient completes the course of prescribed antibiotic therapy. Hospitalization is needed in severe cases there will be progression to gangrene if cellulitis is untreated.

General principles of treatment for bacterial skin infection includes cleansing the skin well and applying an antibiotic. The skin is cleansed with soap and water or with hexachlorophene. Water or saline compresses or heat may be used to dry the horny layer of the skin. Topical antibiotics commonly used, include hydroxyquinilones, such as vioform, neomycin, bactiracin, and gentamycin, or erythromycin. Systemic antibiotics are used only when systemic signs such as fever and malaise are present.

VIRAL INFECTIONS OF THE SKIN

Viral infections of the skin are difficult to treat as viral infection anywhere in the body. When a cell is infected by a virus, a lesion can result. Lesions can also result from an inflammatory response to the viral infections. Herpes simplex, herpes zoster and warts are the common viral infections affecting the skin.

Herpes Simplex

Herpes simplex occurs on two similar yet serologically different strain type 1 and type 2. Herpes simplex virus (HSV) has a DNA containing core surrounded by a phospholipid covering.

Etiology

Factors that may precipitate recurrence of herpes simplex lesion include fever, URI, exhaustion and nervous tension. Lesions also are more common during the menses and after direct exposure to the sun rays.

HSV type generally has oral infections, virus remaining in nerve root ganglion and possibly returning to the skin to produce recurrence when excerbated by sunlight, trauma, menses, stress and systemic infections; contagion to those not previously infected; increase in severity with age, transmission by respiratory droplets or virus containing fluid, such as saliva or cervical secretions. The protection against subsequent infection in other areas with episodes of infection in one area.

HSV type 2 is associated with a lesion of the genitalia, that can be transmitted by sexual contact.

Pathophysiology

There are two phases to HSV infections. Primary infection is acquired by direct exposure to virus, usually through macocutaneous contact with an infected individual. After the initial infection, the virus travels to a sensory nerve ganglion and becomes latent. Reactivation of the virus causes disease recurrence. The HSV remains in the cells of the sensory nerves that supply the affected areas and causes recurrent lesions when the person is subjected to stress. The appearance of vesicles is preceded by several hours by a sensation of burning or itching. A cluster of vesicles on an erythematous basic appears at the macocutaneous junction of the lips or nose or an inflammation of the cornea of one eye with photophobia and tearing. The lesion found on the face and mouth (fever, blister, cold sore), eye (keratitis) (encephalitis).

HSV type 2 virus lesions are painful and may crack open. A crust gradually forms and the lesions heal in about 10 days. HSV can be identified by the Tzanck smear.

Clinical Manifestation

In first episode, symptoms occurring 3-7 days or more after contact; painful local reactions, grouped vesicles on erythmatous base; systemic symptom such as fever and malaise are possible or asymptomatic presentation is possible. In recurrent phase, small recurrence is in similar spot; characteristic grouped vesicle is on erythmatous base.

Management

Treatment includes symptomatic medication; soothing, moist compresses petrolatum to lesions, scarring not usual result; antiviral agents such as acyclovir zovinax. famciclovir (famvir) and valacyclovir (valtrex). Topical use of acyclovir, idoxuridine or vidarabine has been effective in preventing corneal ulceration and visual impairment in herperetic keratitis. Acyclovir is effective in systematically treating primary general herpes simplex and preventing recurrence. Patients with frequent recurrence may benefit from subcutaneous interferon-alfa.

Patient education is the primary nursing intervention needed for the patient with HSV infection regarding etiology, treatment modalities and measures to prevent secondary infection. Topical interferor-alfa, interferor-beta ointment are useful ingenital herpes.

Herpes Zoster

Herpes zoster or shingles is caused by the same virus varicellazoster. that causes varicella (chickenpox). Activation of the varicella zoster virus; frequent recurrence in immunosuppressed patients; potentially contagious to any one who has not had varicella or who is immunosuppressed. It is one of the most persisting and exasperating conditions in elderly persons and leads to discouragement and demoralization.

Pathophysiology

In herpes zoster, clusters of small vesicles usually form in line. They follow the course of the peripheral sensory nerves and often unilateral. Because they follow nerve pathways, the lesions never cross the midline of the body. However, nerves on both the sides of the body can be involved. Two-thirds of persons with herpes zoster develop lesions over the thoracic dermatomes and the remainder show involvement of the trigeminal nerve with lesions on the face, eye and scalp. The rash develops first as macules but progress rapidly to vesicles. The fluid becomes turbid and crusts develop and drop off in about 10 days.

Clinical Manifestation

Linear patches along dermatome of grouped vesicles on erythematous base; usually unilateral and on trunk; burning pain and neuralgia preceding outbreak, mild to severe during outbreak, malaise, fever, itching and pain over the involved area may precede the eruption of lesions. Discomfort from pain and itching is the major problem with herpes zoster. The pain may vary from light burning to deep visceral type pain. Enlargement of the lymph node may occur with rash.

Management

Treatment is symptomatic; antiviral agents such as acyclovir, famciclovir, and valacyclovir; moist compresses, white petrolatum to lesions; analgesia, mild sedation at bed time; Systemic corticosteroids to short course and decrease likelihood of post-herpetic neuralgia (PHN), controversal, usual healing without complication but scarring possible postherpetic neuralgia possible.

Analgesic prescribed for pain. Aspirin without codiene for severe pain. Systemic corticosteroid prednisone are useful.

Local application of capsaicin cream may give some relief.

Verruca Vulgaris

Verruca vulgaris caused by human papilloma virus, spontaneous disappearance in 1-2-years is possible; mildly contagious by autoinoculation, specific response on body part is affected.

Clinical manifestation includes circumscribed, hypertrophic, flesh colored papulae to epidermis, painful on lateral compression.

Multiple treatment includes surgery—scoop removal with scissors and currette; liquid nitrogen therapy; blistering agents—Cantharidin; Keralytic agents—Salicylic acid; CO_2 laser therapy, treatment can result in scarring.

Warts

Warts develop from hypertrophy of epidermal cells as a result of a viral infection. Plantar warts is caused by human papilloma virus. It is seen most commonly in older children and young adults.

Pathophysiology

Warts are benign skin growths that grow in variety of shapes. The common wart is a small circumscribed, painless hyperkerotatic papule usually seen in the extremities, especially the hands. Filiform warts are slender finger—like projections occurring mostly on the face and neck. Plantar warts grow inward from the pressure on the sole of the feet and may be painful. They are differentiated from calluses by lack of skin lines over the surface. Warts that develop in the anogenital region have a lighter-colored surface and a cauliflower-like appearance, and they may cause itching. Anogenital warts may spread either by sexual activity or by other means. Some genital warts in women may predispose the woman in cancer cervix.

Clinical Manifestation

Plantar warts on bottom surface of foot are growing inwards because of pressure of walking or standing; painful when pressure applied; interrupted skin markings; cone shaped with black dot thrombosed vessels when pared.

Management

The most commonly used therapeutic measures for common warts are electrodessiccation and cryosurgery. In electrodesiccation, the top of the wart is seared gently to soften the keratinized surface and then curretted off and the bleeding points cauterized. This method is not used for plantar warts.

Cryosurgery: consists of freezing the lesion with a substance such as liquid nitrogen. Cauterant chemicals—Such as formalin, phenol, nitric acid, canthridin, salicylic acid, or porophyllum may be used. Recalcitrant warts may respond to reciation therapy. Surgical excision is seldom used because of painful scarring may result.

Nursing intervention includes preparing the patient for treatment and assist during treatment.

ALLERGIC CONDITIONS OF THE SKIN

Dermatologic problem associated with allergies and hypersensitivity reactions presents a real challenge to the health care providers. A careful family history and discussion of exposure to possible offending agents provide valuable data. Patch testing involves the application of allergens to the patient skin usually on the back for 48 hours, after which the test sites are examined for erytheme, papules vesicles or all of these. Patch testing is used to determine possible causative agents. This information is valuable to the patient. The best treatment of allergic dermatitis is avoidance of causative agent. The extreme prurits of contact dermatitis is and its potential chronicity make it frustrating problem for the patient, the nurse and the dermatologist.

Dermatitis is a superficial inflammation of the skin, refers to several different conditions resulting in the same type of lesions. Dermatitis is often classified arbitrarily according to special features such as cause, pattern, age or type of treatment required. The term eczema, is often used synonymously with dermatitis but usually refers to the chronic type.

The common allergic conditions of the skin are in brief as follows:

Contact Dermatitis

Contact dermatitis is caused by external agents and may affect various parts of the body. The two types of contact dermatitis are irritant and allergic.

Etiology

1. Irritant contact dermatitis can occur in any person on contact with a sufficient concentration of an irritant:
   - Mechanical irritation may result from wool or glass fibers.
   - Chemical irritants include acids, alkalies, solvents, detergents and oils commonly found in clearing compounds, insecticides and industrial compounds.
   - Biological irritants include urine, feces, and toxins from insects or aquatic plants. People whose hands and feet are constantly wet often develop irritant contact dermatitis.
2. Allergic contact dermatitis is cell-mediated hypersensitivity immune reaction from contact with a specific antigen. Many compounds cause sensitization under specified conditions. Typical antigen includes poison, ivy, synthetics, industrial chemicals, drugs, e.g. sulfanilamide or penicillin, and metals, e.g. Nichel-chromium.

Common causes of contact dermatitis of different areas are as follows:
- *Face/Scalp/Ears:* Cosmetics, haircare producers, jewellery cleansers, sunscreen, contact lens solution, metals nickel glasses.
- *Neck:* Perfumes, clothing especially wool.
- *Trunk:* Deodarants, clothing, perfumes, laundry products.
- *Arms and Hands:* Poison ivy, oak, and sumac, jewellery, nickel, etc. in watch bands, detergents and other cleanser gloves.
- *Legs/Feet:* Medication for "athletes foot" shoes.

Pathophysiology

Characteristic dermatitis lesions appear sooner in irritant contact dermatitis than in allergic type. Manifestations of delayed hypersensitivity, absorbed agent acting as antigen and sensitization after several exposures, appearance of lesions 2-7 days after contact with allergies.

Clinical Manifestation

Red, hive-like papules and plaques; sharply circumscribed with occasional vesicles; exposed areas are more common; usually pruritic; relation of area of dermatitis to causative agent, e.g. metal allergy and dermatitis on ring finger.

Management

- Weeping uninfected lesions respond rapidly to wet dressings with water or burows solution for 20 minutes four times daily.
- Crusts and scales are not removed but are allowed to drop off naturally as the skin heals.
- Systemic antibiotics if infection is present.
- Antihistamines for severe pruritus.
- Plain calamine lotion may be applied for pruritus from poison ivy.
- Elimination of contact allergens.
- Avoidance of irritating affected area.
- Systemic corticosteroid if sensitivity is severe.
- Primary focus of nursing care in prevention includes patient teaching.

Urticaria

Usually allergic phenomena, presence of edema in upper dermis resulting from a local increase in permeability of capillaries usually from histamine.

Clinical manifestation includes spontaneity occurring and rounded elevations, varying size and usually multiple.

Treatment includes removal of source and antihistamine therapy.

Drug Reaction

Any drug that acts as antigen and causes hypersensitivity reaction is possible cause, certain drugs more prone to reaction, e.g. Penicillin. mediated by circulating antibody.

Clinical manifestation includes rash of any morphology, often red, macular and papular, semiconfluent, generalized rash with abrupt onset, appearance as late as 14 days after cessation of drug, possibly pruritic.

Treatment includes withdrawal of drug if possible, antihistamines, local or systemic corticosteroids are possibly necessary.

Atopic Dermatitis

Atopy refers to type I hypersensitivity, which is hereditary and includes asthma, hay fever, eczema and other type of reactions.

Exact cause is unknown, often beginning in infancy and decreasing in incidence with age, association with allergic conditions, costume, hay fever, eczema, elevation, e.g. IgE levels are common, genetically determined, often family history, decreased itch threshold, stress and increased water contact, e.g. frequent hand washing, thumb sucking and other possible agents.

The major symptoms of atopic dermatitis is pruritus, chronic scratching leads to eczematous lesions and subsequent lichenification. There will be scaly, red to redbrown, circumscribed lesions; accentuation of skin marking pruritic and symmetric eruptions common in antecubital and popliteal space in adults. Persons with atopic dermatis are highly susceptible to viral infections Herpes. and bacterial infection staphylococci or beta themolytic streptococci.

There is no cure for atopic dermatitis, but symptoms can be controlled. The focus of therapy in relief of pruritus to break the itch scratch cycle that leads to lesions. For which:

- Topical corticosteroids creams and ointments for localized lesion.
- Topical antibiotic is rarely used.
- Cool compresses with water or burows solution are helpful for acute phases when weeping lesions are present.
- Phototherapy; coaltar therapy, intralesional corticosteroids, lubrication of dry skin.
- Systemic corticosteroids if severe—e.g. eczema.
- Reduction of stress.
- Antibiotic for secondary infection, e.g. penicillin and erythromycin.

Patient education is the major focus of care and should stress prevention of hypersensitivity and control of signs and symptoms. Patient should keep the skin hydrated and avoid temperature extremes and irritating substances. The person with atopic dermatitis will be given education as follows:

- Avoid soap over lesions; soap is an irritant.; use soap minimally over non-affected areas.
- Soak affected areas for 15 to 20 minutes in warm water for hydration; pat skin dry, then immediately apply recommended lotion or cream to seal in moisture.
- Wet wraps may be used in place of soaking; wraps permits evaporation, which cools the skin, thus decreasing pruritus.
- Apply corticosteroids in a thin layer and rub in well; do not use fluonated corticosteroids on the face.
- Avoid wool, furor rough fibers against the skin; they are irritants and cause itching.
- Avoid overheating that increases sweating, leading to itching, wear loose, light clothing in hot weather. Airconditioning promotes comfort sunlight is beneficial to the skin.
- Avoid excessive cold that dries the skin.
- Avoid anything that aggravates the eczema.
- Rinse all garments and bed linen, twice to avoid residue of cleansing agents.
- Consult dermatologist for appropriate laundry agents to prevant irritations from clothing.
- Seek medical care of eczema becomes worse.

Other Type of Dermatitis

- Lichen simplex chronicus (LSC) is a chronic skin condition that results from repeated scratching. Psychological factors are thought to be involved. It may occur without any cause, LCS is more commonly found on the hands, perineum, legs, and occipital region of the scalp. Once itching starts, the itch scratch cycle is initiated and scratching becomes a habit. The skin becomes excoriated and lichenified plaques resulting. Lesion disappears if scratching ceases, but it is difficult for the person to stop scratching. Itching is often worse at night. Topical corticosteroids are the treatment of choice.
- Seborrheic dermatitis may occur primarily in areas of increased sebaccan gland activity on the face, ears, scalp, chest and back. The cause is unknown. Mild seborrheic dermatitis is often seen in the scalp in the form of erythema and dandruff and can be controlled easily by shampooing with selenium sulfide (Selsum blue) shampoo. More extensive seborrheic dermatitis leads to red scaly plaques and is treated with topical hydrocortisone.
- Nummulur dermatitis is chronic condition of uncertain cause occurring most commonly in middle aged or older men. The lesions of nummular dermatitis are corn-shaped and are found on the dorsum of the hands, the extension surfaces of the extremities and the buttocks. Itching is often severe. The skin is usually dry, therefore, frequent bathing is inadvisable. Exposure to sunlight may be helpful. Treatment consists of topical corticosteroids and antibiotic therapy of lacterin isolated by culture.
- Stasis dermatitis is a common skin condition of the lower extremities in older person. It is usually preceded by varicosities and poor circulation. With the reduction in venous return from the legs, substances are normally carried away by the circulation remain in the tissue causing irritation. The skin is often reddened and edematous. Pruritus may be severe. Scratching causes breaks in the skin, which become infected via hands, clothing and other sources. The most important treatment for stasis dermatitis is prevention with careful attention to the treatment of peripheral vascular condition preventing constrictions of the circulation to the extremities. Acute weeping lesions are treated with wet compresses and elevation of the legs.

Skin Reactions

Dermatitis Medicamentosa

Dermatitis medicamentosa or drug rash, can be caused by almost any drug. The rash occurs as a result of gradual accumulation of the drug or because of antibodies that develop in response to a component of the medications. Skin manifestations from drug have a nonallergic or an allergic basis. Commonly seen skin reactions include, erythematous rashes, purpura, vesicles, bullae, ulcers, and urticaria. the reactions may occur at any time but the onset is usually sudden.

Most skin reactions are caused by hypersensitivity reaction to drugs. The following reaction may occur:
- Type I   : Analphylactic urticaria, angioedema.
- Type II : Cytotoxic cell injury.
- Type III : Immune complex serum sickness.
- Type IV : Cell mediated allergic contact dermatitis, allergic photosensitivity.

- Some drugs have combined reactions. For example, Penicillin may produce type I and type III reaction.

Photosensitivity may occur with certain drugs and may take one of two forms: phototoxicity or photoallergy.

1. Phototoxicity may occur in any person taking a photosensitive drug and results from the reaction of the drug chemicals. With radiant energy, particularly ultraviolet light symptoms resemble sunburn erythema, edema, vesicle.
2. Photoallergy reactions are cell mediated type IV. Hypersensitivity reactions, therefore, affect only a small group of persons after several sensitizing exposures of drug and sunlight. Symptoms resemble eczema.

Coaltar derivatives, psoralens, tetracycline, nalidixic acid, sulfalim, dectomycin, chloropromazine, certain dyes, diuretics thiazides phenathiazine oral hypoglycemias and griseofulvin.

The skin reaction to common medications are as follows:
- *Antibiotics,* sulfonamides, thiazide diuretices barbiturates, phenylbutazone.
- *Purpura Ecchymosis:* Petechias, thiazide, sulfonamide, barbiturates, anticoagulants.
- *Mucocutanean lesions:* Sulfanamides, penicillin, barbiturate, phenylbutazone vesicles, bullae ulcers.
- *Urticaria:* Penicillin, streptomycin, tetracyclin, insulin, aspirin, dyes, ACTH and antiserum.

Management of dermatitis medicomentosa include stopping the drug and treating the symptoms with cool moist compresses, antihistamines for pruritus, and topical and systematic corticosteroids. Photosensitivity can be prevented by avoiding direct sunlight on the skin when taking drug with photosensitivity effects. Nursing care include patient education regarding skin reaction to drugs and report and take proper remedial measure.

Explorative Dermatitis

Explorative dermatitis is rare and generalized dermatitis. In most cases, cause is unknown, but the disease may be associated with other types of dermatitis or with a lymphoma or it may be result of drug reaction.

The onset of disease may be rapid or insidious and consist of an elevated temperature and generalized erythema, followed by extensive scaling exfoliation. Pruritus may be present and the lesions often become infected. Loss of large amounts of water and protein from the skin leads to hypoproteinemia, weight loss, and difficulty with temperature control. Heart failure may occur in elderly patient. Death may result from overwhelming infections or circulatory collapse.

Treatment consists of maintaining fluid balance and preventing infection. All drugs are discontinued as potential causative factors although antibiotics may be started after culture and sensitivity tests, and infected lesions. Oral corticosteroids are used for severe case. Daily baths followed by application of petrolatum to the skin promote comfort. Nursing care focuses for management of signs and symptoms and education.

Erythema Multiforme

Erythema multiforme (EM) is self-limiting inflammation of the skin and mucous membranes in genetically susceptecable persons. Although it is mild, it may progress to a toxic epidermal necrolysis type of illness. It can be classified as major and minor. Both forms are thought to be a cell mediated immune response to relevant antigens.

Some medications trigger EM include phenytoin, carbambazepine, sulfonamides NSAIDS, allopurinol and some antibiotics, e.g. cephalosporins. Infection that causes EM include myeoplasmal pneumonia, chickenpox, hepatitis B, infectious mononucleosis and herpes simlex, SLE and leukemia.

Episodes of the disease usually lasts for 1 to 3 weeks. The clinical lesions are characteristically erythematus papulae acrally distributed. The rash is painful and itchy, and it may progress to the bullous variety. The rash occurs on the dorso of the hands, palms, knees, feet and elbows. The oral cavity may be affected by blisters progressing to erosion of the entire oral mucosa and lips. Conjunctivitis may occur it may progress to corneal opacity. If the genital mucosa is involved, adhesions may result as long-term complications. The skin eruptions may be preceded by fever, chest pain and arthralgia. Severe case may be confused with toxic epidermal necrolysis.

A single attack of EM does not usually require treatment. Any suspected triggering agent is discontinued and symptoms treated. Topical steroid may be prescribed to relive itching and burning. Systemic steroids seem to prolong episodes of the disease. A sedatory antihistamine such as hydroxyzine may be of use. The patient with any type of EM needs support and education throughout diagnosic biopsy and treatment as prescribed. Initially other disorders causing blistering must be considered and the patient will require support during this time. Education needed to patient regarding the medication prescribed including administration of dosing and side effects. Nursing intervention is supportive and includes baths, soaks and care.

Infectious Diseases

Skin reactions caused by some communicable diseases such as measle, chickenpox, smallpox, scarlet fever, and accompany severe acute rheumatic fever:
- Measles (rubeola) caused by rubeola virus, incubation period is 8-14. days. Rash appears on the face, they will be pink macular-papular rash and lesions coalesce.
- Germal measles (rubella) caused by rubella virus, incubation period 14-21 days. Rash appears on the

face, they are pink macular-papular rash, lesions usually discretes and it may coalesce.
- Scarlet fever (Scarlatina) caused by hemolytic Streptococcus, incubation period is 1-3 days. Rashes appear on neck and chest. They are bright red scarlet and macules pin point.
- Chickenpox (varicella) caused by varicella zoster virus, incubation period is 14-21 days. Rashes appear on back and chest. They are macule papule, vesicle, crust, lesions at different stages.
- Smallpox (variola) caused by variola virus, incubation period is 7-21 days. Rashes appear on face and chest. They are macule, papule, vesicle, crust, lesions and all at same stage.
- Typhoid fever caused by *Salmonella typhosa*, incubation period is 14 to 7-21. days. Rashes appeal on abdomen. They are macular rash. Treatment includes treating the diseases.

LUPUS ERYTHEMATOSUS

It is one of the tissue diseases that may result in skin condition. There are two forms, systemic lupus erythematosus SLE and discoid lupus erythematosa DLE. SLE has already been discussed in earlier chapter.

DLE is a chronic relative benign skin that has worldwide presence among all races occurring, most often in fourth decade of life. The precipitating factors include physical trauma and stress.

The lesions of the DLE are well demarcated and erythematous, have a characteristic scaly border with an atrophied center and vary in size. The more common sites are the cheeks butterfly pattern, nose, ears, scalp and chest, although other parts of the body including mucous membranes may also be involved. DLE occurs in the absence of other signs and symptoms and nuerological abnormalities of SLE.

There is no cure of DLE. Palliative measures include, topical steroid therapy under occlusive wraps, intralesional steroid therapy, antimalarial therapy with chloroquine, hydroxy chloroquine sulfate or quinacrine hydrochloride. Nursing care is focussed on assisting patients and thus families to live with a chronic incurable disease. Education is necessary regarding palliative and preventive measures. Preventive measures include avoiding physical trauma, using sun screen to prevent sunburn and wearing warm clothing to protect against cold and wind. If stress is a precipitatory factor, measures to reduce stress can be instituted.

PAPULOSQUAMOUS DISEASES

Papulosquamous diseases are characterized by papular, scaly lesions, common disorders are psoriasis, pityriasis rosea and lichen plasius.

Psoriasis

Psoriasis is a genetically determined, chronic, epidermal, proliferative disease. The cause is unknown. There are no specific precipitating factors for the majority of persons. However, some people may develop exacerbations after climatic changes, stressors, trauma, infections, or drugs propranolol, lithium. Pregnant women often experience of remissions of symptoms. It is chronic dermatitis which involves excessively rapid turn over of epidermal cells and family predispositions.

The lesions of psoriasis are elevated, erythematous and sharply circumscribed, with a silvery white scale. Removal of the scale usually results in a characteristic pin-point-bleeding called the 'Auspitz phenomenon'. The primary lesions is a papule; these papules then join to form plaques. Lesions may occur over the entire body but are found more commonly on the scalp, elbows, chins, intergluteal cleft, and trunk. Beefy-red lesions may be observed in an acute flare-up. Nail changes may occur. The nails of persons with psoriasis have characteristic involvement; there may be pitting of the nails, yellowish discoloration, oil drop or salmon patches; leukonychia and whitening of nails, splinter hemorrhage and onycholysis separation of nail from nail bed.

Types of Psoriasis

There are four types of psoriasis viz., psoriasis vulgaris, generalized psoriasis, localized psoriasis and erythematous psoriasis.
- Psoriaris vulgaris may follow streptococcal phanyngitis.
- Generalized postular psoriasis patients require admission to hospital. In generalized and localized postular type, there will be history of plaque type of psoriasis developing pustules on erythmatic base. Other symptoms include fever, chills, arthralgia, hypocalcemia.
- Erythematous psoriasis produces red coloration of the skin with disquamaline scale over most of the body. It is associated with problems of temperature regulation, hypoalbumenia, pedaloedema, and high output cardiac failure caused by inflammatory vasodilation. The complication psoriasis is psoriatic arthritis.

Management

Initially the lesions may be treated with topical keratolytic agents salicylic acid, ammoniated mercury or tropical steroids with occlusive wraps and wet dressing to decrease inflammation. The application of bland emollient petrolatum and mineral oil is important in the treatment of person with psoriasis. These emollients decrease the amount of scale on the psoriatic plaques and the thickness of the plaque. If person is resistent to emollients, coaltar of anthralin products are used. Interlesional injection of corticosteroids for chronic plaques; sunlight, ultraviolet light, alone or with topical or systemic potentiation; no cure is possible, but can be controllable, antimetabolites, methotrexate are used for difficult cases.

The disease is not curable and may wax and wane continuously. Lesions may fade with treatment, only to recur in the same area or elsewhere. Teaching the person with psoriasis will be helpful.
- Nature of psoriasis, non-curable, recurrence of symptoms.
- Reduce episodes of rapidly spreading psoriasis flare-ups. by avoiding skin trauma injuries, sunburn, infections, extremes of temperature, and stress.
- Shampoo hair frequently remove scales of scalps. If scalp has plaques, use a tar shampoo for 10 minutes before rinsing. Press often thick plaques with mineral oil at the night before a morning shampoo; use fine-toothed comb to remove loose scales.
- Avoid self medication, particularly when receiving prescribed therapy.
- Apply topical medication in a thin layer for most lesions, use a thick layer over plaques.
- Monitor for side effects of medication.
- Seek medical follow up during periods of exocerbation.

Pityriasis Rosea

Pityriasis Rosea is a noncontagious skin condition. The cause is thought to be viral. The incidence is higher in winter. The initial symptom is usually a 2 to 10 cm, single, oval lesion herald patch. with a thin scaly border and yellowish centre, appearing most often on the trunk, upper arm or thigh. The herald patch usually precedes other lesions by 1 to 30 days.

A generalized eruptions of multiple erythematous macule follows the herald patch usually followed by papules. A fine scale is usually present. The distribution of lesions often are in long axes, running parallel to each other on the trunk which creates a "Christmas tree" distribution. The skin usually clears in 6 to 8 weeks and the condition does not recur.

Treatment option consists of tropical steroids and colloid baths. Ultraviolet therapy may be used. Exposure to sunlight to the point of minimal erythema. will speed disappearance of the lesions and itching. The patient should be cautious against sunburn. Nursing care is essentially symptomatic and includes assisting patient with topical steroids and colloid baths if itching is present and educating the patient and family.

ACNE

Acne Vulgaris

Acne vulgaris is an inflammatory disorder of sebaceus glands, more common in teenagers but possible development in adulthood. Persistence in adulthood possible. Secondary result of iodides, bromides, cortecosteroids and androgen-dominated birth control pills.

The cause of acne is thought to be multifactorial. Some of the common causes that have been postulated are free fatty acids, endocrine effects, stressors, diet, hereditary and infection.

Pathophysiology

At puberty sabaceous glands undergo enlargement from androgen stimulation. Sebum is released, passed through the follicular canal, and combined with sebacous gland cell fragments, epidermal cells keratin and bacteria. At this time the triglycerides in the sebum and hydrolyzed to glycerol and free fatty acids. The sebum and debris may become plugged in the hair follicle to form an open comedo black head., if it is at the surface or closed comedo white head. The dark color of the blackhead melanin is not dirt and results from passage of melanin from the adjoining epidermal cells. Inflammatory lesions apparently develop from the escape of sebum into the dermis, which then serves as an irritant, causing an inflammatory reaction. Free fatty acids may also be an irritant in the follicle itself.

Clinical Manifestation

Acne occurs mostly on the face and neck, upper chest and back although the upper arms, buttocks and thighs may also be involved. Comedes are the first visible signs, and the skin is characteristically oily. The inflammatory lesions include papules, pustules, nodules, and cysts. Superficial lesions may resolve within 5-10 days without scarring but large lesions last for several weeks and often result scarring ice pick scar.

Management

Treatment of acne may be topical, systemic, intralesional or surgical and includes the following:
- Topical therapy
  - Basic method therapy.
  - Agents: benzoyl peroxide, vitamin A, acid tretin, antibiotics topical erythromycin., sulfur-zinc lotion.
- Removal of comedones with comedoextraction.
- Systemic therapy.
  - Used with topical therapy for severe nodular or dysticacne.
  - Isoretinioc acid accutane.
    * A vitamin A acid ana
    * Side affects: dry lips and conjucative on brittle hair tendernege to finger tips and toe trips, hypertriglyceridaemia birth defects.
  - Systemic antibiotics
  - Estrogen for female patients who have not responded to other therapy.

- Intralesional corticosteroid therapy for cystrs of severe acne.
- Surgery; derm abrasion to remove scars.

Major nursing strategies are counselling and teaching. Stress appears to be one of the causative factors. Therefore, attempts to identify and cope with stressors may be helpful. Acne can be a stressor producing facial disfigurement and sometimes leading to behavior that is hostile aggressive and anxiouis as well as shy and withdrawn. Psychological counsel is desirable. Knowledge of nature of acne helps the person understand the necessary care. Teaching directed towards general health care of skin with the person with acne are as follows:

- Preventive measure:
  - Keep hand and hair away from the face.
  - Avoid constricting clothing over lesions.
  - Shampoo hair and scalp frequently.
  - Avoid exposure to oils and greases.
  - Eat a well-balanced diet and avoid any food that appears to cause skin flare-up.
- General skin care:
  - Keep skin clean; wash face 2 to 3 times daily.
  - Use a medicated soap or agent prescribed by physician.
  - Avoid vigorous rubbing of the skin.
  - Use cosmetics that are water-based, rather than cream-based and avoid those that contain waxesters myristates, palmitates, and stearates.
- During therapy:
  - Follow the prescribed therapy even when immediately improvement is not noted for 2 to 3 weeks.
  - Expect skin desquamation during therapy.
  - Avoid using self-remedies during therapy.
  - Remove cosmetics before applying topical medications.
  - Avoid exposure to direct sunlight if using tretinoin, or taking tetracyclin photosensitivity.
  - Avoid pregnancy if taking accutane possibility of birth defects.

Acne Rosacea

Acne Rosacea is a skin condition that usually affects person over 25 years of age. The cause is unknown. But many causative factors suggested are bacteria, vitamin deficiency, hormonal imbalance, alcohol, caffience, psychological factors and heredity.

Acne rosacea brings with redness over the cheeks and nose, followed by papules, pustules and enlargements of superficial blood vessels. Year of acne rosaea lead to an irregular bulbous thickening of the skin of the distal part of the nose rhinophyma with a red purple discoloration and dilated follicles.

There is no specific treatment for acne rosacea. Some persons respond to tetracyclin and tropical peeling agents. But there is no specific treatment for the vascular component. Rhinophyma may be treated by plastic surgery.

BULLOUS DISEASES

Pemphigus Vulgaris

Pemphigus vulgaris is characterized by an enormous bullae that appears all over the body and on the mucous membrane. The cause of that disease is thought to have an autoimmune basis. Rare but worldwidely occurs primarily in persons between the age of 40 and 60.

Tissue injury results from circulating autoantibodies that bind to the structural proteins within the epidermis. Blister formation occurs above in stratum basalis. Healing is commonly associated with the development of postinflammatory hyperpigmentation rather than scarring.

The disease is characterized by acantholysis cells slip past one another and fluid accumulates between the cells. By placing the thumb firmly on the skin and exerting lateral sliding pressure, the upper epidermis can be dislodged resulting in erosion or blister (Nikolsky's sign). A Tzanck test will identify acantholytic cells. Injection of the crust produces a foul odor and toxemia may result. If the disease is untreated, death usually ensues in about 1 year secondary to sepsis.

Hospitalization is usually required for skin care and monitoring of drug effects. The treatment of choice for severe pemphigus is systemic corticosteroids in large doses, the dose is gradually reduced and improvement is noted. Immunosuppressants—such as methotrexate, cyclophosphamide and azathioprine may be given to reduce the corticosteroid dose. Gold therapy gold sodium thiomalate may be given alone or in combination with corticosteroids for chronic therapy.

Nursing care of the person with severe pemphigus can be a challenge. Stryker frames may be used to help the person's change position painlessly and to prevent weight bearing on row surfaces. Air mattress or flotation system may be used to reduce surface pressure on skin and promote comfort. Dakin's solution compresses may be applied to oozing lesions to help controls odor and infection. Infection is major concern because of the immunosuppressive effect of drug therapy. Special mouth care is required for mouth lesions and bland diets are more easily tolerated. Emotional support and education about general skin lesion care is essential for patient and family.

TUMORS OF THE SKIN

Skin cell growth may develop from the epidermis, from sebacious or sweat glands, from the melanocyte system or from mesodermal tissue. For example, connective or vascular tissue. Most skin tumors are benign even those are malignant with the exception of such tumors of malignant melanoma.

Benign Tumors

The term keratosis refers to any cornification or growth of the horny layer of the skin. Different types of keratosis include corn, and calluses, warts and seborrheic and actinic senile keratosis.

- Corns are due to pressure or ill fitting shoes. In appearance it will be center core that thickness will be inwardly, pain with pressure usually occur on toes. Treatment includes foot pad with center hole to relieve pressure properly fitting shoes, corn will recur if pressure is not relieved.
- Callus are due to constant pressure on plantar surface of foot. It can also occur on palmar surface of hand. In this thickening of horny layer of skin is soon. Treatment includes relief of pressure, regular massage with softening lotion or creams.
- Seborrheic keratosis are benign, genetically determined growths; this care found in increasing number with age and have no association with sun exposure. Normal aging process rarely develops into malignancy, it must distinguish from actinic keratosis which have malignant potential.

  Clinical manifestation includes irregularly round or oval flat-topped papules or plaques, surface is often warty; appearance of being stuck on; increase in pigmentation with age of lesion; usually multiple and possibly itching. Large darkened, greasy warts are usually on trunk, less often on scalp, face and proximal extremities. Sudden increase in number and size may indicate gastrointestinal malignancy.

  No treatment except for cosmetic reasons or constant irritation may be removed by currettage, electrodesiccation, or liquid nitrogen cryosurgery. and eliminate source of irritation minimal scarring.

  Another condition to similar to seborrheic keratosis is dermatosis papulosa nigra is usually seen in Afro-Americans; there will be a small pedunculated and heavily pigmented lesion. Treatment is also similar to seborrhoic keratosis.
- Actinic keratosis is due to chronic exposure to solar radiation; occur on exposed areas of skin; light-skinned persons are most vulnerable. It is premalignant form of squamous cell carcinoma. It is also known as solar keratosis. The clinical appearance will be round or irregular, red brown to gray in color with dry scaly appearance. Treatment includes protective clothing, sunscreens, removal of curettage, liquid nitrogen therapy, dermabrasion, electrodesiccation, large lesions application of 1.5 percent and 5-fluorouracil cream.
- Skin tags are common after midlife, appearance on neck, a small, skin-colored, soft and pedunculated papules. For there is no treatment unless for cosmetic reasons or because of repeated trauma; surgical removal is possible if requested. usually just "clipping off" method anesthesia.
- Lipoma benign tumor of adipose tissue, often encapsulated, most common in 40 to 60 year-old age group. It is a rubbery compressible round mass of adipose tissue, single or multiple variable in size possibly extremely large; most common on trunk, back of neck or foreams. For this, usually there is no treatment, biopsy is used to differentiate from liposarcoma, excision usual treatment when indicated.
- Vitiligo cause is unknown it is genetically influenced, most noticeable is among dark-skinned people and those with summer tan, complete absence of melanocytes the disease is noncontagious. The clinical manifestations include focal amelanosis complete loss of pigment., macular; variation in size and location, usually symmetric and permanent. Treatment includes attempt at repigmentation of pigmented skin with extensive disease 75 percent body involved; cosmetics and strains for camouflage and to de-emphasize vitiligonous area.
- Lentigo in which there is an increased number of normal melanocytes in basal layer of epidermis. Senile lentigo liver spots is related to aging and sun exposure. In the hypopigmented it is brown to black, flat-lesions are seen usually on sun exposed areas. Treatment is only for cosmetic purposes, liquid nitrogen, possible recurrence 1-2 years.

Premalignant Lesions

Skin lesions that may lead to malignancy include actinic keratitis, leukoplakia, Bowens disease and pigmented moles:

- *Leukoplakia:* The exact cause is unknown. It may be caused by external irritants such as poor-fitting dentures, cheek-biting and pipe and cigarette smoking. Chronic maceration, friction, and senile atrophy may lead to vaginal leukoplakia.

  In the mucous membranes develops thickened white patches of keratinized cell, which may eventually lead to squamous cell carcinoma. Erythroplakia red or red and white patches of the mouth has a higher malignancy potential than leukoplakia.

  Treatment includes prevention by removal of causative factor; inspection of mouth, mucus membrane, dental care for rough teeth, proper-fitting dentures. Large lesions are usually surgically excised, and a biopsy is performed. Benign lesions may be removed by electrode siccation.
- *Bowen's disease:* This is due to chemical carcinogens; occurs in old and light-skinned men. It is also called

squamous cell carcinoma *in situ*. Persons affected are at higher risk of developing other malignancies.

The lesions are widely distributed, brown plaques although a single lesion may exist. Treatment includes surgical excision, cryotherapy, curretage and electrodesiccation, carbon dioxide laser therapy and 5-fluorouracil cream or solution.

- Pigmented nevi moles are grouping of normal cells derived from melanocyte like precursor cells. Hereditary predisposition is possible. Most moles are harmless, but others may be dysplectic, precancerous or cancerous.

They appear on most persons regardless of skin color, may be flat, raised, prominant or hairy. Hyperpigmented areas vary in form and color. Color ranges from tank to black. Hyperpigmented areas that vary in form and color ranges from tan to black. They are flat, slightly elevated haloid, verrucoid, polypoid, dome-shaped, sesile or papillomatous and preservation of normal skin markings; hairgrowth is possible. Dysplastic moles usually occur on the upper back in male and on the legs in females.

Changes in mole that require immediate attention which include:
- Development of a ring of new pigment around the base.
- Development of uneven pigmentation.
- Sudden growth, loss of hair and bleeding.

For moles, no treatment is necessary except for cosmetic reasons, skin biopsy for diagnostic decisions and excision of suspicious lesions. To help remember the characteristics of malignant moles, the American Cancer Society has developed the mnemonic ABCD:

A. A symmetry of border.
B. Border irregularity.
C. Color blue-black or variegated.
D. Diameter more than 6 mm.

MALIGNANT LESIONS OF THE SKIN

Malignant tumors of the skin exhibit the characteristics of all malignant conditions. However, skin malignancies are generally growing slowly. The presence of a persistent lesion that does not heal in highly suspicious of malignancy and should be biopsied. Adequate and early treatment can often lead to complete cure. The fact that the skin lesions are so visible to increase the likelihood of early detection and diagnosis. Patient should be taught to selfexamine that skin regular.

The risk factors for skin malignancies include having a fair skin type blonde or red hair and blue or green eyes, history of chronic sun exposure, family history of skin cancer, outdoor occupation and exposure to tar and systemic arsenicals and severe sunburns. The brief description of malignant lesions of the skin is as follows:

- *Squamous cell carcinoma.* The exact cause is unknown; it may arise from acitinic keratoses, Bowen's disease of leukoplakia. This frequently occurres on previously damaged skin, e.g. from sun, radiation, scar. It is malignant tumor of squamous (pricke) cell of epidermis; invasion of dermis surrounding skin and metasis is possible. In early states there is firm nodule with distinct borders with scaling and ulceration and opaque, then later stages, there will be a covering of lesions with scale or horn from keratinization; most commonly found in sunexposed areas such as face and hands. If precursor was premalignant lesion, the lesion will be indurated and surrounded by an inflammatory base. New lesions appear as firm keratotic nodule with an indurated base. Lip or ear lesion may metastasize to regional lymph nodes. Lesions on hair-bearing areas rarely metastasize.

Treatment includes prevention and early detections. Removal by excision, curretage with electrode siccation, irradiation, or chemsurgery or chemical caustics For treatment of tumor without well-defined borders. A dressing size applied with a fixative paste such as zinc chloride, removal of the dressing remain malignant tissue. Reapplication is usually necessary.

- Basal cell carcinoma is a locally invasive malignancy arising from epidermal basal cells. The exact cause is unknown but most common malignant tumor affecting light-skinned persons over age of 40; primarily occurs over hairy areas that contains pilosebacious follicles.

There will be change in basal cells, no maturation or normal keratonization; continuing division of basal cells and formation of enlarging mass; related to excessive sunexposure, genetic skin type, arsenicals, X-ray radiation, scars and some type of nevi; basal cell possibly pigmented but is absent in nevi.

Clinical manifestation includes nodular and ulcerative–small, slowly enlarging papule; borders semitranslucent or "pearly" with overlying telangiectasia, erosion, ulceration and depression of center; normal skin markings, lost. Superficially there will be a erythematous sharply-defined barely elevated multinodular plaques with varying scaling and crusting; similar to eczema but not prurite. Rarely metastatic is treated. If untreated, tumour becomes locally invasive with severe tissue destruction, infection, and haemorrhage. If untreated, metastasizes to bone lung and brain.

Treatment depends on site and extent of tumour; currettage with electrode siccations, excision, irradiations and chemosurgery, electrosurgery, cryosurgery. Ninety-five per cent are slow-growing tumour that invades local tissue.

- *Malignant melanoma:* usually develops from a pigmented nevi, although it may arise from healthy skin.

Three lesions are considered percursors of melanoma; dysplastic nevi; congenital nevi, and lentigo maligns. Chronic exposure is associated with its developments. There is genetic predisposition to melanoma.

Neoplastic growth of melanocytes anywhere on skin, eyes, or mucous membranes, classification according to major histologic mode of spread. There are lentigo malignamelanoma, nodular melanaoma, superficial spreading melanoma and acral-lentiginous melanoma. There will be a potential invasion and widespread metastasis.

Tumours occur most commonly on the head, neck and lower extremities. The lesions vary considerably in appearance and some with deep pigmentation, irregular borders and surrounding erythema, and others with irregular pigmentation yellow, blue, black and irregular surfaces. The rate of growth varies. Late changes include bleeding and ulceration. The incidence of metastasis from maligned melanoma is high and depends on depth of invasion. Metastasis occurs first to the regional lymph nodes and then haematogenous spread to the lungs, liver and other areas.

As in all malignancies, diagnostic is confirmed by biopsy. Metastatic malignant melanoma is resistant to currently available chemotherapeutic agents. Treatment includes wide excision, full thickness, surgical removal, correlation of survival rate with depth of invasion; poor prognosis unless diagnosed and treated early; spreading by local extension, regional lymphatic vessels and blood stream; adjuvant therapy after surgery may be necessary if lesion is greater than 1.5 mm in depth.

- *Kapsosi sarcoma:* The exact cause is unknown. Theories include viral causes, immunosuppression and sexually, transmitted agents, categorized groups affected are elderly men, Jewish and endemic on black Africans and renal transplant recipients and AIDS related.

  Multicentric neoplasm occurs with increasing frequency in HIV-infected individuals; occurs frequently in homosexual men; multiple vascular modules are appearing on the skin, mucous membranes and vescira; severity ranges from minor to fulminant with extensive cutaneous and visceral involvement.

  There will be a slowly progressive red, purple or brown plaques or nodules scattered widely over the body on the skin or mucus membranes, especially on the mouth. Lesions have been found in lymph nodes, gastrointestinal tract and lungs. Lesions do not blanch with pressure and are painless.

  Diagnosis is based upon biopsy of suspicious lesion. Treatment depends upon severity of lesions and patient's immune status; attempt to avoid treatments to further suppress immune system; possible treatment includes localized radiation, intralesional vinblastine, alpha-interferon combination of cryotherapy and chemotherapy. Patients at high-risk should be taught self-assessments for early detection of lesions.

- *Keratoacanthoma* occurs on normal skin areas exposed to sun, tar, oils. It is noninvasive and does not metastasize.

  They are microscopically similar to squamous cell carcinoma grows rapidly to 1-2 cm, remain quiscent for 2-8 weeks, than regresses spontaneously. Dome shaped, shiny, pink lesion contain a keratinous plug, which is expelled as the nodule shrinks. Treatment includes excision and biopsy.

NURSING MANAGEMENT OF DERMATOLOGICAL SURGERY

Treatment of skin lesions by dermatologistic structures include removal of skin lesions. Superficial skin lesions involving only the epidermis which can be removed easily by various means. Deep lesions involving the dermis, such as with some cancers are removed with full thickness and skin excision. The different types of dermatological surgery are:

- *Tangential surgery:* Superficial lesions can be removed by slicing off the lesion with a sharp blade. It is especially useful for removal of flat lesions. The entire lesion may be removed for diagnosis. Hemostasis is obtained with pressure of gelatin foam.
- *Currettage:* Currettage is the scraping or scooping out of a superficial lesions with a currette, a spoon-shaped or sharp-edged instrument. A local anesthetic is usually injected around the lesion before currettage hemostasis is accomplished with a chemical styptic, such a ferric chloride or monsel's solution, with gelatin foam or by electrocoagulation. Lesions which may be removed by currettage include seborrhoeic keratosis, actinic keratosis, basal cell epthelioma, leukoplakia warts and nevi.
- *Punch biopsy:* After the patient received a local anesthetic, a punch is used to remove deep lesions upto 10 mm in diameter. The tissue is then sent for biopsy. Small punch biopsy may be closed with suture. Larger biopsies are partially closed they then heal by secondary insertion. Hemostasis is obtained with gelatin foam packing.
- *Cryosurgery:* Tissue can be destroyed by rapid freezing with substance such as liquid oxygen, carbon dioxide snow or gas, liquid nitrogen, dichlorodifluromethane freon or nitrous oxide. The carbon dioxide snow and liquid nitrogen commonly used the rapid freezing causes formation of intracellular ice, which destroys the cell membranous and produces cell dehydration.

Cryosurgery is commonly used for removing skin tumors, warts and keloids.
- *Electrosurgery:* Electric current may be used in dermatological surgery to remove tissue and to control bleeding.
  - Electrodesciccation is drying of tissue by means of monopolar curretage through the needle electrode.
  - Electrofulguration is a form of electrodesciccation in which needle electrode is held close to, rather than inserted into the tissue that spraying area with sparks.
  - *Electrocoagulation:* Bipolar current is used in which coagulates the tissues, curtailing capillary bleeding and for electrosection, which cuts the tissue.

Preoperative care is as with other patients undergoing any surgery and preoperative teaching about surgery indicated for.

Postoperative care also includes monitoring and taking measures according to type of surgery. The specific points included are:

After superficial skin surgery, the patient is instructed not to remove the crust scalp which acts as a protective healing occurs under the crust. The crust should be kept as dry as possible if it gets wet, it should be patted dry. Alcohol may be applied and allowed to evaporate. Make-up may be used over the crust. The crust may be left uncovered with an adhesive bandage. Signs of redness, edema or pain should be reported to surgeon.

After deep skin surgery, the wound is usually bandaged and patient is given specific instruction for care by the surgeon. Aspirin should be avoided for 7 days before and after surgery because of its anticoagulant property it may lead to postoperative bleeding.

Patient and family will require teaching regarding the care of healthy skin and steps to prevent further damages to the skin which includes:
- Avoiding causative agent.
- Cleansing the skin-bathing.
- Avoiding sunlight.
- Taking balanced nutrients.
- Observation of any change in size, color and any.
- Dangers of self treatment.
- Psychological care.
- Relief of pruritus.
- Temperature control.
- Therapeutic bath and soaks.
- Topical medication.
- Medicated dressing.

Cosmetic surgery on skin may be performed.

PRESSURE ULCERS

Pressure ulcers is localized area of tissues necrosis caused by unrelieved pressure, tissue layers sliding over other tissue layers, shearing and excessive moisture.

Etiology

Factors that put a patient at risk for the development of pressure ulcers include impaired circulation, obesity, elevated body temperature, anemia, contractures, mental deterioration, physical dependence, immobility, incontinence and old age. Systemic illness such as diabetes, collagen diseases, vascular diseases, leprosy, and neurological disorders that affect sensation also result in great risk for ulceration.

Pathophysiology

Unrelieved pressure causes cellular necrosis. The cellular necrosis occurs from vascular insufficiency and causes tissue destruction. Here the pressure is applied to the soft tissue compresses capillaries, distorting structures and occluding blood flow, which leads to ischemia at first, followed by reactive hyperemia. It compensated by increased shunting of capillary circulation to area under pressure; capillaries increased permeability and leakage of fluids into tissues lead to tissue edema and inflammation. Then endothelical cells are disrupted, platelets aggregate and thrombi form in capillaries and lead to cellular death. Cellular death leads to tissue necrosis.

Clinical Manifestation

The clinical manifestation of pressure ulcer depend on the stage of the ulcer as follows:
- *Stage I:* In this stage, pressure ulcer is an observable-pressure related alteration of intact skin, whose indications as compared to an adjacent or opposite area on the body may include changes in one or more of the following:
  - Skin temperature warmth or coolness., tissue consistency firm or boggy feel, sensation pain, itching.
  - The ulcer appears as a defined area of persistent redness in lightly-pigmented skin, whereas in darker skin tones, the ulcer may appear with persistent red, blue or purple hues.

    Here nonblanchable erythema, redness that remain present over an area under pressure 30 minutes after pressure source is removed. Epidermis remains intact.
- *Stage II:* In this stage epidermis is broken, superficial lesion, no measurable depth. Partial thickness, skin loss involving epidermis dermis or both. The ulcer is superficial and presents clinically as an abrasion, blister or shallow crater.
- *Stage III:* In this full thickness skin loss down through dermis include subcutaneous tissue may undermine adjacent skin. Full thickness involving damage to or necrosis of subcutaneous tissue that may extend down to but not through underlying fascia. The ulcer

presents clinically as a deep crater with or without undermining of adjacent tissue.
- *Stage IV:* Full thickness skin loss extending into suppressive structures such as muscle tendon and bone may underline and have various sinus tracts.

If the pressure ulcer becomes infected, the patient may display signs of infection such as leukocytosis and fever. In addition, the pressure ulcer may increase in size, odor and drainage, have necrotic tissue, and be indurated, warm and painful. The most common complication in pressure ulcer is recurrence.

Management

Care of the patient with a pressure ulcer requires local care of the wound and support measures such as adequate nutrition and pressure relief. The current trend to keep a pressure sore slightly moist, rather than dry, to enhance re-epithelialization. In addition to the nurse and other members of the health team they can provide valuable input into the complex treatment necessary to prevent and treat pressure ulcers. Both conservative and surgical strategies are used in the treatment of pressure ulcers depending on the stage and condition of the ulcer.

A holistic approach to nursing management of the patient with pressure ulcers contain four components.
1. Controling the contributing factors by reduction or elimination.
2. Supporting the host.
3. Optimizing microenvironments based on principles of wound healing
4. Providing education for patients and caregivers.

The nursing diagnosis are determined from analysis of patient includes.
- Skin integrity, for impaired, related to nutritional deficits, prolonged immobilization and decreased hemoglobin, and serum albumin.
- Risk for infection.
- Impaired physical mobility.
- Tissue perfusion, altered.
- Self-care deficiency.

Nursing intervention to prevent pressure ulcers are as follows:
- Incontinence
  - Cleanse the skin after each episode of incontinence. Check incontinent patients frequently.
  - Assess causative factors of incontinence.
  - Contain urine and feces in absorbent products that control moisture and exposure to skin; plastic-lined products can contribute to the problem.
  - Minimize moisture next to skin from any source.
- Nutritional Deficits
  - Collaborate with dietitian to assess for optimal nutritional support.
  - Assess for symptoms of nutritional compromise decreased appetite and subsequently less oral intake. Serum albumin level of less than 3-3.5 gm/dl; Hgb level of less than 10 gm/dl; signs and symptoms of dehydration, including thirst, poor skin turgor, and dry mucus membrane, elevated hematocrit and serum sodium level.
- Skin Care and Early Treatment Measures
  - Inspect the skin at regular intervals at least daily.
  - Frequency determined by institutional policy, e.g. every shift instead of daily. and patient degree at risk. A head to toe inspection should be conducted. With attention to intertriginous areas and bony prominences.
  - Bathing schedule should be developed according to patient's preference, institutional policy, and general skin conditions. Use a mild cleansing agent and avoid water temperature extremes.
  - Assess environmental factors such as temperature and humidity for contribution to skin conditions.
  - Lubricate skin with emollient lotions. Avoid lotion with scents or high alcohol contents.
  - Avoid vigorous massage.
- Alteration in mobility/activity
  - Reposition patient at least every 2 hours.
  - Use position pillows or foam wedges to separate skin areas, in contact with each other or to assist with maintaining positions. Use cautiously because these devices can become an additional source of pressure if not properly placed.
  - Heels should be elevated off the bed surfaces with supportive pillows. Heel protectors help reduce friction.
  - Avoid positioning directly on to trochanter, place patient more appropriately with 30 degree side-lying position.
  - Elevating the head of the bed centers all body weight directly over the pelvic triangle. It is best to keep the degree of elevation to less than 45 degree if possible.
  - To reduce friction and shear, use lifting devices to raise patient in bed, rather than dragging patient across the surface of the bed.
  - A pressure reduction or relief device should be used for all patients at risk of pressure ulcer formation.
  - Patients in wheel chairs and other chairs should be taught to shift weight and have pressure-reducing surfaces on which to sit.

BURNS

Burns are a form of traumatic injury caused by thermal, electrical, chemical or radioactive agents. In other words, injuries that result from direct contact or exposure to any thermal, chemical, electrical or radiation source are termed "Burns". Burn injuries occur when energy from a heat source is transferred to the tissues of the body. The depth of injury is related to temperature and the durations of the contact or of exposure.

Types of Burns

Burn injuries are categorized according to the mechanism of injury. It may be thermal, chemical, electrical and radiation.

Thermal Burn Injury

Thermal burns are caused by exposure to or contact with flame, hot liquids, semi-liquids steam, semi-solid tar or objects such as:
- Flame : Example : Clothing ignited with fire.
- Flash : Example : Flame burn associated with explosion combustible fuels.
- Scald : Example : – Hot bath water.
  – Spilled hot beverages.
  – Hot grease or liquids from cooking.
  – Steam burns, pressure workers, microwaved food, automobile radiators.
- Contact : Example : – Hot metal outdoor grill.
  – Hot, sticky tar.

So, the specific examples of thermal burns are those sustained in residential fires, explosive, automobile accidents, scald injuries, clothing ignition and ignition of poorly stored flammable liquids petrol.

Chemical Burn Injury

Chemical injuries are the result of tissue injury and destruction from necrotizing substances. Chemical burns are caused by tissue contact with strong acids, alkalies or organic compounds. The concentration volume, and type of chemical as well as the duration of contact determine the severity of a chemical injury. Chemical injuries to the eyes and inhalation of chemical fumes (e.g. Bhopal Gas Tragedy) are particularly serious.

Chemical burns can result from contact with certain household cleaning agent and various chemicals used in industry, agriculture and the military. More than 25000 chemical products. Chemical can produce respiratory and systemic symptoms as well as skin or eye injuries. For example, when chlorine is inhaled toxic gas produces respiratory distress. Byproducts of burning substances e.g. Carbon are toxic to the sensitive respiratory mucosa. Tissue destruction may continue for upto 72 hours after chemical injury.

As stated earlier, chemical burns are most commonly caused by acids, however, alkali burns also occur. Alkalis are more dangerous than acids, because alkali substances are neutralized by tissue fluids as readily as acid substances. Alkalies adhere to tissues, causing protein hydrolic and liquification. Thus, damages continue even when the alkali is neutralised. An example of alkalies of this type are cleaning agents, drain cleaner and dyes.

Smoke and inhalation of hot air or noxious chemicals can cause damage to the tissues of the respiratory tract. Breathing of hot air may cause damages to the respiratory mucosa.

Examples: inhalation injuries commonly occurring are carbon monoxide poisoning, inhalation injury above the glottis and inhalation injury below the glottis.

Electrical Burn Injury

Electrical injury results from coagulation necrosis that is caused by intense heat generated by the electrical energy as it passes through the body. These injuries can result from contact with exposed or faulty electrical wiring or high voltage power lines. Individuals struck by lightning also sustain electrical injury. It can also result from direct damage to nerves and vessels causing tissues anoxia and death. The extent of the injury influenced by the duration of contact, the intensity of the current voltage, the type of current direct or alternate the pathway of the current and the resistance of the tissues as the electrical current passes through the body. Electrical contact with voltage greater than 40 is potentially dangerous.

Radiation Burn Injury

Radiation burns are the least common type of burn injuries and are caused by exposure to a radioactive service. These types of injuries have been associated with nuclear radiation accidents, the use of ionizing radiation in industry and from therapeutic radiation. A sunburn solar radiation from prolonged exposure to ultraviolet rays is also considered to be a type of radiation burn. The amount of radioactive energy that an individual receives following exposure depends on the strength of the radiative source, the duration of the exposure, the extent of the body area exposed and the amount of shielding between the source and the person. An acute localized injury appears similar to a cutineous thermal injury, and is characterized by skin erythema, oedema and pain. In contrast, the whole body radiation causes radiation sickness that are dose dependent.

Pathophysiology of Burns

Burn wounds occur when there is contact between tissue and energy source on heat, chemicals, electrical current, or radiation. The resulting local effects are influenced by the intensity of the energy, the duration of the exposure, and the type of tissue injured. Immediately after the injury there is an increase in blood flow to the area surrounding the wound. This is followed by release of various vasoactive substances from the burned tissue, which results in increased capillary permeability. Fluid then shifts from the intravascular compartment to the interstitial space producing oedema and hypovolaemia.

The pathophysiologic response that occur immediately following a cutaneous burn injury depends on the extent of size of the burn. For smaller burns, body's response to injury is localized to the injured area. However, with extensive burns, i.e. twenty-five per cent or more of total body surface area (TBSA) the body response to injury is systemic and proportional to the extent of the injury.

Extensive burn injuries affect all major systems of the body. The systemic response to burn injury is topically triphasic, characterized by early hypofunction that is followed later by hyper function of the each organ system.

The physiologic reaction to burns is similar to inflammatory process. Burns may be partial or full thickness. In partial thickness injuries involve the epidermis and upper portion of the dermis. Some of the dermal appendages remain, from which the wound can spontaneously re-epithialize. In full thickness injuries, all layers of the skin and sometimes, underlying tissues are destroyed. In such cases, grafting is required to close the wound.

In addition to changes in the locally burned area, there are alterations and disruptions in the vascular and other systems of the body. Brief description of those changes are given below:

Fluid and Electrolytic Balance

Immediately following a burn injury, vasoactive substances i.e. catecholamines, histamine, serotinin, leukotrienes, kinins and prostaglandins are released from the injured tissues. These substances initiate changes in capillary integrity, allowing plasma to seep into surrounding tissues. Direct heat injury to vessels further increases capillary permeability, which permits sodium ions to enter the cell and potassium ions to exit. Overall, this creates an osmotic gradient, which leads to increase in intracellular and interstitial fluid and further depletes intravascular fluid volume. These substances exert their effect both locally and systematically. The burn injured client's haemodynamic balance, metabolism and immune status are altered.

Haemodynamic alteration leads to inadequate tissue perfusion, which may turn cause acidosis, renal failure, and irreversible burn shock. Hyponatraemia and hyperkalaemia are common electrolyte abnormalities that affect the burn-injured client at different points in the recovery process. Catecholamine release appears to be the major mediator of the hypermetabolic response to burn injury.

Changes in Cardiovascular System

In major burn, heart rate and peripheral vascular resistance increases in response to the release of catecholamines and to the relative hypovolaemia, but initial cardiac output falls hypo-function. At approximately 24 hours after burn injury in persons receiving adequate fluid resuscitation, cardiac output return to normal and that increases 2 to 2.5 times normal to meet the hypermetabolic needs of the body hyperfunctions.

This change in cardiac output occurs even before circulating intravascular volume levels and are restored to normal. Arterial blood pressure is normal or slightly elevated unless severe hypovolaemia exists.

Changes in Respiratory System

Majority of death from the fire are due to smoke and inhalation injury. Without a concomitant inhalation injury, initial findings suggestive of pulmonary insufficiency are rare. Minute ventilation is often normal or slightly decreased early after a burn injury. Following fluid resuscitation and the effects of burn shock on cell membrane potential may cause pulmonary oedema contributing to decreased alveolar exchange. Client may exhibit a rise in minute ventilation or hyperventilation especially if he or she is fearful, anxious or in pain. This hyperventilation is the result of an increase in both respiratory rate and a tidal volume and appears to be the result of the hypermetabolism that is seen after burn injury. Initial respiratory alkosis and respiratory acidosis may associate with hyperventilation and pulmonary insufficiency.

Changes in Urinary System

The body responds initially by shunting blood away from the kidneys as a part of the normal neurohormonal stress response, thus decreasing glomerular filtration race and causing oliguria low uring (output). If fluid resuscitation is delayed or inadequate, hypovolaemia progresses and leads to acute renal failure. However, with adequate fluid resuscitation and a rise in cardiac output, renal blood flow will return to normal. Following resuscitation, the body begins to reabsorb the oedema fluid and to eliminate through diuresis. Urine output then increases.

Changes in Gastrointestinal System

In major burns, blood flows to the mesentric beds is also reduced initially, leading to development of intestinal ileus and gastrointestinal dysfunction. As a result of sympathetic nervous system response to trauma peristalsis decreases, and gastric distension, nausea, vomitting and paralytic ileus may occur. Ischaemia of the gastric mucosa and other aetiological factors put the burn client at risk for duodenal ulcer and gastric ulcer, manifested by occult bleeding and in some cases life-threatening haemorrhage. If the gastrointestinal tract is left untreated and unprotected by antacids, the erosions can progress to ulcer ation i.e. curlings ulcer in burn clients and gastrointestinal bleeding. Following adequate fluid resuscitation, gastrointestinal motility returns, signalled by bowel sounds, flatus, and stool production.

Changes in Immune System

In major burn injuries, immune system function is depressed. The loss of the skin barrier and presence of eschare favours bacterial growth. Hypoxia, acidosis, thrombosis of vessels in the wound area impair host resistance to pathogenic bacteria. Depression of lympocyte activity, a decrease in immunoglobulin production, suppression of complement activities and an alteration in neutrophil and macrophage functioning are evident in following extensive burn injuries. In addition, burn injury disrupts the body's primary barrier to infection. Together, these changes result in some degree of immunosuppression, increasing the risk of infection and life-threatening sepsis, i.e. systemic septicemia.

Changes in Nervous System

The client injured with burns typically suffers no neurologic trauma, (e.g. fall, explosion) impaired perfusion to the brain, hypoxaemia, e.g. close-space fire inhalation injury, e.g. exposure to asphyxiants or other toxic material from the fire., electrical burn injury, or from the effects of the drug present in the body at the time of injury. Burn patient always awake, in hospital. If agitation develops in immediate post burn period, the patient may be suffering from hypovolemia or hypoxemia.

In addition to pathophysiological changes, the burn injured client also shows a myriad of psychological and emotional responses to burn injuries ranging from fear to psychosis. This has been influenced by age, personality, cultural and ethnic backgrouind, extent and location of injuries and the resulting impact on body image.

CLASSIFICATION OF SEVERITY OF BURNS

The treatment of burns is related to the severity of burn injury. The severity of burn injury is classified based on the risk of mortality and the risk of cosmetic or functional disability.

Severity of burns is determined by:
- Burn depth.
- Burn size percentage of TBSA burned.
- Burn location.
- Age of burn victim.
- General health of burn victim.
- Mechanism of injury.

Burn Depth

Burn injuries are classified as a partial thickness or full thickness.
A. Partial thickness burn injuries are classified as first and second degree burns or superficial and deep burns.
   - The cause of *Superficial burns* first degree are superficial first degree are superficial sunburn and quick heat flash. Here only superficial devitalization with hyperexaemia is present. Tactic and pain sensation is intact. In superficial burns, clinical appearance will include erythaema, blanching on pressure, pain and mild swelling. The vescicles or blisters although after 24-hour skin may blister and peel. Discomfort lasts 48-72 hours. Desquamation in 3-7 days.
   - The causes of *deep burns* second degree are flame, flash, scald and contact burns. Here epidermis and dermis involved to varying depth. Some skin elements from which epithethelial regeneration can occur remain viable. The clinical appearance of deep burn will include, fluid-filled vescicles that are red shiny, wet if vescicles have ruptured., severe pain caused by nerve inury, there will be a mild to moderate oedema. Superficial burn heals in less than 21 days. Deep burn require more than 21 days to heal. Healing rates vary with burn depth and presence and absence of infection.
B. *Full thickness* burn injuries are classified as 'third' and 'fourth' degree burns. These are caused by flame, scald, chemicals, tar, electric current. Here all skin elements and nerve endings are destroyed. Coagulation necrosis present. The clinical appearances will be dry, waxy white, leathery or hard skin; visible thrombosed vessels insensitivity to pain and pressure because of nerve destructions. There will be possible involvements of muscles, tendons and bones. 3rd degree requires autografting and 4th degree requires autografting or amputation of extremity.

Burn Size Extent

The size of a burn (percentage of injured skin, excluding first degree burns) is determined by one of the two techniques.
a. The rule of Nine's (9s)
b. An Age-specific burn diagram of Lund-Browder chart.
   Burns size or extent is expressed as a percentage of TBSA (**Fig. 10.1**).
- The rule of '9s' was introduced in the late 1940 as a quick assessment tool for estimating burn size. The basis of this rule is that the body divided into anatomic sections, each of which represents 9% or a multiple of 9% of the TBSA. The method is easy requiring no diagrams to determine the percentage of TBSA injured. Therefore, it has been used in emergency department where the initial assessment occurs.

The Rule of Nine

Head and neck	9%
Arms	9%
Anterior trunk	18%
Posterior trunk	18%
Legs	18%
Perinium	1%
Total	100%

- An age-specific burn diagram of Lund-Browder chart—the percentages for body segments according to age and provides a more accurate estimate of burns. Extent of burn injury is most accurate after initial debridement.

Burn Location

The location of the burn wound has a direct relationship to the severity of the burn injury. Burns of the head, face, neck and circumferential burns of the chest are frequently associated with pulmonary complication it may inhibit respiratory function by virtue of mechanical obstruction secondary to oedema or eschar formation. These injuries may also indicate the possibility of inhalation injury or respiratory mucosal damage.

Burns involving the face often have associated with corneal abrasions. Burns of the ears are prone to auricular chondritis and are susceptible to infections and further loss of tissue. Burns of the hands and joints often require intense physical and occupational therapy and have implications for loss of work time and/or permanent physical and vocational disability. Burns of the hands, feet, joints and eyes are of concern because they make self-care impossible and jeopardize later function. Hands and feet are difficult to manage medically because of superficial vascular and nerve supply system.

Burns involving the perineal area are prone to infection due to autocontamination by urine and focus. The burns of the buttocks or genitalia are susceptible to infection and may be source of emotional conflicts because of the pain involved possible disfigurement.

Circumferential burns of the extremities may produce a tourniquet-like effect and lead to distal vascular compromise i.e., circulatory compromise distal to the burns with subsequent neurologic impairment of the affected extremity. As stated earlier, circumferential thorax burn may lead to inadequate chestwall expansion and pulmonary insufficiency.

Age of the Burn Victim

The client's age affects the severity and outcome of the burn. Mortality rates are higher for children younger than 4 years particularly 0-1 year group, and for clients older than 65 years. Because of an immature immune system and generally poor host defence mechanisms an infant is less able to cope with burn injuries. The older adult heals more slowly and has more difficulty with rehabilitation than a child or younger adult.

Infection of the burn wound and pneumonia are common complications of older patient.

General Health and Burns

Any patient with pre-existing cardiovascular, pulmonary, or renal disease has poorer prognosis for recovery because of the tremendous demands placed on the body by a burn injury. The patient with diabetes mellitus or peripheral vascular disease is at high risk for gangrene and poor healing, especially with foot and leg burns. General physiological debilitation from any chronic disease, including alcoholism, drug abuse, and malnutrition renders the patient less physiologically competent to deal with a burn injury. In addition, the patient who concurrently sustained fractures, head injuries or other trauma has poorer prognosis for recovery from the burn injury.

Mechanism of Burn Injury

Mechanism of burn injury is an important factor used to determine severity. The special consideration is required for electrical and burn injury or any burn injury associated with an inhalation injury.

As stated earlier, in electrical injuries, heat is generated as the electricity travels through the body resulting internal tissue damage. Here, the voltage, type of current, AC or DC, contact site and the duration of contact are important considerations because they affect morbidity. AC is worst than DC because it is associated with cardiopulmonary arrest, ventricular fibrillation, tetanic muscle contractions and long bone or vertebral compression fractures. There will be risk of acute renal failure due to release of myoglobin.

In chemical burns, systemic to all effects from cutaneous absorption of the offending agent may occur. Organ failure and even death have resulted from prolonged contact and absorption of different chemicals.

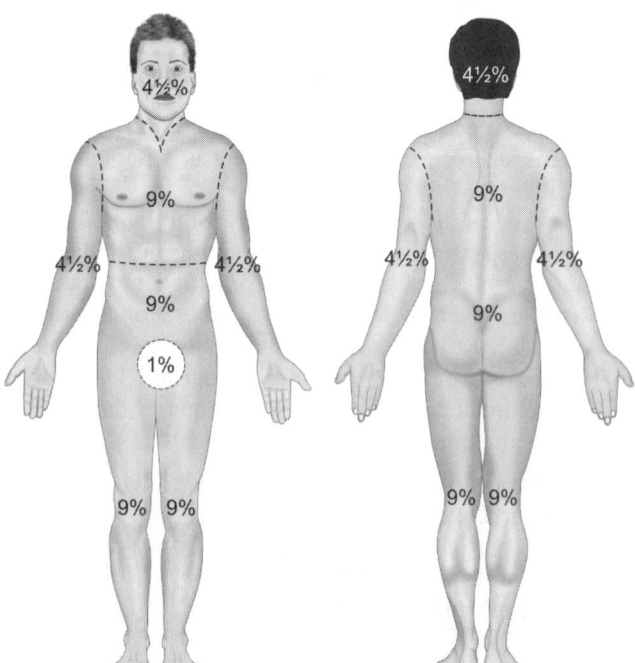

Fig. 10.1: Rule of nines for calculating total burn surface area TBSA.

Management of Minor Burns

A minor burn injury in the adult is generally considered to be less than 15 percent of TBSA in the patients younger than 40 years or 10 percent TBSA in patients older than 40 years without a risk of cosmetic or functional impairment or disability.

Nursing care of minor burn wounds include:
- Wound assessment and initial care of wound.
- Tetanus immunization.
- Pain management.
- Health education.
- Wound assessemnt includes an accurate history of injury i.e., the date and time of accident and the source of the burn and other associated injuries. And also all pertinent pastmedical history which includes drug allergies, medications, illnesses, etc.

    Wound care for minor burns includes cleansing, debridement, removal of any damaging agent, i.e. chemical, tar, etc.) and application of an appropriate topical treatments.

    Generally burn wounds should be washed with mild soap and rinsed thoroughly with warm water. The wounds may be covered with saline-soaked sponges to lessen the discomfort. Loose nonviable tissue should be carefully trimmed away and any hair should be shaved within all" margin around the burn wound.

    A minor chemical burn should be well irrigated with water for at least 20 minutes. Neutralizing agents are not recommended because the neutralizing reaction causes heat, which results in further tissue damage.
- *Tetanus immunization:* Burn wound patients are exposed and are prone to get tetanus. To prevent developing tetanus, the current protocol for tetanus immunization is same for clients with minor burns as for clients with any other type of trauma.
- *Pain management:* is often achieved with small doses of IV morphine followed by oral analgesia in minor burns.
- *Health education:* While providing initial wound care, the nurse is responsible for teaching home wound care, and the clinical manifestations of infections that must require further medical care.

Management of Major Burns

The multiple organ system response that occurs following a major burn injury necessitates an interdisciplinary approach. The nurse, in consultation with other burn team members, is responsible for developing a plan of care that is based on assessment data reflected the physical and psychosocial needs of the client and family or significant other. Burn management can be classified into three phases.

1. Emergent phase (resuscitation)
2. The acute phase and
3. The rehabilitative phase

Emergent Phase

The emergent phase begins at the time of injury, with the prehospital care and concludes when capillary integriy is restored, typically at 48 to 72 hours following injury. The primary goals during the emergent phase of recovery are directed towards sustaining life through prevention of hypovolemia burn shock preservation of vital organ functioning.

Prehospital care of the burn victim begins at the scene of the incident and concludes when institutional emergency medical care is obtained. It should begin with removing the victim from the source of the burn and/or eliminating the source of heat. Prehospital care of the patient with various types of burns are as follows:

Emergency Management of Chemical Burns

The possible causes of chemical burns are exposure to strong acid alkali, corrosive materials or organophosphorous. So the possible assessment finally may include:
- Burning, degeneration of exposed tissues.
- Discoloration of injured exposed skin.
- Localized pain.
- Edema of surrounding tissues.
- Respiratory distress if chemical is inhaled.
- Paralysis, decreased muscle coordination if organophosphorous.

    When managing such cases the caregiver should:
- Wear appropriate protective garb globe.
- Remove the chemical from contact with patient's body.
- Flush chemical from wound and surroundings area with saline solution or water. Brush off lime and other powders.
- Remove clothing including shoes, watches, jewellery and contact lenses if face is exposed.
- Blot, do not rub, skin dry with clean towels.
- Cover all burned area with dry, sterile dressing or clean dry sheet.
- Monitor airway, if airway is exposed to chemicals.
- Attempt to determine type of chemical exposure.

Emergency Management of Inhalation Injury

The possible causes of inhalation burn injuries are exposure of respiratory tract to intense heat, flames, inhalation of noxious chemicals and smoke CO gas. The expected possible assessement findings will include:
- Rapid, shallow respiration.
- Increasing hoarseness.
- Coughing.
- Singed nasal or facial hair.
- Sooty and smoky breath.

- Productive cough, that is black, gray or bloody.
- Irritation of upper airways or burning pain in throat or chest.
- Difficulty in swallowing.
- Restlessness, anxiety.

While managing such cases, the caregiver should:
- Remove patient from toxic environment.
- Establish and maintain airway, anticipates need for intubation of respiratory distress.
- Administer high flow oxygen 100 percent by nonrebreather mark.
- Be prepared to intubate if respiratory distress occurs.
- Remove patient's clothing.
- Establish IV line with larger-guage needle.
- Monitor vital signs including level of consciousness and oxygen saturation.
- Place patient in a high Fowler's position unless spinal injury is suspected.
- Assess for facial and neck burns or other signs of trauma.
- Prepare for emergency, endotrachial intubation if indicated.

Emergency Management of Electrical Burns

The possible causes of electrical burns will be exposure to electric current, i.e. lightening, electric wires, utility wires, etc.

The possible findings of such injury may be:
- Leathery and white charred skin.
- Burn odor.
- Impaired touch sensation.
- Minimal or absent pain.
- Dysrhythmias.
- Depth of wound difficult to visualize; assume injury greater than seen.
- Entrance and exit wounds.

When managing such cases, the caregiver should:
- Remove patient from contact with current source by trained personnel first aider.
- Avoid contact with electric current during rescue.
- Assess for patient airway, breathing and circulation.
- Initiate CPR if necessary.
- Establish and maintain airway.
- Maintain cervical spine precautions.
- Administer high flow oxygen (O_2) by nonrebreather mask.
- Establish IV line with large gauge needle.
- Remove patient's clothing.
- Assess burn areas, especially entrance and exit sites.
- Check pulses distal to burns.
- Monitor heart rate and rhythm.
- Cover burn sites with dry sterile dressing.
- Assess for any other injuries, e.g. fractures
- Monitor vital signs including level of consciousness.

Emergency Management of Thermal Burns

The possible causes of thermal burns include contact with hot liquids or solids, flash flame, open flame, steam or ultraviolet rays. The possible assessment finding may be:
In case of superficial burns:
- Redness.
- Pain.
- Moderate to severe tenderness.
- Minimal edema.
- Blanching with pressure.

In case of deep burns:
- Moist blebs and blisters.
- Mottled white and pink to cherry red.
- Hypersensitive to touich or air.
- Moderate to severe pain.
- Blanching with pressure.

In case of severe full thickness burns:
- Shock, e.g. tachycardia, hypotension.
- Dry leathery eschar.
- White, waxy, dark brown, or charred appearances.
- Strong burn odor.
- Impaired sensation where touched.
- Absence of pain with severe pain in surrounding tissues.
- Lack of blanching with pressure.

When managing such cases, caregiver or nurse should:
- Remove patient from environment and stop the burning process.
- Establish and maintain airway; inspect the face and neck for singed nasal hair, hoarseness of voice, stridor, soot in the sputum, anticipate need for intubation.
- Administer fluid.
- Monitor vital signs including level of consciousness and O_2 saturation.
- Remove clothing and jewellery.
- Examine and treat for other associated injuries, e.g. fractured ribs, pneumothorax, etc.
- Determine depth, extent and severity of burn.
- Anticipate need for analgesic and tetanus prophylaxis.
- Cover large burns with dry and sterile dressing.
- Apply cool compresses or immerse in cool water for minor injuries only less than 10 percent TBSA burn.
- Transport as soon as possible to burn center of hospitals.

In general, the guidelines for prehospital care of burn victims that will be followed are:
- Remove the victim from the sources of the burn:
    - Flame, extinguish burning clothes.
    - Chemical or scald: remove saturated clothing.
    - Chemical: Brush off any dry chemical and begin to copiously irrigate injured areas with water.
    - Hot tar: Cool the tar with water.
    - Electrical: Turn off electricity or remove the electrical source using dry, nonconductive object e.g. a piece of wood.

- Assess the ABCs.
  - Establish airway.
  - Ensure adequate breathing 100 percent O_2 via non-rebreather face mask.
  - Assess circulation.
- Assess for associated trauma.
- Conserve body heat.
- Consider need for IV fluid administration.
- Transfer to hospital or burn unit.

Nursing of Burn Patient in Hospital

Generally an extensive burn patient is referred to hospital and admitted in burn unit or wards. An initial care of such patients includes the following. This phase is considered as acute phase.

- Reassessment of airway, breathing and circulation and associated trauma.
- Initiation of fluid resuscitation/replacement.
- Placement of an indwelling urinary catheter.
- Placement of nasogastric tube.
- Monitoring vital signs and baseline lab studies.
- Pain management.
- Tetanus immunization.
- Data collection.
- Wound care.
- Psychological support.
- Infection control.
- Nutritional support.
- Physical therapy.

- *Reassessment of ABCs:* Some intervention performed in emergency phase may be continued in hospital according to that type of burns. The head of the beds should be elevated to facilitate lung expansion if the patient suffers no hemodynamic instability. Oxygen may be administered if necessary.
- *Initiation of fluid replacement:* For hemodynamic stabilization fluid resuscitation may be initiated immediately on the basis of the percentage of burn injury, i.e. more than 15-20 percent TBSA in adults and more than 10-15 percent in children and patients with electrical burn. The goal of fluid resuscitation is to give sufficient fluid to allow perfusion of vital organs without overhydrating the patient and risking later complication and circulatory overload.

  Generally a crystalloid Ringer's lactate solution is used initially and colloids are used during second day. There, several formulae may be used to determine the amount of fluid to be given in the first 48 hours, which includes the Parkland formula, the Brook's formula and the Evan's formula.

  Among them Parkland formula is commonly used as follows:
  - First 24 hours: 4 ml of Ringer's lactate X weight in kg of X percentage of TBSA is burned.

  Here one-half amount of fluid is given in the first 8 hours calculated from the time of injury. If the starting fluids is delayed, then the same amount of fluid is given over the remaining time. It should be noted that to deduct any fluids given in the prehospital setting, the remaining half of the fluid is given over the next 16 hours.

  For example: Patient weight 70 kg, percentage of TBSA is 80 percent.
  Ist 8 hours = 11,200 ml or 1400 ml/hour.
  IInd 16 hours = 11,200 ml or 700 ml/hour.
  - Second 24 hours = 0.5 ml colloid × 70 kg × 80 percent TBSA/24 hours + 2000 ml 5 percent dextrose in water run concurrently over the 24-hour period.
  For example: 0.5 ml kg × 70 kg × 80 percent = 2800 ml colloid + 2000 ml 5 percent D/W, i.e. 117 ml colloid/hour and 84 ml 5 percent D/W per hour.

- *Placement of Indwelling Catheter:* An indwelling urethral catheter connected to a closed drainage system should be placed to measure hourly urine production.
- *Placement of a Nasogastric Tube:* Placement of a nasogastric tube for the unresponsive patients or for patients with burns of 20 to 25% of more TBSA to prevent emesis and reduce the risk of aspiration.
- *Monitoring Vital Signs:* Provide baseline information as well as additional data for determining the adequacy of fluids resuscitation. Baseline laboratory studies should include blood glucost, blood urea nitrogen, creatinine, serum, electrolytes and hematocrit levels, arterial blood gas and COHb levels should also be obtained in case of inhalation injury.
- *Pain Management:* The nurse must understand the physiologic as well as the psychologic bases of pain. Allowing the patient to ventilate feelings of anger, hostility and frustration serves to assist the patient in depression of the pain. Pain management is achieved through the administration of intravenous narcotic agent, e.g. morphine. In adult, small doses are given intravenously and repeated in 5-10 minutes interval until pain appears to be under control. Extent of pain relief, blood pressure, pulse, respiratory rate and state of consciousness should be assessed after each dose.
- Administration of tetanus toxoid or ATS to prevent tetanus.
- *Data collection* will include all useful information about the incident, time of injury, level of consciousness of patient, any allergies and previous medical history of the patient helps to design the treatment and nursing intervention.
- *Wound Care:* Care of the burn wound is ultimately aimed at promoting wound healing. Daily wound care involves cleansing,, debridement, of eschar devitalized tissue and dressing of the burn wound.

Debridement of burn wound is accomplished through mechanical, enzymatic and surgical means. Wound care also includes typical antibiotic therapy, graft care if done and donor site care. If graft is done, appropriate coverage of the graft, if it is not kept open to air. It should include fine-mesh guage in the closest proximity to the graft before other dressings are applied.

- *Psychological support:* Since the nurse has the most prolonged contact with the patient and family, it is natural that nurse is to be seen as an important source of emotional support. The nurse must assist the patient in maintaining personal worth and re-esetablishing a satisfactory body image. The nurse must have an almost unlimited supply of patience and understanding. The nurse should involve family members for nursing the burn patient.
- *Infection Control:* To prevent infection in the burn patient, nursing care includes vigilant monitoring for clinical manifestation of impending infection, and sepsis, maintenance of clean environment to reduce the reservoir of the microorganisms, use of aseptic technique for all invasive procedures and wound care, and timely administration of prescribed antimicrobial agents systemic and topical. Universal precautions should be followed when caring all clients with burn injuries. The basic principles for infection control should be followed in burns unit.
- *Nutritional Support:* Maintenance of adequate nutrition during the acute phase is essential in promoting wound healing and preventing infection. Based metabolic need may be 40 to 100 per cent higher than normal levels, depending on the extent of the burn. Methods of delivering nutritional support include oral diet restricted in initial stage, till bowel sounds return to normal enteral tube feedings, peripheral parenteral nutrition, total parenteral nutrition and combination of these. The preferred feeding route is oral or enteral; however, the decisions of how to best meet the nutritional needs should be individualized for all clients.
- *Physical Therapy:* The nurse works closely with occupational and physical therapist to identify the rehabilitative needs of the burn clients. An individualized program of splinting, therapeutic, positioning, exercise, ambulation, activities of daily living and pressure therapy should be implemented early in the acute phase of recovery to maximize functional recovery and cosmetic outcome. Patient and family education regarding correct positioning and the need for continued exercise are important.

CHAPTER 11

Nursing Management of Musculoskeletal Disorders

INTRODUCTION

The word "orthopedic" was invented by French Surgeon Nicholas Andry (1743). It is derived from two greek words: 'orthos' meaning straight or correct and 'pedios meaning' of a child, and so can be taken to mean the rearing of straight childrens. Modern orthopedics, however, means much more than that and indeed the word no longer does justice to the vast field of practice in which medicine, surgery, nursing, physiotherapy and many other skills meets and merge in the treatment of disorders of nerves, muscles and skeleton.

Now 'orthopedics' emerged as a branch of surgery dealing with correction of deformities of bone and muscles. 'Orthopedic Nursing' refers to nursing management of disorders of bones and muscles, i.e. diseases and deformities of the muscles and skeleton for thick correction. It can also be called as "musculoskeletal nursing".

Individuals often show the ability to move about freely in the environment. The ability to perform complex and precise movements permits human beings to interact and adapt to environment. Proper functioning of the musculoskeletal system makes such movements possible. The musculoskeletal system consists of bones, muscles, joints, cartilage, ligaments, tendons, fascial and bursal. All the components of the system work together to produce movement and to supply structure. The musculoskeletal system is particularly vulnerable to external forces. Any disturbance in this well-integrated system results in musculoskeletal dysfunction. Problems can arise as a result of disease affecting the nerves, bones, muscles or joints or as a result of trauma to these or surrounding structures. Problems arising outside the musculoskeletal system such as endocrine, or neurological diseases may also directly affect the system resulting in some form of disability. The consequences may be deformity, alteration of body image, alteration in mobility, pain or permanent disability. These problems may produce long-term health problem that interfere with activities of daily living and quality of life.

Individuals with alteration in musculoskeletal functioning requires planning for appropriate interventions. This requires a careful and thorough assessment, based on the nurses' knowledge and understanding of the anatomy and physiology of the musculoskeletal system. Nurse plans for the care of any person with a musculoskeletal system disorders are based on the systemic assessment of needs, capabilities and resources.

Nursing Assessment of the Musculoskeletal System

Correct diagnosis depends on an accurate patient history and a thorough examination. A musculoskeletal assessment can be made on a specific body part, as a part of general physical examination in itself. Decision should be used on the basis of patients' problems in selecting all or part of the components of the musculoskeletal history and physical examination. Accidents often result in trauma to the musculoskeletal system and require a thorough assessment. If the injury is serious or life-threatening, only pertinent information related to the accident is obtained and complete assessment is deferred. A thorough assessment includes subjective data gathered from the patient and family interviews, which includes past health history, medications and other treatment and functional health patterns.

Health History

Symptomatic health information to be obtained are poor health history, i.e. certain illnesses are known to affect musculoskeletal system either directly or indirectly which include tuberculosis, diabetes mellitus, gout, inflammatory or degenerative arthritis, hemophilia, parathyroid problems, rickets, osteomalacia, scurvy, osteomyelitis or soft tissue infection, fungal infection of the bones or joints, and neuromuscular disabilities. If the patient has history of any of these, detailed account of illness should be obtained. In addition, sources of secondary bacterial infections can be obtained.

And obtaining information about medication used by the patient for musculoskeletal problems also are very important, i.e. reason for taking the drug, its name, dose, frequency and length of time it was taken, its effect and side effects. Because some drugs may lead to adverse effects on patient, which include anti-seizures (osteomalacia), phenothiazines (gait disturbances), corticosteroids (abnormal fat distribution) avascular necrosis, and decreased bone and muscle mass), and potassium-depleting diuretics (muscle cramps and weakness), amphetamines and caffein intake can cause increase in motor activity. And any previous surgery or other treatments, musculoskeletal are also obtained.

In addition to medical and surgical history, family history of genetic disorders/abnormalities, congenital abnormalities, also should be obtained. And general history of patients which include patients' age, sex, height and weight, nutritional pattern, occupation, exercise regimen, elimination pattern, ADL, habits like smoking, alcohol, recreational drug use, etc. are also important, for assessment of musculoskeletal system.

Physical Examination

The primary methods used in the physical examination of the musculoskeletal system include inspection and palpation. The data gathered from careful health history will provide the nurse with clues about areas on which to concentrate for examination. The nurse should observe the following.

- Behavior
  - Mental status
    - Orientation to time, place and person.
    - Ability to understand direction.
    - Capacity to retain information.
    - Attention span.
    - Ability to relate to others (is the person's attitude, quiet, talkative, tense, guarded, negative appropriate and inappropriate).
- General appearance:
  - Age, sex may relate to a specific disorder or attitude towards disorder (e.g. elderly susceptible for fall, old women risk for osteoporosis, etc.).
  - Posture may be characteristic of a specific problem (e.g. Scoliosis, Kyphotic posture in ankylosing spondylitis, etc.)
  - Nutritional status:
    - Overweight may indicate diminished ability to perform regular exercise or activity. Excess weight causes increased stress on joints.
    - Underweight may indicate inability to secure or prepare nutritional meals or to carry out feeding activities adequately; may relate to specific systemic conditions causing anorexia, nausea vomiting or malabsorption of food.
- Skin:
  - *Turgor (fullness):* This papery skin may indicate aging, systemic connective tissue disease, or long-term steroid use. Skin is easily broken.
  - *Texture (feel):* Thick leathery patches over forearms, hands, chest, face, indicate scleroderma; ulcerates easily, especially over joints.
  - *Integrity*:
    - Breaks in skin, ulcerations reddened areas
    - Impaired circulation to extremities-breakdown of distal parts.
  - Temperature—Warmth over the painful joints indicative of presence of inflammation or infection.
  - Erythema over joints—indicates inflammation of joint-need for joint to keep rest.
  - Color change on exposure to cold-white (resulting from anterior spasms), blue (cyanosis caused by stagnation of blood), red (warming and reactive vasodilation).
  - Bruising often present in following trauma.
  - Swelling of extremities denote prolonged dependent position, lack of activity, circulatory or renal impairment.
  - May indicate presence of effusion (serous, purulent or blood).
  - Bony enlargement – Indicative of disease process. For example, Hyberden nodes in osteoarthritis (hard, irregular swellings over the distal interphalangeal joints of the fingers) or Bouchard's nodes (cartilaginous or bony enlargement of proximal interphalangeal joint of fingers).
  - Subcutaneous nodules – Indicative of rheumatid arthritis, hard mobile swellings commonly found in subolecranon area.
  - Bursal swellings indicative of bursal inflammation, palpated as soft swelling over the bursae.
  - Synovial cyst – Indicative of hypertrophy of synovial tissue (For example, Baker's Cyst - swelling of the popliteal area often extending to calf).
  - Tophaceous deposits – Indicative of gout, hard translucent swelling over joints as in cartilage such as that of the ear.
  - Tenderness may be elevated by direct pressure and graded by amount of pressure required to produce discomfort. Degree of tenderness is visually in direct proportion to severity of imflammation or trauma. For example, in joint inflammation or injured soft tissue or overlying fracture.
  - General hygiene – Evidence of uncleanliness of body, clothing, may indicate inability to adequately carry out hygiening requirements.
- Nails and hairs:
  - Poorly kept or diseased nails may indicate lack of strength or inability to reach nails to care of nails, change in nail structure may indicate presence of connective tissue disease.
  - Poorly kept hair may indicate inability to lift arms to comb hair.
  - Alopecia, scaling of scalp may indicate connective disease and medications.

    Inspection begins during the nurse's initial contact with the patient. The nurse should observe the patient for any apparent symmetry and for sitting and standing posture, gout, general body build, and configuration of the muscles and signs of any abnormalities of behavior in general appearance, skin, nails, hairs as stated above. And in a head to toe fashion palpate all bones, joints, and soft tissue for temperature, swelling, tenderness, pain or masses. Palpate the spinous processes and intervertebral spaces for tenderness. In addition, assess the sensory function, deep tendon reflex activities, and range of motion. The most common movement that occur at synovial joint includes:

- *Flexion*: Bending of joint that decreases angle between two bones, shortening muscle strength.
- *Extension*: Bending of joint that increases angle between two bones.
- *Hyperextension*: Extension which angle exceeds 180 degrees.
- *Abduction*: Movement of part away from midline.
- *Pronation*: Turning of palm downwards or sole outwards.
- *Supination*: Turning of palm upwards or sole inwards.
- *Circumduction*: Combination of flexion, extension, abduction and adduction resulting in circular motion of body part.
- *Rotation*: Movement about longitudinal axis.
- *Inversion*: Turning of sole inwards towards midline.
- *Eversion*: Turning of sole outward away from midline.

In addition to above, limb length and circumferential measurement of muscle mass are often obtained when subjective problems or length discrepancies are noted and muscle-strength testings performed to know the strength of individual muscles or grasps of muscles is graded in performance of movements during contraction against applied resistance. The muscle strength scale is as follows:

0. No, detection of muscular contraction.
1. A barely detectable flicker or trace of contraction.
2. Active movement of body part with elimination of gravity.
3. Active movement against gravity.
4. Active movement against gravity and some resistance.
5. Active movement against full resistance without evidence of fatigue (normal).

The normal physical assessments of the musculoskeletal system are:
- Full range of motions of all joints.
- No joint swelling, deformity or crepitation.
- Normal spinal curvatures.
- No tenderness on palpation of spine.
- No muscle atrophy or asymmetry.
- Muscle strength of 5.

Assess the person's ability to discern light, touch, gentle pressure, pain and temperature which will evaluate sensory innervation. Perform each test bilaterally and compare results. Check sensation in the dermatomes, which will show abnormalities in spinal nerve innervation. Also evaluate the person's sense of proprioception (position sense) in the extremities.

Absence of reflexes may indicate neuropathy or a lower motor neuron lesion, whereas brisk reflexes indicate an upper motor neuron lesion. Again be sure to compare bilateral responses. The grading of responses of deep tendon reflex activity are as follows (Scale of responses to score DTRA).

0. No response.
1. Sluggish or diminisher.
2. Active or expected response.
3. More brisk than expected, slightly hyperactive.
4. Brisk, hyperactive with intermittent or transient clonus.

The nurse assesses gait by having the patient walk across the room and back. The normal gait cycle will be:
- Stance phase—Begins with heel strike and ends with toe-off.
- Swing phase—Begins with toe off and continues through heel strike.
- Double support—Brief period when both feet are on ground.

Musculoskeletal and neurologic problems can result in gait abnormalities.

In addition, the special assessment techniques for musculoskeletal system are as follows followed by abnormality detected:

- *Limb measurement:* Measurement in centimeters of extremities from a major landmark. Asymmetrical limb length may indicate pelvic obliquity of hip deformities; discrepancies in circumference may indicate atrophy or paresis of muscle groups, less than 1 cm discrepancy is normal in most people.
- *Ballottement:* Compression of the suprapatellar pouch, which is normally snug against the femur. Fluid wave indicates excess fluid in the knee (effusion).
- *Bulge sign:* Stroke the medial aspect of the knee, then tap the lateral side of the patell; a fluid wane or if fluid is present.
- *McMurray's test:* External rotation and valgus stress applied to the knee while the leg is held flexed at the knee and hip (patient is lying supine), normally there is no pain or sound. "Click" or pain indicates meniscal tear.
- *Drawer test (Anteroposterior or mediolateral):* With the patient supine and knee flexed, push forwards and backward on tibia at the joint line; with the patient supine with knee extended, stabilize the femur and ankle while attempting to abduct and adduct the knee; normally there is little or no movement, assess symmetry of responses. Laxity or movement suggests

instability of the anterior or posterior cruciates ligaments or the medial or lateral collateral ligaments of the knee.
- *Straight leg raising (LaSegue) test:* With the patient supine raise the leg straight with the knee extended; normally there is no pain. If the maneuver reproduces sciatic pain, it is considered positive and suggest a herniated disk.
- *Trendelenburg's test:* While the patient stands on one foot and then the other, both iliac crests should appear symmetrical. Asymmetry suggests hip dislocation.
- *Thomas test:* With the patient lying supine and one leg fully extended and other flexed on the chest, observe the ability of the patient to keep extended leg flat on the table. Inability to keep the leg extended suggest a hip flexion contracture in the extended leg that may be masked by increased lumbar lordoses.
- *Phalen's test:* Flex both wrists together at 90 degrees and hold for 60 seconds; normally this produces no symptoms, numbers, tingling or burning in the median nerve distribution suggests carpal tunnel syndrome.
- *Tinel's sign:* Tap over the median nerve where it passes through the carpal tunnel in the wrist; nomally this does not produce any symptom. Tingling along the median nerve distribution is associated with carpal tunnel syndrome.
- *Drop arm test:* Raise the affected arm to - 90 degree of flexion, then have the patient slowly adduct the arm to the side. Inability to lower the arm slowly or smoothly is associated with disruption of the rotator cuff mechanism of the shoulder.
- *Scoliasis Screening:* "Forward bend" test, observe symmetry and height of scapulae, shoulders, iliac crests and rib-cage. A symmetry of scapulae or shoulder height, "winged" iliac crests, demonstrable curve of the spine and rib hump indicates scoliasis.

DIAGNOSTIC STUDIES OF THE MUSCULOSKELETAL SYSTEM

Diagnostic studies provide important information to the nurse in monitoring the patient's condition and planning appropriate intervention. The common diagnostic studies performed and used are as follows:

Radiological Studies

- *Standard X-ray:* An X-ray is taken to determine density of bone. Study evaluates structural or functional changes of bones and joints. In an interoposterior view, X-ray beam passes from front to back, allowing one-dimensional view; Lateral position provides two-dimensional view. Nursing responsibility here is to avoid excessive exposure of patient and self; Before procedure, remove any radio-opaque objects that can interfere with results and explain procedure to the patients.
- *Arthrogram:* This study involves injection of contrast medium or air into joint cavity, which permits visualization of joint structures. Joint movement is followed with series of X-rays. Here nurse has to assess patient for possible allergy to contrast medium including iodine or sea-food. Explain the procedure to patient and prepare the area to be injected aseptically.
- *Diskogram:* An X-ray of cervical or lumbar intervertebral disk is done after injection of contrast dye into nucleus purposes. Study permits visualization of intervertebral disk abnormalities. Preparation of the patient as in arthrogram may be performed in surgery.
- *Sinogram:* An X-ray is taken after injection of contrast dye into sinus tract (deep draining wound). Study visualizes course of sinus and tissues involved. Preparation is as in arthrogram.
- *Tomogram:* Multiple X-ray views of body region are focussed at successively deeper layers of tissue lying in predetermined planes. Study focuses on certain tissues, eliminating or blurring surrounding structures. Technique is useful in locating bone destruction, small body cavities, foreign bodies and lesions overshadowed by opaque structures. Usual preparation includes informing the patient in this procedure is painless.
- *Computed Tomography Scan:* An X-ray beam is used with a computer to provide a three-dimensional picture. It is used to identify soft tissue abnormalities, and various musculoskeletal trauma. Usual preparation plus informing the patient that it is painless, and importance of remaining still during procedure.
- *MRI:* Radio waves and magnetic field are used to view soft tissues. Study is especially useful in the diagnosis of a vascular necrosis, disk disease, tumours, osteomyelitis, ligament tears, and cartilage tears. Patient is placed inside scanning chamber. Gadolinium may be injected into a vein to enhance visualization of the structures. Open MRI does not require the patient to be placed inside a chamber. The nurse's responsibilities here include:
  - Inform that it is painless procedure.
  - Be aware that it is contraindicated in patients with aneurysm clip metaling implants, pacemakers, electronic devices, hearing aids, sharpner and extreme obesity.
  - Ensure that patient has no metal on clothing (e.g. snaps, zippers, jewellery and credit cards).
  - Convert IV to heparin lock.
  - Inform patient about importance of remaining still throughout examination.
  - Inform patients who are claustrophobic that may experience symptoms during examination.
  - Administer anti anxiety agent (if indicated or ordered).

- Open MRI may be indicated for obese patient or patient with large chest and abnormal girth or severe claustrophobia.
- Open MRI may not be available at all facilities.

Bone Mass Measurement

- *Radiogrammetry, radiodensitometry:* Study evaluation bone mass of metacarpals. A very low dose of radiation is used.
- *Single-photon absorptiometry (SPA):* Low dose radiation scanner measures mostly peripheral cortical bone at distal radius or midradius. This study is not useful for follow-up because of slow changes in cortical bone.
- *Dual-photon absorptiometry (DPA):* Technique measures mixed trabecular and cortical bones at sites such as hip and lumbar spine. It can be used to calculate total body calcium concentration.
- *Dual-energy X-ray absorptiometry (DEXA):* Technique measures bone mass of spine, femur, forearm, and total body. Considered to be fast and precise with low dose of radiation.

In these procedures, nurse explains the procedure to patient and inform that the procedures are painless.

Radioisotope Studies

Bone scan: Technique involves injection of radioisotopes, usually sodium pertechnate) that is taken up by bone. Camera scans entire body (front and back) and recording is made on paper. Degree of uptake is related to blood flow to bone. Increased uptake is seen in osteomyelities. Osteoporosis, primary and metastatic malignant lesions of bone, and with certain fracture. Decreased uptake is seen in areas of avascular necrosis.

The nurse's reponsibility includes:

- Give calculated dose of radioistope 2 hours before procedure.
- Ensure the bladder emptied before scan.
- Inform patient that procedure requires 1 hour while patient lies supine and no pain or harm will result from isotope. Be aware that no follow-up scans are required.

Endoscopy

- *Arthroscopy:* The study involves insertion of arthroscope into joint usually knee for visualization of structure and contents. It can be used for exploratory surgery (removal of loose bodies and biopsy) and for diagnosis of abnormalities of meniscus, articular cartilage ligaments of joint capsule. Other structures that can be visualized through the arthroscope include the shoulder, elbow, wrist and ankle. The nurse has to:
  - Inform patient that procedure performed in opening room with strict asepsis and that either local or general anesthesia is used.
  - After procedure, cover wound with sterile dressing.
  - Wrap leg from midthigh to midcalf with compression dressing for 24 hours for knee arthroscopy.
  - Instruct patient to limit activity for few days.
- *Serological studies:* For all the serological studies, nurses have to obtain blood samples by venipuncture and send the sample, to concerned laboratories at right time. Prior to procedure, inform the patient that procedure does not require fasting to some and some need fasting. After procedure, observe the venipuncture site for bleeding or haematoma formation.
  - Mineral metabolism test:
    - *Alkaline phosphatase:* This enzyme produced by osteoblast of bone, is needed for mineralization of organic bone matrix. Elevated levels are found in healing fractures, bone cancers, osteoporosis, osteomalacia rickets, and Paget's disease (normal 20-90 UL).
    - *Calcium:* Bone is primary organ for calcium storage. Calcium provides bone with rigid consistency. Decreased serum levels are found in osteomalacia, renal disease and hypothyroidism rickets. Increase in serum level is immobility and bone demineralization bone cancer, multiple myeloma (Normal 3-4.6 mg/dl).
    - *Phosphorus:* Together with calcium K+ plays vital role in bone metabolism. Decreased level is found in osteomalacia; increased level is found in chronic renal disease, healing fractures, osteolytic metastatic tumour (Normal 2.8-4.5 mg/dl).
- Serum test
  - *Rheumatoid Factor (RF):* Study assesses presence of auto-antibody (RF) in serum. Factor is not specific for rheumatoid arthritis and seen in other connective tissue diseases, as well as in a small percentage of normal population (Normal: negative or less than 1.20).
  - *Erythrocyte Sedimentation Rate (ESR):* This study is non-specific index of inflammation. Study measures rapidity with which RBCs settle out of unclotted blood in 1 hour. Results are influenced by physiologic factors as well as diseases. Elevated levels are seen with any inflammatory process especially rheumatoid arthritis, rheumatic fever, osteomyeltis, and respiratory infections. (Normal less than 20 mm/hr general variation 1-3 m/hr (M), 4-7 mm/hr (P).
  - *Lupus Erythematosus (LE) cells:* Used in the diagnosis and treatment of systemic lupus erythematosus (SLE). Obtain blood from patient and smear made on slide. Normally no LE cells ore present.

- *Antinuclear Antibody (ANA):* Study assesses presence of antibodies capable of destroying nucleus of body's tissue cells, positive in 95 percent SLE cases and may be positive in cases of scleroderma and Rh arthritis.
- *Anti-DNA Antibody:* Study detects serum antibodies that react with DNA. It is the most specific test for SLE cases.
- *Serum complement:* Complement, a normal body protein is essential to both immune and inflammatory reactions, complement components used in these reactions are depleted. Subsequent tests applied to serum yields little or no serum complement components. Complement depletion may be found in patients with Rh arthritis or SLE.
- *Serological Test for Syphilis (STS):* False-positive STS results occur in 10-15 percent of persons with connective tissue diseases. So test may help in diagnosis. FTA-ABS (Fluorescent treponemal antibody absorption) excludes the presence of syphylis.
- *C-reactive Protein (CRP):* Study used to diagnose inflammatory diseases, infections, and active widespread malignancy. CRP is synthesized by the liver and is present in large amounts in serum 18-24 hours after onset of tissue damage (Normal negative).
- *Human Leukocyte Antigen (HLA-B27):* Antigen present in disorders such as ankylosing spondylitis and variants of rheumatoid arthritis.
- *Serum muscle enzyme test:* AST (Serum aspartate aminotransferase transaminase). SGOT (Serum-gutamic-oxaloacetic transminase). Alolase. CPK (Creatinine phosphokinase) isoenzymes MM.MB. Enzymes can be elevated in the presence of primary myopathic (muscle) disease. Elevated levels may result from muscle degeneration or from diffusion., through a muscle membrane that has increased permeability. Enzyme levels are an index of both progress of the myopathic disorder and effectiveness of treatment.
- Higher concentration of CPK is found in skeletal muscle. Increased values are found in progressive muscular dystrophy, polymyositis and traumatic injuries (Normal: 5.5 u/L (M), 5.35 u/L (F)).
- Aldolase study is useful in monitoring muscular dystrophy and dermatomyosites (Normal 1.0–7.5 u/L).
- AST or SGOT enzyme is found in skeletal muscle but primary and enzyme of cardiac and hepatic cell (Normal 1-4.5 u/L (SGOT), AST 8.204/L).

- *Urinary tests:*
    - 24 hour urine for creatine-creatinine ratio. In the presence of muscle disease, the ability of the muscle to convert creatines decreased; the amount of creatine excreted by the kidneys increases, and the ratio of creatine to creatinine increases. Periodic studies are helpful in diagnosis and evaluation of progress of treatment of primary myopathies.
    - Urinary uric acid level (24 hr. collection); End product of purine metabolism is normally excreted in urine. Helpful in diagnosis and decisions regarding treatment modalities for gout. (Normal value should not exceed 900-mg uric acid excretion per day).
    - Urine for deoxypyridinoline (DPD) – First or second morning void. Routine collection – DPD cross links assay provides a quantitative measurement of DPD. which is excreted unmetabolized in the urine during bone resorption.

- *Invasive procedures:*
    - Arthrocentesis is incision or puncture of joint capsule is done to obtain samples of synovial fluid from within joint cavity or to remove excess fluid. Local anaesthesia and aseptic preparation are used before needle is inserted into joint and fluid aspirated. Study is useful in diagnosis of joint inflammation.

        In this, nurse has to inform patient that procedure is usually done at bedside or in examination room. Send sample of synovial fluid to lab examination (if indicated). After procedure, apply compression dressing and have patient rest joint 8-24 hours. Observe for leakage of blood or fluid on dressing.
    - Electromyogram (EMG) study evaluates electrical potential associated with skeletal muscle contraction. Long, small-guage needles are inserted into certain muscles. Needle probes are attached to leads that feed information to electromyogram machine. Recordings of electrical activity of muscles are traced on audiotransmitter, as well as oscilloscope and recording paper. Study is useful in providing information related to lower motor neuron dysfunction and primary muscle diseases. In this procedure, the nurse must inform the patient that the procedure is usually done in electromyogram laboratory while the patients lie supine on special table. Keep patient awake to cooperate with voluntary movement. Inform patient that the procedure involves some discomfort from needle insertion. Avoid administration of stimulants and sedatives 24 hours prior to procedure.

    In addition to this, other procedures are thermography, plethysmography, and somatosensory evoked potential (SSEP).

- Thermography is a technique (noninvasive) uses infrared detector, which measures degrees of heat

radiating from skin surface. Study is useful in investigation of cause of inflamed joints and in following up patient's response to anti inflammatory drug therapy.
- Plethysmography study (noninvasive) records variation in volume and pressure of blood passing through tissues. Test is nonspecific and quantitative.
- SSEP is invasive procedure, it evaluates evoked potential of muscle contractions. Electrodes are placed on muscle and provide recordings of electrical activity of muscle. Study useful in identifying subtle dysfunction of lower motor neuron and primary muscle disease. SSEPT measures nerve conduction along pathways not accessible to EMG. Transcutaneous or percutaneous electrodes are applied to the skin and help identify neutropathy and myopathy. Here, nurse informs the patient that the procedure is similar to EMG, but does not involve needles. Electrodes are applied to the skin.

In addition, biopsies of tissues from a variety of organs are helpful in the diagnosis of disease or disorders affecting the musculoskeletal system.
- Skin biopsy (Punch biopsy).
- Muscle biopsy (Operative procedure).
- Synovium biopsy (closed performed with needle, open performed in surgery).
- Buccal mucosa (Punch biopsy).
- Bone biopsy (operative procedure).

The nurse should prepare the patient according to procedure.

SOFT-TISSUE INJURIES

Soft tissue injuries include sprains, strains, dislocations and subluxation. These common injuries are usually caused by trauma.

Sprains and Strains

A sprain is an injury to ligamentous structures surrounding a joint, usually caused by a wrenching or twisting motion. A sprain is classified according to the amount of ligament fibers torn.
- A first degree involves tears only a few fibers resulting in mild tenderness and slight swelling.
- A second degree sprain is partial disruption of the involved tissue with more swelling and tenderness.
- A third degree sprain is a complex tearing of the ligament. A gap in the muscle may be apparent or felt through the skin of the muscle is torn. Because these areas are nerve endings, the injury is extremely painful.
- The most common areas of sprain occurs in the ankle and wrist.

A strain is a stretching of muscles and its fascial sheath.

Etiology

Acute soft injuries caused by falls, direct blows, crust injury, motor vehicle collisions and sport injuries. The common sport related injuries are:
- *Impingement syndrome:* Entrapment of soft-tissue structures under coracoa cromial arch of the shoulder.
- *Rotator cuff tear:* Tear within muscle or ligaments of shoulder.
- *Skin splints:* Inflammation along tibial shaft from tearing away of tendons caused by improper shoes, overuse, or running on hard pavement.
- *Tendonitis:* Inflammation of tendon in upper or lower extremities as a result of overuse or incorrect use.
- *Ligament injury:* Tearing or stretching of ligament: usually, as a result of direct blow: characterized by sudden pain, swelling and instability.
- *Meniscal injury:* Injury to fibrocartilage of the knee characterized by popping, clicking or tearing sensation and swelling.

Clinical Manifestation

The clinical manifestation of sprains and strains are similar and include pain, edema, decrease in function and bruising. Usually the patient will recount a history of traumatic injury. Possibly of a twisting nature, or recent exercise activity. Minor sprains and strains are usually self-limiting with full function returning within 3 to 6 weeks. A severe sprain can result in an avulsion fracture, in which, ligaments pull loose a fragment of bone. Alternatively the joint structure may become unstable and result in subluxation or dislocation. At the time of injury hemarthrosis (bleeding into a joint space or cavity) or disruption of the lining may occur. An acute strain may involve partial or complete rupture of muscle.

Management

X-rays of the affected part are usually taken to rule out a fracture or widening of the joint structure. Surgical repair may be necessary if the injury is significant enough to produce severe disruption of ligamentous or muscle structures, fracture or dislocation.

To reduce sprains and strains, individuals are encouraged to stretching and warm up exercises before vigorous activity. Pre-conditioning exercises protect an inherently weak joint, because slow stretching is tolerated better by biological tissues than quick stretching. Warm-up exercises "prelengthen" potentially-strained tissues by avoiding the quick stretch often encountered in sports. Warm-up exercise also increases the temperature of muscle, which increases the speed of cell metabolism and the speed of nerve impulse transmission. The increased metabolism contributes to better oxygenation of muscle fiber during work. Stretching also is thought to improve kinesthetic awareness, thus lessening the chance of uncoordinated movement.

In acute soft tissue injury, nurse should assess the patients.

The assessments finding may include:
- Edema.
- Ecchymosis.
- Pain, tenderness.
- Decreased pulse, coolness and capillary refill.
- Decreased sensation with severe edema.
- Decreased movements.
- Pallor.
- Shortening or rotation of extremity.
- Inability to bear weight when lower extremity is involved.
- Decreased function with upper extremity involvement.
- Muscle spasms.

An initial nursing intervention includes:
- Ensure airways, breathing and circulation.
- Assess neurovascular status of involved limb.
- Rest and limitation of movement.
- Application of ice to the injured area.
- Compression of the involved extremity.
- Elevation of the extremity and to prevent edema.
- Analgesia as necessary to relieve pain (Mild analgesic, aspirin, ibuprofen.
- Administer tetanus prophylaxis of skin integrity is broken.

Cold in several forms can be used to produce hypothermia to the involved part. Physiological changes that occur in soft tissue as a result of the use of cold include vasoconstriction, reduction in transmission of nerve impulses, and reduction in conduction velocity. These changes result in analgesia and anesthesia, reduction of muscle spasm without changes in muscular strength or endurance, reduction of local edema and inflammation and reduction of local metabolic requirements. Few unwanted side effects accompany the use of cold to treat a soft tissue injury. Cold is most useful when applied immediately after the injury had occurred. Ice application should not exceed 20 to 30 minutes per application, allowing a warm-down time for 10 to 15 minutes between applications.

Compression also helps in limit swelling, which, if left uncontrolled could lengthen healing time. The elastic compression bandage can be wrapped around the injured part, but it should not be too tight or too loose.

After the acute phase (usually lasting 24 to 48 hours), warm, moist heat can be applied to the affected part to reduce swelling and provide comfort. NSAIDS may be recommended to decrease edema and pain. The patient is encouraged to use the limb provided that the joint is protected by means of casting, taping or splinting. Movement of the joints maintains nutrition to the cartilage, and muscle contraction speeds circulation and resolution of the hematoma.

DISLOCATION AND SUBLUXATION

Dislocation is a severe injury of the ligamentous structures that surround a joint. It results in the complete displacement or separation of the articular surfaces of the joint.

A subluxation is a partial or incomplete displacement of joint surface. The etiology of both are associated with accidents.

Clinical Manifestation

The clinical manifestations of dislocation and subluxation are similar. The most obvious clinical manifestation of the dislocation is asymmetry of the musculoskeletal contour. For example, if a hip is dislocated, the limb is shorter on the affected side. Additional manifestation includes local pain tenderness, loss of function of the injured part and swelling of the soft tissues in the region of that joint. The major complications of a dislocated joint are open joint injuries, intra-articular fractions, fracture dislocation, avascular necrosis and damage to adjacent neurovascular tissues.

Management

X-ray studies are performed to determine the extent and shifting of the involved structures. The joint may also be aspirated to determine the presence of blood (hemarthorosis) or fat cells. Fat cells from the synovial fluid indicate probable intra-articular fracture.

The dislocation requires prompt attention. The longer the joints remain unreduced, the greater the possibility of avascular necrosis (bone cell death due to inadequate blood supply, e.g. hip joint dislocation). The first goal of management is to realign the dislocated portion of the joint in its original anatomic position. This can be accomplished by a close reduction, which may be performed under local or general anesthesia. Anesthesia is often necessary to produce muscle relaxation so that the bones can be manipulated. In some situation surgical open reduction may be necessary. After reduction the extremity is usually immobilized by taping or using a sling to allow the torn ligaments and capsular tissue time to heal. Observation is indicated for the patient with a posterior sternoclavicular dislocation because delayed intrathoracic complications such as pneumothorax or subclavian vessel injury may occur.

Nursing management of subluxation or dislocation is directed towards relief of pain and support and protection of the injured joint. After joint has been reduced and immobilized, motion usually is restricted. A carefully regulated rehabilitation programme can prevent formation of contractures.

CARPAL TUNNEL SYNDROME (CTS)

Carpal tunnel syndrome is a condition caused by compression of the median nerve beneath the transferse carpal ligament within the narrow confines of the carpal tunnel location at wrist.

Etiology

This condition frequently is due to pressure from trauma or edema caused by inflammation of a tendon (tenosynovitis) neoplasm, rheumatoid synovial disease or soft tissue masses such as ganglia. CTS occurs in mostly middle-aged or postmenopausal women. This syndrome is associated with occupations that require continuous wrist movement (e.g. butchers, musicians, hairstylists, secretaries, typists, carpenters and computer operators).

The clinical manifestation of carpal tunnel syndrome are weakness especially of the thumb, pain and numbness or impaired sensation in the distribution of the median nerve and clumsiness in performing hand movements. Numbness and tingling may be present that awaken the patient at night. Holding the wrist in acute flexion for 60 seconds will produce tingling and numbness over the distribution of the median nerve, the palmar surface of the thumb, the index finger, the middle finger, and part of the ring finger. This is known as positive phalen sign. Tapping gently over the area of the inflamed median nerve may reproduce the paresthesia. This is known as a positive Tinel's sign. In late stages there is atrophy of the thenar muscle around the base of the thumb. This syndrome can result in recurrent pain and eventual dysfunction of the hand.

Management

Prevention of carpal tunnel syndrome involves educating employees and employer to identify risk factors. Adaptive devices such as wrist splints may be worn to hold the wrist in slight dorsiflextion to relieve pressure on the median nerve. Special keyboard pads that help prevent repetitive pressure on the median nerve are available for computer operators to help reduce CTS by decreasing tension on the carpal tunnel.

Care of patient with CTS is directed towards relieving the underlying cause of the nerve compression. The early symptoms associated with CTS can usually be relieved by stopping of the aggravating action and by placing the hand and wrist at rest by immobilizing them in a handsling. If the cause is inflammation, injection of hydrocortisone should be given directly in carpal tunnel. If the problem continues the median nerve may have to be surgically decompressed by longitudinal division of the transferse ligament under regional anesthesia. Endoscopic carpal tunnel release is new procedure used for decompression.

REPETITIVE STRAIN INJURY (RSI)

Repetitive strain injury is defined as a comulative trauma disorder resulting from prolonged, forceful or awkward movements. Repeated movements strain tendens, ligaments, and muscles causing tiny tears that become inflamed. If the tissues are not given time to heal properly, scarring can occur. Blood vessels of the arms and hands may become constricted, depriving tissues of vital nutrients and causing an accumulation of factors such as lactic acid. Without intervention, tendons and muscles can deteriorate and nerves become hypersensitive. At this point, even the slightest movement can cause pain.

In addition to the repetitive movements, other factors related to RSI include poor posture and positioning, ill-fitting furniture, a badly designed keyboard, and a heavy workload. The result in damage to the muscles, tendons and nerves of the neck, shoulder, forearm and hand. Symptoms of RSI include pain, weakness, numbness or impairment of motor function. Persons most often affected with RSI are as stated in CTS.

RSI can be prevented through education, ergonomics (consideration of the interaction of humans and their work environment) and appropriate job design. Once diagnosed, the treatment of RSI consists of avoidance of the participating activity, physical therapy, and careful use of analgesia. In most cases, the muscle and tendon damage associated with RSI cannot be surgically repaired.

ROTATOR CUFF INJURIES

The rotator cuff is a complex of four muscles in the shoulder: Supraspinatus, infraspinatus, teres minor and subscapularis. These muscles act to stabilize the humeral head in the glenoid fossa and rotate the humerus.

A tear in the rotator cuff may occur as a gradual degenerative process resulting from aging, poor posture, repulsive stress (especially overhead arm motions) or using arm to break or fall. Young adults are more prone to experience a tear as a result of trauma such as fall, lifting heavy objects or throwing a ball.

Patient with a rotator cuff injury will complain of shoulder pain and cannot initiate or maintain abduction of the areas or shoulder. An X-ray alone cannot benefit in diagnosis, so a tear can be confirmed by arthogram or MRI.

The patient may be treated conservatively with rest, ice and heat, NSAIDs, periodic corticosteroid injections into joint, and physical therapy. If the patient does not respond to conservative treatment or if a complete tear is present, surgical repair may be necessary. This can be performed through arthroscope. If extensive tear or pressure, open repair is indicated. An immobilization device such as sling or more commonly a shoulder immobilizer may be used for several weeks after surgery. Exercises and physical therapy begin within few days of surgery.

MENISCUS INJURY

The meniscus is the fibrous cartilage in the knee and other joints. Meniscus injuries are closely associated with ligament sprains, commonly occurring in athletes engaged in sports such as basket ball, rugby, foot ball, soccer and hockey. These activities produce a rotational stress when the knee is in a flexed position and the foot is fixed. A blow to the knee can cause the menscus to be trapped between the femoral condyles and the plateau of the tibia, resulting in a torn meniscus. A causal relationship exists between occupations that require working in squatting or kneeling position and meniscus injury.

Meniscus injuries alone do not usually cause chronic oedema because cartilage is avascular and aneural. However, a torn meniscus may be suspected when local tenderness or pain is reported. Pain is elicited by abduction or adduction of the leg at the knee. The usual clinical picture is feeling by the patient that knee may click and lock periodically. Quadriceps atrophy is evident if the injury has been present for some time. Degenerative joint disease can occur if a damaged roughened meniscus is not surgically removed.

Management

An arthrogram or arthroscopy or both can diagnose knee problems. MRI also is beneficial before arthroscopy. Because meniscal injuries are commonly caused by sports related activity, athletes should be educated about warm up activities. Proper stretching may make the person less prone to meniscal injury when a fall or twisting occurs.

Examinations of the acutely injured knee should occur within 24 hours of injury. Initial care of this type of injury involves application of ice, immobilization, and partial weight bearing with crutches. Most meniscal injuries are treated in an outpatient setting. The patient should be allowed to ambulate as tolerated. Crutches may be necessary. Use of an immobilizer during first few days protects the knees.

After acute pain has decreased, gradual increase in flexion and strengthening help return the patient to full functioning. Physical therapy may be needed to help the patient strengthen muscles before returning to sport activities. Surgical repair or excision of part of meniscus (menisectomy) may be necessary. Frequently this can be done by arthroscopy. Use of the laser for arthroscopy is undergoing clinical research.

BURSITIS

Bursaes are closed sacs that are lined with synovial membrane and contain small amount of synovial fluid. They are located as sites of friction such as between tendons, bones and overlying joints. A bursac may become inflamed (bursitis) from repeated or excessive trauma or friction, gout, rheumatoid, arthritis or infection.

The primary clinical manifestations of bursitis are warmth, pain and swelling and limited range of motion in the affected part. Since parts of the body at which it occurs include the hand, knee, trochanter, shoulder and elbow.

Management

Attempts are made to determine and correct the cause of the bursitis. Rest is often only the treatment needed. Icing the area will decrease pain and may reduce inflammations. The affected part may be immobilized in a compression dressing or plaster splint. NSAIDS may be used to reduce pain and inflammation. Aspiration and bursal fluid and injection of hydrocortisone may be necessary. If the burn has become thickened and continued to interfering joints' function, require surgical excision (bursectomy).

MUSCLE SPASMS

Local muscle spasms are common conditions often associated with excessive everyday activities and sports activities. Injury to a muscle results in inflammation and edema, which stimulates free nerve endings, resulting in muscle excitation and spasm. The spasms produce additional pain, creating a repetitive cycle.

The clinical manifestation of muscle spasm include pain. Palpable muscle mass in spasm, tenderness, diminished range of motions of affected site, and limitations of the daily activities.

Management

A careful history should be taken and physical examination should be performed to relevant CNS problems. Muscle spasms can be managed with drug therapy (mild analgesics, NSAIDS, skeletal muscle relaxants), physical therapy or both. The physical therapy program might include the use of heat or ice, supervised exercises, massage hydrotherapy, local heat-producing application (oil of Wintergreen) ultrasound (deep heat) manipulation and bracing.

FRACTURES

Etiology

Fractures are disruptions or break in the continuity of the structure of bone. Fractures of bone usually occur as a result of blow to the body, a fall, or another accident. Traumatic injuries account for the majority of the fractures, although some fractures are secondary to a disease (pathological fractures).

The highest incidence of fractures is in males 15-24 years old and in elderly persons especially women aged 65 years or more. Osteoporosis is the most common cause of bone fractures. Neuromuscular instability is an important contributory factor to risk falls, which commonly proceeds a fracture in the elderly ones. Wrist, hip, and vertebral fractures are most common in elderly persons. Persons in high-risk occupations (steel workers and race car drivers and persons with chronic degenerative or neoplastic diseases are also at higher risk for injury).

Pathophysiology

A fracture is a complete or partial interruption of osteous tissue. Fractures can be described and classified according to type, communication or non-communication with external environment and location of the fracture. Fractures are also described as stable or unstable. A stable fracture occurs when some of the perioesteum is intact across the fracture either external or internal fixation has rendered the fragments stationary. Stable fractures are usually transverse, spiral, greenstick. An unstable fracture is grossly displaced during injury and in a site of poor fixation. Unstable fractures are usually comminuted or oblique.

Fracture can be described as complete or incomplete. Complete fractures penetrate both cortexes, producing two bone fragments, by only one cortex is broken in incomplete fracture. A typical complete fracture and incomplete fracture are as follows:

- Typical complete fractures.
  - *Closed (simple) fracture*—Noncommunicating wound between bone and skin.
  - *Open (compound) fracture*—Communicating would be between bone and skin high risk for contamination.
  - *Comminuted fracture*—It is a fracture with more than two fragments. These smaller fragments appear to be floating.
  - *Linear fracture*—Fracture line parallel to the long axis of the bone. The periosteum is not torn away from the bone (Longitudinal fracture).
  - *Oblique fracture*—it is a fracture in which the line of the fracture extends in an oblique direction. Fracture line is 45 degree angle to the long axis bone.
  - *Spiral fracture*—Fracture line encircling bone, in which the line of the fracture extends in a spiral direction along the shaft of the bone.
  - *Transverse fracture*—Fracture line is perpendicular to long axis of bone, in which line of the fracture extends across the bone shaft at a right angle to the longitudinal axis.
  - *Impacted fracture*—Fracture fragments are pushed into each other. It is displaced (overriding) fracture which involves a displaced fracture fragment that is overriding the other bone fragments. The periosteum is disrupted on both sides.
  - *Pathological fracture*—Fracture occurs at a point in the bone weakened by a disease. For example, tumor or oesteoporosis.
  - *Avulsion:* It is a fracture of bone resulting from the strong pulling effect of tendons or ligaments at the bone attachment. A fragment of bone connected to a ligament breaks off from the main bone.
  - *Extracapsular*—Fracture is close to the joint but remains outside the joint capsule.
  - *Intracapsular*—Fractures within the joint capsule.
- Typical incomplete fractures.
  - *Greenstick fracture*—Break on one cortex of bone with splintering of inner bone surface.
  - *Torus fracture*—Buckling of cortex.
  - *Bowing fracture*—Bending of the bone.
  - *Stress fracture*—Microfracture - normal or abnormal, subject to repeated stress such as from jogging or running.
  - *Transochondrial fracture*—Separation of cartilagenous joint surface (articular cartilage) from main shaft bone.

Clinical Manifestation

The clinical manifestation of fractures differ depending on the location and type of fracture and associated with soft-tissue injuries. The common signs and symptoms include the following.

- *Edema and swelling:* Disruption of the soft tissues or bleeding into surrounding tissues. Unchecked edema in closed space can occlude circulation and damage nerves (i.e. there is risk of acute compartment syndrome).
- *Pain and tenderness:* Muscle spasm as a result of involuntary reflex action of muscle, direct tissue trauma, increased pressure on sensory nerve, movement of the fracture parts. Pain caused by swelling at the site, muscle spasm, damage to periosteum. It may be immediate, severe and aggravated by pressure at the site of injury and attempted motion.
- *Loss of normal function:* Due to disruption of bone, preventing functional use, the injured part is incapable of voluntary movement. Fracture must be managed properly to ensure restoration of function.
- *Deformity:* Obvious deformity resulting from loss of bone continuity. Abnormal position of bone as a result of original forces of injury and action of muscles pulling fragment into abnormal position seen as a loss of normal bony contours. Deformity is cardinal sign of fracture. If incorrected, it may result in problems with bony union and restoration of function of injured part.
- *Excessive motion at site:*, i.e. motion when motion does not usually occur.
- *Crepitation:* Crepitus or grating sound occurs if limb is moved gently. Grating or crunching together of bony fragments, producing palpable or audible crunching sensation. Examination of crepitation may increase chance for non-union and bone ends are allowed to move excessively.

- Soft tissue edema in area of injury resulting from extravasation of blood and tissue fluid.
- Warmth over injured area resulting from increased blood flow to the area.
- *Ecchymosis:* Ecchymosis of skin surrounding injured area (may not be apparent for several days). This is discoloration of skin as a result of extravasation of blood in subcutaneous tissue. It usually appears several days after injury and may appear distal to injury. The nurse should reassure patient that process is normal.
- Impairment or loss of sensation or paralysis distal to injury is resulting from nerve entrapment or damage.
- Signs of shock related to severe tissue injury, blood loss or intense pain.
- Evidence of fracture on X-ray film.

Healing of Fracture

It is important to understand the principles of fracture healing to provide appropriate therapeutic interventions. Bone goes through a remarkable reparative process of self-healing (termed union) that occurs in following stages:

- *Fracture hematoma:* When fracture occurs, bleeding and edema create a hematoma, which surrounds the ends of fragments. The hematoma is extravasated blood that changes from a liquid to a semisolid clot.
- *Granulation tissue:* During this stage, active phagocytosis absorbs the products of local necrosis. The hematoma converts to granulation tissue. Granulation tissue (consisting of young blood vessels, fibroblasts and esteoblasts) produces the basis for a new bone substance called 'osteoid'.
- *Callus formation:* As minerals (Calcium, Phosphorous and magnesium) are deposited in the osteoid, it forms an unorganized network of bone that is woven about the fracture parts. Callus is primarily composed of cartilage, osteoblasts, and end of the first week of injury. Evidence of callus formation can be verified by X-ray.
- *Ossification:* Ossification of the callus begins within 2 to 3 weeks after the fracture and continues until the fracture has healed. This stage is marked by ossification of callus that is sufficient to prevent movement at the fracture site when the bones are gently stressed. However, the fracture is still evident on X-ray. During this stage of clinical union, this patient can be converted from skeletal traction to a cast or the cast can be removed to allow limited mobility.
- *Consolidation:* As callus continues to develop, the distance between bone fragments diminishes and eventually closes. This stage is called "Consolidation" and ossification continues. It can be equated with radiograph union.
- *Remodelling:* Excess tissue absorbed in the final stage of bone healing, and union is completed. Gradual return of the injured bone to its preinjury structural strength and shape occurs. Remodelling of bone is enhanced as it responds to physical stress. Initially, stress is provided through exercise. Weight-bearing is gradually introduced. New bone is deposited in sites subjected to stress and resorbed at areas where there is little stress. Radiographic union occurs when there is X-ray evidence of complete bony union.

Many factors, such as age, initial displacement of the fracture, site of the fracture and blood supply to the area, influence the time required for fracture. Fracture healing may not occur in the expected time (delayed union) or may not occur at all (nonunion). The ossification process is arrested by causes such as inadequate immobilization and reduction, excess movement, infection and poor nutrition. Healing time for fractions increases with age. For example, an uncomplicate midshaft fracture of the femur heals in 3 weeks in a new born and requires 20 weeks in an adult. Electrical stimulation is used successfully to stimulate bone healing in some situation of nonunion or delayed union. The complication of fracture healing are delayed union, nonunion, malunion, angulation pseudoarthrosis, posttraumatic osteoporosis, refracture and myositis ossificants.

The major factors that impede bone healing are as follows:
- Excess motion of fracture fragments
  Inadequate immobilization resulting in movement of fragments.
- Poor approximation of fracture fragments:
  - Inaccurate reduction or malalignment of fracture fragments.
  - Excessive bone loss at time of fracture, preventing sufficient bridging of broken ends.
  - Excessive fragmentation of bone, allowing soft tissue to be interposed between bone ends.
  - Inability of patient to comply with restrictions imposed by immobilization, fixation device(s) resulting in movement of fragmentation.
- Compromised blood supply:
  - Damage to nutrient vessels.
  - Periosteal or muscular injury.
  - Severe comminution.
  - Avascularity (type of fracture and result of internal fixation device).
- Excessive edema at fracture:
  - Tissue swelling impedes supply of nutrients to area of fracture.
- Bone necrosis:
  - Injury to blood vessels impedes supply of nutrients to involved bone.
- Infection at fracture side:
  - Infection disrupts normal callus formation.

- Metabolic disorders or diseases (cancer, diabetes, malnutrition, immunodeficiencies—Paget's disease):
  - Retard osteogenesis.
- Soft tissue injury:
  - Disruption of blood supply.
- Medication use, (e.g. steroids, anticoagulants):
  - Steroids can cause osteoporosis, avascular necrosis, long-term use of heparin may cause osteoporosis.

Management of Fracture

Diagnosis of fracture is confirmed by X-ray. Other studies may be indicated if multiple injuries have been sustained. The goals of fracture treatment are:
- Anatomic realignment of bone fragments known as reduction.
- Immobilization to maintain realignment, and
- Restoration of functions of the injured part.

Immediate treatment principles implemented at the time of injury include the following:
- Maintain airway and assess signs of shock.
- Splinting the fracture to prevent movement of the fracture fragments, and further injury to the soft tissues by bony fragments. Splinting and immobilization will also decrease pain.
- Preserve correct body alignment.
- Elevate the injured part to decrease edema.
- Apply cold packs (during first 24 hours) to reduce hemorrhage, edema, and pain.
- Observe for changes in color, sensation, circulation, movement, or temperature of injured part.

Secondary management goals include the following.
- For simple fracture:
  - Optimal reduction (replacing bone fragments in their correct anatomical position).
    * Manual manipulation or closed reduction (moving bone fragments into by applying traction and pressure to distal fragment).
    * Traction.
    * Open reduction (Surgical involvement that may incorporate use of internal fixation device).
  - Immobilization.
    * External fixation cast, splint, external fixator device (wires, external frame).
    * Traction.
    * Internal fixation pins, plates, screws, wires and prosthesis.
    * Combination of the above.
- For compound fracture:
  - Surgical debridement and irrigation of wound to remove dust, foreign material, devitalized tissue and necrotic bone.
  - Wound culture.
  - Pack the wound.
  - Observe for signs of osteomyelitis, tetanus, and gangrene.
  - Wound closure when there is no sign of infection.
  - Reduce fracture.
  - Immobilize fracture.
- Use of bone growth stimulators that use low-voltage electrical impulses to enhance healing in cases of nonunion.

Fracture Reduction

- *Closed reduction (manipulation):* Manipulation is a nonsurgical manual realignment of bone fragments to their previous anatomic position. Traction and countertractions are manually applied to the bone fragments to restore position, length and alignment. Closed reduction or manipulations, the injured part is immobilized by traction, casting, external fixation, splints or orthoses (braces) to maintain alignment until healing occurs.
- *Open reductions:* Open reduction is the correction of bone alignment through a surgical incision. It frequently includes internal fixation of the fracture with the use of wire, screws, pins, plates, intramedullary rods or nails. The type and location of the fractures, age of patient and concurrent disease as well as the result of attempted closed reduction by means of traction, may influence the decision to use open reduction. The main disadvantages of this form of treatment are the possibility of infection, and the complications associated with anesthesia. If open reduction with internal fixation (ORIF) is used, for intra-articular fractures involving joint surfaces, early initiations of ROM of the joint is indicated. Machines that provide continuous passive motion (CPM) to various joints are now available, which help so many ways to prevent certain associated problems.

TRACTION

Traction is the mechanism by which a steady pull is exerted on a part or parts of the body. Traction may be used to accomplish the following:
- Reduce a fracture.
- Maintain correct alignment of bone fragments during healing.
- Immobilize a limb while soft tissue healing takes place.
- Overcome muscle spasm.
- Stretch adhesions.
- Correct deformities.

Types of Traction

Two types of traction are used: Skin traction and skeletal traction.
- *Skin traction* is achieved by applying wide bands of moleskin, adhesive or commercially available devices directly to the skin and attaching weights to them.

The pull of the weights is transmitted indirectly to the involved bone or other connective tissues. Skin traction is generally used for short-term treatment (48 to 72 hours) until skeletal traction or surgery is possible. Tape, boots or splints are applied directly to the skin to maintain alignment, assist in reduction and help diminish muscle spasm in the injured part. The traction weight is usually limited to 5 to 10 lbs (2.3 to 4.5 kg). Commonly in skin traction are as follows with nursing implications.

- *Buck's extension* is used for condition affecting hip, femur, knee, or back. It can be unilateral or bilateral may also be used to correct knee and hip joint contracture while taking care of these patients, nurse has to make all assessments at least on 4th hourly. Assess for altered neurovascular status caused by original injury to or the application of the bandages used. Injury in Buck's traction especially note decreased peripheral vascular flow and peroneal nerve deficit by assessing for ability to dorsiflex toes and foot and for changes in sensation in the first website between the great and second toes. Pressure from the elastic wrap may result in pressure necrosis, especially over the boney prominence and areas prone to pressure. (Anterior tibial border, fibular head, both malleoli, achilles tendon, calcaneous, and dorsum of the foot). In addition, assess for an allergic reaction to the adhesive material, rotation of the extremity, and constant traction and countertraction forces.
- *Russel's traction* used for fracture of femur or hip. Nursing implications are as in Buck's. An additional area prone to pressure necrosis in the area over the hamstring tendons in the popliteal space.
- *Bryant's traction* used for fracture of the femur, fracture in small children and immobilization of hip joints in children and 2 years of 30 lb (14) kg in weight. Nurses should be aware that with traction in place, buttocks just clear the mattress. Check for undue pressure over the outer-head and neck of fibula, dorsum of foot. Achilles tenden, scapulae, and shoulders. Check that bandages or boot has not slipped. Be aware that traction are usually removed for skin care and assessment every 4th hourly.
- *Pelvic belt* (or girdle) used for sciatica, muscle spasm (low back), and minor fractions of the lower spine. Nursing implication include:
    - Check for security of the pelvic belt.
    - Check frequently for skin irritation over iliac crests and in the intergluteal fold.
    - Use measures to prevent skin breakdown.
    - Check and adjust pelvic belt straps so that they are unrestricted and equal in length. Secure the straps with adhesive tape.
    - Use a foot board to prevent foot drop.
    - Maintain correct angle of pull of the traction.
    - Be aware that the physician orders the type fo countertraction.
- *Pelvic sling traction* used for pelvic fractures to provide compression for separated pelvic girdle. Here the sling should keep the pelvis just above the surface of bed. Nurses should assess for pressure necrosis and skin irritation every 4th hourly especially pressure over the iliac crests, intergluteal fold and greater trochanter. Monitor for soiling of the sling and change is needed. Use a fracture bedpan for toileting. Limit use of trapese since it will reduce compressive force from the sling. Use alternating air pressure mattress or other pressure dispersing devices and provide frequent back care.
- *Circumferential:* Head halter used for soft tissue disorders and degenerative disk disease of the cervical spine. It is not commonly used for unstable fractures of the cervical spine. Nursing implications include assessment for alignment with trunk, areas of local pressure over the ears, and mandibular joints and under the chin and occipital area and pain or dysfunction in the temperomandibular joint. Patients may be permitted to remove traction for meals, if not provide a liquid or mechanical soft diet to reduce the temperomandibular joint pain. Since this traction is commonly used in the adults ensure patient can demonstrate safe and effective set up, application and use of the traction before discharge.

- *Skeletal traction* is a traction applied directly to bone. It is generally in place for longer period of time is used to align injured bones and joints or to treat joint contractures and congenital hip dysplasia. It provides long-term pull that keeps the injured bones and joints aligned. To establish skeletal traction the physician inserts a pin or wire into the bone, either partially or completely to align and immobilize the injured part. Weight for skeletal traction ranges from 5 to 45 1b (2.3 to 20.4 kg). The commonly used are:
    - *Overhead arm (90°-96°):* Commonly used for immobilization for traction and dislocation of the upper arm and shoulder. Here, be aware that the shoulder and elbow joint are maintained at 90° angles. Assess for pressure necrois beneath the sling, especially over the bony prominences, assesses distal neurovascular status because of the exposure, skin temperature may be indicative of decreased perfusion. Perform assessment 4th hourly. Inspect the pin sites and perform pin site care according to hospital policies.
    Later arm: Commonly used in immobilization of the fracture and dislocation of the upper arm and

shoulder. Here, inspect the pin site and perform skin care according to hospital policy assess neurovascular status.
- *Balanced suspension traction:* Used for injury or fracture of the femoral shaft of the femur, acetabulum, hip, tibia, or any combination of these. In this traction, nurses should be aware that this traction uses half ring Thomas splint (1) and Pearson attachment (2) and then suspension of the extremities and direct skeletal traction are applied. This allows raising of the buttocks off the bed for bedpan use and skin care without altering the line of traction. Use nursing assessment so that counter-traction is maintained (e.g. position patient high in bed so that feet do not press on foot of bed; do not elevate the head of bed more than 25°, if it causes continual movement toward foot of the bed). Encourage self-help in patients' performances of activities of daily living, movement in bed with help of trapeze, and flexion and extension of affected foot to prevent foot drop. Assess for pressure necrosis, in areas contacted by traction, especially greater trochanter, ischial tuberosity, hamstring tendons, fibular head and both malleolus. Assess distal neurovascular status 4th hourly and inspect pin site and give pin site care accordingly.

The signs and symptoms of neurovascular impairment include pallor, cyanosis, prolonged capillary refill, edema, tissue cold or cool to touch. Patient is unable to move part distal to injury. Patient reports severe pain, decreased sensation or paresthesia in part distal to injury and diminished of absent pulses.

The following guidelines will help to take care of person with traction.
- Patient education:
  - Explain traction in relation to fracture and surgeon's plans of treatment.
  - Explain amount of movement permitted and how to achieve it (e.g. how trapeze can be used to assist with movement).
  - Explain correct body positioning. Maintain proper body alignment.
- Maintain continuous traction, unless indicated otherwise:
  - Inspect traction apparatus frequently to ensure that ropes are running straight and through the middle of the pulleys; that weights are hanging free that bed clothes, the bed or the frame and bars on the bed are not impinging on any part of the traction apparatus.
  - Check ropes frequently to be sure, they are not frayed.
  - Avoid releasing weights or altering the line of pull of the traction.
  - Avoid adding weight to the traction.
  - Check the position of the Thomas splint frequently; if the ring slides away from the groin, read just the splint to its proper position without releasing traction.
  - Avoid bumping into or jarring the bed or traction equipment.
  - Be sure weights are securely fastened to their ropes.
  - Avoid manipulation of pins.
- Maintain countertractions.
- Skin care:
  - Encourage the patient to turn slightly from side-to-side and to lift up on the trapeze to relieve pressure on the skin of the sacrum and scapulae, have the patient lift up for routine skin care to prevent friction and shearing forces.
  - Avoid padding the ring of the Thomas splint, because this will create dampness next to the skin. Bathe the skin beneath the ring, dry it thoroughly and powder the skin lightly.
  - Inspect the skin frequently to be sure it is not being rubbed, contused, or macerated by traction equipment, readjust splints or the extremity in the splint to free the skin from pressure.
  - Keep the skin areas aound pin sites clean and dry; direct care to pin sites (e.g. cleansing with cotton applicators and hydrogen peroxide, povidone iodine, or alcohol) is controversial check with the surgeon regarding method of pin site care.
- Toileting:
  - Use a fracture pan with blanket roll or padding as support under the small of the back.
  - Protect the ring of the Thomas splint with water proof material when female patients are using the bed pan.

FRACTURE IMMOBILIZATION

External fixation of fracture is achieved by a cast or an external fixator.

Casts

The most common external fixation device is the cast. Casting is a common treatment often closed reductions has been performed. It allows the patient to perform many normal activities of daily living. While providing sufficient immobilization to ensure stability. Major cast materials include fiberglass, plaster of paris, polyurethane, thermoplastic resins and thermolabile plastic.
- Plaster of paris, after immersion in water, is wrapped and moulded around the affected part. It is anhydrous calcium sulphate embedded in gauze roll. The strength of the cast is determined by the number of layers of plaster bandage and the technique of application. As the cast dries, it recrystalises and hardens. Heat

is generated during the drying process. Increased edema as a result of the increased circulation may occur as a result of heat produced by the drying cast. After the cast is completely dry, it is strong and firm and can withstand stresses. The plaster is hard within 15 minutes, so the patient can move around without problems. However, it is not strong enough for weight bearing until it is dry (after about 24 to 48 hours).

Thermolabile plastic (orthoplast) and thermoplastic resin (Hexcelite) are moulded to fit the torso extremities after being heated in warm water. Polyurethane, which is formed for polyester and cotton fabric impregnated with a chemical in water activated by immersing in cool water to start chemical process. Casts made by this fiber glass tape are frequently used because they are light weight and relatively waterproof and support earlier mobilization. They are appropriate in cases in which severe edema is not present or when multiple cast changes are not anticipated.

An external fixator is a metallic device composed of metal pins that are inserted into the bone and attached to external rods to stabilize the fracture while it heals. It can be used to apply traction or to compress fracture fragments and to immobilize reduced when the use of a cast or other traction is not appropriate. The external device holds fragments of fractures in place much like surgically implanted internal devices. External fixator devices also used as a part of limb-lengthening process, when indicated. Examples of external fixators include Mini Hoffman's system in use on hand and Hoffman II on the tible (standard system). The other devices for external immobilization and fractures include:
- Braces made of rigid plastic material.
- Plaster or plastic braces that incorporate metal struts attached to pins inserted into bone, such as a helo brace.

The nursing care of the person with a cast will include:
- Patient education
  - Before cast application, explain why and how the cast will be applied.
  - Advise the patient that the plaster cast will feel warm as it dries.
  - Explain the extent to which the patient will be immobilized.
  - Following cast application, explain care of the cast and expectations after discharge.
  - Instruct patient not to insert sharp objects (coat hangers or pencils) under the cast because they may abrade the skin and lead to infection.
  - Cast removal, explain using saw for removal is noisy; saw will not harm skin.
- Handling the new cast
  - Support wet cast with the flat of the hands or on pillows to avoid indentations that will cause pressure on underlying skin.
  - Place cotton blankets or other absorbent material under the cast to aid the drying process.
  - Turn the patient frequently to aid the drying process.
  - Use a fan to circulate air over the cast.
  - Do not apply paint varnish, or shellac to the cast; plaster is porous material that allows air to circulate the skin.
- Skin care
  - Inspect skin at edges of cast and underlying cast for redness or irritation; apply petal-shaped strips of adhesive type or moleskin around rough edges of cast.
  - Remove plaster crumbs from skin with a wash cloth moistered with warm water.
  - Use cream and lotion sparingly, because they may soften the skin and cause the cast to stick to the skin.
  - Apply waterproof material around perineal area to prevent skin irritation and soiling of and damage to cast.
  - Attend to patients report of pain under the cast, particularly over bony prominences, because this may indicate pressure on the skin. If discomfort is not relieved by repositioning, report to physician. Cast pressure may need to be relieved by windowing or bivalving (cutting cast into two halves).
  - Following cast removal, skin care to remove built up exudate to secretions and dead skin. Mineral oil and warm water soaks are helpful.
- Turning
  - Turning to any position is generally permitted, as long as the integrity of the cast is not compromised and the patient is comfortable.
- Toileting (For a long leg or hip spica cast)
  - Use a fracture pan with blanket role or padding as support under the small of the back.
  - Elevate the head of the bed if permitted, or place the bed in reverse Trendenburg position.
- Abdominal discomfort
  - Spice cast may be "windowed" (cut an opening into cast) to provide relief of abdominal distention or as a port for checking bladder distention.
- Mobilization
  - Weight bearing is at the discretion of the surgeon/physician who will prescribe specific limitations.
  - A cast shoe or a walking heel incorporated into a lower extremity cast will permit weight-bearing without damaging the cast.
- Prevention of neurovascular problems
  - Perform neurovascular checks every hour for at least 24 hours after cast application to detect difficulty from swelling or pressure of cast on nerves or vessels. Notify physician of color changes, alterations sensation, or motion unrelieved by

position change, cast may need to be bivalved to relieve pressure.
- Elevate affected extremity on pillows until danger of swelling is over (usually 24 to 48 hours).
- After mobilization of patient with lower-extremity or upper-extremity cast, avoid keeping extremity in dependant position for prolonged periods.
- After lower extremity cast is removed, encourage patient to wear elastic stocking and elevate affected leg at rest until full mobility is regained.

INTERNAL FIXATION

Internal fixation devices are surgically inserted at the time of realignment. Internal fixation is carried out under the most vigorous aseptic conditions, and patients may receive a course of perioporative prophylactic intravenous antibiotics. Example of internal fixation devices include pins, plates and screws. They are biologically inert metal devices such as stainless steel, vitallium or titanium that are used to realign and maintain bony fragments. Proper alignment is evaluated by X-ray studies at regular intervals. A variety of internal fixation devices are also available include:
- Plates and nails.
- Intramedullary rods (ex-Kuntsher nail-Old shaft femur fracture) and Neufeld nail and screw for intrastrachenter fracture).
- Transfixation screws (e.g. Richard's intramedullary hipscrew, for femur. Richard's compression crew and plate for hip frature).
- Prosthetic implants-used particularly fracture is jeopardized, for example fracture through or immediately below the femoral head (e.g. Bipolar modular prosthasis for femurs, and bipolar (left) and unipolar (right) hip prosthesis for hip fracture).

The nursing care of the person with an internal fixation device are as follows:
- Patient Education
  - Prepare the patient for anesthesia.
  - Explain the surgical procedure and general nursing care after surgery.
  - Postoperatively, explain the limits of motion and weight bearing to the affected parts.
- Promoting Mobility:
  - Determine in consultation with the physician, the limits of motion and weight bearing is permitted.
  - Instruct and assist the patients to turn, transfer and ambulate within the prescribed limits (mobilization may begin as early as the day of surgery).
  - Instruct and assist the patients to use an appropriate ambulatory aid if the fracture is of a lower extremity.
- Prevention of Neurovascular Problems:
  - Perform neurovascular checks every hour for the first 24 to 48 hours, notify the physician if any change from preoperative status, because this may indicate pressure from swelling, constricting bandages, or damage to nerves or vessels as surgery.
  - Keep affected extremity elevated.
- Maintenance of immobilization of fracture; considerations for care would be the same as for patients in cast/traction if those devices are used.

Patients with fractures often experience varying degrees of pain associated with muscle spasms. These spasms are caused by involuntary reflexes that result from edema following muscle injury. Muscle relaxants may be prescribed for relief of pain associated with muscle spasm. Common side effects associated with muscle relaxants are drowsiness, lassitude, headache, weakness, fatigue, blurred vision, ataxia, and GI upsets. Reaction includes irritation, rashes, heavy does cause hypotension, tachycardia, and respiratory depression. The nurse has to monitor the same day care.

Proper nutrition is essential component of the reparative process in injured tissue. An adequate energy source is needed to promote muscle strength and tone, build endurance, and enhance ambulation and gait training skills. A diet high in protein and with sufficient calories is necessary to promote bone and tissue healing. Vitamins (D, B & C) and calcium ensure optimal bladder and bowel function. Adequate fluid and high fiber diet with fruits and vegetable will prevent constitipation.

MANAGEMENT OF COMPLICATIONS OF FRACTURE

The majority of fractures heal without complications. If death occurs after a fracture, it is usually the result of damage to underlying organs and soft tissue or from complications of the fracture or immobility complication include problems with bone union, avascular necrosis and bone infections. Indirect complications of fractures associated with blood vessel and nerve damage resulting in conditions such as compartment syndrome, venous thrombosis, fat embolism, and traumatic or hydrovolium, fatembolism and traumatic or hypovolumic shock. Although most musculoskeletal injuries are not life-threatening, open fractures or fracture accompanied by severe blood loss and fractures that damage vital organs (such as the lung and bladder) are medical emergencies requiring immediate attention).

Proper nursing interventions help to prevent complication in appropriate management of fracture are as follows:

Preventing Trauma and Injury/ Promoting Self-care

As health progresses and pain diminishes, patient should be advised to follow the following instructions for preventing trauma and injury and promoting self-care:

- How to move comfortably in bed.
- Safe transfer technique.
- Duration and extent of weight-bearing restriction.
- Type of activity restrictions.
- Proper use of ambulatory or other ADL assistive devices.
- Use and care of immobilization devices (slings, casts, pins)
- Proper positioning of the affected extremity.
- Pain and discomfort relief measures.
- Exercises to maintain strength and enhance circulation.

Maintaining Strength and Mobility/ Promoting Activity

The nurse can use the following intervention to assist the patient to maintain mobility, muscle tone and strength.
- Allow and encourage the patient to move about to the greater extent possible within the restrictions of the fracture reduction and the immobilizing devices.
- Allow and encourage the patient to accomplish as much self-care as possible.
- Encourage the patient to perform muscle toning (isometric) exercises on a regular basis. For example, quadriceps, sitting and glutal sitting.
- Encourage and assist the patient to follow through with exercise program (including ambulation) prescribed by the physician and taught by the physiotherapist and nurse).
- Encourage and assist patient to resume normal functioning of all ADL within limits of immobilization or fixation device) as soon as possible for example using bedside commode or toilet instead of bedpan.

Promoting Comforts

The person with a fracture will often have severe pain in the fracture site, pressure from edema and damage of soft tissues adjacent to the fracture and spasm of the muscles in the fracture area. Measures the nurse can take to help reduce pain include the following:
- During initial stages of treatment, administer prescribed narcotic and non-narcotic analgesics in appropriate doses at timely intervals.
- Instruct the patient about principles of pain management and use of patient-controlled analgesia, if prescribed.
- Administer prescribed agents such as diazepam to reduce muscle spasm.
- Apply ice compress, as ordered to the affected part to reduce swelling and decrease pain.
- Reposition patient frequently with prescribed position or activity limitation to avoid prolonged pressure over bony prominences and to prevent stiffness.
- Instruct patient how to use relaxation techniques (deep-breathing, imagery).
- As pain subsides, negotiate with the patient a reduction in the strength or frequency of analgesic administration.

In addition, positioning is a measure that promotes comfort, provides for adequate ventilation and mobilization of pulmonary secretions, enhance circulation, and relieves pressure on vulnerable skin areas. Before positioning, the nurse should know the location and type of traction, reduction technique, and special activity or positioning restriction according to type of traction, cast, fixation as described earlier.

Maintaining Intact Neurovascular Status and Tissue Perfusion

To maintain an intact neurovascular status and tissue perfusion the nurse has to monitor the neurovascular status of the injured part includes:
- Palpating for warmth.
- Observing color.
- Assessing length of capillary-filling time.
- Questioning patient about pain and paresthesias in injured part.
- Assessing patient's ability to discriminate sensation.
- Observing patient's ability to voluntarily move body part distal to fracture.
- Institute measures to promote venous blood flow:
  - Elevate extremities to level slightly above the heart.
  - Apply elastic stockings or intermittent pneumatic copression devices.
  - Use proper positioning techniques.
  - Avoid external compression on pressure sites.
  - Encourage ROM and isometric exercises.
- Assessing for presence of positive Homan's sign (although not always released).
- Encourage ambulation if possible.
- Obtaining baseline and ongoing measurements of circumferences of both calves for compression.

Preventing Infection

Nursing intervention to promote wound healing include:
- Carefully attending to aseptic technique during dressing changes to prevent infections; assessing wound for signs of healing or presence of infection.
- Monitoring drains for correct placement.
- Assessing pin sites regularly: Perform pin site care as specified to prevent infection.
- Providing and encouraging patient to eat a well-balanced diet to provide the nutritional elements necessary for tissue healing.
- Assessing patient for any systemic signs of infection.
- Monitoring laboratory data (e.g. WBCs, C and S, ESR).
- Assessing patient for therapeutic response to antibiotics if prescribed.

Maintaining Skin Integrity

To prevent skin breakdown, and to promote wound healing, nurse has to take measures to maintain skin integrity which includes:

- Identifying skin areas at risk, particularly areas over bony prominence. For example, heels, sacrum, elbows, scapulae, ischial tuberosities.
- Inspecting the skin (at least every 8 hrly) for signs of pressure (erythema or induration, nonblandible areas).
- Turning at least every 2 hours, while maintaining fracture immobilization using a turning sheet.
- Moving patient from one surface to another with a pull sheet or roller board.
- Rolling patient on to side or lifting patient to place him or her on bedpan rather than sliding pan under the patients.
- For patient who cannot be fully turned because of traction apparatus or other limiting factor, possibly using one or more of the following pressure-relieving devices:
  - Sheep skin pads
  - Flotation pads.
  - Alternating air pressure mattress or alternating air pressure system.
  - Foam mattress.
  - Foam heal or elbow pads.
  - Special bed such as the clinitron, mediscus, or bidyne.
  - Turning frames such as the Foster or Stry Ker frames.
- Regularly inspecting the skin areas in contact with cast edges or traction apparatus and taking appropriate measure to eliminate chafing or rubbing these areas.
- Assisting patient to keep skin clean and dry, especially under casts, slings and traction apparatus.

Promoting Nutrition/Stabilizing Weights

The essentials of nutritions diet including fruits, vegetables, proteins and vitamins are especially important for the persons after a fracture. Nursing intervention to ensure adequate nutrition of the patient include:

- Encourage the patient to eat regular meals.
- Allow the patient adequate time to eat.
- Encourage self-feeding but help the patient whenever needed.
- Attend to patient's need for roughage and fluids and protein.
- Position the patient to facilitate comfortable intake of food and fluids.

Promoting Autonomy and Sense of Control

To promote autonomy the following actions will be helpful:
- Assess and incorporate patient's locus of control (internal or external) into plan of care.
- Explain course of treatment to patient and family.
- Provide opportunities for decision making.
- Incorporate patient preferences into daily plan of care.
- Allow the patient to manipulate the environment wherever needed.
- Involve family and significant others in patient's care.
- Assist patient to set realistic goals.

INFLAMMATORY AND DEGENERATIVE DISORDER—MUSCULOSKELETAL SYSTEM

Rheumatoid Arthritis (RA)

Arthritis, an inflammation of the joint is a common disorder of the musculoskeletal system that causes pain and stiffness in the joint. Rheumatoid arthritis (RA) is a chronic, systemic disease characterized by recurrent inflammation of the diarthrodial joints and related structures and surrounding tissues. The disease process is characterized by recurrent inflammations of the connective tissue throughout the body. Systemic manifestation includes pulmonary, cardiac, vascular, ophthalmological, dermatological, and hematological involvement, showing extra-articular manifestation such as rheumatoid nodules, arteritis neuropathy, scleritis, paricarditis, lymphadenopathy and splenomegaly.

Etiology

The cause of rheumatoid arthritis is unknown. Whether a single causative factor is responsible or multiple factors are involved, several theories have been postulated regarding its pathogenicity.

- *Infection:* Studies continue to probe the possibility of specific infections pathogens, such as Epstein-Barr virus, Par-vovirus and mycobacteria, which may trigger the process.
- *Auto-immunity:* Although no virus particles have been identified, it is likely that an antigenic stimulus such as a virus leads to the formation of an abnormal immunoglobulin G (IgG). RA is characterised by the presence of autobodies against this abnormal IgG. The antibodies to this altered IgG termed as "Rheumatoid Factors" and they combine with IgG to form immune complexes that deposits in the joints, blood vessels and pluera. Complement is activated and an inflammatory response occurs.

The articulations of the cervical spine are also affected.
- *Genetic factors:* A genetic predisposition has also been identified related to certain human leukocyte antigen (HLA) known as the HLA-DR4.
- *Other factors:* Metabolic and biochemical abnormalities, nutritional and environmental factors and occupational and psychosocial influences may play a part in the cause or expression of the disease but their contribution is entirely speculative. RA occurs in young and middle-aged females more often than male.

Pathophysiology

The disease progresses through four stages which include:
- *First State:* The unknown etiologic factor initiates joints imflammation synovitis, with swelling of the synovial lining membrane and production of excess synovial fluid.
- *Second Stage:* Pannel (Inflammatory granular tissue) is formed at the juncture of the synovium and cartilage. This extends over the surface of the articular cartilage and eventually invades the joint capsule and subchondria bone.
- *Third Stage:* Tough fibrous connective tissue replaces pannus, occluding the joint space. Fibrous ankylosis results in decreased joint motion malalignment and deformity.
- *Fourth Stage:* As fibrous tissue calcifies, bony ankylosis may result in total joint immobilization.

Actually disease begins in the synovial membrane within the joint, edema, vascular congestion, fibrin exudate, and cellular infiltrate occur as a result of the inflammatory process. Joint changes are characterized by chronic inflammation with the presence of inflammatory cells and mediators. The infiltrating macrophages are activated and released a variety of cytokines, including interlukin-1 and interlukin-6, tumor necrosis factor (TNF), and colony-stimulating factor. The activity of these cytokines accounts for many of the features of rheumatoid synovity including synovial tissue inflammation, synovial proliferation, cartilage and bone damage and systemic manifestation of rheumatoid arthritis.

Normally synovial tissue secretes synovial fluid that both lubricate the joint and is the medium through which nutrients are supplied to the articular cartilage. Inflammation causes edema, vascular congestion, fibrins exudate and cellular infiltrate to build up around synovium. WBCs move into the synovium, releasing superoxide radicals, H_2O_2, prostaglanding Leukopneou, and callagenases, which manifest synovium thickens particularly at articular junctions. Symptoms of inflammations occur within and overlying the joint (pain, swelling, erythema, warmth). Joint mobility is limited by pain.

Generally articular cartilage covers the ends of articulating bones to provide a smooth surface for movement. When pannus forms at junctions of synovial tissue and articular cartilage, covers the ends of articulating bones to provide a smooth surface for movement. When pannus forms at junctions of synovial tissue and articular cartilage, interfering with nutrition cartilage. Articular cartilage becomes necrotic. Pannus invades subchondrial bone and supporting soft tissue structure (ligaments, tendon destroying them. This leads to joint pain increases at rest and with movement. Destruction of soft tissue structure (ligaments tenden) causes joint to sublux or dislocate. Depending on the amount of articular cartilage destroyed adhesions can develop and the joints can fuse, prohibiting joint motion.

Clinical Manifestations

Rheumatoid arthritis typically develops insidiously. Non-specific manifestations such as fatigue, anorexia, weight loss, fever, malaise, morning stiffness. Pain at rest and with movement, night pain, edematous, erythematous, "boggy" joint. The stiffness becomes more localized after weeks to months. Some patients report a history of precipitating stressful event such as infection, work stress, physical exertion, childbirth, surgery, or emotional upset.

Specific articular involvement is manifested clinically by pain, stiffness, limitation of motion, and signs of inflammation (heat, swelling and tenderness). Joint symptoms are generally, bilaterally symmetric and frequently affect small joints of the hands (proximal interphalangeal) and feet (metatarsophalangeal) as well as larger peripheral joints, including wrists, elbows, shoulders, knees, hips, ankles and jaw. The cervical spine may be affected but axial spine is generally spared. The patient characteristically has joint stiffness on arising in the morning and after periods of inactivity. This morning stiffness may last for 30 minutes to several hours or more depending on disease activity.

Later symptoms of rheumatoid arthritis include:
- Pallor.
- Anemia.
- Color changes of digits (bluish, rubor, pallor).
- Muscle weakness, atrophy.
- Joint deformities.
- Paresthesias.
- Decreased joint mobility.
- Contractures (usually flexion).
- Subluxation.
- Dislocation.
- Increasing pain.

Rheumatoid arthritis may also affect other body systems and rheumatoid nodules takes form in the heart, lungs spleen. The systemic manifestations of RA are as follows:
- **Cardiovascular:** Pericarditis, valvular lesions, myocarditis, vasculitis, Raynaud's phenomenon.
- **Pulmonary:** Pleurisy; rheumatoid nodules in lungs, pneumoconiosis, (Caplan syndrome), interstitial pneumonitis, pulmonary fibrosis, pulmonary hypertension.
- **Neurological:** Compression neuropathy, peripheral neuropathy, cervical myelopathy.
- **Hematological:** Anemia, leukopenia (Felty's syndrome) when accompanied by hepatosplenomegaly).
- **Renal:** Rheumatoid nodules in kidneys.
- **Dermatological:** Rheumatoid nodules, brown lesions, on skin, due to ischemia, ulcers and draining fistulae.

- **Ophthalmological:** Scleritis, Sicca syndrome (Keratoconjunctivitis) Sjögren's syndrome (Keratoconjunctivitis, xerostomia, dryness), glaucoma, scleromalacia.
- **Others:** Fever, malaise and weakness.

Management

Several findings are helpful in diagnosing rheumatoid arthritis in conjunctions with the history and physical examination. The diagnostic criteria for RA includes:
- Morning stiffness: 1 hour and at least 6 weeks duration.
- Symmetric joint swelling.
- Swelling of wrist metacarpophalangeal (MCP) and proximal intraphalangeal (PIP) joints.
- Rheumatoid nodules.
- Positive serum rheumatoid factor test.

According to American Rheumatoid Association, the following presence of four of the seven/nine criteria in nursing for diagnosis of RA, i.e. the diagnostic tests result usually include:
- An elevated erythrocyte sedimentation rate (ESR).
- Positive creactive protein test during acute phases.
- Positive antinuclear antibody test.
- Mild leucocytosis.
- Anemia (hypochromic, nomocytic).
- Positive rheumatoid factor or latex fixation test.
- Narrowing of the joint spaces and erosion of articular surfaces on roentgenographic examination, subluxation and dislocation.
- Inflammatory charges in synovial tissue obtained by biopsy.
- Increased turbidity and decreased viscosity of synovial fluid obtained by arthrocentesis, immune complexes and WBCs present.

Care of the patient with RA begins with a comprehensive program of drug therapy and education. Physical comfort is promoted by NSAIDs and rest. The patient and family are educated about the disease process and have management strategies. Compliance with medications, includes correct administration, reporting of side effects and lab follow up visits. Physical therapy maintains joint motion and muscle strength. Occupational therapy develops upper extremity function and encourages joint inspection through the use of splinting packing techniques and assistive devices.

The purpose of drug therapy is to control inflammation and prevent bone erosion. The common medications used for RA are as follows:
- NSAIDS, Salicylate modify inflammatory process by inhibiting prostaglandin synthetase, analgesics and antipyrotic. For example, Diclofenac, Diflunisal, Etodolac, Fenoprofen, Ibuprofen, Indomethacin. Maproxen, oxaprozin, prioxicam, sulinlac Jolmetin, Diclofenac sodium and misopros are reduces risk of gastric ulcers. In this measure, nurse has to monitor patient for dyspepsia, gastritis, hemorrhage, renal and hepatic function, platelet dysfunction, headache, confusion, (tinnitus with salicylate). Administer with food (check individual drug, food may interfere with absorption). Avoid constant use of salicylates and NSAIDs.
- Corticosteroids are anti-inflammatory, e.g. Prednisone (oral), Hydrocortisone (intra-articular). Patients are advised to take the drug (oral with food or milk; do not abruptly discontinue medication, monitor patient for fluid and electrolytes balance, glucose levels, hypertension, skin lesions (purpura); decreased healing potential, cataract formation; encourage adequate calcium and vitamin D intake to retard osteoporosis; teach patient to avoid sources of infection. The systemic effects are rate with intra-articular use; avoid more than three injections per joint per year.
- DMARD (Disease-modifying anti-rheumatic Drugs) (Table 11.1):
    - Methotrexate (oral or IM) 3 hours
    - Rhematrex.

    Rapid onset of action inhibits degradation of folic acid, which inhibits DNA synthesis of inflammatory cell. In this, before starting therapy renal function should be evaluated. Then monitor patient for hepatic and pulmonary toxicity, leukopenia, anemia, explain to patient that nausea, diarrhoea and stomatitis are common. Advise patient to use birth control while taking medication; check for drug interactions that may increase toxicity risk.
- Hydroxychloroquine (Naqenil); mechanism of this is unclear; acts on DNA synthesis, anti-inflammation. In this, inform patient of need for eye examination before therapy and every 6 months thereafter (Retinal edema may result in blindness); monitor patient for hematological toxicity, gastrointestinal irritation, and hypertension, evaluate renal function.
- Sulfagalazine (Azylfidine) - action is unknown. But anti-inflammatory. Here monitor patient for neurological and gastrointestinal toxicity. Leukopenia, anemia and Stevens-Johnson syndrome; educate patient about need for CBC and liver function test throughout therapy.
- Gold salts (Myochrysine, Ridaura, Joganal). It may be given oral or IM anti-inflammatory mechanism of these drugs is unclear, effect not noted until several months of therapy. Here nurse monitors patient's renal and hepatic damage, dramatitis and mouth ulcerations. Inform patient of need for CBC and urinalysis before and at intervals throughout therapy, stress the need for oral hygiene, therapy, may cause metallic taste in mouth. Oral gold has fewer side effects.
- Azathioprine (Smuran): Action is unknown. It is immune suppressant. In the nursing intervention include monitor patient for blood dyscrasiasis,

Table 11.1: The clinical pharmacology of DMARDS (disease modifying anti-rheumatic drugs).

Drug	Dosage	Adverse effects	Monitoring
A. Monotherapy			
Hydroxychloroquine	200 mg bid for 3 months, then OD	GI symptoms, retinopathy, pruritus paraesthesias, hyperpigmentation, motor neuropathy	Fundus and visual field testing after every 6 months
Sulfasalazine	2–3 g daily (0.5 g bid initially, then increased)	Cytopenias, photosensitivity. Raised transaminases; haemolysis in G6PD deficiency	TLC, DLC and LFT
Methotrexate	7.5–20 mg/week (orally, IM or IV)	GI symptoms, cytopenias, raised transaminases, alopecia, oral ulcers, infections, pneumonias	Blood count, LFT, serum creatinine and serum albumin. Administer folic or folinic acid to reduce side-effects
Leflunomide	100 mg OD × 3 days then 20 mg OD orally	Diarrhoea, alopecia, rash, weight loss, hepatotoxicity, teratogenicity	• Blood count and LFT • Contraindicated during pregnancy
Cyclosporine	2.5–5 mg/kg/day orally	Hair loss, hypertrophy of gums, renal and hepatic dysfunction	TLC, DLC, LFT, creatinine, urine examination initially weekly, then monthly
Gold (sodium aurothiomalate)	10 mg IM stat, 25 mg next week, then 50 mg/week; frequency reduced after 1 g total dose	Stomatitis, colitis, neuropathy, metallic taste, rashes, photosensitivity, pruritus, proteinuria, cytopenias, jaundice	TLC, DLC and urine protein before each injection for 1 month and then before every 4th injection
D-penicillamine	250–1000 mg/day orally on empty stomach	Stomatitis, loss of taste, rashes, photosensitivity, pruritus, proteinuria, cytopenias	TLC, DLC, urine for proteinuria after every 2 weeks for 2 months, then every 2–3 months
Azathioprine	50–150 mg/day (2.5 mg/kg)	GI symptoms, cytopenias, infection, pancreatitis, malignancy	TLC, DLC after every 2 weeks for 2 months, then after every 2 months, then after every 2 months. LFT after every 2 months.
Anakinra	100 mg × 1 daily SC	Headache, infections, neutropenia	Initial, than monthly
TNF-α blockers • Etanercept • Infliximab • Adalimumab	25 mg SC twice a week or 50 mg/week 3–10 mg/kg/IV initially repeated after 2, 6, 10 and 14 weeks 40 mg SC every other week	Infections, e.g. tuberculosis septicaemia and hypersensitivity reactions	Stop the drug, if no response after three months

B. Polytherapy for severe disease, methotrexate is combined with hydroxycholoroquine or sulfasalazine or cyclosporine (the inverted pyramid approach) initially, reducing the number of agents once remission has been achieved.

hepatitis and pancreatitis. CBC necessary as baseline and throughout course of treatment.
- *D-Penicillamine* (Depon, Cuprimine), action is unknown. In this treatment nurse monitors patients for fever, rash, GI upset, blood dyscrasiasis, and delayed wound healing; assess for penicillin allergy; Inform patient of potential for dysgeusia (taste alteration). For interferes with absorption. Rare side effects include polymyositis and Good pasture's syndrome. Urinalysis and CBC counts are needed.
- *Antineoplastics* (Cyclophosphamide-Cytotoxin) suppresses synovitis; retards bony erosions. Here monitor patient for toxic effects including GI distress, bone marrow suppression, alopecia and hemorrhagic cystitis. Inform patients of need for monitoring CBC and urin analysis during therapy; teach patients to increase fluid intake to ensure frequent bladder emptying.

The goal of therapy for persons with RA to relieve symptoms prevent joint destruction, maintain joint functions, and promote independence, and quality of life. In addition to medication, occupation therapy and physical therapy are mainstays of treatment to preserve joint mobility and promote independence, which splints and orthoses (braces) are prescribed by the physician. The purposes of splints and braces are as follows:
- Stabilize or support the joints.
- Protect a joint or body part from external trauma.
- Mechanically correct dysfunction such as foot drop by supporting the joint in its functional position.
- Assists patients to exercise specific joints.

Splints and braces are designed to be as light weight and cosmetically acceptable as possible. The type and function of splints and braces include.

- **Spring-loaded braces:** Oppose the action of unparalyzed muscles and act as partial functional substitue for paralyzed muscles.
- **Resting-splints:** Maintain a limb or joint in a functional position while permitting the muscles around the joint to relax.
- **Functional splints:** Maintain the joint or limb in a usable position to enable the body part to be used correctly.
- **Dynamic splints:** Permit assisted exercises to joints, particularly following surgery of finger joints.

Many assistive devices are available for persons who have impaired upper and/or lower extremity function, which include:
- Utensil with built-up handle
- Utensil with cuffed handle
- Combination knife-fork
- Mug with special handle.
- Long-handled shoe horn.
- Long-handled reacher.
- Stocking guide.

In addition supportive devices or ambulatory aids (walkers, canes and crutches) are usually recommended for persons who cannot bear weight on one or more joints of the lower extremities. Nurses are expected to supervise patient in their use of these devices and encourage patients to use their walking aids correctly.

Other treatment modalities for person with RA include the application of hot and cold packs at the affected joints. It can be achieved by the following:
- Hydrocollator packs (packs containing chemical filter that expands in water and retains heat; may be heated in pot of water or special machines that maintain a constant temperature of 80°C (174°F).
- Paraffin baths.
- Electric heating pads that are approved for use with moist towels.
- Electric heating pads that produce moisture.
- Warm soaks, tub soaks or showers.

The application of cold or ice packs helpful in reducing or preventing swelling (especially after injury) reducing pain, and relieving stiffness.

When conservative therapies are ineffective, surgery is indicated for correction of deformity, relief of pain or restoration of function. The objectives of surgical itervention are as follows:
- Restoration or maintenance of a body part.
- Prevention of deformity.
- Correction of deformity if not already exists.
- Development of the patient's powers of compensation and adaptation of loss of function or permanent deformity is not preventable.

Prior to surgery, the orthopedician considers the procedure best suited to achieve the desired objective for individual clients.

The commonly performed surgical procedures are as follows:
- *Arthroscopy*—Is endoscopic examination of joint, indicated for diagnosis, synovectomy, chondroplasty, removal of bone spurs, osteophytes, and joint mice.
- *Arthrotomy*—Opening of a joint indicated for exploration of joint-drainage of joint and removal of damaged tissue.
- *Arthroplasty*—Reconstruction of a joint, indicated for restore motion, relieve pain, correct deformity and avascular necrosis.
  - *Interposition*—Replacement of part of a joint with a prosthesis or with soft tissue.
  - *Hemiarthroplasty*—Replacement of one articulating surface.
  - *Replacement (total joint)*—Replacement of both articulating surfaces of a joint with prosthetic implants.
- *Synovectomy*—Removal of part or all of the synovial membrane, indicated when delay the progress of RA.
- *Osteotomy*—Cutting a bone to change its alignment indicated in correct deformity (varus or valgus) alters the weight-bearing surface of diseased joint to relieve pain.
- *Arthodesis*—Surgical fusion of a joint by removal of articular hyaline cartilage, introduction of bone grafts, and stabilization with internal or external friction devices. Indicated for stabilizing a joint and relieve pain.
- *Tendon transplants*—Moving tendon from its anatomical position, indicated for substitute one tendon for another that is not working or realign tendon function for example for stability.

In addition to the above, diet, rest, exercises are important in treatment of RA.

Diet: There is no special diet for RA. However, balanced nutrition is important. There is evidence to suggest that ingestion of fish oil (a type of n-3 polyunsaturated fat) as dietary fat is beneficial to persons with RA. A diet containing adequate calories and balanced nutrition is necessary to prevent fatigue and increase energy. If the patient is overweight, a weight reduction diet, combined with exercises, is recommended to decrease the strain on weight-bearing joints.

Rest is a therapy often used with RA. There are two forms of rest viz. Absolute rest or no activity and potential rest of limited activity. This should be decided on the basis of part affected, devices used and so on.

Exercises are advised to accomplish the following:
- Preserve joint mobility (active and passive ROM).
- Maintain muscles tone (active ROM and isometrics).
- Strengthen selected muscle groups (Resistive exercises performed against resistance provided by another person or by weights).

Exercises may be facilitated by the application of heat or cold or the administration of analgesics before exercise period. Exercises are contraindicated in the presence of acute joint or muscle inflammation until it subsides. Exercises may be tailored to the patient's specific needs and capabilities.

Patient and Family Education

As for any chronic illness, patient teaching is perhaps the most important aspect of nursing care and the patient with rheumatoid arthritis. Patient teaching should include the following information:

- Proper balance of rest and activity, assisting the patient in determining his/her activity tolerance.
- Joint protection and energy conservation techniques.
- Proper use of medication (i.e. names of drugs dosages, precautions in administration and side effects or toxic effects).
- Plans for implementation of the exercise program prescribed by the physician and physical therapist.
- Proper application of heat and/or cold packs.
- Proper use of walking aids and other assistive devices.
- Safety measures to prevent injury.
- Application, appropriate use and care of splints and braces.
    - Inspect patient's skin after the orthosis has been applied for short time, to be certain it has caused no skin irritation.
    - Notify orthotist if adjustment needs to be made in orthosis to make it more comfortable or to relieve chafing.
    - Instruct patient in the proper application and care of the orthosis:
        * Metal braces should be stored upright.
        * Leather materials should be treated occasionally with meets foot compound or other leather preservative to prevent cracking and drying.
        * Orthoses fabricated of moulded material should be stored away from sources of heat.
        * If patients fitted with moulded orthoses are braces gain or lose weight, the brace may have to be adjusted or replaced.
    - Assist patient to make the psychological adjustment to wearing the orthoses.
- Basics of good nutrition and the importance of avoiding weight gain.
- Importance of regular following with physician.
- Risks of following programs that promises "cure".
- Joint protection and energy conservative is advised through:
    - Maintaining good posture and proper body mechanism.
    - Maintain normal weight.
    - Use assistive devices if indicated.
    - Avoid positions of deviation and stress.
    - Find less stressful ways to perform tasks.
    - Avoid task that causes pain.
    - Develop organising and pacing techniques.
    - Avoid forceful repetitive movements.

Osteoarthritis (OA)

Osteoarthritis also known as degenerative joint disease (DJD) is a slowly progressive disorder of articulating joints, particularly weight-bearing joints, and is characterized by degeneration of articular cartilage. The damage from osteoarthritis is compared to the joints and surrounding tissues.

Etiology

Osteoarthritis (OA) may occur as a primary OA is unknown. After both primary and secondary OA are influenced by multiple factors (i.e. metabolic mechanical, genetic and chemical). Secondary OA has an identifiable precipitating event, such as previous trauma, fractures, infection or congenital deformities, that is believed to predispose the person to later degenerative changes. Although symptomatic OA is usually seen in the 50-70 years (45-55 years) age-group, it has been observed as early as 20 eyars of age. The other factors that influence the development of OA include congenital structural defects (e.g. Legg-Calve-Perthes disease, i.e. osteochondritis of head of femur in children) metabolic disturbances (e.g. Diabetes Mellitus, Acromegaly), repeated intra-articular hemorrhage (hemophilia) neuropathic arthropathies (e.g. Charcots joints) and inflammatory and septic arthritis.

Specific predisposing factors such as excessive use of stress on joints have been identified as accelerating osteoarthritic changes (e.g. on the knees of football players and the feet and ankle in ballet dancers). Genetic factors influence the development of Heberdensnodes, which involve a single autosomal gene, dominant in women and recessive in men.

Pathophysiology

Although osteoarthritis is generally termed "non-inflammatory", a small amount of low-grade inflammation is observed, and mechanical abnormalities in the joints irritate surrounding soft tissue and bone cause inflammation. Both primary OA and secondary OA affect the articular cartilage. Characteristic of pathological changes include:

- Erosion of articular cartilage.
- Thickening of subchondral bone.
- Formation of osteophytes or bone spurs.

Degenerative changes over time cause the normally smooth, white, translucent joint cartilage to become yellow and opaque with rough surfaces and areas of malacia (softening). As the layers of cartilage become thinner, bony surfaces are drawn closer together. As the cartilage breaks down, fissures may appear and fragments of cartilage becomes loose. Inflammations of the synovial membrane secondary to cartilage causes break down. As the articular surface becomes totally denuded of cartilage, subchondral bone increases in density and becomes sclerotic (eburnated). New bone outgrowth (osteophytes) are formed at joint margins and at the attachment sites of ligaments and tendens. These may break off and appear in the joint cavity as "joint mice".

There are several possible causes for cartilage deterioration, which is an active process. The enzyme hyaluronidase, which is normally found in the synovial fluid, may be responsible for digestion of proteoglycans via cracks in the surface layer of articular cartilage. Another possible cause is that the inadequate nutrition of cartilage may result in cartilage degeneration. Because cartilage is avascular, nutrients are provided by the synovial fluid. DNA synthesis, which is normally absent in the adult articular cartilage is active in OA tissue and appears to be directly proportional to disease severity.

Clinical Manifestation

Clinical manifestation include, joint pain, stiffness and limited range of motion (ROM). Persons generally seek medical help because of pain, i.e. deep aching in the joints. Weather changes and increased activity tend to increase the pain loss of joint motion may be caused by the loss of articular cartilage, muscle spasms, shortening ligaments and osteophytes. Loss of articular cartilage and subchondral bone can lead to joint subluxation and deformity. As the joint degenerates, the person may report decreased mobility and the sensation of grinding and catching.

Arthritis of the hand is more common in women between 65 to 74 years. Hip involvement more common in men; women are more likely to have knee involvement. Arthritic changes in hip cause antalgic gait, and pain usually felt on the aspect of the hip, in the groin, buttocks, inner thigh and knee. OA of the knee are most likely to report pain with motion, stiffness after inactivity and decreased flexion. Neurological symptoms may be caused by osteophytes, foraminal stenosis, disc protrusion and subluxation.

To sum up, clinical manifestation of OA includes:
- *Joint enlargements*—May be from inflammatory exudate, or blood entering in capsule, increasing synovial fluid or fragment of osteophytes in synovium.
- *Crepitus*—May be present on movement.
- Pain increased with weight bearing relieved with rest.
- Limitation of joint motion depends on amount of destroyed cartilage.
- Non inflammatory effusion.
- Morning stiffness less than 1 hour.

And the characteristic changes or symptoms in certain joints include:
- *Knee involvement*—Varus valgus (knocked knees), flexion deformity crepitus and limited ROM.
- *Heberden's nodes*—Bony portuberences occurring on the dorsal surface of the distal interphalangeal joints of the fingers.
- *Bouchard's nodes*—Bony portuberances occurring on proximal interphalangeal joints of the fingers.
- *Coxarthrosis (degenerative joint disease of the hip)*—Pain in the hip on weight bearings, with pain progressing to include groin and medial knee pain and limited ROM.

Management

Diagnosis is made on evaluation of history and physical examination and the results of radiological studies. X-ray of the involved joints. ESR and synovial fluid analysis are also helpful in diagnosis of OA.

There is no specific treatment for OA. Therapy is aimed at symptomatic relief and control of pain, prevention of progression and disability and restoration of joint function. First line of therapy starts with acetaminophen 1 g and upto four times daily. Typical agents, such as Capsaican cream may be used alone or in conjunction with acetaminophen. This cream made from chilli peppers, causes depletion of substance P from nerve endings, thus blocking pain signals to the brain. Low dose of ibuprofen. 400 mg upto Qds may be used.

If acetaminophen is contraindicated (Liver and renal diseases) NSAIDs are the next choice of therapy. Intra-articular injection of corticosteroids are used to treat a symptomatic care of OA. No use of this is restricted, because it may accelerate disease process. A newly approved treatment for OA of knee uses intra-articular injection of synthetic and naturally occurring hyaluronic acid derivatives (orthovise, synvise, and Hyalgan). This is viscosupplementation. Although exact mechanism is unknown but it is beneficial.

Appropriate nutritional intake is encouraged to maintain ideal body weight and avoid weight gain. Weight gain places an unnecessary stress on joints, particularly the hip and knees. Emphasis is placed on the following activities.
- Unloading the stress on painful weight-bearing joints through the use of canes, walkers or crutches.
- ROM exercises to prevent deformities and contractares, muscle strengthening exercises to icrease or maintain muscle, muscle tone and strength.

Aerobic exercise should be included in the regimen to increase endurance and increase overall conditioning. Exercise also is beneficial in reducing fatigue a common complaint of chronic diseased persons.

Surgical Management

When medications and physical therapy have failed, surgery is performed. Surgical management of person with OA is indicated to relieve pain. Improve function, or correct deformity. Surgical procedures include those that preserve or restore articular cartilage and thsoe that realign, fuse or replace joints. Surgical management usually provides the patient with excellent results. However, the patient is at risk for developing surgical complications including infection, nerve and blood vessel injury, deep vein thrombosis and pulmonary fat embolism. The common surgical procedures performed for OA are:

- Abrasion chondroplasty (to stimulate growth of cartilage).
- Osteotomy (to realign joint or to redistribute cartilage).
- Arthrodesis (to relieve pain, to restore stability and alignment).
- Arthroplasty (joint replacement).

Praperatively nurse has to carry out routine assessment procedure collaboratively with other team members as in other surgical procedure with special emphasis on elective surgery. In addition, nursing intervention include preoperative teaching which should focus on assessed risk factors, then may influence his or her case intraoperatively or postoperatively. Major concerns identified by patients with total joint replacement including fear of the unknown, pain, performance, altered body image, dependency depression and fatigue.

Postoperative care of joint replacement surgery includes monitoring vital signs and level of consciousness, coughing and deep breathing, monitoring and recording intake and output, providing adequate nutrition and hydration, managing pain, assessing the surgical site for drainage, and signs of infection, maintaining the position of the operative extremity to prevent dislocation of prosthesis, performing neurovascular checks, providing skin care, encouraging progressive ambulation, preventing infection, teaching and monitoring signs of complication and attending accordingly.

Postoperative Care of the Person with Total Hip Replacement

- Positioning: Positioning will depend on the design of the prosthesis and the method of insertion. Restriction designed to avoid dislocation of the prosthesis usually include the following.
  - Flexion is limited to 60 degrees for 6 to 7 days, then 90 degrees for 2 to 3 months.
  - No adduction is permitted beyond midline for 2 to 3 months. Therefore, no sidelying on operative side unless ordered by the surgeon. Leg is maintained in abduction when lying supine or on non-operative side.
  - No extreme internal or external rotation is permitted.
- Wound care
  - Drains are inserted in wound to prevent formation of hematoma and left in place for 24 to 48 horus.
  - Maintain constant suction through self-contained suction device.
  - Note amount and types of drainage.
  - Use aseptic technique.
  - Following initial dressing change, change dressing once daily and prn, using a septic technique. Observe the incision line for signs of infection. The wound may be left open to air if there is no drainage. Staples are removed 7 to 10 days postoperatively.
- Activity
  - Observe flexion restriction when elevating head of bed.
  - Encourage periodic elevation and lowering of head of bed to provide motion at hip.
  - Instruct patient in use of overhead trapeze to shift weight and lift for bedpan and change of linen.
  - Encourage active dorsiplantar flexion exercise of ankles and quadriceps and gluteal setting exercises to promote venous return, prevent thrombus formation, and maintain muscle tone.
  - Patient may be turned to unoperative side with operative leg maintained in abduction and extension.
  - Begin ambulation as early as possible as the first postoperative day, if tolerated.
    - Observe flexion and adduction restrictions.
    - Observe weight-bearing restrictions prescribed by surgeon (usually partial weight bearing assisted with walker or crutcher).
    - Increase amount of walking each day according to patient tolerance.
  - Begin sitting when patient demonstrates sufficient control of leg to sit within flexion restrictions (usually requires elevation of sitting surfaces, including use of raised toilet seat).
- Medications
  - Prophylactic anticoagulant drug may be prescribed to decrease risk of thrombus formation.
  - Initially control pain with positioning and narcotics, gradually tapered to non-narcotic analgesia according to patient tolerance.
- Discharge instructions
  - Patient must use ambulatory aid, avoid adduction, and limit hip flexion to 90 degree for about 2 to 3 months.
  - A raised toilet seat is to be obtained and used at home until flexation restrictions are removed.
  - Patient may need a long-handled shoehorn and reacher to facilitate ADL within flextion restriction.

- Patient must be made aware of the life-long need for antibiotic prophylaxis when undergoing invasive procedures or dental work to protect prosthesis from bacteremic infection.

Postoperative Care of the Person with Total Knee Replacement

- Positioning:
  - The operative leg(s) is elevated in pillows to enhance venous return for the first 48 hours. Pillows are placed with caution not to flex the knee (s). It is becoming more common for patients who have bilateral total knee replacements at one surgery.
  - The patient may be turned from side to back to side.
- Wound care:
  - Care of drains is as for total hip replacement.
  - Patient is assessed for systemic evidence of loss of blood, (hypotension, tachycardia) if bulky compression dressing is used, since it may hold large quantities of drainage before drainage is visible.
  - Bulky dressings are removed before the patient begins active flexion.
  - Assess wound for heal in and signs of infection. Perform dry sterile dressing change once bulky dressing is discontinued. Leave incision open to air if there is no drainage.
- Activity:
  - Passive flexion in a CPM machine within prescribed flexion-extension limits. Patient's leg may remain in machines as much as tolerated (upto 22 hours per day) to facilitate even healing of tissue.
  - Patient is encouraged to perform active dorsi-plantar flexion of the ankles, quadriceps setting and after the drain is removed, straight leg-raising exercises.
  - Patient begins active flexion exercises three to four times per day on about the third postoperative day. The time when active flexion is permitted varies.
  - Partial weight bearing with an assistive device may be started as early as the first postoperative day and increased as the patient tolerates.
  - Sitting in a chair with leg(s) elevated may be started on the first postoperative day.
  - Patient may be encouraged to wear a resting knee extension spling (immobilizer) on the operative extremity untilable to demonstrate quadriceps control (independent straight leg raising).
- Pain control:
  - Initial control of pain is with narcotics (PCA) and positioning medication is gradually decreased to non-narcotic analgesics as patient tolerates.
  - Ice is usually prescribed to be applied to the knee to reduce swelling and pain.
  - Patient is encouraged to apply ice to knee (1) for 20 to 30 minutes before and after active flexion exercise.
- Discharge instructions:
  - Patient must observe partial weight-bearing restriction and use ambulatory aid for approximately 2 months after discharge.
  - Patient should continue active flexion and straight leg-raising exercises at home.
  - Patient must be made aware of the life-long need for antibiotic prophylaxis before invasive procedure or dental work.

In surgery, total replacement of shoulder, elbow and ankle also performed. Position and other care should be taken accordingly. The complications of total joint arthroplasty are as follows:

- Hip
  - Dislocation.
  - Infection.
  - DVT.
  - Pulmonary embolus.
  - Leg length discrepancy.
  - Pat embolus.
  - Altered gait.
  - Pneumonia.
  - Foot drop.
- Knee
  - Infection.
  - DVT.
  - Pulmonary embolus.
  - Acute compartment
  - Instability.
  - Loosening of prosthesis.
  - Pattellar fracture.
  - Poor patellar tracking.
  - Vascular injury.
  - Reflex sympathetic
  - Nerve damage.
- Shoulder
  - Infection.
  - Loosening of prosthesis.
  - Glenohumeral instability.
  - Dislocation, subluxation.
  - Intraoperative fracture.
  - Rotation cuff tears.
  - Deltoid dysfunction.
  - Nerve damage.
  - Impingement syndrome
  - Pulmonary embolus.
- Elbow
  - Infection.
  - Loosening of prosthesis.
  - Glenohumer instability.
  - Dislocation, subluxation.

- Intraoperative fracture.
- Rotator cuff.
- Elbow
  - Infection.
  - Dislocation.
  - DVT.
  - Pulmonary embolus.
  - Loosening prosthesis.
  - Delayed healing of wound.
- Ankle
  - Infection.
  - Residual pain.
  - Impingement.
  - Loosening prosthesis.

Juvenile Rheumatoid Arthritis (JRA)

JRA is a major rheumatoid disease of youth and is defined as RA beginning before 16 years of age. It may be classified on the basis of the type of onset. Systemic, pauciarticular or polyarticular. Polyarticular resemble adult RA systemic JRA with onset during childhood.

JRA may occur with arthritis confined to one joint (pauciarticular) or several (polyarticular). Children, most often, do not complain of joint pain, but may assume a position of flexion to minimize pain, carefully limit movement or refuse to walk at all. A more constitutional variant known as stills disease (systemic onset) causes high-spiking fever, vague arthralgia, generalized rash, hepatosplenomegally, lymphadenopathy and pleuritis or pericarditis. Complication of JRA includes retarded growth and development, and chronic asymptomatic eye inflammation.

The criterion diagnosis of JRA is persistent athritis of one or more joints for at least 6 consecutive weeks, provided certain other similar disorders are ruled out. High-spiking fever, generalized lymphadenopathy and splenomegaly are more common in children. Leucocytosis is common. JRA can be treated with NSAIDs, if no resposne to NSAIDs use chrystotherapy (treatment with gold sales).

Nursing intervention includes the education of parents and significant ones about the course and prognosis of their child's arthritis according to the onset of classification. Daily participation in planned physical training progress encourages full ROM and muscle strengthening and does not strain affected joints. Swimming, bicycling and dance therapy are better than running, jumping and kicking and routine ophtholmological examinations are advised.

GOUT/GOUTY ARTHRITIS

Gout is characterized by recurrent attacks of acute arthritis in association with increased levels of serum uric acid. It may be classified as primary or secondary.

Etiology

Primary gout occurs predominantly in middle aged men, with almost no incidence in premenopausal women. Gout was considered a disease of the wealthy, associated with rich food and wine. Uric acid is the major end product of the catabolism of purines and primarily excreted by the kidneys. Thus, hyperurecemia may be result of increased purine synthesis, decreased renal excretion or both. There are folklores associated with excess of food and drink with acute attacks of gouty arthritis. Although high dietary intake of purine alone has relatively little effect on uric acid levels, it is clear that hyperurecemia may result from prolonged fasting or excessive alcohol drinking because of increased production of keto acids, which then inhibit normal excretion of uric acid.

The causes of secondary gout include:
Overproduction of uric acid
- Paget's disease.
- Cancer
- Polycythemia vera.
- Multiple myeloma.
- Chronic myelocytic and lymphonytic leukemia.
- Hemolytic anemia
- Cytotoxic drugs.

Under-excretion of uric acid
- Chronic renal insufficiency.
- Ketoacidosis.
- Lactic acidosis.
- Drug ingestion (diuretics, cyclosporine, lovadopa, pyrazinamide). Low dose salicylism.

Unknown etiology
- Hyperparathyroidism.
- Hypoparathyroidism.
- Hypothyroidism.
- Adrenal insufficiency.

Associated condition leading to hyperuricema are acidosis and ketosis, alcoholism, atherosclerosis, cytotoxic drugs, diabetes mellitus, drug-induced renal impairment, hyperlipidemia, hypertension, intrinsic renal disease, malignant disease, myeloproliferation disorder, obesity and sickle cell anemia.

Pathophysiology

Uric acid levels are controlled by diet, purine metabolism and renal clearance. Persons with chronically-elevated uric acid levels will develop gouty arthritis. As stated earlier, gout is classified primary and/or secondary. Undersecretion of uric acid is caused by decreased tubular secretion, increased tubular resorption, or a combination of both. Seventy-five percent cases of primary gout as a result of undersecretion of uric acid, twenty five percent of primary gout are oversecretion of uric acid.

Primary gout is idiopathic, affected persons also tend to have hypertension and obesity.

Secondary gout results from an overproduction of uric acid secondary to increased purine catabolism or impaired excretions of uric acid. Secondary gout usually occurs in the acute care setting. Urate crystals form in the synovial tissue causing severe inflammation.

Clinical Manifestation

In acute phase, gouty arthritis may occur in one or more joints but usually less than four. Affected joint may appear dusky or cyanotic and are extremely tender. Inflammation of the great toe (Podagra) is most commonly the initial involvement. Other joints affected are midtarsal, ankle, knee and wrist joints and olecranon bursa. Acute gouty arthritis is usually precipitated by events such as trauma, surgery, alcohol, ingestion or systemic infection. Onset of symptoms usually are rapid with swelling and pain peaking within several hours. Often accompanied by low grade fever. Individual attacks usually subsides, treated or untreated in 2 to 10 days. They affect joint returns entirely to normal and patients are often free of symptoms between attacks.

Chronic gout is characterized by multiple joint involved and deposits of sodium urate crystals called tophi. These are typically seen in the synovium subchondral done, olecronon burns, and vertebrae; along tendens, and in the skin and cartilage. Tophi are rarely present at the time of the initial attack and generally noted only many years after the onset of disease. Chronic inflammation may result in joint deformity. Destructing the cartilage may predispose the joint to secondary osteoarthritis. Excessive uric acid excretion leads to kidney or urinary tract stone formation.

Management

The diagnosis can be established by finding monosodium urate, monohydrate crystals in the synovial fluid of an inflamed joint or tophus in addition to history and physical examination. Family history of gout, elevated serum uric acid levels, and elevated 24-hour urine for uric acid levels.

Acute gouty arthritis is treated with one of three types of anti-inflammatory agents such as colchicine, NSAIDs, or cortiocosteroids. Corticosteroids should be reserved for cases in the cochicine and NSAIDs are contraindicated or ineffective. Colchicine and NSAIDs are also used as prophylaxis to prevent further attacks of gout **(Table 11.2)**.

Acute gouty arthritis may be prevented by maintenance of the serum uric acid at normal levels. Nursing interventions is directed at supportive care of the inflamed joints—Bedrest may be appropriate, with affected joint properly immobilized. The limitation of motion and degree of pain should be assessed. Treatment effectiveness should be documented. Special care is taken to avoid causing pain so the inflamed joint by careless handling. Involvement of a lower extremity may require use of cradle or footboard to protect the painful area from the weight of bed clothes. In addition, nursing management includes the following:
- Patient teaching
    - Instruct patient on nature of disease.
    - Instruct patient on proper use of prescribed medication.

Table 11.2: Commonly used drugs in treatment of GOUT.

	Colchicine	Allopurinol	Probenecid
Mechanism of action	Inhibits phagocytosis by multiple actions	Xanthine oxidase inhibitor, hence decreases urate formation	Inhibits reabsorption of urate from kidneys (uricosuric agent)
Dose	For acute attack, it is no longer recommended now. It is used: • As prophylactic therapy during interictal period 0.6–1 mg once or twice a day. • Used alongwith uricosuric agents or allopurinol to suppress sudden attacks	Once daily or in divided doses, usually upto 30 mg/day (maximum dose is 800 mg/day)	Start 250 mg twice a day increments upto 1–2 g/day in divided doses
Adverse effects	Nausea, vomiting, diarrhoea, cinchonism, myoneuropathy	Hypersensitivity, drug interactions with azathioprine and mercaptopurine	Rash, convulsions, dyspeptic symptoms, interactions—drug promotes action of furosemide, indomethacin, dapsone, heparin, ampicillin, etc
Uses	• To prevent recurrent attacks of gout. • For polyserositis in Mediterranean fever.	• In symptomatic hyperuricaemia • Used prophylactically in "tumour lysis" or leukaemias. • Acute uric acid nephropathy and urate stones • Tophaceous gout	Symptomatic hyperuricaemia to reduce urate levels
Special remarks	• Dose to be adjusted in renal failure	• Dose to be adjusted in renal failure • Not to be used in acute attack of gout	Contraindicated in presence of renal stones, renal failure and blood dyscrasias

- Encourage patient to lose weight gradually if overweight.
- Encourage lifestyle modification to control hypertension or adherence to pharmocological regimen (medication).
- Encourage patient to take in sufficient fluid to assure daily output of 2000 ml to 3000 ml.
- Advise the patient to avoid excessive intake of purine (sweet bread yeast, heart, herring, herring roe and sardines and excessive alcohol intake).
- Explain to patient that severe dietary purine restriction is not necessary as long as his or her hyperuricemia is well controlled by daily-drug tehrapy.
- Promoting comfort
  - Provide absolute rest until the pain of an acute attack subsides.
  - Avoid touching the joint or moving the affected extremity until the acute pain subsides.

Thorough explanation should be given concerning importance of drug therapy and the need for periodic determination of blood and uric acid levels. The patient should be able to demonstrate knowledge of precipitating factors that may cause an attack, including overindulgence in the intake of calories, purines, and alcohol, starvation (fasting), medication use (aspirin, diuretics) and major medical events (e.g. surgery, MI).

SEPTIC ARTHRITIS

Septic arthritis (infection or bacterial arthritis) is caused by invasion of the joint cavity with micro-organism.

Etiology

Various bacteria are commonly responsible including:
- Neisseria gonorrhoeae (children).
- Meningococci.
- *Streptococcus hemolyticus.*
- *Staphylococcus aureus.*
- Coliform bacteria.
- *Salmonella.*
- *Haemophilus influenzae.*

Hematogenous infection is the most common cause of bacterial arthritis. Persons with an underlying medical illness are at greatest risk. Immunodeficiency, chronic disease intravenous drug abuse, local joint surgery or trauma, intra-articular injections and rheumatoid arthritis also place the person at risk.

Pathophysiology

A site of active infection is often responsible for bacteraemia (micro-organism reaching the bloodstream). Leading to hematogenous seeding joints. Synovial tissue respond to bacterial invasion by becoming:
- Signs and symptoms of septic arthritis.
- Importance of diagnosis and treatment.
- Importance of antibiotic therapy.
- Instructing in care of cast or other immobilizing device.
- Encouraging active joint motion when motion is permitted.
- Instructing about use of crutches or assistive devices.
- Instruct on proper administration of antibiotics if it is continued after discharge.
- Ensuring that patient should be aware of plans for follow-up with physician inflammed. The joint cavity may become involved and pus will be present, in the synovial membrane and the synovial fluid. If allowed to progress, the infection will cause abscesses in the synovium and subchondral done; eventually destroying cartilage. Ankylosis of the joints may result. The patient will report pain, swelling and tenderness of the joint.

Clinical Manifestation

Inflammation of the joint cavity causes severe pain, erythema, and swelling of one or several joints. Large joints, such as the knee and the hip are most frequently involved. Fever or shaking chills often accompany particular symptoms because bacterial entry into a joint is usually by the hematogenous route from a primary site of infection.

Management

Prociss diagnosis is made by aspiration of the joint and culture of the synovial fluid. Blood cultures for aerobic and anaerobic organism, should be obtained. Strict aseptic technique must be followed to avoid introducing additional bacteria into the joint. WBC counts will be high, and X-ray of joint reveals loss of joint space and lythic changes in bones.

Septic arthritis is a medical emergency that requires prompt diagnosis and treatment to prevent joint destructions. Parenteral antibiotic administration is maintained until there are no clinical signs of active synovitis or inflammation in the joint fluid. The treatment of septic arthritis includes:
- Appropriate antibiotic therapy.
- Rest or immobilization of the joint.
- Surgical drainage by needle aspiration arthroscopy, arthrotomy, or a system of irrigation and drainage if injection does not respond to antibiotic therapy or if osteomyelitis, required daily until drainage ceases. Infection of the hip joints must be drained immediately to prevent necrosis of the femoral head.
- Resumption of active range of motion when infection subsides and motion can be tolerated.

Nursing management includes the following.
- Promoting rest of the affected joints.
- Assessment and monitoring of joint inflammation, pain and fever.

- Immobilization of affected joint to control pain is often by resting splints or traction.
- Administering antibiotics on time and as prescribed to maintain blood level.
- Administering prescribed pain medication as necessary.
- Strict aseptic technique should be used during assistance with joint aspiration procedure.
- Support should be offered to the patient requiring repeated arthrocentesis or operative drainage.
- Gentle ROM exercise should be done.
- Patient teaching should be done regarding.

LYME'S DISEASE (LD)

Lyme's disease is tick borne spirochetal infection caused by the "*Borrelia burgdorferi*" and transmitted by the bite of an infected tick. It was first identified in 1975 in Lyme, Connecticut (US) after an unusual clustering of arthritis in children.

Etiology

Lyme's disease is caused by the spirachete (Borrelia burgdorferi). This disease is transmitted by ticks, present most commonly on deer, dogs, cats, raccons, cows and horses. Birds help spread infected ticks by their migratory flights.

Pathophysiology

Lyme's disease has been called "great imitator" because it resembles, mimics other diseases such as influenza, RA multiple sclerosis, chronic fatigue syndrome, and others. Infection with *B. Burgdorferi* stimulates inflammatory cytokines, and autoimmune mechanisms which result in Lyme arthritis. Primarily an extracellular organism *B. Burgdorferi* is thought to invade some cells and cross the blood-brain barrier, resulting in the neurological manifestation of Lyme disease. Infection with this spirochate can be divided into three stages (I, II, III). Not all patients develop all states (See clinical manifestations).

Clinical Manifestation

Stage I (Early localized infection):
- Symptoms appear days to 16 weeks after tick bite.
- Erythema, migraine appear in 50-70% of patients, resolve spontaneously in a few weeks.
- Fatigue.
- Headache.
- Lethargy.
- Myalgia, arthalgia.
- Lymphadenopathy.

Stage II (Early disseminated infection):
- Symptoms occur weeks to months after tick bite.
- Cardiac symptoms—Carditis, dysrhythmias, hear failure, pericarditis, palpitation, dyspnea.
- Neurological symptom—Meningitis, encephalitis, cranial and peripheral neuorpathy and myelitis.
- Musculoskeletal—Arthralgia, myalgia, fibromyalgia.
- Other symptoms—Conjunctivitis, optieneuropathy, Hepatomegaly, hepatitis, generalized lymphadenopathy.

Stage III (Late infection):
Symptoms occur months to years after tickbite.
- Monoarticular or dioarticular arthritis.
- Chronic arthritis.
- Aerodermatitis chronic atrophicans (bluish, red, doughy lesions).
- Ataxia.
- Spastic paresis.
- Periventricular lesions.
- Memory loss.
- Behavioral changes.

Management

Diagnosis is made on the basis of clinical manifestation, history of exposure in an endemic area and a positive serological test for *B. Burgdorferi*. Differential diagnoses also should be made. Serological test includes ELISA (Enzyme linked immunoabsorbent assay, Western blot, and indirect immunofluorence assay.

Patients in Stage I disease should be treated with tetracycline or deoxycycline to prevent development of further symptoms. During Stage II and III, intravenous therapy is indicated, usually cefiaxone (crosses the blood-brain barrier), cefotaxime or penicillin. The patient should be monitored for development of cardiac and neurological sequalae. Persons with musculoskeletal symtoms resulting in impaired mobility require physical therapy and occupational therapy. Nursing interventions are as in RA. Education is the best way to prevent Lyme disease in endemic areas, which include:

- Avoid walking through tall grasses and low bush.
- Avoid tick-infested areas and sitting directly on the ground, stay on paths while hiking.
- Mow grass and remove brush along paths, buildings and camp sites.
- When outdoors in high-risk areas, wear long sleeves and long pants and pants into shoes or sockes.
- Wear closed shoes when hiking.
- Use EPA approved tick repellants on skin and clothing. Wash off repellent thoroughly when returning inside.

Avoid spraying repllents directly on skin of small children:
- Check frequently for ticks crawling from legs to open skin.
- Have pets wear collars, inspect them often, and do not allow them on furniture or beds.
- If a tick is found, use a fine-pointed tweezer to grasp the tick, at the point of attachment, gently pull the tick

straight out, place the tick in a sealed jar and have it tested by a local veterinarian or health department. Don't squeeze the tick, doing so may release infected fluid.
- Dispose off tick in alcohol or flush down toilet. Do not crush with fingers.
- Wash the tick site thoroughly with soap and warm water, apply antiseptic and disinfect the tweezers. Wash hands and clothes properly.
- Ticks are susceptible to dehydration. Reduce humidity by pruning trees, clearing brush, and mowing the lawn on your property.
- Do not have bird feeders or birdbaths in your yard, these attract animals that may have ticks.
- Keep woodpiles away from the house- Move woodpiles and bird-feeders away from house.
- Keep children's play areas away from wooded areas.
- See a doctor or nurse practitioner immediately if flu-like symptoms or bull's-eye rash develop, within a few weeks after removal of tick.

SERONEGATIVE ARTHROPATHIES

Seronegative arthropathies is a term used to describe a group of disease characterized by arthritis (arthropathy) in which the rheumatoid factor is not present in the serum. Diseases included in this category are Ankylosing spondalitis, Psoriatic arthritis, enteropathic arthritis and Reifer's syndrome. These diseases also are known as the 'Spondyle arthritis, and have several characteristics other than a negative rheumatoid factors which include:
- Frequent bouts of spondylitis (inflammation of the vertebrae characterized by stiffness and pain).
- Presence of the cell marker HLA-B27-strong association with H antigen B27.
- Common extra-articular manifestation (eye, heart, skin, mucous membrane).
- Predilection for involvement of sacroiliac joint and spine.
- Oligoarticular asymmetric arthritis.
- Absence enthesitis (inflammation at tendon attachment sites to bone).
- Enthesopathy (plantor facitis and Achilles tendonitis).
- Absence of rheumatoid factor and anti-antibiotics.
- Male predominance.

Ankylosing Spondylitis (AS)

Ankylosing spondylitis is a chronic inflammatory disease that primarily affects the sacroiliac joints, apophysical and costovertebral joints of the spine and adjacent soft tissues.

Etiology

The cause of AS is unknown. The course of disease is marked by remissions and exacerbations. The disease in both sexes, with progressive disease more common in men. Genetic predisposition appears to play an important role in the disease pathogenesis, but the precise mechanisms are unknown. Environmental factors and infection agents are also suspected.

Pathophysiology

Inflammation in joint and adjacent tissue causes the formation of granulation tissue and eroding vertebral margins, resulting spondylitis. Calcification tends to follow the inflammation process, leading to bony ankylosis. Spondylitis means inflammation of the spine. As a result of inflammation, the bones of the spine grow together and ankylose (fuse). The primary site of pathological findings is in the enthesis where ligament tendens and joint capsule insert into bone. In ankylosing, spondylitis, fibrous ossification and eventually fusion of the joint occur. The joint capsule articular cartilage, and periosteum are invaded by inflammatory cells that trigger the development of fibrous scar tissue and growth of new bone. The bony growth changes the contour of the vertebrae and form a new enthesis called a "syndesmophyte" on top of the old one. As the spinal ligaments continue to undergo progressive calcification, the vertebral bodies lose their original contour and appear square, which gives the spine the classic "bamboo" appearance of ankylosing spondylitis. Inflammation usually begins around the sacroiliac joints and progresses up the spine, eventually resulting in fusion of the entire spine. As the inflammatory process involves the costosternal and costovertebral cartilage, it causes the chest pain, which is worse on inspiration.

Clinical Manifestation

The patient typically has lower back pain, stiffness and limitation of motion that is worse during the night and in the morning, but improves with mild activity. General constitutional feature, such as fever, fatigue, anorexia and weight loss are rarely present. Other symptoms depend on the stage of the disease and include arthritis of the shoulders, hips and knees and occasionally ocular inflammation (iritis). Involvement of the costovertebral joints leads to a decrease in chest expansion. Advancing kyphosis leads to a bent-over postage and compensating hipflexion contractures may occur. There is pronounced impairment of neckmotion in all direction. Extraskeletal involvement may include iritis, aortitis, valvular regurgitation and apical pulmonary fibrosis.

Management

Diagnosis is made by history and physical examination and the following findings:
- X-ray films shows that the presence of syndesmophytes and bamboo spine ankylosis of peripheral joints seen. CT and MRI show changes.

- ESR elevated.
- Test by RF is negative.
- HLA-B27 present in the serum.

The objectives of the treatment are to relieve pain, achieve and maintain the best possible alignment of the spine, strengthening the paraspinal muscles and maximal breathing capacity. For which:

- Administration for salicylates, NSAIDs (phenybutazone effective but may cause bone marrow toxicity).
- Sulfasalazine and systemic steroids are avoided except for patients with severe eye disease.
- Exercise is an important component of treatment. Swimming in a warm pool is a good choice for exercise. Rest should be discouraged unless a fracture is present.
- Physical therapy to maintain mobility and reduce severties of deformity. For example, ROM exercises and lying prone (extension) 3 to 4 times per day for 15 to 30 minutes and deep breathing exercises to promote maximum chest expansion (rib cage mobility) is decreased.
- Heat.
- Use of thoracic lumbar sacral orthosis (TLSO).
- Cervical head halter traction to decrease muscle spasms and distractive spine.
- Spinal osteotomy and fusion are usually cervical.
- Hip arthroplasty.
- Value replacement of pace maker insertion if cardiac involvement is present.

Patient teaching is essential. It should focus on the following:

- Facilitating learning.
  - Nature and cause of disease.
  - Prescribed exercises.
  - Appropriate use of prescribed medication.
  - Methods of applying heat to back and hips.
- Promoting maximum ability and reducing severity of deformity:
  - Maintain proper posture and walk erect.
  - Provide firm mattresses and bed board.
  - Encourage patient to sleep without pillow under the head to maintain extension of spine, lying prone or supine is recommended; avoid sidelying.
  - Supervise and encourage regular exercises; assist as necessary.
  - Regular deep-breathing exercises are important to optimize respiratory function. Persons with ankylosing spondylitis should not smoke.
  - Encourage participation in ADL and usual activities to the fullest extent possible.
  - Refer to an occupation therapist for adaptive or supportive devices. Recommend use of long-handled reachers, sponges, and shoe horn, for patient with hip involvement.
- Promoting comfort and relieving pain.
  - Provide heat applications/hydrotherapy and especially prior to exercises.
  - Administer prescribed medications on time.
  - Assess effectiveness of pain relief measures.
  - Promoting acceptance of body image.

PSORIATIC ARTHRITIS

Psoriatic arthritis can be defined as an association of clinically-apparent psoriasis with inflammatory polyarthritis. Psoriatic skin changes may precede or follow articular symptoms. It affects few joints of peripheral, i.e. distal phalanges of hands, feet and metatorsal bones. X-ray findings show asymmetric distribution and resorption of tufts at joints. These patients get spondylitis, Hypauricemia, at present of HLA-B27. Forms of treatment include splinting, joint protection, and physical therapy.

Treating the cases with drug methotrexate is most effective.

REITER'S SYNDROME

Reiter's syndrome is a self-limiting disease associated with arthritis, urethritis, conjunctivitis, and mucocutaneous lesions. The cause of disease is unknown, but it appears to be a reactive arthritis after certain enteric (e.g. *Shigella*) or veneral (e.g. *Chlamydia trachomatis*) infections. This disease usually affects in males, shows HLA-B27 positive, which provides evidence of genetic predisposition.

Diagnosis measures as in ankylosy spondylitis. The arthritis of Reiter's syndrome tends to be asymmetric, frequently involving weight bearing joints of the lower extremities and sometimes lower parts of the back. Arthralgia usually begins 1 to 3 weeks after the appearance of initial infection. The full attack accompanied by fever and other constitutional complaints including anorexia with considerable weight loss and may prove highly debilitating. Soft tissue manifestations cause induced Achilles tendinitis. Treatment is symptomatic and joint inflammation is treated with NSAIDs. Autoimmune is connected two diseases.

SYSTEMIC LUPUS ERYTHEMATOSUS

Systemic lupus erythematosus (SLE) is a chronic multisystem inflammatory disease of connective tissue that often involves the skin, joints, serous membrane (Pleura, Pericardium) kidneys, hematological system and central nervous system.

Etiology

The cause of SLE is unknown. However, factors implicate in the etiology of SLE include genetic predisposition, sex hormones, race, environmental factors (e.g. ultraviolet, radiation, drugs, chemical) viruse and infections, stress

and immunologic abnormalities, SLE is a disorder of immunoregulation.
- Genetic factors may contribute to the development of the disease. Family members of persons with SLE have an increased chance of developing disease.
- Environmental factors associated with cases of SLE. For example, exposure for ultraviolet light is a known cause of exacerbations. Drugs-including procainamide (Pronestyl), isonicosonic acid hydrazial (INH) hydralazine anticonvulsants and chloropromozin are known to induce lupus-like syndromes. Persons with drug-induced lupus do not develop renal and neurological disease. The symptoms usually resolve after the drug is discontinued. Other areas being considered include viral-origin and disturbance is estrogen metabolism (menses and pregnancy).
- Alterations in the immune response may cause immune complexes containing antibodies to be deposited in tissue causing tissue damage.

Pathophysiology

The exact mechanism of is not known. However, several alterations in the immune system are associated with SLE. Numerous cellular antibodies have been identified with it. Antinuclear antibodies, antibodies to DNA, antihistones, and antibodies to ribonucleoprotein (Smith antigen) are strongly associated with SLE.

Abnormalities in both B cells and T cells have been exempted in the persons with SLE. The appearance of B cells is thought to cause an increase in production of antibodies to self and non-self antigen. These antibodies are responsible for the tissue injury seen in SLE. Most visceral lesions are mediated by type III hypersensitivity and antibodies against red blood cells are mediated by type II hypersensitivity. An acute necrotizing vasculitis can occur in any tissue. Most lesions are found in the blood vessels, kidney, connective tissue and skin.

Clinical Manifestation

The clinical manifestation of SLE can be overwhelming. The criteria for classification are remissions and ommissions Fixed erythema, flat or raised, over the molar eminences tending to spare the nasolabial fold.
- *Discord rash:* Erythematus raised patches with adherent keratotic scaling and follicular plugging, atrophic scarring may occur in older lesions.
- *Photosensitivity:* Skin rash as a result of unusual reaction to sunlight by patient history or physician observation.
- *Oral ulcers:* Oral or nasopharyngeal ulceration, usually painless observed by care taken.
- *Arthritis:* Non-erosive arthritis involving two or more peripheral joint characterized by tenderness, swelling of effusion.
- *Serositis:* Plueritis–Plueritic pain or rub hears. Pericarditis–document by ECG or rub.
- Renal Disorders.
  - Persistent proteinuria greater than 0.5 g/dl.
  - Cellular casts–may be RBCs hemoglobin granular, tubular or medial.
- Neurological disorder.
  - Seizures: In the absence of offencing drugs and known metabolic derangements, e.g. anemia, ketoacidosis, or electrolyte imbalances.
  - Psychoses
- Hematological disorders.
  - Hemolytic anemias – with reticulosis or
  - Leukopenia – less than $4.0 \times 10^9/L$ total on two or more occasions.
  - Lymphopenia – less than $1.5 \times 10^9/L$ total on two or more occasions or
  - Thrombocytopenia less than $100 \times 10^9/L$ in the absence of offending drug.
- Immunological disorder
  - Positive lupus erythematous cell preparation or
  - Anti-DNA antibody to negative DNA is abnormal or
  - Anti-Sm - Presence of antibody to Sm nuclear antigen or
  - False positive STS known to be positive for at least 6 months and confirmed by negative. Trepenoma palladium immobilization.
- Antinuclear antibody
  - An abnormal titer of antinuclear antibody by immunofluorescence of an equivalent assay at any point in time and in the absence of drugs known to be associated with drug-induced lupus syndrome, and general constitutional complaints include fever, weight loss, arthralgia, and excessive fatigue and may precede an exacerbation of disease activity.

Management

Diagnosis is made after evaluation of the history and physical examination and results of the laboratory test-lupus cell preparation, antibodies, CBC count, urinalysis, X-ray of the joints, Chest X-ray, complement level CH 50, C3 and ECG.

The following medications are given for SLE:
- NSAIDs to control arthritic symptoms; diclofenic, naproxen, and oxaprozine are effective in treating lupus. Renal function are monitored carefully.
  - Antimalarial drugs, particularly if rasin is extensive.
- Corticosteroids for severe neurological and renal involvement or if NSAIDs or are ineffective.
- Cystotoxic agents if other drugs fail (cyclophosphamide).
- Ointments or skin creams for rash.

Nursing care will depend upon the symptoms manifested. Nursing intervention to maintain musculoskeletal functioning are similar to those for caring for persons with rheumatoid arthritis. Nursing intervention must emphasize health teaching and home management which includes the following:
- Education on the disease process.
- Names of medications and actions, side effects, dosage and administration.
- Energy-conservation and pacing techniques.
- Daily heat and exercise program (for Anthralgia).
- Avoidance of physical and emotional stress, overexposure to ultraviolet light and unnecessary exposure to infection.
- Regular medical and laboratory follow-up.
- Marital counselling if necessary.
- Referral resources to community and health care agency.

All nursing intervention can assist the patient in accepting changes and coping with a chronic disease.

The other autoimmune connective diseases are:
- Scleroderma (Systemic sclerosis).
- CREST syndrome (Limited Cutaneous Scleroderma).
- Sjögren's syndrome.

The brief description of these diseases are as follows.

SYSTEMIC SCLEROSIS

Systemic sclerosis (SS) or scleroderm is a disorder of connective tissue characterized by fibrositic, degenerative and occasionally inflammatory changes in the skin, blood vessels, synovium, skeletal muscle, and internal organ.

It is most common in middle-aged women, causes microvascular damage and fibrous degeneration of tissues in the skin, GI tract, lungs and kidneys. The exact cause is unknown but possible links include environmental toxin, exposure to vinyl chloride, epoxy resins and trichloroethylene. Occupational silica dust exposure increases insidious scleroderma.

Clinical Manifestation

- Raynaud's phenomenon (paraxysmal vosospasm of the digits).
- *GI:* dysphagia, diarrhea and malabsorption.
- *Renal:* Haematuria, proteinuria, renal crisis and hypertension.
- *Cardiopulmonary:* Pericarditis, dysrhythmias, pulmonary hypertension, fibrosis.
- *Dermatologeal:* Hardening, thickening and tightening of the skin, edema.

Management

- Routine diagnostic measures.
- Avoidance of cold; protective clothing.
- Skin care for ulcers.
- Thoracic sympathectomy for Raynaud's phenomenon.
- Metoclopramide, is apride, H_2 blockers and esophageal dilation for gastrointestinal symptoms.
- NSAIDs, calcium channel blockers, prednisone, bronchial lavage, for cardiopulmonary symptoms.
- Splints for contractures and deformities.
- Heat and cold application is needed.
- D-penacillamine and colchicine used to decrease collagen with some success.

CREST SYNDROME

This is variant of scleroderma classified by the extent of skin thickening. It has more favorable prognosis and less organ involvement. Sclerosis may range from a diffuse cutaneous thickening with rapidly progressive and fatal visceral involvement to more benign variant called CREST SYNDROME (Calcinosis, Raynaud's phenomenon, esophageal hypermotility Sclerodactyly) Skin changes of the (fingers) and Telangiectasia (macule-like angioma on the skin).

Clinical Manifestation

- Calcinosis (result of chronic vascular insufficiency): Intracutaneous or subcutaneous calcification on digital pads, particular tissues, extensor surfaces of forearms, olecranon and prepatellar bursae.
- Raynaud's phenomenon.
- Esophageal dysmotility.
- Sclerodactyl.
- Telangiectaria.
- Pulmonary involvement in many patients.

Management

Treatment as for scleroderma. Surgical removal of calcium deposits.

SJÖGREN'S SYNDROME

Sjögren's syndrome is characterizedly autoantibodies to two protein-RNA complexes termed SS-A/Ro and SS-B/La. The clinical manifestations are caused by inflammation and dysfunction of the exocrine glands particularly the salivary and lacrimal glands, which result in dryness of the mouth, eyes and mucus membrane. Lymph nodes, bone marrow and organ involvement is present. RA is 50 percent of patients.

The clinical manifestations include xerostomia, dyspareunia, decreased tearing, gritty sensation in eyes, dysphagia, dental caries, cough, enlarged parotid glands, rheumatoid and antinuclear antibody factor, positive in most patients and anemia.

Ophthalmalogical examination (Schimer's Test) salivary flow rates and lower lip biopsy of minor salivary glands confirm the diagnosis. The treatment is symptomatic including:

- Instillation of artificial tears as often as necessary to maintain adequate hydration and lubrication.
- Vaginal lubrication with a water soluble product such as K-Y jelly may increase comfort during intercourse.
- Surgical punctal acclusion.
- Increased fluid intake, especially with meals.
- Good dental and oral hygiene especially after meals.
- Avoidance of respiratory infections.
- Increased humidity in home and work environment.
- Corticosteroids and immunosuppressive drugs are indicated for treatment of pseudolymphoma.

POLYMYOSITIS/DERMATOMYOSITIS

Polymyositis (PM) is a chronic acquired inflammatory disorder of skeletal muscle. When a characteristic skin rash is present, this disorder is called "dermatomyositis" (DM). Both are diffuse inflammatory myopathies of striated muscle, producing symmetric weakness usually most severe in the proximal muscle (e.g. trunk, shoulder and hip).

Etiology

The etiology of both disorders is unknown, but abnormal reaction of the immune system have been implicated, perhaps triggered by virus. Autoantibodies are found in the serum of affected muscle. These disorders occur twice as frequently in women as in men; usually occurs in the fifth and sixth decades of life.

Pathophysiology

Both polymyositis and dermato/polymyosits are characterised by inflammation of muscle fibers and connective tissues, resulting in extensive tissue necrosis and destruction of muscle fibers. Both cell-mediated and humoral immune mechanisms are associated with the diseases. Inflammatory cells found at the perimysical and perivascular sites contain B cell and helper T cells in dermatomyositis. Less vascular involvement occurs in polymyosites and B and T cells are found in surrounding the muscle fibers and foscicles.

Clinical Manifestation

The initial symptoms of both disorders are similar to those associated with any inflammatory response: Fever, swelling, malaise and fatigue. The diseases which run a course of exacerbations and remissions are usually first noted in proximal muscles in particular, the pelvic and shoulder girdles. The weakness is symmetric. Climbing stairs, raising from a chair and other activities that involve lifting the body becomes increasingly difficult or impossible. Lifting the arm becomes progressively more difficult, and hair combing may be impossible. Other muscles such as the neck flexors and the muscles of swallowing may also be involved. Muscle pain or tenderness is present in some instances in early stages.

Clinical manifestations of both disorders include dysphagia, dyspnea, decreased esophegeal motility, cardiomyopathy and Raynaud's phenomenon. A dusky red lesions may be found in the preorbital region (heliotype) along with preorbital edema in persons with dermatomyositis. This dusky red rash may extend over the face, forehead, neck, upper shoulders, chest and upper back. Scaly lesions on the arms and legs commonly affect the exterior surfaces. Ertythema occurs over the metacarpophalangeal and proximal phalangeal joints. Calcinosis can also occur in dermatomyosisis. The weakness of myositis, if it persits, can lead to contractures and atrophy.

Management

Diagnosis is based on the following:

- History and physical examination including manual muscle test to delineate weakness in specific muscles.
- Electromyogram to delineate a specific pattern of findings to differentiate polymyositis from other types of muscle disease.
- Muscle biopsy to define specific pathological changes in muscle.
- Serum enzyme levels (creatine phosphokinase, lactate dehydrogenase, aldolase) which are elevated in the presence of active disease.
- 24-hour urine test to determine abnormal creatine/creatinine ratio.

Treatment includes high dose corticosteroid therapy (Prednisone upto 60 mg daily). If steroid therapy contraindicated, or ineffective, an immunosuppressant such as methotrexate is prescribed. Cyclophosphamide has been used effectively in some patients and hydroxychloquine may improve rash in persons with dermatomyositis.

Nursing responsibilities include the following:

- *Promoting comfort*
  - During acute episodes, assist with frequent changes of position.
  - Administer prescribed analgesics.
  - Assist with ADL.
  - Provide adequate rest.
- *Promoting mobility*
  - Elevate sitting surfaces to facilitate transfer.
  - Provide appropriate ambulatory device to facilitate comfortable walking.
  - Provide for frequent changes of positive and ROM to prevent contraction.
  - Encourage patient to gradually resume independent ADL as symptoms subside.

- Refer patient to physical therapy for exercise program.
- *Preventing skin breakdown*
  - Reposition patient frequently.
  - Assess skin for integrity.
  - Topical steroids may be prescribed for the rash in persons with dermatomyositis.

In addition, patient should have a thorough understanding of the chronic nature of the disorders, the usefulness and the side effects of all prescribed medications and the importance of regular medical care and serial laboratory testing.

FIBROMYALGIA SYNDROME (FMS)

Fibromyalgia is a musculoskeletal chronic pain syndrome, is characterized by fatigue, stiffness, myalgias, arthralgias, headache, irritable bowel syndrome and sleep disturbance. It has association with arthritis and other rheumatic disorder as discussed earlier. Other generalized pain syndrome affecting musculoskeletal system include polymyalgia rheumatica which often occurs with giant cell arteritis.

Etiology

The etiology is unknown; but there is an association between sleep disturbance and fibromyalgia. Muscle microtrauma and imbalance of neurotransmitters have also been implicated as possible causative factors. Trauma or infection may trigger the onset of symptoms. Symptoms typically occur between the ages of 20-40 years, mainly in women (80%).

Pathophysiology

FMS may appear with RA or SLE or other pain syndrome like polymyalgia rheumatica. Several abnormalities in muscles have been documented in persons with FMS, including lower ATP and ADP levels, higher levels of AMP and changes in the number of capillaries and fiber area. Increased muscle tenderness may be the result of generalized pain intolerance perhaps as a result of CNS abnormalities.

Clinical Manifestations

The characteristic symptom of fibromyalgia is a generalized chronic pain, which may be described as "burning or gnawing". Chronic aching, nonrestorative sleep, morning stiffness and fatigue are commonly reported patients with FMS demonstrate loss of functional abilities similar to patient with RA. Yet no radiographic changes in articular structures are found in FMS. Temporomandibular joint dysfunction, premenstrual symptoms, and mitral valve prolapse may also accompany the disorder. Cognitive disturbances such as memory problems (brain fog) or difficulty in concent rating are common. Depression, anxiety and feelings of hopelessness often result because of the nature of chronic nature of FMS. There is no visible signs of FMS. Headaches, sensitivity to extreme temperature, abdominal pain, paresthesias, menstrual irregularities, irritable bowel and difficulty in concentration may be reported.

Management of FMS

The diagnosis of FMS is made by the presence of typical symptoms and the location of tender points. Eighteen points, tender in normal persons have been identified than one hypersensitive in persons with FM. The diagnostic criterion for FM is a history of widespread pain and the presence of at least pain in 11 of 18 specific tender points sites when palpated (digital palpations) is significant for diagnosis. Bilateral tender point sites are:
- Occiput – Suboccipital muscle insertion.
- Cervical – Low cervical-anterior aspects of the intratransverse spaces C5-C7.
- Trapezius – Midpoint of the upper border.
- Scapular – Supraspinatus-above the medial border of the scapular spine.
- Epicondyle – lateral epicondyle 2 cm distal to the epicondyles.
- Gluteal – Upper outer quadrants of buttocks.
- Trocanter – Greater tochanter-posterior to the trochantic prominence.
- Medial knee–Medial fat pad proximal to the joint line.
- Second rib–Second costochondrial junctions.

FMS may be localized to a specific region of the body (often termed "myofascial pain) or generalized with migratory tender points. Myofascial pain most often involves the posterior neck, lowback, shoulder and chest.

Treatment of FM is symptomatic and requires a high level of patient motivation. The nurse can play a key role in educating the patient to be an active participant in the therapeutic regimen. Pain, aching, and tenderness can be helped by rest and NSAIDs are effective for some patients. Stress, fatigue, and sleep disturbance can be helped by low-dose tricyclin antidepressants (e.g. mitriptyline, imipramine, or trazodone, muscle relaxants, stress management and stress reduction techniques, deep relaxation and a healthful diet. One of the most beneficial approaches to reducing symptom, FM is to encourage patient participation in safe, moderate and exercise programme (e.g. swimming, walking). In addition, gentle stretching exercises, yoga, massage therapy, or tai chai may be helpful. Other treatments that may be effective include heat in the form of whirlpools. Moist packs or hot shower, acupuncture and acupressure.

INFECTIOUS BONE DISEASES

Osteomyelitis

Osteomyelitis is an infection of bone by direct or indirect invasion of an organism. The two types of osteomyelitis are classified by the mode of entry of the pathogen, i.e. exogenous and hematogenous osteomyelitis.

Etiology

- Exogenous osteomyelitis or as described by the Waldragel system as secondary to a contagious source of infection, is caused by a pathogen from outside the body. Examples include pathogens from an open fracture or surgical procedure, involving instrumentation. The infection is also caused by human and animal bites and fist blows to the mouth. The most common organism found in human bite is "*Staphylococcus aureus*" and in animal bites is "*Pasteurella multicida*. The infection spreads from the soft tissues to the bone. Risk factors for developing exogenous osteomyelitis are chronic illness, diabetes, alcohol or drug abuse, and immunosuppression. In diabetes or vascular disease, osteomyletis occur in the feet.
- Hematogenous osteomyelitis is caused by blood-borne pathogen originating from infectious site within the body. Examples include sinus, ear, dental, respiratory and genitourinary infections. In hematogenous osteomyletis the infection spreads from the bone to the soft tissues and can even break through the skin, becoming a draining fistula. This type of osteomyelitis is common in infants, children and elderly persons. The most common organism is *S. aureus* and other organisms are streptococcus B. *Haemophilus influenzae Salmonella* and gram-negative bacteria.

Pathophysiology

In hematogenous osteomyelitis the organisms reach the bone through the circulatory and lympatic systems. The bacteria lodged in the small vessels of the bone, triggering an inflammatory response. Blockage of the vessels causes thrombosis, ischemia and necrosis of the bone. The femur, tibia, humerus and radius are commonly affected. Infections of the pelvic organs frequently spread to the pelvic and vertebrae. Bone inflammation marked by edema, increased vasculature, and leucocytes activity exudate seals the bone canaliculi, extends into the metaphysics and marrow cavity and finally reaches the cortex. New bone laid down over the infected bone by osteoblasts is termed "involucrum". Opening in the involucrum allows infected material to escape into soft tissues. The infectious process weakens the cortex, thereby increasing risk of pathological fracture. 'Bordies abscesses' are characteristics of chronic osteomyelitis. These are isolated encapsulated pockets of micro-organisms surrounded by bone matrix, usually found in long bones. These pockets of virulent organisms are capable of reinfections at any time. The microscopic channels found in bone allow bacteria to proliferate without being affected by body defences. In patient with osteomyelitis the infection begins in the soft tissues disrupting muscles and connective tissues and eventually forming absciss. Acute osteomyelitis left untreated or unresolved after 10 days is termed chronic osteomyelitis.

Clinical Manifestation

Acute oesteomyelitis refers to the initial infection or an infection of less than one month in duration. The clinical manifestation of acute osteomyelitis are both systemic and local. Systemic manifestations include fever, night sweats, chills, restlessness, nausea and malaise. Local manifestation includes severe bone pain that is unrelieved by rest and worse with activity; swelling, tenderness, and warmth at infection site; and restricted movement of affected part. Later signs include drainage from sinus tracts to the skin and fracture site.

Chronic oesteomyelitis refers to a bone infection that persists for longer than 4 weeks or an infection that has failed to respond to the initial course of antibiotic therapy. Chronic type can represent either a continuous, persistent problem or a process of exacerbations and aquiescence. It results from inadequately treated acute osteomyelitis. Pus accumulation causing ischemia of the bone. Over time, granulation tissue turns to scar tissue. This avascular scar tissue provides an ideal site for bacterial grown and is impenetrable to antibiotics.

Management

Diagnosis based on the following:

- A culture and sensitivity test of the drainage (wound) will reveal the causative organisms and identify appropriate antibiotics.
- Blood tests reveal an increase in WBCs, ESR, C-reactive probe levels.
- Blood cultures will determine the presence or absence of septicemia.
- Radiological signs suggestive of osteomyelitis, after the appearance of clinical symptoms.
- MRI, CT scan, Gallium scan are also given usefully to confirm diagnosis.

The goals of treatment of osteomyelitis are:

- Complete removal of dead bone and affected soft tissue.
- Control of infection.
- Elimination of dead space (after removal of necrotic bone).

Many modes of treatment are available. Use of treatment modality is used depends on the area of bone involved. Causative organism, ability to maintain a functional limb, duration of treatment and expected outcomes. Treatment options include:

- Antibiotic therapy: Intravenous antibiotics may be prescribed for upto 6 weeks and oral antibiotic therapy may continue for upto 6 months, e.g. ciprofloxacin and ofloxacin.

- Irrigation and drainage systems: This involves a surgical procedure in which holes are drilled into the cortex of the bone, allowing continuous infusion of antibiotic solution and drainage of inflammatory exudate. Drains are usually removed after a few days to prevent secondary infection.
- Analgesics and antipyretics as necessary.
- Hyperbaric oxygen therapy may be used as an adjunctive therapy.

When conservative modalities fail to control the infection, surgical intervention is indicated. Many types of surgery are possible from simple debridements to amputation.

Nursing management of patient with osteomyelitis includes the following:
- Using aseptic technique during dressing changes.
- Observing the patient for signs and symptoms of systemic infection.
- Encouraging range of motion exercises to prevent contrctures and flexion deformities.
- Administering antibiotics on time and as prescribed.
- Administering analgesics and/or antipyretics as prescribed and monitoring patient for effectiveness.
- Promoting rest of affected joint or limb. The affected limb should be handled carefully to avoid pathological fracure. Splints are often used for immobilization.
- Encouraging participation in ADL to fullest extent.
- Instructing the patient in correct use of assistive devices as needed.

In addition, patient/family education is to be given by the nurse regarding follow up measures of treatment modalities.

LOW BACK PAIN

Low back pain (LBP) is one of the most common conditions a nurse will encounter in practical setting. Although a common disorder, LBP is also a challenge to health care professionals as the problem is worldwide.

Etiology

Several risk factors are associated with low back pain, including lack of muscle tone and excess weight, poor posture, smoking and stress. Jobs that require repetitive heavy lifting, vibration (e.g. Jackhammer operator) and prolonged period of sitting are also associated with LBP. Pain in the lumbar region is common problem because this area:
- Bears most of the weight of the body.
- Is the most flexible region of the spinal column.
- Contains nerve roots that are vulnerable to injury or disease and
- Has an inherently-poor biochemical structure.

Low back pain is most often due to musculoskeletal problem. However, other causes such as metabolic, circulatory, gynecologic, urologic, or psychologic problems, which may refer pain to the lower back, must not be overlooked. The causes for low back pain of musculoskeletal origin include:
- Acute lumbosacral strain.
- Instability of lumbosacral bony mechanism.
- Osteoarthritis of the lumbosacral vertebrae.
- Intervertebral disk degeneration and
- Herniation of the intervertebral disk.

There are two varieties of low back pain, i.e. acute low back pain and chronic low back pain.

Acute Low Back Pain

Acute low back pain is usually associated with some type of activity that causes undue stress on the tissues of the lower back. Often symptoms do not appear at that time of injury but develop later because of gradual increase in paravertebral muscle spasms. Few definitive diagnostic abnormalities are present with paravertebral muscle strain. The straight leg raise test may produce pain in the lumbar area without radiation along the sciatic nerve. If muscle spasms are not severe, the patient may be treated on outpatient basis with a combination of the following:
- Analgesics.
- NSAIDs.
- Muscle relaxants (cyclobenzaprine)
- Use of corset. A corset prevents rotative, flexion and extension of lower back.

If spasms and pain are severe, a brief period of rest at home may be necessary. Since paravertebral muscle spasms are worse when the patient is upright, bed rest is the prime treatment for severe acute low back pain. Bathroom previliges are usually allowed. Bedrest is maintained until patient can move and turn from side to side with minimal discomfort. At this time, gradually increasing activity is initiated. When the patient is comfortable on oral pain medication, a progressive therapy program is begun to regain mobility and strength in lower back structures. If conservative treatment is ineffective, the cause of the pain is nerve root irritation, and epidural corticosteroid infection may be performed.

The nurse should assess the patient' use of body mechanics and offer advice when activities could produce back strains are used. Some 'Do nots' 'Dos' for low back problem are as follows:

Do Nots
- Lean forward without bending knees.
- Lift anything above level of elbow.
- Stand in one position for prolonged time.
- Sleep on abdomen or on back or side with legs outstraight.
- Exceed prescribed amount and type of exercise without consulting health care provider.

Do
- Prevent lower back from straining forward by placing a foot on step or stool during prolonged standing.
- Sleep in a side-lying position, knees and hips bent.
- Sleep on back with a lift under knees.
- Sit on a chair with knees higher than hips and support arms on chair or knees.
- Exercise 15 minutes in the morning and 15 minutes in the evening regularly, begin exercises with a 2 or 3 minutes warm-up period by moving arms and legs, by alternately relaxing and tightening muscles, exercise slowly with smooth movements as directed by the physical therapist.
- Avoid chilling during and after exercising.
- Maintain appropriate body weight.
- Use a lumbar role or pillow for sitting.

Some exercises to strengthen the back as follows:
- Knee to chest lift (to stretch hip, buttocks, lower back muscles).
  - Lie on back on the floor with knees bent and feet flat on floor.
  - Draw both knees upto chest.
  - Place both hands around knees and pull them firmly against chest. Hold for 30 seconds.
  - Lower legs and return to starting position.
  - Repeat 5-10 times.
- Simple leg lift
  - Lie flat on back on floor with left knee bent and left foot flat on floor.
  - Raise right leg as high as comfortably as possible.
  - Hold for counting upto 5.
  - Slowly return leg to floor.
  - Bend right knee and put right foot flat on floor.
  - Raise left leg and hold for 5 counts.
  - Repeat 5-10 times for each leg.
- Double leg lift
  Lie flat on back.
  - Slowly lift legs until feet are 12 inches from the floor.
  - Keep legs straight and hold this position for counting upto 10.
  - Lower legs to floor.
  - Repeat five times.
- Pelvic tilt
  - Lie flat on back on floor with knees bent and feet on the floor.
  - Firmly tighten your buttock muscles.
  - Hold for counting upto 5.
  - Relax buttocks.
  - Repeat 5-10 times.
  - Be sure to keep lower back flat against floor.
- Half sit ups (to strengthem abdominal muscles)
  - Lie flat on floor on back with knees bent, feet flat on floor and hand on chest.
  - Slowly raise head and neck to top of chest.
  - Reach both hands forward and place them on knees.
  - Hold for counting upto 5.
  - Return to starting position.
  - Repeat 5-10 times.
- Elbow Props (to extend lower back)
  - Lie face down with your arms beside your body and your head turned to one side.
  - Stay in this position for 2-5 minutes, making sure that you relax completely.
  - Remain face down and prop yourself on your elbows.
  - Hold this position for 2-3 minutes.
  - Return to starting position and relax for one minute.
  - Repeat 5-10 times.
- Hip tilts
  - Lie flat on back with knees bent.
  - Slowly bend legs and hips to one side as far as possible.
  - Bend to other side.
  - Repeat five times.
- Toe touches
  - Stand straight and relaxed.
  - Lower head and body and try to touch floor with finger tips.
  - Keep knees straight.
  - Do not jerk or lunge towards floor.
  - Bend only as far as you can.
  - Repeat the some for 5 times.

Chronic Low Back Pain

The causes of chronic low back pain include degenerative disk disease, lack of physical exercise, prior injury, obesity, structural and postural abnormalities, and systemic disease.

Pathophysiology

The pathophysiology includes common causes of back pain, such as herniated disc, spinal stenosis, and spondylolisthesis. If disk-herniation is the cause of back pain, the pain comes from the irritated dura and spinal nerves as the nucleus purposes lacks intrinsic innervation can arise from the joint capsule, ligaments, or muscles in the lumb spine. The ligamentous structures of the lumbar spine are richly supplied with pain receptors and are susceptible to tears, sprains and fracture. Muscle sprains and strains are also common causes of backpain.

Clinical Manifestation

The most common feature of a lumbar herniated intervertebral disk in backpain with associated buttock and leg pain along with distribution of the sciatic nerve (radiculopathy). Specific manifestations based on the level of lumbar disk herniation which include:

- L3-L4 – Subjective pain. Back to buttock to posterier thigh to inner calf.
- L4-L5 – Subjective back to buttock to dorsum of foot and beg toe.
- L5-S1 – Subjective back to buttock to sole of foot and heel.

Straight leg raise test may be positive. Back or leg pain may be reproduced by raising the leg and flexing the foot at 90 degrees. Reflex may be depressed or absent, depending on the spinal nerve root involved. Paresthesia or muscle weakness in the legs, feet, or toes may be reported by the patient. If the disk ruptures in the cervical area, the clinical manifestations are stiff neck, shoulder pain radiating to hand, and parasthesias and sensory disturbances of the hand.

Management of Chronic Low Back Pain (CLBP)

Diagnosis made on the basis of the following:
- History and physical examination with emphasis on neurologic deficits and straight leg raising.
- CT Scan-MRI, myelogram, diskogram, EMG. Somato-sensory evoked potential.

Degenerative disk disease is managed by conservatively with rest, limitation of spinal involvement (corset) local heat or ice, ultrasound, transcutaneous electrical nerve stimulation (TENS) and NSAIDS, analgesic muscle relaxants diathermy, thermotherapy, physical therapy. If conservative treatment is unsuccessful, radiculopathy becomes progressively worse, or there is documented loss of bowel or bladder control (Cauda equina), surgery may be indicated. The common surgical procedure includes:
- Laminectomy with or without spinal fusion.
- Diskectomy.
- Percutaneous lateral diskectomy.
- Spinal fusion with or without instrumentation.

Patients who have undergone spinal surgery require vigilant postoperative care. Nursing intervention is aimed at maintaining proper alignment of the spine at all times until healing has occurred.
- Flat bedrest may be maintained for 1 to 2 days depending on the extent of surgery.
- Logrolling patients when turning is essential to maintain proper body alignment.
- Pillows can be used under the thighs of each leg when supine and between the legs when in side lying position to provide comfort and ensure alignment.
- Severe muscle spasms in the surgical area can be managed with medication and with correct turning and positioning.
- The nurse must offer reassurance to the patient that proper technique is being used to maintain body alignment.
- Watch for severe headache or leakage of CSF if it is so reported.
- Frequent monitoring of peripheral neurologic signs of the extremities is a routine postoperative nursing responsibility after spinal surgery. Movements of arms and legs and assessment of sensation be unchanged when compared with preoperative status.

The patient should be instructed to avoid sitting or standing for prolonged periods. Activities that should be encouraged include walking, lying down, and shifting weight from one foot to the other, when standing. The patient should learn to think through an activity before starting any potentially injurious task such as bending, lifting, or stopping. Any twisting movement of spine is contraindicated. A firm mattress or bedboard is essential.

Degenerative Disorders of Spine

Degenerative disease of the spine is a common but difficult problem. The spine has been intervertebral disk joints and 46 posterior facets joints. The intervertebral disks are composed of an outer layer of cartilage called the anulus fibrosus and an inner layer of the cartilage called nucleus pulposure. Several common problems arise with the structures in degenerative disease of the spine. These include degenerative disc disease, herniated vertebral disk, spinal stenosis, spondylolisthesis and spondylosis.

Etiology

Degenerative disc disease develops as a result of biochemical and biomechanical changes in the intervertebral discs. The gelationous mucoid material of the nucleus pulosus is replaced with fibrocartilage as a result of aging. Spinal stenosis, occurs as a result of aging, degenerative disc disease, spondylosis, oesteophyte formation or a congenial condition. The disc space is narrowed, losing its resiliency, and may be unstable at the affected levels. Smoking is a risk factor for the development of disc degeneration and herniation. Other risk factors include sedantary lifestyle and extensive motor vehicle driving. Heredity plays a role in spondylosis, occurring more frequently in conjunction with other congenital spine defects.

Pathophysiology

Pathophysiological changes associated with degenerative disc disease include spinal stenosis (narrowing of the spinal canal), spondylosis (degeneration and stiffness of the vertebral joints), subluxation and vertebral degeneration. Initial disc changes are followed by facet arythropathy, osteophyte formation and ligamentous instability, myelopathy osteophyte formation and ligamentous instability. Myelopathy and radiculopathy (disease involving a spinal nerve root) may follow. The degenerative process usually involves synovitis, which causes cartilage erosion, leading to the formation of osetophytes.

Herniated intervertebral disk is a protrusion of the nucleus purpose through a tear or rupture in the anulus. Herniation occurs anterior, posterior or laterally. Extrusion of the disk material may impinge on a nerve root or on the spinal cord. Herniation occurs in cervical spine (C-5-6, C-6-7), (C4-5), lumbar spine (L5-S1 and L-4-5) levels. It may be the result of trauma, sudden or sharp material or degeneration.

Spinal stenosis is narrowing of the spinal cord or intervertebral foramine at any level, creating pressure on the involved nerve root (s) resulting in neurological symptoms.

Spondylolisthesis is a forward slipping of one vertebra on another. It can be a congenital abnormality or be caused by degenerative changes trauma or bone disease.

Clinical Manifestation

Herniated intervertebral disk shows following possible signs and symptoms.

Cervical

- Decreased range of motions of cervical spine.
- Paresthesia of upper extremities, depending on nerve root involved.
- Weakness or atrophy of upper extremity musculature, depending on level involved.
- Pain in affected nerve root distribution.
- Abdominal reflex activity.
- May have motor or sensory disturbances in lower extremities.

Lumbar

- Sciatica.
- Tenderness or pain with palpation of disk spaces and sciatic notch.
- Painful and/or decreased range of motion of lumbar spine.
- Motor and sensory impairment in affected nerve root distribution (may note discrepancies in calf circumference, weakness in lower extremity, muscle groups, pain and numbness in dermatomal distribution).
- Decreased or absent reflexes.
- Bowel or bladder impairment.
- Positive straight leg raising (Laseques test): Straight leg raising with opposite leg flat will produce a leg pain or radicular symptoms).
- Pain radiating down by in dermatomal distribution.
- Pain relieved by lying down.

Spinal stenosis resulting neurological symptoms. In spondylolisthesis, pain weakness and/or bowel and bladder involvement are seen. The slip may be detected when the spinous processes are palpated.

Management

Diagnostic tests to determine defects in the spine include X-ray films, myelography, CT scanning, and MRI, Conservative management degenerative disorders of spine includes NSAIDs, avoidance of alcohol or aspirins (Leads to GI irritation and bleeding) and prolonged use of narcotic analgesics risk of depending oral corticosteroids helps to relieve pain and skeletal muscle relaxants may be used if necessary.

MANAGEMENT OF SPINAL SURGERY

Postoperative Care of the Patient with Lumbar Spinal Surgery:
- Positioning
  - Head of the bed is kept flat.
  - Patient is encouraged to legroll to change position from side to back to side.
  - Use of turning sheet is advised until patient can assist with turning.
- Neurological checks to assess motor and sensory functions.
- Wound care (drain placed in wound to prevent hematoma formation SOS):
  - Maintain constant suction through drain as required.
  - Maintain drain free of contamination.
  - Monitor excessive output from drains. Output ranges from 20 to 250 ml/8 hours for the first 24 hours, tapers for 12 hours postoperatively and usually is removed 24 to 36 hours postoperatively. Drains that allow reinfusion of serous drainage may be used.
  - Inspect surgical area frequently for evidence of excess drainage or formation of hematoma (bulging of tissues surrounding surgical site).
  - If a spinal fusion has been done, inspect donor site (usually iliac crest) for drainage, hematoma.
- Promoting comfort:
  - Reposition patient frequently.
  - Administer narcotic medications as needed; gradually reduce to non-narcotic analgesics as patient tolerates.
  - Monitor use and effectiveness of PCA pump if ordered.
  - Use fractured bedpan.
- Promoting mobility:
  - Activity out of bed varies. Patient with fusion may need bedrest for 1 to 2 days.
  - Transfer patient out of bed with a little time spent in the sitting position as possible.
    - Start transfer with patient in a side-lying position at the edge of the bed.

- Have the patient push off the bed with the uppermost hand and the lowermost elbow.
- One person assists by guiding the patient's trunk and another assists the patient's leg, over the side of the bed.
- Reverse process for return to bed.
  - The patient may be permitted to walk as much as tolerated with an assistive aid if necessary.
  - Braces or corsets, if prescribed, and applied before the patient gets out of bed.
  - Encourage patient to participate in ADL within prescribed limits of mobility.
- Discharge instructions:
  - Do not lift or carry anything heavier than 2.25 kg (5 lb).
  - Do not drive a car until permitted by surgeon.
  - Avoid twisting motions of the trunk.

Postoperative Care of the Person

Cervical Surgery

- Positioning
  - Keep head of bed elevated 30 to 45 degrees, particularly if anterior surgical approach was used, to decrease swelling in throat and facilitates respirations.
  - If patient is cervical brace, position is not restricted except by patients tolerance.
  - If patient is in cervical traction, patient may be turned side to back to side to patient's tolerance.
- Promoting safety
  - Assess airway and respiratory function frequently. Airway may be compromised by swelling.
  - Provide suction equipment and tracheotomy set in patient's room until swelling in throat subsides and patient is swallowing and breathing normally.
  - Check adjustment screws and straps frequently to ensure there is no loosening of the brace.
  - Advise physician or orthotist of loosening of the brace consequent to decrease in edema, so brace can be readjusted.
- Wound care
  - Inspect surgical areas, including iliac crest donor site, frequently for evidence of excess drainage or formation of hematoma. Use icebag to donor site for comfort.
  - If tong or halo traction is being used, pin care may be required.
- Promoting comfort and reducing pain
  - Provide ice chips to soothe sore throat.
  - Make progressive diet changes slowly; patient will have difficulty in swallowing and will be afraid of smoking. Full liquids or semisolids (ice cream, custards, jelly, nectars) are often better tolerated than clear juice or broth; however, milk products may increase mucous production.
  - Administer analgesics as for any patient having spine surgery. Donor sites often cause more discomfort than does neck incision.
  - Patient may require aerosol treatment or humidifications of air to loosen mucus secretions or make breathing more comfortable.
- Promoting mobility.
  - If a patient is in traction, encourage patient to perform ankle dorsiplanar flexion exercises and quadriceps setting on a regular basis to promote circulation and maintain leg strength.
  - If patient is in brace, out of bed activity, inducting walking, it may begin as soon as patient tolerates.
  - Provide temporary use of walker if donor site pain restricts mobility.
  - Encourage patient to participate in ADL to greatest extent possible.
  - Report any difficulty with brace to physician immediately.
  - Do not drive a car during period that brace must be worn.
  - Report symptoms of graft dislodgingment (dysphagia and a feeling of "fulness" in the throat).

Postoperative Care of the Person with Thoracic Spinal Surgery

Same as for lumbar surgery with the following additions and exceptions.

- Positioning
  - Head of bed may often be elevated to 30 degrees.
- Wound care
  - If pleural cavity entered, a chest tube will be inserted and must be managed postoperatively.
- Promoting comfort.
  - Assist patient to splint chest while coughing.
- Promoting mobility.
  - Encourage and assist patient in vigorous pulmonary hygiene measures.
  - Discourage patient from vigorous pulling or pushing with the arms because weight bearing through the arms poses a threat to the integrity of the graft.
  - Brace is routinely prescribed and must be applied before patient is allowed out of bed.
  - Permit patient to perform whatever activities are comfortable within the limitation of the brace.
  - Encourage patient to participate in ADL within prescribed limits of mobility.
- Discharge instructions.
  - Apply and remove the brace before getting out of bed.

– Wear the brace whenever out of bed, assess skin under brace.

Complications associated with general anesthesia and important consideration after surgery. These include complications such as atelectorsis, paralytic ileus, and urinary retention. Infection is a complication associated with the operative procedure. When instrumentation is used, the risk for infection increases. There is also a risk for hardware failures. Complication of the procedure, postoperative include dural tear, CSF leakage, blood loss, hypovolemia, decreased cardiac output hematoma formation, infection, instruments or graft failure, pseudoarthosis loss of correction deformity, persistent pain, neurological problem, DVT pulmunary embolism, fluid volume overload, and fat embolism.

SCOLIOSIS

There were two types of scoliosis viz. nonstructural and structural.

1. *Nonstructural scoliosis* is also termed postural or functional and is caused by posture pain, leg length inequality and other factors. This form of scoliosis is usually easily corrected either by exercise or by removing the underlying causes. An important distinction is the absence of vertebral rotation. However, untreated nonstructural scoliosis can progress to structural scoliosis.
2. *Structural scoliosis* involves a rotational deformity of the vertebrae. It is further divided into three major categories.
   – Congenital scoliosis (Present at birth) occurs as a result of vertebral malformation in foetal life (accounts for 15 percent).
   – Neuromuscular scoliosis result as a consequence of several diseases.
   – Idiopathic scoliosis has an unknown cause but genetic factors have been lined to the development of disease.

Etiology

- Congenital
- Neuromuscular
  – Cerebral palsy.
  – Charcot-Marie - Tooth disease.
  – Syringomyelia.
  – Spinal cord injury.
  – Poliomyelitis.
  – Myelomenigocele.
  – Muscular dystrophy.
  – Neurofibromatosis.
  – Marfan's syndrome.
- Idiopathic
  – Infantile: 0 to 3 years of age.
  – Juvenile: 3 to 10 years of age.
  – Adolescent: Older than 10 years of age.

Pathophysiology

Scoliosis may develop in localized areas of the spinal column or involve the whole spinal column. Curvatures may be 'S' Shaped or 'C' shaped. The earliest pathological changes begin in the soft tissues. Muscles and ligaments shorten on the concave side of the curve, progressing to deformities of the vertebrae and ribs. In skeletally immature persons, vertebral formations occur as asymmetrical forces are applied to the epiphysis by the shortened and tight soft tissues structures on the concave side of the curve.

Deformities are classified by magnitude, direction, location and etiology. Curve direction is designated by the convex side or the curve. The degree of rotation of the curve is important, because, it determines the amount of impingement on the rib cage. The amount of compression and twisting depends on the position of the vertebrae in the curve. The force of compression is greatest on the apical vertebrae, which becomes the most deformed. Deformity progresses quickly-during skeletal growth and slows later in life, but the greater increase in the curfacture may occur in adult life. Gravity and increase in upper body weight may increase in the deformity in adulthood.

Clinical Manifestation

The person can initially have slight, mild, or severe deformity. Early deformity may not be obvious except on specific examination. In the early stages, the person may note that clothing does not fit correctly or hand evenly, because the height of shoulders is uneven. Pain is not usually an accompanying factor. Persons affected with structural scoliosis may exhibit asymmetry of hip height, pelvic obliquity tilting of the pelvis from the normal horizontal positions; inequalities of shoulder height, scapular prominence; rib prominence; and rip humps which are posterior, unilateral humpings of rib cages visible on forward bending.

In severe cases, cardiopulmonary and digestive functions may be affected because of compression or displacement of internal organs. Total lung capacity, vival capacity and maximum voluntary ventilation are decreased in persons with scoliosis. Cardiac output may be compromised. Significant deviations in the balance of the curve may also affect gait patterns. Right thoracic, right thoracic and lumbar, and right thoracolumbar curves are most common or idiopathic scoliosis. A compensatory durve may develop, allowing the head to be centered over the pelvis. In general, compensatory curves are of less degree, more flexible and less rotated.

Management of Scoliosis

A complete radiological examination of the spine is performed, curve angles, flexibility and degree of vertebal rotation are calculated. Radiographs also help to determine skeletal maturity. In severe case, pulmonary function studies also indicated. Treatment of scoliosis depends on the individual patient and the degree of lateral curvature:

- Early or postural scoliosis may be amenable to postural exercises or exercise combined with traction. Cotrelis traction which is a combination of a cervical head halter with 5 to 7 1b and pelvic traction with 10 to 20 1b may be used.
- When the curve is flexible (less than 40°) and the patient is cooperative, bracing in combination with exercise may be sufficient to correct the deformity (e.g. Milwaukee brace, Rissar Caster, halofemoral or halopelvic traction). Maintaining the ideal weight is consideration in reducing the stress on the spine. The patient should be advised against weight gain, especially if bracing is prescribed, because the brace is specifically fitted and contoured to the individual. The brace can usually accomodate a 10 1b gain or loss.
- Transcutaneous electrical muscle stimulation may be used to stimulate the muscle on the convex side of the curve. Repeated stimulation strengthens the muscle and pulls the spine into alignment. The patient usually uses the stimulator at night.

Surgery is indicated for patients when conservative treatment has failed to halt curve progression for those with severe progressing curves, intractible pain, or compromised pulmonary function or for cosmesis. Many individuals with neuromuscular scoliosis are unable to walk. Surgical corection sometimes performed in these patients to facilitate the ability to transfer or to increase sitting ability or tolerance. Surgical correction is usually involves a posterior approach to the spine with instrumentation and bony fusion. The complication of scoliosis fusion are similar to spinal surgery discussed earlier. Nursing management of the patient with scoliosis correction is similar to spinal surgery discussed earlier.

COMMON HAND AND FOOT PROBLEMS

Hand's Problem

Dupuytren's Contracture

Dupuytren's contracture is a progressive condition maked by hypertrophic hyperplasia of the Palmar fascia that results in a flexion of the distal palm and fingers.

The causes of this contracture is not known. A familar tendency has been noted. And it is associated with diabetes, epilepsy, alcoholism, penile lesions (Peyrobie's disease), and hyperplasia of the plantar fascia (Lederhoses disease). Pathophysiology of this is not completely understood the contracture may take upto 20 years to reach maximum deformity. Depends upon the severity of the deformity and hand dominance, the patient may experience difficulty in gasping objects. Burning pain may accompany attempts at grasping. Usually main complaints are deformity and mild interference with hand function.

Surgery is the preferred method of treatment. Persons with fixed flexion contractures of 30° or more at the metacarpophalangeal or proximal interphalangeal joints are persons for surgery. Surgical repair involves regional fasciectomy or subtotal palmar fasciectomy to allow the patient full motion. Surgical repairs is performed as in outpatient procedure. The most common complication is hematoma and inadequate skin closure. The nursing intervention focuses on postoperative care which includes:

- Elevating hand to control swelling.
- Checking fingers for circulation, sensation and movement of every 1 to 2 hours.
- Administering prescribed analgesics as necessary to maintain comfort.
- Encouraging active extension of fingers.
- Encouraging patient to use hand in self-care activities after 2 to 3 days.

Foot Problem

The foot is the platform that provides support for the weight of the body and absorbs considerable shock in ambulations. It is a complex structure composed of bony structures, muscles, tendons and ligaments. It can be affected by congenital conditions; structural weakness; traumatic injuries; and systemic conditions. Diabetes mellitus, (DM), Rheumatid Arthritis (RA).

Forefoot

- *Hallux valgus (Bunion):* Hallux valgus is the lateral angulation of the proximal phalanx on the metatarsal head of the great toe. It is a painful deformity of great toe consisting of great toe towards second toe, bony enlargement depending upon the degree of angulation, prominence of the medial eminence may occur resulting bunion deformity.
    - Conservative treatment includes wearing shoes with wide forefeet or bunion pocket and use of bunion pads to relieve pressure on bursal sac and NSAIDS for pain relief.
    - Surgical treatment is removal of bursal sac and bony enlargement and correction of lateral angulation of great toe may include temporary or permanent internal fixation.
- Hallux rigidus is a painful stiffness of first metatorsophalangeal joint caused by osteoarthritis or local trauma.
    - Conservmative treatment includes intra-articular corticosteroids and passive manual stretching of first metatorsophalangeal joint. A shoe with a stiff sole decreases pain in the joint during walking.
    - Surgical treatment is joint fusion or arthoplasty with silicone rubber implant.

- *Hammer toe:* It is the deformity of second through fifth toes including dorsiflexion of metatarsophalangeal joint, plantar flexion of proximal interphalangeal joint, and callus on dorsum of proximal interphalangeal joint and end of involved toe complaints related to hammer toe include burning of the bottom of foot and pain and difficulty in walking when wearing shoes.
  - Conservative treatment consists of passive manual stretching of proximal interphalangeal joint and use of metatorsal arch support.
  - Surgical correction consists of resection of base of middle phalanx and head of proximal phalanx and bring raw bone and together. Kirschner wire maintains straight position.
- *Mortons neuroma (Mortons toe or plantar neuroma):* It is neuroma in webspace between third and fourth metatorsal heads causing sharp, sudden attacks of pain and burning sensation. Surgical excision is usual treatment.

Midfoot

- Pes Planus (flat foot) is a loss of metatarsal arch causing pain in foot or leg. Symptoms are relieved by use of resilient longitudinal arch supports. Surgical treatment consists of triple arthrodesis or fusion of subtular joint.
- Pes Cavus is the elevation of the longitudinal arch of foot of arch. Treatment is manipulation and casting (in patients of younger than 6 years of age); Surgical correction is necessary if it interferes with ambulation (in patient older than 6 years of age).

Hindfoot

- Painful heels complaint of heel pain with weight bearing. Common cause plantar bursitis or calcaneal spur in adult. Treatment includes:
  - Corticosteroids are injected locally into inflammed bursa and sponge rubber heel cushion is used.
  - Surgical excision of bursa or spur is performed.

Local Problems

- Corn is a localized thickening of skin caused by continual pressure over bones prominences, especially metatarsal head, frequently causing localized pain. Treatment incldues:

  Corn is softened with warm water or preparation containing salicyl acid and trimmed with razor blade or scalpal. Pressure on bony prominences caused by shoes is relieved.
- Soft corn is painful lesion caused by bony prominences of one toe pressing against adjacent toe; usual location in web space between toes, softness caused by secretions keeping web space relatively moist. Here pain is relieved by placing cotton between toes to separate them. Surgical treatment is excision of projecting bone spur (if present).
- *Callus:* A similar formation to corn but covering of wider area and usual location on weight-bearing part of foot. Treatment is as for corn.
- *Plantar Wart:* A painful papillomatus growth caused by virus that may occur on any part of the skin or sole of foot. Treatment is excision with electrocoagulation or surgical removal is done. Ultrasound may also be used.

Nursing Management of Common Foot Problems

Much of the pain, deformity and disability associated with foot disorders can be directly attributed to or accentuated by improperly fitting shoes, which causes an angulation of the toes and inhibition of the normal movement of foot muscles. The purposes of footwear are to:
- Provide support, foot stability, protection, shock absorptions and a foundation for orthosis.
- Increase friction with the walking surface and
- Treat foot abnormalities.

For which well-constructed and properly fitted shoes are essential for healthy, pain-free feet. Fashion styles especially for women often influence selection of footwear instead of consideration of comfort and support. Patient education should stress the importance of having shoe that comforms to the foot rather than to current fashion trends. To prevent feet problems good foot care is essential. Then education should be given to patient and family by the nurse concerned as follows:

In addition to recognizing common problems, there are many that the person can do to promote healthy feet and prevent feet problems. Nurse has to advise the person, that measures as follows:
- Walk regularly: This will improve circulation. Increase flexibility and encourage bone and muscle development. Walking is very important for maintaining over all foot health.
- Always wear comfortable shoes that provide proper support. The shoes should be sufficiently wide and have low enough heels so that person feels no leg fatigue, leg or foot cramps or pain.
- Advise to massage their (persons) feet to improve circulation and promote relaxation of the feet at least daily.
- If person (Patient) have bunions, wear shoes that are extra-long and wide, this will help ease pressure on thick toes. In addition, used donut shaped bunion cushions, or (mole skin) to take pressure off of the joints.
- Wear heel pads or cushions in the bottom of their (affected persons) shoes to provide theri heels if they walk on hard surfaces for long times.

- Advise to wash their feet every day in warm water. Dry them by blotting with a towel, rather than rubbing.
- If their (affected persons) feet perspire a lot, ask them to dust their feet with talcum or hygienic foot powder. They may also sprinkle some powder into their shoes. Do not use cornscratch powder because it may lead to fungal infection.
- Advise them to trim their nails shortly after they have taken a bath or shower, while they are soft, cut the nail across with a toenail cliper.
- Advise them that they do not go barefoot outdoors especially in area that is not theirs own or a yard. A foreign body may cut or puncture their feet.
- Inspect themselves their feet every day against dust, blisters, and scratches. Provide care as needed and observe for proper heeling.

Many foot problems require surgery. When surgery is performed, the foot is usually immobilized by a bulky dressing shortly cast, slipper (plaster) cast, or a platform shoe that fits over the dressing and has a rigid sole (bunion foot). The foot should be elevated with the head off the bed to help reduce discomfort and prevent edema. Neurovascular status should be assessed postoperatively and routine nursing intervention to be performed accordingly as in other similar surgery.

MUSCULOSKELETAL TUMORS

Tumors may arise from any of the structures of the musculoskeletal system. The type of tumor is determined and classified by the tissue of origin. Tumors can be benign or malignant and can affect both adults and children. The common tumors of musculoskeletal system are:

- *Bone:* Osteoma (benign), osteosarcoma (malignant).
- *Cartilage:* Osteochondroma, enchondroma, periosteal chondroblastomas are benign and chondrosarcomas malignant.
- *Fibrous:* Fibroma (benign) fibrosarcoma (malignant).
- *Bone marrow:* Giant cell (benign). Ewing's sarcoma and myeloma are malignant.
- *Uncertain cell:* Unicameral bone cyst, and aneurysmal bone cyst. Brief description of the common tumors are as follows:
  - Osteosarcoma exhibits a moth-eaten pattern of bone destruction with poorly-defind margins. Osteoid and callus produced by the tumor invades and resorbs normal cortical bone. The tumor erodes through the cortex and periosteum and eventually invades soft tissue. Metastasis to the lungs is common. It mostly affects the long bones of the extremities and pelvis.

    The clinical manifestation of oesteosarcoma are usually associated with a past history of minor injury and gradual onset of pain and selling especially line around the (knee of femur) initial complaint is often described as dull, aching, and intermittent, but the pain rapidly increases in intensity and duration. Night pain is common. Other frequent complaints include generalized malaise, anorexia and weight loss.

    The diagnosis confirmed from biopsies, tissue specimen, elevation of serum alkaline, phosphates calcium levels, X-ray, CT scan and MRI findings.

    Treatment of surgical excision. Preoperative chemotherapy is used to decrease tumor size. Surgical excision (amputation) is the procedure, necessary depending on the size and location of the tumor.
  - Osteochondroma is characterized by
    - Compromise of cancellous bone with cartilaginous cap.
    - Develops during growth periods at metaphysis of bone.
    - Also appears in tendens.
    - May limit joint motion and may recur.

    Surgical excision is choice of treatment.
  - Enchondroma is characterized by:
    - Destruction of cancellous bone.
    - Usually occurs in humerous or fingers.
    - Can cause pathological fracture.
    - May become malignant, especially in long bones or pelvis.

    Surgical excision with wide margin, if not amputation is the treatment.
  - Chondrosarcoma. The characteristics of chondrosarcomas include:
    - Usually affects persons 50-70 years of old.
    - Comprises 20 percent of all bone tumors.
    - Affects males more than females.
    - Slow growing, insidious onset.
    - Most common in humerouses femur and pelvis.
    - Local pain, swelling.
    - May have palpable mass.
    - Serene persistent pain.
    - May infiltrate joint space and soft tissue.
    - May metastasize to lung tissue and may recur.

    Treatment: Surgical excision; amputation.
  - Fibrosarcoma
    - Usually affects persons 30-50 years old.
    - Affects females more than males.
    - Occurs in bony fibrous tissue of femur and tibia.
    - Comprises 4 percent of primary malignant bone tumor.
    - May result from radiation therapy, paget's disease or chronic osteomyelitis.
    - Night pain, swelling possible palpable mass.

- May cause pathological fracture.
- May metastaxises to lungs.

Treatment: wide surgical excision, amputation.

- Gaint Cell Tumour (osteoclastoma)
  - Usually affects ages 20-40 years.
  - Affects females more than males.
  - Comprises 4-5 percent of all benign bone tumors.
  - Appears in epiphysical area, destroys bone matrix and can invade soft tissues.
  - Commonly found in femur, tibia or humerus.
  - Dull aching night pain.
  - Limitation of motions.
  - Swelling.
  - High incidence of recurrence.

Treatment: Wide excision; May require bone graft and amputation.

- Myeloma, Multiple Myeloma (Multifocal)
  - Poor prognosis
  - Common in persons 40 years above.
  - Affects males more than females.
  - Comprises 27-1 bone tumors.
  - Neoplastic proliferation of plasma cells.
  - Causes cortical and medullary bone lysis and infiltrates bone marrow.
  - Aching, intermittent pain in spine, pelvis, ribs, or sternum.
  - Pain increased with weight-bearing.
  - May complain of weight loss, malaise, anorexia.
  - Causes pathological fracture.

Treatment: Palliative treatment. Radiation, chemotherapy.

- Osteoma
  - Usually affects persons of 10-20 years old.
  - Comprises 20 percent of benign tumor of bone.
  - Slow growth.

Treatment is only symptomatic and then excision.

MUSCLE TUMORS

- Leiomyoma: Affects smooth muscles, usually uterus, there will be palpable mass and tenderness. Treated by surgical excision.
- Rhabdomyoma is rare, affects straightened muscle, cause tenderness. Usually treated by surgical excision.
- Leomyosarcoma affects smooth muscle, usually uterus, stomach and small bowel. This radical growth treated by surgical excision with wide margin and radiation and chemotherapy are also used.
- Rhabdosarcoma affects straightened muscle, usually inguinal, popliteal or gluteal areas. There is slow-growing mass and tenderness, treated with radiation, surgical excision and chemotherapy.

NURSING MANAGEMENT OF BONE TUMOR

The patient with bone tumor should be assessed for the location and severity of pain. Weakness caused by anemea and increased debility may be noted. Swelling at the involved site and decreased joint function depending on the tumor site should also be monitored. The possible nursing diagnosis for these patients include:

- Pain related to the disease process, inadequate pain medication or comfort measures.
- Impaired physical mobility related to disease process, pain, weakness and debility.
- Body image disturbance, related to possible amputation, deformity, swelling and effects of chemotherapy.
- Anticipatory grieving related to poor prognosis of the disease.
- Risk for injury (Pathological fracture) related to diseased process and inadequate handling or positioning of the effected body parts.

Nursing care planning and implementation are taken accordingly on the basis of nursing diagnosis in addition to routine preparation and assistance. (Please refer to Oncological Nursing Chapter).

METABOLIC BONE DISEASES

Normal bone metabolism is dependent on adequate intake, absorption and use of calcium, phosphorous, protein, and vitamins. When there is dysfunction in any of these critical factors, generalized reduction of bone marrow may result. Metabolic bone diseases affect the normal hemeostatic functioning of the skeletal system. The etiology of metabolic bone diseases include hormonal, genetic and dietary factors. Common metabolic bone diseases include rickets, osteomalacia, osteoporosis, osteitis, deforman (Paget's disease).

Osteomalacia

Osteomalacia is an uncommon disorder of adult bone associated with vitamin D deficiency, resulting in decalcification and softening of bone. This disease is the same as rickets in children, except that epiphysical growth plates are closed in the adult. Vitamin is required for the absorption of calcium from the intestines. Insufficient vitamin D intake can interfere with the normal minimalization of the bone causing failure or insufficient calcification of bone, which results in softening of bone pain and deformities.

Etiology

Etiological factors development of osteomalacia, include lack of exposure to ultraviolet rays, gastrointestinal malabsorption, extensive burns, chronic diarrhea, pregnancy, kidney disease, medication such as phenytoin (Dilantin).

Clinical Manifestation

- Persistent skeletal pain, especially while bearing weight.
- Low back pain.
- Progressive muscular weakness.
- Weight loss.
- Progressive deformities of the spine (kyphosis) or extremities.
- Fractures are common and demonstrate delayed healing when they occur.
- Decreased serum calcium or phosphorus.
- Elevated serum alkaline phosphates.
- X-rays demonstrate the effects of generalized bone demineralization especially calcium in the bone of the pelvis and pressure associated with bone deformity.
- Looser's transformation zones (ribbons of recalcification in bone found on X-ray).

Management

Collaborative care for osteomalacia is directed towards corrections of the underlying cause. Vitamin D (Cholecalciferol) is usually supplemented, and the patient often shows a dramatic response, calcium or phosphorus intake may also be supplemented.

Paget's Disease (Osteitis Deformans)

Sir James Paget, an English surgeon first described this disorder also called 'osteitis deformans'. It is skeletal bone disorder in which there is excessive bone resorption followed by replacement of normal marrow by vascular, fibrous connective tissue, and new bone that is larger, disorganized and weaker.

Etiology

The etiology of Paget's disease is unknown. But genetic predisposition is identified in 15 to 30 percent. Probably a autosomal dominant pattern of inheritance. And other causative theories include autoimmune dysfunction vascular disorder, vitamin D deficiency in childhood, and mechanical stressors to bone. It may be due to viral infection. The average age (50 to 60 years). It occurs most often after the fourth decade of life and most commonly in men.

Pathophysiology

The axial skeleton is usually affected by Paget's disease, particularly the vertebrae and skull, although the pelvis, femur and tibia are the common sites of disease. Initial changes in this disorder involve an increase in osteoclast mediated resorption of cancellous bone, in addition to an increase in osteoblast mediated bone formation. Bone resorption and formation are increased, resulting in mosaic-like mix of abnormal women and normal lamellar bone. Mineralization may encroach into the marrow and excessive bone formation usually occurs around partially resorbed trabeculae, causing thickening and hypertrophy. Vascularity is increased at affected portions of the skeleton. Lesions may occur in one or more bones, but the disease does not spread bone to bone. Deformities and bony enlargements often occur. Deformities of bone caused by unexplained abnormal focal remodelling with structurally uneven bone. As stated earlier, the region of the skeleton commonly affected are the pelvis, long bones, spine, ribs, sternum and cranium. Bowing of the limbs and spinal curvature may occur in persons with advanced disease.

Clinical Manifestation

In milder forms of Paget's disease, patients may remain free of symptoms and the disease may be discovered incidentally on X-ray or serum chemistry.

The initial clinical manifestations are usually insidious development of skeletal pain (which may progress to severe intractible pain), complaints of fatigue, and progressive development of a waddling pain. Patients may complain that they are becoming shorter or that their heads are becoming larger.

Bone pain is the most common symptom. Degenerative arthritis may occur at adjacent joints. Microfractures, cortical swelling, and lytic bone lesions contribute to the pain. Pain is usually worse with ambulation or activity, but may also occur at rest. Involved bones may feel spongy and warm due to the increased vascularity. Weight-bearing bones such as tubia and femur may become deformed and pressing gait will be affected.

Skull pains usually accompanied by headache, warmth tenderness and enlargement of the head. Flattening of the base of the skull or platybasia may result in serious complication of the obstructive hydrocephalus or brain stem compression. Facial bone involvement may cause deformity or less frequently affect the airway. Conductive and/or sensorineural hearing loss may develop due to otosclerosis or neurological abnormalities.

Pathological fractures are a problem, because of the increased vascularity of invovled bone, bleeding is potential danger. Lytic lesions of the long bones are the most susceptible to fracture.

Longstanding disease may lead to malignate transformation usually osteosarcoma, fibrosarcoma, and benign giant cell tumor. Most common sites for malignancy are the pelvis, femur and humerous.

Features of Paget's Disease and the Bone

Musculoskeletal Manifestation

- Bone and joint pain (may be in a single bone) that is aching, poorly described, and aggraved by walking.
- Low back and sciatic nerve pain.
- Loss of normal spinal curvature.
- Enlarged, thick skull.
- Pathological fracture.
- Osteogenic sacroma.

Skin Manifestation

Flushed, warm skin.

Other Manifestation

- Apathy, lethargy and fatigue.
- Hyperparathyroidism.
- Chronic calcium deficiency
- Urinary or renal stones.
- Heart failure from fluid overload.

Laboratory Finding

- Elevated levels of alkaline phosphates due to osteoblastic activity
- Serum calcium usually normal except with generalized disease immediately.

Management of Paget's Disease

Radiography of individual with Paget's disease will reveal radiolucent areas in the knee, typical fo increased bone resorption. Deformities and fractures may also be present. A bone scan is indicated at diagnosis to determine the extent of disease.

Management of Paget's disease is usually limited to sympatomatic and supportive care and correction of secondary deformities by either surgical implementation or braces. The goals of treatment are to relieve pain and prevent fractures and deformity. Asymptomatic patient generally does not require treatment.

Bone resorption, relief of acute symptoms, and lowering the serum alkaline phosphatase levels may be significantly influenced by administration of calcitonin, which inhibits the osteoclastic activity. Biphosphonates such as alendronates (posamax) tiludronate (skelid), risedronate (actonel), and pamidronate (aredia) are nonhormonal agents are effective in reducing the bone resorption. The biphosphonates and calcitonin are effective agents and effective in reducing the bone resorption. The biphosphonates and calcitonin are effective agents to decrease bone pain and bone warmth, and may analgesic and NSAIDs also be in practice.

Radiation therapy and local surgical procedures such as periosteal stripping may be used for the control of the patient's pain. A firm mattress should be used to provide back support and to releive pan. The patient may be required to wear a corset or light brace to relieve back pain and provide support when in the upright position. The patients should be proficient in the correct application of such devices knowhow to regularly examine areas of the skin for friction damage. Activities such as liffting and twisting should be discouraged. Good body mechanics are essential. Analgesics and muscle relaxants may be administered to relieve pain. A properly balanced nutritional program is important in the management of metabolic disorders of bone, especially pertaining to vitamin D, calcium and protein, which are necessary to ensure the availability of the components for bone formation. Preventive measures such as patient education, use of assistive device, and environmental changes should be actively pursued to prevent falls and subsequent fractures.

OSTEOPOROSIS

Osteoporosis or porous bone is a condition characterized by low bone mass and structural deterioration of bone tissue, leading to increased bone fragility. This metabolic bone disease is the major cause of fractures (especially hip, spine and wrist) in postmenopausal women and older adults in general.

Etiology

The exact etiology of osteoporosis is unknown, several risk factors have been identified as follows:

- *Aging:* Osteoporosis is increasing in incidence, because more people are getting into an older age, usually occurs at over 65 years of age in both sex.
- *Sex:* Osteoporosis is eight times more common in women than men for several reasons:
  - Women tend to have lower calcium intake than men throughout their lives.
  - Women have less bone mass because of their generally smaller frame.
  - Resorption begins at an earlier age in women and is accelerated at menopause.
  - Pregnancy and breastfeeding depletes a woman's skeletal reserve unless calcium intake is adequate
  - Longevity increases the likelihood of osteoporosis and women live lower than men.
- *White race:* Caucasian or Asian-American.
- Family history of osteoporosis.
- Nulliparity.
- *Diet low in calcium:* Chronic calcium deficiency and vitamin D deficiency.
- Sedentary lifestyle: An inactive lifestyle.
- Small frame, low body weight. Thin and small-framed.
- Diet high in protein and fat.

- *Excessive use of alcohol:* Chronic alcohol use.
- Excessive caffeine intake.
- Excessive cigarette smoking.
- Postmenopausal including early or surgically-induced menopause.
- History of anorexia, nervosa or bulimia, chronic liver disease or malabsorption.
- Long-term use of corticosteroids, thyroid replacement and antiseizure medications.

Osteoporosis is redefined as Type I (Postmenopausal) and Type II and further classified as primary or secondary. Primary, osteoporosis is the more common form; has no underlying pathological condition. Secondary osteoporosis results from another cause or medical condition. The causes of secondary osteoporosis are as follows:

- *Endocrine disorder:* Diabetes, Cushing syndrome, hyperparathyroidism, parathyroidism, hypogonadism, prolactinoma.
- *Rh. Arthritis drug-induced:* Glucocorticoids, heparin, chronic use of phosphate binding antacids, loop diuretics, anticonvulsants, barbiturates, lithium and chemotherapy.
- *Disuse:* Prolonged immobilization (Prolonged bedrest, immobilization of limb by casting or splinting), paraplegia, Quadriplegia and lower motor neuron disease.
- *Chronic illness:* Sarcoidosis, cirrhosis, renal tubular acidosis.
- *Cancer:* Multiple myeloma, lymphoma, leukemia.
- Malabsorption syndrome.
- Anorexia nervosa.
- Prolonged parenteral nutrition.
- Alteration in gastrointestinal and hepatobiliary functions.

Pathophysiology

Bone is continually being deposited by osteoblasts and resorbed by osteoclasis, a process called remodelling. Normally, the rate of bone deposition and resorption are equal to each other. So, the total bone mass remains constant, i.e. in the process of normal bone remodelling, bone formation equals bone resorption. An osteoporotic state develops if bone resorption exceeds bone formation (bone deposition). Age-related bone loss begins in both sexes approximately at the age 40 years. Women experience a 35 to 40 percent loss in trabecular bone and upto 60 percent of cancellous bone stores, in contrast; men lose only about two-third of that amount throughout life. By the time a person reaches the age of 75 years, the skeletal mass is reduced 50 percent. From age 30 level, the skeleton continues to lose bone mass at the hip and appendicular skeleton, even after the age of 80 years. Although resorption affects entire skeletal system, osteoporosis occurs most commonly in the bones of the spine, hips and wrists.

Overtime, wedging and fractures of the vertabrae produce gradual loss of height and a humped back known as dowager's hump or khyposis. The usual first signs are back pain or spontaneous fractures. The loss of bone substance causes the bone to become mechanically weakened and prone to either spontaneous fractures from minimal traumas.

Clinical Manifestation

Osteoporosis is often called the "silent thief" and the silent disease, because bone loss occurs without symptoms. People may not know they have osteoporosis until their bones become so weak that a sudden strain, bump, or fall causes a hip, vertebral or waist fracture.

Many fractures related to osteoporosis occur without the patient's knowledge, although some are associated with excrutiating pain. The earliest manifestation of oesteoporosis may be an acute onset of back pain in the mid to low thoracic region as a result of vertebral fracture, occurring at rest with minimal activity. Vertebral fracture can involve the entire vertebrae (compression) or portion, usually the anterior section (wedge). Anterior compression fracture of thoracic vertebrae may cause "dowager's hump" or thoracic khyphosis. Loss of height and protruding abdomen (due to pressure on abdominal viscera) are associated with conditions. Eventually lower rib cage may rest on iliac crest, paravertebral muscle spasm often occurs, but neurological deficits are rare with spontaneous vertebral compression. These postural changes may affect exercise tolerance and food tolerance. The patient will report early satiety and bloatedness. The patient's body image may also be affected as a result of the spinal deformity and collapsed vertebrae may initially be manifested back pain, loss of height, or spinal deformation such as kyphosis or severely stooped posture. Later on, distal radial fractures (Colles' fracture), fracture of the proximal femur and osteoporotic hip fracture occur.

Management

The risk for fracture can be assessed by the patient's risk factors and history and measured precisely with non-invasive diagnostic tools. Measurements of bone mineral deficiency (BMD) and biochemical markers of bone resorption are the basic tools for diagnosis of oesteoporosis.

The goal of pharmacological therapy for persons with osteoporosis is to prevent further bone loss and to decrease risk of fractures which includes:

- Calcium supplements.
- Vitamin D supplements
- Diet high in calcium.
- Exercise program. All four arm/leg lifts, the elbow prop. prone press-ups with deep breathing, standing back band, Isometric posture corrections. Standing and pelvic tilt.
- Oestrogen replacement therapy.
- Calcitonin.
- Biphosphonates—Etidonate (Didronel), Alendronate (Fosamax).
- Raloxifene (Evista).

Surgical intervention is necessary to repair some fractures.

CHAPTER 12

Nursing Management of Immunological Problems

INTRODUCTION

The term immunity refers to the body's specific protective response to an invading foreign agent or organism. In other words, immunity is a state of responsiveness to foreign substance such as microorganisms and tumor proteins. The immune system functions as the body's defense mechanism against invasion and allows a rapid response to foreign substance in a specific manner. Immune response serve three functions:

1. *Defense:* The body protects against invasion by microorganisms and prevents the development of infection by attacking foreign antigen and pathogens.
2. *Homeostasis:* Damaged cellular substances are digested and removed. Through this mechanisms, the body's different cell types remain uniform and unchanged.
3. *Surveillance:* Mutations continually arise in the body but are normally recognized as foreign cells and destroyed.

Immune response occur at genetic and cellular levels. Any qualitative or quantitative change in the components of the immune system can produce profound effect, on the integrity of the human organism. Immune function is affected by a variety of factors such as central nervous system integrity, emotional status, medications, and the stress of illness, trauma or surgery dysfunctions involving the immune system occur across the lifespan. Many are genetically based; others are acquired.

Immune memory is a property of immune system that provides protection against harmful microbial agents despite the timing of re-exposure to the agent. Tolerance is the process by which the immune system is programed to eliminate foreign substances such as microbes, toxins, and cellular mutations but maintain the ability to accept self-antigens. Some evidence is given to the concept of surveillance in which the immune system is in a perpetual state of vigilance, screening and rejecting any invader that is recognized as foreign to the hast.

The term 'immunopathology' refers to the study of diseases than result from dysfunctions within the immune system. Disorders of the immune system may stem from excesses or deficiencies of immune competent cells, alteration in the functions of these cells, immunologic attack on self-antigens, or inappropriate or exaggerated responses to specific antigens.

To gain insight into immunopathology and the growing number of immunologic disorders, and to assess and care of people with immunologic disorders, the nurse needs to understand the immune system and how it functions; to recognize its importance in understanding disease processes, and to apply this knowledge in making appropriate patient care decisions.

Review of Immune System

The immune system is composed of an integrated collection of various cell types, each with a designated functional role in defending against infection and invasion by other organisms. Supporting this system are molecules that are responsible for the interactions, modulations and regulation of the system. These molecules and cells participate in specific interactions with immunogenic **epitopes** (antigenic determinants) present on foreign materials and initiate a series of actions in a host, including the inflammatory response, the lysis of microbial agents, and the disposal of foreign toxins. The major components of the immune system include the bone marrow and the lymphoid tissues, including the thymus gland, the spleen, the lymph nodes, the tonsils and adenoids, and similar tissues in the gastrointestinal, respiratory and reproductive systems.

Bone marrow: The WBCs involved in immunity are produced in the bone marrow. Like other blood cells, lymphocytes are generated from stem cells, which are undifferentiated cells. Descendants of **stem cells** become lymphocytes—the B-lymphocytes (**B-cells**), and the T-lymphocytes (**T-cells**), B-lymphocytes mature in the course bone marrow and then enter the circulation. T-lymphocytes move from the bone marrow to the thymus, where they mature into several kinds of cells with different functions.

Lymphoid tissues: The spleen, composed of red and white pulp, acts somewhat like a filter. The red pulp is the site where old and injured red blood cells (RBCs) are destroyed. The white pulp contains concentrations of lymphocytes. The lymph nodes are distributed throughout the body. They are connected by lymph channels and capillaries, which remove foreign material from the lymph system before it enters the bloodstream. The lymph nodes also serve as centers for immune cell proliferation. The remaining lymphoid tissues contain immune cells that defend the body's mucosal surfaces against microorganisms.

Types of Immunity

There are two general types of immunity: natural (innate) and acquired (adaptive). Natural immunity is a nonspecific immunity that is present at birth. Acquired or specific immunity develops after birth. Natural immune responses to a foreign invader are very similar from one encounter to the next, regardless of the number of times the invader is encountered: in contrast, acquired responses increase in intensity with repeated exposure to the invading agent. Although each type of immunity has a distinct role in defending the body against harmful invaders, the various components usually act in an interdependent manner.

Natural Immunity

The natural (innate) system provides rapid nonspecific immunity and is present at birth. Because of its nonspecificity, it has a broad spectrum of defense against and resistance to infection. Natural (innate) immunity provides a nonspecific response to any foreign invader, regardless of the invader's composition. The basis of this defense mechanism is the ability to distinguish between friend and foe or "self" and "nonself". Natural (innate) immunity co-coordinates the initial response to pathogens through the production of cytokines and other effector molecules, which either activate cells for control of the pathogen (by elimination) or promote the development of the acquired immune response. The cells involved in this response include macrophages, dendritic cells, and natural killer (NK) cells, which have the ability to recognize and respond to a wide variety of pathogens long before the development of antigen-specific acquired immunity. the early events in this immune response are critical in determining the nature of the adaptive immune response. Innate immune mechanisms can be divided into two stages: immediate (generally occurring within 4 hours) and delayed (occurring between 4 and 96 hours after exposure).

White blood cell action: Cellular response is key to the effective initiation of the immune response. WBCs or leukocytes, participate in both the natural and the acquired immune responses. Granular leukocytes, or granulocytes (so called because of granules in their cytoplasm), fight invasion by foreign bodies or toxins by releasing cell mediators, such as histamine, bradykinin, and prostaglandin's, and engulfing the foreign bodies or toxins. Granulocytes include neutrophils, eosinophils, and basophils.

Neutrophils (also called polymorphonuclear leukocytes, or PMNs, because their nuclei have multiple lobes) are the first cells to arrive at the site where inflammation occurs. Eosinophils and basophils, other types of granulocytes, increase in number during allergic reactions and stress responses. Nongranular leukocytes include monocytes or macrophages (referred to as histocytes when they enter tissue spaces) and lymphocytes. Monocytes also function as **phagocytic cells**, engulfing, ingesting and destroying greater numbers and quantities of foreign bodies or toxins than granulocytes do. Lymphocytes, consisting of B-cells and T-cells, play major roles in humoral and cell-mediated immune responses. About 60 to 70% of lymphocytes in the blood are T-cells, and about 10 to 20% are B-cells.

Inflammatory response: The inflammatory response is a major function of the natural immune system that is elicited in response to tissue injury or invading organisms. Chemical mediators assist this response by minimizing blood loss, walling off the invading organism, activating phagocytes, and promoting formation of fibrous scar tissue and regeneration of injured tissue. The inflammatory response is facilitated by physical and chemical barriers that are part of the human organism.

Physical and chemical barriers: Activation of the natural immunity response is enhanced by processes inherent in physical and chemical barriers. Physical surface barriers include intact skin, mucous membranes, and cilia of the respiratory tract, which prevent pathogens from gaining access to the body. The cilia of the respiratory tract, along with coughing and sneezing responses, filter and clear pathogens from the upper respiratory tract before they can invade the body further. Chemical barriers, such as mucus, acidic gastric secretions, enzymes in tears and saliva, and substances in sebaceous and sweat secretions, act in a nonspecific way to destroy invading bacteria and fungi. Viruses are countered by other means, such as interferon. **Interferon**, one type of biologic response modifier, is a nonspecific viricidal protein that is naturally produced by the body and is capable of activating other components of the immune system.

Immune regulation: Regulation of the immune response involves balance and counterbalance. Dysfunction of the natural immune system can occur when the immune components are inactivated or when they remain active long after their effects are beneficial. A successful immune response eliminated the responsible antigen. Immunodeficiencies are characterized by inactivation (e.g., asthma, allergy, arthritis) are characterized by persistent inflammatory responses. The immune system recognition of one's own tissues as "foreign" rather than as self is the basis for many autoimmune disorders. Despite the fact that the immune response is critical to the prevention of disease, it must be well controlled to curtail immunopathology. Most microbial infections include an inflammatory response mediated by T-cells and cytokines, which in excess, can cause tissue damage. Therefore, regulatory mechanisms must be in place to suppress or halt the immune response. This is mainly achieved by the production of cytokines and transformation of growth factor that inhibits macrophage activation. In some cases, T-cell activation is so overwhelming that these mechanisms fail and pathology results. Research on **immunoregulation** holds the promise of preventing graft rejection and aiding the body in eliminating cancerous or infected cells.

Acquired Immunity

Acquired (adaptive) immunity–immunologic responses acquired during life but not present at birth – usually develops as a result of prior exposure to an antigen through immunization (vaccination) or by contracting a disease, both of which generate a protective immune response. Weeks or months after exposure to the disease or vaccine, the body produces an immune response that is sufficient to defend against the disease on re-exposure. In contrast to the rapid but nonspecific innate immune response, this form of immunity relies on the recognition of specific foreign antigens. The two components of the immune response are strongly interrelated. Events occurring early in injection dictate the direction of the adaptive response and activate the acquired immune effector mechanisms, which have a direct feedback on the cells of the innate (natural) system. The acquired immune response is broadly divided into two mechanisms: the cell-mediated response, involving T-cell activation, and effector mechanisms, involving B-cell maturation and production of antibodies.

The two types of acquired immunity are known as active and passive. In active acquired immunity, the immunologic defenses are developed by the person's own body. This immunity typically lasts many years or even a lifetime. Passive acquired immunity is temporary immunity transmitted from a source outside the body that has developed immunity through previous disease or immunization. For example, immune globulin or antiserum, obtained from the blood plasma of people with acquired immunity, is used in emergencies to provide immunity to diseases when the risk for contracting a specific disease is great (e.g., after exposure to hepatitis) and there is not enough time for a person to develop adequate active immunity. Immunity resulting from the transfer of antibodies from the mother to an infant in utero or through breast-feeding is another example of passive immunity. Active and passive acquired immunity involve humoral and cellular (cell-mediated) immunologic responses.

Response to Invasion

When the body is invaded or attacked by bacteria, viruses, or other pathogens, it has three means of defense:
1. The phagocytic immune response
2. The humoral or antibody immune response
3. The cellular immune response

The first line of defense, the phagocytic immune response, involves the WBCs (granulocytes and macrophages), which have the ability to ingest foreign particles. These cells move to the point of attack, where they engulf and destroy the invading agents. Phagocytes also remove the body's own dying or dead cells. Cells in necrotic tissue that are dying release substances that trigger an inflammatory response. Apoptosis, or programmed cell death, is the body's way of destroying worn out cells such as blood or skin cells or cells that need to be renewed. Apoptosis involves the digestion of DNA by endonucleases, which results in targeting of the cells fro phagocytosis. Unlike macrophages, eosinophils are only weakly phagocytic. On activation, eosinophils probably kill parasites by releasing specific chemical mediators into the extracellular fluid. Additionally, eosinophils secrete leukotrienes, prostaglandins, and various cytokines.

A second protective response, the **humoral immune** response (sometimes called the **antibody** response), begins with the B-lymphocytes, which can transform themselves into plasma cells that manufacture antibodies. These antibodies are highly specific proteins that are transported in the bloodstream and attempt to disable invaders. The third mechanism of defense, the **cellular immune response**, also involves the T-lymphocytes, which can turn into special cytotoxic (or killer) T-cells that can attack the pathogens.

The structural part of the invading or attacking organism that is responsible for stimulating antibody production is called an **antigen** (or an immunogen). For example, an antigen can be a small patch of proteins on the outer surface of a microorganism. Not all antigens are naturally immunogenic; some must be coupled to other molecules to stimulate the immune response. A single bacterium or large molecule, such as a diphtheria or tetanus toxin, may have several antigens, or markers, on its surface, thus inducing the body to produce a number of different antibodies. Once produced, an antibody is released into the blood stream and carried to the attacking organism. There, it combines with the antigen, binding with it like an interlocking piece of a jigsaw puzzle. There are four well-defined stages in an immune response: recognition, proliferation, response, and effector.

Recognition stage: Recognition of antigens as foreign, or non-self, by the immune system is the initiating event in any immune response. The body must first recognize invaders as foreign before it can react to them. The body accomplishes recognition using lymph nodes and lymphocytes for surveillance. Lymph nodes are widely distributed internally throughout the body and in the circulating blood, as well as externally near the body's surfaces. They continuously discharge small lymphocytes into the bloodstream. These lymphocytes patrol the tissues and vessels that drain the areas served by that node.

Lymphocytes recirculate from the blood to lymph nodes and from the lymph nodes back into the bloodstream, in a never-ending series of patrols. Some circulating lymphocytes can survive for decades. Some of these small, hardy cells maintain their solitary circuits for a person's entire lifetime.

The exact way in which circulating lymphocytes recognize antigens on foreign surfaces is not known: however, recognition is thought to depend on specific receptor sites on the surface of the lymphocytes. Macrophages play an important role in helping the circulating lymphocytes process the antigens. Both macrophages and neutrophils have receptors for antibodies and complement; as a result, they coat microorganisms with antibodies, complement, or both, enhancing phagocytosis. The engulfed microorganisms are then subjected to a wide range of toxic intracellular molecules. When foreign materials enter the body, circulating lymphocytes come into physical contact with the surfaces of these materials. Upon contact with the foreign material, lymphocytes, with the help of macrophages, wither remove the antigen from the surface or obtain an imprint of its structure, which becomes important in subsequent re-exposure to the antigen.

In a streptococcal throat infection, for example, the streptococcal organism gains access to the mucous membranes of the throat. A circulating lymphocyte moving through the tissues of the throat comes in contact with the organism. The lymphocyte, familiar with the surface markers on the cells of its own body, recognizes the antigens on the microbe as different (nonself) and the streptococcal organism as antigenic (foreign). This triggers the second stage of the immune response – proliferation.

Proliferation stage: The circulating lymphocyte containing the antigenic message returns to the nearest lymph node. Once in the node, the sensitized lymphocyte stimulates some of the resident dormant T- and B-lymphocytes to enlarge, divide, and proliferate. T-lymphocytes differentiate into cytotoxic (or killer) T-cells, whereas B-lymphocytes produce and release antibodies. Enlargement of the lymph nodes in the neck in conjunction with a sore throat is one example of the immune response.

Responses stage: In the response stage, the differentiated lymphocytes function in either a humoral or a cellular capacity. The production of antibodies by the B-lymphocytes in response to a specific antigen begins the humoral response. Humoral refers to the fact that the antibodies are released into the bloodstream and therefore reside in the plasma (fluid fraction of the blood).

With the initial cellular response, the returning sensitized lymphocytes migrate to areas of the lymph node other than those areas containing lymphocytes programed to become plasma cells. Here, they stimulate the residing lymphocytes to become cells that will attack microbes directly rather than through the action of antibodies. These transformed lymphocytes are known as cytotoxic (killer) T-cells. The T-stands for thymus, signifying that during embryologic development of the immune system, these T-lymphocytes spent time in the thymus of the developing fetus, where they were genetically programed to become T-lymphocytes rather than the antibody-producing B-lymphocytes. Vital rather than bacterial antigens induce a cellular response. This response is manifested by the increasing number T-lymphocytes (lymphocytosis) seen in the blood tests of people with viral illnesses such as infectious mononucleosis.

Most immune responses to antigens involve both humoral and cellular responses, although one usually predominates. For example, during transplant rejection, the cellular response predominates, whereas in the bacterial pneumonias and sepsis, the humoral response plays the dominant protective role.

Effector stage: In the effector stage, either the antibody of the humoral response or the cytotoxic (killer) T-cell of the cellular response reaches and connects with the antigen on the surface of the foreign invader. The connection initiates a series of events that is most instances results in the total destruction of the invading microbes or the complete neutralization of the toxin. The events involve interplay of antibodies (humoral immunity), complement, and action by the cytotoxic T-cells (cellular immunity).

Humoral Immune Response

The humoral response is characterized by the production of antibodies by B-lymphocytes in responses to a specific antigen. Although the B-lymphocytes is ultimately responsible for the production of antibodies, both the macrophages of natural immunity and the special T-cell lymphocytes of cellular immunity are involved in recognizing the foreign substance and in producing antibodies.

Antigen recognition: Several theories explain the mechanisms by which B-lymphocytes recognize the invading antigen and respond by producing antibodies. It is known that B-lymphocyte recognize and respond to invading antigens in more than one way.

The B-lymphocytes appear to respond to some antigens by directly triggering antibody formation: however, in response to other antigens, they need the assistance of T-cells to trigger antibody formation. The T-lymphocytes are part of a surveillance system that is dispersed throughout the body and recycles through the general circulation, tissues, and lymphatic system. With the assistance of macrophages, the T-lymphocytes are believed to recognize the antigen of a foreign invader. The T-lymphocyte picks up the antigenic message, or "blueprint", of the antigen and returns to the nearest node with that message.

B-lymphocytes stored in the lymph nodes are subdivided into thousands of clones, each responsive to a single group of antigens having almost identical characteristics. When the antigenic message is carried back to the lymph node, specific clones of the B-lymphocyte are stimulated to enlarge, divide, proliferate, and differentiate into plasma cells capable of producing specific antibodies to the antigen. Other B-lymphocytes differentiate into B-lymphocyte clones with a memory for the antigen. These memory cells are responsible for the more exaggerated and rapid immune in a person who is repeatedly exposed to the same antigen.

Role of Antibodies

Antibodies are large proteins called immunoglobulins (because they are found in the globulin fraction of the plasma proteins). All immunoglobulins are glycoproteins and contain a certain amount of carbohydrate. The carbohydrate concentration, which ranges from approximately 3 to 13%, is dependent on the class of the antibody. Each antibody molecule consists of two subunits, each of which contains a light and a heavy peptide chain. The subunits are held together by a chemical link composed of disulfide bonds. Each subunit has a portion, referred to as the Fab fragment, that serves as a binding site for a site for a specific antigen. The Fab fragment (antibody-binding site) binds to the antigenic determinant similar to a lock-and-key mechanism. The Fab fragment provides the "lock" portion that is highly specific for an antigen. An additional portion, known as the Fc fragment, allows the antibody molecular to take part in the complement system.

Antibodies defend against foreign invaders in several ways, and the type of defense employed depends on the structure and composition of both the antigen and the immunoglobulin. The antibody molecule has at least two combining sites or Fab fragments. One antibody can act as a cross-link between two antigens, causing them to bind or clump together. This clumping effect, referred to as **agglutination**, helps clear the body of the invading organism by facilitating phagocytosis. Some antibodies assist in removal of offending organisms through **opsonization**. In this process, the antigen-antibody molecule is coated with a sticky substance that also facilitates phagocytosis.

Antibodies also promote the release of vasoactive substances, such as histamine and slow-reacting substance, two of the chemical mediators of the inflammatory response. Antibodies do not function in isolation; rather, they mobilize other components of the immune system to defend against the invader. The typical role of antibodies is to focus components of the natural immune system on the invader. This includes activation of the complement system and activation of phagocytosis.

The body can produce five different types of immunoglobulins (Ig). Each of the five types, or classes, is identified by a specific letter of the alphabet: IgA, IgD, IgE, IgG, and IgM. Classification is based on the chemical structure and biologic role of the individual immunoglobulin.

Antigen-antibody binding: The portion of the antigen involved in binding with the antibody is referred to as the **antigenic determinant**. The most efficient immunologic responses occur when the antibody and antigen fit like a lock and key. Poor fit can occur with an antibody that was produced in response to a different antigen. This phenomenon is known as cross-reactivity. For example, in acute rheumatic fever, the antibody produced against *Streptococcus pyogenes* in the upper respiratory tract may cross-react with the patients heart tissue, leading to heart valve damage.

Antigen-antibody binding (Left): A highly specific antigen-antibody complex. (Middle) No match and therefore, no immune response. (Right) Poor fit or match with low specificity, antibody reacts to antigen with similar characteristics, producing cross-reactivity.

Major Characteristics of the Immunoglobulins

IgG (75% of Total Immunoglobulin)
- Appears in serum and tissues (interstitial fluid)
- Assumes a major role in bloodborne and tissue infections
- Activates the complement system
- Enhances phagocytosis
- Crosses the placenta.

IgA (15% of Total Immunoglobulin)
- Appears in body fluids (blood, saliva, tears, breast milk, and pulmonary, gastrointestinal, prostatic, and vaginal secretions)
- Protects against respiratory, gastrointestinal, and genitourinary infections
- Prevents absorption of antigens from food
- Passes to neonate in breast milk for protection.

IgM (10% of Total Immunoglobulin)
- Appears mostly in intravascular serum
- Appears as the first immunoglobulin produced in response to bacterial and viral infections
- Activates the complement system.

IgD (0.2% of Total Immunoglobulin)
- Appears in small amounts in serum
- Possibly influences B-lymphocyte differentiation, but role is unclear.

IgE (0.004% of Total Immunoglobulin)
- Appears in serum
- Takes part in allergic and some hypersensitivity reactions
- Combats parasitic infections.

Cellular Immune Response

The B-lymphocyte are responsible for humoral immunity, and the T-lymphocyte are primarily responsible for cellular immunity stem cells continuously migrate from the bone marrow to the thymus gland, where they develop into T-cells. T-cells continue to develop in the thymus gland, despite the partial degeneration of the gland that occurs at puberty. By spending time in the thymus, these cells are programmed to become T-cells rather than antibody-producing B-lymphocytes. Several types of T-cells exist, each with designated roles in the defense against bacteria, viruses, fungi, parasites, and malignant cells. T-cells attack foreign invaders directly rather than by producing antibodies.

Cellular reactions are initiated by the binding of an antigen to an antigen receptor located on the surface of a T-cell. This may occur with or without the assistance of macrophages. The T-cells then carry the antigenic message, or blueprint, to the lymph nodes, where the production of other T-cells is stimulated. Some T-cells remain in the lymph nodes and retain a memory for the antigen. Other T-cells migrate from the lymph nodes into the general circulatory system and ultimately to the tissues, where they remain until they either come in contact with their respective antigens or die.

Role of T-lymphocytes

T-cells include effector T-cells, suppressor T-cells, and memory T-cells. Two major categories of effector T-cells exist: helper T-cells and cytotoxic T-cells. These effector T-cells participate in the destruction of foreign organisms. T-cells interact closely with B-cells, including that humoral and cellular immune responses are not separate, unrelated processes, but rather, branches of the immune response that interact.

Helper T-cells are activated on recognition of antigens and stimulate the rest of the immune system. When activated, helper T-cells secrete **cytokines**, which attract and activate B-cells, cytotoxic T-cells, NK cells, macrophages, and other cells of the immune system. Separate subpopulations of helper T-cells produce different types of cytokines and determine whether the immune response will be the production of antibodies or a cell-mediated immune response. Helper T-cells produce **lymphokines**, one category of cytokines. These lymphokines activate other T-cells (e.g., interleukin-2 [IL-2]), natural cytotoxic T-cells (e.g., interferon-g), and other inflammatory cells (e.g., tumor necrosis factor). Helper T-cells produce IL-4 and IL-5, lymphokines that activate B-cells to grow and differentiate **(Table 12.1)**.

Cytotoxic T-cells (killer T-cells) attack the antigen directly by altering the cell membrane and causing cell lysis (disintegration) and by releasing cytolytic enzymes and cytokines. Lymphokines can recruit, activate, and regulate other lymphocytes and WBCs. These cells then assist in destroying the invading organisms. Delayed-type hypersensitivity is an example of an immune reaction that protects the body from antigens through the production and release of lymphokines.

Another type of cell, the **suppressor T-cell**, has the ability to decrease B-cell production, thereby keeping the immune response at a level that is compatible with health (e.g., sufficient to fight infection adequately without attacking the body's healthy tissues). **Memory cells** are responding for recognizing antigens from previous exposure and mounting an immune response **(Table 12.2)**.

Roles of Null Lymphocytes and Natural Killer Cells

Null lymphocytes and NK cells are other lymphocytes that assist in combating organisms. These cells are distinct from B-cells and T-cells and lack the usual characteristics of those cells. **Null lymphocytes**, a subpopulation of lymphocytes, destroy antigens already coated with antibody. These cells have special Fc-receptor sites on their surface that allow them to connect with the Fc-end of antibodies; this is known as antibody-dependent, cell-mediated cytotoxicity.

Natural killer cells, another subpopulation of lymphocytes, defend against microorganisms and some types of malignant cells. NK cells are capable of directly killing invading organisms and producing cytokines. The helper T-cells contribute to the differentiation of null and NK cells.

Complement System

Circulating plasma proteins, known as **complement**, are made in the liver and activated when an antibody connects with its antigen. Complement plays an important role in the immune response. Destruction of an invading or attacking organism or toxin is not achieved merely by the binding of the antibody and antigens; it also requires activation of complement, the arrival of killer T-cells, or the attraction of macrophages. Complement has three major physiologic functions: defending the body against bacterial infection, bridging natural and acquired immunity, and disposing of immune complexes and the byproducts associated with inflammation. Complement mediated immune responses are summarized in **Table 12.3**.

The proteins that comprise complement interact sequentially with one another in a cascading or "falling

Table 12.1: Cytokines and their biologic activity.

Cytokines*	Biologic activity
Interleukin – 1 (α and β)	Promotes differentiation of T- and B-lymphocytes, natural killer (NK) cells, and null cells
Interleukin – 2	Stimulates growth of T-lymphocytes and special activated killer lymphocytes (known as lymphocyte activated killer cells [LAK cells])
Interleukin – 3	Stimulates growth of mast cells and other blood cells
Interleukin – 4	Stimulates growth of T- and B-lymphocytes and antibodies
Interleukin – 5	Stimulates antibody responses
Interleukin – 6	Stimulates growth and function of B-lymphocytes and antibodies
Interleukin – 7	Stimulates growth of pre-B, CD4+ and CD8+ T-lymphocytes
Interleukin – 8	Promotes chemotaxis and activation of neutrophils
Interleukin – 9	Stimulates growth and proliferation of T-lymphocytes
Interleukin – 10	Inhibits interferon-gamma and mononuclear cell inflammation
Interleukin – 11	Promotes induction of acute phase proteins
Interleukin – 12	Introduces helper T-lymphocytes
Interleukin – 13	Inhibits mononuclear phagocyte inflammation and promotes differentiation of B-cells
Interleukin – 16	Promotes chemotaxis CD4+ T-lymphocytes and eosinophils
Permeability factor	Increases vascular permeability, allowing white cells into area
Interferon – γ	Activates macrophages; increases expression of class I and II MHC antigen processing and presentation
Interferon – (type 1α and type β)	Exerts antiviral activity in body cells; induces class I antigen expression; activates NK cells
Migration inhibitory factor	Suppress movement of macrophages, keeping macrophages in area of foreign cells
Skin reactive factor	Induces inflammatory response
Cytotoxic factor (lymphotoxin)	Kills certain antigenic cells
Macrophage chemotactic factor	Attracts macrophages into the area
Lymphocyte blastogenic factor	Stimulates more lymphocytes, recruiting additional lymphocytes into the area
Macrophage aggregation factor	Causes clumping to adhere to surfaces more readily
Macrophage activation factor	Allows macrophages to adhere to surfaces more readily
Proliferation inhibitor factor	Inhibits growth of certain antigenic cells
Cytophilic antibody	Binds to an Fc receptor on macrophages, thereby permitting macrophages to bind to antigens
Tumor necrosis factor-alpha	Stimulates inflammation, wound healing, and tissue remodeling
Tumor necrosis factor-beta	Mediates inflammation and graft rejection

* Cytokines are biologically active substances that are released by cells to regulate growth and function of other cells within the immune system. Lymphocytes produce lymphokines, and monocytes and macrophages produce monokines. This table lists some of the cytokines that play a role in immune system functioning.
(MHC = Major histocompatibility complex)

domino" effect. The complement cascade is important to modifying the effector arm of the immune system. Activation of complement allows important events, such as removal of infectious agents and initiation of the inflammatory response, to take place. These events involve active parts of the pathway that enhance chemotaxis of macrophages and granulocytes, alter blood vessel permeability, change blood vessels diameters, cause cells to lyse, alter blood clotting, and cause other points of modification. These macrophages and granulocytes continue the body's defense by devouring the antibody coated microbes and by releasing bacterial products.

There are several ways to activate the complement system: the classic pathway, the alternative pathway, and the lectin pathway.

Classic Pathway of Complement Activation

The classic pathway (the first method discovered) is activated by antigen–antibody complexes; it begins when antibody binds to a cell surface and ends with lysis of the cell. This involves the reaction of the first of the circulating complement proteins (C1) with the receptor site of the Fc portion of an antibody molecule after formation of an antigen–antibody complex. The activation of the first

Table 12.2: Lymphocytes involved in immune responses.

Type of immune response	Cell Type	Function
Humoral	B-lymphocyte	Produces antibodies or immunoglobulins (IgA, IgD, IgE, IgG, IGM)
Cellular	T-lymphocyte	
	Helper T	Attacks foreign invaders (antigens) directly. Initiates and augments inflammatory response.
	Helper T1	Increases activated cytotoxic T-cells
	Helper T2	Increases B-cell antibody production
	Suppressor T	Suppresses the immune response
	Memory T	Remembers contact with an antigen and on subsequent exposures mounts an immune response
	Cytotoxic T	Lyses cells infected with virus; (killer T) plays a role in graft rejection
Nonspecific	Non-T or non-B lymphocyte	
	Null cell	Destroys antigens already coated with antibody
	Natural killer (NK) cell (granular lymphocyte)	Defends against microorganisms and some type of malignant cells; produces cytokines

Table 12.3: Complement-mediated immune responses.

Response	Complement products	Effects
Cytolysis	C5b-C9	Lysis and destruction of cell membranes of body's cells or pathogens
Opsonization	C3b, C5b	Targeting of the antigen so that it can be easily engulfed and digested by macrophages and other phagocytic cells
Chemotaxis	C3a, C5a	Chemical attraction of neutrophils and phagocytic cells to the antigen
Anaphylaxis	C3a, C5a	Activation of mast cells and basophils with release of inflammatory mediators that produce smooth muscle contraction and increased vascular permeability

complement component then activates all the other components, in the following sequence: C4, C2, C3, C5, C6, C7, C8 and C9. (The components are named in the sequence in which they were discovered).

Alternative and Lectin Pathways

The alternative and lectin pathways of complement are activated without the formation of antigen-antibody complexes. These pathways can be initiated by the release of bacterial products, such as endotoxins. When complement is activated without the formation of antigen-antibody complexes, the process bypasses the first three components (C1, C4 and C2) and begins with C3. Regardless of the method, once activated, the complement system destroys cells by altering or damaging the cell membrane of the antigen, by chemically attracting phagocytes to the antigen (chemotaxis), and by rendering the antigen more vulnerable to phagocytosis (opsonization). The complement system enhances the inflammatory response by releasing vasoactive substances. The alternative and lectin pathways of complement are activated without the formation of antigen-antibody complexes. These pathways can be initiated by the release of bacterial products, such as endotoxins. When complement is activated without the formation of antigen-antibody complexes, the process bypasses the first three components (C1, C4 and C2) and begins with C3. Regardless of the method, once activated, the complement system destroys cells by altering or damaging the cell membrane of the antigen, by chemically attracting phagocytes to the antigen (chemotaxis), and by rendering the antigen more vulnerable to phagocytosis (opsonization). The complement system enhances the inflammatory response by releasing vasoactive substances.

Complement components, prostaglandins, leukotrienes and other inflammatory mediators all contribute to the recruitment of inflammatory cells, as do chemokines, a group of cytokines. The activated neutrophils pass through the vessel walls to accumulate at the site of infection, where they phagocytose complement-coated microbes. This response is usually therapeutic and can be lifesaving if the cell attacked, by the complement system is a true foreign invader, such as streptococcal or staphylococcal organism. However, if that cell is actually part of the person—for example, a cell of the brain or liver, the tissue lining the blood vessels, or the cells of a transplanted organ or skin graft—the result can be devastating disease and even death. This vigorous and deadly attack on the material identified as foreign is underscored by the resulting purulent material (the remains of microbes, granulocytes, macrophages, T-cells, plasma proteins, complement, and antibodies) that accumulates in wound infections and abscesses. In addition, many autoimmune diseases (e.g., systemic lupus erythematosus) and disorders characterized by chronic infection (e.g., myocardial infarction, stroke) are thought to be caused in part by continued or chronic activation of complement, which in turn results in chronic inflammation.

The RBCs (erythrocytes) and platelets (thrombocytes) also have a role in the immune response. RBCs and platelets have complement receptors and, as a result, play an important role in the clearance of immune complexes that consist of antigen, antibody and components of the complement system.

Role of Interferons

Biologic response modifiers, such as the interferons, continue to be investigated to determine their roles in the immune system and their potential therapeutic effects in disorders characterized by disturbed immune responses (Korholz & Kiess, 2003). Interferons have antiviral and anti-tumor properties. In addition to responding to viral infection, interferons are produced by T-lymphocytes, B-lymphocytes, and macrophages in response to antigens. They are thought to modify the immune response by suppressing antibody production and cellular immunity. They also facilitate the cytotytic role of macrophages and NK cells. Interferons are undergoing extensive testing to evaluating their effectiveness in treating tumors and acquired immunodeficiency syndrome (AIDS). Some interferons are already used to treat immune-related disorders are already used to treat immune-related disorders (e.g., multiple sclerosis) and chronic inflammatory conditions (e.g., chronic hepatitis).

Genetic Engineering

One of the more remarkable evolving technologies is **genetic engineering**, which uses recombinant DNA technology. Two facets exist with this technology. The first permits scientists to combine genes from one type of organisms with genes of a second organisms. This type of technology allows cells and microorganisms to manufacture proteins, monokines, and lymphokines, which can alter and enhance immune system function. The second facet of recombinant DNA technology involves gene therapy. If a particular gene is abnormal or missing, experimental recombinant DNA technology may be capable of restoring normal gene function. For example, a recombinant gene is inserted onto a virus particle. When the virus particle splices its gene, the virus automatically inserts the missing gene, and theoretically corrects the genetic anomaly. Extensive research into recombinant DNA technology and gene therapy is ongoing.

Stem Cells

Stem cells are potentially immortal cells that are capable of self-renewal and differentiation; they continually replenish the body's entire supply of both RBCs and WBCs. Some stem cells, described as totipotent cells, have tremendous capacity to self-renew and differentiate. Embryonic stem cells, described as pluripotent, give rise to numerous cell types that are able to form tissues (Porth, 2005). Research has shown that stem cells can restore an immune system that has been destroyed. Stem cell transplantation has been carried out in humans with certain types of immune dysfunction, such as severe combined immunodeficiency (SCID); clinical trials using stem cells are underway in patients with a variety of disorders having an autoimmune component, including systemic lupus erythematosus, rheumatoid arthritis, scleroderma, and multiple sclerosis. Research with embryonic stem cells has enabled investigators to make substantial gains in developmental biology, gene therapy, therapeutic tissue engineering, and the treatment of a variety of diseases. However, along with these remarkable opportunities, many ethical challenges arise, which are largely based on concerns about safety, efficacy, resource allocation, and human cloning.

PRIMARY IMMUNE ABERRATIONS AND DISEASE

The immune response is protective inhealthy individuals; however, that protection depends on an intact immune system. Four primary immune aberrations can lead to disease: (1) a deficiency of one or more immune components (**immunodeficiency**), (2) an abnormal production of antibodies (**gammopathy**), (3) an exaggerated or inappropriate immune response (**hypersensitivity**), and (4) immunologic attacks on host cells (**autoimmunity**).

Immunodeficiencies

The four components of the immuno system—Humoral (B cell mediated) immunity, cellular (T-cell) immunity, phagocytosis, and complement—act together and independently to protect the host from infection and disease. Both primary (congenital) and secondary (acquired) immunodeficiencies produce chronic or recurring infections that can, without effective treatment, lead to death.

Primary Immunodeficiencies

Primary immunodeficiencies (PIs) are a group of disorders that occur from congenital genetic defects that block or prevent the maturation or function of immune cells. Most PIs arte autosomal, or X-linked, and have both dominant and recessive inheritance patterns. They commonly occur in persons under the age of 20 and, because of inheritance patterns, affect males in 70% of cases. The most common immunodeficiencies are secondary or acquired. Most people are born with a normal immune response, but secondary factors or occurrences affect the immune system, causing dysfunction. Immunosuppressive agents; malignancies; chronic diseases; nutritional deficits; age; and some viral infections, such as human immunodeficiency virus (HIV), can cause secondary immunodeficiency.

Pathophysiology of Primary Immunodeficiencies

PI disorders are characterized by defects in immunologic cell development or function that result in B-lymphocyte (also known as B cell). T cell, complement, or phagocytic cell deficiency. Recurrent infections or repeated infection treatment failures generally prompt the clinician to suspect the presence of immunodeficiency. Without treatment, most individuals suffering from these deficiencies die of overwhelming infectious early in life.

Immunodeficiencies produce a variety of clinical manifestation based on the type of deficiency. Not all patients experience all manifestations listed. Common manifestations include:
- Frequent bacterial and viral infections
- Infection with unusual or opportunistic organisms
- Associated autoimmune disease
- Painful, swollen, wrist, elbow, ankle, or knee joints
- Digestive problems, nausea, or vomiting
- Chronic skin or mucous membrane infections
- Blood disorders
- Diarrhea
- Fever
- Fatigue
- Weakness
- Enlarged lymph noses or spleen.

Antibody Deficiencies

Selective immunoglobulin A (IgA) deficiency is the most common PI and has both autosomal dominant and recessive inheritance traits. The exact defect that leads to low serum IgA levels in unknown, but may be related to impaired B cell differentiation and subsequent loss of immunoglobulin secreting ability. The disorder is associated with increased incidence of infections, autoimmunity, allergies, gastrointestinal disorders, and cancer. B-lymphocytes produce *antibodies* that recognize mark foreign antigens so that other immune components will react and destroy them. X-linked agammaglobulinemia is an example of an inherited, B cell immunodeficiency that results from failure of pre-B cells to differentiate into mature B cells. This disorder occurs exclusively in males and is usually diagnosed within the first 3 years of life. Individuals with agammaglobulinemia are particularly susceptible to infections from pyrogenic bacteria such as *Streptococci, Staphylococci, Pseudomonas* organisms, and *Haemophilus influenzae*; infections of the eyes, sinuses, ears, nose, and lungs, and viruses such as hepatitis and polio.

Combined B and T Cell Deficiencies

Stem cell immunodeficiency (severe combined immunodeficiency, or SCID) refers to the complete absence of both T cell (cellular) and B cell (humoral) immunity. This disorder has many variants. In the most severe form the common stem cell for white blood cells is absent, resulting is subsequent loss of B cells, T cells, and phagocytic cells. Infants with this condition generally die in utero or soon after birth. A less severe form of SCID results from impaired stem cell maturation, which interferes with T and B cell development. T and B cells are significantly reduced or absent even though other white blood cells are present in normal numbers. People with SCID are at high risk for developing nearly every type of infection because of pancytopenia. Thymic hypoplasia (DiGeorge syndrome) is a cellular immunodeficiency resulting from thymus gland hypoplasia and inability to assist in the maturation of T cells. Even though B cells are normal, children with total loss of thymic function are at increased risk for infection and may not live more than 5 to 6 years without treatment.

Phagocytic Defects

Phagocytes (neutrophis and macrophages) are white blood cells that engulf and destroy antibody-coated antigens. Phagocytic defects may interfere with their ability to move to the site of an infection or destroy pathogens. Chronic granulomatous disease is the most severe form of phagocytic cell deficiency. It involves a deficiency in the molecules needed by neutrophils to destroy foreign antigens. Individuals with phagocytic disorders are at risk for developing mild to severe bacterial infections. Signs and symptoms depend on the site of infection and type of infecting organism.

Complement System Defects

The complement system is composed of proteins that attach themselves to antibody coated antigens and facilitate destruction of the antigen. Persons with complement deficiency have a diminished ability to destroy invading pathogens and are at increased risk for infection. A common complement deficiency. C2 deficiency, is associated with an increased incidence of autoimmune disease, such as glomerulonephritis or rheumatoid arthritis, and severe infection such as meningitis.

Secondary Immunodeficiencies

Secondary immunodeficiencies result from numerous factors. Generalized **immunosuppression** is often induced therapeutically to decrease unwanted immune reactions, such as hypersensitivity reactions, autoimmune diseases, neoplasia, or organ rejection.

Immunosuppressive Therapies

Corticosteroids have both anti-inflammatory and immunosuppressive properties. They inhibit movement of leukocytes and alter cellular and humoral immunity. when infection is present in a person receiving corticosteroids, the severity of the infection may increase despite the induced minimization of symptoms. Cyclosporine, a primary immunosuppressant drug used after organ transplantation, acts by inhibiting helper T cells and facilitating development of suppressor T cells.

Cytotoxic drugs and other cancer chemotherapeutic agents (alkylating agents, antifolates, and antimetabolites) destroy replicating cells. Consequently, they produce immunosuppression by destroying rapidly dividing immunologically stimulated cells. They also interfere with basic cellular metabolic processes in which B and T cell numbers are reduced.

Specific immunosuppression may be induced in people with hypersensitivities by administration of antigens in small amounts over time. This antigenic stimulation forms circulating immunoglobulin G (IgG) antibodies (immunoglobulins) that combine with the offending antigen to block contact with immunocompetent cells or immunoglobulin E (IgE)–coated mast cells, thus suppressing the immune response and preventing hypersensitivity reactions. Allergists use an adaptation of this method to desensitize persons who are allergic to antigens such as pollens or dust mites. A slightly different method of immunosuppression involves administration of a specific antibody, which then combines with the antigen to block contact with the immunocompetent cell. This method is used successfully in obstetrics in preventing the sensitive Rh-negative mother from reacting to an Rh-positive fetus during pregnancy.

Antilymphocytic globulin and antithymocytic globulin are antisera prepared by isolating the active globulin fraction from the serum of horses, goats, or rabbits that have been immunized with human lymphocytes or thymocytes. These antisear produce immunosuppression by decreasing all lymphocytes, although T cells are more affected than B cells. Because these globulins are xenogeneic (from another species), serum sickness may occur, and this limits their use to short-term therapy.

Monoclonal antibodies (MoAbs) are also used to suppress immunity. because they are derived from a single cell line (monoclonal), they are very specific and can be targeted against subpopulations of lymphocytes, such as helper T cells. Monoclonal antibodies are useful in treating cancers, autoimmune disorders, and renal allograft rejection.

Many chemicals have immunosuppressive effects in exposed humans. T lymphocytes seem to be affected more severely than other immune cells. Examples of potentially damaging environmental chemicals are asbestos, dioxin, insecticides, and heavy metals. Irradiation also suppresses immunity by suppressing both primary and secondary immune responses, although primary suppression is more effective. Irradiation destroys lymphocytes either directly or through depletion of precursor stem cells.

Other factors: Prolonged physical and psychosocial stress stimulates the production of corticosteroids, which suppress immunity and increase the risk for infections and tumors. T and B cells are reduced for up to a month after surgery, most likely because of stress. Chronic conditions such as diabetes mellitus are common causes of secondary immunodeficiency. Malnutrition and subsequent protein and calorie deficiencies result in reduced T cell numbers. The immune systems of older adults are less efficient, with decreased Y cell function, variable ability to respond to antigenic stimulation, and decreased proliferation of immune cells. HIV causes a serious secondary immunodeficiency, acquired immunodeficiency syndrome (AIDS).

Complications: Frequent acute and chronic bacterial, viral and fungal infections and repeated infection treatment failures are the complications of primary and secondary immunodeficiencies. Without adequate treatment, these complications can lead to weight loss, fatigue, poor quality of life, sepsis, septic shock, and death.

Management of Immunodeficiency Disorder

The primary goals of collaborative management for patients with suspected immunodeficiency disorders are to (1) identify those at risk for the disorder, (2) prevent infection or effectively treat existing infections, (3) replace missing humoral or cellular immunologic factors as possible.

Diagnosis is based on patient history, physical examination, and laboratory findings; however, there is no one specific test fro all diseases.

Antimicrobial agents to treat existing and prevent new infections are key to the successful management of both primary and secondary immunodeficiencies. Immmunoglobulin replacement therapy, which contains intravenous immunoglobulin (IVIG), is accepted treatment for patients with antibody deficiencies. The optimal dose of immunoglobulin, which is usually between 400 and 500 mg/dl, is maintained by monitoring the trough of immunoglobulin levels in the blood. Immunoglobulin are usually given intramuscularly or intravenously on a monthly basis. Reactions to immunoglobulins can include back or abdominal pain, nausea and vomiting, chills and fever, headache, myalgia, or fatigue. Fortunately, anaphylactic reactions to immunoglobulins are rare.

Other chemotherapeutic treatments for immunodeficiency include (1) injections of interferon gamma, a cytokine that activates phagocytes; (2) injections of growth factors,, which increase neutrophil production; and (3) granulocyte-macrophage colony stimulating factor or granulocyte colony-stimulating factor, both of which stimulate the production of granulocytes (white blood cells).

Bone marrow transplantation may be used for patients with T cell deficiencies. The major risk of this therapy is graft-versus-host disease. Bone marrow cells from family members with identical human leukocyte antigens have been used successfully in treating patients with combined immunodeficiencies.

Patients with immunodeficiency diseases have no specific dietary restrictions. A well-balanced, nutritious diet that includes all food groups and has adequate calories and protein to support tissue healing and growth is recommended, since it helps support immunity. Efforts should be made to prevent the transfer of food-borne microbes that may be potential sources of infection by thoroughly washing or cooking fruits and vegetables, thoroughly cooking meat products, and avoiding placing cooked foods on surfaces where raw meat was prepared.

Nursing Management

The nurses has to assess for:
- Frequency and length of any chronic bacterial or viral infections
- Bacterial infections of the ears, sinuses, lungs, bronchi
- Painful joints of the wrist, elbows, ankles, or knees
- Digestive problems, nausea, or vomiting
- Frequent bouts of diarrhea
- Chronic skin infections
- Blood disorders
- Enlarged lymph nodes or spleen
- Fever
- Poor skin turgor, bruising, lesions on the skin or mucous membranes
- Swollen joints
- Decreased weight for height

Problems usually associates with immunodeficiency disorder was includes the following.

Risk for Infection

Common nursing objective for the patient with a diagnosis of risk for infection are:

Patient will:
- Recognize signs of new infections and report for treatment early
- Use precautions to prevent new infections
- Maintain treatment regimens for treatment or prevention of infections.

For which the nurse consistently monitors patients who have immunodeficiencies or are undergoing immunosuppression therapy for indications of systemic infection, such as fever, changes in vital sign pattern, irritability, fatigue, or cough. Meticulous skin an perineal care and a clean environment reduce the patients potential for contact with infectious organisms. Injections are avoided and invasive lines kept to a minimum to prevent a portal of entry for microbes. When invasive lines are necessary, the nurse carefully monitors insertion sites for signs of localized infection. The nurse cultures suspicious drainage and monitors laboratory data to detect new infections and to determine the effectiveness of medications and other treatments. Live immunizations and oral polio vaccines are avoided in immunocompromised patients because of the risk of contracting infections via the immunization.

Immunodeficient or immunosuppressed patients and their families need to know the nature of the immunodeficiency and how to avoid infection. Many patients do not require hospitalization, but they do need to be taught about infection control measures to follow at home. They need to be able to recognize the signs and symptoms of infection and which symptoms to report to the health care provider. Teaching includes information about the use of protective strategies such as hand washing techniques and asking people with infections such as colds or chickenpox not to visit. Frequent turning and deep breathing exercises are encouraged to prevent atelectasis and pneumonia. Careful attention should be given to older adults because of their increased risk for infection resulting from a decline in T cell function and immune response efficiency.

There are no specific activity restrictions; however, the nurse counsels patients about the need to avoid becoming overly fatigued. Patients with immunodeficiency disorders need to understand the importance of ongoing follow-up care. Referrals to community or home health nurses for continued assessment and treatment of infections may be necessary. Hospice care may be appropriate for patients with terminal primary or secondary immunodeficiency disorders.

Patient teaching should include information about the nature of immunodeficiency and prescribed medications, as well as the following instructions regarding the preventions and management of the infection:
- Avoid persons with infections (especially colds)
- Inspect skin daily for lesions or breaks
- Avoid bumping, breaking, or tearing skin
- Eat a well-balanced diet with sufficient calories to maintain ideal weight
- Drink at least six glasses of fluid daily
- Avoid becoming overly fatigued
- Try to get sufficient sleep every night
- Decrease environmental contaminants:
- Take prophylactic antibiotics before any manipulative or invasive procedures (dental procedures, biopsies, endoscopies, arteriograms).
- Keep scheduled follow-up appointments with health care provider
- Report signs of infection immediately (increased temperature, redness of swelling of skin or mucous membranes, change in color of sputum, unusual drainage, diarrhea).

Gammopathies

Gammopathies, also known as hypergammaglobulinermias, refer to elevated levels of serum gamma globulin resulting from overproduction. The blood normally contains a large number of different proteins collectively called plasma proteins. One type of protein, gamma globulin, combines to make varying types of antibodies for fighting different infections. When the majority of protein produced is an identical type of gamma globulin, the abnormally produced protein is called *monoclonal gammopathy or plasma* cell dyscrasia. Multiple myeloma and macroglobulinemia are plasma cell dyscrasias that have distinctive clinical patterns.

Polyclonal gammopathies involve the overproduction of virtually all classes of immunoglobulins in response to inappropriate antigenic stimulation. High levels of dysfunctional immmunoglobulins depress the synthesis of normal immunoglobulins, leaving the patient susceptible to infection. IgG and IgM are most commonly involved. The immunoglobulin levels reflect the severity of disease produced. Polyclonal gammopathies are associated with chronic bacterial infections and connective tissue diseases such as lupus erythematosus and rheumatoid arthritis.

Multiple Myeloma

Multiple myeloma, which is plasma cell cancer, is the most serious and prevalent of the monoclonal gammopathies. The cause of multiple myeloma is unknown, but studies have shown possible associations with genetic factors, a decline in immune function, exposure to chemicals or radiation, and more recently a viral origin.

Pathophysiology: Multiple myeloma is a type of bone marrow cancer, which occurs from uncontrolled growth of plasma cells. Normally the bone marrow contains less than 5% plasma cells. Patients with multiple myeloma have bone marrow that contains between 10 to 90% plasma cells. The malignant plasma cells are most often monoclonal, originating from one single defective cell. The cancerous plasma cells collect in many bones, where they may form tumors, weaken bones, and cause pain and fractures. Calcium is released from damaged bones, causing hypocalcaemia and resultant fatigue, muscle weakness, or confusion. The increased numbers of myeloma cells within bone marrow prevent the formation of white blood cells, erythrocytes, and normal plasma cells, leading to anemia and increased susceptibility to infections. The kidneys are also affected and at increased risk for damage because of the excretion of excess antibodies and calcium.

Patients with multiple myeloma are staged to determine treatment options and prognosis. Staging is based on the estimated number of myeloma cells calculated from the amount of abnormal monoclonal immunoglobulin in the urine and blood; the amount of calcium in the blood; the degree of bone destruction noted on X-ray examination; and the amount of hemoglobin in the blood.

Early in the disease process patients may be symptom free. When manifestations do occur, they may consist of back or rib pain, weight loss, fatigue, weakness, or repeated infections. Later stages of the diseases are associated with nausea, vomiting, anemia, renal damage, or extremity weakness. By the time of diagnosis, bone lesions are typically present in the skull, spine, and pelvis. The major problems encountered by patients with multiple myeloma are related to the complication of pathologic fractures, renal failure, and infection.

Clinical Manifestations

- *Pain (an early symptom):* Plasma cells accumulate within the bone marrow, causing destruction of bone, which results in fractures
- *Renal compromise:* Excessive amounts of protein excreted in the urine and hypercalcemia adversely affect renal function
- *Infections:* Abnormal plasma cells accumulate in the bone marrow, decreasing the production of normal white blood cells (WBCs). Decreased WBCs result in increased bacterial infections
- *Weakness:* The accumulation of abnormal plasma cells in the bone marrow prevents red blood cells production and results in anemia

Management: Collaborative management of multiple myeloma is directed at improving the quality of the patients life by controlling symptoms, reducing tumor cell burden, and preventing complications. Chemotherapy prolongs the survival for patients with stage I disease for 40 to 46 months, stage II disease for 35 to 40 months, and stage III disease for 24 to 30 months.

Various laboratory and other diagnostic tests are completed when patients are symptomatic. summarizes common diagnostic tests for multiple myeloma include the following:

- Urine and serum protein electrophoresis to determine the presence of abnormal proteins and number of normal immunoglobulins
- Bone marrow biopsy to determine the presence and number of cancerous plasma cells
- Computed tomography scans and radiography that show a "punched-out" type of bone lesion or generalized osteoporosis of the axial skeleton
- Complete blood count to determine the presence of anemia, leukopenia or thrombocytopenia
- Magnetic resonance imaging to detect the presence of bone abnormalities and fractures
- Blood chemistries to detect the presence of hypercalcemia and elevated uric acid levels
- Estimated myeloma cell mass to estimate the tumor burden

Combination drug therapy has proven to be a more effective treatment for multiple myeloma than single chemotherapeutic agents. Oral melphalan combined with prednisone is the treatment of choice to reduce tumor load. Other chemotherapy combinations are (1) vincistine sulfate, doxorubicin, cyclophosphamide, and carmustine; (2) vincristine, doxorubicin and dexamethasone; and (3) thalidomide and dexamethasone. Interferon-alpha therapy has been shown to prolong the duration of initial remission once achieved. Glucocorticoids and calcitonin reduce the lytic bone destruction of hypercalcemia. Erythropoietin stimulates the production of red blood cells and helps correct anemia.

The type of combination therapy or other agents used depends on several factors, including the patients age, the stage of the disease, and the patients kidney function. If cell transplantation is being considered, drugs with increased risk for bone marrow damage are avoided.

For patients who have a solitary skeletal lesion (plasmacytoma) but are otherwise asymptomatic and have fewer than 50% plasma cells in their bone marrow, radiotherapy has been shown to increase survival rates. When bone damage to the spine is extensive, orthopedic fixation devices may be used for stabilization and to prevent cord compression. For patients in renal failure, dialysis may be necessary to correct azotemia and hypercalcemia. Plasmapheresis, a process that filters the blood, may be useful in removing accumulated myeloma proteins that thicken blood and impede circulation to the brain.

Adequate hydration is necessary to prevent renal complications related to the excretion of increased amounts of urates and calcium in the urine. Fluid intake needs to be sufficient to ensure a minimal urinary output of 1500 ml/day to maintain renal function. If the patient is unable to maintain adequate fluid intake orally or requires nothing-by-mouth status for diagnostic or surgical procedures, intravenous fluids need to be administered. The nurse weighs the patient daily to assess for fluid retention, and monitors the patients blood urea nitrogen and serum creatinine levels to evaluate renal function. A well-balanced diet is encouraged, but there are no specific dietary restrictions unless renal failure occurs.

Nursing Management
The nurses to assess for:
- Back or rib pain
- Excessive fatigue or weakness
- Increased incidence of bacterial infections, urinary tract infections, or shingles
- Changes in urinary pattern or output
- Recent or frequent fractures
- Increased thirst, nausea, loss of appetite.

And also assess for:
- Weight gain and edema
- Pale skin or mucous membranes
- Cough
- Abnormal lung sounds

The main problem associated with multiplex is Pain (Acute or chronic)

Common examples of nursing objective for the patient with a diagnosis of pain are:

Patient will:
- Use nonanalgesic measures to control pain (e.g., relaxation)
- Rate pain as 3 or less on a scale of 1 (no pain) to 10 (severe pain)
- Verbalize satisfactory control of pain.

For pain in the early stages of multiple myeloma, patients may experience little pain or discomfort. During the advanced stage of disease, pain is likely due to fragile bones and fractures. General comfort measures, such as back care, fresh linens, or a quiet environment, may reduce the patients discomfort. Analgesic medications may include nonsteroidal anti-inflammatory agents or narcotic analgesics. Ambulation is encouraged to prevent further bone demineralization associated with immobility, but skeletal pain may be a deterrent to ambulation. A light-weight spinal brace, analgesics, local radiotherapy, and nonanalgesic pain control methods such as distraction may be of benefit.

Safety is of vital importance because of the risk of fractures. Area rugs should be removed from the home to eliminate a potential source of falls. If the patient is completely immobile, careful turning is important. Even a tug on the arm or a turn toward the bed rail can cause a fracture. A lift sheet and the assistance of several people are necessary to facilitate moving the patient gently and safely without causing extensive pain.

Hypersensitivities

The immune system is always ready to respond to foreign antigens. Under certain circumstances, however, this response may bring harm as well as protection. Hypersensitivity diseases may be related to two abnormalities: the immune response to antigens may be unrestrained, producing tissue injury; or the immune response may be directed toward self-antigens because of a loss of self-tolerance, which is known as autoimmunity.

Hypersensitivity diseases are broadly divided into five categories based on the immunologic mechanisms involved in the reaction. Immediate hypersensitivity (type I) is mediated by IgE and causes injury from the release of histamine from mast cells. Antibody-mediated (type II) hypersensitivity exists when anti-bodies are directed against self-antigens. When antigen-antibody complexes collect in blood vessels or other tissues, immune complex disease (type III) hypersensitivity disease exists. T cell mediated hypersensitivity (type IV or delayed) exists when T cells are directed against self-antigens in tissues. Another relatively new hypersensitivity, known as stimulatory (type V), involves the binding the autoantibodies to hormone receptors that mimic the hormone itself, which stimulates target cells.

Immediate Hypersensitivity

Immediate or type I hypersensitivity is an exaggerated immune response occurring in persons who have been previously sensitized to the specific antigen. The antigen producing the reaction is referred to as an *allergen*, and the reaction itself is called allergy or atopy. Immediate hypersensitivities are characterized by inappropriate, rapid and exaggerated responses mediated by IgE antibodies and mast cells. People who tend to produce IgE in response to antigens such as pollen or dust mites are said to be atopic. A severe, potentially lethal systemic form of immediate hypersensitivity reaction is known as systemic anaphylaxis or *anaphylactic shock*.

The onset of allergic diseases generally occurs between the ages of 2 and 15 years, although they can begin at any age. Atopic dermatitis is the most common skin disease, but allergic rhinitis accounts for the majority of visits to health care providers each year. It is estimated that 8% of children under the age of 6 and 1 to 2% of adults have food allergies. Allergic reactions account for 5 to 10% of all above drug reactions.

The tendency to become hypersensitive and produce IgE antibodies in response to inhaled or ingested substances is inherited as a dominant trait. If both parents have allergies, their children have a 50% probability of also having allergies. The specific substances that an individual develops hypersensitivity to, however, are determined by the allergens to which that individual is exposed. A person does not inherit a specific allergy, only the predisposition to develop allergies. No association has been found between gender, race, or geographic area and an increased risk of anaphylaxis.

Allergens are primarily characterized by their route of exposure. Inhaled allergens such as pollens, dust mite fecal matter, fungal hyphae or spores, animal dander are main casual agents of hayfever, chronic rhinitis, and asthma. Common food allergens, such as peanuts, eggs, milk, soy, chicken and shellfish, are thought to trigger mast cell degranulation in the gut after entering the circulation. Whether an allergic response occurs and to what degree depends on a combination of interrelated factors.

Pathophysiology: Immediate hypersensitivities are medicated by the IgE class of immunoglobulins. In generally predisposed people, initial exposure to an allergen prompts the activation of TH2 cells, which are not produced by normal individuals. TH2 cells stimulate the production of IgE antibodies that sensitize the person to the allergen. This initial contact with the allergen is known as the *sensitizing dose*. In some cases it may take several doses of allergen before the persons immune system is fully sensitized. Once sensitization is complete, subsequent exposure (termed the *challenging dose*) results in the allergen combining with IgE and binding to receptor sites on mast cells and basophils. This antigen-antibody reaction results in a rapid release of potent vasoactive mediators such as histamine, kinins, chemotactic factors, and active products of arachidonic acid metabolism (leukotrienes, prostaglandins, and thromboxanes).

Vasoactive mediators produce the clinical manifestations associated with immediate hypersensitivity, which includes smooth muscle contraction, increased vascular permeability and increased mucous gland secretion. These changes may occur locally or at the site of the antigen-antibody reaction. Atopic allergens generally produce localized tissue reactions that remain confined to a specific area such as the skin, nasal passages, or lungs. Hives (urticaria) are pruritic lesions characterized by a pale pink elevated edge (wheal) on an erythematous background. Skin exposed to latex can precipitate contact urticaria. Chronic urticaria that occurs in response to heat, cold, or various light waves is not an IgE-mediated hypersensitivity. Angioedema is a form of urticaria that involves the subcutaneous tissue rather than the skin. It can affect an entire anatomic part, such as the eyelid, thumb, or lip. Swelling is present, but not pruritus. Atopic diseases are not usually life threatening, but the symptoms can be uncomfortable and may cause the individual to miss school or work. A mosquito bite is a classic example of this type of reaction; the intradermal injection of the mosquito anticoagulants produces a wheal-flare type of reaction within minutes.

Clinical manifestations immediate (Type I) hypersensitivity include the following:

Respiratory	*Dermal*
Rhinorrhea	Hives
Watery, itching eyes	Rash
Obstruction of Eustachian tubes	Angioedema
Sneezing	
Sinusitis	*Abdominal*
	Nausea
Headache	Vomiting
Facial pain	Cramping
Bronchospasm	Diarrhea
Dyspnea	
Stridor	*General*
Tachypnea	Fever
Wheezing	Diaphoresis
Cyanosis	Malaise
Use of accessory muscles for breathing	Joint pain
Flaring of nare	Hematopoietic suppression
	Anxiety
	Anaphylaxis

Anaphylaxis

Anaphylaxis may be localized or widespread. Localized anaphylaxis produces hives and angioedema. If widespread mast cell degranulation occurs, producing systemic effects such as decreased blood pressure, bronchial obstruction, and edema in many tissues, systemic anaphylaxis or anaphylactic shock is said to exist. It is the most sever form of immediate hypersentivity in humans. Apprehension and sneezing are two of the earliest symptoms of systemic anaphylaxis. Edema and itching may also occur at the site of antigen entrance. These mild reactions are rapidly followed, sometimes in a matter of seconds or minutes, by severe manifestations that lead to vascular collapse shock, and death unless rapid action is taken. Insect or snake venoms; foods; and drugs such as penicillin, streptokinase, or amphotericin B are most often associated with anaphylaxis, although almost any antigen to which a person is hypersensitive has the potential for producing a systemic reaction.

Clinical Manifestations
Localized
Hives
Angioedema

Systemic
Apprehension
Edema of the face, hands, or other parts of the body
Wheezing
Dyspnea
Respiratory collapse

Vascular collapse with shock:
- Rapid, weak pulse
- Falling blood pressure
- Cyanosis
- Death

The factors that determine a hypersensitivity response will include the following:
- *Responsiveness of the host to the allergens:* If the host is highly sensitive to the antigen, a greater than normal chance exists that a tissue-damaging reaction will occur
- *Amount of allergen:* Generally the greater the amount of allergen contracted, the more severe the reaction
- *Nature of the allergen:* Any foreign protein or protein-containing component can serve as an allergen when coupled with a normal tissue protein carrier. Examples include pollens, foods, animal dander, house dust, and feathers
- *Route of entrance of the allergen:* Allergens may gain host entry via the respiratory tract, through epidermal or mucosal surfaces, by injection, or through the digestive tract
- *Timing of exposure to the allergens:* If the host's contacts with the allergen ma are widely separated by time, the immunologic mediators may be so dilute that little responses occurs. Conversely, if frequent contact is made with the allergen, reactions are more likely to occur.
- *Site of the allergen immune mediator reaction:* A reaction can occur in the tissues with little consequence; however, the same reaction occurring in the bloodstream can lead to a severe reaction
- *Host's threshold of reactivity:* The host's immune system can be changed by factors such as stress, fatigue, or infection, all of which can decrease the immune system's responsiveness to potential allergens

Latex hypersensitivity, which has a high potential for producing anaphylaxis, has become a universal concern among health care workers, since numerous medical products such as gloves, catheters, and tubes contain latex. The prevalence of latex allergy is estimated at about 6% for the general population. Signs of latex allergy depend largely on the route of exposure. When latex particles are aerosolized, wheezing, rhinitis, and conjunctivitis may occur. Mucosal exposure frequently results in angioedema. There is no cure for latex hypersensitivity, and avoidance is the principal treatment.

Management of Hypersensitivity

The health history, including an environmental assessment, is one of the most valuable diagnostic tools for the health care provider evaluating the patient for immediate hypersensitivities. Intradermal skin testing and the radioallergosorbent test (RAST) may be helpful in identifying antigens and determining therapy for persons with allergens. Eosinophilia (increased eosinophil count) is associated with antigen-antibody reactions and occurs in persons with allergies, and drug hypersensitivity.

Medications

Symptom relief is the primary aim of drug therapy for allergies. Urticaria and angioedema are usually self-limiting; therefore treatment is often not required. Anaphylaxis is treated with epinephrine to shorten its duration and prevent relapse. When intravenous access is not available, epinephrine is administered by intramuscular injection to provide the highest level of absorption. Antihistamines, such as diphenhydramine (Benadryl), are given to block histamine receptors. Short-term corticosteroid therapy, either oral or inhaled (cromolyn sodium), may be useful for decresign the inflammation associated with allergic responses. Leukotriene-mediated bronchoconstriction is treated with leukotriene receptor blocking agents such as montelukast (singulair) or zafirlukast (Accolate). Aminophylline or inhalants such as isoproterenol (terbutaline, albuterol) may also provide symptomatic relief from bronchoconstriction.

Avoidance therapy, in which the patient is taught to reduce exposure to triggering antigens, is the most effective treatment to decrease allergic attacks, especially for food, drug, and animal dander, but it can be useful in treating seasonal allergies. For instance, limiting outdoor activities and staying in air-conditioned settings when the pollen counts are high decrease seasonal allergy symptoms.

Immunotherapy is often useful in reducing symptoms in patients who cannot avoid antigens such as dust mites or pollen. The health care provider injects an extract of the allergen subcutaneously starting with the dose at which the person was found to be sensitive by skin testing. Over time, serum IgE-specific antibody levels fall, IgG blocking antibodies increase, and lymphocyte responsiveness to the antigen is reduced. Increasing amounts of allergen are injected at weekly intervals. If large local reactions occur during therapy, the dose is lowered until better tolerated. Systemic reactions, although uncommon, may occur within 30 minutes of injection of the allergen extract. Treatment includes placing the person in a supine position and administering epinephrine. If the nurse notes signs and symptoms of systemic anaphylactic shock, oxygen is administered and intravenous fluids infused rapidly to support blood pressure. Because of its potential for anaphylaxis and death, the patient and primary caregiver must be certain that the symptoms warrant the risk, expense, and inconvenience of immunotherapy.

Clinical manifestations immunotherapy reactions include the following:

Localized
Redness   Edema
Pruritus   Tenderness

Systemic
Nasal stuffiness   Sneezing
Reddening of conjunctiva   Chest tightness
Wheezing   Fainting
Apprehension   Anaphylactic shock

The future of immediate hypersensitivity treatment appears to lie in learning how to more effectively modulate the immune response. Possible therapies include manipulating IgE response by using IgE-specific suppressor T cells; using antibodies against IgE idiotopes; or using cytokines to suppress IgE synthesis.

Diet: The diet may be altered in patients with food allergies to avoid those foods precipitating the response. Suspected foods fare eliminated to see if allergy symptoms disappear. They may be reintroduced to see if they again cause symptoms. Foods suspected of causing systemic anaphylaxis are not reintroduced or only reintroduced under supervision in a hospital setting.

Nursing Management of the Patient with Immediate Hypersensitivity (Type 1)

Assess for:
- History of allergic reactions (type, frequency, or perceived causes)
- Familial history of allergies
- Recent exposure to sensitizing substances (chemicals, drugs)
- Changes in living, working, or environmental conditions
- Characteristics of present environment (house, clothing, plants, trees, or animals)
- Symptoms experienced: respiratory, dermal, gastrointestinal, or general
- Alleviating factors, either prescribed, herbal or over the counter.

And also assess for:
- Rashes (location, color).
- Mouth breathing (nasal obstruction).
- Flaring nares.
- Difficulty hearing (plugged Eustachian tubes).
- Pale bluish turbinates that are edematous with clear secretions.
- Tearing or dark areas under eyes (venous dilation of skin).
- Scleral or conjunctival infections.
- Increased respiratory rate.
- Use of accessory muscles for breathing.
- Audible wheezing.
- Anxious expression.

Problem Associated with Hypersensitivity

Risk for Latex Allergy Responses

Common nursing objectives for the patient with a diagnosis of risk for latex allergy response (or other allergy responses) are:

Patient will:
- Verbalize understanding of approaches for avoiding allergen (all latex-containing products).
- Plan to alter habits or environment to reduce exposure to antigens
- Verbalize understanding of prescribed and alternative approaches to symptom relief

Here, an important aspect of nursing care for the patient with allergies is helping the patient identify and adjust to lifestyle changes to reduce exposure to allergens and maintain health. In many cases this involves few lifestyle changes, and the patient and family readily adjust. In other cases the patient may need to adjust to a complex medication schedule, give up a beloved pet, or move to another climate. Patients may have a change employment to avoid allergens such as chemicals, molds, or fibers. These changes may place emotional or financial burdens on the patient and family, especially if the job market or patients skills are limited. The nurses role is to help the patient explore alternative solutions and make the best choices possible to maintain health.

Teaching the patient and family about the disorder and methods to avoid the allergen is another important nursing interventions for the patient with allergies. The nurse reviews results of allergy testing, assessment findings, and patient history so the patient and family understand which allergens need to be controlled or avoided. The nurse teaches patients the importance of controlling their living and working environments to reduce exposure to antigens and, hence, the risk of reactions. If animal dander is a source of allergy and removal of a family pet is unacceptable to the patient or family, they may explore ways to decreases the pets impact on the allergic patient, such as keeping the pet outdoors or away from the room where the patient sleeps or spends large amounts of time.

The nurse emphasizes the need for total avoidance for patients who are latex sensitive. Patients are taught about prescribed medications, including desired actions, dosage schedules, and potential side effects. The nurse stresses the importance of maintaining drug schedules for prophylactic drugs, such as cromolyn, and reminds the patient and family that these drugs are of no value during an acute allergic attack.

Anaphylaxis can occur after exposure to offending antigens or from immunotherapy; consequently, the nurse teaches the patient and family about symptoms that need to be reported, potential reactions that necessitate emergency measures, and use of emergency care kit. If the patient chooses to undergo immunotherapy, the nurse discusses the risks and benefits, schedules, and costs. The nurse informs the patient that immunotherapy can be reinstituted if symptoms recur.

Patients with immediate hypersensitivities need to be aware of situations in which their specific allergens are likely to be present. The nurse gives those with insect sting sensitivity information about where to obtain and how to use emergency kits for insect stings. The nurse teaches both the patient and family how to use the self-injecting syringe to administer epinephrine. If the patient is unable to use the syringe, an inhalation of high-dose epinephrine may be taken from a metered dose aerosol, which is found in some emergency kits.

Ineffective Airway Clearance

Common nursing objective for the patient with a diagnosis of *ineffective airway clearance* are:

Patient will:
- Maintain a patent airway
- Correctly demonstrate the use of emergency anaphylactic equipment
- Verbalize the need to have emergency anaphylactic equipment available at all times
- Verbalize the need to inform all health care providers regarding his or her latex sensitivity

Death from anaphylaxis occurs from asphyxiation because of upper airway edema and congestion, irreversible shock, or a combination of these factors (see the section on clinical manifestation of systemic anaphylaxis). The primary concern during an anaphylactic reaction is ensuring that the patient's airway is patent. The nurse positions the patient in a high Fowler's position to maximize ventilation; inserts an oral airway if necessary; and removes secretions by suction or by encouraging the patient to cough. Oxygen therapy is initiated in accordance with facility protocols. The nurse encourages slow, deep breathing to facilitate the intake of oxygen and decrease anxiety. The administration of epinephrine or bronchodilators such as aminophylline may be necessary to decrease bronchospasm. In severe cases, tracheostomy may be necessary to maintain a patent airway. The nurse closely monitors the patient both during and after anaphylaxis, since recurrence is possible.

Respiratory compromise can lead to impaired cardiac function and death within minutes. At the first sign of anaphylaxis, the nurse gives the patient epinephrine, 1:1000 solution, 0.3 to 0.5 ml subcutaneously or intramuscularly. If shock continues, the nurse may administer albuterol (Ventolin) or epinephrine through aerosol treatments. Vasopressors such as dopamine may be prescribed for severe shock to assist in maintaining blood pressure and cardiac output.

Since drug allergies are a significant cause of anaphylaxis, the nurse questions all patients about allergies and drug sensitivities before initiating drug therapy. High-risk persons are instructed to wear an identification bracelet or necklace at all times that indicates the known allergy. Such devices may be obtained from Guinine or other commercial sources. Persons with known drug allergies are advised to alert heath care workers of their allergies when animal sera, allergenic extracts, or contrast media containing iodide need to be given for any reason, so that epinephrine can be readily available. The nurse monitors the patient for at least 30 minutes after administration of such substances. Any reaction that occurs within a few minutes forewarns of an impending emergency.

Nurses need to recognize the potential for drug cross-sensitivity what administering alternative drugs to allergic patients. For example, cephalosporins are frequently administered to patients who are sensitive to penicillin. A small percentage of patients will, however, also be sensitive to cephalosporin because it has a cross sensitivity with penicillin. The yellow dye contained in some tablets has cross sensitivity with aspirin and may cause anaphylaxis in aspirin-sensitive patients.

Health Education Patient with Allergies

Patient teaching should include information about the allergy and prescribed medication, as well as the following instructions on avoiding allergens.

Animal Dander
- Avoid fur bearing pets if possible, or keep pets outdoors.
- Avoid furniture stuffed with horsehair or feathers.

Pollen Spores

Use air conditioning if possible; keep windows closed at night; if using air condition in car, start car, roll down windows, and allow air conditioner to run for 10 to 15 minutes before entering car.
- Limit time outdoors between sunset and sunrise, especially when windy.
- Do not hang wash outside to dry (pollen and molds stick to wet wash).
- Avoid gardening, raking leaves, mowing lawn, or being near freshly cut grass.
- Keep car windows closed when driving.
- Minimize number of indoor plants.
- Vacation in selected geographic areas, such as beach or sea, that are free of specific allergen during seasonal height, if possible.

House Dust
- Use synthetic materials; avoid wool and cotton
- Use a minimum of lint-producing articles.
- Put away items that are difficult to dust.
- Dust with damp cloth daily.
- Use air conditioner if possible.
- Change furnace filter every month when in use.
- The Patient with Immediate Hypersensitivity: Sting
- Patient teaching should include:
  - Emergency care for the specific allergy
  - Availability and use of commercially prepared emergency kit
  - Concentration and route of emergency use epinephrine (1:1000 epinephrine injection)
  - Use of self-injection syringe of epinephrine supplied with kit (spring loaded; can be given through clothing).

Also include the following instructions about the emergency procedure if sting occurs:
- Immediately swallow the uncoated antihistamine tablet
- Inject the epinephrine
- If unable to self inject, inhale high dose epinephrine from metered dose aerosol (if included in kit).

Tissue-specific Antibody Hypersensitivities

In antibody-mediated hypersensitivity, also known as cytotoxic hypersensitivity, antibodies are directed against specific target cells or tissues; thus the damage is restricted to those cells or tissues that bear the specific antigen, such as platelets. These reactions differ from immune-complex (type III) reactions in that type III reactions involve circulating antigen-antibody complexes.

A classic example of a specific antibody-mediated (type II) hypersensitivity reaction occurs with the infusion of mismatched blood. *Acute hemolytic transfusion reaction* (ABO incompatibility) is the most serious adverse reaction to blood transfusions and results in approximately 1 death per 1,00,000 units of blood infused. The reaction occurs within the first 30 minutes of blood administration. Studies of **hemolytic** reactions have shown that mistakes in specimen collection and labeling or inadequate patient identification are the primary errors responsible.

Another type of antibody-mediated hypersensitivity occurs when the mother is sensitized to antigens on the infant's erythrocytes and makes antibodies against those antigens. This condition is known as *hemolytic disease of the newborn*. The Rhesus D (RhD) factor is the most commonly involved antigen of the antigen RhD is present; the term Rh-negative means that the RhD antigen is absent. Approximately 85% of the population has Rh-positive blood. Between 10 and 15% of Caucasian infants and approximately 5% of African-American infants experience Rh incompatibility.

Tissue-specific hypersensitivities injure host cells by binding IgG or IgM to an antigen on the surface of a target cell, such as a platelet. Once binding occurs, the cell is destroyed by phagocytic attack, nonspecific lymphocytic attack or lysis of the cell through the activation of the full complement cascade.

Immunologic Transfusion Reactions

Acute hemolytic reaction are caused by antigen-antibody complexes on the erythrocyte membrane. These complexes activate Hageman factor (coagulation factor XII) and the complement cascade. The Hageman factor initiates the kinin system, causing increased capillary permeability, arteriole vasodilation, and hypotension. The complement system initiates intravascular hemolysis, as well as histamine and serotonin release from the mast cells. Hageman factor also combines with free compatible erythrocytes, activating the intrinsic clotting cascade, which causes disseminated intravascular coagulation (DIC).

Febrile nonhemolytic reactions are among the most common transfusion reactions. They occur when the recipient becomes sensitized to the donor's white blood cells, platelets, or plasma. Symptoms usually begin 30 minutes after the start of the infusion. Although this reaction is not usually serious, it is uncomfortable.

Allergic transfusion reactions are due to the recipient's sensitivity to foreign plasma proteins. Common symptoms include hives, rash, and urticaria. If the symptoms are mild, the patient is treated with antihistamines and the transfusion is restarted slowly. Anaphylaxis can occur but fortunately is rare.

Delayed hemolytic reactions occur 7 to 14 days after the transfusion and are thought to be the result of sensitization of the recipient's immune system to the transfused erythrocyte antigens. The recipient may also have been previously sensitized but have antibody titers that are undetectable at the time of transfusion.

Post-transfusion graft versus host disease, which was once relatively rare, is occurring more frequently because of increased use of purposeful immunosuppression as treatment (e.g., bone marrow transplantation). The donor lymphocytes begin to reject the patient's host cells 4 to 30 days after the infusion of blood.

Noncardiac pulmonary edema is thought to be caused by a high titer of leukocyte antibodies in either the donor or recipient plasma. These antibody-to-granulocyte reactions cause granulocyte aggregates that are filtered out by the lung. The antibodies attached to the initiate the complement cascade and promote histamine release, causing an influx of inflammatory cells into the lung.

Hemolytic Disease

Hemolytic disease, most commonly seen in newborns, occurs when the Rh-negative mother is first exposed to the fetus's Rh-positive blood. Rh antibodies are formed against the Rh-positive blood. On subsequent exposures to Rh-positive blood, such as a second pregnancy, the Rh antibody binds to its corresponding antigen on the surface of the erythrocyte containing Rh factor. The Rh-antibodies do not usually fix complement; therefore hemolysis does not occur immediately as it does in the ABO system. Instead, the Rh-factor erythrocytes are rapidly broken down by macrophages in the spleen, with conversion of hemoglobin to bilirubin, resulting in jaundice.

Nonimmunogenic transfusion reactions. The administration of blood can cause reactions that are not immunologic. These include circulatory overload, sepsis, and transmission of disease. The clinical manifestations of nonimmunogenic transfusion reactions:

- *Circulation overload:* This can occur when blood is given to rapidly or in large quantities. Older adults are particularly vulnerable. Patients develop signs of fluid overload and pulmonary congestion. The transfusion is stopped and oxygen and diuretics may be administered.
- *Sepsis:* Bacterial contamination can occur at time during the collection or handling of blood. Signs of sepsis being almost immediately. The transfusion is stopped, and the patient receives antibiotics and treatment for shock if it occurs.
- *Disease transmission:* Hepatits, cytomegalovirus, and humanimmunodeficiency virus are the most common diseases transmitted by blood transfusions. Hepatitis A and B are effectively identified with current screening capabilities, but hepatitis C is still readily transmissible.

Management: Prevention is the key to management of transfusion reactions. Blood received from volunteer donors through the blood banks is carefully screened and labeled. Most of the serious reactions that occur from transfusions are the result of human error. Typing, screening and cross-matching of blood in the laboratory must be accurate. Typing is established by testing the recipients serum against commercial A and B cells to detect isoaglutinins. The recipient's serum is then screened for all antibodies that were not found in the typing. The goal of cross-matching is to ensure the recipient's blood does not contain antibodies that will attack and destroy the transfused erythrocytes.

One method for preventing immunologic blood transfusion reactions and disease transmission is planned autologous transfusion, which involves using the persons own blood for replacement. Health care providers collect blood at regular intervals before anticipated use, such as forthcoming surgery, and store and freeze the blood until needed. This method is especially useful for persons with rare blood types, for those whose religious beliefs preclude receiving donor blood, or for those expected to need several units of blood during surgery (e.g., selected heart surgeries or joint replacements).

Auto transfusion, which consists of collecting, filtering, and immediately reinfusing the persons own blood, may be performed in the emergency department, the operating room suite during surgery, the post anesthesia care unit, or the critical care unit. Blood draining from the surgical site is suctioned into a bag and passes through a filter to remove microaggregates. When the bag is full, it is disconnected from the system and the blood is infused into the patient with an administration set, using a standard or microembolic filter.

Blood components are often administered rather than whole blood. Blood can be fractionated into red blood cells, platelets, and plasma either by centrifuge or automated cell separators. Blood can also be withdrawn from a donor, a portion separated out, and the remainder returned to the donor (apheresis). Using blood components rather than whole blood is a more efficient use of a scarce commodity for more recipients, prevents fluid overload, and decreases the risk of adverse effects.

The nurse administering blood or blood products carefully monitors it and follows strict institutional protocols. If a patient reports any of the symptoms associated with transfusion reaction, the nurse stops the stops transfusion immediately, maintains venous patency by administering normal saline, and notifies the primary care provider immediately. Patients who exhibit any sign of anaphylaxis or hemolytic reaction receive frequent vital sign monitoring and are assessed for signs of impending shock, renal failure, or DIC. The blood and tubing are returned to the laboratory for analysis, and a first voided urine specimen is collected to analyze for signs of hemolysis. The patients hemoglobin and hematocrit levels are carefully monitored to determine the extent of the reaction. Patients who experience mild allergic reactions to blood may receive premedication with an antihistamine if they should need transfusion in the future.

Persons with any of the following are not permitted to donate blood:

- History of infectious diseases such as hepatitis, human immunodeficiency virus infection, acquired immunodeficiency syndrome (AIDS), tuberculosis, or malaria
- Malignant diseases
- Allergies of asthma
- Polycythemia vera
- Abnormal bleeding tendencies
- Hypotension (current)
- Anemia (current)
- Recent pregency or major surgery
- Men with at least one homosexual or bisexual contact since 1975 (concern for AIDS)
- International travel to malarial areas or high-risk countries (concern for AIDS)
- Blood transfusion during past 6 months
- History of jaundice
- Disease of the heart, lung, or liver
- Immunizations or vaccinations with attenuated viral vaccine rubella or rabies vaccine
- Hemoglobin level below 13.5 gm/dl for men or 12.4 gm/dl for women
- Abnormalities in vital signs, particularly fever.

Treatment for hemolytic disease of the newborn involves the administration of Rh-immunoglobulin (RhoGAM) to mothers who have not been sensitized by a former pregnancy. The immunoglobulin is given by injection at about 28 weeks of pregnancy or within 72 hours after birth, amniocentesis, or interrupted pregnancy because of miscarriage or abortion. The immunoglobulin contains antibodies that destroy any of the fetus's red blood cells that have entered the mother's blood, preventing sensitization and Rh incompatibility during the next pregnancy.

Antigen-Antibody Complex Hypersensitivities

Antigen-antibody complex (type III) (also known as immune-complex) hypersensitivities are caused by the formation or deposition of antigen-antibody complexes in various tissues, which results in complement activation and inflammation. These reactions generally occur several hours after exposure to the antigen. Unlike antibody mediated (type II) responses, these reactions tend to be systemic and characterized by widespread vasculitis, arthritis, or nephritis. Systemic lupus erythematosus, post-streptococcal immune complex glomerulonephritis and serum sickness are examples of antigen-antibody hypersensitivity diseases.

Guidelines for Safe Practice of Blood Transfusion

Patient Receiving Blood Transfusion

Carefully check all of the following:
- Obtain baseline vital signs and check at frequent intervals throughout the procedure.
- Administer all blood products through micron mesh filters.
- Assess patient for any unusual sensations felt throughout the transfusion. (This information may help with early identification of any reactions).
- Infuse blood within 4 hours after it is taken from the blood bank (to prevent bacterial growth).
- If blood cannot be infused within 4 hours, return it to the blood bank for proper refrigeration.
- Follow facility guidelines for proper disposal of empty blood bag and tubing.
- Record patients response to the infusion.
- Report any adverse effect to the primary care provider immediately.
- Return the blood bag and tubing to the laboratory for testing if a reaction occurs.

Serum Sickness

Serum sickness develops within 1 to 3 weeks after administration of a foreign serum, such as horse or rabbit serum. It may also occur after administration of certain drugs (e.g., antimicrobials such as penicillin and sulfonamides). Classic serum sickness is rarely encountered today because large doses of foreign sera are rarely administered.

The pathogenesis of serum sickness involves the attachment of foreign serum proteins to IgM and IgG. These antigen-antibody complexes bind to complement, initiating the complement cascade and resulting in chemotaxis, vasodilation, and cell lysis. These chemotactic factors lead to an influx of phagocytes, which tend to intensify the inflammatory response.

The antigen-antibody reactions of serum sickness occur in many organs, but the kidneys, choroids plexus, joints, skin and lungs are primarily affected. Itching and discomfort at the injection site are usually the first symptoms, followed by lymphadenopathy, fever, urticaria or erythematous rash, angioedema of the face, and joint pain. Splenomegaly, abdominal pain, headache, nausea, and vomiting may also occur.

Treatment of antigen-antibody hypersensitivity depends on the cause. Serum sickness is a self-limiting disease. Mild symptoms respond well to antihistamines salicylates. More sever symptoms are treated with steroids such as prednisone, and symptom relief is often achieved within hours. Epinephrine is given if an anaphylactic reaction occurs.

T Cell-Mediated Hypersensitivity

T cell-mediated (type IV) hypersensitivity, also known as delayed hypersensitivity, is mediated by T cells rather than antibodies. Graft rejection, contact dermatitis, and hypersensitivity induced by chronic infection (e.g., tuberculosis) are examples of T cell-mediated hypersensitivity reactions.

T cell-mediated hypersensitivity generally occurs within 12 to 72 hours after a sensitized individual comes in contact with the offending antigen. The reaction occurring from an inactivated or purified protein derivative (PPD) tuberculin test is a classic example. People who have undergone sufficient exposure to *Mycobacterium tuberculosis* to be sensitized to the organism, whether or not they have the disease, develop redness and in duration in response to the injection within 8 to 12 hours.

Allergic contact dermatitis is an inflammatory response confined to the skin that results from repeated exposure of a sensitized person to an allergen. Environmental substances such as cosmetics, hair dyes, detergents, poison ivy or oak, or latex may serve as the offending antigen in these reactions.

Another important T-cell mediated hypersensitivity reaction occurs when organs or tissues are transferred from one person to another. Transplantations have been performed for many years, but they remain limited because of the rejection process resulting from this type of hypersensitivity.

Pathophysiology: T cell-mediated hypersensitivities do not involve antibodies such as IgE. Rather, macrophages identify the antigen as foreign, encode it, and present it to T cell lymphocytes, which become sensitized lymphocyte forms cytotoxic T cells or activates nonspecific phagocytic cells (macrophages and polymorphonuclear leukocytes) through release of lymphokines. The cytotoxic T cell lymphocytes destroy the antigen directly by breaking down the cell membrane, causing lysis and cell death.

Allergic contact dermatitis is one of the most commonly encountered T cell-mediated hypersensitivities and type of allergic disease. Dermal contact with the antigen produces sensitization and the clinical manifestations associated with the reaction. The allergen attaches to skin proteins, which function as haptens to stimulate the proliferation of a T cell population sensitized to the allergen. After sensitization, subsequent exposure to the contact allergen leads to formation of an erythematous, vesiculated (blistered) lesion. The inflamed area is red, swollen, and warm and may itch, burn or sting. The location of the lesions often provides data but the causative allergic agent.

The tubercle bacillus *(M. tuberculosis)* itself is not directly toxic to human cells or tissues. The organism invades the tissues of a nonsensitized host and establishes residence in the host tissues, causing virtually no damage. However, in time, as the organism sheds antigenic material, the T cell-mediated response is triggered. The sensitized lymphocytes and activated macrophages attack not only the organism but also the tissues surrounding the organism. This process is aimed at destroying the foreign organism, but tissue destruction may result. The lesions associated with tuberculosis (such as caseation necrosis cavitations) and general toxemia are results of the hypersensitivity. After the initial sensitization with the infectious organism, subsequent contact with the tuberculosis organism or an extract of a purified protein from the organism elicits a hypersensitivity reaction. This is the basis of the Mantoux tuberculin skin test. The skin rashes of smallpox and measles and the lesions of herpes simplex virus are all examples of microbially induced T cell hypersensitivities.

In organ transplantation the foreign tissue or organ serves as the allergen against which the cell mediated response is directed. Cytotoxic T lymphocytes attack and destroy the tissues directly, resulting in destruction of transplanted tissues. Discussions of specific types of transplants are found in chapters dealing with the disorders for which they are used as treatment.

Management: Treatment for contact dermatitis includes elimination of known allergens, decreased exposure, or both. Topical anti-inflammatory agents such as corticosteroid creams may be useful in reducing the discomfort associated with itching and in decreasing healing time. For severe reactions, systemic corticosteroids and antihistamines may be necessary. There is no specific treatment, other than treatment of the underlying infection, for hypersensitivity reactions to infective agents. If secondary infection develops as a result of the patient scratching the area, antibodies may be prescribed. Immunosuppression therapy is used to control transplant rejection.

Stimulatory Hypersensitivity

Stimulatory hypersensitivity is a B cell-mediated response that occurs when auto-antibodies bind to target cell surface receptors and cause inappropriate stimulation of the cell, such as the thyroid gland. The usual feedback mechanism is lost; consequently the cell continuously secretes its hormone in an uncontrolled manner. Thyrotoxicosis (Graves disease) is thought to be induced by this mechanism. It is believed that thyroid-stimulating immunoglobulin and thyrotoxicosis (Grave's disease) is thought to be induced by this mechanism. It is believed that thyroid-stimulating immunoglobulin and thyroid-stimulating hormone binding inhibitory immunoglobulin stimulate the secretion of thyroid hormone. Signs and symptoms of hyperthyroidism are produced even though the actual condition is not present and the thyroid gland itself is completely normal.

The causes of stimulatory reactions are unknown but may be related to loss of self-tolerance. Treatment of stimulatory hypersensitivity involves removing the focus of the abnormal secretion when only one organ is involved, such as the thyroid gland. If multiple tissues are involved, immunosuppression is used in an attempt to suppress the production of autoantibodies, halt over secretion of the hormone, and prevent associated symptoms.

Autoimmune Diseases

The cause of autoimmunity, or the loss of self-tolerance, is not clearly understood. Autoimmune diseases occur more frequently in women, especially during the childbearing years, than in men. Some autoimmune diseases affect certain populations more than others. For example, rheumatoid arthritis and scleroderma are more common among Native Americans than in the general population. Lupus erythematosus affects African-American and Hispanic women more than Caucasian women.

Pathophysiology: Autoimmunity refers to the formation of antibodies against self cells. The principal factors in the development of autoimmunity are genetic predisposition, environment, and viral infections. Antibodies produced against one's own cells are referred to as *autoantibodies*. When produced against deoxyrinonucleic acid (DNA), they are called anti-DNA antibodies. These self-reactive immunoglobulins are often associated with pathologic states in the body; however, they can also be isolated from the serum of disease-free individuals and are present in about half of adults over the age of 70 years.

Several theories exist about the mechanism of autoimmunity:

- *Release of sequestered antigens:* If an antigen does not come into contact with the immune system during fetal development when self tolerance normally develops, the antigen remains antigenic. Later, as a result of trauma or infection, the antigen may be exposed to the immune system, eliciting an autoimmune response (e.g., autoantibodies against heart muscle after acute myocardial infarction).
- *Defective suppressor T cells:* Suppressor T cell function may be lost or altered so that autoantibodies are allowed to proliferate without control.
- *Synthesis of cross reactive antibodies:* Antibodies synthesized in response to certain foreign antigens may have cross-reactivity with similar antigenic components within human tissues.
- *Alteration of self-antigens:* Normal body proteins may be altered by chemicals, infectious organisms, or therapeutic drugs and present new antigenically active groups to the immune system. Autoimmune hemolytic anemia may result from alteration of the Rh antigens of the red blood cells, rendering it antigenic. Certain antibodies can have a similar effect.

Autoimmune disorders are grouped into categories according to the body part or tissues involved. *Organ-specific* diseases produce chronic inflammatory changes in a specific organ, such as the kidney or heart. *Nonorgan-specific* autoimmune disorders are characterized by chronic inflammatory changes in many different organs and tissues throughout the body.

Classifications of autoimmune disorders organ specific

Blood
Autoimmune hemolytic anemia
Idiopathic thrombocytopenic purpura

Heart

Rheumatic fever

Central Nervous System
Multiple sclerosis
Guillain-Barr'e syndrome
Muscles
Myasthenia gravis
Endocrine System
Addison's disease
Autoimmune thyroiditis (Hashimoto's disease)
Graves disease
Hypothyroidism

Eye
Uveitis

Gastrointestinal System
Pernicious anemia
Ulcerative colitis
Kidneys
Glomerulonephritis
Goodpasture's syndrome
Skin
Pemphigus vulgaris

Nonorganspecific
Systemic lupus erythematosus
Rheumatoid arthritis
Progressive systemic sclerosis

Treatment for autoimmune disorders consists of immunosuppression and control of clinical manifestations, primarily through systemic corticosteroid therapy. Initial doses of 60 mg of oral prednisone often bring about a noticeable decrease in symptoms. Once symptoms are controlled, dosages are slowly decreased and then discontinued until the next exacerbation. Cytotoxic drugs such as cyclophosphamide, azathioprine, and methotrexate are sometimes prescribed for patients with severe or persistent manifestations.

Patients with autoimmune disorders are encouraged to eat well balanced diets, maintain daily exercise patterns without becoming excessively fatigued, and get adequate rest and sleep. The nurse explains the anticipated benefit of prescribed medications, dosage schedules, and adverse effects, especially when patient are taking corticosteroids or other immunosuppressive drugs. The nurse cautions patients against abruptly withdrawing steroid medications, since abrupt cessation can result in adrenal insufficiency or crisis. Close follow-up care is emphasized for all patients taking immunosuppressive agents.

Chronic Fatigue Syndrome

Chronic fatigue syndrome (CFS) is a condition of unexplained fatigue that lasts 6 months or longer and eventually leads to disability. CFS may follow a cold, influenza, bronchitis, or mononucleosis. In other instances CFS develops gradually, with no clear initiating event. Accompanying manifestations, such as muscle and joint discomfort, headache, loss of concentration, weakness and tender lymph nodes, may go unnoticed because they are similar to the flu. Unlike the flu, however, the fatigue and other symptoms remain or reappear frequently. CFS is now recognized in people of all ages, races, and socioeconomic groups. The primary clinical manifestations of CFS is prolonged, debilitating fatigue accompanied by any or all of the symptoms listed in the below:

- Clinically evaluated, unexplained, persistent or relapsing chronic fatigue that is of new or definite onset (i.e., not lifelong), is not the result of ongoing exertion, is not substantially alleviated by rest, and results in substantial reduction in previous levels of occupational, educational, social, or personal activities.
- The concurrent occurrence of four or more of the following symptoms:
  - Substantial impairment in short-term memory or concentration
  - Sore throat
  - Tender lymph nodes
  - Muscle pain
  - Multijoint pain without swelling or redness
  - Headaches of a new type, pattern, or severity
  - Unrefreshing sleep
  - Postexertional malaise lasting more than 24 hours.

These symptoms must have persisted or recurred during 6 or more consecutive months of illness and must not have predated the fatigue.

Conditions That Exclude a Diagnosis of Chronic Fatigue Syndrome

- Any active medical condition that may explain the presence of chronic fatigue, such as untreated hypothyroidism, sleep apnea and narcolepsy, and iatrogenic conditions such as side effects of medication
- Some diagnosable illnesses that may relapse or may not have completely resolved during treatment. If the persistence of such a condition could explain the presence of chronic fatigue, and if it cannot be clearly established that the original condition has completely resolved with treatment, the such patients should not be classified ads having chronic fatigue syndrome. Examples of illnesses that can present such a picture include some types of malignancies and chronic cases of hepatitis B or C virus infection.
- Any past or current diagnosis of a major depressive disorder with psychotic or melancholic features; bipolar affective disorders; schizophrenia of any subtype; delusional disorders of any subtype; dementias of any subtype; anorexia nervosa; or bulimia nervosa.
- Alcohol or other substance abuse, occurring within 2 years of the onset of chronic fatigue and any time afterward.
- Severe obesity as defined by a body mass index [body mass index = weight (kg)/height (m)^2] equal to or greater than 45. (NOTE: Body mass index values vary considerably among different age groups and populations. No "normal" or "average" range of values is meaningful. The range of 45 or greater was selected because it clearly falls within the range of severe obesity.)

The exact cause of CFS remains unknown. Conditions that may trigger its development are genetic and environmental factors, viral infection, transient traumatic conditions, toxins, or stress. The clinical course of CFS varies considerably among patients, and it is difficult to diagnose because the same symptoms occur with many other conditions and diseases. CFS often follows a cyclic course, alternating between illness and relatively symptom-free intervals, which is similar to that of autoimmune disorders such as lupus erythematosus or multiple sclerosis. About 50% of patients recover within the first 5 years after onset. No characteristics of the disease or persons with the disease have been identified to show that one person is more likely to recover than another.

Management: Treatments for CFS have included antiviral agents, antidepressants, and immune modulators, but none have proven effective. Consequently, treatments are aimed at controlling symptoms and helping patients return to a normal or near-normal lifestyle. Non-steroidal anti-inflammatory drugs may be beneficial in reducing body aches or fever, and nonsedating antihistamines have been useful for relieving allergy symptoms. No cure for this disease exists at this time.

Patient care focuses on self-management of fatigue to improve function and quality of life. The nurse helps the patient identify potential triggers to fatigue and encourages them to avoid situation or activities adversely affect their energy levels. Periods of activity are scheduled at times when patients feel better and are alternated with rest periods. Exercise may seem contradictory in the presence of fatigue, but exercise improves conditioning and can restore energy. Patients are assisted with developing individualized exercise programs that incorporate a gradual increase in exercise intensity and duration. Exercise beds to be incorporated in a manner that does not exacerbate fatigue, yet promotes regular participations.

A well balanced diet is essential to promote adequate energy stores. Nighttime sleep should be as free of interruption as possible, and daytime naps are avoided if they interfere with night-time sleep. The patient may also benefit from relaxation, meditation, massage, imagery, therapeutic touch, music, or biofeedback.

Chronic fatigue syndrome is disease with overwhelming subjective symptoms, and health care providers commonly treat patients experiencing persistent debilitating fatigue with over skepticism, if not direct accusations of malingering. Symptoms of CFS may be attributed to life stress, unhappiness, female hormone imbalances, or simply psychocomaticism. The nurse plays an important role in reassuring the patient about the validity and severity of the symptoms. Family members should be included in discussions and teaching sessions about disease etiology and management. Family support is critical to the patient because many occupational and family roles may have to be reduced or eliminated in the face of overwhelming fatigue. Patient and families may be encouraged to contact local or national CFS support groups to establish networks of information and support for dealing with this debilitating chronic disease.

Human Immunodeficiency Virus Infection (HIV)

Human immunodeficiency virus (HIV) infection is an acquired infection in which the HIV integrates itself into CD4 (helper T4) cells, causing severe immune dysfunction. HIV infection renders the person unusually susceptible to other life-threatening infections and malignancies. In its most serious form, HIV results in acquired immunodeficiency syndrome (AIDS).

Etiology: The origin of HIV is still largely unknown. Evidence suggests an African origin, since an AIDS-like illness in Central Africa has been known to exist the early 1960s. Some researches hypothesize that the most likely source of human infection was from nonhuman primates. The causative agent of HIV infection is HIV, a **retrovirus** belonging to the *Lentivirus* subfamily. Several human retroviruses have been identified. Two of them, HIV-1 and HIV-2 are associated with depletion of helper T4 cells and subsequent loss of cellular immunity.

HIV is a blood borne, sexually transmitted disease (STD). The routes of viral transmission are well documented: (1) direct transmission from person to person by sexual contact, (2) direct inoculation with contaminated blood products, needles, or syringe, and (3) infection from mother to her fetus or newborn. Sexual practices, including vaginal or anal penetration without a condom and oral sexual practices, are associated with a high risk for infection. The use of contaminated needles for subcutaneous, intramuscular, or IV injection is another source of infection. Women who are HIV infected may pass the virus onto their newborns via three potential routes: gestation, delivery, and rarely, breast milk.

Blood, semen and vaginal secretions are primary sources for infection, and epidemiologic studies indicate that transmission via saliva, tears, and breast milk is sufficient and unlikely to produce infection. HIV is not transmitted by casual contact, including sneezing; coughing; spitting; hand shaking; and contacting potential secretions in toilet seats, bathtubs, showers, swimming pools, utensils, dishes, or linens used by infected persons. HIV is not transmitted by biting or blood-sucking insects.

Blood transfusions are not a significant source of HIV infection today. In each unit of donated blood is tested of HIV infection, as well as several other blood borne infections, such as hepatitis B. HIV screening of blood products has been conducted since 1985, only recipients of transfusions before that time were at significant risk for infection via the blood supply. It is possible for a contaminated unit of blood to test negative for HIV if the donor has not yet formed antibodies to the virus at the time of donation. As a result, the risk of exposure to HIV via blood supply is estimated to be 1 in 1.4 to 1.8 million units of blood. Since 1985, seven cases have been reported of organ transplant recipients contracting HIV. In all cases, problems prevented the identification of the donor's HIV status before harvesting of organs.

The risk for HIV transmission to health care workers prompted the CDC to implement Universal Precautions. Those precautions, now known as Standard Precautions, apply to all patients regardless of their medical diagnosis. The Standard Precaution protocol acknowledges that recognized and unrecognized microorganisms can exist in any body fluid, and the use of appropriate precautions reduces the risk for transmission within the hospital environment.

Risk Factors of HIV

- Sexual practices:
  - Unprotected sex
  - Multiple sexual partners
  - Anal or oral sexual activity
- Improper condom use or condom breakage.
- Open sores, lesions, or irritation in the genital area.
- Contaminated blood.
- Contaminated needles.
- Occupational exposure.
  - All health care workers – Acute care, long-term care, and home care.
  - Dental workers.
  - Corrections officers and law enforcement personnel.
- Perinatal exposure (during pregnancy, birth, or breast-feeding).

Transmission of HIV

HIV is a fragile virus. It can only be transmitted under specific conditions that allow contact with infected body fluids, including blood, semen, vaginal secretions, and breast milk. Transmission of HIV occurs through sexual intercourse with an infected partner, exposure to HIV infected blood or blood produces, and perinatal transmission during pregnancy, at the time of delivery, or through breastfeeding.

HIV infected individuals can transmit HIV to others within a few days after becoming infected. After that, the ability to transmit HIV is lifelong. Transmission of HIV is subject to the same requirements as other microorganisms (i.e., a large enough amount of the virus must enter the body of a susceptible host). Duration and frequency of contact, volume of fluid, virulence and concentration of the organism, and host immune status all affect whether infection is established after an exposure. The viral load (or the number of viruses) in the blood, semen, vaginal secretions, or breast milk of the "donor" is an important variable. Large amounts of HIV can be found in the blood during the first 6 months of infection and again during the late stages of the diseases. Unprotected sexual or blood exposure to an infected individual is more risky during these periods, although HIV can be transmitted during all phases of the disease.

HIV is not spread casually. The virus cannot be transmitted through hugging, dry kissing, shaking hands, sharing eating utensils, using toilet seats, or attending school or working with an HIV infected person. It is not transmitted through tears, saliva, urine, emesis, sputum, feces, or sweat. Repeated studies have failed to demonstrate transmission of the virus by respiratory droplets, enteric routes, or casual encounters in any setting. Health care workers have a very low risk of acquiring HIV at work, even after a needle-stick injury.

Sexual Transmission

Unprotected sexual contact with an HIV-infected partner is the most common mode of transmission. Sexual activity provides an opportunity for contact with semen, vaginal secretions, and/or blood, all of which have lymphocytes that may contain HIV.

Although men who have sex with men (MSM) still account for most cases of HIV in the United States and Canada, heterosexual transmission has become more prevalent and is now the most common method of infection for women. The riskiest sexual activity is unprotected anal intercourse. During any form of sexual intercourse (anal, vaginal, or oral), the risk of infection is greater for the partner who receives the semen, although infection can also be transmitted to an inserting partner. This occurs because the receiver has prolonged contact with infected fluids, and helps explain why women are more easily infected than men during heterosexual intercourse. Sexual activities that involve blood, such as during menstruation or as a result of trauma to local tissues, also increase the risk of transmission. In addition, the presence of genital lesions caused by other sexually transmitted disease (e.g., herpes, syphilis) significantly increases the likelihood of infection.

Contact with Blood and Blood Products

HIV can be transmitted during exposure to blood through drug-using equipment. Used equipment may be contaminated with HIV and other blood-borne organisms, and sharing that equipment can result in disease transmission.

It has been reported that transfusion of infected blood and blood products has caused only 1% of adult AIDS cases. In 1985, routine screening of blood donors to identify at-risk individuals and testing donated blood for the presence of HIV were implemented, thereby improving the safety of the blood supply. HIV infection as a result of blood transfusions is now unlikely, but still possible because blood donated during the first few months of infection may not test positive for HIV antibodies. Clotting factors used by people with hemophilia are now treated with heat or chemicals that kill HIV and other blood born viruses, thus eliminating that risk.

Puncture wounds are the most common means of work-related transmission. The risk of infection after a needle-stick exposure to HIV-infected blood is 0.3 to 0.4% (or 3 to 4 out of 1000). The risk is higher if the exposure involves blood from a patient with a high viral load, a deep puncture wound, a needle with a hollow bore and visible blood, a device used for venous or arterial access, or a patient who dies within 60 days. Splash exposures of blood on skin with an open lesion present some risk, but it is much lower than from a puncture wound.

Perinatal Transmission

Perinatal transmission is the most common route of infection for children. Transmission from an HIV-infected mother to her infant can occur during pregnancy, at the time of delivery, or after birth through breastfeeding. On average, 25% of infants born to untreated HIV-infected women will be born with HIV. This means that 75% of these infants would not have been infected even without treatment.

Pathophysiology

The **human immunodeficiency virus (HIV)**, a ribonucleic acid (RNA) virus, was discovered in 1983. RNA viruses are called **retroviruses** because they replicate in a "backward" manner (going from RNA to deoxyribonucleic acid [DNA]). Like all viruses, HIV cannot replicate unless it is inside a living cell.

The natural history of HIV infection is associated with an unpredictable course of disease progression. Patients may undergo a prolonged period of clinically silent infection, often lasting more than 10 years, during which the virus remains dormant. Although the virus is consistently detected throughout this time, patients may exhibit only subtle immunologic alterations. Once viral replication begins, which can occur rapidly, **CD4 lymphocytes** are destroyed and the patient becomes symptomatic.

The life cycle of HIV is similar to that of the other retroviruses. HIV interacts with a CD4 glycoprotein found on the membrane of CD4 lymphocytes. CD4 refers to the particular protein expressed on the surface of the helper T4 lymphocyte. The CD4 glycoprotein is also found on the surface of several other cells, including some monocytes, macrophages, glial fells, and gastrointestinal (GI) cells. Presence of the CD4 glycoprotein allows the virus to fuse to the host cell. Once fused, the virus is infected into the cell cytoplasm, where it sheds its two outer coats, releasing two ribonucleic acid (RNA) copies, which are subsequently transcribed into proviral deoxyribonucleic acids (DNA). The proviral DNA is then integrated into the CD4 cell by the retroviral enzyme reverse transcriptase.

HIV has GP120 glycoprotiens that attach to CD4 and chemokine CXCR4 and CCR5 receptors on the surface of CD4 T cells. Viral RNA then enters the cell, produces viral DNA in the presence of reverse transcriptase, and incorporates itself into the cellular genomein the presence of integrase, causing permanent cellular infection and the production of new virions. New viral RNA develops initially in long strands that are cut in the presence of protease and leave the cell through a budding process that ultimately contributes to cellular destruction.

The virus may remain dormant in the CD4 cells, or replicate by using the host cell's genetic machinery to assemble and release new viral particles. Viral replication eventually depletes the host's CD4 cells, resulting in a dramatic loss of immune protection. Infections that were once disarmed by the healthy immune system, are eventually able to cause serious and potentially life-threatening disease. HIV escapes the host's immune system may be thought that viral entry into host cells occurs before the host's virus-specific immune response is initiated. Once HIV gains entry into T cells, the virus reshapes the host's immune system, impairing antigen-processing function, humoral neutralizing response, the production of new CD4 cells, and HIV-specific CD8 cells.

Several potential cofactors, which may be viral, host, or environmental, are thought to directly influence the replication of HIV or the severity of its pathogenic effects. Viral cofactors may include herpes simplex virus, cytomegalovirus (CMV), and Epstein-Barr virus. Host cofactors may include a variety of cytokines and intracellular mediators. Environmental cofactors may include repeated exposure to HIV, which may induce hyper activation of the immune system, resulting in an expansion of the pool of HIV-replicating cells.

The spectrum of HIV infection ranges from asymptomatic primary infection to overt AIDS, which is characterized by potentially life-threatening opportunistic infections. Early in the AIDS epidemic, it was believed that HIV infection could be divided into four separate processes: acute HIV infection, latent infection, AIDS-related complex, and AIDS. It is now known that the infection is one continuous disease process with three stages: primary HIV infection, chronic asymptomatic disease, and AIDS. The CDC uses a case definition for AIDS surveillance and reporting, which has evolved over time and incorporates both laboratory and clinical stages. However, it is more useful to discuss the disease in terms of staging.

Primary HIV-1 infection: symptoms of primary HIV infection generally occur within 2 to 4 weeks after HIV exposure and last between 2 and 10 weeks. Symptoms are similar to the flu or mononucleosis, consisting of fever, sore throat, fatigue, nausea, vomiting, headache, rash, or lymphadenopathy. Most of these manifestation go away without intervention; however, the lymphadenopathy usually persists throughout the course of the disease. During this time there is a corresponding rapid rise in serum HIV RNA copies, which may reach 1 million copies/ml or more; a decrease in CD4 cell numbers; and a large increase in CD8 cell numbers. The decline in viral copies coincides with the resolution of clinical manifestations. Antibodies to HIV-1 are usually negative during the primary HIV-1 phase of infection.

Chronic Asymptomatic Infection

The initial phase of infection may be followed by a period of latency that can last from several months to 10 years or more. During this time the person may be completely **asymptomatic** or experience only mild symptoms such as fatigue, headache, or lymphadenopathy. Over time, however, active viral replication begins. As viral load increases, CD4 cell counts gradually decline. The actual rate of decline varies among individuals and can be altered by antiretroviral therapy. Generally, by 12 weeks after infection, anti- HIV antibodies have been produced and can be detected by immunoassay even when the patient is asymptomatic.

AIDS

As viral replication continues and more CD4 cells are destroyed, the immune system becomes further compromised. Clinical manifestations associated with AIDS are primarily those of opportunistic infections, which are discussed later in this chapter. The clinical manifestations box summarizes other manifestations. AIDS is the end stage of HIV infection. Without treatment death occurs within 3 to 5 years.

Clinical Manifestations of HIV/AIDS

- Chills and fever
- Night sweats
- Dry, productive cough
- Dyspnea
- Lethargy
- Confusion
- Stiff neck
- Seizures
- Headache

- Malaise
- Fatigue
- Oral lesions
- Skin rash
- Abdominal discomfort
- Diarrhea
- Weight loss
- Lymphadenopathy
- Progressive generalized edema.

Complications: AIDS and its associated opportunistic infections can affect every organ and body system. *Opportunistic* infectious are those pathogens that take advantage of decreased immunity to produce disease. Pulmonary infection from a variety of organism is a constant threat and is often the first manifestation of AIDS. Such infections can rapidly leas to severe hypoxemia. Numerous GI problems are associated with opportunistic infections or antiretroviral therapy. Other common problems include granulomatous hepatitis, drug toxicity hepatitis, or coinfection with a hepatitis virus; masses or lesions from lymphomas and Kaposi's sarcoma; cholangitis eating or swallowing or may experience dyspepsia, diarrhea, and weight loss. Loss of lean muscle mass is common.

HIV crosses the blood HIV-brain and blood-cerebrospinal fluid (CSF) barriers and infects microglia and possibly other cells, resulting in encephalopathy. This process results in loss of cognitive and motor function. Many of the opportunistic infections also can affect the central nervous system. Peripheral neuropathy with loss of motor function often occurs. The eyes are vulnerable to CMV, which can result in blurred vision and decreased acuity. The lesions are progressive and may lead to total blindness unless early and aggressive treatment is instituted.

Thrombocytopenia, anemia, and neutropenia may be present with AIDS. The causes of these problems are not precisely known, but it is thought that HIV deceases red blood cell production. Drug side effects also affect the hematologic system and can cause impaired production and increased destruction of red blood cells.

Opportunistic infections can affect the heart by producing pericarditis or myocarditis. Severe pulmonary hypertension associated with multiple episodes of *Pneumocystis carinii* pneumonia can cause right ventricular failure.

Although not as common as other system dysfunctions, all endocrine glands can be infiltrated with HIV. The adrenal gland is most commonly affected. Adrenal insufficiency may result from invasion by infective organism, tumor growth, or drug therapy.

Musculoskeletal manifestations of HIV are common and may be mild or severe. Arthralgia is seen with acute infection and may also result from drug therapy. Myalgia, weakness, and wasting may also occur secondary to decreased appetite.

Fluid and electrolyte and acid-base imbalances occur from a variety of causes, including renal, GI, or endocrine changes or drug therapy. Renal dysfunction may occur from acute kidney failure secondary to hypovolemia, interstitial nephritis caused by invasion of renal tissue by tumors or infective organisms, or glomerulosclerosis from HIV-associated nephropathy. Specific opportunistic infections are discussed later in the chapter.

Management of HIV

Diagnostic tests of HIV/AIDS includes the following:

Antibody Assays

Antibody assays measure the immune system's response from exposure to a specific antigen. When an antigen enters the host, the immune system recognizes the antigen and produces specific antibodies against it. Antibody assay tests depend on antibody formation, but a patient's serum may not have detectable levels of antibody during the initial stage of infection. Approximately 90% of the population forms antibodies in response to HIV and the production of detectable antibodies is known as the "window period". Newborns maintain maternal antibodies for as long as 18 months; therefore antibody testing is unreliable until the infant is 18 months of age.

Enzyme-linked Immunosorbent Assay (ELISA)

The ELISA is a highly specific test that is close to 99.6% sensitive for HIV-1 antibodies. If the patients serum is reactive, the patient is considered seropositive for HIV antibodies. False-positive tests are possible and may occur from recent influenza or hepatitis B vaccines; in multiparous women; after multiple blood transfusion; or with multiple myeloma, alcoholic hepatitis, or biliary cirrhosis.

Western Blot

If a patient has a positive ELISA, as it confirmed by the Western blot technique, another more sensitive test for HIV-1 antibodies. The Western blot test for antibodies to four major HIV antigens, two of which must be present for a positive result. Like the ELISA, the Western blot test relies on the production of antibodies and, therefore, may not detect antibodies during the early stages of infection.

Rapid Tests

The ELISA and Western blot tests have been the most widely used tests to determine the presence of antibodies to HIV-1. However, these tests are technically demanding and require sophisticated equipment. Rapid HIV antibody tests are being more widely used today because of ease of use and convenience. Many have comparable sensitivities to the ELISA and Western blot.

Viral Load

Plasma HIV RNA levels indicate the amount of virus in the persons serum, which is a reflection of active viral replication, or viral load. The steeper the rate of increase in plasma HIV RNA, the greater the risk of disease progression unless antiretroviral therapy is started. HIV RNA viral load is measured by one of three assays: quantitative RNA-PCR, branched DNA(bDNA) assay, or nucleic acid sequence-based amplification (NASBA). These tests are greater than 98% sensitive and can detect as few as 40 HIV RNA copies/ml. another test, the p24 antigen assay, detects the viral protein p24 in the blood of HIV-infected patients. Since the assay is only about 50% sensitive, it is used less often than the quantitative tests for HIV RNA.

Viral load is measured periodically in HIV-positive persons to assess their disease progression and to monitor the effectiveness of antiretroviral therapy. Therapy is aimed at reducing plasma HIV RNA levels of below the limit of detection by assay. For accuracy, two HIV RNA assays are completed within 1 to 2 weeks, and both values are used to establish a baseline for the infected person. It is important for nurses to understand that suppression of HIV RNA levels to below the limits of detection does not mean that HIV infection has been eliminated or that viral replication has been halted completely. It simple means that HIV levels have been reduced to such a degree that they cannot be measured by present methods.

CD4 Cell Counts

CD4 cell counts are used to measure the extent of immune damage that has occurred as a result of HIV infection and its complications, and to monitor the immunologic benefit of antiretroviral therapy. CD4 cell counts are obtained on all newly diagnosed patients to establish a baseline and every 3 to 4 months thereafter if counts are above 350/mm3 and the patient is asymptomatic and not receiving drug therapy. Once drug therapy is initiated, counts are monitored every 2 to 4 weeks initially and then every 3 to 4 months if the patient stabilizes.

CD4 cell counts are used in conjunction with viral load to predict the possibility of disease progression, determine when to start antiretroviral therapy, and monitor the effectiveness of treatment. Patients with plasma HIV RNA levels of less than 7000 copies/ml and CD4 counts of greater than 350/mm^3 have less than a 2% likelihood of progressing to AIDS within 3 years without treatment. Conversely, those with viral loads greater than 55,000 copies/ml and CD4 counts of less than 200/mm^3 have an 85% likelihood of progressing to AIDS within 3 years.

Other Tests

Other diagnostic studies are obtained to establish baselines, monitor patient progress, and identify possible coinfections.

Medications for HIV/AIDS

Recent drug developments have decreased the speed of disease progression in many HIV-infected individuals and increased the life span of those living with AIDS. In 1995 the US food and Drug administration approved a class of drugs named protease inhibitors. When a protease inhibitor is combined with two other drugs (reverse transcriptase inhibitors), a highly active antiretroviral therapy (HAART) "cocktail" is created that reduces HIV viral load to undetectable levels. Those drug combinations are the mainstay of HIV treatment.

HAART works by disrupting HIV at different stages during its replication process. The nucleoside and nucleotide reverse transcriptase inhibitors (NRTIs), abacavir (ABC), zidovudine (AZT), didanosine (ddI), stavudine (d4T), lamivudine (3TC), zalcitabine (ddC), and tenofovir, act through two mechanisms. They competitively bind to reverse transcriptase, and they block the elongation of the DNA chain, both of which interfere with the early stages of HIV viral replication. The nonnucleoside reverse transcriptase, and they block the elongatin of the DNA chain, both of which interfere with the early stages of HIV viral replication. The nonnucleoside reverse transcriptase inhibitors (NNRTIs, or nucleoside analogs), nevirapine (NVP), efavirenz (EFV), and delavirdine (DLV), prevent viral replication through competitive binding of reverse transcriptase, but they do not terminate DNA chains.

The protease inhibitors (PIs) indinavir (IDV), ritonavir (RTV), amprenavir (APV), saquinavir (SAQ), lopinavir (LPV), and nelfinavir (NFV) prevent HIV from making the long protein molecules necessary to create new viruses, thus halting replication toward the end of viral replication. Enfuvirtide is a class of drugs known as a fusion inhibitor. It is the first agent of its class to be approved for treatment of HIV. It binds the glucoprotein region of the HIV envelope and prevents viral fusion with the CD4 target cell membrane.

The goals of HAART treatment are to maximally suppress plasma HIV RNA levels of below detectable levels on assay, restore or preserve immunologic function by preventing the destruction of CD4 cells for as long as possible, improve the quality of life, and reduce mortality. Clinical trials are ongoing to find more effective drug therapies with fever side effects.

In 2004 the CDC revised their guidelines for use of antiretroviral agents in HIV-infected adults and adolescents. The guidelines include recommendations for initiating antiretroviral therapy in persons who are asymptomatic, as well as those with established disease. The recommendations were derived from studies designed to identify the risks versus benefits of treatment. Clinical trials indicated that patients whose Cd4 T cell counts fell below 200 cells/mm^3 were at significantly increased risk for opportunistic infections and should be offered antiretroviral therapy.

No optimal time to initiate anteroviral therapy has been identified for HIV-infected patients with CD4 cell counts grater than 200 cells/mm³ who are asymptomatic, although many clinicians offer therapy when CD4 counts are less than 350 cells/mm³. The available drug regimen are potent, complex, and challenging for adherence. Thus the decision to initiate therapy must be a joint decision between the patient and practitioner.

Patients are likely to experience drug toxicity and numerous side effects. They must be compliant with large pill burdens and tightly prescribed administration regimens; be able to financially withstand the cost of therapy; and be prepared for the possibility of drug resistance, which may limit future therapy options. Drug resistance can develop if viral replication is not sufficiently suppressed or the person is already infected with a resistant strain of HIV. On the other hand, patient who delay therapy run the risk of permanent immune system damage, inability to effectively inhibit vital replication at a later stage in the disease, and increased risk of HIV transmission.

At present HIV infection and AIDS have no vaccine or cure, although the number of potential HIV vaccines in clinical trails supported by the International AIDS Vaccine Initiative and other agencies has doubled since 2000. Although many trials show promise, more research and funding are needed. In addition, ethical questions regarding testing of potential vaccines on healthy subjects must be addressed as trials go forward.

No special treatments exist for the early stages of HIV infection. Respiratory treatments may become necessary as the patients disease progresses. Standard precautions are necessary during hospitalization and at home. Treatments associated with maintenance and improvement of nutritional status usually become necessary. Specific treatments related to opportunistic infections are discussed in **Table 12.4**.

Surgery does not play a role in the standard management of HIV. Patients may undergo surgical biopsy of skin lesions, surgical treatment of internal Kaposi's sarcoma lesions that do not respond to chemotherapy, or drainage of abscesses or other sites of infection. Those all represent management of AIDS complications, however, and are not primary therapies for HIV disease.

Diet: Although no particular diet is indicated for persons with HIV, nutritional deficits commonly develop from both the disease itself and the opportunistic infections associated with the disease. Anorexia, nausea, and diarrhea are commonly associated with antiretroviral therapy, further contributing to nutritional alterations. Many persons with AIDS develop wasting syndrome, especially late in the disease. Wasting syndrome involve involuntary weight loss in excess of 10 to 15% of normal baseline weight. It is related to decreased nutrient intake, decreased nutrient absorption, and metabolic disturbances.

Patients must be carefully monitored to evaluate the adequacy of intake and food intolerances. A high-protein diet is encouraged to prevent weight loss and potential cachexia. In the later stages of disease, when infections and muscle wasting prevent adequate food intake, IV nutritional support may be necessary.

Nursing Management HIV Infection

Nursing assessment for individuals not known to be infected with HIV should focus on behaviors that could put the person at risk for HIV infection and other sexually transmitted and blood born diseases. All patients should be assessed for risky behaviors on a regular basis. The assumption should not be made that someone is without risk because he is too young or because she is married or sings in the church choir. Nurses can help individuals assess risk by asking four basic questions: (1) Have you ever had a blood transfusion or used clotting factors? If so, was it before 1985?, (2) Have you ever shared drug-using equipment with another person?, (3) Have you ever had a sexual experience in which your penis, vagina, rectum, or mouth? and (4) Have you ever had a sexually transmitted disease (STD)? These questions provide the minimum data needed to initiate a risk assessment. A positive response to any of these questions requires an in-depth exploration of issues related to the identified risk.

Specific assessments are needed when an individual has been diagnosed with HIV infection. Repeated nursing assessments over time are essential because people's circumstances change. Early recognition and treatment of problems can decrease the progression of HIV infection an prevent new infections. A complete history and thorough systems review can help the nurse identify and address problems in a timely manner.

Nursing Diagnoses

Nursing diagnoses related to HIV infection are indicated by several variables: the stage (e.g., Is prevention of HIV infection the issue? Are there concerns related to ongoing infection? Is the patient dying?); the presence of specific etiologic problems (e.g., respiratory distress, depression, pain); and psychosocial factors (e.g., issues related to self-esteem, sexuality, family interaction, finances). Because HIV infection is a complex and individually experienced disease, a broad spectrum of nursing diagnoses may include, but are not limited to, those presented below:

- Acute pain
- Anxiety
- Caregiver role strain
- Chronic low self-esteem
- Decisional conflict
- Diarrhea
- Disturbed body image
- Disturbed thought processes
- Fatigue

Table 12.4: Manifestations and treatment of common opportunities diseases associated with HIV infection.

Organism/disease	Clinical manifestations	Prophylaxis and treatment
Candida albicans	Thrush, esophagitis, vaginitis; whitish yellow patches in mouth, esophagus, GI tract, vagina	Treatment: fluconazole (Diflucan), clotrimazole (Lotrimin), nystatin (Mycostatin), itraconazole (Sporanox); if fluconazole refractory; amphotericin B (Fungizone) 2°Prophylaxis: only if subsequent episodes are frequent or severe recurrences: fluconazole (Diflucan), itraconazole (Sporanox)
Coccidioides immitis	Pneumonia/fever, weight loss, cough	Treatment: amphotericin B (Fungizone), fluconazole (Diflucna), itraconazole (Sporanox) 2°Prophylaxis: to prevent recurrence of documented disease: fluconazole (Diffucan), amphotericin B (Fungizone), itraconazole (Sporanox)
CNS lymphoma	Cognitive dysfunction, motor impairment, aphasia, seizures, personality changes, headache	Treatment: radiation, chemotherapy
Cryptococcosus neoformans	Meningitis, cognitive impairment, motor dysfunction, fever, seizures, headache	Treatment: amphotericin B (Fungizone), fluconazole (Diflucan), itraconazole (Sporanox) 2°Prophylaxis: to prevent recurrence of documented disease: fluconazole (Diflucan), amphotericin (Fungizone), itraconazole (Sporanox)
Cryptosporidium muris	Gastroenteritis, watery diarrhea, abdominal pain, weight loss	Treatment: antidiarrheals, nitazoxanide (Alinia), paromomycin (Humatic)
Cytomegalovirus (CMV)	Retinitis–retinal lesions, blurred vision, loss of vision Esophagitis/stomatitis – difficulty swallowing; colitis/gastritis – bloody diarrhea, pain, weight loss Pneumonitis – respiratory symptoms Neurologic disease – CNS manifestations	Treatment: ganiclovir (Cytovene), foscarnet (Forcavir), cidofovir (Vistide), valganciclovir (Valcyte) 2°Prophylaxis: to prevent recurrence of documented disease: ganciclovir (Cytovene), foscarnet (Foscavir), cidofovir (Vistide), valganciclovir (Valcyte)
Hepatitis B virus (HBV)	Jaundice, fatigue, abdominal pain, loss of appetite, nausea, vomiting, dark urine; 30% may have no signs or symptoms	1°Prevention: Hepatitis B vaccine series; screen and vaccinate those with no evidence of previous HBV infection; encourage for IDU, sexually active MSM, sexual partners or household contacts of HBV-infected individuals, and those with hepatitis C virus; hepatitis A vaccine series should be given to prevent additive effects and advanced liver damage; screen and vaccinate those without evidence of previous HAV infection Treatment: adefovir dipivoxil (Hepsera), α-interferon, lamivudine (Epivir), entecavir (Baraclude)
Hepatitis C virus (HCV)	Jaundice, fatigue, abdominal pain, loss of appetite, nausea, vomiting, dark urine; 80% may have no signs or symptoms	Prophylaxis: None for HCV. Hepatitis A and B vaccine series should be given to prevent additive affects and advanced liver damage; screen and vaccinate those without evidence of previous HAV/HBV infection. Treatment: α-interferon, ribavirin (Virazole)
Herpes simplex	HSV1 (type 1): orolabial and mucocutaneous vesicular and ulcerative lesion; keratitis – visual disturbances; encephalitis – CNS manifestations HSV2 (type 2): gential and perianal vesicular an ulcerative lesions	Treatment: acyclovir (Zovirax), famciclovir (Famvir), valacyclovir (VAltrex), foscarnet (Foscavir), cidofovir (Vistide) 2°Prophylaxis: only if subsequent episodes are frequent or severe: acyclovir (Zovirax), famciclovir (Famvir), valacyclovir (Valtrex)
Histoplasma capsulatum	Pneumona–fever, cough, weight loss Meningitis–CNS manifestations; disseminated disease	Treatment: amphotericin B (Fungizone), itraconazole (Sporanox), fluconazole (Diflucan) 2°Prophylaxis: to prevent recurrence of documented disease: itraconazole (Sporanox), amphotericin B (Fungizone).
Influenza virus	Fever (usually high), headache, extreme tiredness, dry cough, sore throat, runny or stuffy nose, muscle aches; nausea, vomiting, and diarrhea can occur	1°Prevention: Inactivated trivalent influenza virus vaccine; provide annually, before influenza virus season; revaccinate if initial vaccine was given when CD4+ T cell count was <200 µl treatment: supportive therapy

- Fear
- Grieving
- Hyperthermia
- Imbalanced nutrition: less than body requirements
- Impaired oral mucous membrane
- Ineffective coping
- Ineffective denial
- Ineffective therapeutic regimen management
- Insomnia
- Interrupted family processes

- Noncompliance
- Powerlessness
- Relocation stress syndrome
- Risk for disuse syndrome
- Self-care deficit
- Situational low self-esteem
- Social isolation
- Spiritual distress.

Planning

Prevention of HIV infection presents a number of challenges for the patient, many of which are related to the difficulties of behavior change. Nurses can be instrumental in this process. Nursing interventions to prevent disease transmission depend on assessment of the patients individual risk behaviors, knowledge, and skills. Nursing orders based on these assessments can encourage the patient to adopt, healthier, and less risky behaviors.

Infection with HIV affects the entire of a person's life from physical health to social, economic, and spiritual well-being. Once infected, no known treatment can eliminate HIV from the body. Therefore the overriding goals of therapy are to keep the viral load as low as possible for as long as possible, maintain or restore a functioning immune system, improve the patients quality of life, prevent opportunistic disease, reduce HIV-related disability and death, and prevent new infections. Nursing interventions can assist the patient to (1) adhere to drug regimens; (2) promote a healthy lifestyle that includes avoiding exposure to additional sexual and blood-borne disease; (3) protect others from HIV; (4) maintain or develop healthy and supportive relationships; (5) maintain activities and productivity; (6) explore spiritual issues; (7) come to terms with issues related to disease, disability, and death; and (8) cope with the frequent symptoms caused by HIV and its treatments. Goals are individualized and change as new treatment protocols develop and/or as HIV disease progresses.

Implementation

The complexity of HIV disease is related to its chronic nature. As with most chronic and infectious diseases, primary prevention and health promotion are the most effective health care strategies. When prevention fails, disease results. HIV has no cure, continues for life, causes increasing physical disability, contributes to impaired health, and ultimately leads to death.

Nursing interventions at every stage of HIV disease can be instrumental in improving the quality and quantity of the patients life. Nurses who emphasize a holistic and individualized approach to care as well-suited to provide optimal care to these patients.

A major goal of health promotion is to prevent disease. Even with recent successes in the treatment of HIV, prevention is crucial for control of the epidemic. In addition, health promotion encourages early detection of disease so that, if primary prevention has failed, early intervention can be implemented. HIV infection is preventable. Avoiding and/or modifying risky behaviors are the most effective prevention tools. All patients should be provided with education and behavior change counseling that is specific to the patient's need, culturally sensitive, language appropriate, and age specific. Nurses are excellent resources for this type of education, but they must be comfortable with and know how to talk about sensitive topics such as sexuality and drug use.

Prevention behaviors have been known and recommended since the mid 1980s. It is important to remember that a range of activities can reduce the risk of HIV infection and that individuals will choose methods that best fit their life circumstances. The goal is for the person to develop safer, healthier, and less risky behaviors. These techniques can be divided into *safe activities* (those that eliminate risk) and *risk-reducing* activities (those that decrease risk, but do not eliminate it). The more consistently and correctly prevention methods are used, the more effective they are in preventing HIV infection.

Research shows that the majority of new HIV infections were transmitted by individuals who were not aware that they were infected. CDC develop four strategies in the *Advancing HIV Prevention (AHP)* initiative: (1) HIV testing should be a part of routine health care based on risk assessment and clinical need; (2) rapid HIV testing should also be used to diagnose HIV outside of traditional care settings (e.g., in community-based organizations and at health fairs), (3) providers should work with HIV-infected patients and their partners to change risky behaviors and decrease the risks of HIV transmission, and (4) perinatal transmission should be further reduced by universally offering HIV tests to pregnant women and appropriate treatment to those found to be infected.

Decreasing Risks Related to Sexual Intercourse

Safe sexual activities eliminate the risk of exposure to HIV in semen and vaginal secretions. Abstaining from all sexual activity is the most effective way to accomplish this goal, but there are safe options for those who cannot or do not wish to obtain. Limiting sexual behavior to activities in which the mouth, penis, vagina or rectum does not come into contact with a partners mouth, penis, vagina or rectum is safe because there is no contact with blood, semen or vaginal secretions. Safe activities include massage, masturbation, mutual masturbation ("hand job"), telephone sex, and other activities that meet the "no contact" requirements. *Insertive sex* between partners who are not infected with HIV or not at risk of becoming infected with HIV is also considered to be safe.

Risk reducing sexual activities decrease the risk of contact with HIV through the use of barriers. Barriers should be used when engaging in insertive sexual activity (oral, vaginal or anal) with a partner whose HIV status is not known or with a partner who is known to have HIV. The most commonly used barrier is the male condom. The efficacy (protection provided under ideal circumstances) of male condom is essentially 100%; their effectiveness (protection provided in actual or "real life" circumstances) is 80 to 90%. Correct use of male condoms, increased effectiveness. Female condoms provide an excellent alternative to male condoms. Female condom efficacy is also close to 100% and effectiveness is 94 to 97% against HIV and STD transmission. Use can be complicated, so careful instruction and practice are required. In addition, squares of latex (known as dental dams) or plastic food wrap can be used to cover the external female genitalia during oral sexual activity.

Proper Use of the Male Condom

- Use only condoms that are made with latex or polyurethane. "Natural skin" condoms have pores that are large enough for HIV to penetrate.
- Store condoms in a cool, dry place and protect them from trauma. The frictioncaused by carrying them in a back pocket, for instance, can damage the latex.
- Do not use a condom if the expiration date has passed or if the package looks worn or punctured
- Lubricants used in conjunction with condoms must be water soluble. Oil-based lubricants can weaken latex and increase the risk of tearing or breaking.
- Nonlubricated, flavored, or unflavored condoms can provide protection during oral intercourse.
- The condom must be placed on the erect penis before any contact is made with the partner's mouth, vagina, or rectum to prevent exposure to preejaculatory secretions that may contain HIV.
- See proper instructions and proper steps in male condom placement written on packet of condom.
- Remove the penis and condom from the partner's body immediately after ejaculation and before the erection is lost. Hold the condom at the base of the penis and remove both from the partner's body at the same time. This keeps semen from leaking around the condom as the penis becomes flaccid.
- Remove the condom after use, wrap in tissue, and discard. Do not dispose in the toilet, as this can cause plumbing problems.
- Condoms are not reusable! A new condom must be used for every act of intercourse.

Decreasing Risks Related to Drug Use

Drug use, including alcohol, is harmful. It can cause immuno suppression and malnutrition, as well as a host of psychological problems. However, drug use in and of itself does not cause HIV infection. The major risk for HIV infection is related to sharing equipment and/or having unsafe sexual experiences while under the influence of drugs. Basic risk reduction rules are: (1) do not use drugs; (2) if you use drugs, do not share equipment; and (3) do not have sexual intercourse when under the influence of any drug (including alcohol) that impairs decision-making ability.

The safest mechanism is to abstain from drugs. Although this is the best option for those who do not currently use drugs, it may not be a viable option for users who are not prepared to quit or for those who have no access to drug treatment services. The risk of HIV for these individuals can be eliminated if they do not share equipment. Injecting equipment ("works") includes needles, syringes, cookers (spoons or bottle caps used to mix the drug), cotton, and rinse water. Equipment used to snort (straws) or smoke (pipes) drugs can also be contaminated with blood. None of this equipment should be shared. Access to sterile equipment is an important risk elimination tactic. Some communities have needle and syringe exchange programs (NSEPs) that provide sterile equipment to users in exchange for used equipment. Opposition to these programs is supported by the fear that ready access to injecting supplies will increase drug use. However, studies have shown that, in communities where exchange programs have been established, drug use does not increase, rates of HIV and other blood-borne infections are controlled, and an overall cost benefit results. Cleaning equipment before use is a risk-reducing activity. It decreases the risk for those who share equipment, but cleaning requires equipment, takes time, and may be difficult for a person in drug withdrawal.

Decreasing Risks of Perinatal Transmission

The best way to prevent HIV infection in infants is to prevent HIV infection in women. Women who are already infected with HIV should be asked about their reproductive desires. Those who choose not to have children need to have family planning methods discussed in detail. Should they become pregnant, abortion may be desired and should be discussed in conjunction with other options.

Proper Use of Female Condom

- Female condoms consist of a polyurethane sheath with two spring-form rings.
    1. The smaller ring is inserted into the vagina and holds the condom in place internally. This ring can be removed if the condom is to be used for anal intercourse. It should not be removed if the condom is to be used for vaginal intercourse.
    2. The larger ring surrounds the opening to the condom. It functions to keep the condom in place while protecting the external genitalia.

- Use only water soluble lubricants with female condoms
  - Female condoms come prelubricated and with a tube of additional lubricant
  - Lubrication is needed to protect the condom from tearing during sexual intercourse and can also decrease noise that results from friction of the penis against the condom.
- Some men have reported that the female condom better than the male condom. Other men like male condoms better. The only way to find out which type of condom works best is to try them both.
- Practice inserting the female condom. Lubrication makes the condom slippery, but do not get discouraged, just keep trying.
- During sexual intercourse, ensure that the penis is inserted into the female condom through the outer ring. It is possible for the penis to miss the opening, thus making contact with the vaginal or rectal mucosa, and defeating the purpose of the condom.
- Do not use a male condom at the same time as a female condom as this is unnecessary and could result in less adherence to consistent condom use.
- After intercourse, remove the condom before standing up.
- Twist the outer ring to keep the semen inside, gently pull the condom out of the vagina or rectum and discard
- Do not dispose in the toilet, as this can cause plumbing problems
- Do not reuse a female condom.

If HIV-infected pregnant women are appropriately treated during pregnancy, the rate of perinatal transmission can be decreased from 25% to less than 2%. The current standard of care is that all women who are pregnant or contemplating pregnancy should be counseled about HIV infection, informed of their choices, routinely offered access to voluntary HIV-antibody testing, and, if infected, offered optimal ART.

Decreasing risks at work: The risk of infection from occupational exposure to HIV is small but real. Precautions and safety devices decrease the risk of direct contact with blood and body fluids. Should exposure to HIV-infected fluids occur, **postexposure prophylaxis (PEP)** with combination ART based on the type of exposure, the volume of the exposure, and the status of the source patient can significantly decrease the risk of infection. The possibility of treatment makes reporting of all blood exposures even more critical.

HIV Testing and Counseling: Testing is the only sure way to determine if a person has HIV infection. Any individual who is at risk for HIV should be encouraged to be tested. When negative, testing can relieve anxieties about past behaviors and provide opportunities for prevention education. When positive, testing provides the needed impetus to seek treatment and to prevent sexual and drug-using partners. HIV testing should be accompanied by pretest and posttest counseling as given below:

General Guidelines

- People who are being tested for HIV frequently fearful about the test results:
  - Establish rapport with the patient
  - Assess patients ability to understand HIV counseling
  - Determine the patients ability to access support systems.
- Explain the benefits of testing:
  - Testing provides an opportunity for education that can decrease the risk of new infections
  - Infected individuals can be referred for early intervention and support programs.
- Discuss negative aspects of testing
  - *Confidentiality issues:* breaches of confidentiality have led to discrimination
  - A positive test affects all aspects of the patients life (personal, social, economic, etc) and raise difficult emotions (anger, anxiety, guilt and thoughts of suicide).

Pretest Counseling

- Determine the patients risk factors and when the last risk occurred. Counseling should be individualized according to these parameters
- Provide education to decrease future risk of exposure
- Provide education that will help the patient protect sexual and drug-sharing partners
- Discuss problems related to the delay between infection and an accurate test. Testing will need to be repeated at intervals for up to 6 months after each possible exposure. Discuss the need to use measures to decrease the risks to the patient and the patients partners during that interval
- Discuss the possibility of false-negative tests, which are most likely to occur during the window period
- Assess support systems. Provide telephone numbers and resources as needed
- Discuss patients personally anticipated responses to test results (positive and negative)
- Outline assistance that will be offered if the test is positive.

Post-test Counseling

- If the test is negative, reinforce pretest counseling and prevention education. Remind patient that test needs to be repeated at intervals for up to 6 months after the most recent exposure risk.
- If the test is positive, understand that the patient may be in shock and not hear much of what you say

- Provide resources for medical and emotional support and help the patient get immediate assistance.
- Remind patient that effective treatments are available: HIV is not a death sentence.
- Review health habits that can improve the immune system.
- Arrange for patient to speak to HIV-infected people who are willing to share with and assist newly diagnosed patients during the transition period
- Reinforce that a positive HIV test means that the patient is infected, but does not necessarily mean that the patient has progressed to AIDS.
- Educate to prevent new infections. HIV-infected people should be instructed to avoid donating blood, organs, or semen; to avoid sharing razors, toothbrushes, or other household items that may contain blood or other body fluids; and to protect sexual and needle sharing partners from blood, semen, and vaginal secretions.

Acute Intervention

Early intervention: Early intervention after detection of HIV infection can promote health and limit disability. Because the course of HIV is variable, assessment is very important. Nursing interventions are based on and tailored to patient needs noted during assessment. The nursing assessment in HIV disease should focus on early detection of symptoms, opportunistic diseases, and psychological problems.

Initial response to diagnosis of HIV: Reactions to a positive HIV-antibody test are similar to the reaction of people who are diagnosed with any life-threatening, debilitating, or chronic illness. They include anxiety, panic, fear, depression, denial, hopelessness, anger, and guilt. Unfortunately all of these emotions are overlaid with the stigma and discrimination that continue to pervade social reactions to HIV. Many of these reactions are also seen in the patient's family members, friends, and caregivers. As time passes, patients and their loved ones must confront common issues associated with any life-threatening illness. These include complex treatment decisions; feelings of loss, anger, powerlessness, depression and grief; social isolation imposed by self or others; altered concepts of the physical, social emotional, and creative self; thoughts of suicide; and the possibility of death.

Antiretroviral therapy: Multidrug-therapy protocols have been shown to significantly reduce viral loads and reverse clinical progression of HIV. However, nurses must be aware that the protocols can be complex, the drugs have side effects and potential interactions with other medications, and ART does not work for everyone. All of these factors contribute to problems with adherence to treatment, a dangerous situation because of the risk of developing drug resistance. Frequently, nurses are the clinicians who work most closely with patients who are trying to cope with these issues. Interventions include education about (1) the advantages and disadvantages of new treatments, (2) the dangers of nonadherence to therapeutic regimens, (3) how and when to take each drug, (4) drug interaction to avoid, and (5) side effects that must be reported to the health care provider.

Health Teaching Guide Use of Antiretroviral Drugs

Resistance to antiretroviral drugs is a major problem in treating HIV infection. To decrease the risk of developing resistance:

- Take at least three different antiretroviral drugs from at least two different drug classes; discuss options with your health care provider to find the best regimen for you.
- Know what you are taking and how to take them (some have to be taken with food, some must be taken on an empty stomach, some cannot be taken together). If you do not understand, ask. Get your nurse to write the instructions clearly for you.
- Take the full dose prescribed and take it on schedule. If you cannot take the drug because of side effects or other problems, report it to your health care provider immediately.
- Take all of the drugs as prescribed. Do not quit taking one drug while continuing the others. If you cannot tolerate one of your drugs, talk to your health care provider, who will recommend a new set of drugs.
- Many of the antiretroviral drugs interact with other drugs, including a number of common drugs you can buy without a prescription. Be sure your health care provider and pharmacist know all of the drugs that you are taking, and do not take any new drugs without checking for possible interactions.
- The goal of antiretroviral therapy is to decrease the amount of virus in your blood. This is called your *viral load*. The best result is to get your viral load below detectable levels. Most health care providers will check for possible interactions.
- Two to 4 weeks after you start on drug therapy (or change your therapy), your health care provider will test your viral load to find out if the drugs are working. These results are reported in absolute numbers or in logarithms (a mathematical concept). All you need to know is that you want to see the viral load drop. If reports are in logarithms, you want to see a drop of at least 1 unit, which means that 90% of your viral load has been eliminated. If your viral load drops by 2 units, your viral load will have decreased by 95%. If your viral load drops by 3 units, your viral load will have decreased by 99%.
- An undetectable viral load means that the amount of virus is extremely low and viruses cannot be found in the blood using the current technology. It does

not mean that the virus is gone because much of the virus will be in lymph nodes and organs that the tests cannot detect. It also does not mean that you are no longer able to transmit HIV to others; you will need to continue protecting call of your sexual and drug-using partners from HIV.

When to start antiretroviral therapy: ART has evolved continuously since the first antiretroviral drug was released in 1987. When new drugs were developed, clinicians had the ability to combine and substitute medications. For a while, the preferred treatment strategy was known as "hit it early, hit it hard". This was thought to be appropriate because decreasing the viral load provides for better health outcomes. However, side effects and treatment "burnout" often led to non-adherence, which increased the risk of developing resistance to medications. For this reason, federal guidelines now suggest that treatment can be delayed until greater immune suppression is observed. The most important consideration for initiating therapy is patient readiness. Nurses can provide in-depth education and counseling for patients as they struggle to make this decision.

Adherence: Adherence is the accurate and consistent fidelity to a treatment regimen. Adherence to drug regimens is a critical component of drug therapy for people with HIV infection and an area when nurses are uniquely well prepared to provide assistance. Taking drugs as ordered (right dose and time) every day is important for all drug therapy. The difference with HIV is that missing even a few doses can lead to viral mutations that allow HIV to become resistant to the drug.

The difficulty of adhering consistently is probably clear to anyone who has tried to take a 10-day course of antibiotics. Patients with HIV infection to take anywhere from 2 to 20 pills a day, at precise times during the day. This process must be repeated every day for the rest of their lives even though they often suffer uncomfortable side effects. Nurses have learned that helping people adhere to difficult treatment regimens requires a number of things. The most important is to remember that each patient is a unique individual with unique ways of dealing with therapy. Patients may be helped with technologies such as electronic reminders, beepers, or timers on pillboxes. Group support and individual counseling can also help, but the best approach is to learn about the patient's life and assist with problem solving within the confines of that life. The strategies proven to assist with adherence to antiretroviral.

Antiretroviral therapy includes the following:
- Establish the patients readiness to start therapy
- Provide education on dosing of medication
- Review potential side effects of drugs
- Anticipate and treat side effects
- Use educational aids, including pictures, pillboxes, and calendars
- Engage family and friends in the education process
- Simplify regimens, dosing, and food requirements
- Use team approach with nurses, pharmacists, and peer counselors
- Provide accessible and trusting health care team
- Integrate medication doses into patients life and work schedules

Health promotion: HIV disease progression may be delayed by promoting a healthy immune system whether the patient choosers to use ART or not. Useful interventions for HIV-infected patients include (1) nutritional support to maintain lean body mass and ensure appropriate levels of vitamins and micronutrients; (2) moderation or elimination of alcohol, tobacco, and drug use; (3) keeping recommended vaccines up to date; (4) adequate rest, exercise, and stress reduction; (5) avoiding exposure to new infectious agents; (6) mental health counseling; and (7) getting involved in support groups and community activities.

Patients should be taught to recognize symptoms that may indicate disease progression and/or drug side effects so that prompt medical care can be initiated. Nurse provides an overview of symptoms that patients should report. In general, patients should have as much information as needed to make the informed decisions that guide appropriate nursing intervention.

Acute exacerbations: Chronic diseases are characterized by acute exacerbation of recurring problems. This is especially true in HIV disease where infections, cancers, debility and psychosocial/economic issues may interact to overwhelm the patients ability to cope. Nursing care becomes more complex as the patients immune system deteriorates and new problems arise to compound existing difficulties. When opportunistic diseases or difficult side effects of treatment develop, symptom management, education, and emotional support are necessary.

Nursing care assumes primary importance in helping patients prevent the many opportunistic diseases associated with HIV infection. The best prevention of opportunistic disease is adequate treatment of the underlying HIV infection. In addition to assisting the patient with the medication prescribed for these diseases, the nurse will need to provide appropriate supportive care. If the patient has *Pneumocystis jiroveci* pneumonia, for example, nursing interventions will be required to assure adequate oxygenation. If the patient has cryptococcal meningitis, an important nursing concern will be to maintain a safe environment for a confused patient.

Ambulatory and Home Care

Ongoing care: HIV-infected patients share problems experienced by all individuals with chronic diseases, but these problems are exacerbated by negative social constructs surrounding HIV. In HIV, the stigma of illness is compounded by several factors. HIV-infected people may be seen as lacking control over urges to have sex or use drugs. It is then easy to jump to the conclusion that they brought the disease on themselves and therefore deserve to be sick. Behaviors associated with HIV infection may be viewed as immoral (e.g., homosexuality, having many sexual partners) and are sometimes illegal (e.g., using drugs, sex work). The fact that infected individuals can transmit HIV to others increases stigma, and stigma leads to discrimination in all facets of life. For example HIV-infected people have lost jobs, homes and insurance, even though these forms of discrimination are illegal according to the Disabilities Act. Unfortunately, this problem occurs all over the world and is often more severe for women.

Discrimination related to HIV infection can lead to social isolation, dependence, frustration, lowered self-image, loss of control, and economic pressures. It is of interest that all of these variables may have contributed to the patients infection in the first place. Low self-esteem, searching for social contact, frustration, and economic difficulties can all contribute to drug use and risky sexual behaviors.

Disease and drug side effects: Physical problems related to HIV and/or the treatment of HIV can interrupt the patients ability to maintain a desired lifestyle. HIV-infected patients frequently experience anxiety, fear, depression, diarrhea, peripheral neuropathy, pain, nausea, vomiting, and fatigue. These are symptoms that nurses deal with routinely. Interventions for these symptoms do not change significantly based on the primary diagnosis. Individual considerations will, of course, influence the way that the nurse approaches each patient. Nursing management of diarrhea, for instance, still includes helping patients collect specimens, recommending dietary changes, encouraging fluid and electrolyte replacement, instructing the patient about skin care, and managing skin breakdown around the perineal area. Nursing approaches for fatigue in HIV include teaching patients to assess fatigue patterns, determine contributing factors, set activity priorities, converse energy, schedule rest periods, exercise, and avoid substances such as caffeine, nicotine, alcohol, and other drugs that may disturb sleep.

Report the following signs and symptoms immediately to health care provider:
- Any change in level of consciousness: lethargy, hard to arouse, unable to arouse, unresponsive, unconscious.
- Headache accompanied by nausea and vomiting, changes in vision, changes in ability to perform coordinated activities, or after any head trauma.
- Vision changes: blurry or black areas in vision field, new floaters, double vision.
- Persistent shortness of breath related to activity and not relieved by a short rest period.
- Nausea and vomiting accompanied by abdominal pain.
- Vomiting blood.
- Dehydration: unable to eat or drink because of nausea, diarrhea, or mouth lesions; severe diarrhea or vomiting; dizziness when standing.
- Yellow discoloration of the skin.
- Any bleeding from the rectum that is not related to hemorrhoids or trauma (from anal sexual intercourse).
- Pain in the flank with fever and unable to urinate for more than 6 hours.
- Blood in the urine.
- New onset of weakness in any part of the body, new onset of numbness that is not obviously related to pressure, new onset of difficulty speaking.
- Chest pain not obviously related to cough.
- Seizures.
- New rash accompanied by fever.
- New oral lesions accompanied by fever.
- Severe depression, anxiety, hallucinations, delusions, or thoughts of causing danger to self or others.

Report the following signs and symptoms within 24 hours:
- New or different headache; constant headache not relieved by aspirin or acetaminophen.
- Headache accompanied by fever, nasal congestion, or cough.
- Burning, itching, or discharge from the eyes.
- New or productive cough.
- Vomiting 2-3 times a day.
- Vomiting accompanied by fever.
- New, significant, or watery diarrhea (more than 6 times a day).
- Painful urination, bloody urine, urethral discharge.
- New, significant rash (widespread, painful, itchy, or following a path down the leg or arm, around the chest, or on the face).
- Difficulty eating or drinking because of mouth lesions.
- Vaginal discharge, pain or itching.

Some HIV-infected patients, especially those who have been infected for a long time and who have been on ART, develop a set of metabolic disorders that include changes in body shape (fat deposits in the abdomen, upper back, and breasts along with fat loss in the arms, legs, and face) due to lipodystrophy, hyperlipidemia (elevated triglycerides and decreases in high density lipoproteins), insulin resistance and hyperglycemia, bone disease (osteoporosis, osteopenia, avascular necrosis), lactic acidosis, and cardiovascular disease. It is still not clear why these disorders develop, but it is probably a combination of factors such as long-term infection with HIV, side effects of ART, genetic predisposition, and chronic stress.

Management of metabolic disorders currently focuses on detecting problems early, dealing with the symptoms, and helping the patient cope with new problems and changes to treatment regimens. It is important to recognize and treat these problems early, especially since cardiovascular disease and lactic acidosis are potentially fatal complications. A frequent first intervention is to change ART medications because some drugs are more often associated with these problems. Lipid abnormalities are generally treated with lipid lowering drugs, dietary changes, and exercise. Insulin resistance is treated with hypoglycemic drugs and weight loss. Bone disease may be improved with exercise, dietary changes, and calcium and vitamin D supplements.

Body changes that combine fat accumulation and wasting are major problems for patients with this syndrome. There is little evidence that exercise or dietary changes make any difference. Human growth hormone, testosterone, and anabolic steroids have been used to help resolve these changes, but they frequently are not effective or even available. Some patients have had plastic surgery to reduce areas of fat and to build up sunken areas of the face, but access to these procedures is limited. Nursing interventions can focus on helping the patient to make treatment decisions and cope with negative changes in body image.

Terminal care: Despite exciting new developments in the treatment of HIV infection, many patients eventually experience disease progression, disability, and death. Sometimes these occur because treatments do not work for the patient. Sometimes the patients HIV becomes resistant to all available drug therapies. In other cases, a patient may make a calculated decision to forego further treatment, allowing the disease to progress toward death. Nursing care during the terminal phase of any disease needs to focus on keeping the patient comfortable, facilitating emotional and spiritual acceptance of the finite nature of life, helping the patients significant others deal with grief and loss, and maintaining a safe environment. Nurses become pivotal care providers during the terminal phase of illness, especially when patients and families choose terminal care at home.

CHAPTER 13

Nursing Management of Infectious Diseases

INTRODUCTION

An infectious disease is any disease caused by the growth of pathogenic microbes in the body. It may or may not be communicable (i.e., contagious). Modern science has controlled, eradicated, or decreased the incidence of many infectious disease. However, increase in other infections, such as those cause by antibiotic-resistant organisms and emerging infectious disease, are of great and growing concern. Examples of these infectious diseases are presented in this chapter. It is important to understand infectious causes and the treatment of contagious, serious, and common infections. **Table 13.1** presents an overview of many infectious diseases, their causative organisms, mode of transmission, and usual incubation periods (time between contact and development of the first signs and symptoms).

The nurse plays in important role in infection control and prevention. Education patients may decrease their risk of becoming infected or may decrease the sequelae of infection. Using appropriate barrier precautions, observing prudent hand hygiene, and ensuring aseptic care of intravenous (IV) catheters and other invasive equipment also assists in reducing infections.

Table 13.1: Infectious disease, causative organisms, modes of transmission, and usual incubation periods.

Disease or condition	Organism	Usual mode of transmission	Usual incubation period (Infection to first Symptom)
Acquired immuno-deficiency syndrome (AIDS)	Human immunodeficiency virus (HIV)	Sexual; percutaneous; perinatal	Median of 10-year
Amebiasis	Entamoeba histolytica	Contaminated water	2–4 week
Anthrax	Bacillus anthracis	Airborne or contact	2–60 days
Chancroid	Haemophilus ducreyi	Sexual	3–5 days
Chickenpox	Varicella zoster	Airborne or contact	About 14 days
Cholera	Vibrio cholerae	Ingestion of water contaminated with human waste	A few hours to 5 days
Cryptosporidiosis	Cryptosporieium species	Ingestion of contaminated water; direct contact with carrier	Probably 1–12 days
Cytomegalovirus (CMV) infection	Cytomegalovirus	Transfusion and transplantation; sexual; perinatal	Highly variable: 3–8 week after transfusion, 3–12 week after delivery a newborn
Diarrheal disease (common causes)	Campylobacter species Clostridium difficile	Ingestion of contaminated food fecal-oral	3–5 days Variable; in part related to the influence of antibiotics
	Salmonella species	Ingestion of contaminated food or drink	12–36 hours
	Shigella species	Ingestion of contaminated food or drink; direct contact with carrier	1–3 days
Ebola	Ebola virus	Contact with blood or body fluids	2–21 days
Gonorrhea	Neisseria gonorrhoeae	Sexual; perinatal	2–7 days
Hand, foot, and mouth disease	Coxsackievirus	Direct contact with nose and throat secretions and with feces of infected people	3–5 days
Foodborne hepatitis	Hepatitis A virus	Ingestion of contaminated food or drink; direct contact with carrier	15–50 days
	Hepatitis E virus	Ingestion of contaminated food or drink; direct with carrier	Unclear

Contd...

Contd...

Disease or condition	Organism	Usual mode of transmission	Usual incubation period (Infection to first Symptom)
Bloodborne hepatitis	Hepatitis B virus	Sexual; perinatal; percutaneous	45–160 days
	Hepatitis C virus	Sexual; perinatal; percutaneous	6–9 months
	Hepatitis D	Sexual; perinatal; percutaneous	Unclear
	Hepatitis G	Percutaneous	Unclear
Herpangina	Coxsackievirus	Direct contact with nose and throat secretions and feces of infected people	3–5 days
Herpes simplex	Human herpes virus 1 and 2	Contact with mucous membrane secretions	2–12 days
Histoplasmosis	Histoplasma capsulatum	Inhalation of airborne spores	5–18 days
Hookworm disease	Necatar americanus; Ancyclostoma duodenale	Contact with soil contaminated with human feces	A few weeks to many months
Impetigo	Staphylococcus aureus	Contact with S. aureus carrier	4–10 days
Influenza	Influenza virus A, B, or C	Droplet spread	24–72 hour
Listeriosis	Listeria monocytogene	Foodborne; perinatal	Unclear; probably 3–70 days
Lyme disease	Borrelia burgdorferi	Tick bite	14–23 days
Lymphogranuloma venereum	Chlamydia inguinale	Sexual	Weeks to years
Malaria	Plasmodium vivax; Plasmodium malariae; Plasmodium falciparum; Plasmodium ovale	Bite from Anopheles species mosquito	12–30 days
Meningococcal meningitis or bacteremia	Neisseria meningitides	Contact with pharyngeal secretions; perhaps airborne	2–10 days
Mononucleosis	Epstein-Barr virus	Contact with pharyngeal secretions	4–6 weeks
Mycobacterial diseases (nontuberculosis Mycobacterium species)	Mycobacterium avium; Mycobacterium fortuitum; Mycobacterium gordonae; other Mycobacterium species	Variable; probably contact with soil, water, or other environmental source, water, or other environmental sources; none is transmissible person-to-person	Variable
Mycoplasma pneumoniae	Mycoplasma pneumoniae	Droplet inhalation	14–21 days
Pediculosis	Pediculus humanus capitis (head louse); Phthirus pubis (crab louse)	Direct contact	1–2 week
Pinworm disease	Enterobius vermicularis	Direct contact with egg-contaminated articles	4–6 weeks life cycle; often takes months of infection before recognition
Pneumocystis jiroveci pneumonia	Pneumocystis jiroveci	Unknown; not transmitted person-to-person	Infants: 1–2 month; adults unclear
Pneumococcal pneumonia	Streptococcus pneumoniae	Droplet spread	Probably 1–3 days
Rabies	Rabies virus	Bite from rabid animal	2–8 weeks
Respiratory syncytial disease	Respiratory syncytial virus	Self-inoculation by mouth or nose after contact with infectious respiratory secretions	3–7 days
Ringworm	Micorporum species; Trychophyton species	Direct and indirect contact with lesions	4–10 days
Rocky mountain	Human herpes virus 6	Saliva	10–15 days

Contd...

Contd...

Disease or condition	Organism	Usual mode of transmission	Usual incubation period (Infection to first Symptom)
Rotavirus gastroenteritis	Rotavirus	Fecal-oral-route	About 48 hours
Rubella	Rubella virus	Droplet spread; direct contact	14–21 days
Scabies	*Sarcoptes scabei*	Direct skin contact	2–6 weeks
Severe acute respiratory syndrome (SARS)	SARS-associated coronavirus (SARS-CoV)	Droplet; direct contact; occasionally	2–10 days
Smallpox	*Variola major*	Airborne and contact	7–14 days
Syphilis	*Treponema pallidum*	Sexual; perinatal	10 days to 10 weeks
Tetanus	*Clostridium tetani*	Puncture wound	4–21 days
Trichinosis	*Trichinella spiralis*	Ingestion of insufficiently cooked foods, especially pork and beef	10–14 days
Tuberculosis	*Mycobacterium tuberculosis*	Airborne	4–12 week sto the formation of primary lesion
West Nile virus	West Nile virus	Bite of infected mosquitoes; from transfusions and transplants; perinatal	3–14 days

THE INFECTIOUS PROCESS

The Chain of Infection

A complete chain of events is necessary for infection to occur. The necessary elements for infection to occur are the follow:
- A causative organism.
- A reservoir of available organisms.
- A portal or mode of exit from the reservoir.
- A mode of transmission from reservoir to host.
- A susceptible host.
- A mode of entry to host.

Causative Organism

The types of micro organisms that cause infections are bacteria, rickettsiae, viruses, protozoa, fungi, and helminthes.

Reservoir

Reservoir is the term used for any person, plant, animal, substance, or location that provides nourishment for micro-organisms and enables further dispersal of the organism. Infections may be prevented by eliminating the causative organisms from the reservoir.

Mode of Exit

The organism must have a mode of exit from a reservoir. An infected host must shed organisms to another or to the environment before transmission can occur. Organisms exit through the respiratory tract, the gastrointestinal tract, the genitourinary tract or the blood.

Route of Transmission

A route of transmission is necessary to connect the infectious source with its new host. Organisms may be transmitted through sexual contact, skin-to-skin contact, percutaneous injection, or infectious particles carried in the air. A person who carries or transmits an organism but does not have apparent signs and symptoms of infection is called a carrier.

It is important to recognize that specific organisms require specific routes of transmission for infection to occur. For example, *Mycobacterium tuberculosis* is almost always transmitted by the airborne route. Health care providers do not "carry" *M. tuberculosis* bacteria on their hands or clothing. In contrast, bacteria such as Staphylococcus aureus are easily transmitted from patient to patient on the hands of health care providers.

When appropriate, the nurse should explain routes of disease transmission to patients. For example, a nurse may explain that sharing a room with a patient who is infected with human immunodeficiency virus (HIV) does not pose a risk because intimate contact (i.e., sexual or parenteral) is necessary for transmission to occur.

Susceptible Host

For infection to occur, the host must be susceptible (not possessing immunity to a particular pathogen). Previous infection or vaccine administration may render the host immune (not susceptible) to further infection with an agent. Although exposure to potentially infectious microorganisms occurs essentially on a constant basis, our elaborate immune systems generally prevent infection from occurring. A person who is immunosuppressed has much greater susceptibility to infection than a healthy person.

Portal of Entry

A portal of entry is needed for the organism to gain access to the host. Again, specific organisms may require specific portals of entry for infection to occur. For example, airborne. *M. tuberculosis* does not cause disease when it settles on the skin of an exposed host; the only entry route for *M. tuberculosis* is through the respiratory tract.

Colonization, Infection, and Infectious Disease

Relatively few anatomic sites (e.g., brain, blood, bone, heart, vascular system) are sterile. Bacteria found throughout the body usually provide beneficial normal flora to complete with potential pathogens, to facilitate digestion, or to work in other ways symbiotically with the host.

Colonization

The term colonization is used to describe microorganisms present without host interference or interaction. Organisms reported in microbiology test results often reflect colonization rather than infection. The nurse and other members of the patient's health care team must interpret microbiology test results accurately to ensure appropriate treatment.

Infection

Infection indicates a host interaction with an organism. A patient colonized with *S. aureus* may have staphylococci on the skin without any skin interruption or irritation. However, if the patient had an incision, *S. aureus* could enter the wound, resulting in an immune system reaction of local inflammation and migration of white cells to the site. Clinical evidence of redness, heat, and pain and laboratory smear suggest infection. In this example, the host identifies the staphylococci as foreign. Infection is recognized by the host reaction (manifested by signs and symptoms) and by laboratory-based organism identification.

Infectious Disease

It is important to recognize the difference between infection and infectious disease. **Infectious disease** is the state in which the infected host displays a decline in wellness due to the infection. When the host interact immunologically with an organism but remains symptom free, the definition of infectious disease has not been met. For example, when a person is first infected with *M. tuberculosis*, infection can be detected by a positive tuberculin skin test, which demonstrates immunologic recognition. Most people who are infected with *M. tuberculosis* have latent infection, but few people (approximately 10%) actually become ill and advancing pneumonia.

The primary source of information about most bacterial infections is the microbiology laboratory report. The microbiology laboratory report should be viewed as a tool to be used along with clinical indicators to determine whether a patient is colonized, infected, or diseased. Microbiology report from clinical specimens usually show three components: the smear and stain, the culture and organism identification, and the antimicrobial susceptibility (i.e., sensitivity). As a marker for the likelihood of infection, the smear and stain generally provide the most helpful information because they describe the mix of cells present at the anatomic site at the time of specimen collection. Culture and sensitivity results specify which organisms are recognized and which antibiotics affect the bacteria.

Preventing Infection in the Hospital

Isolation Precautions

Isolation precautions are guidelines created to prevent transmission of microorganisms in hospital. The firs tier, called standard Precautions, is designed for the care of all patients in the hospital and is the primary strategy for preventing HAIs. The second tier, called transmission-based precautions, is designed for care of patients with known or suspected infectious diseases spread by airborne, droplet or contact route.

STANDARD PRECAUTIONS

The tenets of Standard Precautions are that all patients are colonized or infected with microorganisms, whether or not there are signs or symptoms, and that a uniform level of caution should be used in the care of all patients. The elements of Standard Precautions include hand hygiene, use of gloves and other barriers (e.g., mask, eye protection, face shield, gown), proper handling of patient care equipment and linen, environmental control, prevention of injury from sharps devices, and patient placement (i.e., room assignments) within health care facilities. Hand hygiene, glove use, needlestick prevention, and avoidance of splash or spray of body fluids are discussed in the following sections.

Hand Hygiene

The most frequent cause of infection outbreaks in health care institutions is transmission by the hands of health care workers. Hands should be washed or decontaminated frequently during patient care. The recommended hand hygiene methods are as follows:

- **Hand decontamination with alcohol-based product**
  - After contact with body fluids, excretions, mucous membranes, nonintact skin, or wound dressings as long as hands are not visibly soiled.
  - After contract with a patient's intact skin (as after taking pulse or blood pressure or lifting a patient).

- In patient care, when moving from a contaminated body site to a clean body site.
- After contact with inanimate objects in patient's immediate vicinity
- Before caring for patients with severe neutropenia or other form of severe immune suppression.
- Before donning sterile gloves when inserting central catherters.
- Before inserting urinary catheters or other devices that do not require a surgical procedure
- After removing gloves.
- **Hand washing**
  - When hands are visibly dirty or contaminated with biologic material from patient care.
  - When health care workers do not tolerate waterless alcohol product.

When hands are visibly dirty or contaminated with biologic material from patient care, hands, should be washed with soap and water. In intensive care units and other locations in which virulent or resistant organisms are likely to be present, antimicrobial agents (e.g., chlorhexidine gluconate, iodophors, chloroxyleno, and triclosan) may be used. Effective hand washing requires at least 15 *seconds of vigorous scrubbing*, with special attention to the area around nail beds and between fingers, where there is a high bacterial load. Hands should be thoroughly rinsed after washing.

If hands are not visibly soiled, health care providers are strongly encouraged to use alcohol based, waterless antiseptic agents for routine hand decontamination. These solutions are superior to soap or antimicrobial handwashing agents in their speed of action and effectiveness against microorganisms. Because they are formulated with emollients, they are usually better tolerated than other agents, and because they can be used without sinks and towels, health care workers have been found to be more compliant with their use. Nurses working in home health care or other agents, and because they can be sued without sinks and towels, health care workers have been found to be more compliant with their use. Nurses working in home health care or other settings where they are relatively mobile should carry pocket-sized containers of alcohol-based solutions.

Normal skin flora usually consists of coagulase-negative staphylococci or diphtheroids. In the health care setting, workers may temporarily carry other bacteria (i.e., transient flora) such as *S. aureus, Pseudomonas aeruginosa*, or other organisms flora are superficially attached and are shed with hand hygiene and skin regeneration.

Hand washing or disinfection reduces the bacterial load and decreases the risk of transfer to other patients. All health care setting should have mechanisms to evaluate compliance with hand disinfection by all who care for patients.

Nurses should not wear artificial fingernails or nail extenders when providing patient care. These items have been epidemiological linked to several significant outbreaks of infections. Natural nails should be kept less than 0.25 inches (0.6 cm) long, and nail polish should be removed when chipped, because it can support increased bacterial growth.

Glove Use

Glove provide an effective barrier for hands from the microflora associated with patient care. Gloves should be worn when a health care worker has contact with any patient's secretions or excretions and must be discarded after each patient care contact. Because microbial organisms colonizing health care workers' hands can proliferate in the warm, moist environment provided by gloves, hands must be thoroughly washed with soap or an antimicrobial agent after gloves are removed. As patient advocates, nurses have an important role in promoting hand washing and glove use by other hospital workers, such as laboratory personnel, technicians, and others who have contact with patients.

Latex gloves are often preferred over vinyl gloves because of greater comfort and fit and because some studies indicate that they afford greater protection from exposure. However, their increased use in recent years has been accompanied by increased reports of allergic reactions to latex among health care workers. Reactions range from local skin irritation to more severe reactions, including generalized dermatitis, conjunctivitis, asthma, angioedema, and anaphylaxis.

The nurse who experiences irritation or an allergic reaction associated with exposure to latex should report symptoms to an occupational health specialist or physician. Suggested methods for reducing the incidence of such reactions include the use of vinyl gloves, powder-free gloves, or "low-protein" latex gloves.

Needlestick Prevention

The most important aspect of reducing the risk of blood-borne infection is avoidance of percutaneous injury. Extreme care is essential in all situations in which needles, scalpels, and other sharp objects are handled. Used needles should not be recapped. Instead, they are placed directly into puncture-resistant containers near the place where they are used. If a situation dictates that a needle must be recapped, the nurse must use a mechanical device to hold the cap or use a one handed approach to decrease the likelihood of skin puncture.

Avoidance of Splash and Spray

When the health care provider is involved in an activity in which body fluids may be sprayed or splashed, appropriate barriers must be used. If a splash to the face may occur, goggles and a face mask are warranted. If the health care worker is handling material that may soil clothing or is involved in a procedure in which clothing may be splashed with biologic material, a cover gown should be worn.

TRANSMISSION-BASED PRECAUTIONS

Some microbes are so contagious or epidemiologically significant that precautions in addition to the Standard Precautions should be used when such organisms are recognized. The CDC recommends a second tier of precautions, called **transmission-based precautions.** The additional isolation categories are Airborne, Droplet, and Contact Precautions.

Airborne precautions are required for patients with presumed or proven pulmonary TB, chickenpox, or other airborne pathogen. Airborne precautions are also advised if a patient is infected with smallpox (e.g., as result of a bioterrorist attack). When hospitalized, patients should be in rooms with negative air pressure; the door should remain closed, and health care providers should wear an N-95 respirator (*i.e.* protective mask) at all times while in the patient's room.

Droplet precautions are used for organisms that can be transmitted by close, face-to-face contact, such as influenza or mentingococcal meningitis. While taking care of patient requiring Droplet Precautions, the nurse should wear a face mask, but because the risk of transmission is limited to close contact, the door may remain open.

Contact precautions are used for organisms that are spread by skin-to-skin contact, such as antibiotic-resistant organisms or *Clostridium difficile*. Contact Precautions are designed to emphasize cautious technique and the use of barriers for organisms that have serious epidemiologic consequences or those easily transmitted by contact between health care worker and patient. When possible, the patient requiring contact isolation is placed in a private room to facilitate hand hygiene and decreased environmental contamination. Masks are not needed, and doors do not need to be closed.

DISINFECTING SKIN

The patient's own flora, traversing the exterior of peripherally inserted inserted catheter or contaminating the central catheter hub, is the most common bacterial source of catheter related bacteremia. Rarely, IV fluid itself can become contaminated and serve as a source of infection. The preferred solution for disinfection of the insertion site is chlorhexidine gluconate (CHG). Alternative solutions are povidone-iodine or alcohol. Triple-antibiotic ointment should not be use on the insertion site because it has been shown to lead to increased colonization with *Candida* species.

There is no apparent difference in risk or benefit when comparing transparent polyurethane dressings and gauze dressing. However, if blood is oozing from the catheter insertion site, a gauze dressing should be used. Most importantly, the dressing should be applied using aseptic technique and should be sealed along into entire perimeter.

CHANGING INFUSION SETS, CAPS, AND SOLUTIONS

Infusion sets and stopcock caps should be changed no more frequently than every 3 days, unless an infusion set is used for the delivery of blood or lipid solutions. Infusion sets and tubing for blood, blood products, or lipid emulsions should be changed within 24 hours of initiating the infusion. Blood infusions should finish within 4 hours of hanging the blood; lipid solutions should be completed within 24 hours hanging. There are no guidelines for the appropriate intervals for the hang time of other solutions. Injection ports should be cleaned with 70% alcohol or an iodophor before accessing the system.

Preventing Infection in the Community

The state and local health departments has responsibility for prevention and control of infection in the community. Methods of infection prevention include sanitation techniques (e.g., water purification, disposal of sewage and other potentially infectious materials), regulated health practices (e.g., the handling, storage, packaging, and preparation of food by institutions), and immunization programs. The immunization programs have markedly decreased the incidence of infectious diseases.

The goal of vaccination programs is to use wide-scale efforts to prevent specific infectious diseases from occurring in a population. Public health decisions about vaccine campaign implementation efforts are complex. Risks and benefits for the person and the community must be evaluated in terms of morbidity, mortality, and financial cost and benefit.

The most successful vaccine programs have been those for the prevention of smallpox, measles, mumps, rubella, polio, diphtheria, pertussis, and tetanus.

Vaccines are suspensions of antigen preparations, intended to produce a human immune response to protect the host from future encounters with the organism. Because no vaccine is completely safe for all recipients, contraindications on package inserts of a vaccine must be heeded. These guidelines provide details about studied experiences with allergy and other complications and provide crucial information about refrigeration, storage, dosage, and administration. The most common adverse effects are allergy to the antigen or carrier solution and the occurrence of the actual disease (often in modified form) when live vaccine is used. (Note: For details of all infectious/communicable diseases, please refere authors text on Community Health Nursing, 3rd edition)

THE PATIENT WITH AN INFECTIOUS DISEASE

Assessment

The health history and physical examination and the use of diagnostic tests are important for determining the presence of infection and infectious diseases.

Symptoms of infectious diseases vary significantly between and within diseases. For some infections, visible symptoms such as rash, redness, or swelling provide early warnings of infection. In other infections, such as TB and HIV, asymptomatic latency is prolonged, and infection must be determined through diagnostic procedures.

The goals of history taking are to establish the likelihood and probable source of infection as well as the degree associated pathology and symptoms. The patient's previous medical record is reviewed when possible. In obtaining a health history, some of the following questions may be asked:

- Does the patient have a history of previous or recurrent infections?
- Has there been fever? How high has the patient's temperature been? What is the fever pattern? Is the temperature constant, or does it rise and fall? Has fever been associated with chills? Has the patient taken medication to relieve fever?
- Is there cough? Is the cough chronic or acute? Is it associated with shortness of breath? Does the cough produce sputum? Is the sputum bloody? Has the patient had a tuberculin skin test (TST) recently? If so, what were the result? Ha the patient been given isoniazid (INH) Prophylaxis for TB infection? Has the patient been treated for TB in the past?
- Is there pain? Where is the pain? What is the nature of the pain? Does the patient have sore throat, headache, myalgias, or arthralgias? Is there pain on urination or other activity?
- Is there edema? Is there drainage associated with the edema? Is the edematous area warm to touch?
- Is there a draining lesion? Is the drainage associated with trauma or a previous procedure? Is the drainage purulent or clear?
- Does the patient have diarrhea, vomiting, or abdominal pain?
- Is there rash? What is the nature of the rash – is it flat, raised, red, crusted, purulent, or lace-like?
- What is the patient's vaccination history?
- Has the patient taken medications that could induce rash?
- Has there been exposure to another person who has an identified infectious disease or rash?
- Has there been an insect or animal bite? Has there been an animal scratch or other exposure to pets, farm animals, or experimental animals?
- What medications are used? Have antibiotics been taken recently or long term? Is the patient being treated with corticosteroids, immunosuppressive agents, or chemotherapy?
- Is there a history of substance abuse?
- Has the patient been treated in past for other infectious diseases? Has the patient been hospitalized for infectious disease?
- If sexual history is pertinent, has there been sexual exposure to another person with a known sexually transmitted disease (STD)? Has the patient been treated for STDs in the past? Is the patient pregnant, or has she recently been pregnant? Has the patient been tested for HIV?
- Has the patient traveled to or form a developing country or abroad? What was the immunization or antimicrobial prophylaxis used for protection while traveling?
- What is the patient's occupation? What are the patient's recreational activities? Hobbies?

Because infection may occur in any body system, physical examination may reveal signs of infection at any body site. Generalized signs of chronic infection may include significant weight loss or pallor associated with anemia of chronic diseases. Acute infection may manifest with fever, chills, lymphadenopathy, or rash. Localized signs vary by source of infection. Purulent drainage, pain, edema, and redness are strongly associated with localized infection. Cough and shortness of breath may be caused by influenza, pneumonia, or TB, as well as many noninfectious causes.

Diagnosis

Nursing Diagnoses

Based on assessment data, the patient's major nursing diagnoses related specifically to infection may include the following:

- Risk for infection transmission
- Deficient knowledge about the disease, cause of infection, treatment, and prevention measures
- Risk for inffective thermoregulation (fever) related to the presence of infection

Infection may interrupt the normal function of any affected body system.

Collaborative Problems/Potential Complications

Based on the assessment data, potential complications that may develop include the following:

- Septicemia, bacteremia, or sepsis
- Septic shock
- Dehydration
- Abscess formation
- Endocarditis
- Infectious disease-related cancers
- Infertility
- Congenital abnormalities.

Planning and Goals

Major goals for the patient may include prevention of spread of infection, increased knowledge about the infection and its treatment, control of fever and related discomforts, and absence of complication.

Nursing Interventions

Preventing Infection Transmission

Preventing the spread of infection requires and understanding of the usual routes of transmission of the organism. The hospitalized patient may pose a contagious risk to others if the disease is easily spread (such as *C. difficile*) or is spread through an airborne route (such as TB). In these situations, strict adherence to isolation measure is important in reducing the opportunity for spread. Preventing transmission of organisms from patient to patient usually requires participation of the health care team. Transmission of organisms on the hands and gloves of health care workers remains a common source of cross-infection in the hospital or clinic setting.

Nurses serve an important role in preventing the transfer of organisms in two ways. First, as the health professionals who often spend the most time with patients, nurses have a greater opportunity for spreading organisms. It is imperative that nurses disinfect there hands before and after contact with patients and after performing a potentially hand-contaminating activity. Hands must be disinfected each time gloves are removed. For example, the nurse who has performed endotracheal suctioning should remove the gloves, was the hands, and put on a new pair of gloves before performing wound care on the same patient.

The second way that nurses reduce hand-to-hand spread is to serve as patient advocates. With the number of health care workers involved in patient care each day, there is a significant opportunity for breaks in hand-hygiene technique. To the degree feasible, the nurse should observe the hand-hygiene activities of other professionals and discuss with them any lapses in technique that are observed.

Teaching about the Infectious Process

Interruption of transmission requires diagnosis and patient compliance with the treatment regimen. The nurse's role is to educate the patient and, in some situations, to report the case to public health officials for contact tracing and verification of follow-up.

The nurse must stress the importance of immunization to parents of young children and to others for whom vaccines are recommended, such as patients who are elderly, are immunosuppressed, or have chronic illnesses or disabilities. Nurses should recognize their personal responsibility to receive the hepatitis B vaccine and an annual influenza vaccine to reduce potential transmission to themselves and vulnerable patient groups.

Infectious diseases often seem mysterious and frequently are socially stigmatizing. Patient teaching efforts require empathy and sensitivity. For example, in the past, TB was a stigmatizing disease. The nurse may need to provide core information to the patient who needs INH prophylaxis to promote understanding and allay guilt that the patient may feel.

Controlling Fever and Accompanying Discomforts

Fever must always be investigated to determine whether infection is the source. Evidence indicates that fever, mediated by the hypothalamus, may potentiate beneficial functions in the syndrome of reactions known as *acute-phase reaction*. These reactions include changes in liver protein synthesis; alternations in serum metals, such as iron; and increased production of certain classes of white blood cells and other cells of the immune system. Most fevers are physiologically controlled so that the temperature remains below 105.8°F (41°C). However, severe fever, as occur with meningococcal meningitis, may cause heat stroke and other complications. Even milder fevers accompanied by fatigue, chills, and diaphoresis are often uncomfortable for the patient. Whether fever is treated or untreated, adequate fluid intake is important during febrile episodes.

Monitoring and Managing Potential Complications

The patient with a rapidly progress infectious ease should have vital signs and level of consciousness closely monitored. X-ray finding and mocrobiologic, immunologic, hematologic, cytologic and parastilogic laboratory values must be interpret the context of other clinical findings to assess the course of the infectious disease.

Antibiotic therapy is frequently complex, and cations are necessary because of sensitivity test rest and disease progression. It is important to initiate biotic therapy as soon as it is prescribed rather waiting until routine medication scheduling times ensure that therapeutic blood levels can be attain as quickly as possible.

Evaluation

Expected Patient Outcomes

Expected patient outcomes any include the followed:
- Used appropriate outcomes may include the specific infection.
- Acquire knoeledge about the infectious pro
- Exhibits absence of elevated body temperature.

(*Note:* For details description of certain infectious disease, please read authors title on "Community Health Nursing", 3rd edition)

CHAPTER 14

Perioperative Nursing

INTRODUCTION

The word 'surgery' comes from the 'kheirurgos', which means working by hand. Surgery is defined as "the branch of medicine dealing with manual and operative procedures for correction of deformities and defects, repair of injuries".

Surgery long back became a medical speciality, because often the treatment of a wide variety of illness and injuries include some types of surgical intervention. Surgery is an invasive method of treatment that may be planned or unplanned, major or minor, and that may involve any body part or system. Care for the client during all phases of the surgical experience needs to be continuous, and integrated surgical procedures require physical and psychosocial adaptations and are stressors for both the client and the family. The client's recovery from a surgical procedure requires skillful and knowledgeable nursing care whether the surgery is of outpatient or in the hospital setting. Nurses working in both settings must understand the principles of caring for surgical clients.

As stated earlier, a client faces variety of stressors when confronting surgery. Anticipatory surgery leads to fear and anxiety for clients who associate surgery with pain, possible disfigurement, dependence, and perhaps even loss of life. Family members often fear a disruption in lifestyle and experience a sense of powerlessness as the surgery approaches. The trauma sustained during surgery creates physical needs requiring close supervision and skilled intervention by the nurse and surgeon. Nurses use all phases of nursing process used perioperatively to make assessment and provide interventions necessary to promote the recovery of health, prevent further injury or illness, and facilitate coping with alterations in physical structure and function.

DEFINITION OF PERIOPERATIVE NURSING AND NURSE

Perioperative nursing refers to the role of nurse during the perioperative, intraoperative and postoperative phases of a clients surgical experience. The concept of perioperative nursing stresses the importance of providing continuity of care.

- Perioperative nursing refers to the role of the nurse during the preoperative, intraoperative and postoperative phases of a client's surgical experience. The concept of perioperative nursing stresses the importance of providing continuity of care.
- A perioperative nurse is defined as the registered nurse, who, using the nursing process, designs, coordinates and delivers care to meet the identified needs of the clients whose protective reflexes or self-care abilities are potentially compromised because they are under the influence of anesthesia during operative or other invasive procedures.
- Perioperative nurse, possesses and applies knowledge of the procedure and the client's intraoperative experience throughout the client-care continuum. And also they assess, diagnose, plan, intervene and evaluate the outcome of interventions based on criteria and support of a standard care targeted towards the population
- The perioperative nurse addresses the changing physiological, pathophysiological, sociocultural and spiritual responses of the client that have been initiated by the prospect of performance of the invasive procedure.

SCOPE OF THE PERIOPERATIVE NURSING

The scope of perioperative nursing practice consists of three phases:

1. *Preoperative phase:* It begins where the decision for surgical intervention is made and ends with transference of the client to the operative site. Nursing activities range from a baseline assessment of the client during the preoperative interview and continues with assessment in the pre-admission unit, client room, holding area, or induction room on the day of surgery. Before surgery, the nurse prepares the client and family for the surgery, performs diagnostic tests, and assesses the client in preparation for the operation.
2. *Intraoperative phase:* It begins where the client is transferred to the operating room bed and ends when the client is transferred to an area of recovery from anesthesia. In this phase, nursing interventions range from communicating the client's plan of care, identifying nursing activities, necessary for expected outcome and establishing priorities for nursing actions. During surgery, the nurse assists surgeons and other operating room nurses to ensure that the client

receives optimal care. The nurse also coordinates client needs with team members and personnel's from other disciplines, coordinates the use of the supplies and equipment, controls the environment, prepares for potential emergencies, and communicates and documents the client's plan of care.

3. *Postoperative phase:* It begins with the client's transfer to an area for recovery and ends with client's recovery from surgery. Nursing activities range from communicating pertinent information about the client's surgery, to assist the client to be physical stability and wakefulness and institute measures to help the client achieve maximum recovery.

Classification of Surgical Procedure

Surgery can be defined as the art and science of treating diseases, injuries and deformities by operation and instrumentation. The surgical procedure involves the interaction of the patient, the surgeon, and the nurse. Surgical procedures usually are classified on the basis of urgency degree of risk, and purposes.

Based on Urgency

Surgery may be classified as elective surgery, urgent surgery and emergency surgery.

Elective surgery: It is preplanned and performed on the basis of client's choice. It is not essential and may not be necessary for health and delay in surgery has no ill effects, can be scheduled in advance based on the choice of client. The purposes of elective surgery are as follows:
- To remove or repair a body part
- To restore function
- To improve health
- To improve self-concept

For example, tonsillectomy, hernia repair, cataract extraction and lens implant, hip prosthesis, hemorrhoidectomy, etc.

Urgent surgery: In which the surgery is the necessity for the client's health, but not an emergency. This is performed for the purposes as in elective surgery and to prevent further tissue damage. For example, removal of gallbladder, coronary artery, removal of tumor, etc.

Emergency surgery: When surgery must be done immediately to preserve the client's life, remove or repair body part, restore function, improve health and self concept. For example, perforated ulcer, intestinal obstruction, tracheostomy, cesarean section, etc.

Based on Degree of Risk or Seriousness

Surgery has been classified as major or minor on the basis of risk for the client:

Major surgery: It involves extensive reconstruction or alteration in body parts poses great risks to well-being. It requires hospitalization usually belonged to well-being; has a high degree of risk; involves major body organs, life-threatening situations and potential postoperative complications. Major surgery may be elective, urgent, or emergency. For example, nephrectomy, cholecystectomy, colostomy, hysterectomy.

Minor surgery: It is primarily elective; it is usually a brief, carries low risk and results in few complications. It can be performed in clinics, outpatient clinic and minor operation theaters. For example, teeth extraction, removal of warts, skin biopsy, laparoscopy, dilatations and curettage.

Based on Purpose

Surgical procedures based on purpose include diagnostic, ablative, palliative, reconstructive, transplant, constructive.

Diagnostic: It is surgical exploration that allows physician to make or to confirm diagnosis, may involve removal of tissue for further diagnostic testing. For example, breast biopsy, laparoscopy, bronchoscopy, exploratory laparotomy (incision in peritoneal cavity to inspect abdominal organs).

Ablative: It is excision or removal of diseased body part. For example, appendicectomy, subtotal thyroidectomy, partial gastrectomy, colon resection, amputation, cholecystectomy, etc.

Palliative surgery: It is performed to relieve or reduce intensity of an illness or disease symptoms will not produce cure. For example, colostomy, nerve root resection (rhizotomy) debridement of necrotic tissue, balloon angioplasty, arthroscopy, etc.

Reconstructive surgery: It is performed to restore function to traumatized or malfunctioning tissues and to improve self-concept. For example, scar revision, plastic surgery, skin graft, internal fixation of fractures, breast reconstruction.

Transplant: It is performed to replace organs or structures that are diseased or malfunctioning. For example, kidney, cornea, liver, heart, joints, total hip replacement.

Constructive surgery: It is performed to restore function lost or reduced as a result of congenital anomalies. For example, repair of cleft palate, closure of a trial defect in heart.

Sometime combination of several surgery explained above also are performed as and when needed.

The common prefixes and suffixes used to explain the types of surgical procedures are described in **Table 14.1**.

ROLE OF NURSE IN PERIOPERATIVE CARE

General Care

Each surgical client responds differently in surgery, when he/she enters the healthcare setting in different stages of health. Many variables influence a person's physiologic and psychological responses to the surgical experience. These include physical and mental status, extent of

Table 14.1: Common prefixes and suffixes in surgery.

Prefixes		Suffixes	
Terms	Definitions	Terms	Definitions
Supra-	Above, beyond	-oma	Tumor, swelling
Artho-	Joint	-ectomy	Removal of organ
Chole-	Bile or gall	-rrhapy	The suturing or stitching of part of an organ
Cysto-	Bladder	-scopy	Looking into
Endocephalo-	Brain	-ostomy	Making an opening or stoma
Hystero-	Uterus	-otomy	Cutting into
Mast-	Breast	-plasty	To repair or restore
Menigo-	Membrane	-cele	Tumor, hernia, swelling
Myo-	Muscle	-itis	Inflammation
Nephro-	Kidney		
Oophor-	Ovary		
Pneumo-	Lung		
Pyelo-	Pelvis, kidney		
Salpingo-	Fallopian tube		
Thoraco-	Chest		
Viscero-	Organ especially abdomen		

disease, magnitude of the surgery, social and financial resources and psychological and physiological preparation for surgery. When considered effectively, these variables reveal the degree of risk for a client undergoing surgery.

While making physiological assessment before surgery, nurse elicits information about age; presence of pain; nutritional status; fluid and electrolyte balance; presence of infections; physical mobility, skin integrity, cardiovascular; pulmonary, renal, gastrointestinal, liver, endocrine, neurologic and hematologic function; sensory medication history, abnormalities, injuries and previous surgeries, health habits, and sociocultural history and note any abnormalities and report to the concerned and take suitable measures to correct and sending the client to operating room.

The possible preoperative tests include the following and reasons for those tests and normal ranges stated are as follows:
- Complete blood count and picture should be tested.
- Serum potassium (normal 3.5–5 mEq/L) to identify hyperkalemia or hypokalemia.
- Serum sodium (normal 136 to 145 mEq/L) to identify hypernatremia, dehydration or overhydration.
- Serum chloride (normal 96-100 mEq/L) to identify hyperchloremia, hypochloremia, or metabolic disorder.
- Glucose (normal 60-100 mg/dL) to identify hypoglycemia or hyperglycemia.
- Creatinine (normal 0.7–1.4 mg/dL) to identify acute or chronic renal disease.
- Blood urea nitrogen (BUN) (10-20 mg/dL) to identify impaired liver or kidney function or excessive protein or tissue catabolism.
- Hemoglobin (Hb) (Female) (12 to 15 gm/dL; male 13–17 gm) to identify the presence and extent of anemia.
- Hematocrit (Hct) (Female 36%; Male 39–51%) to identify the presence and extent of anemia.
- Prothorombin time (PT) or clotting time (CT) (11–18 seconds) to identify dysfunction of blood clotting (prothrombin level).
- Partial thromboplastin time (PTT) to identify deficiencies of coagulation factors.
- Chest X-ray (No abnormal heart of lung lesion) to determine size and contour of heart, lungs, and major vessels.
- Electrocardiogram (ECG) (Normal rate and rhythm) to determine the electrical activity of the heart.
- Urine analysis to identify abnormalities.

Any deviations from the normal, should be noted and reported to take precautions during surgery. And the common medical conditions that increase the high risk in surgery will include bleeding disorders, diabetes mellitus, heart diseases, upper respiratory infection, liver diseases, fever, chronic respiratory diseases, and immunological disorders. A special precaution should be taken on these cases before, during and after surgery.

PREOPERATIVE CARE

Persons who require surgical intervention and nursing care enter the healthcare settings in a variety of situations, ranging from essentially healthy people who have planned elective procedure to emergency admissions for treatment of trauma. Surgical client may be of any age and at any point on the health-illness continuum. It is the nurse's responsibility to identify factors that affect risk from a surgical procedure, assess physical and psychosocial needs of the client and family and establish a plan of care, based on appropriate nursing diagnoses, that includes interventions to meet needs and facilitate recovery as the client progresses through the perioperative period. Nurse has to perform preoperative assessment and Teaching as discussed below:

Preoperative Assessment

The nurses make preoperative assessment by taking history, conducting physical examination, performing diagnostic tests as required preoperatively according to client's status/requirements, and takes informed consent in preoperative phase. Informed consent is very essential for anyone is undergoing any invasive procedure like surgery. A consent form is the legal document which signifies the client's informed consent for the procedure. The consent form guards the client against unwanted invasive procedure. It also protects the healthcare facility and healthcare professional (use consent form as per Policy of Hospital).

In addition, preoperative teaching is an important component in the client's operative experience. Teaching about postoperative phase is the nurse's responsibility. Clients and families need to know about surgical events, and sensations, how to perform physical activities necessary to decrease postoperative complications and facilitate recovery. The teaching-learning process is individualized to meet both specific and common client needs. Preoperative teaching allays anxiety and encourages clients to participate actively in their own care. The basic areas that must be covered in preoperative teaching are the following:

Preoperative nursing interventions are derived from the nursing assessment and must reflect each individual patients specific needs. Physical preparations will be determined by the pending surgery and the routines of the surgery setting. Preoperative teaching may be minimal or extensive. General information for surgery should be given. Nursing assessment includes following:

Cardiovascular System

- Identify acute or chronic problems; focus on presence of angina, hypertension, heart failure, recent history of myocardial infarction.
- Auscultate and palpate baseline pulses; apical, radial, and pedal for rate and characteristics (compare one side to the other).
- Inspect and palpate for presence of edema (including dependent areas) noting location and severity.
- Inspect and palpate neck veins for distention.
- Take baseline blood pressure in both arms.
- Identify any drug or herbal product that may affect coagulation (e.g. aspirin, ginkgo, ginger).
- Review laboratory and diagnostic tests for cardiovascular function.
- Identify patients with pacemakers and/or implantable debrillators.

Respiratory System

- Identify acute or chronic problems; note the presence of infection or chronic obstructive pulmonary disease (COPD), asthma.
- Assess history of smoking, including the time interval since the last cigarette and the number of pack-years. (Remember that although smoking should be discouraged preoperatively, it may be difficult for patients to stop during this time of anxiety).
- Auscultate lungs for normal and adventitious breath sounds.
- Determine baseline respiratory rate and rhythm, and regularity of pattern.
- Observe for cough, dyspnea and use of accessory muscles of respiration.

Neurologic System

- Determine orientation to time, place, and person.
- Identify presence of confusion, disorderly thinking, or inability to follow commands.
- Identify past history of strokes, transient ischemic attacks or nervous system diseases (e.g. Parkinson's disease, multiple sclerosis).

Urinary System

- Identify any preexisting disease.
- Determine ability to void. Prostate enlargement may affect catheterization during surgery and ability to void postoperatively.
- If necessary, note color, amount, and characteristics of urine.
- Review laboratory and diagnostic tests for renal function.

Hepatic System

- Inspect skin color and sclera of eyes for any signs of jaundice.
- Review past history of substance abuse, especially alcohol and IV drug use.
- Review laboratory and diagnostic tests for liver function.

Integumentary System

- Assess mucous membranes for dryness and intactness.
- Determine skin status; note drying, bruising, or breaks in surface.
- Inspect skin for rashes, boils or infection, especially around the planned surgical site.
- Assess skin moisture and temperature.
- Inspect the mucous membranes and skin turgor for dehydration.

Musculoskeletal System

- Examine skin/bone pressure points.
- Assess for presence of any pressure ulcers.
- Assess for limitations in joint range of motion and muscle weakness.
- Assess mobility, gait and balance.
- Assess for presence of joint pain.

Gastrointestinal System

- Determine food and fluid intake patterns and any recent weight loss.
- Weigh and measure patient.
- Assess for the presence of dentures and bridges (loose dentures or teeth may be dislodged during intubation).

Immune System
- Identify any immunodeficiency or autoimmune disorders
- Assess for use of corticosteroids or other immunosuppressant drugs.

Preoperative Teaching

The patient has a right to know what to expect and how to participate effectively during the surgical experience. Preoperative teaching increases patient satisfaction and may reduce postoperative fear, anxiety, and stress. Teaching may also decrease complication, the duration of hospitalization. And the recovery time following discharge. In most surgical settings, patients often arrive only a short time before surgery is scheduled. This includes patients arriving for ambulatory surgery and patient who will be hospitalized postoperatively. Preoperative teaching for these patients is generally done in the surgeon's office or preadmission surgical clinic and reinforced on the day of surgery. The patient usually goes home several hours after ambulatory surgery, the patient usually goes home several hours after recovery depending on the patient's progress and procedure-specific needs. If ambulatory patients have not hade preoperative teaching in an outpatient setting before surgery, teaching must address needs of the highest priority and include information that focuses on the safety of the patient. Written materials must be provided for patient to use for review and reinforcement at home. When providing preoperative teaching for a patient several days before surgery, the nurse must provide a balance between telling so little that the patient is unprepared and explaining so much that the patient is overwhelmed. The nurse who observes carefully and listen sensitively to the patient can usually determine how much information is enough in each instance, remembering that anxiety and fear may decrease leaning ability. The nurse must also assess what the patient wants to know right away and give priority to his or her concerns.

Generally, preoperative teaching concerns three types of information: sensory, process and procedural. Different patients, with varying cultures, backgrounds, and experience may want different types of information. With *sensory information*, patients want to know what they will see, hear, smell and feel during the surgery. For example, the nurse may tell them that the OT (Operation Theatre) will be cold, but they can ask the OT nurse for a warm blanket; the lights in the OT are very bright; or there will be lots of sounds that are unfamiliar and there may be specific smells present. Patients wanting *process information* may not want specific details but desire the general flow of what is going to happen. This information would include the patient's transfer to the OT, and waking up in the POCU (Postoperative Care Unit). Patients may also be informed that as soon as they are awake, their family may come in to visit them. With *procedural information*, desired details are more specific. For example, this information would include that an IV line will be started while patients are in the holding area and the surgeon may mark the operative site with an indelible marker to verify site and side. Other procedural information includes that when patients are transferred to the OR (Operating Room), they will be asked to move onto the narrow bed and a safety strap will be put over their thighs.

Preoperative teaching provided to the patient must be communicated to the nurses providing postoperative care so that learning can be nurses providing postoperative care so that learning can evaluated and duplication of teaching can be prevented. Because the nurse has limited time for teaching, the team approach is usually used. Nurses in offices, homes, or clinics may initiate the teaching. The perioperative nurses continue teaching and evaluate the patients understanding of the content. The discharge nurse provides written instructions and additional information for reinforcement. Community nurses may also be involved if the patient has continuing learning needs that these nurses can address during home visits after patients are discharged.

All teaching should be documented in the patient's medical record. A patient and family teaching guide for preoperative preparation is presented as follows:

Sensory Information
- Holding area may be noisy.
- Drugs and cleaning solutions may be smelled.
- Operation theatre (OT) can be cold; warm blankets are available.
- Talking may be heard in the OT but may be distorted because of masks. Questions should be asked if something is not understood.
- OT bed will be narrow. A safety strap will be applied over the knees.
- Lights in the OT may be very bright.
- Monitoring machines (ticking and pinging noises) may be heard when awake. Their purpose is to monitor and ensure safety.

Procedural Information
- What to bring and what type of clothing to wear to the ambulatory surgery center.
- Any changes in time of surgery.
- Fluid and food restrictions.
- Physical preparation required (e.g. bowel of skin preparation).
- Purpose of frequent vital signs assessment.
- Pain control and other comfort measures.
- Why turning, coughing, and deep breathing postoperatively is important; practice sessions need to be done preoperatively.

- Insertion of intravenous lines.
- Procedure for anesthesia administration.
- Expected surgical site and/or side to be marked with indelible ink or marker.

Process Information

Information About General Flow of Surgery

- Admission area.
- Preoperative holding area, OR, and recovery area.
- Families can usually stay in holding area until surgery.
- Families may be able to enter recovery area as soon as patient is awake.
- Identification of any technology that may be present on awakening, such as monitors and central lines.

Where Families Can Wait during Surgery

- Patients and family members need to be encouraged to verbalize concerns.
- OR staff will notify family when surgery is completed.
- Surgeon will usually talk with family following surgery.

All patients should receive instruction about deep breathing, coughing, and moving postoperatively. This is essential because patients may not want to do these activities postoperatively unless they are taught the rationale for them and practice them preoperatively. Patients and families should be told if there will be tubes, drains, monitoring devices, or special equipment after surgery, and that these devices enable the nurse to safely care for the patient. Examples of individualized teaching may include how to use incentive spirometers or postoperative patient-controlled analgesia pumps. The patient should also receive accurate surgery specific information, such as a patient having an immobilizer following a total joint replacement, a patient having an epidural catheter for postoperative pain control, or the patient being told about waking up in the intensive care unit following extensive surgery.

The ambulatory surgery patient or the patient admitted to the hospital the day of surgery will need to receive information before admission. Some ambulatory surgical centers have the staff telephone the patients the evening before surgery to answer last-minute questions and to reinforce teaching. Each surgical center has policies and procedures that direct and enable this communication in a timely manner.

The patient will need basic information such as time to arrive at the surgery center and the time of surgery. Arrival time is usually 1 to 2 hours before the scheduled time of surgery to allow for the completion of the preoperative assessment and paperwork preparation. Information can also include the day-of-surgery events such as patient registration, parking, what to wear, what to bring, and the need to have a responsible adult present for transportation home after surgery. To provide for general hygiene and preparation of surgical areas the surgeon may order a preoperative shower, an enema, and food and fluid restrictions. Historically, patients having elective surgery were usually instructed by the Anaesthesia Care Provider (ACP) to have nothing by mouth (NPO) starting at midnight on the night before surgery. Protocols may vary if the patient is having local anesthesia or the surgery is scheduled for late in the day. The NPO protocol of each surgical facility should be followed because varying NPO protocols exist. Providing the patient with the rationale for adhering to NPO orders can significantly increase the patient's perception of their importance. Restriction of fluids and food is designed to minimize the potential risk of aspiration and to decrease the risk of postoperative nausea and vomiting. The patient who has not followed this instruction may have surgery delayed or cancelled, so it is critical that the surgical patient understands and adheres to these restrictions.

Legal Preparation

Legal preparation for the client undergoing surgery consists of checking that all required forms have been correctly signed and are present on the chart, and that the patient and family clearly understand what is going to happen. Standard consent forms include those for the surgical procedure and blood transfusions. Other forms may include those that have been completed for advance directives and power of attorney. Before nonemergency surgery can be legally performed, the patient must voluntarily sign an **informed consent** form in the presence of a witness. Informed consent is an active, shared decision-making process between the provider and the recipient of care. Three conditions must be met for consent to be valid. First, there must be *adequate disclosure* of the diagnosis; the nature and purpose of the proposed treatment; the risks and consequences of the proposed treatment; the probability of a successful outcome; the availability, benefits, and risks of alternative treatments, and the prognosis if treatment is not instituted. Second, the patient must demonstrate clear *understanding and comprehension* of the information being provided before receiving sedating preoperative medications. Third, the recipient of care must *give consent voluntarily*. The patient must not be persuaded or coerced in any way by anyone to undergo the procedure.

Although the surgeon is ultimately responsible for obtaining the patients consent for surgical treatment, the nurse may be responsible for witnessing the patient's signature on the consent form. At this time the nurse can be patient advocate, verifying that consent for surgery is truly voluntary. If the patient is unclear about operative plans, the nurse should contact the surgeon about the patients need for additional information. The patient also should be aware the consent, even when signed, can be withdrawn at any time if the desire to give permission for the procedure changes. If the patient is a minor, is unconscious, or is mentally incompetent to sign the permit, the written permission may be given by a legally appointed representative or responsible family member. Procedures for obtaining consent, especially from minors and patients who are mentally incompetent, vary among states and institutions. Therefore the nurse should follow specifics required by the states nurse practice act and the institutional or agency policies that apply to an individual situation.

A true medical emergency may override the need to obtain consent. When immediate medical treatment is needed to preserve life or to prevent serious impairment to life and the individual patient is incapable of giving consent, the next of kin may give consent. If reaching the next of kin is not possible, the physician may institute treatment without written consent. A note is written in the chart documenting the medical necessity of the procedure. In the case of emergency where consent cannot be obtained, the intraoperative nurse will usually need to complete an incident report because it is an occurrence that is inconsistent with routine facility operations.

The nurse discusses a patients impending surgery in the preoperative holding area. It becomes obvious that this competent adult patient was not fully informed of the alternatives to this surgery. She has signed the consent form but clearly was not fully informed about her treatment options. An important points to be considered here are as given below:

- Informed consent requires that patients have complete information about the proposed treatment and its possible consequences, as well as alternative treatments and possible consequences
- Risks and benefits of each treatment option must also be explained in order for patients to weigh treatment options
- An opportunity to have questions answered about the various treatment options and their possible outcomes is also an important element of informed consent
- Informed consent is an ongoing process that needs periodic assessment and discussion, not an event where a person signs a document
- Paternalism results when health care providers do not provide complete information for patients to make fully informed decisions or when they decide what is best for patients

Nursing Responsibilities in the Day of Surgery

Day of surgery preparation will vary a great deal depending on whether the patient is an inpatient or an outpatient. The nursing responsibilities immediately before surgery include final preoperative teaching, assessment and communication of pertinent findings, ensuring that all preoperative preparation orders have been completed, and ensuring that records and reports are present and complete to accompany the patient to the OR. It is especially important to verify the presence of a signed operative consent, laboratory data, a history and physical examination report, a record of any consultations, baseline vital signs, and nurses notes complete to that point. In addition, the site and side of the anticipated surgery may be marked with an indelible marker and documented to indicate agreement with the patient.

If the patient is an inpatient, the hospital nurse is responsible to ensure that the patients is ready and appropriately prepared for surgery. If the patient is an outpatient, the patient or family member will share the responsibility for preoperative preparation. Hospitals may require that a patient wear a hospital gown with no underclothes, whereas surgery centers may allow the patient to wear underwear, depending on the surgical procedure to be performed. The patient should not wear cosmetics because observation of skin color will be important. Nail polish and artificial nails should be removed so that capillary refill and pulse oximetry can be assessed. An identification band is put on the patient and, if applicable, an allergy band. All patient valuables are returned to a family member or secured according to institutional protocol. If the patient prefers not to remove a wedding ring, the ring can be taped securely to the finger to prevent loss. All prostheses, including dentures, contact lenses, and glasses, are generally removed to prevent loss or damage to them. Hearing aids may be left in place to allow the patient to better follow instructions. Glasses and hearing aids must be returned to the patient as soon as possible following surgery.

The patient should be encouraged to void before preoperative medications are administered if the medications will interfere with maintaining balance and increase the risk for a fall when ambulating to the bathroom. The patient should have an empty bladder on transfer to the OT to prevent involuntary elimination under anesthesia and reduce the possibility of urinary retention during early postoperative recovery. The use of preoperative checklist ensures that all preoperative preparations have been completed before the patient is given any sedating medications.

Preoperative Medications

Preoperative medications are used for a variety of reasons. A patient may receive a single drug or a combination of drugs. Benzodiazepines and barbiturates are used for their sedative and amnesic properties. Anticholinergics are given to reduce secretions. Opioids may be given to decrease intraoperative anesthetic requirements and to decrease pain. Antiemetics may be given to decrease nausea and vomiting. It identifies common preoperative medications and the purposes of their use preoperatively.

Other medications that may be administered preoperatively include antibiotics, eye drops, and routine prescription drugs. Antibiotics may be administered throughout the perioperative period for a patient with a history of congenital or valvular heart disease to prevent the development of infective endocarditis. Antibiotics may also be ordered for the patient undergoing surgery where wound contamination is either a potential risk (e.g., gastrointestinal surgery) or where wound infection could have serious postoperative consequences (e.g., cardiac and joint replacement surgery). Antibiotics are most commonly administered intravenously (IV) and may be started either preoperatively or in the OT (Operation Theatre).

Eye drops commonly ordered and administered preoperatively for the patient undergoing cataract and other eye surgery. Many times the patient will require multiple sets of eye drops administered at 5-minute intervals. It is important to administer these drugs as ordered and on time to adequately prepare the eye for surgery.

Medications that patients routinely use for health maintenance or disease management may or may not be used on the day of surgery. To facilitate patient teaching and eliminate confusion about which medications should be taken, the nurse should carefully check written preoperative orders and clarify the orders with the surgeon and/or ACP if there is any question.

Premedications may be administered orally (PO), IV, substaneously (SC), or intramuscularly (IM). Oral medications are given 60 to 90 minutes before the patient goes to the OR unless otherwise ordered. Because patients are fluid restricted before surgery, the patient should swallow these medications with a minimal amount of water. IM and SC injections are usually to be given 30 to 60 minutes before arrival at the OT (minimally 20 minutes). Intravenous medication are usually administered to the patient after arrival in the preoperative holding area or operating room. The patient should be informed about the expected effects of the medications, such as relaxation, drowsiness, and dryness of the mouth.

Transportation to the Operation Theatre

If the patient is an impatient, the OT staff sends transport personnel to the patients room with a cart or trolley to transport the patient to surgery. The nurse assists the patient in transferring from the hospital bed to the OR cart, and the side rails of the cart are raised and secured. The nurse should ensure that the completed chart goes with the patient, as well as any ordered preoperative equipment, such as antiembolism devices or the patient's inhaler. In many institutions the family may accompany the patient to the holding area.

In an ambulatory surgical center, the patient may be transported to the OT by cart or wheelchair, or, if no sedatives have been administered, the patient may even walk accompanied to the OT. In all cases it is important for the nurse to ensure patient safety during transport. The method of transportation and the person who transported the patient should be documented by the nurse responsible for the transfer.

The family should be instructed where to wait for the patient during surgery. Many hospitals have a surgical waiting room where OT personnel communicate the status of the patient to the family. It is in this waiting room that the surgeon can locate the family after surgery and where families can be notified that the surgery is complete. Some hospitals provide pagers to waiting family members so that they may eat or do errands during the surgery.

While the patient is in surgery the inpatient nurse should have the patients room prepared for the postoperative arrival.

Any additional necessary equipment, including IV poles, oxygen, suction, and additional pillows for positioning, should also be placed in the room. The room also is organized to facilitate entry of the transport cart.

In addition, preoperative teaching is an important component in the client's operative experience. Teaching about postoperative phase and is the nurse's responsibility. Clients and families need to know about surgical events, and sensations, how to perform physical activities necessary to decrease postoperative complications and facilitate recovery. The teaching-learning process is individualized to meet both specific and common client needs. Preoperative teaching allays anxiety and encourages clients to participate actively in their own care. The basic areas that must be covered in preoperative teaching are the following:

Deep breathing exercises and coughing exercises: These help expand collapsed lung and prevent postoperative pneumonia atelectasis. Coughing exercise help to guard the suture.

Turning exercises: These help prevent venous stasis, thrombophlebitis, decubitus ulcer formation, and respiratory complications.

Extremity exercises: These help prevent circulatory problems, such as thrombophlebitis, by facilitating venous return to the heart.

Ambulation: Early ambulation when appropriate, helps prevent postoperative complications.

Pain control: Regarding medication (IV or IM) or NPO (nothing per oral), relaxation technique are advisable. In addition, TENS and PCA are taught for pain control measure.

Postoperative equipment: Client may be instructed about equipments that may be used postoperatively. Depending upon the surgery, various tubes, drains, and IV lines are used.

Physical preparation: The physical preparation of the client for surgery may vary, depending on the client's physical status and special needs, type of surgery to be done and surgeon's order. Certain nursing interventions are appropriate for all surgical clients in the areas of hygiene and skin preparation, elimination, nutrition, and fluids and rest and sleep. The nurse is responsible for the preparation and safety of the client on the day of surgery.

- *Skin preparation:* The skin is cleaned by scrubbing the operative site one or more times with an antiseptic soap or solution to remove bacteria. This can be done by the client while taking a bath or shower. Ideally, a shower is taken in the evening before the morning of surgery. Shampooing the hair and the cleaning of the fingernails also help to reduce number of organism present. The incisional area usually is shaved before surgery because hair serves as a reservoir of bacteria. Usually the operative area is washed before surgery with an antiseptic such as povidoneiodine (Betadine) to clean and disinfect the skin.
- *Elimination:* The gastrointestinal tract needs special preparation on the evening before surgery to:
    - Reduce the possibility of vomiting and aspiration during anesthesia
    - Reduce the possibility of a bowel obstruction, and
    - Prevent contamination from fecal material during intestinal tract or bowel surgery.

    Emptying the bowel of feces in no longer routine procedure before surgery, but the nurse should use preoperative assessment to determine the need for an order of bowel elimination. If the client is scheduled for surgery of the GI tract, cleansing enema usually ordered.

    Insertion of an indwelling urinary catheter may be ordered before surgery, especially in clients having pelvic surgery, to prevent bladder distention or accidental injury. If an indwelling catheter is not in place, the client should void immediately before receiving premedication to ensure an empty bladder during surgery.
- *Nutrition and fluids:* Preparation involves restricting food and fluid. If a client undergoing surgery is to receive a general anesthesia, foods and fluids are restricted 8 to 10 hours before the operation. This restriction significantly reduces the possibility of aspirations of gastric contents, which can cause aspiration pneumonia. Most clients have an NPO status after midnight.
- *Rest and sleep:* These are important components in reducing stress before surgery and in healing and recovery after surgery. The nurse can facilitate rest and sleep in the immediate preoperative period by meeting psychological needs, carrying out teaching, providing a quiet environment, and administering prescribed bedtime sedative medication.

To sum up immediate preoperative preparations begin at least 1 to 2 hours before surgery in the hospital. The nurse's responsibility on the day of surgery will include the following:

- Note allergies according to institutional policy.
- Take and record the vital signs, assess and report the abnormalities for elevated temperature.
- Check the identification band to make sure it is legible, accurate and securely fastened to the client.
- Be sure that informed consent has been obtained and is clearly documented.
- If a skin preparation has been ordered, check that it has been completed accurately and thoroughly.
- Check for the carry out any special orders, such as administering enema or starting on IV line, recurred previous records, inserting nasogastric tube, giving medications.
- Verify that the client has not eaten for the last 8 hours. Check that fluids have been restricted although sometimes the physician will order clients to take their usual oral medication with a small sip of water.
- Ask the client to void, measure and record the amount of urine (if indicated).
- Assist the client with oral hygiene if necessary
- Help the client to remove jewellery to prevent loss or injury from swelling, during or after surgery. Many facilities allow the client to keep wedding band or *mangala suthra (tali)* on as long as they are taped securely. If jewellery is removed, it should be stored according to policy or given to authorized member of their family.
- Remove all hairpins or hairpieces. This prevents injury to the client during surgery as well as possible loss or hairpieces or wigs.
- Remove colored nail polish from at least one nail for the pulse oximeter to allow intraoperative and postoperative assessment of skin and nailbeds for circulation and oxygenation of tissues.
- If the client is wearing hearing aid, notify the operating room nurse. Leave it in place so that operating room personnel know it is there and can communicate with the client.
- Remove all prosthesis, such as dentures, or partial plates, eye glasses, contact lenses and artificial limbs and store them safely (dentures may cause respiratory, distress).
- Give the preoperative medications that are prescribed, either at a scheduled time or "on call". The commonly ordered medications are:
    - Sedatives and tranquilizers to alleviate anxiety and facilitate anesthesia induction, e.g. nembutol, chlorpromozen, or diazopen.

- ♦ Anticholenesterase to decrease pulmonary and oral secretions to prevent laryngospasm, e.g. atropine.
- ♦ Narcotic analgesics to facilitate client's sedation and relaxation and to decrease the amount of anesthetic agent need, e.g. morphine.
- ♦ Neurolephanalegiscs agents to cause a general state of calmness and sleepness.

  To prevent omissions and preoperative nursing intervention, most facilities supply nurses with a preoperative checklist. As each intervention on the list is completed, the nurse initials it. Documents through checklists and narrative charting, the nursing intervention carried out.
- Assist in moving client from the bed to the operating room stretcher when it is time to transport the client to surgery, ensuring accurate identification.

INTRAOPERATIVE CARE

Intraoperative phase begins when the client enters the surgical suite and ends with admission to the recovery area. Nursing care during this phase focuses on the client's emotional well-being, as well as on physical factors such as safety positioning, maintaining asepsis and controlling the surgical environment. The nurses are the client's advocates upon induction of anesthesia.

In the surgical holding area, the nurse is responsible for reviewing the record for completeness, ensuring proper identification of the client, client's safety and providing emotional support. It is important to deal with the fears and concerns of a frightened or agitated client. A relaxed client undergoes anesthetic induction easier than who is anxious. If the client still seems anxious despite sedation and reassurance, notify the surgeon or anesthesia personnel. Here the anesthetologist sees the client, IV fluids starts by him or her or nurse-anesthetist. Nurse anaesthetist also can administer medication needed during surgery. The procedures vary among institutions of health care. Nurse has to perform following activities during intraoperative phase.

The preoperative assessment of the surgical patient establishes baseline data for intraoperative and post-anesthesia care. Assessment data provided by the patient and family in the holding area and data from the inpatient nursing units are verified and used to develop a plan of care for the patient.

Psychosocial Assessment

The perioperative nurse who cares for the patient in the OT is knowledgeable about the activities that occur when a patient is transferred into the surgical suite. This knowledge allows for informative and reassuring explanations, especially to the anxious patient. General questions regarding surgery or anesthesia can usually be answered by the perioperative nurse. Examples of these questions include, "When will my I go to sleep?" "Who will be in the room?" "When will may doctor arrive?" "How much of my body will be exposed and to whom?" "Will I be cold?" "When will may I wake up?" Specific questions relating to details of the surgical procedure and anesthesia may be referred to the surgeon or ACP.

Cultural assessment is essential to understanding the patient's response to the surgical experience. For example, members of the Jehovan's Witness community may refuse blood transfusions. For Muslims, the left hand is considered unclean, so the nurse should use the right hand to administer forms, drugs, and treatments. Some patients may request that surgically removed body tissue be preserved so that it may be ritually buried. Some body piercings may also have cultural meaning. An interpreter may be necessary if the patient does not speak local language or English. Spiritual considerations, attitudes, and expression regarding pain and health beliefs and practices should individualize the plan of care.

Physical Assessment

A thorough physical assessment should be made during the preoperative preparation of the patient. Physical assessment data that are specifically important to intraoperative nursing care include baseline data such as vital signs, height, weight, and age; allergic reactions to food, drugs and latex; condition and cleanliness of skin; skeletal and muscle impairments; perceptual difficulties; level of consciousness; nothing by mouth (NPO) status; and any sources of pain or discomfort. Vital signs are important as baseline data to evaluate the effects of intraoperative medications and body positioning. Height and weight of the patient guide the nurse regarding the width and length of the OR bed. The need for extra warmth is indicated by the patient's age, metabolic problems, and planned surgical procedures.

Some allergic reactions may be avoided with such simple measures as a change in "pepping" solutions or the type of tape used with dressings. Catastrophic reactions can possibly be avoided if latex sensitivity is determined before the procedure begins. The condition and cleanliness of the skin determine the amount and type of intraoperative skin preparation solutions, and will alert the team to the potential for infection as a result of open or closed skin lesions. Knowledge of skeletal and muscle impairments helps prevent injury during positioning. Knowledge of the presence of piercings will allow jewelry to be removed to prevent site burns when using electrosurgery. Perceptual difficulty, such as vision or hearing impairment, will guide the nurse in adapting communication techniques to individual needs. An altered level of consciousness necessitates increased safety and protection techniques.

Communicating identified sources of pain to other health team members prevents subjecting the patient to unnecessary discomfort.

Transferring the Patient

Before transferring the patient into the scheduled OT, the nurse spends significant time preparing the room to ensure privacy, safety, and prevention of infection. Surgical attire (pants and shirts, masks, protective eyewear, and caps or hoods) is worn by all persons entering the OT suite. All electrical and mechanical equipment is checked for proper functioning. Aseptic technique is practiced as each surgical item is opened and placed systematically on the instrument table. Sponges, needles, and instruments are counted to ensure accurate retrieval at the close of the procedure.

During room preparation and during the procedure the functions of the team members are delineated. The scrub person will scrub hands and arms, don sterile gown and gloves, and touch only those items in the sterile field. The circulating nurse remains in the unsterile field and implements those activities that permit touching all unsterile items and the patient. Every person on the surgical team must share the responsibility for monitoring aseptic practice and initiating corrective action when a sterile field is compromised.

Once the patient has been properly identified and the OT has been adequately prepared, the patient is transported into the room for the surgery. Each time a patient is transferred from one bed to another, the wheels of the stretcher should be locked, and a sufficient number of personnel should be available to lift, guide, and prevent accidental falling. Once the patient is on the OT bed, safety straps should be snugly placed across the patients thighs. At this time the monitor leads (e.g., ECG leads), blood pressure cuff, and pulse oximeter are usually applied and an IV catheter is inserted if it was not in place when the patient arrived from the holding area.

Scrubbing, Gowning and Gloving

Surgical hand antiseptics is required of all sterile members of the surgical team (scrub assistant, surgeon, and assistant). This is done to eliminate dirt, skin oil, and transient microorganisms, to decrease the microbial count as much as possible; and to inhibit rapid rebound growth of microorganisms. The agent used for antisepsis should be an effective antimicrobial agent. It should significantly reduce microorganisms on the skin; contain a nonirritating; antimicrobial preparation; be broad spectrum and fast acting; and have a persistent effect. The procedure should be standardized for all personnel. When the procedure of scrubbing is the chosen method for surgical hand antisepsis, the team members fingers and hands should be scrubbed first with progression to the forearms and elbows. The hands should be held away from surgical attire and higher than the elbows at all times to prevent contamination from clothing or detergent suds and water from draining from the unclean area above the elbows to the clean and previously scrubbed areas of the hands and fingers. Waterless, alcohol-based agents are replacing traditional soap and water in many facilities. When a waterless hand rub product is chosen, the team member should first wash and dry hands and forearms with soap and water.

Once surgical hand antisepsis is completed, the team members enter the OT to put the surgical gowns and gloves. Because the gowns and gloves are sterile, it is permissible for the scrubbed people to manipulate and organize all sterile items for use during the procedure.

Basic Aseptic Technique

To prevent infections, aseptic technique is practiced in the OT. This is implemented through the creation and maintenance of a sterile field. The center of the sterile field is the site of the surgical incision.

There are specific principles that the team members should understand to practice aseptic technique. Unless these principles are followed, the safety of the patient is compromised, and the potential for postoperative infection is increased. It presents basic principles of aseptic technique.

- All materials that enter the sterile field must be sterile
- If a sterile item comes in contact with an unsterile item, it is contaminated.
- Contaminated items should be removed immediately from the sterile field.
- Sterile team members must wear only sterile gowns and gloves; once dressed for the procedure, they should recognize that the only parts of the gown considered sterile are the front from chest to table level and the sleeves to 2 inches above the elbow.
- A wide margin of safety must be maintained between the sterile and unsterile fields.
- Tables are considered sterile only at tabletop level; items extending beneath this level are considered contaminated.
- The edges of a sterile package are considered contaminated once the package has been opened.
- Bacteria travel on airborne particles and will enter the sterile field with excessive air movements and currents.
- Bacteria travel by capillary action through moist fabrics and contamination occurs
- Bacteria harbor on the patients and the team members hair, skin, and respiratory tracts and must be confined by appropriate attire.

In addition to following the principles of aseptic technique, the surgical team is responsible for following the guidelines to protect the patient and the team from exposure to blood-borne pathogens. These guidelines emphasize standard and transmission-based precautions; engineering and work practice controls; and the use of personal protective equipment such as gloves, gowns, aprons, caps, face shields, masks, and protective eyewear. This is especially important in the OT environment because of the high potential for exposure to blood born pathogens.

Assisting the Anesthesia Care Provider

While the perioperative nurse checks the OT to complete its preparation, the anesthesia care provider (ACP) prepares the patient for the administration of the anesthetic. The nurse must understand the mechanism of anesthetic administration and the pharmacologic effects of the agents. The nurse should know the location of all emergency drugs and equipment in the OT area.

The circulating nonsterile perioperative nurse may be involved in placing monitoring devices to be used during the surgical procedure (e.g. urinary catheter, ECG leads). If the patient is to have a general anesthetic, the nurse remains at the patient's side to ensure safety and to assist the ACP. These responsibilities may include obtaining blood pressure measurements and assisting in the maintenance of the patient's airway. During the surgical procedure, the circulating nonsterile perioperative nurse also provides a vital communication link for the ACP to ancillary departments such as the laboratory or blood bank.

Maintenance of Safety

All surgical procedures, regardless of where they take place, can put the patient at risk for injury. These injuries can be infections, physical trauma from positioning or equipment used, or physiologic effects of surgery itself. The perioperative nurse must be alert to all safety issues as the patient in the OT is often compromised from the effects of anesthesia. Smoke particles produced during laser procedures may contain trace hydrocarbons, including acetone, isopropanol, toluene, formaldehyde, and cyanide. These airborne contaminates can cause respiratory irritation and have mutagenic and carcinogenic potential. Smoke evacuators may be used to minimize this exposure. Care must be taken with correct placement of the grounding pad and all aspects of the electrosurgical equipment to prevent injury from burns of fire. All members of the surgical team stop what they are doing during a *surgical time-out* just before the procedure is started to verify patient identification, surgical procedure, and surgical site.

Positioning the Patient

Positioning the patient is a critical part of every procedure and usually follows administration of the anesthetic. The ACP will indicate when to begin the positioning. The position of the patient should allow for accessibility to the operative site, administration and monitoring of anesthetic agents, and maintenance of the patients airway. When positioning for the surgical procedure, care must be used to (1) provide correct skeletal alignment; (2) prevent undue pressure on nerves; (3) provide for adequate thoracic excursion; (4) prevent occlusion of arteries and veins; (5) provide modesty in exposure; and (6) recognize and respect individual needs such as previously assessed aches, pains, or deformities. It is a nursing responsibility to secure the extremities, provide adequate padding and support, and obtain sufficient physical or mechanical help to avoid unnecessary straining of self or patient.

Various positions in which the patient may be placed include supine, prone, Trendelenburg, lateral, kidney, lithotomy, jackknife, and sitting. The supine is the most common used. It is suited for surgery involving the abdomen, heart, and breast. The prone position allows easy access for back surgeries (e.g., laminectomies). The lithotomy position is used for some types of pelvic organ surgery (e.g., vaginal hysterectomy).

Whatever position is required for the procedure, great care is taken to prevent injury to the patient. Because anesthesia has blocked the nerve impulses, the patient will not feel pain or discomfort, or stress being placed on the nerves, muscles, bones, and skin. Improper positioning could potentially result in muscle strain, joint damage, pressure ulcers, nerve damage, and other untoward effects.

General anesthesia causes peripheral vessels to dilate. Position changes affect where the pooling of blood occurs. If the head of the OT bed is raised, the lower torso will have increased blood volume and the upper torso may become compromised. Hypovolemia and cardiovascular disease can further compromise the patient's status. Consequently the perioperative nurse, working with the entire surgical team, carefully plans and implements the patients positioning, and then closely monitors the patient throughout the surgical procedure.

Preparing the Surgical Site

The purpose of skin preparation, or "prepping", is to reduce the number of organisms available to migrate to the surgical wound. The task of prepping is usually the responsibility of the circulating nurse.

The skin is prepared by mechanically scrubbing or cleansing around the surgical site with antimicrobial agents identified as being nonallergic to the patient. Hair that will interfere with the surgical procedure is removed. The area is then scrubbed in a circular motion. The principle of scrubbing from the clean area (site of the incision) to the dirty area (periphery) is observed at all times. A liberal area is cleansed to allow for added protection and unexpected occurrences during the procedure.

Patient After Surgery

Through constant observation of the surgical progress, the ACP anticipates the end of the surgical procedure and uses appropriate types and doses of anesthetic agents so that their effects will be minimal at the end of the surgical procedure. This also allows greater physiologic control of the patient during the transfer to the post anesthesia care unit (PACU) or postoperative care unit (POCU). The patient's response to nursing care is evaluated by the OR nurse based on outcome criteria established during the development of the patients plan of care. The ACP and the perioperative nurse or another member of the surgical team accompany the patient to the PACU. A report of the patient's status and the procedure is communicated to the nurse receiving the patient in the PACU to promote safe, continuing care.

Anesthesia Administration

Anesthesia means the absence of pain (Greek: an=without + aisthesis = feeling). Anaesthesia is an artificially-induced state of partial or total loss of sensation, with or without loss of consciousness. Anesthesia produces muscle relaxation, blocks transmission of nerve impulses and suppresses reflexes.

There are two types of anesthesia, i.e., general and regional anesthesia.

General Anesthesia

General anesthesia is a drug induced depression of the central nervous system (CNS) that is reverted either by metabolic elimination in the body or by pharmocologic means. General anesthetic agents produces analgesia, amnesia and unconsciousness, characterized by loss of reflexes and muscle tone.

There are four stages of anesthesia. Brief explanation and nursing intervention in these stages are as follows:

Onset: Starts from anaesthetic administration to loss of consciousness. In this stage, client may be drowsy or dizzy and may experience auditory or visual hallucinations. Nursing action in this stage will include, close operating room doors, keeping room quiet, and standby to assist client.

Excitement: Starts from loss of consciousness to loss of eyelid reflexes. Here there will be increase in automatic activity, irregular breathing, client may struggle. In this stage, nurse has to remain, quitely at client's side, assist anaesthetists if needed.

Surgical anesthesia: This stage starts with loss of eyelid reflexes, to lose of motor reflexes and depression of vital function. Here client is unconscious, muscles are relaxed and no blink or gag reflexes. In this stage, begin preparation (if indicated) only when anaesthetists indicate stage III has been reached and client is under good control.

Danger (death) stage experiences: Vital functions too depressed may lead to respiratory and circulatory failure. In this stage, client is not breathing and he may or may not have a heartbeat. If arrest occurs, nurse responds immediately to assist establishing airway, provide cardiac arrest tray, drugs, syringes, long needles, assist surgeon with closed or open cardiac massage.

General anesthesia can be administered by inhalation or intravenously. An inhalation agent will include nitrous oxide, halothene (fluothene) enflurane (ethrane) and isofluorane (porane) and the intravenous drugs are thiopental sodium (penthathol), fentanyl citratedroperidol (innovar) and ketamine hydrochloride. The selections of anaesthetic agents are according to decision of the anesthesiologist. But continuous monitoring of side effects of the drugs, vital signs are essential.

Regional Anesthesia

Regional anesthesia blocks the pain stimulus at the origin and along afferent neurons of along the spinal cord. Regional anesthesia produces a loss of painful sensation in only one region of the body and does not result in unconsciousness. The client may receive sedative that produces drowsiness. The Regional anesthetic agents block the conduction of impulses in nerve fiber without depolarizing the cell membrane are: Local agents and topical agents. An example of local agents are Bupivacaine HCl (Marcaine HCl) (xylocaine) and examples of topical agents will include benzocaine, ethylchloride spray, tetracain HCl. All these agents have their own side effects. Contraindication for children, test dose can be given prior to use of these agents to know any allergies to these agents.

The types of regional anesthesia are:
- Topical anesthesia
- Local infiltration anesthesia
- Field block anesthesia
- Peripheral nerve block anesthesia
- Spinal anesthesia
- Epidural anesthesia
- Caudal anesthesia.

The other types of anesthesia are used in modern drugs acupuncture, cryothermia and hypnoanesthesia. The type of anesthesia chosen depends on the surgery performed and level of unconscious desired.

Nursing care during surgery will include providing emotional care, assessing the client with positioning (as required for type of surgery) maintaining safety, maintaining surgical asepsis, prevent client heat loss, monitoring malignant hyperthermia, assisting with surgeon to perform surgery by providing proper equipments and supplies, assisting with wound closure, assessing drainage, and transferring client to recovery room.

Anesthetists and anesthesiologists use the Physical (P) Status classification system to describe the patients general status and identify potential risks surgery. There are six classes of physical status.

- P1. A normal healthy patient.
  Example: No systemic abnormality, localized infection without fever, benign tumor, hernia
- P2. A patient with mild systemic disease, without functional limitations.
  Example: Well-controlled hypertension, well-controlled diabetes mellitus, chronic bronchitis, obesity, age over 80 years
- P3. A patient with severe systemic disease associated with functional limitations.
  Example: Severe disease, compensated heart failure, myocardial infraction more than 6 months ago, angina pectoris, severe dysrhythmia, cirrhosis, poorly controlled diabetes or hypertension, ileus
- P4. A patient with an incapacitating systemic disease that is a constant threat to life.
  Example: Sever heart failure, myocardial infarction less than 6 months ago, severe respiratory failure, advanced liver or renal failure.
- P5. A moribund patient who is not expected to survive for 24 hours with or without operation.
  Example: Unconscious patient with traumatic head injury and agonal respirations.
- P6. Patient is brain dead and is being prepared as an organ donor.

Surgical Asepsis Maintenance

Surgical asepsis prevents the contamination of surgical wounds. The patients natural skin flora or a previously existing infection may cause postoperative wound infection. Rigorous adherence to the principles of surgical asepsis by OT personnel is basic to preventing surgical site infections. All surgical supplies, instruments, needles, sutures, dressings, gloves, covers and solutions that may come in contact with the surgical wound or exposed tissues must be sterilized before use. Traditionally, the surgeon, surgical assistants, and nurses prepared themselves by scrubbing their hands and arms with antiseptic soap and water, but this traditional practice is being challenged by research investigating the optimal length of time of scrub and the best preparation to use. In some institutions, an alcohol based product or scrubless soap is used to prepare for surgery.

Surgical team members wear long-sleeved, sterile gowns and gloves. Head and hair are covered with a cap, and a mask is worn over the nose and mouth to minimize the possibility that bacteria from the upper respiratory tract will enter the wound. During surgery, only personnel who have scrubbed, gloved, and gowned touch sterilized objects. Nonscrubbed personnel refrain from touching or contaminating anything sterile. An area of the patients skin considerably larger than that requiring exposure during the surgery is meticulously cleansed, and an antiseptic solution is applied. If hair needs to be removed, this is done immediately before the procedure to minimize the risk of wound infection. The remainder of the patient's body is covered with sterile drapes.

In addition to the protocols described previously, surgical asepsis requires meticulous cleaning and maintenance of the OT environment. Floors and horizontal surfaces are cleaned frequently with detergent, soap, and water or a detergent germicide. Sterilizing equipment is inspected regularly to ensure optimal operation and performance. All equipment that comes into direct contact with the patient must be sterile. Sterilized linens, drapes, and solutions are used. Instruments are cleaned and sterilized in a unit near the OT. Individually wrapped sterile items are used when additional individual items are needed.

To decrease the amount of bacteria in the air, standard OT ventilation provides 15 air exchanges per hour, at least 3 of which are fresh air. A temperature of 20° to 24° C (68° to 73°F), humidity between 30 to 60%, and positive pressure relative to adjacent areas are maintained. Staff members shed skin scales, resulting in about 1000 bacteria-carrying particles (or colony-forming units [CFUs]) per cubic foot per minute. With the standard air exchanges, air counts of bacteria are reduced to 50 to 150 CFUs per cubic foot per minute. Systems with high-efficiency particulate air (HEPA) filters are needed to remove particles larger than 0.3 µm. Unnecessary personnel and physical movement may be restricted to minimize bacteria in the air and achieve an OT infection rate no greater than 3 to 5% in clean, infection-prone surgery. Some OTs have laminar airflow units. These units provide 400 to 500 air exchanges per hour. When used appropriately, laminar airflow units result in fewer than 10 CFUs per cubic foot per minute during surgery. The goal for a laminar airflow-equipped OT is an infection rate of less than 1%. An OR equipped with this unit is frequently used for total joint replacement or organ transplant surgery.

Despite these precautions, wound contamination may occur during surgery but may only become apparent days or weeks later in the form of a surgical site infection that results in a longer hospital stay. Constant surveillance and conscientious technique in carrying out aseptic practices are necessary to reduce the risk of contamination and infection.

All practitioners involved in the intraoperative phase have a responsibility to provide and maintain a safe environment. Adherence to aseptic practice is part of this responsibility. The basic principles of aseptic technique follow:

- All materials in contact with the surgical wound or used within the sterile field must be sterile. Sterile surfaces or articles may touch other sterile surfaces or articles

and remain sterile; contact with unsterile objects at any point renders a sterile area contaminated.
- Gowns of the surgical team are considered sterile in front from the chest to the level of the sterile field. The sleeves are also considered sterile from 2 inches above the elbow to the stockinette cuff.
- Sterile drapes are used to create a sterile field. Only the top surface of a draped table is considered sterile. During draping of a table or patient, the sterile drape is held well above the surface to be covered and is positioned from front to back.
- Items are dispensed to a sterile field by methods that preserve the sterility of the items and the integrity of the sterile field. After a sterile package is opened, the edges are considered unsterile. Sterile supplies, including solutions, are delivered to a sterile field or handed to a scrubbed person in such a way that the sterility of the object or fluid remains intact.
- The movements of the surgical team are from sterile to sterile and from unsterile to unsterile areas. Scrubbed persons and sterile items contact only unsterile items contact only unsterile areas.
- Movement around a sterile field must not cause contamination of the field. Sterile areas must be kept in view during movement around the area. At least a 1-foot distance from the sterile field must be maintained to prevent inadvertent contamination.
- Whenever a sterile barrier is breached, the area must be considered contaminated. A tear or puncture of the drape permitting access to an unsterile surface underneath renders the area unsterile. Such a drape must be replaced.
- Every sterile field is constantly monitored and maintained. Items of doubtful sterility are considered unsterile. Sterile fields are prepared as close as possible to the time of use
- The routine administration of hyperoxia (high levels of oxygen) is not recommended to reduce surgical site infections. In a study of 165 patients undergoing general surgery, the rate of surgical site infection was higher in patients who received 80% oxygen during surgery than in those who received 35% oxygen.

Nursing Intervention of Intraoperative Patient

Nursing assessment of the intraoperative patient involves obtaining data from the patient and the patients record to identify variables that can affect care and serve as guidelines for developing an individualized plan of patient care. The intraoperative nurse uses the focused preoperative nursing assessment documented on the patient record. This includes assessment of physiologic status (e.g., health-illness level, level of consciousness), psychological status (e.g., anxiety level, verbal communication problems, coping mechanisms), and physical status (e.g. surgical site, skin condition, and effectiveness of preparation; immobile joints), and ethical concerns.

Based on the assessment data, some major nursing diagnoses may include the following:
- Anxiety related to expressed concerns due to surgery or OR environment.
- Risk for perioperative positioning injury related to positioning in the OR (Operating Room).
- Risk for injury related to anesthesia and surgery.
- Disturbed sensory perception (global) related to general anesthesia or sedation.

Based on the assessment data, potential complications may include the following:
- Nausea and vomiting.
- Anaphylaxis.
- Hypoxia.
- Unintentional hypothermia.
- Malignant hyperthermia.
- DIC.
- Infection.

Goals for care of the patient during surgery include reducing anxiety, preventing positioning injuries, maintaining safety, maintaining the patients dignity and avoiding complications. To achieve goals of care following nursing intervention are performed.

Reducing Anxiety

The OT environment can seem cold, stark, and frightening to the patient, who may be feeling isolated and apprehensive. Introducing yourself, addressing the patient by name warmly and frequently, verifying details, providing explanations, and encouraging and answering questions provide a sense of professionalism and friendliness that can help the patient feel secure. When discussing what the patient can expect in surgery, the nurse uses basic communication skills, such as touch and eye contact, to reduce anxiety.

Attention to physical comfort (warm blankets, position changes) helps the patient feel more comfortable. Telling the patient who else will be present in the OR, how long the procedure is expected to take, and other details helps the patient prepare for the experience and gain a sense of control.

Preventing Intraoperative Positioning Injury

The patient's position on the operating table depends on the surgical procedure to be performed as well as on the patients physical condition. The potential for transient discomfort or permanent injury is present, because many positions are awkward. Hyperextending joints, compressing arteries, or pressing on nerves and bony prominences usually results in discomfort simply because the position must be sustained for a long period of time. Factors to consider include the following:

- The patient should be in as comfortable a position as possible, whether conscious or unconscious.
- The operative field must be adequately exposed.
- An awkward position, undue pressure on a body part, or use of stirrups or traction should not obstruct the vascular supply.
- Respiration should not be impeded by pressure of arms on the chest or by a gown that constricts the neck or chest.
- Nerves must be protected from undue pressure. Improper positioning of the arms, hands, legs, or feet can cause serious injury or paralysis. Shoulder braces must be well padded to prevent irreparable nerve injury, especially when the Trendelenburg position is necessary.
- Precautions for patient safety must be observed, particularly with thin, elderly, or obese patients and those with a physical deformity.
- The patient may need light restraint before induction in case of excitement.

The usual position for surgery, called the dorsal recumbent position, is flat on the back. One arm is positioned at the side of the table, with the hand placed palm down; the other is carefully positioned on an armboard to facilitate IV infusion of fluids, blood, or medications. This position is used for most abdominal surgeries except for surgery of the gallbladder or pelvis.

The Trendelenburg position usually is used for surgery on the lower abdomen and pelvis to obtain good exposure by displacing the intestines into the upper abdomen. In this position, the head and body are lowered. The patient is held in position by padded shoulder braces.

The lithotomy position is used for nearly all perineal, rectal, and vaginal surgical procedures. The patient is positioned on the back with the legs and thighs flexed. The position is maintained by placing the feet in stirrups.

The Sims or lateral position is used for renal surgery. The patient on the nonoperative side with an air pillow 12.5 to 15 cm (5 to 6 inches) thick under the loin, or on a table with a kidney or back lift.

Other procedures, such as neurosurgery or abdoino-thoracic surgery, may require unique positioning and supplemental apparatus, depending on the operative approach.

Protecting the Patient From Injury

A variety of activities are used to address the diverse patient safety issues that arise in the OR. The nurse protects the patient from injury by providing a safe environment. Verifying information, checking the chart for completeness, and maintaining surgical asepsis and an optimal environment are critical nursing responsibilities. Verifying that all required documentation is completed is one of the first functions of the intraoperative nurse. The patient is identified, and the planned surgical procedure, correct surgical site, and type of anesthesia are verified. It is important to review the patients record for the following:

- Correct informed surgical consent, with patients signature.
- Completed records for health history and physical examination.
- Results of diagnostic studies.
- Allergies (including latex).

In addition to checking that all necessary patient data are complete, the perioperative nurse obtains the necessary equipment specific to the procedure. The need for nonroutine medications, blood components, instruments, and other equipment and supplies is assessed, and the readiness of the room, completeness of physical setup and completeness of instrument, suture and dressing setups are determined. Any aspects of the OT environment that may negatively affect the patient are identified. These include physical features, such as room temperature and humidity; electrical hazards; potential contaminants (dust, blood, and discharge on floor or surfaces, uncovered hair, faculty attire of personnel, jewelry worn by personnel); and unnecessary traffic. The circulating nurse also sets up and maintains suction equipment in working order, sets up invasive monitoring equipment, assists with insertion of vascular access and monitoring devices (arterial, Swan-Granz, central venous pressure, IV lines), and initiates appropriate physical comfort measures for the patient.

Preventing physical injury includes using safety straps and side rails and not leaving the sedated patient unattended. Transferring the patient from the stretcher to the OR table requires safe transferring practices. Other safety measures include properly positioning the grounding pad under the patient to prevent electrical burns and shock, removing excess antiseptic solution from the patient's skin, and promptly and completely draping exposed areas after the sterile field has been created to decrease the risk for hypothermia.

Nursing measures to prevent injury from excessive blood loss include blood conservation using equipment such as a cell-saver (a device for recirculating the patients own blood cells) and administration of blood products. Few patients undergoing an elective procedure require blood transfusion, but those undergoing higher-risk procedures (such as orthopedic or cardiac surgeries) may require an intraoperative transfusion. The circulating nurse anticipates this need, checks that blood has been cross matched and held in reserve, and is prepared to administer blood.

Serving as Patient Advocate

Because the patient undergoing general anesthesia or moderate sedation experiences temporary sensory/perceptual alteration or loss, he or she has an increased need for protection and advocacy. Patient advocacy in the OR entails maintaining the patients physical and emotional comfort, privacy, rights, and dignity. Patients, whether conscious or unconscious, should not be subjected to excess noise, inappropriate conversation, or, most of all, derogatory comments. As surprising as this sounds, banter in the OR occasionally includes jokes about the patients physical appearance, job, personal history, and so forth. Cases have been reported in which seemingly deeply anesthetized patients recalled the entire surgical experience, including disparaging personal remarks made by OR personnel. As an advocate, the nurse never engages in this conversation and discourages others from doing so. Other advocacy activities include minimizing the clinical, dehumanizing aspects of being a surgical patient by making sure the patient is treated as a person, respecting cultural and spiritual values, providing physical privacy, and maintaining confidentiality.

Monitoring and Managing Potential Complications

It is the responsibility of the surgeon an the anesthesiologist or anesthetist to monitor and manage complications. However intraoperative nurses also play an important role. Being alert to and reporting changes in vital signs and symptoms of nausea and vomiting, anaphylaxis, hypoxia, hypothermia, malignant hyperthermia, or DIC and assisting with their management are important nursing functions. Each of these complication was discussed earlier. Maintaining asepsis and preventing infection are responsibilities of all members of the surgical team.

Expected patient outcomes may include the following:
- Exhibits low level of anxiety while awake during the intraoperative phase of care
- Remains free of perioperative positioning injury
- Experiences no unexpected threats to safety
- Has dignity preserved throughout OR experience
- Is free of complications (nausea and vomiting, anaphylaxis, hypoxia, hypothermia, malignant hyperthermia, or DIC) or experiences successful management of adverse effects of surgery and anesthesia should they occur.

POSTOPERATIVE CARE

The postoperative phase of surgery is final phase of the surgical experience. Nursing plays a critical role in returning the client to an optimal level of functioning. The postoperative period can be divided into two phases, i.e. immediate postanesthesia and postoperative period, and later in postoperative phase.

Immediate Postoperative Phase

Immediate postoperative phase is the first few hours after surgery when the client is recovering from the effect of anesthesia. Here the nurse has to keep all emergency equipment and drugs, etc. for the use of patient's recovery from anesthesia and on admission to postoperative unit, the nurse performs the following:
- Assess airway patency and support as needed, cramp, strider, wheezes or decreased breath sounds.
- Applies humidified oxygen via nasal cannula or facemask (unless otherwise ordered).
- Records vital signs (blood pressure, heart rate, strength and regularity, respiratory rate and depth, oxygen saturation, skin color, and temperature).
- Assess the client's level of consciousness, muscle strength and ability to follow commands.
- Observe the client's IV infusions, dressings, drains and special equipment.
- Remain at the client's bedside, continuing close observations of the client's conditions.

After the client has been positioned safely and baseline vital signs status has been ascertained, the nurse receives verbal report regarding surgery in detail, i.e. type of surgery, time of incision, patient's condition during surgery, type of anesthesia, sedative, all untoward incident happened and everything about surgery and documents the reliable and retainable information for further care that follow surgeon's and anesthetist's instructions for patient's recovery.

It is very important that nursing intervention associated with immediate recovery (ABCs) are as follows:

Airway (A)

- Maintain Patency, keep head tilted up and back may position on side with the face down and neck slightly extended
- Note presence or absence of gag / swallowing reflex
- Suction until awake and alert
- Provide oxygen if necessary.

Breathing (B)

- Evaluate depth, rate, sounds, rhythm and chest movement
- Assess color of mucous membrane
- Place hand above nose to detect respirations if shallow
- Initiate coughing and deep breathing as soon as able to respond
- Chart time oxygen is discontinued.

Consciousness (C)

- Able to extubate airway
- Responds to commands
- Verbalizes responses
- Reacts to stimuli.

Circulation (C)

- Monitor IPR every 15 minutes; to take axillary or rectal temperature, if necessary

- Assess rate, rhythm, quality of pulse
- Evaluate color and warmth of skin and nailbeds
- Check peripheral pulse if indicated
- Monitor IVS solution, rate, site.

System Review (S)

- Assess neurological functions
- Monitor drains, tubes, color and amount of output
- Evaluate pain response, may need to give analgesics
- Observe for allergic reactions
- Assess urinary output, if Foley's catheter is in place.

For remaining postoperative period, nurse has to take following measures (**Table 14.2**):
- Continuous assessment of respiratory and circulatory assessment
- Ensure optimal respiratory function –deep breath and coughing exercises
- Relieving postoperative discomforts by relieving pain, restlessness nausea and vomiting, abdominal distention, hiccups, etc.
- Maintaining normal body temperature
- Avoid injury by providing proper positioning in bed
- Maintaining normal nutritional status by IV fluids, total parenteral nutrition
- Promoting normal urinary functions
- Promoting bowel elimination – preventing paralytic ileus, and constipation
- Restoring mobility by proper positioning
- Early ambulation – bed exercises
- Prevent and treatment of complication like shock, hemorrhage, deep venous thrombosis (DVT), pulmonary embolism, respiratory complication like undetected hypoxemia, atelectasis, bronchitis, bronchopneumonia and lobar pneumonia, hypostatic pulmonary congestion, pleuracy, etc. and gastric complication like nutritional anemia, intestinal
  - obstruction and postoperative psychosis

Potential Postoperative Problems and its Management

Respiratory Problems and their Management

In the immediate postanesthetic period, the most common causes of airway compromise include obstruction, hypoxemia, and hypoventilation. Patients at risk include those who have had general anesthesia, are older, smoke heavily, have lung disease, are obese, or have undergone airway, thoracic, or abdominal surgery. However, respiratory problems may occur with any patient who has been anesthetized

Airway obstruction is most commonly caused by blockage of the airway by the patients tongue. The base of the tongue falls backward against the soft palate and occludes the pharynx. It is most pronounced in the supine position and in the patient who is extremely sleepy after surgery. Less common causes of airway obstruction include laryngospasm, retained secretions, and laryngeal edema.

Hypoxemia, specifically a partial pressure of arterial oxygen (PaO_2) of less than 60 mm Hg, is characterized by a variety of nonspecific clinical signs and symptoms, ranging from agitation to somnolence, hypertension to hypotension, and tachycardia to bradycardia. Pulse oximetry will indicate a low oxygen saturation (less than 90 to 92%). Arterial blood gas analysis should be used to confirm hypoxemia if the pulse oximetry indicates a low oxygen saturation.

The most common cause of postoperative hypoxemia is atelectasis. **Atelectasis** (alveolar collapse) may be the result of bronchial obstruction caused by retained secretions or decreased respiratory excursion. Atelectasis occurs when mucus blocks bronchioles or when the amount of alveolar surfactant (the substance that holds the alveoli open) is reduced. As air becomes trapped beyond the plug and is eventually absorbed, the alveoli collapse. Atelectasis may affect a portion or an entire lobe of the lungs. Hypotension and low cardiac output states can also contribute to the development of atelectasis.

Other causes of hypoxemia that may occur include pulmonary edema, aspiration, and bronchospasm. *Pulmonary edema* is caused by an accumulation of fluid in the alveoli and may be the result of fluid overload; left ventricular failure; or prolonged airway obstruction, sepsis, or aspiration. Pulmonary edema is characterized by hypoxemia, crackles on auscultation, decreased pulmonary compliance, and the presence of infiltrates on chest X-ray.

Aspiration of gastric contents into the lungs is a potentially serious airway emergency. Symptoms include bronchospasm, hypoxemia, atelectasis, interstitial edema, alveolar hemorrhage, and respiratory failure. Gastric aspiration may also cause laryngospasm, infection, and pulmonary edema. Because of the serious consequences of gastric aspiration, prevention, as opposed to treatment, is the goal.

Bronchospasm is the result o fan increase in bronchial smooth muscle tone with resultant closure of small airways. Airway edema develops, causing secretions to build up in the airway. The patient sured that these activities will not cause the incision to separate. Adequate hydration, either parenteral or oral, is essential to maintain the integrity of mucous membranes and to keep secretions thin and loose for easy expectoration.

Please refer **Table 14.2** for common immediate postoperative problem, and their mechanism, manifestation and nursing intervention.

Cardiovascular Problems and their Management

In the immediate postanesthetic period, the most common cardiovascular problems include hypotension,

Table 14.2: Common immediate postoperative respiratory complications care.

Complication and causes	Mechanisms	Manifestations	Nursing interventions
Airway obstruction			
Tongue falling back	Muscular flaccidity associated with ↓ consciousness and muscle relaxants	Use of accessory muscles Snoring respiration ↓ Air movement	Patient stimulation Jaw thrust Chin lift Artificial airway
Retained thick secretions	Secretion stimulation by anesthetic agents. Dehydration of secretions	Noisy respirations Coarse crackles	Suctioning Deep breathing and coughing IV hydration Chest physical therapy
Laryngospasm	Irritation from endotracheal tube or anesthetic gases. Most likely to occur after removal of endotracheal tube	Inspiratory stridor (crowing respiration) Sternal retraction Acute respiratory distress	O_2 Positive pressure ventilation IV muscle relaxant Lidocaine Corticosteroids
Laryngeal edema	Allergic drug reaction Mechanical irritation from intubation Fluid overload	Similar to laryngospasm	O_2 Antihistamines Corticosteroids Sedatives Possible intubation
Hypoxemia			
Atelectasis	Bronchial obstruction caused by secretions or ↓ lung volume	↓ Breath sounds ↓ O_2 saturation	Humidified O_2 Deep breathing Incentive spirometry Early mobilization
Pulmonary edema	↑ Hydrostatic pressure ↓ Interstitial pressure ↑ Capillary permeability	Crackles Infiltrates on chest X-ray Fluid overload ↓ O_2 saturation	O_2 therapy Diuretics Fluid restriction
Pulmonary embolism	Thrombus dislodged from peripheral venous system; lodged in pulmonary arterial system	Acute tachypnea Dyspnea Tachycardia Hypotension ↓ O_2 saturation	O_2 therapy Cardiopulmonary support Anticoagulant therapy
Aspiration	Inhalation of gastric contents	Wheezing Dyspnea Tachynea ↓ O_2 saturation	O_2 therapy Cardiac support Antibiotics
Bronchospasm	↑ Smooth muscle tone with closure of small airways	Wheezing Dyspnea - O_2 saturation	O_2 therapy Bronchodilators
Hyperventilation			
Depression of central respiratory drive	Medullary depression from anesthetics/opioids/sedatives	Shallow respirations ↓ Respiratory rate/apnea ↓ PaO_2 ↑ $PaCO_2$	Stimulation Reversal of opiodis/benzodiazepines Mechanical ventilation
Poor respiratory muscle tone	Neuromuscular blockade Neuromuscular disease	As above	Reversal of paralysis Mechanical ventilation
Mechanical restriction	Tight casts, dressings, positioning, and obesity preventing lung expansion	As above	Elevate head of bed Repositioning Loosen dressings
Pain	Shallow breathing to prevent incisional pain	As above Complaints of pain Guarding behavior	Opioid analgesic therapy in reduced dose

hypertension, and dysrhythmias. Patients at greatest risk for alterations in cardiovascular function include those with alterations in respiratory function, those with a history of cardiovascular disease, the elderly, the debilitated, and the critically ill.

Hypotension is evidenced by signs of hypoperfusion to the vital organs, especially the brain, heart, and kidneys. Clinical signs of disorientation, loss of consciousness, chest pain, oliguria, and anuria reflect hypoxemia and the loss of physiologic compensation. Intervention must be timely to prevent the devastating complications of cardiac ischemia or infarction, cerebral ischemia, renal ischemia, and bowel infarction.

The most common cause of hypotension in the POCU is unreplaced fluid and blood loss, which may lead to hypovolemic shock. Hemorrhage is always a risk of surgery, and marked blood loss is possible when cauterization or ligatures fail. Hemorrhage most often occurs internally, requiring assessment for changes in level of consciousness and vital signs. If changes are detected, treatment will be directed toward restoring circulating volume. If there is no response to fluid administration, cardiac dysfunction should be considered to be the cause of hypotension.

Primary cardiac dysfunction, as may occur in the case of myocardial infarction, cardiac tamponade, or pulmonary embolism, results in an acute fall in cardiac output. Secondary myocardial dysfunction occurs as a result of the negative chronotropic (rate of cardiac contraction) and negative inotropic (force of cardiac contraction) effects of drugs, such as β-adrenergic blockers, digoxin, or opioids. Other causes of hypotension include decreased systemic vascular resistance, dysrhythmias, and measurement errors that may occur if a blood pressure cuff is incorrectly sized.

Hypertension, a common finding in he POCU is most frequently the result of sympathetic nervous system stimulation that may be result of pain, anxiety, bladder distention, or respiratory compromise. Hypertension may also be the result of hypothermia and pre-existing hypertension. It may be seen after vascular and cardiac surgery as a result of revascularization.

In the POCU, *dysrhythmias* are often the result of an identifiable cause other than myocardial injury. The leading causes include hypokalemia, hypoxemia, hypercarbia, alterations in acidbase status, circulatory instability, and preexisting heart disease. Hypothermia, pain, surgical stress, and many anesthetic agents are also capable of causing dysrhythmias.

In the clinical unit, postoperative fluid and electrolyte imbalances are contributing factors to cardiovascular problems. Such imbalances may develop as a result of a combination of the body's normal response to the stress of surgery, excessive fluid losses, and improper IV fluid replacement. The body's fluid status directly affects cardiac output. Fluid retention during the first 2 to 5 postoperative days can be the result of the stress response. This response serves to maintain both blood volume and blood pressure. Fluid retention results from the secretion and release of two hormones by the pituitary—antidiuretic hormone (ADH) and adrenocorticotropic hormone (ACTH) and activation of the renin-angiotensin-aldosterone system. ADH release leads to increased water reabsorption and decreased urinary output, increasing blood volume. ACTH stimulates the adrenal cortex to secrete cortisol and, to a lesser degree, aldosterone. Fluid losses resulting from surgery decrease kidney perfusion, stimulating the renin-angiotensin-aldosterone system and causing marked release of aldosterone. Both of the mechanisms that increase aldosterone lead to significant sodium and fluid retention, increasing blood volume.

Fluid overload may occur during this period of fluid retention when IV fluids are administered too rapidly, when chronic (e.g., cardiac, renal) disease exists, or when the patient is an older adult. Conversely, fluid deficit may be related to slow or inadequate fluid replacement, which leads to decreases in cardiac output and tissue perfusion. Untreated preoperative dehydration or intraoperative or postoperative losses from vomiting, bleeding, wound drainage, or suctioning may be contributing factors to fluid deficits.

Hypokalemia can be a consequence of urinary and gastrointestinal (GI) tract losses, and it results when potassium is not replaced in IV fluids. Low serum potassium levels directly affect the contractility of the heart and thus may also contribute to decreases in cardiac output and in overall body tissue perfusion. Adequate replacement of potassium is usually 40 mEq/day. However potassium should not be given adequate renal function has been established. A urine output of at least 0.5 ml/kg/hr is generally considered indicative of adequate renal function.

Cardiovascular status is also affected by the state of tissue perfusion or blood flow. The stress response contributed to an increase in clotting tendencies in the postoperative patient by increasing platelet production. Deep vein thrombosis (DVT) may form in leg veins as a result of inactivity, body position, and pressure, all of which lead to venous stasis and decreased perfusion. DVT, especially common in the order adult, obese individual, and immobilized patient, is a potentially life-threatening complication because it may lead to pulmonary embolism. Patients with a history of DVT have a greater risk for pulmonary embolism. Pulmonary embolism should be suspected in any patient complaining of tachypnea, dyspnea, and tachycaradia, particularly when the patient is already receiving oxygen therapy. Other manifestations may include chest pain, hypotension, hemoptyis, dysrhythmias, and heart failure. Superficial thrombophlebitis is an uncomfortable but less ominous complication that may develop in a leg vein as a result of venous stasis or in the arm veins as a result of irritation from IV catheters or solutions. If a piece of a clot becomes dislodged and travels to the lung, it can cause a pulmonary infarction of a size proportionate to the vessel in which it lodges.

Nursing Management of Cardiovascular Problems

The most important aspect of the cardiovascular assessment is frequent monitoring of vital signs. They are usually monitored every 15 minutes in Phase I, or more often until stabilized, and then at less frequent intervals. Postoperative vital signs should be compared with preoperative and intraoperative readings to determine when the signs are stabilizing at a level that is normal for the patient's condition. The ACP or surgeon should be notified if the following occur:
- Systolic BP is less than 90 mm Hg or greater than 160 mm Hg.
- Pulse rate is less than 60 beats per minute or greater than 120 beats per minute.
- Pulse pressure (difference between systolic and diastolic pressures) narrows.
- BP gradually decreases during several consecutive readings.
- There is a change in cardiac rhythm.
- There is a significant variation from preoperative readings.

Cardiac monitoring is recommended for patients who have a history of cardiac disease and for all older adult patients who have undergone major surgery, regardless of whether they have cardiac problems. The apical-radial pulse should be assessed carefully, and any irregularities should be reported.

Assessment of skin color, temperature, and moisture provides valuable information in detecting cardiovascular problems. Hypotension accompanied by a normal pulse and warm, dry, pink skin usually represents the residual vasodilating effects of anesthesia and suggests only a need for continued observation. Hypotension accompanied by a rapid pulse and cold, clammy, pale skin may be caused by impending hypovolemic shock and requires immediate treatment.

Nursing diagnoses and collaborative problems related to potential cardiovascular problems for the postoperative patient include, but are not limited to, the following:
- Decreased cardiac output
- Deficient fluid volume
- Excess fluid volume
- Ineffective tissue perfusion
- Activity intolerance
- Potential complication: hypovolemic shock
- Potential complication: thromboembolism.

Nursing interventions in the POCU are designed to prevent and treat cardiovascular problems. Treatment of hypotension should always begin with oxygen therapy to promote oxygenation of hypoperfused organs. Volume status should be assessed as described, and errors of BP measurement should be ruled out. Because the most common cause of hypotension is fluid loss, IV fluid boluses will be given to normalize BP. Primary cardiac dysfunction may require drug intervention. Peripheral vasodilation and hypotension may require vasoconstrictive agents to normalize systemic vascular resistance.

Treatment of hypertension will center on addressing the cause of sympathetic nervous system stimulation and eliminating the precipitating cause. Treatment may include the use of analgesics, assistance in voiding, and correction of respiratory problems. Rewarming will correct hypothermia-induced hypertension. If the patient has preexisting hypertension or has undergone cardiac or vascular surgery, drug therapy designed to reduce BP will usually be required.

An accurate intake and output record should be kept during the postoperative period, and laboratory findings (e.g., electrolytes, hematocrit) should be monitored. Nursing responsibilities relating to IV management are critical during this period. In particular, the nurse should be alert for symptoms of too slow or too rapid a rate of fluid replacement. Assessment should also be made of the hazards associated with the IV administration of potassium, such as cardiac dysrhythmias and pain at the infusion site.

Leg exercises should be encouraged 10 to 12 times every 1 to 2 hours while awake. The muscular contraction produced by these exercises and by ambulation facilitates venous return from the lower extremities. When confined to bed, the patient should alternately flex and extend the legs. When the patient is sitting in a chair or lying in bed, there should be no pressure to impede venous flow through the popliteal space. Crossed legs, pillows behind the knees, and extreme elevation of the knee gatch of the bed must be avoided.

Early ambulation is the most significant general nursing measure to prevent postoperative complications. The exercise associated with walking (1) increases muscle tone; (2) improved GI and urinary tract function; (3) stimulates circulation, which prevents venous stasis and speeds wound healing; and (4) increases vital capacity and maintains normal respiratory function.

Currently the most effective means of preventing DVT and pulmonary emboli in surgical patients is use of subcutaneous heparin or low-molecular-weight heparin (LMWH) in combination with antiembolism stockings. One recent study indicated that the combination LMWH and thigh-length stockings was the best method to decrease the risk for developing a DVT.

The nurse may prevent syncope by making changes slowly in the patients position. Progression to ambulation can be achieved by first raising the head of the patients bed for 1 to 2 minutes and then by assisting the patient to sit on the side of the bed while monitoring the radial pulse for rate and quality. If no changes or complaints are noted, ambulation can be started. If faintness occurs, the nurse can help the patient sit on the edge of the bed while continuing of feeling faint during ambulation, the nurse should provide assistance to a nearby chair or ease the patient to the floor. The patient should remain in either location until recovery is evidenced by BP stability, and then be helped back to the bed. If faintness occurs, it is often frightening for the patient and for the unprepared nurse, but syncope poses no real physiologic danger, although injury can result from a fall.

Syncope (fainting) is another factor that reflects the cardiovascular status. It may indicate decreased cardiac output, fluid deficits, or defects in cerebral perfusion. Syncope frequently occurs as a result of postural hypotension when the patient ambulates. It is more common in the older adult or in the patient who has been immobile for long periods of time. Normally when the patient quickly moves to a standing position, the arterial press receptors respond to the accompanying fall in blood pressure with sympathetic nervous system stimulation, which produces vasoconstriction and thereby maintains blood pressure. These sympathetic and vasomotor functions may be diminished in the older adult and the immobile or postanesthetic patient.

Neurologic Problems

Postoperatively, emergence delirium is the neurologic **alteration** that causes the most concern. **Emergence** delirium, or *waking up wild*, can include behaviors such as restlessness, agitation, disorientation, thrashing, and shouting. This condition may be caused by anesthetic agents, hypoxia, bladder distention, pain, electrolyte abnormalities, or the patients state of anxiety preoperatively. Hypoxia should be suspected first.

Delayed emergence may also be a problem postoperatively. Fortunately, the most common cause of delayed emergence is prolonged drug action, particularly of opioids, sedatives, and inhalational anesthetics, as opposed to neurologic injury. Normal awakening can be predicted by the ACP based on the drugs used in surgery.

Two types of postoperative cognitive impairment are seen in surgical patients: delirium and postoperative cognitive dysfunction (POCD). POCD is almost exclusively seen in the older surgical patient. While postoperative confusion and delirium are also more commonly seen in the older patient, they may occur in patients of any age. Confusion or delirium may arise from a variety of psychologic and physiologic sources, including fluid and electrolyte imbalances, hypoxemia, drug effects, sleep deprivation, and sensory deprivation or overload.

Anxiety and depression may also occur in postoperative patients. Any patient may experience these responses as part of grieving for lost body parts or function or for decreased independence during the recovery and rehabilitation process. Radical surgeries leading to changes in body function or surgical findings that suggest a poor prognosis may cause more pronounced psychologic reactions.

Alcohol withdrawal delirium may also occur as a result of alcohol withdrawal in a postoperative patient. Alcohol withdrawal delirium is a reaction characterized by restlessness, insomnia and nightmares, irritability, and authority or visual hallucinations.

The nurses in the POCU, should assess the patients level of consciousness, orientation, and memory and his or her ability to follow commands should be assessed. The size, reactivity, and equality of the pupils should be determined. The patients sleep/wake cycle and sensory and motor status should also be assessed. If the neurologic status is altered, possible causes should be determined. If the patient was mentally alert before surgery and becomes cognitively impaired postoperatively, the nurse should suspect delirium.

Nursing diagnoses related to potential neurologic or psychologic problems for the postoperative patient include, but are not limited to, the following:
- Disturbed sensory perception
- Risk for injury
- Disturbed thought processes
- Impaired verbal communication
- Anxiety
- Ineffective coping
- Disturbed body image
- Fear.

The most common cause of postoperative agitation in the POCU is hypoxemia. As a result, attention must focus on evaluating respiratory function. Once hypoxemia has been ruled out as the cause of postoperative delirium and all potentially known causes have been addressed, sedation may prove beneficial in controlling the agitation and providing for patient and staff safety. Emergence delirium is usually time limited and will resolve before the patient is discharged from the POCU. Because the most common cause of delayed emergence is prolonged drug action, delays in awakening usually spontaneously resolve with time. If necessary, benzodiazepines and opioids may be pharmacologically reversed with antagonists.

Until the patient is awake and able to communicate effectively, it is the responsibility of the POCU nurse to act as a patient advocate and to maintain patient safety at all times. This includes having the side rails up, securing IV lines and artificial airways, verifying the presence of identification and allergy bands, and monitoring physiologic status.

To prevent or manage postoperative delirium, the nurse should address factors that are known to contribute to the condition. Maintenance of normal physiologic function is important and includes fluid and electrolyte balance, adequate nutrition, pain management, proper bowel and bladder function, an dearly mobilization. The nurse can also use environmental aids, such as clocks, calendars, and photographs, to help orient the patient.

The nurse should attempt to prevent psychologic problems in the postoperative period by providing adequate support for the patient. Supportive measures include taking time to listen to and talk with the patient, offering explanations and genuine reassurance, and encouraging the presence and assistance of significant others. The nurse must observe and evaluate the patients behavior to distinguish a normal reaction to the stress situation from one that becoming abnormal or excessive.

The nurse should discuss the patients expectations regarding activity and assistance needed following discharge. The patient must be included in discharge planning and should be provided with the information and support to make informed decisions about continuing care.

The recognition of alcohol withdrawal delirium in a patient not previously known to be an alcoholic presents a particular challenge. Any unusual or disturbed behavior should be reported immediately so that diagnosis and treatment may be instituted.

Pain and Discomfort and their Management

Despite the availability of analgesic drugs and pain-relieving techniques, pain remains a common problem and a significant fear for the patient in the POCU and during the postoperative period. Postoperative pain is caused by the interaction of a number of physiologic and psychologic factors. The skin and underlying tissues have been traumatized by the incision and retraction during surgery. In addition, there may be reflex muscle spasms around the incision. Anxiety and fear, sometimes related to the anticipation of pain, create tension and further increase muscle tone and spasm. Positioning during surgery or the use of internal devices such as an endotracheal tube or catheters may also result in pain. The effort and movement associated with deep breathing, coughing, and ambulating may aggravate pain by creating tension on the incision area. Pain can contribute to complications such as dysfunction of the immune system and blood clotting, and delayed return of normal gastric and bowel function. It also increases the risk of atelectasis and impaired respiratory function. When the internal viscera are cut, no pain is felt. However, pressure in the internal viscera elicits pain. Therefore deep visceral pain may signal the presence of a signal the presence of a complication such as intestinal distention, bleeding, or abscess formation.

The patients self report is the single most reliable indicator of pain. Since this is not always possible in the POCU, the patient should be observed for other indications of pain (e.g., restlessness, increased heart rate, diaphoresis). Identifying the location of the pain is important. Incisional pain is to be expected, but other causes of pain, such as a full bladder, may be present.

Nursing diagnoses for the patient experiencing pain and discomfort include, but are limited to the following:
- Acute pain
- Anxiety.

The most effective interventions for postoperative pain management include using a variety of analgesics. Intravenous opioids provide the most rapid relief. Drugs are administered slowly and titrated to allow for optimal pain management with minimal to no adverse drug side effects. More sustained relief may be obtained through the use of epidural catheters, patient controlled analgesia, or regional anesthetic blockade.

Postoperative pain relief is a nursing responsibility because the surgeons orders for analgesic medication and other comfort measures are usually written on an as-needed as basis. During the first 48 hours or longer, opioid analgesics (e.g., morphine) are required to relieve moderate to severe pain. After that time, nonopioid analgesics, such as nonsteroidal anti-inflammatory agents, may be sufficient as pain intensity decreases.

Analgesic administration should be timed to ensure that it is in effect during activities that may be painful for the patient, such as ambulating. Although opioid analgesics are often essential for the postoperative patients comfort, there are undesirable side effects. Side effects such as constipation, nausea and vomiting, respiratory and cough depression, and hypotension are most common with the opioids. Before administering any analgesic, the nurse should first assess the nature of the patients pain, including location, quality, and intensity. If it is incisional pain, analgesic administration is appropriate. If it is chest or leg pain, medication may simply mask a complication that must be reported and documented. If it is gas pain, opioids can aggravate it. The nurse should notify the physician and request a change in the order if the analgesic either fails to relieve the pain or makes the patient excessively lethargic or somnolent.

Patient-controlled analgesia (PCA) and epidural analgesia are two alternative approaches for pain control. The goals of PCA are to provide immediate analgesia and to maintain a constant, steady blood level of the analgesia agent. PCA involves self-administration of predetermined doses of analgesia by the patient. The route of delivery may be IV, oral, or epidural. Some advantages of PCA are early ambulation, improved wound healing, and earlier hospital discharge.

Epidural analgesia is the infusion of opioid analgesics through a catheter placed into the epidural space surrounding the spinal cord. The goal of epidural analgesia is delivery of medication directly to opiate receptors in the spinal cord. Administration methods include intermittent bolus dosing, continuous infusion, and patient-controlled epidural analgesia (PCEA). The overall effectiveness and the technique of administration result in a constant circulating level and a reduced total dose of medication. The use of epidural analgesia for postoperative pain is increasing based on research that has demonstrated superior pain relief and improved functional outcomes after major surgery in patients who receive epidural analgesia compared with patients receiving IV PCA.

The acute pain of surgery almost always requires the use of analgesics. However, nonpharmacologic approaches such as repositioning, massage, distraction, relaxation, and deep breathing can enhance pain management. Music and educational interventions have also been shown to be effective adjuncts to pain medication.

Alterations in Temperature and its Management

Hypothermia, a core temperature of less than 96.8°F (36°C), occurs when heat loss exceeds heat production. In addition to the usual heat loss mechanisms of radiation, convection, conduction, and evaporation, heat loss may occur in the perioperative setting because of infusion of cool IV fluids and ventilation with dry gases.

Although all patients are at risk for hypothermia, the older, debilitated, or intoxicated patient is at an increased risk. Long surgical procedures and prolonged anesthetic administration lead to redistribution of body heat from the core to the periphery. This places the patient at increased risk for hypothermia. Complications from hypothermia may include compromised immune function, postoperative pain, bleeding, myocardial ischemia, impaired wound healing, and delayed drug metabolism.

Another complication of hypothermia is shivering. Shivering can increase oxygen consumption, carbon oxide production, and cardiac output, as well as significantly affect the patient's comfort level.

Temperature variation in the postoperative period provides valuable information about the patient's status. Fever may occur at anytime during the postoperative period. A mild elevation (up to 100.4°F [38°C]) during the first 48 hours usually reflects the surgical stress response. A moderate elevation (higher than up to 100.4°F [38°C]) is caused more frequently by respiratory congestion or atelectasis and less frequently by dehydration. After the first 48 hours, a moderate to marked elevation (higher than 99.9°F [37.7°C]) is usually caused by infection.

Wound infection, particularly from aerobic organisms, is often accompanied by a fever that spikes in the afternoon or evening and returns to near-normal levels in the morning. The respiratory tract may be infected secondary to stasis of secretions in areas of atelectasis. The urinary tract may be infected secondary to catheterization. Superficial thromhbophlebitis in the leg veins may produce a temperature elevation between 7 and 10 days after surgery.

Nosocomial infectious diarrhea caused by *Clostridium difficile* may be signaled by fever, diarrhea, and abdominal pain. Surgical patients who receive antibiotics for a period of time are at risk.

Intermittent high fever accompanied by shaking chills and diaphoresis suggests septicemia. This may occur at any time during the postoperative period because microorganism may have been introduced into the blood stream during surgery, especially in GI or genitourinary (GU) procedures, or picked up later from the site of a wound or from a urinary tract or vein infection.

The nurses in POCU, should perform frequent assessment of the patient's temperature is important to detect patterns of hypothermia and/or fever that may be present in the postoperative period. Temperature may be taken orally, or via the tympanic membrane or axilla. The color and temperature of the skin should also be assessed. The nurse should observe the patient for early signs of inflammation and infection that may precede a fever so that any complications that arise may be treated in a timely manner.

Nursing diagnoses for the patient with an altered temperature include, but are not limited to, the following:
- Hyperthermia
- Hypothermia
- Risk for imbalanced body temperature.

The nursing intervention for altered temperature will include the following:

Passive rewarming in a patient with hypothermia (i.e., shivering) raises basal body metabolism. *Active rewarming* requires the application of external warming devices, including warm blankets, heated aerosols, radiant warmers, forced air warmers, and heated water mattresses. When using any external warming device, body temperature should be monitored at 15-minute intervals, and care should be taken to prevent skin injuries. In addition, oxygen therapy via nasal prongs or mask is used to treat the increased demand for oxygen accompanying the increase in body temperature. Shivering is usually quickly suppressed by opioids.

The nurse's role with respect to postoperative fever may be preventive, diagnostic, and therapeutic. The patient's temperature is usually measured every 4 hours for the first 48 hours postoperatively and then less frequently if no problems develop. Meticulous asepsis is maintained with regard to the wound and the IV site, and airway clearance is encouraged. If fever develops, chest X-rays may be taken, and depending on the suspected cause, cultures of the wound, urine, or blood are obtained. If infection is the source of the fever, antibiotics are started as soon as cultures have been obtained. If the fever rises above 103° F (39.4°C), antipyretic drugs and body-cooling measures may be employed.

Gastrointestinal Problems and their Management

Postoperative nausea and vomiting occur in 20 to 30% of adult patients. These problems are responsible for unanticipated hospital admission of day-surgery patients, increased patient discomfort, delays in discharge, and patient's dissatisfaction with the surgical experience. Numerous factors have been identified as contributing toe ht development of nausea and vomiting, including gender (female), history of motion sickness or previous postoperative nausea and vomiting, and action of anesthetics or opioids, as well as duration and type of surgery. Delayed gastric emptying and slowed peristalsis that result from handling of the bowel during abdominal surgery also contribute to nausea and vomiting, as does the assumption of oral intake too soon after surgery.

Abdominal distention is another common problem caused by decreased peristalsis as a result of handling of the intestine during surgery and limited dietary intake before and after surgery. Following abdominal surgery, motility in the large intestine may be reduced for 3 to 5 days, although motility in the small intestine resumes within 24 hours. Swallowed air and GI secretions may accumulate in the colon, producing distention and gas pains.

Hiccups (singultus) are intermittent spasms of the diaphragm caused by irritation of the phrenic nerve, which innervates the diaphragm. Postoperative sources of direct irritation of the phrenic nerve may be gastric distention, intestinal obstruction, intra-abdominal bleeding, and a subphrrenic abscess. Indirect irritation of the phrenic nerve may be produced by acid-base and electrolyte imbalances. Reflex irritation may come from drinking hot or cold liquids or from the presence of a nasogastric tube. Hiccups usually last a short time and subside spontaneously; occasionally they may be persistent, but they are rarely debilitating.

The nurses in POCU should perform following activations. The patient should be questioned about feelings of nausea. If vomiting occurs, it is important to determine the quantity, characteristics, and color of the vomitus. The abdomen should be assessed for distention and the presence of bowel sounds. Because bowel sounds are frequently absent or diminished in the immediate postoperative period, all four quadrants should be auscultated to determine the presence, frequency, and characteristics of the sounds. The return of normal bowel motility is usually accompanied by the passage of flatus in addition to normal bowel sounds and the absence of distention.

Nursing diagnoses for the patient experiencing GI problems include, but are not limited to, the following:
- Nausea.
- Risk for aspiration.
- Risk for deficient fluid volume.
- Imbalanced nutrition: less than body requirements.
- Potential complication: fluid and electrolyte imbalance.
- Potential complication: hiccups.

Postoperative nausea and nausea are treated with the use of antimetic or prokinetic drugs. Other methods of decreasing nausea and vomiting are being tested, such as giving carbohydrate-rich fluid to patients before laparoscopic cholecystectomy. In the POCU, oral fluids should be given only as indicated and tolerated. Intravenous fluids will provide hydration until the patient is able to tolerate oral fluids. Care should be also be taken to prevent aspiration if the patient vomits while still sleepy from anesthesia. Having suction equipment readily available at the bedside and turning the patients head to the side will help protect the patient from aspiration. Other nonpharmacologic nursing interventions that may be effective include biofeedback, hypnosis, relaxation, guided imagery, music therapy, distraction, and acupressure.

Depending on the nature of the surgery, the patient may resume oral intake as soon as the gag reflex returns. The patient who had abdominal surgery is usually allowed nothing by mouth (NPO) until the presence of bowel sounds indicates the return of peristalsis. When the patient is NPO, IV infusions are given to maintain fluid and electrolyte balance. A nasogastric tube may be used to decompress the stomach to prevent nausea, vomiting, and abdominal distention. Regular mouth care is essential for comfort and stimulation of salivary glands when the patient is NPO or has a nasogastric tube. When oral intake is allowed, clear liquids are offered first and the IV infusion is continued, usually at a reduced rate. If oral intake is well tolerated by the patient, the IV infusion is discontinued, and the diet is advanced until a regular diet is tolerated.

Abdominal distention may be prevented or minimized by early and frequent ambulation, which stimulates intestinal motility. The nurse should assess the patient regularly to detect the resumption of normal intestinal peristalsis as evidenced by the return of bowel sounds and the passage of flatus. The nasogastric tube must be clamped. Resumption of a normal diet after bowel sounds have returned will also enhance the return of normal peristalsis.

The patient may need to be encouraged to expel flatus and assured that expulsion is necessary and desirable. Gas pains, which tend to become pronounced on the second or third postoperative day, may be relieved by ambulation and frequent repositioning. Positioning the patient on the right side permits gas to rise along the transverse colon and facilitates its release. Bisacodyl (Dulcolax) suppositories may be ordered to stimulate colonic peristalsis and expulsion of flatus and feces.

Urinary Problems and their Management

Low urine output (800 to 1500 ml) in the first 24 hours after surgery may be expected, regardless of fluid intake. This low output is caused by increased aldosterone and ADH secretion resulting from the stress of surgery, fluid restriction before surgery, and fluid loss through surgery, drainage, and diaphoresis. By the second or third day, the patient will begin to have increasing urinary output after fluid has been mobilized and the immediate stress reaction subsides.

Acute urinary retention can occur in the postoperative period for a variety of reasons. Anesthesia depresses the nervous system, including the micturition reflex arc and the higher centers that influence it. This allows the bladder to fill more completely than normal before the urge to void is felt. Anesthesia also impedes voluntary micturition. Anticholinergic and opioid drugs may also interfere with the ability to initiate voiding or to empty the bladder completely.

Retention is more likely to occur after lower abdominal or pelvic surgery because spasms or guarding of the abdominal and pelvic muscles interferes with their normal function in micturition. Pain may alter perception and interfere with the patient's awareness of bladder filling. Voiding ability is probably impaired to the greatest extent by immobility and the recumbent position in bed. The supine position reduces the ability to relax the perineal muscles and external sphincter.

Oliguria (the diminished output of urine) can be a manifestation of renal failure and is a less common, although more serious, problem after surgery. It may result from renal ischemia caused by inadequate renal perfusion or altered cardiovascular function.

The nurses in the POCU should monitor the following:

The urine of the postoperative patient should be examined for both quantity and quality. The color, amount, consistency, and odor of the urine should be noted. Indwelling catheters should be assessed for patency, and urine output should be at least 0.5 ml/kg/hr. Most patients urinate within 6 to 8 hours after surgery. If no voiding occurs, the abdominal contour should be inspected and the bladder assessed for distention.

Nursing diagnoses and collaborative problems related to potential urinary problems for the postoperative patient include, but are not limited to, the following:
- Impaired urinary elimination
- Potential complication: acute urinary retention

The nurse may facilitate voiding by normal positioning of the patient – sitting for women and standing for men. Providing reassurance to the patient regarding the ability to void and the use of techniques such as providing privacy, running water, having the patient drink water, or pouring warm water over the perineum may also be of assistance. Ambulation, preferably to the bathroom, and the use of a bedside commode are additional helpful measures to assist in voiding.

The surgeon often leaves an order to catheterize the patient in 6 to 8 hours if voiding has not occurred. Because of the possibility of infection associated with catheterization, the nurse should first try other measures to induce voiding and validate that the bladder is actually full. In assessing the need for catheterization, the nurse should consider fluid intake during and after surgery and determine bladder fullness (e.g., palpable fullness above the symphysis pubis, discomfort when pressure is applied over the bladder, or the presence of the urge to void). Straight catheterization is preferred because of the possibility of infection associated with an indwelling catheter.

Integumentary Problems and their Management

Surgery generally involves an incision through the skin and underlying tissues. An incision disrupts the protective skin barrier. Therefore, wound healing is one of the major concerns during the postoperative period.

An adequate nutritional state is essential for wound healing. Amino acids are readily available for the healing process because of the catabolic effects of the stress-related hormones (e.g., cortisol). The patient who was well nourished preoperatively can tolerate the postoperative delay in nutritional deficits that occur with chronic disease (e.g., diabetes, ulcerative colitis, alcoholism) is more prone to problems of wound healing. Abdominal wound healing is affected by obesity. Wound healing is also a concern for the older adult. The patient who is unable to meet nutritional needs postoperatively may be provided with enteral nutrition or parenteral nutrition to promote healing.

Wound infection may result from contamination of the wound from three major sources: (1) exogenous flora present in the environment and on the skin. (2) oral floral, and (3) intestinal flora. The incidence of wound sepsis is higher in patients who are malnourished, immunosuppressed, or older, who have had a prolonged hospital stay or a lengthy surgical procedure (lasting more than 3 hours). Patients undergoing bowel surgery, particularly following a traumatic injury, are at particularly high risk. Infection may involve the entire incision and may extend downward through the deeper tissue layers. An abscess may form locally, or the infection may spread throughout entire body cavities, as in peritonitis. Evidence of wound infection usually does not become apparent before the third to the fifth postoperative day. Local manifestations include redness, swelling and increasing pain and tenderness at the site. Systemic manifestations are fever and leukocytosis.

An accumulation of fluid in a wound may create pressure, impair circulation and wound healing, and predispose to infection. For these reasons, the surgeon may place a drain in the incision or make a stab wound adjacent to the incision to allow for drainage. These drains may be firm catheters attached to a Hemovac or other source of gentle suction.

Nursing assessment of the wound and dressing requires knowledge of the type of wound, the drains inserted, and expected drainage related to the specific type of surgery. A small amount of serous drainage is common from any type of wound. If a drain is in place, a moderate to large amount of drainage may be expected. For example, an abdominal incision with an accompanying drain is expected to have a moderate amount of serosanguineous drainage in the first 24 hours. In contrast, an inguinal herniorrhaphy should have only minimal serous drainage during the postoperative period.

In general, drainage is expected to change from sanguineous (red) to serosanguineous (pink) to serous (clear yellow). The drainage output should decrease over hours or days, depending on the type of surgery. Wound infection may be accompanied by purulent ously joined wound edges) may be preceded by a sudden discharge of brown, pink, or clear drainage.

Nursing diagnoses related to surgical wounds of the postoperative patient include, but are not limited to, the following:
- Risk for infection
- Potential complication: impaired wound healing

When drainage occurs on the dressing, the type, amount, color, consistency, and odor of drainage should be noted and recorded. The effect of position changes on drainage should also be assessed. The surgeon should be notified of any excessive or abnormal drainage and significant changes in vital signs.

The incision may be covered with a dressing immediately after surgery. If there is no drainage after 24 to 48 hours, the dressing may be removed and the incision left open to the air. If the initial operative dressing is saturated, institutional policy determines whether the nurse may change the dressing or simply reinforce it.

When a dressing is changed, the number and type of drains present should be noted. Care should be taken to avoid dislodging drains during dressing removal. When the dressing is changed, the incision site should be examined carefully. The area around the sutures may be slightly reddened and swollen, which is an expected inflammatory response. However, skin around the incision should be of normal color and temperature. Clinical manifestations of infection include redness, swelling, pain, fever, and increased white blood cell count. If healing is by primary intention, little or no drainage is present, and no drains are in place, a single-layer dressing or no dressing is sufficient. When drains are in place, when moderate to heavy drainage is occurring, or when healing occurs other than by primary intention, a multiple-layer dressing is needed.

DISCHARGE FROM THE POCU

The choice of discharge site is based on patient acuity, access to follow-up care, and the potential for postoperative complications. The decision to discharge the patient from the POCU is based on written discharge criteria. Examples of discharge criteria are provided in as given below:

Postanesthesia Discharge Criteria (Phase I)

- Patient awake (or baseline)
- Vital signs stable
- No excess bleeding or drainage
- No respiratory depression
- Oxygen saturation >90%
- Report given.

Ambulatory Surgery Discharge Criteria (Phase II/III)

- All POCU discharge criteria met
- No IV opioid drugs for last 30 minutes
- Minimal nausea and vomiting
- Voided (if appropriate to surgical procedure/orders)
- Able to ambulate if age appropriate and not contraindicated
- Responsible adult present to accompany patient
- Discharge instructions given and understood.

Discharge to the Clinical Unit

Before discharging the patient from the POCU to the clinical unit, the POCU nurse provides a verbal report about the patient to the receiving nurse. The report summarizes the operative and postanesthetic period.

The nurse who receives the patient on the clinical unit assists POCU transport in transferring the patient from the POCU cart onto the bed. Care must be taken to protect IV lines, wound drains, dressings, and traction devices. The use of a draw sheet or transfer board and sufficient personnel facilitates transfer of the patient.

Vital signs should be obtained, and patient status should be compared with the report provided by the POCU. Documentation of the transfer is then completed, followed by a more in-depth assessment. Postoperative orders and appropriate nursing care are then initiated.

Nursing Assessment and Care of Patient on Admission to Clinical Unit

- Record time of patients return to unit.
- Take baseline vital signs.
- Assess pain and discomfort.
    - Note last dose and type of pain control.
    - Note current pain intensity.

- Assess airway and breath sounds.
- Assess neurologic status, including level of consciousness and movement of extremities.
- Assess wound, dressing, and drainage tubes:
  - Type and amount of drainage.
  - Connect tubing to gravity or suction drainage (per orders).
- Assess color and appearance of skin.
  - Time of voiding.
  - Presence of catheter, patency, and total output.
  - Bladder distention or urge to void.
- Assess urinary status.
- Position for airway maintenance, comfort, and safety (bed in low position, side rails up).
- Check IV infusion:
  - Type of solution
  - Amount of fluid remaining
  - Flow rate
  - Integrity of insertion site and size of catheter
- Attach call light within reach, and orient patient to use of call light.
- Ensure that emesis basin and tissues are available.
- Determine emotional condition and support.
- Check for presence of family member or significant other: Orient patient and family to immediate environment
- Check and carryout postoperative orders.

CHAPTER 15

Nursing Management of Disorders of Eye

INTRODUCTION

Person's orientation to the world is primarily visual. People will learn much about their environment and themselves through their eyes. Practically every behavior is affected by the visual sense.

Visual systems consist of the internal and external structures of the eyeball, the refractive media, and the visual pathways. The internal structures are the iris, lense, ciliary body, choroid and retina. The external structures are the eyebrows, eyelids, eyelashes, lacrimal system, conjunctiva, cornea, sclera, and extraocular muscles. The entire visual system is important for visual function. Light reflected from an object in the field of vision passes through the transparent structures of the eye, and, in doing so, is refracted (bent) so that clear image can fall on the retina. From the retina, the visual stimuli travels through the visual pathway to the occuplital cortex, where they are perceived as an image. Vision contributes meaning and pleasure to the human experience.

NURSING ASSESSMENT OF THE VISUAL SYSTEM

Assessment of the visual system is an integral part of the nurse's role, Visual screening is conducted with persons of all ages and in all settings, and most life disorders are identified by nurses, physician, in schools, industry, outpatient clinics or ophthalmologists. Admission to the hospital is usually limited to medical and surgical treatment that cannot routinely be accomplished on an outpatient basis. Because, persons with eye problems usually are managed on an outpatient basis. Visual impairment is usually not the major diagnosis of persons for whom the nurse is providing care. However, visual impairment is frequently present and may be undiagnosed. Therefore, nurses should routinely assess visual ability, especially in persons who have systemic diseases that affect vision or who are taking medication with known visual side effects.

A complete visual assessment consists of a careful patient interview combined with physical assessment of the eye structures. General areas explored during the interview includes the patient assessment of his or her vision and any recent changes in visual acuity, whether glasses for contacts are used on the date of the last professional eye examination. The presence of severity of common eye symptoms, such as blurred vision, "floaters" dry, scratchy eyes, burning or chronic headaches are explored. The interview allows the nurse also to explore the person's health promotion practices and request to use of protective eye wear, particularly for occupational exposure. Any history of head trauma, loss of consciousness, or direct trauma or infections is important to explore.

Since many eye disorders are inherited, a family history is essential. Questions are directed especially to a family history of cataracts, glaucoma, diabetes, hypertension, STDs, AIDs, cancer poor vision glasses or blindness. A person's medical that could not be corrected with history is also obtained with particular attention to all medications in current use.

The tissues of the eye are for the most part transparent, making abnormalities easily detectable. Ocular manifestation of systemic disease also can be identified. In addition, the vascular system (retinal vascular system) and cranial nerve (optic nerves) of the eye can be visualized on examination. Assessment includes inspection of the external structure and gross measures of visual acuity. A basic assessment of the eye and vision are as given below:

- *Facial and ocular expression:* Prominence of eyes: alert or dull expression.
- *Eyelids and conjunctiva:* Symmetry, presence of edema, ptosis, itching, redness, discharge, blinking, equality and growths.
- *Lacrimal system:* Tears, swelling and growths.
- *Sclera:* Color.
- *Cornea:* Clarity.
- *Anterior chamber:* Depth, presence of blood and pus.
- *Iris and pupils:* Irregularities in color, shape and size.
- *Pupillary reflex:*
  - *Light:* Constriction of pupil in response to light in that eye (direct light reaction); equal amount of constriction in the other eye (consensual light reaction).
  - *Accommodation:* Convergence of eyes and constriction of pupil as gaze shifts from far to near object.
- *Lens:* Transparent or opaque.
- *Peripheral vision:* Ability to see movement and objects well on both sides of field of vision.
- *Acuity with and without glasses:* Ability to read newsprint, clocks on wall, and name tags and to recognize faces at bed-side and at door.
- *Supportive aids:* Glasses, contact lenses, prosthesis.

The normal physical assessment of the visual systems include the following:
- Visual acuity 20/20 ou; no diplopia.
- External eye structures are symmetric without lesions or deformities.
- Lacrimal apparatus is nontender without drainage.
- Conjunctiva clear; sclera white.
- Perrla. Pupil normally equal, round and react to light and accommodation.
- Lense clear.
- EOMI.
- Disc margin sharp.
- Retinal vessels are normal with no hemorrhage or spots.

Common Assessment Techniques

There are related to vision include the following.
- *Visual acuity testing* is performed to determine patient's distance and near visual acuity. In this, patient reads for Snellen chart and 20 ft. (distance vision test) or Jaoeger's chart at 14 in (near vision test). Examiner notes smallest print patient can read on each chart. Examples of visual acuity measurement are as follows:
  20/20 Normal
  20/40-2 Missed two letters of the 20/40 line.
  10/400 At 10 ft. reads line than normal eye sees at 400 ft.
  CF/2 ft. Counts fingers at 2 feet.
  HM/3 ft. Sees hand movement at 3 feet.
  LP/Proj. Light perception with projection.
  NLP No light perceptions.
- *Extraocular muscle testing* is performed to determine if the patient's extraocular muscles are functioning in a normal manner, with no underaction or overaction. In this the examiner makes patient follow a light source or other fixation object through a complete field of gaze, in the cover-uncover test, examiner covers patient's eye then uncovers it to see if eye has deviated under the cover.
- *Confrontation visual field test* is done to determine if patient has a full field of vision without obvious scotomas. Here patient faces examiner, covers one edge, fixates on examiner's face and counts number of fingers that the examiner brings into patient's field of vision.
- *Pupil function testing* is performed to determine if patient has normal pupillary response. In this, the examiner shines light into the patient's pupil and observes pupillary response, each pupil is examined independently, examiner also checks for consensual and accommodative response.
- *Tonometry* is to measure intraocular pressure (normal pressure is 10–21 mm Hg). In this applanation, tonometer is gently touched to the anesthesized corneal surface; examiner looks through ocular of slit lamp microscope, adjusts pressure dial until mires are aligned, and notes intraocular pressure reading.
- *Slit-lamp microscopy* provides magnified view of the conjunctiva, sclera, cornea, anterior chamber, iris, lens and vitreous. In this the patient is seated with chin placed in chin rest, slit beam illuminate ocular structures, examiner looks through magnifying occular assess various structures.
- *Ophthalmoscopy* provides magnified view of the retina and optic nerve head. Here examiner holds ophthalmoscope close to the patient's eye, shining light into back of eye and looking through aperture on ophthalmoscope, examiner adjusts dial to select one of the lenses in ophthalmoscope that produces desired amount of magnification to inspect ocular fundus.
- *Color vision testing* is performed to determine patient ability to distinguish colors. Here patient identifies numbers or paths formed by pattern of dots in series of color plates.
- *Stereopsis testing* is performed to determine patient ability to see objects in three dimensions; to test depth perceptions. From a series of plates patient identifies geometric pattern or figure that appears closer to patient when viewed through special spectacles that provides three-dimensional view.
- *Keratometry* is done to measure the coreneal curvature often done before fitting contact lenses, before doing refraction surgery or after corneal transplantation.

The terms describing refractions are:
- Accommodation—Ability to adjust between far and near objects.
- Emmetropia—Normal eye, light rays focus on retina.
- Ametropia—Refractive error, light rays do not focus on retina.
- Myopia—Near sightedness, light rays focus in front of retina.
- Hyperopia—Far sightedness, light rays focus behind retina.
- Presbyopia—Hyperopia from loss of lens elasticity because of aging.
- Astigmatism—Irregular curvature of cornes, light rays do not focus at same point.

Common assessment abnormalities found in the visual system

1. **General findings**
- *Pain:*
  - Foreign body sensation may be due to superficial corneal abrasion, it can result from contact lens wear or trauma; conjunctival or corneal foreign body are usually lessened with lid closure.
  - Severe, deep and throbbing pain is due to anterior uveitis, acute glaucoma, infection; acute glaucoma associated with nausea, and vomiting.
- Photophobia refers to abnormal intolerance to light may be due to inflammation or infection of cornea or anterior uveal tract (iris and ciliary body).

- Blurred vision is gradual or sudden inability to see clearly. This may be due to refractive errors, corneal opacities, cataracts, retinal changes, (detachment, macular degeneration), optic neuritis, or atrophy, central retinal vein or artery thrombosis, refractive changes related to fluctuations in serum glucose.
- Scotoma refers to blind or partially blind area in the visual field. This may be due to disorders of optic chiasm, glaucoma, central serous chorioretinopathy age and related macular degeneration; injury, migraine headache.
- Spots, floaters, i.e. patient describes seeing spots, "spider webs" "curtain" or floaters within the field of vision. The most common cause lies in vitreous liquification (benign phenomenon); other possible causes include hemorrhage into vitreous tumor, retinal holes, or tears, impending retinal detachment, visions detachment, intraocular hemorrhage and chorioretinitis.
- Dryness is discomfort, sandy, gritty, irritation or burning. It is due to decreased tear formation or changes in the tear composition because of aging or various systemic diseases.
- Halo around lights is a presence of a halo around light. It may be due to refractive changes, corneal edema as a result of a sudden rise in intraocular pressure in angle-closure glaucoma or secondary glaucoma.
- Glare headache, ocular discomfort, reduced visual acuity. It is related to corneal inflammation or to opacities in the cornea, lens, or vitreous that scatter the incoming light; can also result from light scatter around edges of an intraocular lens, worse at night, when pupil is dilated.
- Diplopia double vision. It may be due to abnormalities of extraocular muscle action related to muscle or cranial nerve pathology.

2. **Organ-wise findings**
a. **Eyelids**
- *Allergic reactions:* Redness, excessive tearing, and itching of lid margins. There are many possible allergens; associated eye trauma can occur from rubbing itchy eyelid.
- *Hordeolum (Stye):* Refer to small, superficial white nodules along lid margin. This is due to infection of a sebaceous gland of eyelid and causative organism usually bacterial (most commonly staphylococcus aureus).
- *Chalazion* refers to reddened, swollen area in eyelid, involves deeper tissues than hordeolum can be inflamed and tender. This may be due to granuloma formed around to sebacious gland occurs as a foreign body reaction to sebum in the tissue can develop from a hordeolum or from rupture of a sebaceous gland with resulting sebum in the tissue.
- *Blepharitis,* i.e. redness, swelling and crusting along lid margin. It is due to bacterial invasion of lid margins; often chronic.
- *Dacrocystitis* redness, swelling and tenderness of medial area of lower lid (in region of lacrimal sac). It is due to blockage of nasolacrimal duct and subsequent infection.
- *Xanthelasma* raised, yellowish plaques on eyelids usually on nasal portion. It may be due to lipid disorders and may be normal fingings.
- *Ptosis* dropping of upper lid margin, unilateral or bilateral. It is due to mechanical causes as result of eyelid tumors or excess skin; myogenic causes attributable to condition involving the levator muscle or myoneural function; such as myasthenia gravis; neurogenic causes affecting third cranial nerve that innovates the levator muscle.
- *Entropion* is inward turning of upper or lower lid margin, unilateral or bilateral. It is due to congenital causes resulting in development, abnormalities, involutional entropion related to horizontal eyelid laxity can cause irritation and tearing.
- *Ectropion* is outward turning of lower lid margin. This is due to mechanical causes as a result of eyelid tumors, herniated orbital fat, or extravasation of fluid; paralytic ectropian occurs when orbicularis muscle functions is disturbed as with Bell's palsy.
- *Lid lag* slower or absent closing of one lid. It is due to possible involvement in cranial nerve VII.
- *Blepharospasm* increased blink rate when severe spasms occur, it is found unable to open eyelids. It may be due to inflammation, involvement of cranial nerves V and VII, can occur as a response to bright lights.
- *Decreased blink* decreased rate of eyelid closure. It may be due to decreased corneal sensation; possible involvement of CN VII; dry eye and corneal damage may result if blink rate significantly decreased.

b. **Conjunctiva**
- *Conjunctivitis:* Redness and swelling of conjunctiva may be itchy. It is due to bacterial or viral infection may be allergic response or inflammatory response to chemical exposure.
- *Subconjunctival hemorrhage:* Appearance of blood spot on sclera, may be small, it can affect entire sclera. It may be due to conjunctival space caused by coughing, sneezing, eyerubbing or minor trauma, generally it does not require any treatment.
- *Pinguecula:* Raised area (growth) on conjunctiva, horizontally oriented in medial area of bulbar conjunctiva. This was due to degenerative lesion related to chronic ultraviolet light or other environmental exposure.
- *Jaundice:* Yellowish color of entire sclera. Jaundice is related to liver dysfunction: Yellow color is normal after diagnostic study requiring intravenous fluorescein injection.

c. **Cornea**
- *Corneal abrasion:* Localized painful disruption of the epithelial layer of cornea can be visualized with fluorescein dye. It may be due to trauma, overwear or improper fit of contract lenses.
- *Corneal opacity:* Whitish area of cormally transplant cornea; may involve entire cornea. It may be result of scar tissue formation related to inflammation, infection, trauma, degree of visual acuity deficit depends on location and size of opacity.
- *Pterygium:* Triangular, horizontally oriented thickening of bulbar conjunctiva that extends post cornea-ocleral border onto cornea. It is commonly thought to be or extension of a pinguecula; degenerative lesion is related to chronic ultraviolet light or other environmental exposure; surgical removal is necessary if progression to central cornea.

d. **Globe**
- *Exophthalmos:* Protrusion of globe beyond its normal position within bony orbit; sclera is often visible above iris when eyelids are open. This may be the result of intraocular or periorbital tumors; thyroid eye disease; swelling or tumors of the frontal sinus; dry eye and corneal damage may occur as a result of inability to close eye normally.

e. **Pupil**
- *Mydriasis:* Pupil is larger than normal (dilated). It may be due to emotional influences, trauma, acute glaucoma (fixed middilated), systemic or local drugs and head injury.
- *Miosis:* Pupil is smaller than normal. It may be due to iritis, morphine or similar drugs, glaucoma is treated with miotic agents.
- *Anisocoria:* Pupils are unequal (constricted). It is due to CNS disorders, slight difference in pupil size is normal in a small percentage of the population.
- *Dyscoria:* Pupil is irregularly shaped. It may be due to congenital causes (e.g. iris coloboma); acquired causes (e.g. trauma, iris-fixated intraocular lens implant and posterior synechiae surgery on iris).
- *Abnormal response to light or accommodation:* Pupils respond asymmetrically or abnormally to light stimulus or accommodation. It is due to CNS disorders; general anesthesia.

f. **Iris**
- *Heterochromia:* Iris are different colors. It is result of congenital causes (Honer's syndrome); acquired causes (Chronic iritis, metastatic carcinoma, diffuse iris nevus or melanoma).
- *Iridokinesis:* Iris appears to shake on movement of eye. It is due to aphakia.

g. **Extraocular muscles**
- *Strabismus:* Deviation of eye position in one or more directions. It is result of overaction or underaction of one or more extraocular muscles; it can be congenital or acquired; neuromuscular involvement, CN III, IV or VI involved.

h. **Visual field defect**
- *Peripheral:* Partial or complete loss of peripheral vision. It may be due to glaucoma, complete or partial interruption of visual pathway migraine headache.
- *Central:* Loss of central vision may be due to macular disease.

i. **Lens**
- *Cataract* is opacification of lens, pupil can appear cloudy or white. When opacity is visible behind pupil opening, it is due to aging, trauma, electrical shock, diabetes, chronic system, corticosteroid therapy and congenital.
- *Subluxation or dislocation:* Edge of lens may be seen through pupil. "Setting sun" sign. It is due to trauma and systemic disease (e.g. Marfan's syndrome).

Diagnostic Studies of Visual System

Diagnostic studies provide important information to the nurse in monitoring the patient condition and planning appropriate intervention. The common basic diagnostic studies of vision and their description and nursing responsibilities are as given below:

- *Retinoscopy* is an objective (though inexact) measure of refractive error, handheld retinoscopy directs focussed light into the eye, refractive error distorts the light. Distortion is neutralized to determine refractive error, useful for the patient unable to cooperate during process of subjective refraction (e.g. confused patients). The procedure is painless, it may need to help patient hold head still. Pupil dilation will make it difficult to focus on nearby objects, dilation may last for 3-4 hours.
- *Refractometry* is subjective measure of refractive error, multiple lenses are mounted on rotating wheels; patient sits looking through apertures at Snellen acuity chart, lenses are changed; patient chooses lenses then make acuity sharpest; cycloplegic drugs used to paralyse accommodation during refraction process. Nursing responsibilities is as in retinoscopy.
- *Visual field perimetry* is detailed mapping of the visual field; study uses semicircular, bowl-like instrument that presents patient with a light stimulus in various parts of the bowl. Specific pattern of visual field loss is used to diagnose glaucoma and certain neurologic deficit. Procedure is painless but may be fatiguing, elderly or debilated patient may need rest period; patient must fixate on center target for accurate testing.
- *Ultrasonography* A-scan probe is applanated against patient's anesthesized cornea; it is used primarily for axial length measurement for calculating power of intraocular lens implanted after cataract extraction.

B-Scan probe is applied to patient closed lid; used more often than A-Scan for diagnosis of ocular

pathology such as intraocular foreign bodies or tumors, vitreous opacities, retinal detachments. The procedure is painless (Cornea is anesthized for A-Scan).
- *Indirect ophthalmoscopy* indirect ophthalmoscopy is worn on examiner's head; light is projected through a handheld lens into patient's eyes, stereoscopic view is larger and provides a better view of peripheral retina, always used when some retinal abnormalities are suspected. Light source is bright, patient may be uncomfortably photophobic especially because pupil is dilated.
- *Fluorescein angiography* fluorescein (a nonradioctive, noniodine dye) is intravenously injected into anticubital or other peripheral vein, followed by serial photographs (over 10 min period) of the retina through dilated pupil; provides diagnostic information about flow of blood through pigment epithelial and retinal vessels; often it is used in diabetic patients to accurately locate areas of diabetic retinopathy before laser destruction of neovascularization.

  If extravasation occurs, fluorescein is toxic to tissue, systemic allergic reactions are rare, but nurse should be familiar with emerging equipment and procedure, tell the patient that dye can sometimes cause transient vomiting, all nausea, yellow discoloration of urine and skin in normal and transient.
- *Amsler grid test* is self administered using a handheld card printed with a grid of lines (similar to graph paper); patient fixateous center dot and records any abnormalities of the grid lines such as wavy, missing, or distorted areas used to monitor macular problems. Regular testing is necessary to identify any changes in mucular function.
- *Schirmer tear test* study measures tear volume produced throughout fixed time period; one end of a strip for filter paper is placed in lower lid culdesac; area of tear saturation is measured after 5 minutes is useful in diagnosing keratoconjunctivitis sicca. Test may be done with closed or open eyes.

In addition there are four electrophysiology examinations performed in ophthalmology, electroretinogram (ERG), electro-oculogram (EOG), dark adaptometry, and visual evoked potential. The main purpose of these examinations is to assess the function of the visual pathway from the photoreceptors of the retina to visual cortex of the brain. They are useful in diagnosing retinal vascular occlusions, toxic drug exposure, inherited retinal diseases and intraocular foreign body. Patient education regarding the purpose and method of testing is a nursing responsibility for all diagnostic procedures.

VISUAL IMPAIRMENT

Visual impairment ranges in severity from diminished visual acuity to total blindness. The patient may be categorized by the level of visual loss:

- Total blindness is defined as no light perception and no usable vision.
- Functional blindness is present when the patient has some light perception but no usable vision.

The patients with either total or functional blindness is considered legally blind and may use vision substitutes such as guide dogs and cones for ampulation and braille for reading. Vision enhancement techniques are not helpful.

Legal blindness is defined as central visual acuity for distance 20/200 or worse in the better eye (with correction) and/or a visual field no greater than 20° in its widest diameter or in the better eye (compared with a normal range of about 180°).

Etiology

Visual impairment has numerous causes and preventable blindness is a major health problem.

- Refractive errors (myopia, hyperopia, presbyopia, astigmatism) are the most common visual problems, but numerous other nutritional, infections metabolic and systemic disorders adversely affect the function of the eye.
- *Nutritional deficiencies:* A lack of vitamin A and B complex can cause changes within the retina, cornea, and conjunctiva. Night blindness is caused by vitamin A deficiency. Optic neuritis can result in vitamin B deficiency especially in alcoholics.
- Infection of trachoma, is common cause of visual impairment.
- Macular degeneration, is a disease of the aging retina.
- Cataract and glaucoma.

In addition, the eye can also be adversely affected by variety of systemic diseases which include the following:

Vascular Disorders

- *Hypertension:* Persistent uncontrolled hypertension can cause hemorrhage, edema, and exudates in the retina. Retinal asterics narrow, causing degenerative changes.
- *Cardiovascular accident:* Depending on the location of the stroke, the patient may experience hemianopsin or blindness.
- *Sickle cell disease:* This can cause neovascularization, arterial occlusions or retinal hemorrhage.

Neurological Disorders

- *Multiple sclerosis:* Demyelination can result in optic neuritis diplopia and nustagmus.

Endocrine Disorders

- *Graves disease:* Accumulation of fat and fluid in the retroocular tissue can produce exophthalmos (protrusion of eye) and lid retraction.
- *Diabetic retinopathy:* Retinal capillary walls thicken and develop microaneurysms. Retinal veins widen

and become tortuous. Small hemorrhages occur which leave scars that decrease vision. As the disease worsens, neovascularization occurs and the new vessels grow into the vitreous tumor. These vessels are vulnerable to both obstruction and rupture. Vision decreases as "floaters" are perceived in the eye.

Connective Disorders

- *Rheumatoid arthritis, SLE:* Neovascularizations, inflammations of the cornea, sclera, or uveal tract occur.

AIDS-related Disorders

- *Herpes zoster ophthalmicus:* Herpes can invade the cornea and create ulceration that is potentially blinding.
- *Cytomegalovirus (CMV):* CMV affects AIDS patients. It spreads rapidly through the cells of the retina and the blood vessels and can totally destroy the retina.
- *Kaposis sarcoma:* The lesions of Kaposis sarcoma can affect the skin of the eyelids and conjunctiva or the orbit itself.

Pathophysiology

Refractive Disorders

Refractive disorders include irregularities of the corneal curvature length and shape of the eye as well as the focusing ability of the lens. The common refractive errors include the following:

- *Myopia* (near sightedness) causes light rays to be focussed in front of the retina. Myopia may occur because of excessive light refraction by the cornea and lens or because of an abnormally long eye. Myopia may also occur because of lens swelling that occurs when blood glucose levels are elevated, as in uncontrolled diabetes. This type of myopia is transient and variable and fluctuates with blood glucose level. During childhood especially during adolescence when the child growth rate increases, myopia may progress rapidly and require frequent changes in the patient's glass. This excessive lengthening of the eye is often attributable to genetic factors.
- *Hyperopia* (far-sightedness) causes the light rays to focus behind the retina and requires the patient to use accommodation to focus the light rays on the retina for near and far objects. This type of refractive error occurs when the cornea or lens do not have adequate focussing power or when the eyeball is too short.
- *Presbyopia* is the loss of accommodation because of age. As the eye ages the crystalline lens becomes larger, firmer and less elastic. These changes decrease the eyes accommodative ability. The accommodative ability continues to decline with each decade of life and by approximately by the age of 70 years, the accommodative power of the lens declines to zero. When this occurs, the patient cannot focus on near objects without some form of visual aid.
- *Astigmatism* is caused by an unequal corneal curvature. This irregularity causes the incoming light rays to be bent unequally. Consequently the light rays do not come to a single point of focus on the retina.
- *Aphakia* is defined as the absence of the crystalline lens. The lens may be absent congenitally or it may be removed during cataract surgery. A lens that is traumatically dislocated results in functional aphakia, although lens remains in the eye.

Macular Degeneration

Degenerative changes occur in the thin layer of blood vessels that arise in the retina and extend into the choroid and their membrane cover. Both neovascular (exudative or wet) and non-neovascular (non-exudative or dry) forms occur. In neovascular degenerations there is a sudden proliferation of new fragile blood vessels in the macular area that tend to leak and damage macula. Scarring occurs and functional losses progress rapidly. It occurs in 5% persons, responsible for 80% severe vision loss. The non-neovascular degenerative form of macular degeneration occurs from the deposit of waste products and slow atrophy of the choroid, retina and pigment epithelium.

Clinical Manifestation

In refractive errors/disorders, there is defect of the refracting media of the eye prevents light rays from converging into a single focus on the retina. Defects are the result of irregularities of the cornea curvature, the focusing power of the lens or the length of the eye. The major symptom is blurred vision. In some cases, the patient may also complain of ocular discomfort, fatigue, eye strain or headaches.

Macular degeneration causes a variety of symptoms including visual blurring and distortion and usually causes some degree of central vision loss and a decreased ability to distinguish colors. Early signs and progression of the disease can be readily detected with the use of the Amsler grid. The individual perceives dark spots, missing areas and distorted wavy lines. Intravenous fluorescein angiography may be used to visualize or confirm the extent of neovascularization of vessel leakage is suspected.

Management

Visual impairment caused by refractive errors is usually diagnosed as a part of routine eye examination. The patient with refractive errors uses corrective lenses to improve the focus of light rays on the retina. Eye glasses and contact lenses are widely used to correct common refractive errors and restore visual acuity, includes the following:

- *Emmetropia:* Normal vision. Light focuses on retina without accommodation for distance vision and

with accommodation for near vision. Spectacles and contact lenses are not indicated.
- *Myopia:* Spectacle: Concave (minus) lens bends light rays outward.
  Contact lens: Rigid, soft, daily wear or extended wear.
- *Hyperopia:* Spectacle: Convex (plus) lens binds light rays inward.
  Contact lens: Rigid or soft, daily wear or extended wear.
- *Astigmatism*
  Spectacle: Cylinder lens, bends light rays in different directions to align in a focussed point.
  Contact lens: Rigid or soft toric; daily wear or extended wear.
- *Presbyopia*
  Spectacle: Convex for near vision, can be reading glasses or bifocals with reading correction in lower part of lens.
  Contact lens: Bifocal rigid or soft, monovision (one eye corrected for distance, one for near).
- *Aphakia*
  Spectacle: Thick, convex, virtually never used after cataract extraction.
  Contact lens: Rigid, soft, daily wear or extended, not used after cataract extractions.

Refractive surgery, defined as any operative procedure performed for the purpose of elimination of refractive error, it has become an increasingly viable alternative to glasses and contact lenses for persons with visual impairment related to refraction error. The common refractive surgery includes the following:
- Radial keratotomy (RK).
- Incisional keratotomy (IK).
- Photorefractive keratotomy (PRK).
- Laser in situ keratomileusis (LASIK).
- Intraocular lens (IOL) implantation.

All these procedures are performed in ambulatory surgery centers. Careful preoperative teaching is provided to the nurse according to procedure and its advantages. Patients are permitted to gradually resume activities and usually experience a slow improvement of vision over a period of weeks or months. The nurse administers analgesics as needed to keep the patient comfortable and administer antibodies to decrease the incidence of infection.

There is no adequate treatment currently available for the non-neovascular form of macular degeneration. Oral zinc may reduce the progression of the disease. A small percentage of patients with neovascular degeneration can benefit from laser therapy to coagulate the abnormal vessels.

Nurse's Role in Prevention of Visual Impairment

Some forms of visual impairment are preventable and most forms can be slowed or treated with early diagnosis and appropriate therapy. Regular eye examinations by competent professionals are an important health promotion measure throughout life, especially as a person's age advances.

The nurse's role as a health educator with individuals, groups and communities is vital in preventing health problems, that the potential for visual impairment. In addition to health education, the nurse can promote visual health by early recognition of conditions or situations that carry a high risk of visual impairment. The following is information about those adult conditions and situation amenable to nursing interventions:
- *Glaucoma* is a significant cause of preventable visual impairment. Early recognition of glaucoma is extremely important in promoting visual health. The nurse can advocate and provide assistance for screening programs. In addition, nurse should provide health information regarding the importance of regular ophthalmic examination, especially the patient at high risk for this disorder. The nurse can provide this information to an individual patient, groups of patients or the general community.
- *Ocular trauma* can lead to blindness or severe visual impairment. Many injuries can be prevented by identifying and correcting situations that may lead to eye injuries such as:
  - Failure to properly use eye protection during potentially hazardous work, hobby, or sports activities.
  - Improper handling or storing of chemicals and especially storing alkalies or acids.
  - In appropriate response to ocular injuries, particularly failure to institute prompt, continuous ocular irrigation after exposure to a potentially toxic substance; and
  - Failure to properly use seat belts or infant and child vehicle-restraint devices.

  The nurse should take an active role in educating the patient about these potentially harmful situations.
- As *contact lens* wear becomes increasingly common and contact lens companies continue to market directly to consumers. Many people have become casual about wearing and caring for their lenses. Although contact lenses are generally safe and effective, they can be a significant potential source of ocular problems when the patient does not use or care for the lenses properly. The nurse should promote ocular health by teaching the patient correct wearing and cleaning techniques and recommending appropriate ophthalmic follow-up. Nurse should stress for using only approved contact lens solutions.
- *Women* of child bearing age should be immunized against rubella (GM) to prevent congenital blindness in infants, which can result from rubella infection, in the mother during first timester of pregnancy. Person who comes in contact with this group of women especially those who work in health care agencies must be immunized as well.
- *Genetically* transmitted syndromes and conditions often have ocular manifestations. The nurse working with

the patients of child bearing age should be prepared to make referral for genetic counseling when appropriate.

EYE INFECTIONS AND INFLAMMATION

Infections and inflammation can occur in any of the eye structures and may be caused by microorganism, mechanical irritations, or sensitivity to some substances. Inflammation of the eye is the most acute condition affecting the eye. The common infection and inflammation of the external eye or extraocular disorder include the following:

- *Hordeolum* (Sty) is common infection of the sebaceous glands in the lid margins, caused by staphylococcus. It creates a red, swellen, circumscribed and acutely tender postules that gradually resolves or ruptures. The nurse should instruct the patient to apply warm, moist compresses at least four times a day until the abscesses drains. Antibiotic ointment. If severe, incision of postule if it does not resolve spontaneously. If there is a tendency for recurrence, the patient should perform lid scrubs daily. In addition, appropriate ointments or drops may be indicated.
- *Chalazion* is an inflammation of a sebaceous gland in the lids. It may evolve from a hordeolum or may occur in a primary inflammatory response to the material released into the lid tissue when a blocked gland ruptures. It is sterile cyst located in the connective tissue in the free edges of the eyelid. Lump is small, hard and nontender, but may put pressure on the eye and affect vision. The chalazion appears as a swollen nonpainful reddened area, usually on the upper lid. It may disappear spontaneously become infected or require local excision of impairing vision. Initial treatment is similar to that for a hordeolum.
- *Trachoma*, a chronic infectious form of conjunctivitis believed to be caused by *Chlamydia trachomatis*, is one of the leading causes of blindness. It can be effectively treated early in the disease with antibiotics, hard to eradicate once chronic.
- *Keratitis* is an inflammation, or infection of the cornea, it can be superficial or deep, acute or chronic. Staphylococcus and streptococcus bacteria and herpes simplex viruses are common causes. Pain, photophobia or blepharospasm are common. It can result in visual loss. In this, steroids are used to control inflammation, antibiotics, cycloplegics to rest the eye, corneal transplant may be necessary.
- *Uveitis* is an acute inflammation of the uvea from infection, allergy, toxic agents and systemic disorders. It causes eye pain, swelling photophobia and visual impairment. It may be self-limiting, treatment of underlying cause plus cycloplegics to rest the eye. Warm moist compresses to reduce inflammation and increase comfort.
- *Blepharitis* is a common chronic bilateral inflammation of lid margins. Inflammation of the eyelids frequently begin in childhood and recurs causing redness and scaling of the upper and lower lid at the lash orders. The lids are red rimmed with many scales or crusts on the lid margins and lashes. The patient may primarily complain of itching but may also experience burning, irritation, and photophobia. Conjunctivitis may occur simultaneously.

  Daily facial cleaning and shampoo to remove scales, local antibiotics may be helpful. If the blepharitis is caused by a staphylococcal infection, care includes the use of an appropriate ophthalmic antibiotic ointment. Seborrheic blepharitis, related to seborrhea of the scalp and eyebrows is treated with antiseborrheic shampoo for the scalp and eyebrows. Often blepharitis caused by both staphylococcal and seborrheal micro-organism and the treatment must be more vigorous to avoid hordeolum, keratitis and other eye infections. Conscientious hygienic practices involving skin and scalp must be emphasized. Gentle cleansing of the lid margins with baby shampoo can effectively soften and remove crusting.
- *Corneal ulcer* infection of the cornea is not common but it can readily lead to ulceration. Ulcers typically cause pain, tearing and spasms of the eyelid. A greyish white corneal opacity is seen with fluorescein evaluation. Minor abrasions heal spontaneously and without scarring; comfort measures critical as the pain can be severe possible need for antibiotics and corticosteroids.
- *Conjunctivitis* is an infection or inflammation of the conjunctiva. It may result from mechanical trauma such as that caused by sunburn or from infection with organisms such as *Staphylococcus*, streptococci or *Haemophilus influenzae*. Two sexually transmitted agents that cause conjunctivitis are *Chlamydia trachomatis* and *Neisseria gonorrheae*. It is often caused by allergic reaction with the body or by external irritants (e.g. poison ivy or cosmetics). Viral agents include human adenovirus and herpes simplex virus. Acute mucopurulent conjunctivitis (pink eye) is usually seen among school children but occur at any age and it is highly infectious.

The symptoms of conjunctivitis may vary in severity. Hyperemia and burning are common initial symptoms that progress rapidly to mucopurulent exudates, which crusts on the base of the eyelashes and easily transfer red to unaffected eye. Viral infections produce minimal exudate. The conjunctiva are grossly reddened and inflamed. Inflammation of the cornea can result in ulceration and even perforation usually in response to virulent organisms such as *Neisseria gonorrheae*. Involvement of the cornea, although rare, is extremely serious and can even result in the loss of the eye. The corneal ulceration is usually identified on slit lamp examination and may be outlined with the use of sterile fluorescein dye.

Treatment of conjunctivitis includes careful cleansing of the eyelids and lashes and the use of topical antibiotics.

Warm moist compress may be used to gently remove from adherent crusts from the eyes, especially in the morning. The procedure for applying warm moist compress includes the following:
- Use sterile technique when infection or ulceration is present. Clean technique may be used for allergic reactions.
- Use separate equipment for bilateral eye infections.
- Wash hands before treating each eye.
- Temperature of compress should not exceed 49°C (120°F).
- Change compress frequently every 5 minutes as ordered. Always wash hands first.
- Do not exert pressure on the eyeball.
- Sterile petroleum may be used on skin around eyes, if desired to protect the skin.
- If sterile is not required, moist heat may be applied by means of a clean face cloth.
- Since the drainage material is infectious, it should be disposed carefully.

Common ophthalmic drugs used to treat infection or inflammation includes the following:
- Antibiotics and antiviral drugs
    - Polymyxin B, bacitracin (polysporin).
    - Polymyxin B, neomycin, bacitracin (neosporin).
    - Bacitracin.
    - Idoxuridine (IDU).
    - Gentamicin sulfate (garamycin).
    - Chloramphenical (chloromycin).
- Steroids
    - Prednisone.
    - Prednisolone acetate.
    - Methyl prenisolone (depomedrol).
    - Triamcinolone.
    - Dexamethasone.
    - Fluorometholone.
- Cycloplegic and mydriatic action
    - Atrophin sulphate.
    - Cyclopentolate hydrochloride (cyclogyl).
    - Homatrophine hydrobromide (isopromide).
    - Scopolamine hydrobromide.
    - Tropicamide (mydriacyl).

The antibiotic may be used in the form of ointment or drop form. Ointment remains in contact with the eye much longer, giving a prolonged effect. There is also less absorption into the lacrimal passages than with eye drops. Eye ointment can, however, produce a film in front of the eye that may blur vision.

The nurse teaches the patient about the disease and its treatment. Since diseases are infectious, avoid crowded environment and to keep the hand away from the eyes. Frequent handwashings are encouraged. The nurse instructs the patient about how to instill the ophthalmic ointment or drops. The ointment is gently placed directly on to the exposed conjunctiva from the inner to the outer canthus. Care should be taken to avoid the eyelashes or any part of the eye that would contaminate the tip of the tube. The nurse warns the patient against possible blurring of vision. If both ointment and drops are used, ointment is applied last. Treatment at bed time minimizes the adverse effects of blurred vision.

EYE TRAUMA AND INJURY

Eyes are protected by the bony orbit and by fat pads but sometimes everyday activities can result in ocular trauma. Ocular injuries can involve the ocular adnexa, the superficial structures or the deeper ocular structures. Eye injuries can result in permanent blindness. Most of the injuries are considered to be preventable.

Etiology

The types of ocular trauma include blunt injuries, penetrating injuries or chemical exposure injuries. Cause of ocular injuries include automobile accidents, accidental occurrences such as falls, sports and leisure activity injuries, assaults, or work-related situation which include the following:
- *Blunt injury:* It is due to hit by fist and other blunt objects. Mechanical trauma can include lacerations of the eyelids as well as direct injury to the eye itself. Contusions can cause bleeding into the anterior chamber (hyphema).
- *Penetrating injury:* It is due to fragments such as glass, metal, wood and knife, stick or other large objects.
- *Chemical injury:* It can occur in the home, school and industrial setting, and may involve either an acid or an alkali substance. Prompt treatment is essential to prevent permanent eye damage.
- *Thermal injury:* Direct burn from curling iron, or other hot surface. Indirect burn for ultraviolet light (e.g. welding, torch, sun ultraviolet burns are also concerned and may occur from excess sun exposure (skiing, outdoor work, or sunbathing) or the use of heat lamps and tanning beds.
- *Foreign bodies* on the surface of the cornea can cause eye injury, which include particles of glass, wood and metal.
- Trauma due to blunt and penetrating objects.
- Burns chemical or thermal injuries already explained above.

Pathophysiology

Although the eyes are vulnerable to trauma, the natural protective mechanism of eyes both prevent and minimize minor eye injuries. The heavy orbit bone protects the eye from most blunt mechanical injuries. The 'eyes' natural lubricating system is augmented by tears to help flush away chemicals and other foreign bodies and the blink reflex protects from the most low-impact forces.

Acid causes coagulation in the cornea which although produces significant local trauma actually prevents the substance from penetrating and damaging the deeper structures of the eye. Alkaline substance, however, penetrates the corneal epithelium and release proteas and collagenases that can cause corneal necrosis and perforation.

Penetrating injuries or retained foreign bodies can result in sympathetic ophthalmia, a serious inflammation of the ciliary body, iris and choroid that occurs in the uninjured eye. The cause of the acute inflammations is unknown, but it is believed to be some type of autoimmune response. The inflammation can spread rapidly from uvea to the optic nerve. The uninjured edge becomes inflamed, painful and photophobic with a decline in visual acuity.

Clinical Manifestation

After the injury or trauma, the following signs and symptoms are found depending upon the extent of injury or trauma.
- Pain
- Absent eye movement
- Photophobia
- Fluid drainage from eye (e.g. blood CSF, aqueous tumor)
- Redness-diffuse or localized
- Abnormal or decreased vision
- Swelling
- Visible foreign body
- Ecchymosis
- Prolapse bleb
- Tearing
- Abnormal intraocular pressure
- Blood in the anterior chamber.

Management

Prompt professional assessment and care, perhaps, are the most important aspects of management of eye injuries and may protect eyes from serious visual impairment. First aid measures for the injury could be widely taught and posted clearly in all settings in which injuries are significant risks.
- *Chemical burns:* Are immediately treated with copious flushing of the eye with water. A litmus paper may be applied to the conjunctiva to determine the pH if the substance is unknown. Irrigation is continued for at least 15 minutes before the patient is transferred for further evaluation and treatment. The purpose of eye irrigation is to remove chemical irritants, foreign bodies and secretions, and cleanse the eye postoperatively (may be done preoperatively). The eye irrigation procedure is performed as follows:
    - Prepare solutions: Physiological solutions of sodium chloride or Lactated Ringers' solution are most commonly used.
    - Position person comfortably go towards one side so that fluid cannot flow into the other eye.
    - Use appropriate means (e.g. kidney basin, large towel) to catch irrigatory fluid.
    - Use appropriate amounts of solution:
        - If small amounts are needed (cleanse eye postoperatively) sterile cotton balls moistened with solution can be used.
        - If moderate amounts of fluids are needed (removing secretions) plastic squeeze bottle is used to direct irrigating fluid along with the conjunctiva and over the eyeball from inner to outer canthus.
        - If copious amounts of fluids are needed (i.e. for removing chemical irritants) bags of solutions such as intravenous bags along with the tubing to direct the flow onto the eye can be used.
    - Avoid directing a forceful stream onto the eye.
    - Avoid touching any eye structures with irrigating equipment.
    - If there is drainage, wrap a piece of gauze around the index finger to raise the lid and ensure thorough cleansing.
- *Mechanical trauma:* Also requires prompt professional assessment and care. The risk of infection is accompanied by the risk of losing the eye. Antibiotics, wound suture, cycloplegic agents and cold compresses are all possible interventions depending on the exact nature of the injury.

The first aid of eye injuries includes the following.
- *Burns, chemical, flame*: Flush eye immediately for 15 minutes with cold water or any available nontoxic liquid; seek medical assistances.
- *Loose substance on conjunctiva, dirt, insects*: Left upper lid over lower lid to dislodge substance, produce tearing, irrigate eye with water if necessary; do not rub eye; obtain medical assistance if these interventions fail.
- *Contact injury; contusion, ecchymosis, laceration*: Apply cold compressor if no laceration is present; cover eye if laceration is present and seek medical assistance.
- *Penetrating objects*: Do not remove object; place protective shield over the eyes (For example paper cup); cover the uninjured eye to prevent excess movement of injured eye and seek medical assistance.

Trauma is often a preventable cause of visual impairment. The nurse's role is individual and community education is extremely important in reducing the incidence of ocular trauma. The efforts concerning eye safety and the first aid for eye injuries should be taken.

The body's natural eye defenses can be appropriately augmented by the use of goggles, shields and safety lenses for sports and high risk activities. Children need to be taught about the risks associated with BB guns, slingshots, and even rubber bands. The use of protective sunglasses may also be important, depending on the patient's

occupation and leisure time sun exposure. The rules for eyes safety are as follows:
- Spray aerosols away from eyes.
- Wear protective glasses during active sports such as racquetball.
- Slowly release steam from ovens, pots, pressure cookers and microwave popcorn bags.
- Gaze at solar eclipses only through adequate filters.
- Wear safety goggles whenever hazardous work is being done or if you are in a work place area where such hazards exist.
- Fit all machinery with safeguards.
- Keep dangerous items and chemicals away from children.
- Store sharp objects safely.
- Pick up rocks and stones rather than going over them with a lawn mower.

GLAUCOMA

Glaucoma is an eye disease characterized by progressive optic nerve atrophy and loss of vision. It is not one disease but rather group of disorders characterized by:
- Increased intraocular pressure and the consequences of elevated pressure.
- Optic nerve atrophy, and
- Peripheral visual loss.

Etiology

The etiology of glaucoma deals primarily with the consequences of elevated intraocular pressure (IOP). A proper balance between the rate of aqueous production (referred to as inflow) and the rate of aqueous reabsorption (referred to as outflow) is essential to maintain the IOP within normal limits. The term glaucoma refers to a group of disorders as given below:
- *Primary open angle glaucoma (POAG):* Is chronic or simple usually caused by obstruction trabecular meshwork.
- *Secondary open angle glaucoma (SOAG):* Occur from an abnormality in the trabecular meshwork or an increase in venous pressure.
- *Primary angle-closure glaucoma (PACG):* Narrow angle, acute PACG outflow impaired as a result of narrowing or closing of angle between iris and cornea. Intermittent attacks—pressure normal when angle open, if persistent, acute ocular emergency.
- *Secondary angle-closure:* Can result from ocular inflammations, blood vessel changes and trauma.
- *Congenital glaucoma:* Is an abnormal development of filtration angle, can occur secondary to other systemic eye disorders.

Pathophysiology

The normal balance of production and drainage of aqueous humor allows IOP to remain relatively constant within the normal range of 10 to 21 mm Hg with a mean pressure of 16 mm Hg. Normal diurnal variations are limited to about 5 mm Hg. Obstruction in any part of the outflow channels for aqueous humor results in a back up of fluid and an increase in IOP. A sustained elevation gradually damages the optic nerve and impairs vision, IOP POAG, the changes occur slowly and the damage is insidious. The process can also occur more rapidly in response to injury or infections or as complications of surgery.

Clinical Manifestation

POG (Primary Open Angle Glaucoma)
- Frequently no signs or symptoms in the early stages.
- IOP typical elevated is greater than 24 mm Hg.
- Slow loss of vision.
- Peripheral vision lost before central.
- Tunnel vision.
- Persistent dull eye pain.
- Difficulty in adjusting to darkness.
- Failure to detect color changes.

PACG (Primary Angle Closure Glaucoma)
- *Acute:* Severe ocular pain, decreased vision, pupil enlarged and fixed-colored halos around lights, eye red, steamy cornea, may cause nausea and vomiting.
- IOP usually dramatically elevated, may exceed 50 mm Hg.
- Permanent blindness if marked increase in IOP for 24 to 48 hours.

Congenital Glaucoma

Enlargement of eye, lacrimation, photophobia, blepharospasm.

Management

Number of diagnostic tests are used to diagnose and monitor glaucoma. These include:
- Visual acuity measurement.
- *Tonometry:* Measurement of IOP.
- *Tonography:* Estimation of the resistance in the outflow channels by continuously recording the IOP over 2 to 4 minutes.
- *Ophthalmoscopy:* Evaluation of color and configuration of the optic cup.
- *Visual field permietry:* Measurement of visual function in the central field of vision.
- *Gonicoscopy:* Examination of the angle structures of the eye, where the iris ciliary body and cornea meet.
- *Fundus photography.*

Drug therapy is the foundation of treatment for most forms of glaucoma. The goal of therapy is to keep the IOP low enough to prevent the patient from developing optic nerve damage. Common medication for glaucoma include the following (from a tonic drops or oral).

- *Miotics:* Constrict the pupil (miosis) by directly stimulating the spinter muscle (e.g. cholinergics, pilocarpine HCl carbachol). They increase outflow of aqueous humor by ciliary muscle pull on trabecular meshwork. Here nursing intervention includes: evaluate the effectiveness of drug; monitor frequency of use; inform the patient that blurred vision and poor night vision may occur due to a small pupil; other side effectiveness of drug; monitor frequency of use; inform the patient that blurred vision and poor night vision may occur due to a small pupil and other side effects include eyebrow or lid discomfort, burning sensation with drop instillation.
- *Cholinesterase inhibition:* Constricts ciliary muscle and iris sphincter; iris is pulled away from anterior chamber angle, allowing drainage of aqueous humor and lowering IOP (e.g. Physiostigmine, Isoflurophate, Demercarium Bromide, echothiophate iodide). Here nursing intervention includes advice to avoid use of isoflurophate and demercarium during pregnancy. Inform patient that blurred vision, watering eyes, browache, and change in vision may occur.
- *Beta adrenergic antagonists:* Decreases aqueous humor production and increase the outflow thereby decreasing IOP (e.g. Timolol maleate, Betaxolol, Levobunolol. Carteolol, Metipronolol). Here evaluate effectiveness, use caution when administering NSAIDs be to patient, who have pulmonary or cardiac disease—can cause spasms.
- *Carbonic anydrase inhibitors:* Decreases aqueous humor production by inhibiting carbonic anhydrase in ciliary processes (an enzyme necessary to produce aqueous humor) (e.g. Acetazolamide Diamox), Ethoxzolamide, Dichlorophenamide, Methazolamide, Darzolamide). In the treatment, evaluate the effectiveness, monitor tingling sensation as extremities, tinnitus, gastric upset, or hearing dysfunction.
- *Adrenergic agents:* Reduce aqueous humor formation and increases outflow (e.g. Epinephryl borate, Epinephrine HCl, Epinephrine bitartrate Dipivefrin Apraclonidine). Here, evaluate the effectiveness, monitor side effects, headache, browache, blurred vision, tachycardia, pigment deposits in cornea, conjunctiva and lids.
- *Osmotic agents:* Move water from the intraocular structures, resulting in a marked ocular hypotonic effect, thereby decreasing IOP. (e.g. Glycerine, monitor electrolytes for depletion, monitor glucose levels in patients with type diabetes. Drugs can cause hyperglycemia.
- *Prostaglandin agonists:* Increase outflow of aqueous humor. It is used primarily with patient intolerance to or unresponsive to other glaucoma agent (e.g. Latanoprost). Nursing intervention includes monitor renal and hepatic function during treatment. Teach patient about adverse side effects of burning on administration, blurred vision, itching and photophobia.

Surgical intervention indicates when conservative treatments fail to control the IOP. The common surgical procedures are:
- Argon laser trabeculoplasty (ALT).
- Trabeculectomy with or without filtering implant.
- Cyclocryotherapy destruction of ciliary body.

Nursing care for the patient after trabulectomy includes the following.
- Routine postanesthesia care.
- Protection of operative eye with patch or shield positioning the patient on back or unoperative side and safety measures.
- Maintaining comfort in the operative eye.
- Assessment as appropriate, of the IOP, appearance of the bleb, and anterior chamber depth.
- Administration of medications such as a cycloplegic, a mydriate, and a combination of antibiotic and steroids.

An acute care for PACG includes the following:
- Topical cholinergic agent.
- Hyperosmotic agent.
- Laser peripheral iridotomy.
- Surgical iridectomy.

Postoperative care includes relieving pain, and patient/family education and supporting selfcare including self-administration of eyedrops.

The self-administration of eyedrops include the following:
- Wash the hands throughly before administering the medication.
- Tilt the head back and look up towards the ceiling.
- Pull the lower lid gently down and out to expose the conjunctiva and create a sac.
- Bring the dropper from the side and apply the eye drops. Avoid touching the eyelashes, conjunctiva, or surface of the eye with the dropper. Resting the thumb on the forehead can help to stabilize the hand.
- Close both eyes gently. Do not squeeze them tightly to prevent the medication spilling over.
- Apply slight pressure at the inner canthus of the eye to decrease systemic absorption of the medication.
- If more than one drop is to be administered, wait 2–5 minutes before administering the second drop.

CATARACT

A cataract is a clouding or opacity within the crystalline lens that leads to gradual painless blurring and eventual loss of vision. The patient may have a cataract in one or both eyes. If present in both eyes, one cataract may affect the patient's vision. The cataracts are third leading cause of preventable blindness.

Etiology

Cataracts are generally classified as senile (associated with aging), traumatic (associated with injury), congenital (present at birth) and secondary (occurring after other diseases). These include blunt or penetrating trauma, congenital factors such as maternal rubella, radiation or ultraviolet light exposure, certain drugs such as systemic corticosteroids or long-term topical corticosteroids and ocular inflammation. The risk factors associated with cataract include the following:

- *Age:* The incidence increases dramatically after the age of 65.
- *Sex:* Cataracts are slightly more common in women than men.
- Ultraviolet light exposure:
  - More common in persons living in warm sunny climates.
  - More common in persons who have worked out door extensively.
- High dose radiation exposure.
- *Drug effects:* Use of corticosteroids, phenothiazines and selected chromotherapeutic agents.
- Poorly-controlled diabetes mellitus accumulation of sorbitol (byproduct of glucose).
- Trauma to the eye.

Cataracts may result from the ingestion of injurious substances, such as dinitrophenol or naphthalene, or systemic absorption of hair dyes. Cataracts may also occur secondary to eye diseases such as uveitis or eye trauma, or with systemic diseases, such as diabetes mellitus, galactosemia, or sarcodiosis.

Pathophysiology

Cataract development is mediated by a number of factors. In senile cataract formation, it appears that altered metabolic processes (decrease in protein, an accumulation of water and an increase in sodium content) within the lens that cause an accumulation and disrupts the normal lens fibre structure. These changes affect lens transparency, causing vision changes. The cause of these pathological changes is not known. Cataracts usually develops bilaterally, but at different rate. The primary symptom of cataract is a progressive loss of vision. The degree of loss depends on the location and extent of the opacity. Person with an opacity in the center portion of the lens can generally be better in dim light when the pupil are dilated. The person with presbyopia may find that reading without glass is possible in the early stages of cataract formation, because the greater convexity of the lens creates an artificial myopia.

Clinical Manifestation

The patient with cataracts may complain of a decrease in vision, abnormal color perception and glare. There is a gradual painless blurring and loss of vision. Peripheral vision may be affected first. Near vision may initially improve. Glare is due to light scatter caused by lens opacities, and it may be significantly worse at night and in bright light, when the pupil dilates. There will be halos around lights, loss of ability to discriminate between hues and cloudy white opacity on the pupil.

The visual decline is gradual, but rate of cataract development varies from patient to patient. Some patients may complain of a sudden loss of vision because they inadvertently cover their unaffected eye and the decreased acuity of the eye with cataracts becomes "suddenly apparent". Secondary glaucoma can also occur if the enlarging lens causes increased intraocular pressure.

Management

Diagnosis of cataract based on decreased visual acuity or other complaints of visual dysfunction. The diagnostic tests of cataract include the following:

- Visual acuity measurements.
- Ophthalmoscopy (direct or indirect).
- Slit lamp microscopy.
- Blood testing and potential acuity testing in selected patients.
- Keretometrics and A-Scan ultrasound (if surgery is planned).
- Visual field perimetry.

Medications do not play a role in the management of cataract. Anesthetics, anti-inflammatory agents and antibiotics are used after surgery. The presence for cataract does not necessarily indicate a need for surgery, although surgery is the choice of treatment, nonsurgical therapy may postpone the need for surgery, which includes, change, prescription of glasses, strong reading glasses or magnifiers, increased lighting, life adjustment and reassurance.

Surgery is the definitive treatment for cataracts. It is indicated when palliative measures no longer provide an acceptable level of visual function. Common surgical procedure for cataract includes:

- Removal of lens
  - Phacoemulsification.
  - Extracapsular extraction.
- Correction of surgical aphakia.
- Intraocular lens implantation (most frequent type of correction).
- Contact lens.

Most cataract surgery is performed in the ambulatory surgery centers, few patients require hospitalization. Routines for preoperative care vary with the setting and the eye surgeon. The patient may be asked to perform a face scrub before admission and the eyelashes may be cut. The pupil of the operative eye is dilated and paralyzed before surgery and sedation may be initiated. The drugs used for this purpose are mydriatics (Phenylephrine HCL) and cycloplegics (e.g. Atrophin). The nurse will instil dilating drops and nonsteroidal inflammatory eyedrops to reduce inflammation and to help maintain pupil dilation. The nurse ensures that the patient has understood all explanation about the surgery and expected postoperative care and restrictions. The nurse also ensures that plans are in place for someone to transport the patient home and hopefully to assist with patient care during the first ten postoperative days.

Most of the patients are discharged within a few hours. Immediate care of the person after cataract surgery includes the following:

- Position patient on back or unoperated side to prevent pressure in operated eye.
- Keep siderails up as necessary for protection.
- Place bedside table onside of unoperated eye (Patient then turns towards the unoperated side).
- Place call light within reach.
- Stress avoidance of actions that increases IOP (for example, sneezing, coughing, vomiting, straining, or sudden bending over with the head below the waist).

The nurse instructs the patient to be careful to prevent soap or water from entering the operative eye during face or hair-washing. The nurse also instructs the patient to avoid heavy lifting, active exercises, isometric exercises, or straining during defecation until cleared by the surgeon to prevent abrupt fluctuation in IOP. The nurse reviews plans for following care and provides patient and family teaching as given below:

- Teach patient and family proper hygiene and eye care techniques to ensure that medications-dressing, and/or surgical wound are not contaminated during necessary eye care.
- Teach patient and family about signs and symptoms of infection and how to report those to allow early recognition and treatment of possible infection.
- Instruct patient to comply with postoperative restrictions on head positioning, bending, coughing and valsalvas manoeuvre to optimize to visual outcomes and prevent increased IOP.
- Instructs patient to instil eye medications using aseptic techniques and to comply with prescribed eye medications routine to prevent infection.
- Instruct patient to monitor pain and take prescribed medication for pain as directed and to report pain not relieved by prescribed drug.
- Instruct patient about the importance of continued follow-up as recommended to maximize potential visual outcomes.

RETINAL DETACHMENT

A retinal detachment is a separation of the sensory retina and the underlying pigment epithelium, with fluid accumulation between the two layers.

Etiology

Retinal detachment occurs when the outer pigmented layer and the inner sensory layer of the retina separates. Inflammation and bleeding are common contributors to the detachment. The risk factors for retinal detachment includes:

- *Hish myopia:* Premature, accelerated rate of vitreous detachment, increases incidence of lattice degeneration.
- *Aphakia:* Retinal tears that presumably occur because of surgical disturbance of the vitreous.
- *Proliferative diabetic retinopathy:* Vitreous remain attached to areas of neovascularization as normal process of vitreal contraction occurs.
- *Retinal lattice degeneration:* Retinal holes common in lattice degeneration, vitreous remains attached to area of degeneration as the normal process of vitreal contraction occurs.
- *Ocular trauma:* Retinal breaks after blunt or penetrating trauma allow fluid to accumulate in the subretinal space.

Pathophysiology

The retina is a smooth unbroken, multilayered surface. Degenerative holes or tears in the retina can allow vitreous humor to pass through and initiate a detachment (rhegmatogenous detachment). The presence of an inflammatory mass, blood clot, or tumor can also separate the retina layers (exudative detachment). The vitreous also undergoes some determination with aging and can fall forward exerting a traction pull on the inner lining of the retina causing detachment (traction detachment).

Clinical Manifestation

Rational detachment may occur suddenly or develop slowly. Symptoms include floating spots or opacities before the eyes, flashes of light and progressive loss of vision in one area. Patient with a detaching retina describes symptoms that include photopsia (light flashes) floaters and a "cobweb" "hairnet" or ring in the field of vision. The floating spots are blood and retinal cells that are freed of the time of tear, they cast shadows on the retina as they drift about the eye. The flashes of light are caused by the vitreous traction on the retina. The area of visual loss depends entirely on location of detachment.

Once the retina has detached, the patient describes a painless loss of peripheral or central vision "like a curtain" coming across the field of vision. If the detachment extends to include the macula, blindness results. When the detachment is extensive and occurs quickly, the patients may have sensation that a curtain has been drawn before the eyes but there is no pain associated with the detachment.

Management

The diagnosis of retinal separations is established by ophthalmoscopic examination of the retina to identify the location and extent of the retinal tear. B-Scan ultrasonography may be used to improve the accuracy of the diagnosis of the vitreous in opaque. The assistance of nurse is required for diagnosis.

Detachment that compromises vision is repaired surgically. Common surgical techniques to seal retinal breaks and relieve traction on retina includes the following:
- Photocoagulation.
- Cryoretinoplexy.
- Scleral buckling procedure.
- Draining of subretinal fluid.
- Vitrectomy.
- Intravitreal bubble.

In most cases, retinal detachment is an urgent situation and the patient is confronted suddenly with the need for surgery. The patient needs emotional support, especially during the immediate preoperative period when preparations of the surgery produce additional anxiety. The nurse administers mydriatics or cycloplegics if ordered. When the patient experiences postoperative pain, the nurse should administer prescribed pain medication and the patient to take the medication as necessary after being discharged. The patient may go home within a few hours after surgery or may remain in the hospital for several days. Patient and family teaching provided as in discussion made earlier after eye surgery.

The nurse attempts to increase the patient's physical and emotional comfort, administering topical antibiotics, topical corticosteroids, analgesic, mydriatics as ordered. Follow the positioning and activity as preferred by patient's eye surgeon.

The patient is discharged within a few days. The nurse ensures the patient that family care giver can correctly administer all medications and eyedrops. The nurse reinforces the need to limit activity, avoid bending over below the level of the waist and to avoid constipation and straining. Activities that require close vision such as reading, needle work or writing are limited because they require rapid eye movements and accommodations. Watching television and walking are appropriate, although patients with gas bubbles may still have restrictions on positioning their heads. An eye shield is worn during the sleep for about 2 weeks. The nurse instructs the patient to contact surgeon immediately if acute eye pain develops, eye discharge increases, or turn yellow or green, and if symptoms of detachment recur.

STRABISMUS

Strabismus is a condition in which the patient cannot consistently focus two eyes simultaneously on the same objective. It is an ocular misalignment that results from an imbalance in the intraocular muscles. One eye may deviate in (estotropia) out (exotropia) up (hypertropia) or down (hypotropia).

Etiology

The eyes may be misaligned in any direction, e.g. esotropia (turning in) exotropia (turning out), hypertropia (turning up) and hypotropia (turning down). Strabismus is usually associated with childhood. But it can also be a lifelong disorder. Strabismus in the adult may be caused by thyroid disease, neuromuscular problems of the eye muscles, entrapment of the extraocular muscles in orbital floor fractures, retinal detachment repair or cerebral lesion, i.e. brain tumor, head injury, stroke and thyroid ophthalmopathy.

Pathophysiology

The ability to move the eyes in all directions and fixate on an object is the function of the six pairs of extraocular muscles. Strabismus are frequently able to compensate for the confused images and avoid diplopia. Adults with new-onset strabismus are rarely able to compensate. In the adult, primary complaint with strabismus is double vision.

Management

Strabismus is diagnosed through a standard visual field assessment. A variety of treatment options exists.
- Glasses with prisms may successfully realign the eyes and restore binocular vision.
- Eye exercises have been widely prescribed for patients with strabismus to "strengthen" the weak muscles but there is little evidence of their effectiveness.
- Surgical correction is the standard treatment. The extraocular muscles are selectively weakened (recession), tightened (resection) or physically shifted (transposition) to achievebalanced eye movement. Adjustable sutures can be used to achieve an even more accurate alignment. A slip knot is attached during surgery. Once the anesthetic has worn off, the patient ocular alignment is checked and minor correction can be made tightening or loosening the knot.
- Drug therapy with botulinum nurotoxin A (Botox) may eliminate the need for surgery or be used in conjunction with surgery. Botox is injcted into the extraocular muscle and interfere with the release of acetylcholine at the neuromuscular junctions. The toxin appear to strengthen the antagonistic muscle and wakens the injected muscle over a period of weeks to months.

Most strabismus surgery is performed on an outpatient basis under either local or geneal anesthesia. Postoperative care focuses on careful monitoring and preparation of the patient for self-care at home. The eyes may be patched initially for protection, especially if an adjustable suture was used. Patients are instructed to avoid strenous exercises and heavy lifting until approved by the surgeon. Slight redness, swelling and irritation are expected and the nurse instructs the patient to use cold compress for comfort. Dust and heavy pollen can irritate the eye and should be avoided. The nurse instructs the patient to monitor the eye for healing and to promptly report any sign of infection.

EYE TUMORS

Tumors (benign and malignant) may affect the eye and related structures. They may originate within the eye or metastasize from another primary site.
- Benign neoplasm includes lymphomas, hemangiomas and mucocells from the sinus.
- Malignant tumors threaten both the patient vision and life as extention frequently involves vital structures within the brain.

The eyelids are vulnerable to any of the standard tumors that affect the skin including nevi and xanthelasma (lipid deposits near the corner of the eye). Positive outcomes frequently require early diagnosis and prompt treatment. Treatment usually involves surgical excision but may also include various forms of radiotherapy.

Malignant Melanoma

A melanoma involving the eye is rare, but it is the most common form of intraocular tumor in adults. Retinoblastoma is the most common form of eye tumor, but it is congenital and is typically diagnosed in childhood. Usually melanoma occurs unilaterally.

Malignant melanoma occurs in the choroid, ciliary body and iris. They are slow-growing, but they metastasize early due to the vascularity of the choroid. Vision may not be affected until tumor becomes large or affects the macule.

Intraocular malignant melanoma are frequently diagnosed with an ophthalmoscope examination. Ultrasonography and fundus photography may be useful in documenting the size and placement of tumor. Fluorescein angiography may be used to document the vascular involvement the tumor.

Surgery is the primary treatment for an intraocular melanoma. Treatment is based on the exact size, shape and location of the tumor. Every effort is made to preserve the patient's vision if possible. Small tumor that involves the iris may be successfully treated with iridectomy, often with the removal of the ciliary body as well.

Large melanoma of the choroid is usually treated with enucleation of the eye, which involves surgical removal of the entire eye including sclera. Evisceration is removal of the contents of the eye with retention of the sclera. Extenteration involves removal of the entire eye and all other soft tissues in the bony orbit.

Nonsurgical treatment includes radiation therapy, photocoagulation and trachytherapy in which radioactive plaques are sutured into sclera.

Role of Nurse in Enucleation

Enucleation is the removal of the eye. The primary indications for enucleation is blind painful eye. This may result from absolute glaucoma, infection or trauma and ocular malignance.

The diagnosis of the eye malignancy and the need to undergo enucleation create a crisis situation for the patient and family. The virulence of the malignancy may necessitate immediate surgery with little time to prepare for the loss of the eye either physically or emotionally.

The nurse plays an important role in providing support and counseling to the patient during this difficult time. Both the patient and family need to be encouraged to talk about their feelings and concerns and to be helped to adjust their lives when confronted by this serious situation.

The surgical procedure includes severing the extraocular muscles close to their insertion on the globe, inserting an implant to maintain the intraorbital anatomy, and suturing the ends of the extraocular muscles over the implant. The conjunctiva covers the joined muscles and a clear conforming is placed over the conjunctiva until the permanent prosthesis is fitted. A pressure dressing helps prevent postoperative bleeding.

Postoperatively the nurse observes the patient for signs of complications including excessive bleeding or swelling, increased pain, displacement of implant, or temperature elevation. Patient education should include the instillation of tropical ointments or drops and wound cleansing. The nurse should also instruct patient in the method of inserting the conformer into the socket in case it falls out. The patient is often devastated by the loss of an eye. Even when enucleation occurs following a lengthy period of painful blindness, the nurse should recognize and validate the patient's emotional response and provide support to the patient and family.

Approximately 6 weeks following surgery, the wound is sufficiently healed for the permanent prosthesis. The prosthesis is fitted by an ocularist and designed to match the remaining eye. The patient should learn how to remove, cleanse and insert the prosthesis. Special polishing is required periodically to remove dried protein scretions. The measures to take care of prosthetic eye is as follows:
- Remove prosthesis, gently depress the lower lid and exert a small amount of pressure under lower edge of prosthesis.
- Wash prosthesis with soap (For example: Ivory) and water. Soap is less irritating than detergents and rinse throughly.
- Reinsert prosthesis: Place upper portion under upper lids. Pull down lower lid and slip lower edge behind lower lid. With finger or thumb, gently pull down on lower lid and slide prosthesis in place.
- Do not expose the plastic eye to alcohol, ether or any other solvent, they can damage the eye beyond repair.
- If rubbing the eye, rub towards the nose. Wiping away from the nose may cause the eye to fall out.
- Wear a protective patch or goggles when swimming, diving, or water skiing or removal the eye and store it.
- If the eye is left out of the socket, store it in water or contact lens solution.
- Add cornal grafting.

CHAPTER 16

Nursing Management of Disorders of Ear, Nose and Throat

INTRODUCTION

Hearing is one of the five senses and both hearing (auditory function) and balance (vestibular function) are important in activities of daily living. Hearing helps us interact with the environment and adds aesthetic pleasure as well as warning danger. Hearing also is essential for the normal development and maintenance of speech. The organs of balance are contained within the ear and relay information about the body's position to the brain.

Nurses are involved in every aspect of the care of the patient with a auditory and vestibular problems including prevention, detection and treatment. Auditory problems are common and can interfere with the person's activities of daily living, which can occur at any age and may require immediate attention. Every nurse needs to be skilful in examining the outer ear and grossly assessing the patient's hearing and equilibrium. Nurses frequently participate in case findings of person with hearing and balance disorders. Detection of hearing impairment and or a balance problem is an important nursing responsibility and the nurse is frequently the first member of the health care team to be approached by the patient regarding problems with hearing and balance.

NURSING ASSESSMENT OF AUDITORY SYSTEM

Assessment of the auditory system includes assessment of the vestibular system because two systems are so intimately related. It is often difficult to separate the symptomatology between two systems. The nurse must help the patient describe symptoms and problems in order to differentiate the source of the problems.

Subjective Data

Prior to health history, the nurse attempts to determine if the patient hears well and seeks to validate the patients functional status with the family members or significant others. Generally common behavior cues suggesting the loss of hearing which include that any adult may exhibit one or more of the following traits:

- Is irritable, hostile or hypersensitive in interpersonal relations.
- Has difficulty in hearing upper frequency consonants.
- Complain about people's mumbling.
- Turns-up volume on television.
- Asks for frequent repetition or misunderstandings.
- Answers questions inappropriately.
- Loses sense of humour, becomes grim.
- Leans forward to hear better, face looks serious and strained.
- Appears aloof and "stuck up".
- Complains of ringing in the ears.
- Has an unusually soft or loud voice.
- Has garbled speech.

The individual may also focus on the speaker's face and lips, rather than making eye contact. If the patient has a hearing loss, it is important for the nurse to face the patient directly and speak clearly. If the patient wears a hearing aid, the nurse ensures that it is in use functioning properly.

The patient should be questioned about previous problems regarding the ears, especially problems experienced during childhood. The frequency of acute middle ear infections (otitis media); perforations of the eardrums, drainage, complications and history of mumps, measles, or scarlet fever should be recorded. Congenital hearing loss can result from infectious diseases (rubella, influenza or syphilis), terotogenic medications or hypoxia in the first trimester of pregnancy. The nurse also assesses the patient for any incidence of pain (earache), drainage (otorrhea), tinnitus or vertigo. An environmental and work history is also obtained, i.e. occupational exposure; history of old trauma (blow to ears or a foreign body).

The nurse completes a thorough medication history as a variety of drugs are potentially ototoxic. Ototoxic agents directly affect the eighth cranial nerve or the organs of the hearing and balance. These drugs can cause symptoms such as tinnitus, headache, dizziness, vertigo, nausea, ataxia, nystagamus or a discernible change in hearing.

The common ototoxic drugs include the following:

- Aminoglycosides (gentamycin, chloramycin, streptomycin, amikacin, neomycin and kanamycin).
- Vancomycin, viomycin, polymixin B, polymixin E.
- Loop diuretics: Furosemide, Torsemide, Bumetamide, Ethacrynate acid sodium diamox (acetazolamide).
- Erythromycin.
- Salicilates: Aspirin.
- NSAIDs: Nemocylin.
- Quinine Sulphate: Chloroquin and quinidine.

The patient is questioned regarding self-care of the ears. Determining the frequency of hearing tests are the method and frequency of cleaning the ears, helps the nurse plan appropriate health teaching. Incorrect method of cleaning the ears such as the use of cotton-tripped applicators can lead to impacted cerumens and hearing loss. The nurse asks the patient about any history of ear infection and method of treatment. A history of chronic ear infections alerts the nurse to the possibility of sequela.

Dizziness hearing loss can have devastating effects on the patient's quality of life. The nurse carefully explores the extent of disruptions of the patients lifestyle caused by the symptoms and evaluates the patient's emotional response to these disruptions. If the ability to communicate is impaired, the patient may feel socially isolated. The nurse carefully explores the nature and effectiveness of the patient coping mechanisms. When either balance or hearing is affected, the patient's risk for injury increases, and safety measure are carefully explored.

Objective Data

The external ear is inspected and palpated before examination of the external canal and tympanum. The auricle, peratricular area, and mastoid area are observed for equality of conformation of both ears, color of skin, nodules, swelling, redness and lesions. The auricle and mastoid areas are then palpated for tenderness and nodules. Grasping auricles may elicit pain, especially if inflammation of the external ear or otitis.

Visualization of tymphanic membrane is difficult and requires illumination. In addition magnifications allow a more accurate assessment of the ear. An otoscope consists of a handle, a light source a magnifying lens and an attachment for visualizing the ear canal and eardrum. The tymphanum is observed for color, landmarks, contour and intactness.

Assessment of the inner ear for balance is accomplished by observation of gait, the Gaze test for nystagmus and the Rombert test.

Diagnostic Studies of Auditory System

Routine blood and urine tests rarely provide significant information related to diseases of the ears. The common diagnostic studies of auditory systems include the following:

- Auditory
  - *Pure tone audiometry*: Sounds are presented through earphones in sound proof room. Patient responds nonverbally when sound is heard. Response is recorded on an audiogram. Purpose is to determine hearing range of patient in terms of dB and Hz for diagnosing conductive and sensorineural hearing loss. Tinnitus can cause inconsistent results.
  - Bone conduction: Vibrator (Vibrating tuning fork) is placed on mastoid process, and hearing by bone conduction is recorded. It diagnoses conductive hearing loss.
  - One syllable and two syllable work lists: Words are presented and recorded at comfortable level of hearing to determine percentage correct and word understanding.
  - Auditory evoked potential (AEP): Procedure is similar to EEG. Electrodes are attached to patient in a darkened room. Electrodes are placed typically at the vertex, mastoid process, or earlobes and forehead. A computer is used to isolate the auditory from other electrical activity to the brain.
  - Electrocochleography: Test is useful for uncooperative patient or patient who cannot volunteer useful information. Test records electrical activity in the cochlea and auditory nerve.
  - Auditory Brainstem Response (ABR): Study measures electrical peaks along auditory pathways of inner ear to brain and provides diagnostic information related to acoustical neuroma, brainstem problems and CVA.
- Vestibular
  - *Caloric test stimulus*: Endolymph of the semicircular canals is stimulated by irrigation of cold (68°F or 20°C) or warm (97°F or 36°C) solution into ear. Patient is seated in supine position, observation of type of nystagmus, nausea and vomiting, falling or vertigo produced is helpful in diagnosing diseases of labyrinth.

    Decreased function is indicated by decreased response and indicates disease of vestibular system. Other ear is tested similarly and results are compared.
  - *Electronystagmography (ENG)*: Electrodes are placed near patient's eyes and movement of eyes (nystagmus) is recorded in graph during specific eye movements and when ear is irrigated. Study diagnosis diseases of vestibular system.
  - *Posturography*: Balance test that can isolate one semicircular canal from others to determine site of lesion. Here inform that test is time consuming and uncomfortable; test can be discontinued at any time at patient's request.
  - *Rotatory chair testing*: The patient is seated in a chair driven by a moto under computer control. It evaluates peripheral vestibular system.

HEARING IMPAIRMENT (HEARING LOSS)

Hearing loss is one of the main problems. Hearing impairment and dizziness (major symptoms of inner ear problem) can hinder communication with others, limit social activities, and negatively impact employment.

Hearing loss diminishes the individual aesthetic enjoyment of major aspects of daily living and can adversely affect quality of life.

Etiology

Hearing loss is a symptom rather than a specific disease or disorder and can be the result of mechanical, sensory or neural problems. The major types of hearing loss includes the following:

- Conducting hearing loss: Loss of the hearing from mechanical problem.
- Sensorineural hearing loss: Loss of hearing involving the cochlea and auditory nerve; bone and air conduction equal but diminished.
- Neural hearing loss: A sensorineural hearing loss originating in the nerve or brainstem.
- Fluctuating hearing loss: A sensorineural hearing loss that varies with time.
- Sensory hearing loss: A sensory neural hearing loss originating in the cochlea and involving the hair cells and nerve endings.
- Sudden hearing loss: A sensorineural hearing loss with a sudden onset.
- Central hearing loss: Loss of hearing from damage to the brain auditory pathways or auditory center.
- Functional hearing loss: Loss of hearing for which no organic lesion can be found.
- Mixed hearing loss: Elements of both conduction and sensorineural hearing loss.

Pathophysiology

Conductive hearing loss results from any interference with the conduction of sound impulses through the external auditory canal, the eardrum, or the middle ear. Conductive hearing loss may be caused by anything that blocks the external ear, such as wax, infection or a foreign body, a chickening, retraction, scarring or perforation of the tymphanic membrane; or any pathophysiological changes in the middle ear affecting or fixing one or more of the ossicles.

Sensorineural hearing loss results from disease or trauma to the inner ear, neural structure, or nerve pathways leading to the brainstem. Some of the causes of "nerve" deafness are infectious diseases, (measles, mumps and meningitis), arteriosclerosis, ototoxic drugs, neur of cranial nerve VIII, otospongiosis (form of progressive deafness) caused by the formation of new abnormal sponges bone in labyrinth, trauma to the head or ear, or degeneration of the organ of corti occuring most commonly from an advancing age (Presbycusis). Central deafness is also known as central auditory dysfunction, results from the inability of the CNS to interpret normal auditory stimuli may be due to tumour or CVA.

Presbycusis is a hearing loss associated with aging that becomes more common after the age of 50, changes in the delicate labyrinthine structures over the decades cause a hearing loss predominently in the higher frequencies.

Hearing loss is frequently accompanied by tinnitus, which is defined in a ringing or any other noise in the ear. Tinnitus accompanies most sensorineural hearing losses and is often a warning of impending or worsening hearing loss. Persistent tinnitus is extremely annoying and the only cure for tinnitus is to correct the underlying cause/condition.

Clinical Manifestation

If the hearing loss is congenital and significant, the young child will have significant speech and language problems. Rehabilitation must be started early. Deafness is often called the "unseen handicap" because it is until conversation is started with a deaf adult that the difficulty in communication is not realized. It is important that the health professionals be aware of the need for thorough validation of deaf persons understanding of health teaching. Descriptive visual aids can be helpful. Because of the difficulty in communication, deaf person always or often seeks relationship with other deaf person. The person who develops hearing loss later in life varies in the amount of loss.

Interference in communication and interaction with others can be the source of many problems for the patient and family. Often the patient refuses to admit or may be unaware of impaired hearing. Irritability is common because of the concentration which the patient must listen to understand speech. The loss of clarity of speech in the patient with sensorineural, hearing loss is most frustrating. The patient may hear what is said, but not understand it. Withdrawal, suspicion, loss of self-esteem and insecurity are commonly associated with advancing hearing loss.

Management

Hearing loss is often first detected by a family member rather than by the affected person. All possible hearing test can be performed for knowing the extent of hearing loss.

Hearing aids offers assistance to many individuals with hearing impairments. Hearing aids amplify sound in a controlled manner and are used by both hard-of-hearing and deaf persons. Hearing aids make sound louder, but do not improve the ability to hear and the amplication of background noise can be confusing especially in crowded settings.

Regardless of the type, the hearing aid consists of the following parts:

- Microphone to receive sound waves from the air and changes sound waves from the air and changes sounds into electrical signals.
- Amplifier to increase the strength of electrical signals.

- Battery to provide the electrical energy needed to operate the hearing aid.
- Receiver (loudspeaker) to change electrical signals back into sound waves.

Speech reading commonly called lip reading can be helpful in increasing communication. The patient is able to use visual cues associated with speech such as gestures and facial expression to help clarify the spoken message. This helps in verbal and nonverbal communication.

There are three types of implanted hearing devices which are either available for use or underdevelopment. They are cochlear implants, bone conduction devices, and semiplantable heavy devices. Now there are numerous assisting devices available to assist the hearing-impaired persons. Direct amplification devices, amplified telephone receivers, alerting systems that flash when activated by sound, an infrared system for amplifying the sound of the TV and combination of FM receiver and hearing aid are all aids that can be explored by the nurse based on the individual patient needs.

Role of Nurse in Dealing with Hearing Problem

Hearing loss is a major health problem to be concerned. The nurse has an important role in preservation of hearing. To fulfil this role, the nurse has many responsibilities, which include educating the patient about keeping the defects out of ears, environmental noise control, ototoxic drugs, risk for heavy loss and detection of hearing loss.

- *Keeping the objects out of ears:* The nurse instructs the patient to keep objects out of the ear. Ears should be cleaned only with a wash cloth and finger. Bobby pins and cotton tipped applicators should especially be avoided. Penetration of the middle ear by a cotton-tipped applicator can cause serious injury to the eardrum and ossicles and may result in facial paralysis as a result of nerve damage. These applicators can also impact cerumen against the eardrum and impair hearing. People should be taught to avoid inserting hard articles into the ear canal, obstructing the ear canal with any object, inserting unclean articles or solutions to the ear or swimming in poluted water.
- *Environmental noise control:* Support environmental noise control. Hearing impairment can be caused by an acute loud noise (acoustic trauma), or by cumulative effects of variation intensities, frequencies and duration of noise (noise-induced hearing loss). Sensorineural hearing loss as a result of increased and prolonged environmental noise such as amplified sound is occurring in young adults at an increasing rate. Health teaching regarding avoidance of continued exposure to noise 85 to 95 decibel (dB) is essential. Continued exposure to noise causes some persons to be more irritable and tense. The range of sounds audible to humans are as follows:

Decibel (dB)
0 : Lower sound audible to the human ear.
30 : Quiet library, soft whisper are the examples.
40 : Living room, quiet office, bedroom away from traffic.
50 : Light traffic at a distance, refrigerator and gentle breeze.
60 : Airconditioner at 20 ft., conversation, sewing machine.
70 : Busy traffic, noisy restaurant. At this dB level, noise may begin to affect hearing if exposure is constant.
Hazardous zone for hearing loss (Hz)
80 : Subway—Heavy city traffic, alarm clock at two feet, factory noise. These noises are dangerous, if exposure to them lasts for more than 8 hours.
90 : Truck traffic—Noisy home appliances, shop tools and lawn mowers. As loudness increases, the "safe" time exposure decreases, damages can occur in less than 8 hours.
100 : Chain saw—Stereoheadphones, pneumatic drill. Even 2 hours of exposure can be dangerous at this dB level. Such 5 dB increases the safe time is cut in half.
120 : Rockband concert in front of speakers, sand blasting, thunder clap. The danger is immediate; exposure to 120 dB can injure ears.
140 : Gunshot blast, jet plane. Any length of exposure time is dangerous; noise at this level may cause actual pain in the ear.
180 : Rocket launching pad. Without air protection, noise at this level causes irreversible damage; hearing loss is inevitable.

The nurse should participate in hearing conservation program in work environment and advise precaution against hearing loss.

The nurse explores the patient's understanding of the role of the noise in hearing loss and encourage moderation of music levels, especially with the use of headphones. The use of protective ear covers in noisy environments is strongly recommended.

- Immunization: Promote childhood and adult immunization including the measles, mumps and rubella (MMR). Various viruses can cause deafness as a result of fatal damage and malformation affecting the ear. Deafness occurs following exposure to rubella in first trimester of pregnancy. Women should be tested for immunity and taken care accordingly.
- Ototoxic drugs can cause ototoxicity in damage to hearing. Monitor the patient reaction to drugs known for ototoxity as drugs list shown earlier.
- Identify the person who has risk for potential of hearing loss.

- Detection of hearing loss: The nurse should be observant of symptoms that indicate hearing loss at all ages.

When communication with the person with hearing impaired, follow the undermentioned guidelines:
- Get the patient's attention by touching him or her lightly, flickering the room light, or raising an arm or hand.
- Stand facing the patient with the light on your face; this will help the person's speech (lip) read.
- Speak slowly and clearly, but do not overaccentuate words.
- Speak in normal tone; do not shout. Shouting overuses normal speaking movements and may cause distortion. If the person has a conductive loss making the voice louder without shouting may be helpful.
- If the person does not seem to understand what is said, express it differently. Some words are difficult to "see" in speech reading, such as white and red.
- Do not smile, chew gum, or cover the mouth when talking to a person with limited hearing.
- Use phrases to convey meaning rather than one-word answers. Supplement words with body language.
- Do not show annoyance by careless facial expression. Persons who are hard of hearing depends more on visual cues.
- Write out proper names or any statements that you are not sure that the patient understood.
- Encourage the use of hearing aid if the person has one; allow him or her to adjust it before speaking.
- Avoid the use of the intercom when communicating with the patient.
- Do not avoid conversation with a person who has hearing loss.
- Post a note at the bedside and nurse's station alerting personnel that the person is hard of hearing.

The nonverbal and verbal aids for communicating with the patient with impaired hearing are summarized as given below and follow the same:
- Nonverbal aids:
  - Draw attention with hand movement.
  - Have speakers face in good light.
  - Avoid covering mouth or face with hands.
  - Avoid chewing, eating, smoking while talking.
  - Maintain eye contact.
  - Avoid distracting environemnt.
  - Avoid careless expression that patient may misinterpret.
  - Use touch.
  - Move close to better ear.
  - Avoid light behind speaker.
- Verbal aids:
  - Speak normally and slowly.
  - Do not overexagerate facial aggressions.
  - Do not overenunciate.
  - Use simple sentences.
  - Rephrase sentences and use different words.
  - Write name or difficult words.
  - Avoid shouting.
  - Speak in normal voice directly into better ear.

The person with a hearing aid should know how to take care for the aid and what to do if the aid does not work. The nurse must also have basic knowledge of the hearing aid to assist persons who are unable or unwilling to do this when ill. The person is encouraged to use hearing aid and store it safely in its case when it is not in use.

The care of the hearing aid includes the following:
- Turn the hearing aid off when not in use.
- Open the battery compartment at night to avoid accidental drainage of the battery.
- Keep an extra battery available at all times.
- Wash the ear mold frequently (daily if necessary) with mild soap and warm water and use a pipe cleaner to cleanse the cannula.
- Do not wear the hearing aid if an ear infection is present.

When hearing aids fail to work, do the following:
- Check the on-off switch.
- Inspect the earmold for cleanliness.
- Examine the battery for correct insertion.
- Examine the cord plug for correct insertion.
- Examine the cord for breaks.
- Replace the battery cord or both, if necessary. The life of batteries varies according to amount of use and power requirements of the aid.

Batteries last from 2 to 14 days.
- Check the position of the earmold in the ear of the hearing aid.
- Whistles, the earmold probably is not inserted properly into the ear canal or the person needs to have a new earmold made.

DISORDERS OF EXTERNAL EAR

The external ear may be affected by masses, trauma, wax impaction, and infection. Most common disorders of the external ear are as follows:
- *Masses:* Masses may be cysts, exostosis (bony protrusions) infection polyps and malignant tumors. Most cysts arise from sebaceous glands. Polyps typically arise from the middle ear or lympatic membrane. Malignant tumors are usually basal carcinomas on the pinna and squamous cell carcinoma in the canal.
  Masses of all types are fairly rare and if treatment is indicated, surgical excisionis performed. Squamous cell carcinoma can invade the underlying tissue and spread throughout the temporal bone and it needs further treatment and follow-up.

- *Trauma:* Both sharp and blunt injuries are common. Penetrating injury can damage hearing but infection and cosmetic appearance are more common concerns. Trauma to the external ear can cause injury to the subcutaneous tissue that may result in a hematoma. If the hematoma is not aspirated, inflammation of the membranes of the ear cartilage (Perichondritis) can result. Antibiotics are given to prevent infection. Supportive care and protection from infection are indicated. Cosmetic surgery may be needed.
- *Foreign bodies:* Many options exist. Insects, cotton pieces, nuts and seeds are the most common. Remove carefully aided by microscopic visualization. Insects are removed by filling canal with mineral oil.
- *Pruritus:* This frequent complaint in elders results from sebaceous gland atrophy and dry epithelium. Dry cerumen worsens the itching. Daily application of glycerine or mineral oil drops decreases dryness and softens cerumen.
- *Impacted cerumen:* This may result from use of cotton-tipped applicator or other object to clean the ear. Age related drying of cerumen increases incidence. Impacted wax is softened and loosened with alternating instillation of glycerine to soften and hydrogen peroxide to loosen the cerumen for removal by warm water irrigation. The clinical manifestation of cerumen impaction includes hearing loss, otalgia, tinnitis, vertigo, cough, cardiac depression (vasal stimulation).
- *External otitis:* External otitis involves inflammation or infection of the epithelium of the auricle and ear canal. The infection begins in the skin lining of the ear canal and can include the canal.

Etiology

External otitis occurs more frequently in summer than in winter. It may be caused by infection, dermatitis or both. Bacteria and fungi may be cause. The bacteria most commonly cultured are *Pseudomonas aeruginosa, Proteus vulgaris, Eucherichia coli,* and *S. aureus.* The most common fungi are *Candida albicans* and *Aspergillus.* Fungi are often causative agents of external otitis, especially in warm, moist climates. The warm, dark environment of the ear canal provides good medium for the growth of microorganism. The localised form of the infection is an ear canal furuncle or abscess. In the presence of a systemic disease such as diabetes, the external otitis can spread wildly through cartilage and bone is then termed as "malignant external otitis". The most common form of external otitis is called "swimmer's ear" because, it is prevalent when water remains in the ear canal. Occasional perichondritis occurs resulting in necrosis of the cartilage and loss of distinctive shape of the auricle.

Pathophysiology

Local trauma, contamination or ongoing exposure to moisture produces an environment conducive to the overgrowth of normal flora. Pain in the external ear is most common symptom. Painful sites are tender because of the close proximity of the bone (a hard surface), when palpating the ear. A clue to early external otitis is tenderness when gently pulling on the pinna. A freeunner of pain is external otitis itching in the ear canal.

Clinical Manifestation

- Pain (otalgia) is one of the first signs of external otitis.
- Drainage from the ear may be serosangineous or purulent. The drainage will be green and have a musty smell.
- Temperature elevation occurs when there is extensive involvement of tissue.
- The swelling of the ear canal can block hearing and cause dizziness.

Management

Diagnosis of external otitis is made by observation with the otoscope light using the largest speculum of the year will accommodate without causing the unnecessary discomfort. Culture and sensitivity studies can be done.

Treatment for an external ear infection depends on the stage of the infection. Local/topical antibiotics are the mainstay of the treatment. If the ear canal is swollen and shut, a "wick" may be inserted to allow the antibiotic drops to penetrate canal. Irrigation may be performed to remove infection and debris. Cotton wicks should be used with caution in young patients, and psychotic patients who may push them farther into the ear. Aspirin or codiene usually controls the pain. Topical antibiotics include polymyxin B. colistin, neomycin, and chloromphenicol Nystretin used for fungal infection. Corticosteroids may also be used unless the infection is fungal. If the surrounding tissue is involved, systemic antibiotics are prescribed. Warm, moist compresses or heat may be applied. Improvement should occur in 48 hours but 7 to 14 days are required for complete resolution. In belief, management or external otitis includes:
- Diagnostic: Otoscopic examination, culture and sensitivity
- Treatment by: Analgesics (depending on severity)
    - Warm compress
    - Cleansing of the canal
    - Ear wick
    - Antibiotic otic drops
    - Systemic antibiotics.

The nurse instructs the patient/family in the safe administration of ear drops as follows:
- Wash hands before and after procedure.

- Warm the ear drops to body temperature before administration. Dizziness may occur from insertion of drops that are too warm or too cold.
- Instruct the patient to tilt his/her head so that the ear to be treated is up.
- Straighten the ear canal by pulling the external ear up and back.
- Instil prescribed number of drops to run along ear canal.
- Press gently several times on the tragus of the ear to ensure proper instillation or hold the head in position for 2 to 3 minutes.

As an ointment is prescribed to control itching or inflammation it is applied using a cotton-tipped applicator. The applicator is inserted any deeper into the ear than cotton and a new applicator used each time.

The nurse instructs the patient to avoid getting water in the ear plugs or cotton with vaseline. If earplugs are used, thorough cleansing with alcohol or mild detergent between uses is recommended to prevent reinfection. The patient should not go swimming during this time.

PROBLEMS OF MIDDLE EAR AND MASTOID

Infection with its associated complications is the most common disorders of the middle ear, but masses, trauma and other conditions may occur. The less common disorders of the middle ear are perforated tympanic membrane, otostenosis and mastoiditis, the more common disorder is otitis media (acute or chronic).

Perforated Tympanic Membrane

Perforation may occur acutely after trauma or as the result of chronic infection. Damage may extend to the osscicles and worsen the hearing loss.

Acute perforation may heal spontaneously. Infection is treated with appropriate systemic antibiotics. Surgical corrections of the perforations may be performed; myringoplasty for the membrane or tympanoplasty if repair includes the middle ear structures. Crafts may be taken from the muscle fascia, a vein, or perichondrium. Success rate is high.

Otosclerosis

Etiology

Otosclerosis, an autosomal dominant disease, is the fixation of the foot plate of the stapes in the oval window. It is common cause of conductive hearing loss in youth, especially women and accelerates during pregnancy. It is common finding in children who have a rare disease known as osteogenesis imperfection. Problem involves the stapes, sclerotic bone forms on the stapes limiting its movement and resulting conductive hearing loss. The underlying cause is unknwon.

Pathophysiology

This spongy bone develops from the bony labyrinth, causing immobilization of the foot plate of the stapes, which reduces the transmission of vibration to the inner ear fluids. Although, hearing loss is typically bilateral one ear may show greater hearing loss progression. The patient often unawares of the problem until the loss becomes so severe, that communication is difficult. Loss of hearing usually becomes increasingly severe.

Management

Otoscopic examination may reveal a reddish bluish of the tympanum (Schwarz's sign) caused by the vascular and bony changes within the middle ear. Tuning fork tests help identify the conductive component of the hearing loss. On the Rinne test, bone conduction will be better than air conduction if hearing loss is greater than that of 25dB. An audiogram demonstrates good hearing by bone conduction.

A hearing aid may initially be prescribed. Advanced diseases is treated surgically through stapedectomy in which a prosthesis replaces the otosclerotic footplate. The success rate is high.

Nursing management of the patient undergoing stapedectomy is similar to that the patient who has undergone a tympanoplasty. Postoperatively the patient may experience dizziness, nausea, and vomiting as a result of stimulation of the labyrinth intraoperatively. Some patients demonstrate nystagmus on lateral gaze because of disturbance of perilymph. Care should be taken to decrease sudden movements by the patient that may bring on to exacerbate dizziness. Actions (coughing, sneezing, lifting, bending, straining during bowel movements) should also be minimized.

To brief the management of otosclerosis includes:
- Diagnosis by otoscope examination, Rinne Test (512 H2 tuning fork), Webers' test, Audiometry and Tympanometry.
- Treatment by hearing aid, stapedectomy, analgesics, antiemetics, antibiotics and antimotion drugs.

Mastoiditis

Chronic otitis media can result in the extension of the infection into the mastoid cavity. The volume of drainage from the middle ear increases.

Antibiotic therapy is the foundation of care, possibly supplemented by irrigations. Aggressive treatment is appropriate to prevent serious complications. Surgical mastoidectomy may be necessary in rare situations.

Otitis Media

Otitis media is a general term that refers to inflammation of the mucous membranes of the middle ear, eustachian tube and mastoid. The mucous membranes are continuous with those of the respiratory tract and infection can easily ascend to the ear.

Etiology

Otitis media is caused by various types of bacteria.
- Acute otitis media: Occurs in childhood is associated with colds, sore throat, and blockage of the eustachian tube. The earlier the initial episode, the greater the risk of subsequent episode. Risk factors include young age, congenital abnormalities, immune deficiencies, passive smoke inhalation, eustachian tube damage from viral infections, family history of otitis media, recent upper respiratory infections, male gender, participation in day care, bottle feeding and allergic rhinitis. Although most patients have mixed infections, bacteria are the predominant aetiologic agents.
- Chronic otitis media: Untreated or repeated attacks of acute otitis media may lead to a chronic condition. This is more common and persons who experience episodes of acute otitis media in early childhood. Organism involved in chronic otitis media include S. aureus, *Streptococcus, Proteus mirabilis, P. aeruginoss* and *E. coli*.
- Serous otitis media: Recurrent infection usually causing drainage and perforation of the tympanic membrane is called chronic otitis media. Between the episodes of infection, fluid may collect in the middle ear (Serous Otitis Media). Blockage in the eustachian tube creates a vacuum that causes fluid formation. When the inflammation accompanying infection subsides and the residual fluid may be too thick to drain.
- Adhesive otitis media: Otitis media is also found in conjunction with upper respiratory infections or allergies. If fluid is present within the ear for a protracted period of time, the tympanic membrane retracts and adhesive otitis media may develop.

Likewise, any long-term blockage of eustachian tube can also lead to adhesive otitis media and result in hearing loss.

Pathophysiology

Since the middle ear transmits sound from the tympanic membrane to the inner ear, middle ear infection frequently causes conductive hearing loss from pressure behind the tympanic membrane. The hearing loss is usually correctable with resolution of the infection. Common additional symptoms include throbbing pain in the affected ear, inflammation, fever and drainage and bulging of the eardrum with possible perforation. Blood, pus, and other material may be present when perforation occurs. A thick yellow purulent discharge is common finding with chronic otitis media.

Tympanosclerosis: A deposit of collagen and calcium within the middle ear can also result from repeated infection. The deposits can harden around the ossicles and contribute to a worsening of any conductive, hearing loss. Because of the anatomy of the temporal bone, middle ear infection can, in rare cases, lead to a life-threatening brain abscess.

Clinical Manifestation

Throbbing pain, fever, malaise, headache and reduced hearing are signs and symptoms of acute otitis media. Chronic otitis media is characterized by clear, bloody or purulent, mucoid or serous discharge accompanied by hearing loss and occasionally by ear pain, nausea and episodes of dizziness. The patient may complain of hearing loss and occasionally by earpain, nausea and episodes of dizziness. The patient may complain of hearing loss, that may be a result of distruction of the ossicles, a tympanic membrane perforation or the accumulation of fluid in the middle ear space. Occasionally, facial palsy or an attack of vertigo may alert the patient to this condition. Chronic otitis is usually painless but if pain is present, it indicates fluid under pressure. Untreated condition can result in perforation of the eardrum and the formation and the formation of cholesteatoma (an accumulation of keratanizing squamous epithelium and the middle ear). It is enlarging tumor behavior which may destroy adjacent bones including ossicles.

Unless removed surgically a cholesteatoma can cause extensive damage to the structures of the middle ear, can erode the bony protection of the facial nerve, may create a labyrinth fistula, or even invade the dura threatening the brain.

In addition, other complication of the chronic otitis media include, sensorineural hearing loss, facial nerve dysfunction, lateral sinus thrombosis, brain or subdural abscess, and meningitis. In otitis media with effusion, patient complains of a feeling of fullness of the ear, "pluged feeling" or popping and decreased hearing.

Management

The diagnosis of otitis media is usually made, based on the patient's symptoms of acute ear pain and fever. Otoscopic examination of the ear canal readily reveals the inflamed bulging tympnic membrane and perforator or drainage if present. Mastoid X-ray may be useful. The aim of treatment is to clear the middle ear infection.

Antibiotic therapy is the key to treatment of otitis media. The common medication for treatment of otitis media include the following:
- Antibiotics inhibit cell wall synthesis bacteriocidal (e.g. Amoxicillin trimethoprim sulphate, methoxazole, amoxicillin clavulanate and cefaclor). During this treatment, nurse assesses for allergies or sensitivities; instructs patient to take medication round the clock,

not to miss any doses and to finish prescriptions completely; assess for super infection.
- Analgesics act as CNS depressant, analgesic, antipyretic, anti-inflammatory (e.g. analgesics, antipyretics, narcotic, acetominaphen with codes. Here nurses assess vital signs, especially temperature; caution patient not to drive or operate machinery if taking codeine; also not to take other CNS depressants, including alcohol, while taking medication; teach patient to increase fluid and roughage intake to avoid constipation, take medication with meals to decrease possible nausea; do not increase dose assess effectiveness of pain relief.
- Antihistamines (e.g. chlorpheniramine) act on H1 receptor antagonist, antiemetic, antitursive, anticholenergic, and local anesthetic action. During this treatment nurse monitors blood pressure (BP) in hypertensive patients. Avoid driving car or operating machinery until drug effects are determined; caution against alcohol use which may cause an additive effect or drowsiness.
- Decongestants (e.g. Pseudoephedrine) is sympathominetic acts directly on smooth muscle; produce little congestive rebound that occurs with nasal sprays. During this treatment the nurse:
    - Monitors heart rate, and BP especially in patient with cardiac history.
    - Teaches patient not to take medications before bedtime because of stimulant effect.
    - Withhold medication if restlessness or tachycardia occurs.
    - Teach patient to avoid other over the counter medications, which may contain ephedrine.

The systemic antibiotic therapy based on the culture and sensitivity results is initiated. In addition, patient may need to undergo frequent evaluation of drainage and debris in OPDs. Antibiotic ear drops and acetic acid ear drops are also used to reduce infection. When the eustachian tube is chronically obstructed, it may be necessary to remove fluid from the middle ear. Myringotomics, with or without tubes are performed to regain normal middle ear and eustachian tube function. Myringotomy involves making tiny incision in the tympanic membrane through which the fluid can be suctioned. To keep the incision open and prevent reaccumulation of fluid, various types of transtympanic tube can be inserted with incision. These tubes fall out by themselves in 3 to 12 months.

Surgical interventions may be necessary if attempts to control the infection medically are unsuccessful. The ossicles become neurotic. Repairing the damage of middle ear infection requires difficult microsurgical procedure, which includes tympano-ossiculoplasty and mastoidectomy. The surgical therapy for chronic ear infected includes:

- *Myringoplasty:* Surgical reconstruction is limited to repair of tympanic membrane perforation.
- *Tympanoplasty without mastoidectomy:* An operation to eradicate disease in the middle ear and to reconstruct the hearing mechanism without mastoid surgery, with or without tympanic membrane grafting.

The nurse will assist in all the aspects of management of otitis media which include ear irrigation, instillation of otic drops, powders, acetic acid drops, and administration of analgesics, antiemetics, systematic antibiotics and preoperation and postoperation care for patients who are under grave surgical trauma.

The nurse instructs the patient against having water in the ear during treatment. This includes showering and shampooing as well as swimming. Commercial plugs or other barriers may be used as temporary protections during shampooing. If an ear wash is prescribed, the nurse teaches the patient and designated family caregiver how to perform ear wash safely at homes. It should be noted that:

- The procedure should be performed by a family member or significant other if possible. It cannot be performed effectively by the patient alone. The following guidelines are helpful for performing earwash.
- Wash hands before and after the procedure.
- Fill a 2 to 3 ounce ear syringe with the solution, warmed to body temperature.
- Position the patient lying on his or her side with the affected ear up.
- Place the tip of the syringe gently into the ear canal. Do not be afraid to insert it into the ear.
- Pump the solution from the syringe back and forth into the ear. Do this vigorously and repeatedly. The fluid must actively move in and out of the ear canal to be effective.
- Assist the patient to lean over the side and let the solution run out of the ear at the end of the procedure.
- Apply ear drops if instructed.
- Continue to use the ear wash solution as instructed for about 2 weeks or until the ear is dry and without drainage.

Most patients undergoing ear surgery have very short-term hospitalization. The nurse teaches the patient what to expect after discharge and how to promote healing during the recovery period. The nurse informs the patient that decreased hearing is expected initially from the presence of swelling and packing in the ear. Cracking or popping noises are commonly heard in the affected ear and are expected. Minor earache and discomfort in cheek and jaw are common, but should be managed effectively with mild analgesics. Dizziness or light-headedness may also be present, initially the patient should be cautious when getting out of the bed and walking. Bleeding and drainage are negligible. A cotton ball frequently provides

adequate dressing. In addition, patient teaching after surgery includes the following:
- Sneezing or coughing, with the mouth open or needed for the first week after surgery.
- Blow the nose gently as needed, one side at a time.
- Avoid vigorous activity until approved by the surgeon.
- Change cotton ball dressing as prescribed.
- Report any drainage other than a slight amount of bleeding to the surgeon.
- Keep ear dry for 6 weeks after surgery.
    - Do not shampoo the hair without barrier.
    - Protect the ear when necessary with two pieces of cotton counter piece saturated with petrolatum.
    - Avoid loud noisy environment. Do not fly until approved by surgeon.
- Balance ear pressure as needed by holding nose, closing mouth and swallowing.

PROBLEMS OF INNER EAR

Sensorineural hearing loss is most common. Inner disorder and may occur in conjunction with an identified ear problem or an isolation. The hearing loss usually is incomplete but it is frequently progressive. The loss of discrimination (understanding words) is characteristic feature of sensorineural hearing loss. The inner part of the ear is so delicate that it does not lend itself to surgical correction or repair. Three symptoms that indicate the disease of inner ear are vertigo (whirling), sensorineural hearing loss, and tinnitus (ringing) in the ear. Symptoms of vertigo arise from the vestibular labyrinth, wherein hearing loss and tinnitus arise from the auditory labyrinth. There is an overlap between manifestation of inner ear problems and CNS disorder.

Acoustic Neuroma

Etiology

It is slow-growing lesion that can occur at any age and usually occurs unilaterally. The tumor typically grows at point where CN VIII enters the internal auditory canal, the temporal bone and may extend to the brainstem. The tumor is more common in women and tends to occur in person between 30 and 60 years of age.

Pathophysiology

The tumor arises from the neurilemma sheath (sheath of Schwann) along the vestibular branch of the nerve and spreads to the cochlear brands. Early diagnosis is important because the tumor can grow and compress the facial nerve and arteries within the ear canal. It is important the tumor should be diagnosed before it becomes intracranial. In rare cases, the pressure of the tumor can become life-threatening symptoms include tinnitus, vertigo, and a progressive unilateral loss of ability to hear high-pitched sound. Disorders of the facial nerve may emerge if the tumor is compressing the structure as well.

Clinical Manifestation

Early symptoms are associated with VIII cranial nerve compression and destruction. They include unilateral, progressive, sensorineural hearing loss, unilateral tinnitus and mild intermittent vertigo. One of the earliest symptoms of an accoustic neuroma is reduced touch sensation in the posterior ear canal.

Management

Diagnostic tests include neurologic audiometric and vestibular tests and CT scan and MRI with gadolinium enhancement. Acoustic neuroma are treated surgically, usually by a neurosurgeon. Surgery to remove small tumors performed through the middle cranial fossa or retrolabyrinthine approach, which preserves hearing and vestibular function. A translabyrinthine approach is usually used for medium sized tumor and when hearing is minimal. Although hearing is destroyed by this approach, advantages include good access to the tumor and preservation of the facial nerve. Retrosigmoid (suboccipital) or transotic approaches are used for large tumors (greater than 3 cm). It is almost impossible to preserve hearing when the tumor is greater than 2 cm.

Menier's Disease

Menier's disease (idiopathic endolymphatic hydrops) is characterized by symptom caused by inner ear disease; episodic vertigo, tinnitus, fluctuating sensorineural hearing loss and aural fullness. It causes significant disability for the patient because of sudden, severe attacks of vertigo with nausea and vomiting.

Etiology

Exact aetiology is unknown. A virus believed to play a role in aetiology, but this has not been proven. This disease occurs when the normal fluid and electrolytic balance of the inner ear is disrupted. It may be result in an excessive accumulation of endolymph in the membranous labyrinth.

Pathophysiology

The underlying pathological changes of Menier's disease include overproduction and defective absorption of endolymph, which increases volume and pressure within the membranous labyrinth until distension results in rupture and mixing of the endolymph and perilymph fluids. The two fluids have significantly different compositions and the mixture disrupts the fluid and electrolyte balance within the labyrinth. Then symptoms of disease develop and exhibit.

Clinical Manifestation

The classic Menier's disease attacks last from 2 to 3 weeks approximately; the time is required to close the rupture and restore fluid balance. The symptoms range from mild to incapacitating and include vertigo, tinnitus, and fluctuating sensorineural hearing loss from degeneration of the hair cells.

Prodromal symptoms include tinnitus, earfullness and hearing loss. Most of the patients experience vertigo associated with nausea, vomiting and ataxia.

Management

The diagnosis is based on the presence of classic triad of symptoms plus a prodromal symptoms of fullness or pressure in the involved ear. The triad includes episodic true vertigo, sensorineural hearing loss and tinnitus and other disorder can also result in vertigo and balance disturbances. To maintain balance, the brain must integrate data from vestibular visual and proprioceptive system. The glyceral test may help in the diagnosis in Menier's disease.

There is no known cure for Menier's disease and the management focusses on controlling symptoms. A variety of medication may be used in the management of this disease, primary and the attempt to control disabling symptom which includes the following:

Acute Care (One or More)

- Sedatives (diazepam, valium)
- Anticholenergic (atropine)
- Vasodilators.
- Antihistamine (diphenhydramine-Benadryl).

Surgery may be performed when the patient symptoms cannot be satisfactorily controlled with medical intervention, which include:
- Conservative surgical interventions
  - Endolympathic shunt.
  - Vestinodular nerve section.
- Destructive surgical intervention
  - Labyrinthotomy.
  - Labyrinthectomy.

Nursing Management

During the acute attack, antihistamines, anticholenergics and benzodiazepam can be used as suppressants for the labyrinth. Acute vertigo is treated symptomatically with bedrest, sedation and antiemetics or drugs for lotion sickness administered orally, rectally or intravenously. The patient requires reassurance and counselling that the condition is not life-threatening. Management between attacks may include vasodilation, diuretics, antihistamines, a low-sodium diet and avoidance of caffeine and nicotine, diazepam used to reduce dizziness. Over a time, patient responds to the prescribed medication.

Diet therapy is frequently quite helpful in controlling the symptoms associated with Menier's disease. The nurse encourages the patient to follow low-salt diet and avoid the excess use of caffeine, sugar, monosodium glutamate and alcohol. The intake of food and fluids over the course of the day, some patients are able to achieve significant symptom improvement from diet modification alone.

Patient needs clear instructions about how to manage in acute attack of vertigo. The nurse instructs the patient to immediately lie down on a firm surface if possible, loosen the clothing, and close the eyes until the acute vertigo stops. Driving and operating machinery should not be attempted during attack. Between the attacks the patient can resume normal activities but should avoid swimming underwater which may cause a loss of orientation.

Loss of balance places the patient with vertigo at high risk for falls. The nurse assists the patient to explore ways to increase the safety of the home environment. The nurse reminds the patient of the importance of sitting or lying down at the onset of dizziness to reduce the risk of falls. The nurse advises the patient to avoid ladders, work on roof or trees or climbing on high places until the vertigo is controlled. Balance therapy can be extremely helpful in supporting the balance network in the brain, and the nurse reinforces the importance of daily practice with these exercises.

Other Vestibular Disorders

- Vestibular neuronitis is the infection of the vestibular nerve with sudden onset commonly caused by virus. First attack of vertigo is most severe and subsequent attacks are less severe.
- Labyrinthitis infection of the labyrinth of inner ear is caused by virus or bacteria. It will have severe vertigo diminishing with time and tinnitus may not be present. There is no permanent sensorineural hearing loss.
- Benign paraxysmal positioned vertigo is degenerative debris free floating in the endolymph. Many theories suggest the cause is idiopathic, (In this, positional vertigo is with quick head movements or position change).
- Presbyastasis (Presbyvertigo) this is balanced disorders of aging due to degenerative changes of the vestibule. Vertigo attack leads to imbalance when standing/walking, leading to falls and injuries.

Presbycusis of the hearing of old age includes the loss of peripheral auditory sensitivity a decline in word recognition ability, and associated psychologic and communication issues. The cause of presbycusis is related to degenerative changes in the inner ear such as loss of hair cells, reduction of blood supply, diminution of endolymph production, decreased basilar membrane flexibility and loss of neurons in the cochlear nuclei. Noise exposure is though to be a common factor related to presbycusis.

Procedure 20.7: Irrigating the External Auditory Canal

Purposes
- To remove discharge from the canal.
- To facilitate removal of cerumen or foreign body.

Nursing Focus

Ask if the patient has a history of draining ears or has ever had a perforation or other complications from a previous ear irrigation. If the reply is "Yes" check with the health care provider before proceeding with the irrigation.
- Equipment: Kind and amount of solution desired (usually warm water).
- Solutions:
  - Ear Syringe or irrigating container with tubing, clamp and catheter.
  - Protective towels.
  - Cotton balls and cotton-tipped applicators.
  - Solution bowl and emesis basin.
  - Bag for disposable items.

Procedure: Preparatory Phase
- After explaining procedure to the patient, place in a position of sitting or lying with head tilted forward and toward affected ear.
- Position protective towels.

DISORDERS OF NOSE AND SINUSES

Deviated Septum

Deviated septum is deflection of the normally nasal septum. It is most commonly caused by trauma to the nose or congenital disproportion, a condition in which the size of the septum is not proportioned to the size of the nose.

On inspection, septum is to one side, altering the air passage symptoms are variable. The patient may experience obstruction to nasal breathing, nasaledema, or dryness of the nasal mucosa with crusting and bleeding (epistaxis). A severely deviated septum may block drainage of mucus from the sinus cavities, resulting in infection (sinusitis). Nasal breathing is subjective and only the patient can gauge the degree of obstruction and amount of discomfort it causes.

Health promotion is aimed at prevention of precipitating factors such as accidental falls in childhood. Medical management of deviated septum includes the use of decongestants or a nasal corticosteroid only to reduce nasal edema. Before using the inhaler, ask the person to gently blow their nose, making sure that their nostrils are clear. Then follow these steps:
- Remove the cap from the nasal inhaler.
- Shake the container well.
- Hold the inhaler between the thumb and forefinger.

Nursing action	Rationale
Performance phase	
Use a cotton applicator to remove any discharge on outer ear	To prevent carrying discharge deeper into canal
Place basin close to the patient's head and under the ear	To provide a receptacle to receive irrigating solution
Test temperature of solution it should be comfortable to the inner aspect of wrist area *Gerontologic alert*: Take special care not to irrigate an older adult's ear with cold water, as dizziness may be happened	Solutions that are hot or cold are most uncomfortable and may start a feeling of dizziness
Ascertain whether impaction is due to a foreign hydroscopic (attracts or absorbs moisture) body before proceeding	If water contacts such a substance, it may cause it to swell and produce intense pain
Gently pull the outer ear upward and backward (adult) or downward and outward (child)	To straighten the ear canal (See figure)
Place tip of syringe or irrigating catheter at opening of ear, gently direct stream of fluid against sides of canal	To decrease direct force of irrigation against eardrum and possibility fo rupturing it
If an irrigating container is used, elevate only high enough to remove secretions or no more than 15 cm (6 in) above patient's ear	To provide safe and effective pressure of fluid, if height is more than 15 cm (6 in) pressure will be too great and may damage tissue
Observe for signs of pain or dizziness	Discontinue treatment if they occur
If irrigating does not dislodge the wax, instil several drops of prescribed glycerin. Carbamide peroxide (Debrox) or other solutions as directed 2 or 3 times daily for 2–3 days	To soften and loosen impaction

Note: This is more effective in dislodging cerumen than if the flow of solution were directed straight into the canal.

Follow-up phase
- Dry external ear.
- Remove soiled equipment and make the patient comfortable.
- Patient should lie on irrigated (affected) side for a few minutes after procedure to allow any remaining solution to drain out.
- Record time of irrigation, kind and amount fo solution, nature of return flow, and effect of treatment.

- Tilt the head back, slightly and insert the end of the inhaler into the nostril, painting it slightly towards the outside nostril wall. Hold the nostril closed with one finger.
- Press down the container to release one dose and at the same time inhale gently.
- Ask patient to hold the breath for a few seconds then breathe out slowly through the mouth.
- Withdraw the inhaler from the nostril and repeat the process for the other nostril if more than one puff is prescribed for nostril repetition.
- Replace the protective cap on the inhaler.

Surgery is an option for patient with severe symptoms. A nasal septoplasty is performed to reconstruct and properly align the deviated septum. Nasal septoplasty can be performed alone or with a rhinoplasty.

Nasal Fracture

Nasal fracture is most often caused by trauma of substantial force to the middle of the face. Complications of the fracture include airway obstruction, epistaxis and cosmetic deformity. Nasal fractures are classified unilateral, bilateral or complex. A unilateral fracture typically produces little or no displacement. Bilateral fractures, the most common fractures, give the nose a flattened look. Powerful frontal blows cause complex fractures, which may also shatter frontal bones. Diagnosis is based on the health history, direct observation and X-ray finding.

On inspection, nurse should assess the patient's ability to breathe through each side of the nose and note the presence of edema, bleeding, or hematoma. There may be ecchymosis under one or both eyes. The nose is inspected internally for evidence of septal deviation, hemorrhage or clear drainage, which suggest leakage of CSF. If clear drainage is observed, a specimen may be sent for determining CSF. Injury of sufficient force to fracture nasal bones results in considerable swelling of soft tissues. With extensive swelling, it may be difficult to verify the extent of deformity or the repair the fracture until several days later when edema is subsiding.

The goals of nursing management are to reduce edema, prevent complications, educate the patient and provide emotional support. Ice may be applied to the face and nose to reduce edema and bleeding. When a fracture is confirmed, the goal of management is realignment of the fracture using closed or open reduction (septoplasty, or rhinoplasty). These procedures re-establish cosmetic appearance and proper function of the nose and provide an adequate airway.

Nursing management of nasal surgery (rhinoplasty, septoplasty, or nasal fracture reductions) includes the following:
- Before surgery, the patient should be instructed to avoid taking aspirin containing drugs for 2 weeks to reduce bleeding.
- In post operative period, include assessment of respiratory status, pain management, and observation of the surgical site for hemorrhage and edema.
- Health teaching is important, because, these procedures involve a short hospital stay and the patient must be able to detect early and late complications. The problem of patient undergoing surgery may have certain problems needing nursing care.
- *Altered health maintenance* r/t Lack of knowledge of the procedure, for which nurse has to explain the procedure, expected post-operative course, and required self-care to decrease anxiety and increase patient cooperation. Answer questions as needed and assess the patient perception about body image and expectation of surgery to obtain information to use in patient care.
- *Ineffective breathing pattern related to presence of packaging*, nasal edema, intranasal splints, as manifested by complaints of shortness of breath, alterations in respiration rate, rhythm or depth. Here, the nurse has to assess for respiratory distress, elevate head of bed, provide supplemental oxygen (if prescribed).

  Instruct the patient to blow nose, open mouth when sneezing, and coughing to maintain correct position of packing. Apply cold compress to incisional area to promote vasoconstriction and reduce edema. Instruct the patient to call nurse for any untoward effects.
- *Pain related to edema* from surgical procedure, for which nurse should teach patient correct analgesic schedule, describe to patient the amount of pain expected, and teach patients non-pharmacological measures (elevation of head, cold compress) and avoid using aspirin on NSAIDs. Teach patient gentle cleaning techniques such as use of cotton swabs, with hydrogen peroxide to clean crusting and application of water soluble jelly to lubricate when packing has been removed to promote cleanliness and prevent infection and promote use of bedside humidifier to decrease drying of mucosa and promote comfort and management of nasal hemorrhage or epistaxis.

Simple first aid measures should be used first to control epistaxis. The nurse should keep the patient quiet, position the patient in a sitting stature, leaning forward, or if not possible, in a reclining position with head and shoulders elevated; apply direct pressure by pinching the entire soft laven portion of the nose for 10 to 15 minutes; apply ice compresses to the nose, and have the patient suck on ice; partially insert a small guaze pad into the bleeding nostril and apply digital pressure if bleeding continues and obtain medical assistance, if bleeding does not stop. When first aid measure is not effective, management involves localisation of the bleeding site and application of a vasoconstrictive agent cauterization or anterior packing indicated. Anterior packing may consist of ribbon guaze impregnated with antiseptic ointments that is wedged firmly in the desired location and remain in place for 48 to 72 hours. If posterior packing is required, the patient should be hospitalised. Inflatable balloons may be used as the nasal pack on gauze rolls may be inserted. Stringes attached to the packaging are brought to the outside and taped to check for ease of removal. A nasal sling (folded 2 × 2 in gauze pad) should be taped over the nares to absorb drainage. Since packing is painful, mild narcotic analgesic is administered.

Failure of posterior packing indicates surgical correction.

Rhinitis

Rhinitis refers to inflammation of the mucous membrane of the nose. It may be acute or chronic or allergic rhinitis. All forms of rhinitis cause sneezing, nasal discharge with nasal obstruction and headache. Etiology, pathophysiology and diverse manifestations are according to this type as follows:

Acute Rhinitis

Etiology: Acute rhinitis (coryza, common cold) is caused by viruses that invade the upper respiratory tract. It is an inflammatory, condition of the mucous membrane of the nose and accessory sinuses caused by a filterable virus. It affects almost everyone at some time and occurs most often in winter with additional high incidences in early rain fall and spring. Some of the known causes of the common cold are 100 serotypes of rhinoviruses, coronoviruses, adenoviruses, echoviruses, influenza and parainfluenza viruses and coxsackieviruses.

It is the most prevalent infectious disease and is spread by airborne droplet sprays emitted by the infected person while breathing talking, sneezing or coughing or by direct hand contact. Frequency increases in winter months, when people stay indoors and overcrowding is more common. Other factors such as chilling, fatigue, physical and emotional stress and the patient compromised immune status, may increase susceptibility.

Clinical manifestations: The patient with acute viral rhinitis typically first experiences tickling, irritation, sneezing or dryness of the nose or nasopharynx followed by copious nasal secretions, some nasal obstruction, watery eyes, elevated temperature, general malaise, and headache. After the early profuse secretions, the nose becomes more obstructed and the discharge is thicker, within few days, the general symptoms improve, nasal passages reopen, and normal breathing is established. Secondary invasion by bacteria may cause pneumonia, acute bronchitis sinusitis and otitis media.

Management: No specific treatment exists for the common cold. The goals of treatment are to:
- Relieve symptoms
- Inhibit spread of infections, and
- Reduce the risk of bacterial complications.

Rest, fluids, proper diet, antipyretics and analgesics are helpful. Complications of acute rhinitis include pharyngitis, sinusitis, otitis media, tonsilitis, and chest infection. Treat with proper antibiotic therapy. Antibiotics have no effect on virus if taken unjudiciously, may produce resistance organisms.

Allergic Rhinitis

Etiology: Allergic rhinitis (hayfever) is a type I-hypersensitive reaction. It is the reaction of the nasal mucosa to a specific antigen (allergen). Attacks of seasonal rhinitis usually occur in spring and fall and are caused by allergy to pollens from trees, flowers or grasses or weeds. Inhaled allergens are classified as outdoor (seasonal) also called acute or indoor (perennial), also called chronic. The outdoor allergens are pollen of trees, grasses or weeds. Inhaled allergens are classified as outdoor (seasonal) also called acute or indoor (perennial lasting for long time), also called chronic. The outdoor allergens are pollen of trees, grasses or weeds. The indoor allergens are spores of molds, dustmites, and animal danders.

Clinical manifestation: Manifestations of allergic rhinitis are nasal congestion, sneezing, watery, itchy eyes and nose, altered sense of smell and thin watery nasal discharge. The nasal turbinates appear pale, boggy and swollen. The turbinates may fill the air space and press against the nasal septum. The posterior ends of the turbinates can become so enlarged that they obstruct sinus aeration or drainage and result in sinusitis. With chronic exposure to allergens the patient responses include, headache, congestion, pressure and postnasal drip. The patient may complain of cough, hoarseness, or the recurrent need to clear throat. Congestion may be sufficient to cause snoring. Nasal polyps may be present if the allergy has persisted for a long time.

Management: There are several measures used in management of allergic rhinitis. The measures to reduce symptoms of allergic rhinitis are:
- Avoidance is the best treatment.
- *Avoid house dust:* Use the approach "less is best". Focus on the bedroom. Remove carpeting. Limit furniture. Enclose the pillows, mattresses and springs in airtight, zipper-sealed, vinyl cloth bags, install an airfilter if possible. Close the airconditioning vent into the room.
- *Avoid house dust-mites:* Wash building in hot water (130°F) weekly. Wear a mask when vacuuming. Double bag the vacuum-cleaner. Install a filter on the outlet post of the vacuum cleaner. Avoid sleeping or lying on upholstered furniture. Remove carpets that are laid down on concrete. If possible, have someone else for cleaning the house.
- *Avoid mold spores:* The three 'D's that promote growth of mold spores are darkness, dampness, and drafts.

Avoid places where humidity is high (e.g. basements, camps on the lake, clothe hampers, greenhouses, stables, barns).

Dehumidifiers are rarely helpful. Ventilate closed rooms, open doors and install fans. Consider adding windows to dark room. Consider keeping lights on in closets. A basement light with a timer that provides light several hours a day decreases mold growth:

- *Avoid pollens:* Stay inside with closed doors and windows during high pollen season. Avoid the use of fans. Install an airconditioner with a good airfilter. Wash filter weekly during high pollen season. Put the car air conditioner on "recirculate" when driving.
- *Avoid pet allergens:* Remove pets from the interior of the home. Clean the living area thoroughly. Do not expect instant relief. Symptoms usually do not improve significantly for 2 months following pet removal.
- *Avoid smoke:* The presence of a smoker will sabotage the best of all possible symptoms reduction programme. The drug therapy involves the use of antihistamines, decongestants and nasal sprays. An oral antihistamine or oral decongestant is typically used first. If therapy is not effective, a nasal corticosteroid spray may be used to decrease inflammation. Corticosteroid administered by a nasal spray are purely absorbed in the system in circulation.
    - *Antihistamines* bind with H1 receptors on target cells, block of histamine binding. Relieve acute symptoms of allergic response (itching, sneezing, excessive secretions, mild congestions) may cause sedation (diminished alertness, slow reaction time, somnolence) and stimulation (restlessness, nervous insomnia) and may cause palpitation tachycardia, urinary retention or frequency. So, the nurse warns the patient regarding side effects and teaches the patient to report palpitations, change in heart rate, change in bowel, bladder habits and instruct the patient not to use alcohol with antihistamines because of additive depressive effects.

    An example of antihistamine includes first generation agents such as ethanalamines (e.g. benzedrine) ethylenediamines, alkylamins (chlorpheniramine) piperazines, piperidine, phenothazine (phenergan), etc. The second generation agents such as Astemizole, Loratadine, Cetrizone, etc.
    - *Decongestants* stimulate adrenergic receptors on blood vessels promote vasoconstriction and reduce nasal edema and rhinorrhea. Example, oral pseudoephedrin (sudafed), topical-nasal-spray: e.g. oxymetazoline, phenylephrine. The side effects include CNS stimulation causing insomnia, excitation, headache, irritability, increased blood and ocular pressure, dysuria, palpitations, tachycardia. Here the nurse advises patient of adverse reactions. Advise some preparations are contraindicated for patients with cardiovascular diseases, hypertension, diabetes, glaucoma, prostate hyperplasia, hepatic and renal disease. Teach patient that these drugs should not be used for more than 3 days or more than 3-4 times a day. Longer use increases risk of rhinitis medicamentosa.
    - *Corticosteroids* nasal spray inhibits inflammatory response. At recommended dose, systemic side effects are unlikely because of low systemic absorption. If used greater than prescribed dose, mild transient nasal burning and stringing occurs. Here nurse should teach patient correct use instruct patient to use on regular basis and not p r n reinforce that spray acts to decrease inflammation, and discontinue the use of nasal infection to develop.
    - *Mast cell stabilizer*, i.e. nasal spray (cromolyn spray, nidocromia spray) inhibits degranulation of sensitized mast cells which occurs after exposure to specific antigen. Has minimal side effects. Teach patient correct use, explain occurrence of nasal irritation or burning.
    - *Anticholinergic* nasal spray (ipratropium bromide), blocks hypersecretory effects by competing in binding sites on the cell. Reduces rhinorrhea and common cold, allergic and non-allergic rhinitis. The side effects include dryness of mouth and nose. Does not cause systemic side effects.

Chronic rhinitis is a chronic inflammation of the mucous membrane with increased nasal mucosa caused by repeated acute infections, by an allergy or by vasomotor rhinitis. The cause of vasomotor rhinitis is unclear but this condition may result from an instability of the autonomic nervous system caused by stress, tension or some endocrine disorders. Rhinitis may also be caused by the overuse of nose drops.

In addition to measures of management of rhinitis suggestion is made in acute allergic rhinitis, that the patient should be taught to self administration of nose drops as given below:

- Wash hands
- Assume a position that will facilitate flow of medication:
    - Sit on chair and tip head well backward, or
    - Lie down with head extended over the edge of bed, or
    - Lie down with pillow under shoulders and head tipped backwards.
- Turn head to side that will receive the drops.
- Place no more than three drops of solution into each nostril at one time (unless otherwise prescribed).
- Remaining position with head tilted backward for 3 to 5 minutes to permit solution to reach posterior nares.

- If marked congestion is still present 10 minutes after nose drop insertion, another drop or two of solutions may be administered (nasal constriction from first insertion may facilitate additional drops reaching posterior nares).
  And advise the person with rhinitis regarding:
  - Obtain additional rest.
  - Drink at least 2 to 3 litres of fluid daily
  - Medications: Use nasal spray or nose drops two or three times per day as ordered.
- Prevention of further infection:
  - Blow nose with both nostrils open to prevent infected matter from being forced into eustachian tube.
  - Cover mouth with disposable tissues when coughing and sneezing to prevent droplet nuclei from contaminating the air.
  - Dispose of used tissues carefully.
  - Avoid exposure when possible (i.e., avoid crowds, people with cold specific allergens). Elderly persons and those with chronic lung diseases are particularly vulnerable and should have a flu shot yearly.
  - Wash hands frequently and especially after coughing, blowing the nose, sneezing, and so on. Evidences suggest that several types of colds are transmitted from person to person by hand contact and from touching objects handled by persons with a cold.
  - Seek medical attention if the following are present.
- High fever, severe chest pain, earache.
- Symptoms lasting longer than 2 weeks.
- Recurrent cold.

Sinusitis

The sinuses are airfilled cavities lined with nucleus membranes. Any inflammation of the mucous membrane of the sinuses is termed as "Sinusitis".

Etiology

Sinusitis develops when the ostia (exit) from the sinuses is narrowed or blocked by inflammation or hypertrophy (swelling) of the mucosa. The secretions that accumulate behind the obstruction provide a rich medium for growth of bacteria, viruses and fungi all of which cause infections.
- Bacterial sinusitis is most commonly caused by *Streptococcus pneumoniae, Haemophilus influenzae,* or *Moraxella catarrhalis,* beta-hemolytic streptococcus, Klebsiella pneumoniae, anareobic organism.
- Viral sinusitis follows an upper respiratory infection in which the virus penetrates the mucous membrane and decreases ciliary transports, e.g. rhinovirus, parainfluenza, adenovirus.
- Fungal sinusitis is uncommon and is usually found in patients who are debilated or immunocompromised.

Acute sinusitis usually results from an URI, allergic rhinitis, swimming or dental manipulations all of which cause inflammatory changes and retention of secretions. Chronic sinusitis generally results from repeated episodes of a acute sinusitis that result in irreversible loss of the normal ciliated epithelium lining the sinus cavity.

Pathophysiology

The first symptom of acute bacterial sinusitis is usually a stuffy nose followed by slowly developing pressure over the involved sinus. Other signs and symptoms include general malaise and toxicity, persistent cough, postnasal drip, headache slightly elevated or normal temperature and mild leukopnea. Symptoms worsen over 48 to 72 hours culminating in severe localised pain and tenderness over the involved sinus. The patient often believes that the pain is due to an infected tooth.

In acute frontal and maxillary sinusitis pain usually does not appear until 1 to 2 hours after awakening. It increases for 3 to 4 hours after awakening and then becomes less severe in the afternoon and evening. There may be bloody or blood-tinged discharge from the nose in the first 24 to 48 hours. The discharge rapidly becomes thick, green and copious, blocking the nose. The throat may become inflamed and sore on one side, because of the purulent discharge.

Clinical Manifestation

Acute sinusitis causes significant pain over the affected sinus purulent nasal drainage, nasal obstruction, congestion, fever and malaise. The patient looks and feels sick. Assessment involves inspection of the nasal mucosa and palpation of the sinus points for pain. Findings that indicate acute sinusitis include a hyperemic and edematous mucosa, enlarged turbinates and tenderness over the involved sinuses. Pain is caused by the accumulation of pus and absorption of air behind a blocked ostium. The patient also experiences recurrent headaches that change in intensity with position or when secretions drain.

Management

For most patients, diagnosis is made without any studies. Certain cases of radiographic studies are indicated particularly chronic sinuses, conventional sinus X-rays, computed tomography (CT) and MRI. Fibrocystic examination of the nose (Rhinoscopy) may also be used. Management of acute bacterial sinusitis centers on relief of pain and shrinkage of the nasal mucosa. Ibuprofen and oral decongestant such as pseudoephedrine are commonly prescribed. In some patients, codeine may be required for pain relief. The antibiotic of choice is limited for 10 days.

If patient does not improve after 5 days of amoxicilline a changes of antibiotics may be necessary, which includes Loracarbef amoxicillin clavulanate potassium (Augmentin), cefaclor, doxycycline, trimethoprim, and sulfamethoxazole, clarithromycin, azithromycin (5 days).

Patient may obtain relief from saline nasal sprays steam, from a shower, or a humidifier. Hot wet packs applied to the face over the infected sinus (es) either continuously or for 1 to 2 hours at a time for four times a day may provide symptomatic relief. A washcloth wrung out in hot water is convenient way to provide wet pack.

Acute frontal sinusitis with pain, terness and edema of the frontal or sphenoid sinus may require hospitalization because of the risk of intracranial complications and osteomyelitis. High dose of intravenous antibiotic and nasal congestants orally or spray may be ordered.

Fungal sinusitis can range from mild infections resembling chronic sinusitis to severe life-threatening invasive infections, needs prolonged and necessary antibiotics or surgical drainage of sinuses.

Invasive fungal sinusitis is most likely to occur in transplant patients, patients on chemotherapy, patients with AIDS, or persons with controlled diabetes. Aspergillus and Mucor are two types of fungi most prone to cause invasive disease. Symptoms include facial fullness, cranial neuropathies, and pain.

Proptosis of the eye, facial swelling and blood-stinged discharge may be present. These patients need hospitalization. Treatment includes IV amphoterun B, aggressive surgical management are required.

The types of sinus surgery are:
- *Functional endoscopic sinus surgery (FESS):* Here sinus endoscope enters sinus and removes diseased mucosa and opens ostia. It is used for chronic sinusitis and removal of polyps.
- *Caldwell-Luc (Radical Antrum perforation):* Here clearing out of maxillary sinus through incision under upper lip, It is used as chronic maxillary sinusitis.
- *Transnasal external or transantral ethimoidectomy:* Various approaches used to excise inject ethmoid and sphenoid cells. It is used in chronic ethimoid and sphenoid sinusitis.
- *Frontal sinusotomy:* A complete removal of diseased mucosa of both frontal sinus, space packed with subcutaneous fat from abdomen. Performed in chronic frontal sinusitis.
- *Ethimoid sinus surgery:* Ethmoid sinus removed and anterior wall of sphenoid sinus opened. Performed in chronic sphenoid sinusitis.

The nurse has to perform preoperative teaching for the person undergoing sinus surgery, which includes: Determine patients' understanding about the surgical procedure. Clarify misconceptions and answer patients' and family questions. Explain that the patient will:

- Have nothing to eat or drink for 6 to 8 hours preoperatively.
- Receive a sedative before surgery.
- Feel pressure, not pain during surgery.
- Have a nasal pack for 24 to 48 hours postoperatively and may feel like he or she has a "head cold".
- Have "black eyes" and swelling around the nose and eyes for 1 to 2 weeks postoperatively.
- Have prescription for pain medication as needed.

Postoperative care of the person undergoing sinus surgery will include:
- After general anesthesia, position patient well into the side to prevent swelling of aspiration of blood drainage.
- Administer cool mist via face tent or collar, or provide humidifier.
- When the patient is awake, remind him or her to expectorate secretions and not swallow them.
- Encourage mid Fowler's position when fully awake to promoted drainage and decrease edema.
- Apply ice compresses over nose (or ice bag over nose, (or ice bag over maxillary and frontal sinuses) in the early postoperative period.
- Monitor patient for:
  - Excessive bleeding from nose (may be evidence of repeated swallowing).
  - Decreased visual acuity, especially diplopia, indicating damage to optic nerve or muscles of globe of eye.
  - Complaint of pain over the individual sinus, which may indicate infection or inadequate drainage.
  - Fever–Take temperature rectally.
- Give frequent mouth care using a soft toothbrush. If there is an oral incision, mouthcare is given before meals to improve appetite and after meals to decrease danger of infection.
- Change nasal pad when it is soiled.
- Apply ice compresses to ecchymosis areas to constrict blood vessels, decrease oozing and edema, and help relieve pain.
- Encourage liberal fluid intake. Patient may be very thirsty because of dry mouth from mouth breathing.
- Teach patient to:
  - Avoid blowing nose for at least 48 hours after packing is removed to prevent bleeding.
  - Avoid sneezing: If the patient must sneeze he or she should keep mouth open.
  - Avoid lifting heavy objects.
  - Report signs of infection–fever, purulent discharge to surgeon.
  - Expect tarry stools from swallowed blood for a few days.
  - Avoid constipation (Valsalvas manoeuvre i.e., straining can cause bleeding).
  - Expect that ecchymosis of nose and eyes will begin to change color over next 1 to 2 weeks.

– Take prophylactic antibiotics as prescribed. Do not stop until all medication is taken.

In addition, patients are advised to take more rest to heal; precaution to be given blowing and sneezing. Keep head elevated for proper breathing, small dressing pad around dressing to absorb drainage, and instruct the patient not to take aspirin or any product containing aspirin, which can cause bleeding and caution with oral hygiene to avoid injury to the incisions.

DISORDERS OF THROAT

Acute Pharyngitis

Acute pharyngitis is an acute inflammation of the pharyngeal walls. It may include the tonsils, palate, and uvula.

Etiology

It may be caused by hemolytic streptococci, staphylococci, other bacteria, filterable virus or fungi. Acute follicular pharyngitis (strep throat) results from beta hemolytic streptococcal invasion. *Neisseria gonorrhoeae* and *Corynebacterium diphtheriae* and other bacteria causing pharyngitis. Fungal pharyngitis caused by candidiasis can develop prolonged use of antibiotics or inhaled corticosteroids as in immunosuppressed patient (e.g. AIDS).

Pathophysiology

Dryness of the throat is common complaint. The throat appears red, and soreness may range from slight scratchiness to severe pain with difficulty in swallowing. A hacking cough may be present. Children often develop a very high fever, whereas adults may have only a mild elevation of temperature, symptoms usually precede or occur simultaneously with the onset of acute rhinitis or acute sinusitis.

Clinical Manifestation

In follicular pharyngitis uniform infection of pharyngeal walls, purulent exudate, edema of lymphoid tissue of palate, tonsils uvula, occur and show sore throat, slightly elevated temperature, and malaise.

In gonococcal or viral pharyngitis, vesicles may be present on pharyngeal walls and tonsils occur. There will be minimal discomfort, fever, diffuse sore throat.

In infectious mononucleosis (Epstein-Barr virus), exudate on pharyngeal walls and tonsils, spleen may be enlarged. There will be a sore throat, cervical lymphadenopathy, and fever.

Fungal pharyngitis (e.g. especially cardiases-Thrush) develop in patient who is immune suppressed and in prolong antibiotics. There will be pus, dysphagia, white plaque, in mouth or on pharyngeal walls.

Management

Acute pharyngitis is usually relieved by hot saline throat gargles. An ice collar may make the person feel more comfortable. For adults acetylsalicylic acid administered orally. Aspergum may be prescribed. Lozenges containing a mild anesthetic may help relieve local soreness. Moist inhalations may help relieve local soreness. A liquid diet usually is better tolerated than solid food and fluids to at least 2.5 litre per day is encouraged.

Oral hygiene may prevent drying and cracking of the lips and usually refreshes the mouth. If the temperature is elevated, the person should remain in bed and even if ambulatory and a febrile, should have extra rest.

A throat culture is necessary to identify the offending organism. For follicular pharyngitis, the choice of antibiotic is penicillin. If person is allergic to penicillin, erythromycin or other antibiotic is prescribed. Candida infections are treated with nystatin and antifungal, antibiotic.

The goals of nursing management are infection control, symptomatic relief and prevention of secondary complications. The patient should be encouraged to increase fluid intake, cool, bland liquids and gelatin will not irritate pharynx. Citrus fruits juice should be avoided because they irritate the mucous membrane. And make the patient understand the need to take prescribed antibiotic until the course is completed.

Acute Follicular Tonsillitis

Acute follicular tonsillitis is an acute inflammation of the tonsils and their crypts. It is usually caused by the streptococcus organism. It is more likely to occur when the persons's resistance is low, and it is common in children.

Pathophysiology and Clinical Manifestation

The onset is almost always sudden, and symptoms include sore throat, pain on swallowing, fever, chills, general muscle aching and malaise. These systems often last for 2 to 3 days. The pharynx and tonsils appear red, and the peritonsillar tissues are swollen. Sometimes a yellowish exudate drains from crypts in the tonsils. A throat culture usually is taken to identify the offending organism.

Complications of untreated tonsillitis include heart and kidney damage, chorea and pneumonia. Incidence of these complications is decreasing with early diagnosis and widespread use of penicillin. Recurrent attacks of tonsillitis need to undergo tonsillectomy. This procedure is usually performed from 4 to 6 weeks after an acute attack is subsided.

Peritonsillar abscess typically occurs as a complication of acute pharyngitis and acute tonsillitis if bacterial invasion of one or both tonsils. The tonsils may enlarge sufficiently to threaten airway patency. Infections extend from the tonsils to form an access in the surrounding tissues. The presence of pus behind the tonsils causes difficulty in swallowing, talking and opening the mouth, the difficulty in swallowing may be so great that the person is unable to swallow. Pain is severe and may extend to the ear on the affected side. The patient will experience high fever, leukocytosis and chills.

Management

The patient with acute tonsillitis is encouraged to rest and take generous amounts of fluid orally. Warm saline throat gargle (irrigation) may be ordered, and antibiotics are given for streptococcal pharyngitis, acetaminophen (tyclerol) and codeine sulfate may be ordered for pain and discomfort. An ice collar applied to the neck may relieve discomfort.

Early detection and treatment with IV antibiotic therapy may clear the infection and prevent abscess development. If antibiotics to which the offending organism is sensitive are administered early, infection subsides. If the peritonsillar abscess caused by anerobic organisms hydrogen peroxide (an oxidizing agent) in the form of mouthwash may help to relieve symptoms. If an abscess develops incision and drainage are required. An emergency tonsillectomy may be performed, or an elective tonsillectomy may be scheduled after the infection subsided.

Chronic Enlargement of Adenoids and Tonsils

Tonsils and adenoids are lymphoid structures located in the oropharynx and nasopharynx. They reach full size in childhood and then begin to atrophy during puberty. When adenoids enlarge, usually results of chronic infections but sometimes for no known reason they cause nasal obstructions. The person breathes through mouth, snores loudly, may have a dull facial expression and may have reduced appetite, because the blocked nasopharynx can interfere with swallowing. Hypertrophy of the tonsils does not usually block the oropharynx but may affect speech and swallowing and cause mouth breathing.

Pathophysiology

The tonsils are red and swollen with yellow or white exudate found mainly in the crypts of the tonsils. Signs and symptoms include fever, dry throat, malaise, dysphagia, otalgia, and a feeling of fullness in the throat. Lymph nodes in upper part of the neck is swollen and palpable.

Management

The tonsils and adenoids are removed when they become enlarged and cause symptoms of obstruction, when they are chronically infected. When the person has repeated attacks of tonsillitis or after repeated peritonsillar abscess. Chronic infections of these structures usually do not respond to antibiotics and may become foci of infections by spreading organisms to other parts of the body such as heart and kidney.

Tonsillectomy is performed with either general or local anaesthesia. After tonsils are removed, pressure is applied to stop superficial bleeding. Bleeding vessels are tied off with sutures or by electrocoagulation. The person is monitored carefully for hemorrhage, especially when sleeping, because a large amount of blood may be lost without any external evidence of bleeding. The person who is bleeding excessively often is returned to the operating room for surgical treatment to stop the hemorrhage. If sutures are used, the person will have more pain and discomfort than that occurring after simple tonsillectomy and may be unable to take solid food for several days.

The tough, yellow, fibrous membrane that forms over the operative site begins to break away between the fourth and eight postoperative days and haemorrhage may occur. The separation of the membranes accounts for throat being more painful at this time.

Pink granulation tissue soon becomes apparent and by the end of the third postoperative week, the area is covered with normal mucous membrane.

The following points to be kept in mind while taking care of a person after tonsillectomy:
- Position patient on side until fully awake after general anesthesia of in mid-Fowler's position when awake.
- Monitor for hemorrhage:
  - Frequent swallowing (inspect throat).
  - Bright red vomitus
  - Rapid pulse
  - Restlessness.
- Comfort
  - Give 30 percent cool mist via collar
  - Apply ice collar to neck (will also reduce bleeding by vasoconstriction).
  - Use acetamonephin in place of aspirin (in tendency on bleeding).
- Food and fluids:
  - Give ice-cold fluids and bland foods during initial period (e.g. ice chips, popsicles, jella)
  - Milk is usually not given, because it may increase mucus and cause the patient to clear the throat.
  - Advance to normal diet as soon as possible.
- Patient and family teaching:
  - Avoid attempting to clear throat immediately after surgery (may initiate bleeding).
  - Avoid coughing, sneezing, vigorous nose blowing and vigorous exercise for 1 to 2 weeks.
  - Drink fluids (2 to 3 L/day) until mouth odor disappears.
  - Avoid hard, scratchy foods such as pretzels, popcorn or toast, until throat is healed
  - Report signs of bleeding to physician immediately.

- Expect more throat discomfort between 4th and 8th postoperative days because of membrane separation.
- Expect stool to be black or dark for a few days because of swallowed blood.
- Resume normal activity immediately as long as it is not stressful and does not require straining.

Acute Laryngitis

Acute laryngitis is an inflammation of the mucous membrane lining of the larynx accompanied by edema of the vocal cords. It may be caused by cold, by sudden changes in temperature or by irritating fumes.

Pathophysiology/Clinical Manifestation

Symptoms vary from a slight huskiness to complete loss of voice. The throat may be painful and feel scratching, and a cough may be present.

Management

Laryngitis management requires only symptomatic treatment. The person is advised to remain indoors in an even temperature and to avoid talking for several days or weeks, depending on the severity of the inflammation. Steam inhalation may be soothing and cough syrups or home remedies for cough to provide relief to some patients. Smoking should be avoided. Additional fluids by mouth help prevent dehydration and drying of throat.

The nursing role is mainly patient teaching, which could include the following:
- Need to take antibiotics as prescribed (Full course as prescribed).
- Need to increase fluid intake.
- Need to stop smoking for smokers.
- Need to avoid smoky environment.
- Refferral to a support group of persons wanting to stop smoking.
- Precautions to be observed in using steam inhalations.

Chronic laryngitis may occur in persons who use their voices excessively, who smoke a great deal or who work continuously where there are irritating fumes. Hoarseness usually is worse in early morning and evening. There may be dry, harsh cough. Treatment of chronic laryngitis includes removal of irritants, voice test, correction of faulty voice habits, steam inhalation. Additional fluid by mouth care are encouraged.

Laryngeal Paralysis

Laryngeal paralysis may result from disease or injury of either the laryngeal nerves or the vagus nerve.

Etiology

Laryngeal paralysis may be caused by:
- Aortic aneurysm
- Mitral stenosis
- Laryngeal cancer
- Subglottic or cervical esophageal tumors
- Bronchial carcinoma
- Neck injury
- Severing or stretching of the recurrent laryngeal nerve during thyroidectomy
- Prolonged intubation of patients in intensive care units.

Pathophysiology

Either one or both vocal cords may be paralyzed. If only one cord is affected, the airway is adequate and now the voice may be affected. Efforts to improve the voice in persons with unilateral cord paralysis have been accomplished by injecting a small quantity of Gelfoam or Teflan into paralyzed cord. This swells the cord and pushes it towards the midline where the other cord can approximate it better during phonation.

Bilateral paralysis causes a poor airway that results in incapacitating dyspnea, stridor on exertion and a weak voice. A sudden bilateral vocal cord paralysis is not common and usually a result of massive cerebrovascular accident or blunt trauma both of which are incompatible with life.

Management

Diagnostic tests performed include:
- Indirect laryngoscopy to diagnose vocal cord abnormality
- Videostroboscopy (observe vocal cords vibration during phonation). Here fibreoptic laryngoscope is attached to videotape to record actual cord motion. This is to diagnose abnormal vibrations of cord.
- Electromyography to determine innervation and thus movement of vocal cords.
- CT scan to determine cause of vocal cord paresis or paralysis such as tumor or aneurysm along course of recurrent laryngeal nerve.

Treatment of laryngeal paralysis is symptomatic.
- Antacids are used if patient experiencing gastroesophageal reflux which neutralize gastric acid.
- H2 inhibitor, used to reduce the amount of gastric acid produced.
- Antibiotics are used for infection.
- Tracheostomy may be necessary to maintain airway
- Other procedures are followed according to causes.

Laryngeal Edema

Acute laryngeal edema may be caused by anaphylaxis, urticaria, acute laryngitis, scream inflammatory diseases to the throat or edema after intubation. It causes the airway to narrow or close and required immediate restoration of the airway.

Treatment of acute laryngeal edema consists of administration of an adrenocorticosteroid or epinephrine. Intubation or tracheostomy may be necessary.

Airway Obstruction

Airway may be complete or partial. Complete airway obstruction is medical emergency. Partial airway obstructions may occur as a result of aspiration of food as foreign body. In addition, partial airway obstruction may result from laryngeal edema following extubation laryngeal or tracheal stenosis, and neurologic depression.

Symptoms include stridor, use of accessory muscles, suprasternal and intercoastal retractions, wheezing, restlessness, tachycardia and cyanosis.

Management

Prompt assessment and treatment are essential because partial obstructions may quickly progress to complete destruction. Interventions to maintain a patient airway include use of obstructed airway (Heimlich) manoeuvre, endotracheal intubation and tracheostomy.

An endotracheal tube is usually chosen initially as a means of providing airway, tracheostomy is performed only if airway maintenance is necessary for longer than 10 to 14 days or if trauma to the airway prevents the use of an endotracheal tube.

In endotracheal intubation, a tube is passed through either the nose or mouth into the trachea, whereas in a tracheostomy, an artificial opening is made in the trachea into which a tracheostomy tube is inserted. The procedures are used to:
- Establish and maintain patent airway
- Prevent aspiration by sealing off the trachea from digestive tract in the unconscious or paralysed person
- Permit removal of tracheobronchial secretions in the person who cannot cough adequately, and
- Treat the patient who requires positive pressure mechanical ventilation that cannot be given effectively by masks.

The endotracheal tubes is made of plastic with an inflatable cuff so that a closed system with the ventilator may be maintained. The tube is inserted via the mouth or nose through the larynx into the trachea. If an oral endotracheal tube is used, a rubber airway or bite block is often necessary to prevent the patient from biting down on the tube and obstructing the airway.

Tracheostomy

A tracheostomy is a surgical incision into the trachea for the purpose of establishing an airway. It is the stoma (an opening) that results from the tracheostomy. Indications for a tracheostomy are to:
- Bypass an upper airway obstruction
- Facilitate removal of secretions
- Permit long-term mechanical ventilation
- Permit oral intake and speech in the patient who requires long-term mechanical ventilation.

Nursing Care

Before the procedure the nurse should explain to the patient and the family the purpose of the procedure and inform them that the patient will not be able to speak if an inflated cuff is used.

The patient and family should be informed the normal speech will be possible as soon as the cuff can be deflated.

A variety of tubes are available to meet individual patient needs, which include:
- Tracheostomy tube with cuff and inflated balloons: When properly inflated, lower pressure, high-volume cuff distributes cuff pressure over large areas, minimizing pressure on tracheal wall.
- Fenestrated tracheostomy tube with cuff and inner cannula and decannulation plug: When inner cannula is removed, cuff deflated, and decannulation plug inserted, air flows around the tube through fenestration in outer cannula and up over vocal cords. Patient can then speak.
- Speaking tracheostomy tube (Portex, National) with cuff, two external tubings; It has two tubings, one leading to cuff and second to opening above the cuff. When port is connected to air source, air flows out of opening and up over the vocal cords, allowing speech in the cuff inflated.
- Tracheostomy tube (Bivona Fome-cuff) foam filled cuff: This cuff is filled with plastic foam. Before insertion, cuff is deflated. After insertion, cuff is allowed to fill passively with air. Pilot tubing is not capped and no cuff pressure monitoring is required.

All tracheostomy tubes contain a face plate or flange, which rests on the neck between the clavicles and outer cannula. In addition, all tubes have an obturator, which is used when inserting the tube. During insertion of the tube, the obturator is placed inside the outer cannula with its rounded tip protruding from air end of the tube to ease insertion. After insertion, the obturator must be immediately removed so that air can flow through the tube. The obturator should be kept in an easily accessible place at the bedside (e.g. taped to the wall) so that it can be used quickly in case of accidental decannulation.

Nursing Management of Endotracheal or Tracheostomy Tube

An endotracheal or tracheostomy tube provides a direct route for introduction of pathogen, into the lower airway, increasing the risk of infection. It is essential that the following preventive nursing intervention be consistently implemented.

Minimize Infection Risk
- Endotracheal airways irritate the trachea resulting in increased mucus production. Assess the patient regularly for excess secretions and suction as often as necessary to maintain a patent airway.
- Provide constant airway humidifications. Endotracheal airways bypass the upper airway which normally humidifies and warms inspired air. An external source of cool, humidified air must be provided to avoid thickening and crusting of bronchial secretions.
- All respiratory therapy equipment should be changed every 6 hours. In addition:
  - Replace any equipment that touches the floor,
  - Remove water that condenses in equipment tubing. Do not pour condensed water back into humidifier reservoir, because it may contain pathogens.
- Provide frequent mouth care. Secretions tend to pool in the mouth and in the pharynx, particularly if the cuff of the tube is inflated. An endotracheal tube or oral airway increases the risk of ulceration or abrasion of the lips and oropharynx.
  - Gently suction oropharynx as needed
  - Inspect the lips, tongue and oral cavity regularly
  - Clean the oral cavity with swab soaked in saline
  - Apply moisturising agent to cracked lips.
- Maintain adequate nutrition levels:
  - The person with endotracheal tube is allowed nothing by mouth. Nourishment will be given parenterally or gastrointestinal feedings. Gastrointestinal supplemental feedings are preferred because they maintain the function of the gut, proposeless infection risk, and more economical than IV fluids. While administering GI feeding to the intubated patient, nurse will:
    - Assess for bowel sounds and tube placement
    - Elevate head of the bed at least 45 degrees
    - Inflate the tracheostomy tube cuff.
      - If using a Salem sump nasogastric tube, check the amount of residual feeding. If the half volume of the feeding to be given remains, the tube feeding is withheld.
      - Administer the tube feeding over 20-30 minutes.
      - Keep head of bed elevated for 45-60 minutes after feeding.
      - Assess at regular intervals for aspiration.
      - Regularly assess for tube placement and residual stomach contents.
  - The patient with a tracheostomy tube is usually able to swallow and have a normal oral intake. Some experts prefer that the cuff on the tracheostomy tube be inflated while the patient is eating to prevent aspiration. Others believe that cuff bulges into esophagus and make swallowing more difficult, and they therefore prefer that cuff be deflated. Nursing assessment will determine which technique to be used. Methyline blue dye can be swallowed before each feeding or mixed with tube feeding. If the dye does not appear in tracheal secretions, it is safe to proceed with the meal.

Ensure Adequate Ventilation and Oxygenation
- Assess lung sounds regularly. Unless the individual's underlying pathology alters lung ventilations, sounds should be heard bilaterally, and chest expansion should be symmetrical. If an endotracheal tube is inserted too far it will slip into one of the mainstems of bronchi (usually the night) and occlude the opposite bronchus and lung resulting in atelectasis on the obstructed side. Even if the endotracheal tube is still in the trachea, airway obstruction will result if the end of the tube is located on the carina. This will result in dry secretions that obstruct both bronchi. So the tube is pulled back until it is positioned below the larynx and above the carina. The tube is then fastened securely in place.
- Turn and reposition the patient every 2 hours for maximum ventilation and lung perfusion.
- Assess respiratory frequency, tidal volume and viral capacity
- Perform postural drainage, percussion and vibration as appropriate

Provide Safety and Comfort
- Most endotracheal and tracheostomy tubes have cuffs for the following reasons:
  - To provide a sealed airway for positive pressure mechanical ventilation, and
  - To prevent aspirations in the unconscious person during tube feedings
- Assess tube placement in regular intervals:
  - The tube is secured around neck with tape or specially designed ties, and
  - The endotracheal tube is marked to establish a landmark for position comparison and to measure and document the length of the tube that extends beyond the patient lips.
- Change tapes or ties whenever soiled to decreased skin irritation.
- Always keep a spare tube at the bedside.
- Minimize sensory deprivations. Because patients with these tubes with cuff-inflated cannot talk. Therefore, an acceptable communication mode must be established as follows:
  - Organise questions so that patient can use a simple 'Yes' or 'No' response (nodding head, using hand signals, or squeezing the nurse's hand)
  - The patient may be able to use an erasable board or note pad to communicate

- Always talk to the patient and explain all procedures,
- Reorient the patient frequently,
- Encourage family and friends to talk to patient and offer encouragement,
- Keep call light (or tap bell) within the patient's reach
- Reinforce that the ability to speak will return when the tube is removed.

Observe Special Precautions during the Immediate Extubation Period

- Monitor for signs such as increased respiratory distress, increased restlessness, hoarseness and laryngeal stridor indicating upper airway obstruction secondary to laryngeal edema.
- Assess for adequacy of cough and gag reflex
- After removal of a tracheostomy tube there is a temporary air leak at the incision site. To speak, the patient will have to occlude the opening with a finger.
- The tracheal stoma can be suctioned. However, frequent use of the stoma for suctioning can delay closure and healing of tracheostomy incisions.

Procedure for Suctioning a Tracheostomy Tube

- Assess the need for suctioning 4th hourly. Indications include coarse crackles or rhonchi over large airways, moist cough, increase in peak inspiratory pressure and mechanical ventilator and restlessness or agitation if accompanied by decrease in SPO_2 or PaO_2. Do not suction routinely or if patient is able to clear secretion with cough.
- If suctioning indicated, explain the procedure to the patient.
- Collect necessary equipment; suction catheters no larger than half the lumen of the tracheostomy tube), gloves, water, cup, and drape. If a closed tracheal suction is used, the catheter is enclosed in a plastic sleeves and reused for 24 hours. No, additional equipment is needed.
- Check suction source and regulator. Adjust suction pressure until the dial reads 120 to 150 mm Hg pressure with tubing occluded.
- Wash hands, put on goggles and gloves.
- Use sterile technique to open package, fill cup with water, put on gloves, and connect catheter to suction. Designate on hand as contaminated for disconnecting, bagging and operating the suction control. Suction water through the catheter to test the system.
- Assess SPO_2 heart rate and rhythm to provide baseline for detecting change during suctioning.
- Provide preoxygenation by: (i) adjusting ventilator to deliver 100 per cent O_2, (ii) using reservoir equipped manual resuscitate bag (MRB) connected to 100 per cent O_2; or (iii) asking patient to take 3-4-deep breaths.

While administering oxygen, the method chosen will depend on the patient's underlying disease and ability or illness. The patient who has tracheostomy for an extended period of time and is not acutely ill, may be able to tolerate suctioning without use of an MRB or the ventilator.

- Gently insert the catheter without suction to minimize the amount of oxygen removed from the lungs. Insert the catheter approximately 5-6 inches. Stop if any obstruction is met.
- Withdraw the catheter 1-2 cm and apply suction intermittently, while withdrawing catheter in a rotating manner. If secretion volume is large, apply suction continuously.
- If the patient develops mucous plugs or thick secretions a 3-5 ml bolus of normal saline may be instilled into the airway to loosen secretions sufficiently to clear the airway either through coughing or suctioning.
- Limit suction time to 10 seconds. Discontinue suctioning if heart rate decreases from baseline by 20 beats, increases from baseline by 40 beats per minute, an arrhythmias or SPO_2 decreases to less than 90 per cent.
- After each suction-pass, oxygenate with 3-4 breaths by ventilator, MRB or deep breaths with oxygen.
- Rinse catheter with sterile water.
- Repeat procedure until airway is clear. Limit insertions of suction catheter to three passes.
- Return oxygen concentration to prior setting.
- Rinse catheter and suction the oropharynx or use mouth suction.
- Dispose of catheter by wrapping it around fingers of gloved hand and pulling glove over catheter. Discard equipment in proper waste container.
- Auscultate to assess changes in lung sounds. Record time, amount and character of secretions and response to suctioning.

Tracheostomy Care

Although nursing care of persons with either endotracheal or tracheostomy tube is similar, patients with tracheostomies have additional nursing care needs. Nursing care includes maintaining air humidification, providing nourishment, and weaning for the tracheostomy tube. The care of the tracheostomy tube. The care of the tracheostomy is as follows:

- Explain procedure to the patient.
- Collect necessary sterile equipment (e.g. suction catheter, gloves, water, basin, drape, tracheostomyties, tube brush or pipe cleaners, 4 × 4s, hydrogen peroxide 3 per cent, sterile water and tracheostomy dressing (optional)

Note: Clean rather than sterile technique is used at home.

- Position patient in semi-Fowler's position.

- Assemble needed materials on bedside table next to patient.
- Wash hands, put on goggles and gloves.
- Auscultate chest sounds. If rhonchi or coarse crackles are present suction the patient if unable to cough up secretions.
- Unlock and remove inner cannula, if present. Many tracheostomy tubes do not have inner cannula. Care for these tubes includes all steps except for inner cannula care.
- If disposable inner cannula is used, replace with new cannula. If non-disposable cannula is used:
  - Immerse inner cannula in 3 per cent hydrogen peroxide and clean inside and outside of cannula using tube brush or pipe cleaner,
  - Drain hydrogen peroxide from cannula. Immerse cannula in sterile water and shake to dry.
  - Insert inner cannula into outer cannula with the curved part downward and lock in place.
- Remove dried secretions from stoma using 4 × 4 soaked in sterile water. Gently pat area around the stoma dry. Be sure to clean under the tracheostomy face plate, using cotton swabs to reach this area.
- Maintain position of tracheal retention sutures if present, by taping above and below the stoma.
- Change tracheostomy ties. Tie tracheostomy ties securely with room for one finger between ties and skin. To prevent accidental tube removal, secure the tracheostomy tube by gently applying pressure to flange of the tube during the tie changes. Do not change tracheostomy ties for 24 hours after the tracheostomy procedure.
- As an alternative some patients prefer tracheostomy ties made of velero, which are easier to adjust, other patients use plastic IV tubing because it is easily cleaned and dries without need to replace the ties.
- Unless excessive amounts of exudate are present avoid using a tracheostomy dressing since this keeps the site moist and may predispose to infection.
- If drainage is excessive, place dressing around tube. A tracheostomy dressing or unlined gauze should be used. Do not cut the guaze because threads may be inhaled or wrope around the tracheostomy tube. Change the dressing frequently. Wet dressings promote infection and stoma irritation.
- Repeat care three times a day and as needed and also follow manufacturers' instructions.

CHAPTER 17

Nursing Management of Neurological Disorders

NURSING ASSESSMENT OF THE NERVOUS SYSTEM

The human nervous system is a highly-specialized system responsible for the control and integration of the body's activities. The ability to conduct an accurate neurological assessment depends on the nurse's knowledge of neuroanatomy and neurophysiology and skill in recognizing and interpreting subtle deviations from normal. Although neurological assessment usually is complete in phases and depends on the condition of the person and the urgency of the situation, assessment of mental status, level of consciousness, language and speech, perceptual status and sensory status.

History

A careful history, i.e. a skillfully taken history often holds the key to diagnosis. The person is asked to give a time to time account of the14 illness including the onset and progression as well as the nature of the symptoms. It is particularly important to note the speed of onset, frequency of remissions, (if any), and any diurnal patterns or intensity changes in symptoms. Symptoms that require further assessment are complaints of pain, headache, seizures, vertigo, numbness, visual changes, and weakness. Identification of specific patterns of symptoms may provide pertinent diagnostic information about the pathological process.

When eliciting data about health history, the nurse should ask the patient specific questions about diabetes mellitus, pernicious anemia, cancer, infections, thyroid disease, substance abuse, and hypertention, because these conditions can affect the nervous system. Any hospitalization, injuries, or surgeries related to nervous system and use of medications, especially sedatives, narcotics, tranquilizers, mood-elevating drugs and their side effects should also be asked about.

In addition, information is collected about family members and their relationships and interactions, ethnic background, housing, recreational interests, occupation, education, coping mechanisms, dependence-independence characteristics, and how the person manages usual activities of daily living. Particular attention should be paid to reports of any recent changes in the patient's usual behaviors such as increased irritability or memory loss. A family health history and developmental history also are included.

Mental Status

While determining the presence of organic brain disease, specific abnormalities of higher cerebral functions are very significant for which clinical observation of mental function is important change in the level of consciousness (LOC) it can be most sensitive indicator of neurological function. The functional components of consciousness are aroused (alertness) and awareness (consent) of self and environment. Arousal is mainly controlled by brainstem activity including the reticular activating system (RAS). Awareness requires an intact cerebral cortex and association fibers. Thus, the state of consciousness depends on the interaction between the brainstem and cerebral hemisphere.

Arousal is determined by eye opening. A spontaneous opening of the eyes occurs where a person is spoken to by the examiner. A painful stimulus may be applied to determine whether the arousal mechanism is intact if eye opening does not occur with verbal and auditory stimulus.

Awareness is assessed by determining the patient's orientation to self and environment, which includes assessment of person, place, and time (day, month, year) is the most effective method.

Assessment of mood and behavior also includes in the mental examination, because of a particular mood may be associated with a specific disease. For example:

- Emotional liability is often seen in bilateral (diffuse) brain disease where the mood shifts easily and quickly from one extreme to the other.
- Euphoria is a superficial elevation of mood accompanied by unconcern even in the presence of threatening events. It needs to be determined whether the persons mood is appropriate to the topic of conversation.
- Personality change with the appearance of violent temper and aggressive behavior may occur with destructive lesions of the inferior frontal parts of the limbic system.

Nurse should assess mental status. The components of the mental status examination will include:

- General appearance; which includes motor activities, body posture, dress and hygiene, facial expression, and speech.
- State of consciousness: Which includes orientation to place, person, and situation, as well as memory, general knowledge, insight, judgement, problem-solving and calculation.

- Mood and affect which includes noting agitation, anger, depression, euphoria and the appropriateness of these states. Questions should be directed to bring out the feelings of the patient.
- *Thought content:* Which includes noting illusions, hallucinations, delusions or paronia.
- Intellectual capacity, i.e. noting retardation, dementia, and intelligence.

Language and Speech

Language ability is concentrated on a cortical field includes parts of the temporal lobe, the temporo-parieto-occipital junction (TPO), the frontal lobe of the dominant (usually left) hemisphere and occipital lobe. Lesion in any of these areas will produce some impairment in language ability aphasia or dysarthria.

- Aphasia is the impairment of language functions. There were different types of aphasias what had been identified as follows:
  - Motor expression aphasia is the impairment of ability to speak and write. Patient can understand written and spoken words. This may be due to lesions in the insular and surrounding region including Broca's motor area.
    In the anomic, fluent, and non-fluent aphasia are as follows:
  - Anomic refers to inability to name objects, qualities, and conditions although speech is fluent due to lesion in area of angular gyrus.
  - Fluent refers to speech in well-articulated and grammatically correct but lacking in content and meaning.
  - Non-fluent aphasia refers to problems in selecting, organizing and initiating speech patterns, may also affect writing. It is due to lesion and motor cortex at Broca's area.
    - Sensory (peceptive) aphasia refers to impairment of ability to understand written or spoken language, is due to disease of auditory and visual word centers. Wernicke's aphasia is also the same as sensory aphasia due to lesion lying in Wernicke's area of left hemisphere.
    - Mixed aphasia refers to combined expressive and receptive aphasia deficits due to damage to various speech and language areas.
    - Global aphasia refers to total aphasia involving all functions that make up speech and communication. Few if any imbibe language skills. This is due to severe damage to speech area.
    - Dysarthria is an indistinctness in word articulation or enunication resulting from interference with the peripheral speech mechanisms (e.g. the muscles of the tongue, palate, pharynx or lips).

Dysarthria may be manifested by a single alteration or a variety of alterations and there are characteristic changes in particular diseases. For example in crebellar disease, speech is often thick with prolongation of speech sounds occurring at intervals. In Parkinsonism, speech is characterized by a decrease in loudness and a change in vocal emphasis patterns that makes sound seem monotonous.

Perception

Sensation is integrated and interpreted in the sensory cortex, especially in the parietal lobe. It is important for the nurse to recognise perceptual problems, because they can be more difficult to deal with the changes in the patient's ability to move or sense. Disorders of perceptions commonly involve spatial-temporal relationships or the perception of self.

The ability to recognize objects through any of the special senses is known as "gnosia". Lesions involving a specific association area of the cortex produces a specific type of agnosia (absence of the ability). One type of ability often tested is stereognosis, the ability to perceive—an object's nature and form by touch. This is assessed by asking the person to identify familar objects placed in the hand at a time, while keeping his eyes closed.

Apraxia is another perceptual problem, refers to the inability to perform skilled, purposeful movements in the absence of motor, sensory or coordination losses. The different types, of apraxia are as follows:

- Constructional apraxia is an impairment in producing designs in two or three dimensions, involves copying, drawing, or constructing. This is due to lesion in occipitoparietal lobe of either hemisphere.
- Dressing apraxia is an inability to dress oneself accurately. Makes mistakes as putting clothes on backwards, upside down, inside out, or putting both legs in the same pantleg. This is due to lesion in occipetal or parietal lobe usually in nondominant hemisphere.
- Kinesthetic apraxia is a loss of kinesthetic memory pattern, which result in patient inability to perform a purposeful motor task although it is understood. This is due to lesion in frontal lobe of either hemisphere or precentral gyrus.
- Idiomotor apraxia is an inability to imitate gestures or perform a purposeful motor task on command. May be able to do spontaneous. This is due to lesions in parietal lobe of dominant hemisphere and supramarginal gyrus.
- Ideational apraxia is an inability to carry out activities automatically or on command, because of inability to understand the concepts of the act. This is due to lesion in parietal lobe of dominant hemisphere or diffuse brain damage as in arteriosclerosis.

Sensory Status

Accurate assessment of sensory function depends on the person's cooperation, alertness, and responsiveness. The person should be relaxed and have the eyes closed during all portions of the sensory examination to avoid recovering visual clues. Also, sensation should be tested side by side and distally to proximity. Both superficial and deep sensations are tested on trunk and extremities. Areas of sensory loss or abnormality are mapped out on a body diagram according to the distribution of the spinal dermatomes and peripheral nerves.

PAIN

- Superficial pain perception is assessed by stimulating an area by pinprick and asking the person to report discomfort. Sharp and dull objects can be alternated for increased discrimination.
- Deep pain can be assessed by multiple means, some of which have the potential of causing tissue injury. It is necessary to assess deep pain only when the person has a decreased level of consciousness. Deep pain can be assessed by applying pressure over the nail beds or supraorbitally. Pressure may also be applied over bony areas, such as sternum. Nail bed pressure is applied by placing a pin or similar object on the nail bed and squeezing it between the examiner's thumb and forefinger. Deep pain may also be elicited by squeezing the trapezius muscle. Pinching and pricking may damage tissues and are avoided wherever possible.
- Crude touch may be assessed by touching area with cotton and requesting that the person indicate when the touch is felt.
- Temperature is tested by touching particular areas with warm to hot and cold to cold object and asking the person to state the sensations felt.

Motion and Position

Proprioceptive fibers transmit sensory impulses from muscles, tender ligaments, and joints. This results in an awareness of the position of one's limbs in space (Kinesthetic sense). Proprioception is tested by the examiner's grasping the sides of the person's distal phalax and moving it up and down. If proprioception is intact, the person reports correctly the direction in which the joint is being moved. Proprioceptive ability can also be assessed by the Remberg test, in which the person is asked to stand erect with the feet together and the eyes closed. A positive test occurs where the person loses balance which indicates a pathological condition.

Vibration is tested by placing a low frequency tuning fork on a bony prominence of each extremity and assessing the person's ability to feel it.

Neurological Examination

Generally neurological examination assesses six categories of functions and reflex function. The primary purpose of the nursing neurologic examination is to determine the effects of the neurologic dysfunction on daily living in relation to the patients and the family's ability to cope with the neurologic deficits, for which the medical model of examination also used for nursing purposes. The mental status examination already discussed. The nurse has to use or keep ready following equipment needed to perform a neurological examination which include:

- Compass.
- Cotton applicators.
- Dermatomes.
- Dynomemeter.
- Flash light.
- Miscellaneous items of varied shape and size (coin, key, marble).
- Ophthalmoscope.
- Otoscope.
- Colored pencil.
- Pins with sharp and blunt ends.
- Printed page.
- Reflex hammer.
- Tape measure.
- Tongue depressor.
- Tuning fork.
- Snellen chart.
- Stoppered vials containing:
  - Peppermint, oil of cloves, coffee and soap (small).
  - Sugar, salt, vinegar and quinine (taste).
  - Cold and hot water (temperatures).
- Watch with second hand.

Cranial Nerves

Testing of each cranial nerve (CN) is an essential component of the neurological examination. The 12 cranial nerves may be tested in numbered sequence. Some nurses prefer to test at the same time with those cranial nerves with similar function such as voluntary motor function visceral motor function, and special sensory or general sensory functions. However, some cranial nerves have both motor and sensory functions. Prior to the test the CN, it is better to review.

The cranial nerves and their functions are as follows:

Olfactory	• Sensory	• Smell reception and interpretation
Optic	• Sensory	• Visual acuity and visual fields
Oculomotor	• Motor	• Raise eyelids, most extraocular movements

Trochlear	• Motor	• Downward, inward eye movements
Trigeminal	• Motor	• Jaw opening and clenching, chewing and mastication
	• Sensory	• Sensation to cornea, iris, lacrimal glands, conjunctiva, eyelids, forehead, nose, nasal and mouth mucosa, teeth, tongue, ear facial skin
Abducens	• Motor	• Lateral eye movement
Facial	• Motor	• Movement of facial expression of muscles except jaw, close eyes, labial speech sounds (bmw and rounded vowels)
	• Sensory	• Taste-anterior two-thirds of tongue-sensation of pharynx • Parasympathetic-secretion of salivary glands and carotid reflex
Vagus	• Motor	• Voluntary muscles of phonation (guttural speech sounds) and swallowing
	• Sensory	• Sensation behind ear and parts of external ear canal
Spinal	• Motor	• Turn-head. shrug shoulders, accessory some action for phonation
Hypoglossal	• Motor	• Tongue movement for speech sound articulation (l, t, n) and swallowing

Testing Cranial Nerves

- *Olfactory nerve:* Special receptors located within the superior or uppermost part of each nasal chamber transmit neural impulse over the olfactory bulbs to the olfactory nerves in the area of central cortex concerned with olfaction. When testing thus CN, the nurse asks the patient to close one nostril, close both eyes and sniff from a bottle containing coffee, spice, soup, or some other readily recognised odor. If yes, the patient is asked to name the odor. Awareness of an odor must be differentiated from the ability to name a specific substance. The same may be repeated in other nostril. Anosmia (absence of smell) or hypotmia (decreased sensitivity of the sense of smell) is often associated with complaints of lack of taste, even though test may demonstrate sense to be intact. Anosmia caused by varied lesion involving any part of the olfactory pathways.

- *Optic nerve:* When retina is stimulated, nerve impulses are transmitted over the optic nerves (extending from the optic disk to the chiasm) and the optic tracts with radiation terminating in the visual cortex of the occipital lobes. Optic nerve function is assessed in relation to visual acuity, visual fields and the appearance of fundus. Each eye is tested separately.

  Visual acuity is mediated by the cones of the retina. Central vision is grossly tested by reading newspaper print. Distance visual activity is assessed through the use of the 'Snellen chart'. Individuals with vision impairment are tested to determine light perception (LP), hand movement (Hm), and finger count (fc).

  Visual fields are assessed grossly by confrontation techniques. The examiner, positioned directly opposite to the patient asks the patient to close one eye, look directly at the bridge of the examiner's nose and indicate when an object (finger, pencil tip, head of pins) presented from periphery of the four visual quadrants. The same test is repeated for the other eye. Visual field defects may arise from lesions of the optic nerve, optic chiasma, or tracts that extend through the temporal, parectal or occipital lobe. Visual charges resulting from brain lesion are hemianopsia (one-half of the field affected) a quadrantanopsia (one-fourth of visual field affected) or monocular.

  The ocular fundus is defined as that portion of the interior of the eyeball, that lies posterior to the lens. It includes optic disk, blood vessels, retina and macula. Funduscopy reveals the physical condition of the optic disk (head of the optic nerve) as well as the retina and blood vessels.

- *Oculomotor, trochlear and abducens nerves:* Cranial nerves III, IV and VI are motor nerves that arise from the brainstem and innervate the six extraocular muscle attached to the eyeball. These muscles function as a group in the coordinated movement of each eyeball is the six cardinal fields of gaze, giving the eye both straight and rotary movement. The four straight or rectus, muscles are the superior, inferior, lateral and medial rectus muscles. The two slanting or oblique muscles are the superior and inferior. Since these three cranial nerves all help move the eye, they are tested together. The patient is asked to follow the examiner's finger as it moves horizontally and vertically (making cross) and diagonally (making an X). If there is weakness or paralyses in one of the eye muscles, the eyes do not move together, and the patient has a disconjugate gaze. The presence and direction of nystagmus (fine, rapid, jerking movements of the eyes) is observed at this time even though it is most often indicated to vestibula cerebellar problems.

Double vision (diplopia) squint (strabismus) and involuntary rhythmic movement of the eye balls (nystagmus) may indicate weakness of some of the extraocular muscles because of deficits of these motor nerves. Ptosis or drooping of the upper eyelid over the globe may be caused by damage to the oculomotor nerve. Other functions of the oculomotor nerve are tested by checking for pupillary constriction and for convergence (eye turning inward) and accommodation (Pupils constricting with near vision).

- *Trigeminal Nerve:* Cranial nerve V is a mixed nerve with motor and sensory components. It is the largest cranial nerve. The motor part innervates the temporal and masseter muscles, the sensory part supplies the cornea, face, head, and mucus membranes of the nose and mouth.

  The sensory component of the trigeminal nerve is tested by having the patient identify light touch (cotton) and pinprick in each of the three divisions (ophthalmic maxillary and mandibular) of the nerve on both sides of the face. The patient's eyes should be closed during this part of the examination.

  The corneal reflex test evaluates trigeminal nerves and facial simultaneously. It involves applying a cotton wisp strand to the cornea. The sensory components of this reflex (corneal sensation) is innervated by the ophthalmic division of VCN. The motor component (eye blink) of thin reflex is innervated by facial nerve. Normally, the person blanks laterally. This is especially important reflex to assess in persons with decreased level of consciousness because the absence of the blink reflex can result in corneal damage.

- *Facial nerve:* It is a mixed nerve that is concerned with facial movement and sensation of taste. It innervates the muscles of facial expression. The inability to smile, close both eyes slightly look upward wrinkle the forehead, show the teeth, purse the lips, and blow out the cheeks constitutes weaknesses or paralysis of the facial muscle innervated by this nerve. Its function is tested by asking the patient to raise the eyebrows, close the eyes tightly, purse the lips, draw back the corners of the mouth in an exaggerated smile, and frown. The examiner should note any asymmetry in the facial movements, because they can indicate damage to the facial nerve. The sensation of taste is tested by placing salty sweet, bitter and sour substances, in turn on the side of the protruded tongue for identification. A loss of task over the anterior two-third of the tongue is present when this nerve is diseased, as occurs in mastoid canal lesions.

- *Acoustic nerve:* Cranial nerve VIII is composed of a cochlear division related to hearing and a vestibular division related to equilibrium. The conchlear portion of this nerve is tested by having the patient close the eyes and indicate when a ticking watch or the rustling of the examiner's finger tips is heard as the stimulus is brought closer to the ear. Each ear rested individually and the distance from the patient's ear to sound source when first hand is retarded. A more complete examination, including bone and air conduction of sound involves assessment with a tuning fork and audiometric testing.

  The vestibular portion of this nerve is not routinely tested unless the patient complains of dizziness, vertigo, or unsteadiness or has auditory dysfunctioning. There are variety of ways in testing this portion of the nerve. In the past-pointing test, the person is asked to raise the arms and bring the index fingers down on the examiner's finger with the arm outstretched, first with the eyes open and then with the eyes closed. Normally, the person's fingers touch the examiner's without difficulty. In vertibular disease, the finger points to one side or the other consistently. The person is also assessed for nystagmus.

- *Glossopharyngeal and vagus nerves:* These two cranial nerves are tested together because both innervate the pharynx. Both nerves supply the posterior pharyngeal wall and normally when the wall is touched, there is contraction of these muscles on both sides, with or without gagging. This test is unreliable for either nerve alone, because the vagus nerve is chief motor nerve and the soft palatal, pharyngeal and laryngeal muscles assessment includes testing voice and cough sounds. In unilateral movement of the motor portion of the vagus nerve the voice is harsh and nasal. Bilateral involvement produces more severe speech problems, swallowing difficulty and fluid regurgitation through nose. Sensory function of the vagus is usually not tested.

- Spinal accessory nerve is motor nerve that supplies the sternocleidomastoid and the upper part of the trapezius muscles. This nerve tested by asking the patient to shrug the shoulders against resistance and to turn the head to either side against resistance. There shall be smooth contraction of the above-said muscles. Symmetry, atrophy or fasciculation of the muscle should be noted.

- Hypoglossal nerve is purely motor nerve. The person's tongue is first inspected at rest. Any asymmetry unilaterally decreased bulk, deviations, or fasciculation (fine twitching) are noted. When the nerve is involved, the tongue deviates towards the side of the lesion. In an upper motor neuron lesion, the tonge is affected on the side opposite the lesion (contralateral). Atrophy of the tongue shown through wrinkling and loss of substance on the affected side.

Motor Status

Function of the nerve system assessed through gait and stance, muscle strength, muscle tonus, coordination, involuntary movement and muscle stretch reflexes.

- Gait and stance are compelx activities that require muscle strength, coordination balance, proprioception, and vision. Ataxia is general term meaning lack of coordination in performing planned, purposeful motion such as walking or gait. It is caused by disturbance of position sense or by cerebellar or other diseases. To evaluate the gait, the person is asked to walk freely and naturally and then walk heel to toe in a straight line, tandem walk, because this exaggerates abnormality. To evaluate stance, the person is asked to perform the Romberg standing with the feet close together, first with eyes open and then with eyes closed. Patients with problem and proprioception have difficulty in maintaining balance with their eyes closed. Patients with cerebellar disease have difficulty even with their eyes open. A variety of distinctive gait characterizes specific neurological disorder (e.g. Parkinsonism).
- Muscle strength or power is assessed systematically-including trunk and extremity muscles. One common assessment of muscle strength is asking the patient to grasp both hands of the nurse or doctor and squeeze them simultaneously. The nurse or doctor compares the squeezing ability of one hand to another. Assessment of muscular strength of the feet can be performed by plantar flexion and dorsiflexion.
- To test muscle tonus, the nurse passively moves the person's limbs through a full range of motion. A skilled examiner can differentiate hypertonic from hypotonic muscles, Hypertonic extremities are in fixed positions and feel firm; hypotonic extremities assume a position governed by gravity over extension and overflexion found in hypertonic.
- Coordination can be tested in several ways. The finger to nose test involves having the patient alternately touch the nose with index finger then touch the examiner's finger. Other tests include asking the patient to pronate and supinate both hands rapidly and to do a shallow knee bend, first on one leg and then on another. Dysarthria—a sign of uncoordination of speech muscles.

Involuntary movement: It is important to observe the location of muscle involved amplitude of movement, speed of onset, duration of contraction and relaxation and rhythm. The effects of posture, rest, sleep, distraction, voluntary movement and emotional stress on involuntary movement are determined. Emotional stress usually increases involuntary movement and they may subside during sleep. Abnormal movement may be the result of organic disease or psychosomatic in origin. Example: involuntary movements are tremor, chorea and arthrosis.

Reflexes

The reflex is a predictable response that results from a nerve input over a reflex arc. Tendons attached to skeletal muscles have receptors that are sensitive to stretch. A reflex contraction of the skeletal muscles occurs when the tendon is stretched. A simple muscle stretch reflex is initiated by briskly tapping the tendons of a stretched muscle, usually with reflex hammer. Assessment of reflexes requires an experienced examiner, a reflex hammer and a relaxed patient. The reflex is elicited by striking the hammer onto the muscle insertion tendon. Comparison of right and left sides should reveal equal responses. The reflex response graded as subjective, four point scale that requires clinical practice to use accurately (as follow).

0 = Absent	0 = Areflexia
1 = Weak response	1+ = Hyporeflexia
2 = Normal response	2+ = Normal
3 = Exaggerated response	3+ = Brisker than normal
4 = Hyperreflexia with clonus	4+ = Hyper reflexia

Clonus, an abnormal response, is a continued rhythmic contraction of the muscle after the stimulus has been applied. In general the biceps, triceps, brachioradialis and patellar and Achilles tendon reflex are tested. Some common diagnostic reflexes of the CNS are as follows:

- *Brachioradialis reflex* strimulats C5-C6 section of spiral card
- *Abdominal reflex* is an anterior stroking of the sides of lower torso causes contraction of the abdominal muscles. Absence of reflex indicates lesions of peripheral nerves or in reflex centers in lower thoracic segments of spinal cord; may also indicate multiple sclerosis.
- *Achilles* reflex (ankle jerk) refers to tapping of calcaneal (Achilles) tendon of soleous and gastronemius muscle cause both muscles to contract, producing plantar flexion of food. Absence of reflex may indicate damage to nerves innervating posterior leg muscles or to lumbosacral neurons; may also indicate chronic diabetes, alcoholism syphilis, subarachnoid hemorrhage.
- *Biceps reflex* refers to tapping of biceps tendon in elbow produces contracton of brachialis and biceps muscle, producing flexion at elbow. Absence of reflex may indicate damage at the C5 or C6 vertebral level.
- *Brudzinski's* reflex refers to forceful flexion of neck produces flexion of legs, thighs. This indicates irritation of meninges.

- *Kernig's reflex* refers to flexion of hip, with knee straight and patient lying on back, produces flexion of knee. This reflex indicates irritation of meninges or herniated intervertebral disc.
- *Patellar reflex* (knee jerk) refers to tapping of patellar tendon-causes contraction of quadriceps femoris muscle, producing upward jerk of leg. Absence of this reflex may indicate damage at the L2, L3, or L4 vertebral level; may also indicate chronic diabetes and syphilis.
- Plantar reflex refers to stroking of the lateral part of sole-causes toes to curl down. If corticospinal damage, great toe flexes upward and other toes fan out (Babinskie's sign). This reflex indicates damage to upper motor neuron. Normal in children less than 1-year old.
- Triceps reflex refers to tapping of triceps tendon at elbow-causes contraction of triceps muscle, producing extension at elbow. Absence of reflex may indicate damage at C6, C7 or C8 vertebral level.

DIAGNOSTIC STUDIES OF THE NERVOUS SYSTEM

Diagnostic studies provide important information to the nurse in monitoring the patient's condition and planning appropriate interventions. The common diagnostic studies and the nurse's responsibility in particular diagnostic studies of the nervous system are as follows:

Cerebrospinal Fluid (CSF) Analysis

CSF is a clear fluid that is formed in the third, fourth and lateral ventricles of the brain. Samples are obtained through either a lumbar puncture or cisternal puncture and examined for any increase or decrease in its normal constituents and foreign substances such as pathogenic organism and blood. The normal CSF values are as given below:

- Specific gravity : 1.007
- pH : 7.35
- Appearance : Clear, colorless
- RBCs : None
- WBCs : 0–8/μl (0.0.008/L)
- Opening pressure with LP : 60–150 mm H_2O
- Pressure : 75 to 180 mm H_2O
- Protein : Lumbar : 15–45 mg/dl
  Cisternal : 15-25 mg/dl
  Ventricular : 5-15 mg/dl
- Glucose : 45-75 mg/dl.
- Microorganisms : None

Generally CSF is aspirated by needle insertions in L3-4 or L4-5 interspace to assess many CNS diseases. Nurse's responsibility while obtaining specimen through LP includes:

- Assist patient to assume and maintain lateral recumbent position with knees flexed.
- Ensure maintenance of strict aseptic technique.
- Ensure labelling of CSF specimen in proper sequence.
- Keep patient flat for at least a few hours depending on physician's preference.
- Encourage fludis.
- Monitor neurologic and vital signs.
- Administer analgesia as needed.

Radiological Tests

- *Skull and spine:* X-rays of the skull and spinal column is done to detect fractures, bone erosion, calcification and abnormal vascularity. Here nurse has to explain that procedure is non-invasive. Explain position to be assumed during X-ray.
- *Cerebral angiography:* Involves the injection of contrast medium into the cerebral arterial circulation which assists in determining etiology of strokes, seizures, headaches and motor weakness. A catheter is inserted into the femoral artery (the most common entry site) and advanced to the carotid and cerebral vessels. Serial films are taken as the dye circulates through the cerebral circulation.

  The nurse informs the patient that the procedure takes one to two hours.
  - Keep patient withhold preceding meal 6 to 10 hours prior to procedure.
  - Explain that patient will have hot flush of head when dye is injected.
  - Administer premedication as ordered.
  - Explain need to be absolutely still during procedure.
  - Monitor neurologic and vital signs every 15-30 minutes for first hours.
  - Maintain pressure dressing and ice to injection site.
  - Maintain bedrest until patient is alert and vital signs are stable.
  - Report any sign of change in neurologic status.
- *Computed tomograph (CT) scan:* Computer assisted X-ray of several levels of thin cross sections of body parts are done to detect problems such as hemorrhage, tumor, cyst, edema, infarction, brain atrophy and hydrocephalus. In this procedure, the nurse:
  - Explains the procedure is noninvasive (if no dye is used).
  - Observe for allergic reactions and note puncture site (if dye is used).
  - Explain appearance of scanner.
  - Instruct the patient on need to remain absolutely still during procedure.
- *Myelography* refers to X-ray of spinal cord and vertebral column after injection of dye into subarchnoid space is used to detect spinal lesions (e.g.) ruptured disk, tumor). In this, the nurse's responsibilities are to:
  - Administer pre-procedure sedation as ordered.
  - Instruct patient to empty bladder.

- Inform patient that test is performed with patient on tilt in table that is moved during test.
- Encourage fluids.
- Monitor neurologic and vital signs.
- *MRI*—In MRI internal body parts are visualized by means of magnetic energy. No invasive procedures are required unless contrast material is used. Here, there is need for nurse to screen patient for metal parts and pace maker in the body. Instruct patient to be on knee to lie very still for upto 1 hour. Sedation may be necessary if patient is claustophobic.
- Positron Emission Tomography (PET) measures metabolic activity of brain regions to assess cell death or damage by using radioactive compounds. In this procedure, nurse:
  - Explains procedure to patient.
  - Explains that two IV line will be inserted.
  - Instruct patient not to take sedatives or tranquilizers.
  - Empty bladder before procedure.
  - May be asked to perform different activities during test.

Electrographic Studies

- *Electroencephalography (EEG):* In this, electrical activity of brain is recorded by scalp electrodes to evaluate cerebral disease, CNS effects of systemic diseases and brain death. In this procedure, the nurse:
  - Informs patient that procedure is painless and without danger of electric shock.
  - Withhold stimulants.
  - Informs that patient may be asked to perform various activities such as hyperventilation during test.
  - Determines whether any medication (e.g. tranquilizer, antiseizures) should be withheld.
  - Resume medications after test.
  - Assist patient to wash electrode paste out of hair.
- *Electromyography:* Nerve conduction is an electrical activity associated with nerve and skeletal muscles is recorded by insertion of needle electrodes to detect muscle and peripheral nerve disease. Here inform patient of slight discomfort associated with insertion of needle.
- *Evoked potentials* refer to electrical activity associated with nerve conduction along sensory pathways is recorded by electrodes placed on skin and scalp. Stimulus generates the impulse. Procedure is used to diagnose disease, locate nerve damage, and monitor function intraoperatively. This needs explaining procedure to patients.
- *Visual evoked potentials* refer to electrical activity in visual pathway is recorded with rapidly reverting checkerboard pattern on television screen. One eye is tested at time. Needs explaining the procedure to patients.
- *Braunstem auditory evoked potentials* refer to electrical activity in auditory pathway is recorded with earphones that produce clicking sounds. One ear is tested at time.
- *Somatosensory evoked potentials* refer to electrical activity in certain nerve pathways is recorded with mild electrical pulse (several per second). This procedure needs to inform patient that stimulus may cause mild discomfort or muscle switch.

Ultrasound

- *Carotid duplex studies:* In which sound waves determine blood flow velocity, which indicates presence of occlusive vascular disease.
- *Transcranial doppler:* Same technology as carotid duplex, but evaluates intracranial vessels. In these procedures, the nurse needs to explain the procedure to the patient.

INTRACRANIAL PROBLEMS

Altered Level of Consciousness (LOC)

Consciousness and coma (unconsciousness) exist as opposite ends of a spectrum. Full consciousness is a state of awareness and ability to respond optimally to one's environment. Coma is the opposite, a state of total abscence of awareness and ability to respond, even when stimulated. Unconsciousness is an abnormal state in which the patient is unknown of self or environment. It can range from brief episode, such as the prolonged unconsciousness of coma from which the person cannot be roused, even with vigorous external stimuli. Between these two extremes are degrees of unconsciousness varying in length and severity. A wide range of awareness and responsiveness exists between these extremes are shown as follows:

Alert → confused → lethargic → obtunded → stuporous → comatase.

The terminology used in this figure (continuum of consciousness).

- *Alert:* Attends to environment, responds appropriately to commands and questions with minimal stimulation.
- *Confused:* Disoriented to surroundings, may have impaired judgement, may need cues to respond to commands.
- *Lethargic:* Drowsy, needs gentle verbal or touch stimulation to initiate response.
- *Obtunded:* Responds slowly to external stimulation, needs repeated stimulation to maintain attention and response to the environment.
- *Stuporous:* Responds only minimally with vigorous stimulation may only mutter or moan as a verbal response.
- *Comatose:* No observable response to any external stimuli.

The labels used to identify the various points along the continuum are arbitrary and do not reflect any universal agreement as to the nature of consciousness. Consciousness has two primary components—arousal and content.

- Arousal is a function of the brainstem pathways that govern wakefulness, particularly the reticular activating system (RAS) i.e., a network of nerve fibers and cell bodies that is located in the reticular formation in the central part of the nervous system. An intact RAS can maintain a state of wakefulness, even in the absence of a functioning of cortex.
- Content refers to the ability to reason, think and feel and to react to stimuli with purpose and awareness. Content is the sum of multiple interconnected cerebral hemisphere functions, including thought, behavior, language and expression. These activities are mediated by the higher centers. Intellect and emotional functions are also controlled by these centers.

Disruptions in arousal, content or both can alter the individual level of consciousness (LOC). Interruptions of impulses from the RAS or alterations of the functioning of the cerebral hemisphere can cause unconsciousness. Any condition that markedly alters the functions of the hemispheres or that depresses or destroys the upper brainstem results in impaired consciousness.

Etiology

The two general causes for altered LOC are structural and metabolic as follows:

Structural Causes

- *Trauma:* Concussion, contusion, traumatic intracranial hemorrhage subdural hematoma, epidural hematoma, cerebral edema intracerebral hematoma.
- *Vascular disease:* Cerebral infarction, intracerebral hemorrhage, subarachnoid hemorrhage, brainstem infarction, brainstem hemorrhage, cerebellar hemorrhage.
- *Infections:* Meningitis, encephalitis, brain abscess, cerebellar abscess.
- *Neoplasms:* Primary brain tumors, metastatic tumors, brainstem tumors.

Metabolic Causes

- *Systemic metabolic derangements:* Hypoglycemia, diabetic ketoacidosis, hyperglycemic nonketonic hyperosmalar states, uremia, hepatic encephalopathy, hyponatremia, myxedema.
- *Hypoxic or anoxic encephalopathies:* Severe congestive heart failure, chronic obstructive pulmonary disease with execerbation, severe anemia, prolonged hypertension, postictal states and concussions.
- *Toxicity:* Exogenous toxins-drug overdose (opiates, barbiturates and alcohol)
  - Alcohol intoxication.
  - Lead poisoning.
  - Heavy metals.
  - Carbon monoxide.
- Endogenous toxins: Hypoglycemia, uremia, hepatic encephalitis, thiamine deficiency.
- Extremes of body temperature: Heat stroke, hypothermia.
- Deficiency states: Wernicke's encephalopathy.
- Seizures.

Pathophysiology

Full consciousness is a product of many delicate interactions within the nervous system. Arousal is a function of the RAS. Fibres from the upper brainstem, thalamus, and hypothalamus receive input from sensory pathways in the brain and peripheral nervous system. The RAS fibres supply stimulation to the cerebral hemispheres to initiate and maintain arousal. When a person is aroused, or awake, he or she is ready to respond to the environment. The cerebral cortex also provides feedback to the RAS to modulate and regulate the information sent to the cortex. The ability to consciously respond to the environment is a function of cerebral hemispheres. The cerebral cortex, diencephalon, and upper brain stem act together to control voluntary motor function, language, memory and emotion. These higher level cognitive functions represent the content portion of consciousness. A person needs both arousal, or wakefulness, content to be considered fully conscious.

Many specific aetiologic events can result in unconsciousness. Above-stated causes can be grouped according to the pathophysiologic mechanisms such as supratentorial mass lesions, subtentorial mass lesions, destructive lesions, or metabolic and diffuse cerebral disorders. Psychic disorders such as depression, catotonia and schizophrenia can result in failure to respond to the environment.

Supratentorial mass lesions generally interfere with consciousness by compressing and shifting the cerebral contents and causing pressure on the upper brainstem containing the RAS. These lesions, occuring above the tentorium may include those resulting from trauma, subarachnoid hemorrhage, intracerebral hemorrhage or infarction, tumors, and abscesses. The most serious consequence of supratentorial mass lesion is herniation of the cerebral hemisphere through the tentorial notch, causing compression of the brainstem. Another form of herniation occurs if the brain shifts laterally, forcing the cingulate gyrus under the falx and compressing the blood vessels and brain tissue of the opposite hemisphere. The end result herniation is ischemia and irreversible infarction.

Subtentorial masses or destructive lesions that occur below the tentorium interfere with consciousness by compressing or destroying the RAS above the midpons. Pontine or cerebellar hemorrhage, infarction, tumor, or abscess can affect the subtentorial area of the brain through direct brain compression, upward herniation into the foramen magnum.

Metabolic or diffuse cerebral disorders of either intracranial or extracranial origin can cause alterations in the conscious state. These disorders can disturb cerebral metabolism and thus alter the regulation of cellular nutrition, electrolyte balance, oxygen and carbon dioxide regulation, and enzymatic functions. Specific metabolic problems that can cause unconsciousness include uremia, diabetic mellitus, hypoglycemia alcohol intoxication, drug overdose, and lead poisoning. Regardless of the cause of the unconscious state, two pathophysiologic processes that affect cerebral metabolism generally occur which include, cerebral ischemia, anoxia and cerebral edema. In which cerebral ischemianoxia managed by instituting measures to ensure adequate systemic circulation and cerebral edema treated by hyperosmotic drugs and corticosteroids, e.g. 50 percent dextrose IV with cortisone.

Clinical Manifestation

The clinical manifestation associated with altered LOC are as follows:
- Decreased wakefulness.
- Decreased attention to surrounding environment.
- Confusion.
- Hallucinations.
- Illusions.
- Disorientation.
- Agitation
- Poor memory.
- Decreased ability to carry out activities of daily living.
- Decreased mobility.
- Incontinence.

Management

Diagnostic tests: Diagnostic evaluation of altered LOC include searching for the structural or metabolic aetiology of the changes. The work-up includes a detailed history, extensive neurological examination, radiological examination and laboratory testing, which include the following:

Structural tests	Metabolic tests
Skull X-rays	Complete blood count
Electroencephalography	Urinalysis
Computerized tomography	Electrolytes (glucose, bun, creatinine)
Cerebral angiogram	Calcium
Magnetic resonance imaging	Liver function studies
Evoked potential	• Cardiac enzymes • Serum osmolarity • Lumbar puncture • Arterial blood pressure • Toxicology serum for drug abuse

While diagnostic test results are pending, or tests are being scheduled, a detailed history is obtained from the patient, when possible and also from family, significant others and physical examination. The detailed neurological examination provides the foundation for assessment of the patient with altered LOC, but health care providers including nurses use a variety of scales to standardize the ongoing evaluation of a patient's functioning. Example includes Glasgow Coma Scale (GCS), the Rancho Los Amigo Scale (RLAS) and mini-mental state examination.

- Glasgow Coma Scale (GCS): The GCS was developed to evaluate head injured patients but can be used with a wide variety of neurological patients. GCS does not take place comprehensive neurological examination, but the results (scores) can be graphed and used to identify trends in the patient's overall function and predict outcomes. The GCS is as given below:

1. **Glasgow Coma Scale**

   Category and response   *Score*
   - Eye opening:
     - Spontaneously open   4
     - Open to verbal request   3
     - Open with painful stimuli   2
     - No opening   1
   - Best verbal response:
     - Oriented to time, place, person,
     - converse appropriately   5
     - Converse, but confused   4
     - Words spoken, but conversation not sustained   3
     - Sounds made, no intellible words   2
     - No response   1
   - Best motor response:
     - Obeys commands   6
     - Localizes to painful stimuli   5
     - Withdraws to painful stimuli   4
     - Abnormal flexion to pain (decorticates posturing)   3
     - Abnormal extension to pain (decerebrate posturing)   2
     - No response   1

2. **Rancho los amigos scale (RLAS)**

RLAS was developed as a behavioral rating scale to aid in the assessment and treatment of brain injured patients. It assesses the progressive recovery of cognitive abilities as demonstrated through behavioral changes and is most commonly used in subacute and rehabiliative setting.

RLAS is used to know the level of cognitive functioning as follows:
- *No response:* Patient is completely unresponsive to any stimuli.
- *Generalized response:* Patient reacts inconsistently and nonpurposefully to stimuli in non-specific manner.

- *Localized response:* Patient reacts specifically but inconsistant.
- *Confused-agitated:* Patient is heightened state of activity with severely decreased ability to proess information.
- *Confused-inappropriate:* Patient appears alert and is able to respond to simple commands fairly consistently.
- *Confused-appropriate:* Patient shows goal-directed behavior but depends on external input for direction.
- *Automatic-appropriate:* Patient appears appropriate and oriented within hospital and homesetting, goes through daily routine automatically with minimal to absent confusion and has shallow recall of actions.
- *Purposeful-appropriate:* Patient is alert and oriented, is able to recall and integrate past and recent events, and is aware of end responsive to culture.

Nursing Assessment

Nursing assessment begins with patient's detailed history and the specific factors to assess in a patient experiencing altered LOC are subjective data which include:
- When the change in LOC was not noticed.
- Onset-sudden or slowly progressive.
- Patient and family awareness and understanding of the symptoms.
- Ability to think, think abstractly, calculate and make every day decisions.
- Recent history of falls, infection or other trauma.
- Medication in use—Prescription and over-the-counter drugs, alcoholism.
- Visual changes.
- Other symptoms, pain, fever, nausea, headache and objective data which includes:
- Motor status, presence of posturing.
- Sensory status.
- Cranial nerve assessment, protective reflexes.
- Breathing pattern.
- Oxygen status.
- Laboratory results (electrolytes, HB percent blood glucose, BUN, creatinine.
- Drug level.

Nursing Diagnosis

The possible nursing diagnosis is altered LOC will be:
- Ineffective breathing pattern r/t neuromuscular impairment, cognition.
- Altered tissue perfusion, cerebral r/t decreased or altered blood flow.
- Altered thought process r/t structural or metabolic imbalance.
- Ineffective thermoregulation r/t impaired regulatory function.
- Risk for injury r/t sensory/motor deficits, loss or integrative function.
- Impaired physical mobility r/t neuromuscular impairment.
- Altered nutrition (body requirement r/t decreased alertness, chewing/swallowing difficulty.
- Bowel incontinence r/t perceptual or cognitive impairment.
- Altered urinary elimination r/t perceptual or cognitive impairment.
- Altered urinary elimination r/t neuromuscular impairment.
- Impaired health maintenance r/t perceptual or cognitive impairment.
- Risk for impaired skin integrity r/t impairment mobility, nutrition pressure.
- Ineffective family company r/t temporary family disorganization.
- Knowledge deficit r/t disorder, plans of treatment, etc.

Objectives

Patient with altered LOC should achieve the following:
- Maintain effective breathing pattern.
- Maintain adequate systematic blood pressure to perfuse the brain.
- Maintain coherent thought process, is not confused.
- Maintain body temperature within normal limits.
- Safety precautions in place does not experience injury.
- Maintains highest possible mobility with use of assistive devices and assistance of others.
- Consume adequate balanced nutrients to maintain stable body weight.
- Maintain regular pattern of bowel elimination without constipation, diarrhea or incontinence.
- Maintain urinary incontinence with or without external continence device.
- Participate in self-care to the maximum degree possible.
- Skin integrity maintained, no evidence of redness or injury.
- Family activity participates in all decision-making and planning for patient care, use coping strategies to adapt family role changes.
- Patients and family indicate understanding of diagnosis of LOC.

Nursing Intervention

The following measures to be taken to achieve the above objectives of the patient with altered LOC.
- Protect the airway and promote gas exchanges.
  - Turn side to side 4th hourly.
  - Encourage coughing and deep breathing every hour while awake.
  - Suctions oral and pharyngeal airway promptly if necessary.
  - Monitor oxygen saturation and blood gases.

- Promote cerebral tissue perfusion.
  - Maintain hydration, prevent hypovolemia.
  - Monitor effects of antihypertensive, other medication and promote adequate cardiac output and systemic blood pressure.
- Promote tissue perfusion.
  - Turn patient 4th hourly.
  - Perform passive or active range of motion to enhance circulation at least once per shift.
  - Apply elastic stockings or intermittent compression devices to prevent deep vein thrombosis.
- Promote sensory-perceptual function.
  - Provide meaningful stimuli.
  - Speak to patient before touching.
  - Orient patient to surroundings.
  - Provide adequate lighting.
  - Have calender and clock within patient's view.
  - Have familiar objects in patient's view.
- Maintain normal body temperature.
  - Hyperthermia
    * Remove excess bed coverings.
    * Maintain a cool room temperature.
    * Administer antipyretic medication.
    * Provide tepid bath.
  - Hypothermia
    * Apply warmed blankets.
    * Use heat lamps with caution
    * Increase room temperature.
- Prevent Injury.
  - Keep a call bell within the reach of patient.
  - Implement seizure precautions as needed.
  - Provide eye care to prevent corneal damage at least once per shift.
  - Apply restraints only as last resort at physician's order.
- Promote mobility.
  - Perform active or passive range of motion every shift.
  - Assist patients with ambulation at position changes.
- Maintain nutrition.
  - Record intake to assess quantity and quality.
  - Assist patient with feeding and swallowing safely with instruction to take small bites and chew carefully.
  - Administer enteral feedings at recommended rate for needs.
  - Weigh patient daily or weekly to assess gain or loss.
- Maintain regular bowel function.
  - Provide adequate hydration.
  - Ensure adequate fiber in diet or tube feedings.
  - Administer stool softener as needed.
- Maintain bladder continence.
  - Remove indwelling catheters as soon as possible.
  - Provide, regular toileting to prevent incontinence.
- Maintain hygiene.
  - Assist patient with ADL as needed.
  - If patient is unable to care for self, provide bath, mouth, eye and skin care regularly.
  - Shampoo patient's hairs as needed.
- Maintain skin integrity.
  - Reposition patient at least at every 2 hours' interval.
  - Use lotion or other skin moisturizers to prevent dry skin.
  - Keep sheets dry, free of wrinkles.
  - If skin breakdown is present or if patient is at high risk use pressure relief device.
  - Avoid shearing and friction when moving patient.
- Supporting family coping.
  - Assess family for usual coping skills and resources used.
  - Introduce family to new resources available for support.
  - Listen and address family concerns and provide needed information.
  - Teach patient care skills needed for home care to family.

In addition, the patient with confusion or disorientation may be taken care by using following measures.

- Promote communication.
  - Touch may be useful to establish communication.
  - Use calm, quiet and unhurried voice to talk to patient.
  - Talk slowly and distinctly and use short sentences.
  - Face patient when talking and stay with conversational range.
- Promote orientation.
  - Explain procedure in advance.
  - Environment should be well-lighted.
  - Keep large calender and clock in view.
  - Introduce self when caring for patient.
  - Keep sensory stimulation to a minimum.
  - Provide consistency in staff caring for patient.
  - Keep decision making to a minimum.
- Support family.

Increased Intracranial Pressure (ICP)

Normal intracranial pressure (ICP) is the pressure exerted by the total volume from the three components within the skull: brain tissue, blood and CSF. ICP can be measured in the ventricles, subarachnoid space, subdural space, epidural space, or brain paranchymal tissue using a water manometer or a pressure transducer. With the patient in the lateral recumbent position, the pressure is generally recorded at 60 to 150 mm H_2O with the use of the water manometer. When the patient is lying with a 30-degree elevation of the head and the pressure is measured intracranially, it is 0 to 15 mm Hg with the use of the pressure transducer. A sustained pressure above the upper limit is considered abnormal.

Increased ICP is a life-threatening situation that results from an increase in any or all of the three components, i.e. brain tissue, blood and CSF. It is a pathological process common to many neurological conditions. The intracranial volume composed of brain tissue (85%) intracranial blood volume (5%) and cerebrospinal fluid (10%). Any increase in the volume of any of these contents singly in combinations, results in an increase in ICP, because the cranial vault is rigid and nonexpandable.

Etiology

Any lesion that increases one or more of the intracranial content is called a space-occupying lesion. Cerebral edema is the important factor contributing to increased ICP. Conditions associated with cerebral edema are as follows:

- Mass lesions
  - Neoplasms (primary and materialistic).
  - Abscess hydrocephalus.
  - Hemorrhage (intracerebral and extracerebral hematoma).
- Head injuries (hemorrhage, contusion, post-traumatic brain swelling).
- Brain surgery.
- Brain infections.
- Vascular insult.
  - Infarction (thrombolic and embolic).
  - Venous thrombosis.
  - Anoxic and ischemic episodes.
- Toxic or metabolic encephalophatic conditions.
  - Lead and arsenic intoxication.
  - Renal failure and liver failure.
  - Reye's syndrome.

Contributory factors are increased ICP will include:

- Hypercapnia ($PaCO_2$ 45 mm Hg)
- Hypoxemia (PaO_2 60 mm Hg)
- Cerebral vasodialatory agents (e.g. alothane, antihistamine)
- Valsalva manuoever.
- Body positioning (prone, flexion of neck, extreme hip flexion).
- Isometric muscle contractions
- Coughing or sneezing
- Rapid eye movement sleep
- Emotional upsets
- Noxious stimuli
- Arousal from sleep
- Clustering of actions.

Pathophysiology

The cranial vault is a rigid, closed compartments. The intracranial contents of the brain, blood and CSF occupy the skull fully and exists in a dynamic equilibrium under normal conditions. The Monro-Kellie hypothesis states that conditions that increase one or more of the intercranial conent must cause a reciprocal change in the remaining contents or an increase in ICP will occur. As the intercranial volume increases, compensatory mechanisms take place. CSF-filled spaces can be compressed and CSF redistributed to the lumbar cistern to reduce intracranial CSF volume. Intracranial blood vessels, especially the veins can be compressed by surrounding brain tissue and displace intracranial blood volume. These compensatory mechanisms initially are able to accommodate a growing intracranial volume without significant increases in ICP, but these mechanisms are quickly exhausted if the intracranial volume continues to increase. When the volume within the skull overwhelms, the compensatory mechanisms and intracranial pressure begins to rise. Small increase in pressure occurs in response to initial increase in volume. As compensatory mechanisms fail, additional increase in volume causes dramatic increase in ICP. Normal ICP between 0 to 15 mm Hg. pressure over 20 mm Hg are considered to be increased ICP.

As pressure within the skull increases, the cerebral blood vessels may be compressed, causing a reduction in cerebral blood flow (CBF). CBF is the amount of blood in millilitres passing through 100 gms of brain tissue in 1 minute. The global CBF is approximately 50 ml per minute per 100 gram of brain tissue. There is a difference in flow between the white and gray matter of the brain. The white matter has a slower blood flow (25 ml/m/100 g brain tissue) and the gray matter has a faster blood flow (75 ml/minute/100 g. brain tissue). The maintenance of blood flow to the brain is critical because the brain requires a constant supply of oxygen and glucose. The brain uses 20 percent of the body's oxygen and 25 percent of its glucose. Inadequate perfusion initiates a vicious cycle, causing the partial carbon dioxide pressure (PCO_2) to increase and the partial oxygen pressure (PO_2) and pH to decrease cerebral arterioles have the ability to autoregulate, which allows them to dilate or constrict to maintain a constant blood supply to the brain. Changes such as an increasing PCO_2 or decreasing pH cause vasodilatation of the cerebral blood vessels and an increase in ICP. Autoregulation works when the mean arterial pressure (MAP) is between 50 mm Hg and 150 mm Hg and when the metabolic environment of the brain is normal. Severe anoxia and hypotensive state cause autoregulation to fail, subjecting the brain blood supply to the wide variations of systolic blood pressure (SBP).

Cerebral perfusion pressure (CPP) is a parameter used to monitor the adequacy of blood flow to the brain in the face of increased ICP. As ICP increases, blood vessels may be compressed, reducing blood flow to the brain in the face of increased ICP. As ICP increases, blood vessels may be unpressed, reducing blood flow to the brain. SBP needs to be high enough to overcome the ICP and deliver sufficient oxygen and glucose to brain tissues. The CPP measured by subtracting ICP from MAP. The formula is:

CPP = MAP - ICP   SBP + 2 (DBP)
MAP = DBP + 1/3 (SBP–DBP) or 3
       (DBP = Diastolic Blood Pressure.)
For example, SBP = 122/84
   MAP = 97, ICP = 12 mm Hg
       CPP = 85 mm Hg.

The actual brain structure can also be affected by increased ICP. The brain is surrounded and divided into compartments within the skull by the dura matter. The presence of edema or space-occupying lesions may cause brain tissue to shift or herniate. Subfalcial or cingulate herniation occurs when the brain is forced under the falx-cerebri that separates the cerebral hemispheres. Uncal herniation occurs when the uncal portion of the temporal lobes shift over the edge of the tentorium cerebelli. Transformental herniation occurs when the brainstem is forced downward through the foramen magnum.

Clinical Manifestations

The clinical manifestations of increased ICP can take many forms, depending on the cause, location and rate at which the pressure increase occurs. The common clinical manifestation of increased ICP are as follows:

Early Signs

- Decreasing level of consciousness in the earlier and most sensitive sign.
- Headache that increases in intensity with coughing and straining.
- Pupillary changes:
  – Dilation with slowed constrictions.
  – Visual disturbances such as diplopia and ptosis.
- Contralateral motor or sensory losses:
  – Decrease in motor function.

Late Signs

- Further decrease in level of consciousness.
- Changes in vital signs:
  – Rise in systolic blood pressure.
  – Decrease in distolic blood pressure.
  – Widened pulse pressure.
  – Slow pulse.
- Respiratory dysrhythmias:
  – Shallow, slowed respirations.
  – Irregular patterns or periods of apnea.
  – Hiccups.
- Fever without clear source of infection.
- Vomitting (more common in children).
- Decerebrate (Extensor or decorticate (flexor) posturing).

It is often difficult to identify increased ICP as the cause of comaloss of consciousness also confuses the interpretation of clinical signs making it difficult to follow the progression of the increasing ICP.

Diagnostic Studies

- History and physical examination.
- Vital signs, neurologic checks, ICP measurements (via intraventricular catheter, subdural bolt or epidural transducer) every hour.
- Skull, chest and spinal X-rays.
- MRI, CT scan, EEG, angiography.
- Cerebral blood flow and velocity studies, PET.
- Lubricating studies including CBC, coagulation profile, electrolytes creatinine, ammonia level, general drug and toxicology screen, CSF protein, cells and glucose, arterial blood gas analysis.
- ECG.

The nurse has to assist in carrying out these diagnostic studies.

Management

- The goals of management are to identify and treat the underlying cause of increased ICP and to support brain function. A careful history is an important diagnostic aid that can direct the search for the underlying cause. The possible causes of unconsciousness may be:
- *Trauma:* Head and neck trauma.
- *Infection:* Meningitis and encephalitis.
- *Poison:* Drug overdose, toxic exposure and carbon monoxide.
- *Metabolic:* Diabetic coma, insulin shock, liver failure, uremia, cardiac arrest and CVA.

An assessment finding (possible) over dose of drug and others elicited are:

- Unresponsive to voice and pain.
- Dilated or pinpoint pupils may be unreactive.
- Involuntary movements.
- Flaccidity or rigidity of muscles.
- Depressed or hyperactive reflexes.
- Decerebrated or decorticate posturing.
- Diaphoresis.
- Hyperthermia.
- Flushed dry skin.
- Glasgow Coma Scale score < 12.
- Abnormal vital signs.
- Arrythmias.
- Odor of alcohol, acetone on breath.
- Track marks.
- Signs of trauma.
- Petechae or rash.

An intervention included in emergency management of unconscious patient will indicate:

In Initial Stages

- Ensure patent airway
- Administer oxygen via nasal cannula or nonrebreather mask.

- Establish IV access with one large bore catheter and normal saline.
- Administer IV naloxine if narcotic overdose suspected.
- Administer thiamine to malnourished or known alcoholic patient to prevent Wernicke's encephalopathy.
- Administer one vial 50% dextrose if blood glucose < 60 mg/dl (3.3 mm 01/L).
- Prepare for IV insulin administration of glucose > 400 mg/dl (22.2 mm 01/L).
- Elevate head of bed or position on side to prevent aspiration (unless trauma involved).

And Ongoing Monitoring Instituted to

- Monitor vital signs, level of consciousness, oxygen saturation, cardiac rhythm, Glasgow Coma Score, pupil size and reactivity, respiratory status.
- Anticipate need for intubation if gag reflex is absent.
- Anticipate gastric lavage if drug overdose is suspected.

The nursing intervention to be continued along with collaboration management of patient with increased ICP are:

- Elevation of head of bed to 30 degrees with head in a neutral position to facilitate reduction of cerebral edema.
- Intubation and controlled ventilation to $PaCO_2$ of 30 to 35 mm Hg because CO_2 is a potent cerebral vasodilator and hyperventilation reduces $PaCO_2$.
- Good pulmonary toilet to improve ventilation and prevent pulmonary complication by removing accumulated secretions, which helps to reduce risk of aspiration and ensure patent airway.
- Maintenance of fluid and electrolyte balance and assessment of osmalality.
- Maintenance of systolic arterial pressure between 100 and 160 mm Hg.
- Maintenance of CPP > 70 mm Hg.
- Maintenance of PaO_2 at 100 mm Hg or greater.
- Maintenance of normothermia.
- Adequate sedation.
- Drug therapy as prescribed.
  - Osmotic diuretics (mannitol).
  - Loop diuretics fursomide (lasix), ethacrynic and (Edecrin).
  - Corticosteroids (methylprednisone, dexamethosone (Decadran).
  - GI ulcer prophylactic (H2-Receptor antagoinst, e.g. Cimetedine).
- ICP monitoring.

HEAD INJURY

Head injury includes any trauma to the scalp, skull, or brain tissues either singly or collectively. The term head trauma is used primarily to signify craniocerebral trauma, which includes alteration in consciousness, no matter how brief. Head trauma has a high potential for poor outcome. Death from head injury trauma occurs at three time points after, injury, immediately after injury, within 2 hours after injury, and approximately 3 weeks after injury. The majority of deaths after a head injury occur immediately after the injury, either from the direct head trauma or from massive hemmorrhage and shock. Death occurring within a few hours of the trauma caused by progressive worsening of the head injury or from internal bleeding. An immediate note of change in neurologic status and surgical intervention are critical in the prevention of deaths at this point. Death occurring 3 weeks or more after injury results from multisystem failure. Expert nursing care in the weeks following the injury are crucial in decreasing mortality. Factors that predict a poor outcome include the presence of an intracranial hematoma, increasing age of the patient, abnormal motor responses, impaired or absent eye movement or pupil light refluxes, early sustained hypertension hypoxemia, or hypercapnia and ICP level higher than 20 mm Hg.

Etiology

The variables that influence the extent of the injury to the head include the following:

- Status of the head at impact moving or still.
- Location and direction of the impact.
- Rate of energy transfer.
- Surface area involved in the energy transfer.

Blunt head injuries will occur due to motor vehicle collision, pedestrian event, fall, assault and sports injury. Penetrating head injuries are due to—Gunshot wound arrow and such types.

Pathophysiology

Mechanisms of trauma to the head are of general types, deformation, acceleration deceleration and rotation.

- *Deformation* results from the transmission of energy to the skull of the energy is sufficient, the skill is deformed of fractured.
- *Acceleration*-deceleration injuries typically occur when the acceleration skull moving in a motor vehicle, suddenly decelerates when it hits an immobile object as the steering wheel or windshield.
- *Rotational* forces also distort the brain and can cause tension, stretching and diffuse shearing of brain tissues. Often the forces of acceleration, deceleration and rotation occur together, affecting both the brain and spinal cord.

Injuries vary from minor scalp wound to concussion and open skull fractures with severe brain injury.

- *Scalp lacerations* are the most minor of the head trauma, because the scalp contains many blood vessels with poor constructive abilities. Most scalp lacerations associated with profuse bleeding. The major complication associated with it is infection.

- *Skull fractures* are a common form of primary craniocerebral trauma. Fracture of the skull may be linear or depressed, simple or communuted, or combine and closed or open.
  – Linear fractures caused by low-velocity injuries in which break is continuity of bone without alteration of relationship of parts.
  – Depressed fractures caused by powerful blow, in which inward dentation of skull is seen.
  – Simple fractures are caused by low to moderate impact in which linear or depressed fracture without fragmentation or communicating lacerations are present.
  – Communuted fractures are caused by direct high momentory impact, in which multiple linear fractures with fragmentation of bone into many places are seen.
  – Compound facture is a severe head injury in which there will be a depressed skull fracture and scalp laceration with communicating pathway to intra-cranial cavity.

The location of the fracture alters the presentation of the clinical signs and symptoms. Clinical manifestation of the skull fractures by location are as follows:

Location	Syndrome or sequelae
Frontal Fracture	• Exposure of brain to contaminatants through frontal air sinus • Possible association with air in forehead tissue • CSF rhinorrhea or pneumocranium
Orbital fracture	• Periorbital ecchymosis (raccoon eyes)
Temporal fracture	• Boggy temporal muscle because of extravasation of blood, benign oval-shaped bruise behind ear in mastoid region (Battles sign) • CSF otorrhea
Parietal fracture	• Deafness • CSF or brain otorrhea • Bulging of tympanic mem-brane caused by blood or CSF • Facial paralysis • Loss of taste • Battle's sign
Posterior fossa fracture	• Occipital bruising resulting in fracturecortical blindness end visual field defects • Rare appearance of ataxia or other cerebellar signs
Basillar skull fracture	• CSF or brain otorrhea, bulging of tympanic mem-brane caused by blood or CSF • Battle's sign • Tinnitus or hearing difficulty • Facial paralysis • Conjugate deviation of gaze • Vertigo

The major potential complication of skull fractures are intracranial infections and hemotoma, as well as meningeal and brain tissue damage.

Brain injuries are categorized as being minor or major.

- *Minor head injury:* Concussion is considered as minor head injury. Concussion refers to a sudden transient mechanical head injury with disruption of neural activity and a change in level of consciousness. Signs of concussion include:
  – Brief disruption in LOC.
  – Amnesia regarding the event (retrograde amnesia) and
  – Headache.

  The manifestations are generally of short duration. A loss of consciousness may occur that is instant or delayed, and the person usually recovers rapidly. Any person who exhibits alteration in consciousness after a blow to the head should be closely observed, after the injury, because the extent of the damage is not always immediately apparent. The postconcussions syndrome is seen anywhere from 2 weeks to 2 months after concussion. The symptoms include:
  – Persistent headache, dizziness and fatigue.
  – Lethargy.
  – Personality and behavioral changes.
  – Shortened attention-span-impaired concentration.
  – Decreased short-term memory and memory impairment.
  – Changes in intellectual ability.

- *Major head injury:* Major head injury includes contusions and laceration. Both injuries represent severe trauma to the brain. Contusion and laceration associated with closed injuries.

  A *contusion* is the bruising of the brain tissue within a focal area that maintains integrity of the piamater and archnoid layers. It is structural alteration characterized by extravasation of blood into the brain. A contusion develops areas of necrosis, infarction, hemorrhage and edema. A contusion frequently occurs at the site of the fracture. It may be at the site of impact or on the opposite side of a camp contra camp injury. Contusions often damage cerebral cortex. Bleeding around the contusion site is generally minimal, and the blood is reabsorbed slowly. Neurologic assessment demonstrates focal findings and generalized disturbance in the LOC. Seizures are a common complication of brain contusion.

  Lacerations involve actual bearing of the brain tissue and occur frequently in association with depressed and compound fractures and penetrating injuries. Tissue damage is severe, and surgical repair of the laceration is impossible., because of the texture of the brain tissue. If bleeding is deep into the brain parenchyma, focal and generalized signs are noted.

When major head injury occurs, many delayed responses are seen including hermorrhage, hematoma formation, seizures and cerebral edema. Intracerebral hemorrhage is generally associated with cerebral laceration. This hemorrhage manifests as a space-occupying lesion accompanied by unconsciousness, hemeplegia on the contralateral side and dilated pupil on the ipsilateral side. As the hematoma expands, syptoms of increased ICP become more severe. Prognosis generally poor with a large intracerebral hemorrhage.

Diffuse axonal injury (DAI) caused by rapid movement of the brain during which delicate axons are stretched and damaged. This damage interferes with nervous transmission and can cause extensive diffuse deficits.

Complications

Secondary injury occurs as a result of the body response to the initial trauma, which include cerebral edema, increased ICP and hematoma formation.

Cerebral edema: In response to local injury, bleeding and systemic disturbances in circulation that result in hypoxia, the brain becomes edematous. Cell damage and systemic hypoxia cause cell membranes to fail, leading to cytotoxicoedma, cell lining the blood vessels are damaged and capillaries become more permeable, allowing fluid to leak out into the interstitial space. This is called vasogenic edema.

Increased ICP, vasogenic edema contributes to increased ICP.

Hematoma Formation

- An epidural hematoma results from bleeding between the dura and the inner surface of the skull.
- A subdural hematoma occurs from bleeding between the duramater and the arachnoid layer of the meningeal covering of the brain. It results from injury to brain substance and its parenchymal vessels (venous brain).
- Intracerebral hematoma occurs from bleeding within the parenchyma.

This usually occurs within the forntal and temporal lobes possibly from the rupture of intracerebral vessels at the time of injury. A burst lobe in an intracerebral or intracerebellar hematoma that is in extension of subarchnoid hemorrhage. This type of intracerebral hematoma is thought to result from hemorrage of supra-cortical vessels.

Nursing Management During Emergency

Assessment may be done as with other naurological assessment procedures, and diagnostic studies. Accordingly, findings of the assessment during emergency management will include.

- *Surface findings:*
  - Scalp laceration.
  - Fracture or depression in skull.
  - Bruises or contusions on face, Battle's sign (Bruising behind ears).
  - Reccon eyes (dependent bruising around eyes).
- *Respiratory findings:*
  - Central neurogenic hyperventilation.
  - Cheyne stokes respirations.
  - Decreased oxygen saturation.
  - Pulmonary edema.
- *Central nervous system:*
  - Unequal or dilated pupils.
  - A symmetric facid movements.
  - Garbled speech and abusive speech.
  - Confusion.
  - Decreased level of consciousness.
  - Combativeness.
  - Involuntary movements.
  - Seizures.
  - Bowel and bladder incontinence.
  - Flaccidity.
  - Depressed or hyperactive reflexes.
  - Decerebrate or decorticate posturing.
  - Glasgow Coma Scale 12.
  - CSF leaking from ears or nose.

The nursing intervention during initial stage and ongoing monitoring are as follows:

In an initial stage:

- Ensure patent airway.
- Stabilize cervical spine.
- Administer oxygen via nasal cannular or non-rebreather mask.
- Establish IV access with two large bore catheters to infuse normal saline or lactated Ringer's solution.
- Control external bleeding with sterile pressure dressing.
- Assess for rhinorrhea, scalp wounds.
- Remove patient's clothing.

Ongoing monitoring includes:

- Maintain patient warmth using blankets, warmth IV fluids, overhead warming lights and warm humidifying oxygen.
- Monitor vital signs, level of consciousness, oxygen saturation, cardiac rhythm, Glasgow Coma Score, pupil size, and reactivity.
- Anticipate need for intubation if gag reflex is absent.
- Assume neck injury with head injury.
- Administer fluids cautiously to prevent fluid overload and increasing ICP.

Nursing Management

Assessment: The patient with head injury is always considered to have potential for development of increased

ICP. The data collected generally include information gathered for unconscious patient, which include Glasgow Coma scales, monitory neurological status and determining the leakage of CSF, etc.

Nursing Diagnosis

- Altered tissue perfusion, cerebral related to interruption and cerebral blood flow associated with cerebral hemorrhage, hemotomy and edema.
- Hyperthermia related to increased metabolism, infection and loss of cerebral integrative function secondary to possible hypothalmic injury.
- Sensory/perceptual alteration related to cerebral injury and ICU environment.
- Pain related to headache, nausea and vomiting.
- Impaired physical mobility r/t decrease LOC and treatment imposed and bedrest.
- Risk for eye injury r/t loss of protective reflexes.
- Risk for infection r/t and environmental contamination.
- Anxiety r/t abrupt charges in health status, hospital environment.
- Self-esteem disturbance r/t altered appearance of head and face.

Planning: The voerall goals are that the patient with an acute head injury will:
- Maintain adequate cerebral perfusion.
- Remain normothermic.
- Be free from pain, discomfort and infection and
- Attain maximum cognitive, motor and sensory function.

Nursing Intervention

The following nursing intervention to be installed when taking care of person with closed head injury.
- Promote rest
  - Provide with quiet environment.
  - Observe frequently.
  - Administer anticonvulsants as ordered.
  - Medication for pain as necessary.
- Maintain temperature
  - Give tepid sponge bath if hyperthermic.
  - Administer antipyretic as ordered.
  - Use hypothermia blanket if ordered.
  - Reduce or increase temperature in patient's room as needed.
- Promote adequate respiration
  - Suction only as necessary to provide adequate airway.
  - Elevate head of bed to 30 degrees.
  - Administer supplemental oxygen if ordered.
  - Place patient in side lying position.
- Observe for drainage from ears and/or nose
  - Make no attempt to clean out orifice.
  - Do not suction nose if drainage is present.
  - Test drainage for presence of CSF and refer immediately if present.
- Control of cerebral edema
  - Administer diuretics as ordered.
  - Elevate head of bed to 30 degrees.
  - Perform neurological checks as ordered.
- Maintain electrolyte balance
  - Observe for inappropriate hydration or dehydration.
  - Monitor electrolytes.
- Maintain elimination
  - Keep accurate intake and output record.
  - Restrict fluid if ordered.
  - Monitor output.
  - Remove catheter as soon as possible.
- Provide emotional support
  - Give specific guidelines for appropriate behavior.
  - Give positive feedback.
  - Allow patient adequate time to complete tasks.

INFECTIONS AND INFLAMMATION OF BRAIN

Meningitis

Meningitis is an acute inflammation of the pia mater and the arachnoid membrane surrounding the brain and spinal cord. Therefore, meningitis is always cerebrospinal infection.

Etiology

Bacterial meningitis affects the leptomeninges, the pia and arachnoid layers and the CSF. The most common pathogens causing meningitis are *Haemophilus influenzae*, *Neisseria meningitidis*, and *Streptococcus pneumoniae*. The causative organism is very significantly at different ages. *Haemophilus* is common in young children, and often follows an upper respiratory infection or ear infections.

Neisseria has its highest incidence in children and young adults and can cause an overwhelming septicemia. *Streptococcus pneumonia* causes pneumococcal form of meningitis which is common in adults. Viral meningitis also called septic meningitis caused by viral and nonviral sources.

Pathophysiology

Organisms and viruses reach the nervous system by many routes. The most common route is the bloodstream and bacteria in the nasopharynx may enter the bloodstream during an upper respiratory infection. Once the organism reaches the brain, the CSF in the subarachnoid space and the arachnoid membrane become infected. The infection then spreads rapidly throughout the meninges and eventually invades the ventricles. The inflamatory response to the infection tends to increase CSF production with a moderate increase in pressure. In bacterial meningitis, the purulent secretion produced quickly spreads to other areas of the brain through the CSF. If this process extends into the brain parenchyma or if concurrent encephalitis is present, cerebral edema and increased ICP become more problem. Pathological alteration includes hyperemia of the meningea vessels, edema of brain tissue, increased ICP and generalized inflammator reactions with exudation of white blood cells into the subarachnoid. Hydrocephalus may be caused by exudate blocking the small passages between ventricles.

Clinical Manifestation

- Fever.
- Severe headache.
- Nausea and vomiting.
- Nuchal rigidity (resistance to flexion of the neck).
- Positive Kerning's sign (inability of the patient to extend the legs when the knee is flexed at the hip).
- Positive Brudzinski's sign (the hip and knee flex when the neck of patient's neck is flexed).
- Photophobia.
- A decreased LOC.
- Signs of increased ICP.
- Coma is associated with poor prognosis.

Headache becomes progressively worse and may be accompanied by vomiting and irritability. If the organism is meningococcus, a skin rash is common and petechiae may be seen.

Complications

The most common complications of meningitis is residual neurologic dysfunction. Cranial nerve dysfunction (III, IV, VI, VII or VIII) and cranial nerve irritation (II, III, IV, VI, VII, VIII). Accordingly, sensory loss occurs. And hemiparesis dysphasia and hemianopia may also occur. These signs usually resolve. If resolution does not occur, a cerebral abscess, subdural empheyema, subdural effusion, or persistent meningitis is suggested. Acute cerebral edema may occur with bacterial meningitis causing seizures, CN III palsy, bradycardia, hypertensive coma and death. And non-communicating hydrocephalus may occur if the exudate causes adhesions that prevent the normal flow of the CSF from the ventricles. A complication of the menigococcal meningitis is the Waterhouse-Friderichsen syndrome.

Diagnostic Studies

- History and physical examination.
- Analysis of CSF.
- CBC, coagulation profile, electrolyte levels, glucose, platelet count.
- Routine urinalysis.
- Blood culture (twice).
- Urine specific gravity (4th hourly).
- CT scan, MRI, EEG, skull X-Ray studies, brain scan.

Management

Meningitis can cause a medical emergency. When meningitis is suspected antibiotic therapy (Penicillin, ampicillin, ceftriaxone, cefotaxime) is instituted after the collection of specimens for culture, even before the diagnosis is confirmed. Diagnostic measures include lumbar puncture and analysis of CSF. The fundus of the eye should be examined via opthalmoscope for Papilledema before lumbar puncture for identification of possibly-increased ICP.

Treatment of bacterial infections consist of antibiotic therapy for the causative organism and determine by culture of CSF. Parenteral antibiotic at least 10 days. Antibiotic may be given direct, i.e. intrathecally. Steroids may be given to reduce edema.

General treatment measures include suggestive care to control and reduce fever, balance fluids and electrolytes and promote comfort. The patient with meningitis is usually actualy ill. The fever is high and head pain is severe. Irritation of the cerebral cortex may result in seizures. The changes in mental status and LOC depend on the degree of increased ICP. Assessment of vital signs, neurologic evaluation, fluid intake and output and evaluation of the lung field and skin should be performed at regular intervals based on the patient's condition and recorded carefully.

Encephalitis

Encephalitis is an acute inflammation of the brain and is usually caused by virus, can also be caused by bacteria or fungi.

Etiology

Viral infection is the most common, typically caused by the arbovirus or Herpes Simplex (HSV). Many different viruses have been implicated in encephalitis, some of them are associated with certain seasons of the year and endemic to certain geographic area. Epidemic encephalitis is transmitted by ticks and mosquitos. Nonepidemic encephalitis may occur as a complication of measles, chickenpox and mumps.

Pathophysiology and Clinical Manifestations

Encephalitis causes degenerative changes in the nerve cells of the brain and produces scattered areas of inflammation and necrosis. Some inflammation of the meninges is also typically present. The symptoms vary significantly from virus to virus. But often include fever, headache, seizures, stiff neck and a declining level of consciousness that can progress from lethargy and restlessness to coma. Manifestations resemble those of meningitis. A wide variety of local neurological signs can also be present. The mortality rate for encephalitis also varies subsequentally, but most of the patients experience some degree of residual deficit. Deficits include decreased cognitive functioning, personality changes, paralysis, and dementia. Patients can also be left deaf and blind.

Diagnosis and Treatment

Early diagnosis and treatment of viral encephalitis are essential for favourable outcomes. Brain imaging techniques such as MRI, and PET along with polymerase chain reaction tests for the HIV, DNA levels in CSF allow for earlier detection of viral encephalitis.

Collaborative and nursing management is symptomatic and supportive. Cerebral edema is a major problem and diuretics (mannitol) and corticosteroids (dexamethasone) are used to control it. The decrease is characterized by diffuse damage to the nerve cells of the brain. Perivascular cellular infiltration, proliferation of glial cells and increasing cerebral edema. The sequelae of encephalitis include mental deterioration, amnesia, personality changes and hemiparesis.

Acyclovir (20 Virax) and vidarabine (Vire-A) are used to treat encephalitis caused by HIV infection. Long term symptoms, memory impairment, epilepsy, anosmia, personality changes, behavioral abnormalities and dysphasia. For maximal benefit, antiviral agents should be started before the onset of coma.

BRAIN ABSCESS

Brain abscess is an accumulation of pus within the brain tissue that can result from a local or a systemic infection.

Etiology

Direct extension from ear, tooth, mastoid, or sinus infection is the primary cause. Other causes for brain abscess formation include spetic venous thrombosis from a pulmonary infection, bacterial endocardities, skull fracture, and nonsterile neurologic procedure. Streptococci and staphylococci are the primary infective organisms.

Clinical Manifestation

Manifestations are similar to those of meningitis and encephalitis and include headache and fever. Signs of increased ICP may include drowsiness, confusion, and seizures. Focal symptoms may be present and reflect the local area of the abscess. For example visual field defects or psychomotor seizures are common with temporal lobe abscess, whereas an occipital abscess may be accompanied by visual impairment and hallucinations.

Management

Antimicrobial therapy is the primary treatment for brain abscess. Other manifestations are treated symptomatically. If drug therapy is used effective, the abscess needs to be drained, or removed if it is encapsulated. In untreated, treated cases, mortality rate is 100 percent. Seizures occur in 30 percent cases.

Nursing measures are similar to those for management of meningitis or increased ICP for surgical drainage or removal is the treatment of choice, nursing care is similar to that described under cranial surgery.

Other infections of the brain include subdural empheyema, estiomyelitis of the cranial bones, epidural abscess and venous sinus thrombosis after periorbital cellulitis.

INTRACRANIAL TUMORS

Tumors of the brain may be primary, arising from tissues within the brain or secondary, resulting from a metastasis from malignant neoplasm elsewhere in the body. Brain tumors are generally classified according to the tissue from which they arise. If malignant, the tumor is graded according to general cancer staging procedures.

Classification of Intracranial Tumors

Brain tumors may be classified as those arising inside the brain substance as follow:
- *Gliomas*
  - *Astrocytoma*: arises from supportive tissue, glial cells and astrocytes. Usual location is the white matter of frontal and temporal lobes in adults, lateral and cerebellar lobes in children. This is and moderately malignant grades I and II.
  - *Glioblastoma multiforme*: arises from primitive stem cell (glioblast) usual location is cerebral hemisphers. This is highly malignant and invasive and grades III and IV.
  - *Oligodendroglioma*: arises from glial cells and dendrites. Usual location are cerebral hemispheres, most in frontal lobe, some in basal ganglia and cerebellum. Most are benign (encapsulation and calcification).
  - *Ependymoma*: arise from ependymal epithelium usually occurs in lateral and fourth ventricles in children and young adults. They are benign to highly malignant, most benign and encapsulated.
  - *Medulloblastoma*: Arise from supportive tissue, usually at posterior fossa, fourth ventricle, brainstem in children. They are highly malignant and invasive, metastatic to spinal cord and remote areas of brain.
- *Menigioma:* Arise from endothelial cells, fibrous tissues elements, transitional cells and angioblasts. Usual locations are arachnoid villi dura, half over convexity of hemisphere and half at base of hemisphere. They are usually benign, encapsulation outside brain substance.
- *Acoustic neuroma* (*neurofibroma*): Arise from Schwann cells inside auditory meatus on vestibular (sheath of vestibular portion of III CN) occurs at site between pons and cerebellum. They are usually benign or low grade malignancy encapsulation.

- *Pituitary adenoma:* Arise from pituitary glandular tissue, located at pituitary gland, usually benign.
- *Vascular tumors:* (Hemangioblastoma, arteriovenous malformation) Arises from overgrowth of arteries and veins enlarging from feeder vessels. Usual location is parietal cortex near middle cerebral vessels. They are benign.
- *Metastatic tumors:* Due to cancer cells spread to the brain via circulatory system from lungs, breast, kidney, thyroid and prostate. Usual location is cerebral cortex and diencephalone. They are malignant.

Pathophysiology

The clinical manifestation of intracranial tumors are generally caused by the local destructive effects of the tumors, the resulting accumulation of metabolites, the displacement of structures, the obstruction of CSF or, and the effects of edema and increased ICP on cerebral function. The rate of growth and the appearance of manifestations depend on the location, size and miotic rate of the cells of the tissue of origin.

Clinical Manifestations

A wide range of possible manifestations are associated with brain tumors with the classic feature being progressive manifestations of clinical symptoms. Symptoms can be generalized as well as specific to the tumor location and the structures of the brain that are compressed. The general symptoms are:
- "Pressure" headache (generalized or periorbital).
- Nausea and vomiting unrelated to food intake.
- Symptoms of increased ICP.
- Visual changes:
  - Blurred vision.
  - Diplopia (with III, IV and VI nerve compression).
  - Visual field alteration (with tumor compression of the optic chasam or optic pathways).
  - Enlarged blind spot related to papilledema.
- Seizures.
- Speech difficulty (when the tumor affects the language area in the dominant hemisphere).
- Weakness or hemiparesis (when the tumor affects the motor cortex).
- Alteration in level of consciousness (with a midbrain tumor).
- Personality changes (with frontal tumors).
  Tumor location and associated presenting symptoms are as given below:
  Each area of the brain controls a particular activity.
  - *Cerebral hemispheres*
    - Frontal lobe (unilateral): unilateral hemiphlagia, seizures, memory deficit, personality and judgment changes; visual disturbances.
    - Frontal lobe (bilateral): Symptoms associated with unilateral frontal lobe, and ataxic gait, aphasia (Motor dysfunction).
    - Parietal lobe: Speech disturbance (if tumor is in the dominant hemisphere, inability to write, inability to replicate pictures, spatial disorders, unilateral neglect). Loss of right-left discrimination, seizures, paresthesic sensory-perceptual deficits.
    - Occipital lobe: Visual disturbances (blindness), headache and seizures.
    - Temporal lobe complex or partial seizures, with automatic behavior.
    - Halluciations (Olfactory, visual or gustatory), Aphasia (receptive, sensory).
  - *Subcortical:* Hemiplegia, other symptoms may depend on are of infiltration.
  - *Meningeal tumors:* Symptoms associated with compression of the brain and depends on tumor location.
  - *Metastatic tumors:* Headache, nausea or vomiting because of increased ICP other symptoms depend on location of tumour.
  - *Thalamus and sellar tumors:* Headache, nausea, or and papilledema, nystagamus occur from an increased ICP diabetes incipedus may occur.
  - *Fourth ventricle and cerebellar tumors:* Headache, nausea, and papilledema mystagamus, occur from an increased ICP, ataxic gait and changes in coordination.
  - *Cerebellopontine tumors:* Tinnitus and vertigo deafness.
  - *Brainstem tumors:* Headache upon awakening, drowsiness, vomiting, ataxic gait, facial muscle weakness, hearing loss, dysphagia, dysarthria, "Crossed eyes" or other visual changes and memiparesis.

SPINAL CORD TUMORS

Depending upon the nerves involved:
- *Cervical:* Pain, weakness or muscle wasting in arms, back, neck or legs.
- *Thoracic:* Pain accentuated with deep breathing and coughing, lack of bowel or bladder control may occur depending on tumor location.

Management of Intracranial and Spinal Cord Tumors

The nurse works collaboratively with other members of the health care team to implement the prescribed medical therapy. Because the nurse has a major role in discharging planning and patient teaching. Nurses also has the responsibilities to assist in diagnostic studies.

Diagnostic Studies

An extensive history and a comprehensive neurologic examination must be done in the work-up of a patient with a suspected brain tumor. A careful history and physical examination may provide data with respect to location. Diagnostic studies are similar to those used for a patient with increased ICP. The sensitivity of MRI allows detection of very small tumors. Other diagnostic studies include CT scan, skull X-rays, cerebral angiography EEG, brain scan, PET and lumbar puncture myelogram.

An initial nursing assessment similar to that of unconscious patriot. In addition, assessment should be structured to provide baseline data of neurologic status and the information LOC. Areas to be assessed include the LOC and content consciousness, motor abilities, sensory perception, integrated function (include bowel and bladder functions, balance and proprioception and coping abilities of the patient and family. Watching a patient perform ADL and listening to the patient conversation are convenient ways are to perform part of neurological assessment. *The possible nursing diagnosis are:*

- Altered tissue perfusion: cerebral related to cerebral edema.
- Pain (headache) r/t cerebral edema and increased ICP.
- Self-care deficit r/t altered neuromuscular junction.
- Anxiety r/t diagnosis and treatment.
- Potential for seizures r/t abnormal electrical activity of brain.
- Potential for increased ICP r/t presence of tumor.

The overall goals are that the patient with brain tumor will:

- Maintain normal ICP.
- Maximize neurological functioning.
- Be free from pain and discomfort and
- Be aware of the long-term implication with respect to prognosis and cognitive and physical function. Determination of the presence of seizures, syncope, nausea and vomiting pain and headache or other pain is important in planning care for the patient.

Drug therapy is used in the management of brain tumor, both to treat the tumor with chemotherapy and to manage symptoms. The common medication used and nursing intervention are as follows:

- Phenytoin (Dilantin) used to prevent seizures. In this, the nurse has to assess for gingival hyperplasia, administer drug on schedule and assess for signs of toxicity and rash.
- Dexamethasone (Decadran), used to reduce cerebral edema. In this the nurse has to monitor for increased blood glucose, taper dosage after long-term therapy.
- Laxatives/stool softener are used to prevent constipation. The nurse should monitor fecal impaction and instruct patient not to strain.
- Ranitidin or Famotidin are used to decrease gastric acid secretion. This is usually safe and without significant side effects.
- Radiation therapy lengthens survival in patient with malignant gliomas especially when it is combined with partial surgical removal.

Diet therapy: No special diet is prescribed for the patient with brain tumor. Regular diet may be recommended with modification according to condition of the patient.

Surgical therapy, i.e., surgical removal is the preferred treatment for brain tumor.

INTRACRANIAL SURGERY

A surgical opening through the skull is known as craniotomy. This procedure is used to treat any pathology requiring surgical intervention within the cranial cavity. Person with tumors, strokes, subarachnoid hemorrhage and trauma requiring surgical repair may also undergo craniotomies. The basic preparation of the patient before surgery and care in the immediate postoperative period are virtually the same, regardless to underlying conditions:

Indication for cranial surgery are as follow:

- *Intracranial infections:* Caused by bacteria. In these early findings, include stiffneck, headache, fever, weakness, seizures, and later finding include seizures, hemiplegia, speech disturbances, occular disturbances, changes in LOC. Surgical procedure is excision of drainage of abscess.
- *Hydrocephalus:* Due to overproduction of CSF, obstruction to flow, defective reabsorption. In these early findings are, mental changes, disturbance in gait later findings are memory impairment. Urinary incontinence, increased tendon reflexes and Surgery will be on placement of ventriculaterial or ventriculopenitoneal shunt.
- *Intracranial tumors:* Due to benign or malignant cell growth. Manifestation included are change in LOC, pupillary changes, sensory or motor deficit, papilloedoma, seizures, personality changes. Surgical procedure will be excision or partial resection of tumour.
- *Intercranial bleeding:* Due to repture of cerebral vessels because of trauma or cardiovascular accident. In epidural hemorrhage, there will be momentary unconsciousness, lucid period, then rapid deterioration. In subdural, there will be headache, seizures and pupillary changes, for which, is surgical evaluation through burr holes or cranotomy.
- *Skull fractures:* Due to trauma to skull. Here we find headache, CSF leakage, cranial nerve deficit. Surgical procedure performed here are debridement of fragments and necrotic tissue, elevation and realignment of bone fragments.

- *Arteriovenous malformation*: May be due to congenital tangle of arteries and veins (frequently in middle cerebral artery). Symptoms are headache, intracranial hemorrhage, seizures, mental deterioration. Excision of malformation is the surgical procedure.
- *Aneurysm repair*: Due to dilatation of weak area in arterial wall, (usually near anterior portion and circle of Willis). Manifestation before rupture are headache, lethargy, visual disturbance. After rupture, violent headache, decreased LOC, visual disturbances, motor disturbances. Here dissection and clipping of aneurysm is the surgical procedure.

The types of cranial surgery performed are:

- *Burr hole:* It is the opening into cranium with a drill, used to remain localized fluid and blood beneath the dura.
- *Craniotomy:* Opening into the cranium with removal of a bone flap and opening the dura to remove lesion, repair a damaged area, drainblood or relieve increased ICP.
- *Craniectomy:* Excision into the cranium to cut away a bone flap.
- *Cranioplasty:* Repair of a cranial defect resulting from trauma, malformation, or previous surgical procedure: artificial material used to replace damaged or lost one.
- *Stereotaxis:* Precision localization of a specific area of the brain using a frame or a frameless system based on 3-dimensional coordination: procedure is used for biopsy, radiosurgery, or dissection.
- *Shunt procedures:* Provide an alternative pathway to redirect CSF from one area to another using a tube or implanted device. Examples include ventriculoperitoneal shunt and CSF reservoir.

The following guidelines are used for preoperative care of the patient having intracranial surgery:

- Baseline data of neurological and physiological status are recorded.
- Patient and family are encouraged to verbalize fears.
- Treatment and procedures are explained fully, even if unsure whether patient understands.
- If head is shaved, it usually is done in the operating room.
- An antiseptic shampoo may be ordered at the night before the surgery.
- If hair is shaved, it is saved and given to patient or family.
- Family is prepared for appearance of patient after surgery:
  - Head dressing.
  - Edema and ecchymosis of face common.
  - Possible decrease in mental status.

And following guidelines of care should be used for postoperative care of patient after intracranial surgery.

- Perform monitoring:
  - Assess neurological status, including ability to move, level for orientation and alertness and pupil checks.
  - Assess degree and character of drainage.
    - Amount of drainage and bleeding should be minimal.
    - Initial head dressing can be reinforced as necessary.
    - Often incision is left open to air after first several days.
- Promote mobility:
  - Turning to either side is permitted.
  - If supratentorial surgery was performed, the head of the bed is kept elevated at least 30-degrees.
  - Early ambulation is encouraged to prevent complications of bedrest. Observe carefully for signs of postural hypotension; raise head of bed gradually; patient should always sit on edge of bed before standing.
- Promote decreased intracranial pressure:
  - Space nursing activities to allow patient to rest between them.
  - Coughing and vomiting shall be avoided.
  - Suctioning should be performed only as necessary and then gently and cautiously.
- Protect safety of patient:
  - Use soft hand restraints if restraints are necessary.
  - Use mittens as alternative to restraints. Change Mitt. fourth hourly provide range of motions to hand at this time.
  - Keep side rails up at all times.
- Promote electrolyte balance:
  - Perform accurate intake and output with measurement of specific gravity. Do frequent testing for blood glucose.
  - Have patient resume oral diet as soon as possible, assess for difficulty in swallowing or absence of gag reflex.
  - Monitor electrolytes for evidence of abnormality.
- Promote comfort:
  - Medicate for comfort with codeine sulphate or non-narcotic analgesic.
  - Ice cap for headache may be helpful.

CEREBROVASCULAR ACCIDENT/STROKE

Cerebrovascular accident refers to any pathological process involving the blood vessels of the brain. Cerebrovascular accident (CVA) also referes to as stroke or brain attack, is a broad term that includes a variety of disorders that influence blood flow to the brain and results in neurologic deficits. Proper functioning of the brain depends on an adequate blood supply to deliver oxygen and glucose for neuronal activity and to remove the end product of metabolism. CVA results when there is inadequate supply of blood to the brain (cerebral ischemia) or cerebral hemorrhage within the brain. Regardless of the cause, the damaged brain no longer performs cognitive, sensory, motor or emotional functions. The effects of CVA may vary from minor to severe disability.

Etiology

CVA can be defined as a neurological deficit that has a sudden onset and lasts over 24 hours. Ischemic strokes account for an estimated 85% of the total and this percentage can be further broken down into strokes resulting from atherosclerolic (20 percent), cardiogenic (20 percent), idiopathic (30 percent) and other causes (15 percent). Brief descriptions of these ischemic strokes are as follows:

- *Atherosclerotic:* Atherosclerosis affects both the large extracranial and intracranial arteries. The lumen of the vessel narrows and can be a target site for thrombus formation. Transient ischemic attacks (TIA) occur in about half of patients before the stroke.
- *Small penetrating artery thrombosis/lacuna/lacunar:* Thrombosis of a small penetrating brain artery causes a small damaged area of tissues in the deep white matter structures of the brain, called a lacuna. Lacunae typically occur in the basal ganglia, internal capsule, pons or thalamua.
- *Cardiogenic/embolic:* Most of these strokes are the result of emboli, usually of cardiac origin, that break off and travel in the arterial circulation until they reach a vessel that is too narrow to allow further passage. Atrial fibrillation is the most common cause of the emboli.
- *Other:* Ischemic strokes can also result from vasospasm, in inflammation coagulation disorders, and the effects of drug abuse, particularly cocaine.
- *Idiopathic:* No identifiable cause is establisehd in upto 30 percent of all ischemic strokes.

The risk factors associated with strokes can be divided into nonmodifiable and potentially modifiable. The nonmodifiable include gender, age, race, hereditary. Modifiable are lifestyles, habits including excessive alcohol consumption, cigarette smoking, obesity, diet high in fat content, and drug abuse, increase the risk for stroke. Many pathologic conditions also increase the risk for stroke includes cardiac disease, diabetes mellitus, hypertension, migraine, headache, hypercoagulability states (e.g. high serum fibrinogen levels, increased hematocrit), polycethemia, and sickle cell anemia.

Pathophysiology

The cerebrovascular system is highly adaptive. It maintains constant blood flow to the brain in spite of significant changes in the systemic circulation. Blood flow must be maintained at 750 ml/min (55 ml/100 g) brain tissue or 20 percent of the cardiac output to ensure optimal cerebral functioning of blood flow to the brain in totally interrupted (e.g. cardiac arrest), neurologic metabolism is altered in 30 seconds, metabolism stops in 2 minutes, and cellular death occurs in 5 minutes. The factors that affect cerebral blood flow can be divided into extracranial (Systemic blood pressure, cardiac output and viscosity of the blood) and intracranial (Metabolic alteration, conditions of blood vessels supplying the brain, and intracranial pressure). Both extracranial and intracranial factors may be involved in a stroke. The initial insult may be related to one or more of these factors. For example, when an intracranial hemorrhage occurs, the continuity of the vascular system is interrupted. The lost blood and cerebral edema secondary to the inflammatory process contribute to an increase in intracranial pressure. This interferes with cerebral perfusion, and carbon dioxide and hydrogen ion concentration increase, leading to further dilation of cerebral vessels and increased ICP. Atherosclerosis is common pathophysiologic process in stroke is usually involved in the development of a thrombosis and is often implicated in strokes caused by emboli.

Clinical Manifestations

A CVA ultimately affects many body functions including neuromotor activity, elimination, intellectual function, spatial-perceptual alterations, personality and affect, sensation and communication. The specific neurological defects that are produced by stroke reflect the location and severity of the ischemia and the adequacy of the collateral circulation in the region. Many of the features overlap with other forms of brain injury.

Clinical manifestations of specific cerebral artery involvements are as follows:
- *Middle cerebral artery involvement:*
  - Blockage of main stem
    * Contralateral paralysis (hemiplegia).
    * Contralateral anesthesia loss of proprioreception, fine tough, localization (hemiperesis).
    * Dominant hemisphere: Aphasia.
    * Nondominant hemisphere: Neglet of opposite side, dysmetria.
    * Homonymous hemianopsia and conjugate gaze paralysis.
- *Anterior cerebral artery involvement*
  - Occlusion of stem.
  - Occlusion distal to anterior to communicating artery.
    * Contralateral sensory and motor deficit of foot and leg.
    * Contralateral weakness of proximal upper extremity.
    * Urinary incontinence (possibly unrecognized by patient).

- Apraxia.
- Personality change: flat affect, loss of spontaneity and distractability.
- Possible cognitive impairment.
- *Posterior cerebral artery involvement*
  - Thalamogeniculate branch occlusion.
  - Contralateral sensory loss.
  - Temporary hemiparesis.
  - Homonymous hemianopsia.
  - Paramedian branch occlusion: Central midbrain and thalamus.
    - Weber's syndrome: oculomotor nerve palsy.
    - Contralateral hemiplegia.
  - Cortical occlusion: temporal and occipital lobe.
    - Incomplete homonymous hemianopsia.
    - Dominant hemisphere: dysphasia and anaemia.
    - Nondominant hemisphere: disorientation.
  - Upper basical occlusion (bilateral)
    - Visual disturbances (blindness, homonymous, hemianopsia, visual hallucinations, apraxia of ocular movements)
    - Anemia: objects and inability to count.
    - Possible memory loss.
- *Vertebrobasilar artery involvement.*
  - Bilateral motor and sensory deficits of all extremities.
  - Ipsilateral Horner's syndrome: miosis, ptosis, decreased sweating.
  - Hoarseness.
  - Dysphagia.
  - Nystagmus, diplopia and blindness.
  - Nausea, vomiting.
  - Ataxia.

The term stroke commonly evokes a classic mental picture of specific disabilities, but a wide variety of presentations can occur commonly encountered symptoms are as follows:

- *Motor*
  - Hemiparesis or hemiplegia of the side of the body opposite the site ischemia, initially flaccid, progressing to spastic.
  - Dysphagia: swallowing reflex may also be impaired.
  - Dysarthria.
- *Bowel and bladder*
  - Frequency, urgency and urinary incontinence. Potential for bladder retraining is good if cognitively intact.
  - Constipation related more to immobility than to the physical effects of stroke.
- *Language*
  - Nonfluent aphasia (also known as motor/expressive aphasia)—difficulty or inability to comprehend speech.
  - Fluent aphasia (also known as sensory/receptive aphasia)—difficulty or inability to comprehend speech.
  - Alexia—inability to understand the written word.
  - Agraphia—inability to express self in writing.
- *Sensory-perceptual*
  - Diminished response to superficial sensation—touch, pain, pressure, heat and cold.
  - Diminished proprioception—knowledge of position of body parts in the environment.
  - Visual defects—decreased acuity, diplopia, homonymous hemoanopsia.
  - Perceptual deficits.
    - *Unilateral neglect syndrome:* A distortion in body image in which the patient ignores the affected side of the body (distorted body image).
    - *Apraxia inability:* To carry out learned voluntary acts, i.e. loss of ability to carry out a learned sequence of movement or use objects correctly when paralysis is not present.
      Constructional: May not be able to sequence a planned act necessary for activities of daily living (e.g. dressing, brushing teeth and combing hair).
    - *Agnosia:* Inability to recognize a familar object by use of the senses, through senses sight (visual A) sound (auditory-A), touch (tactile A).
    - *Anosognosia:* Inability to recognize or denial of a physical deficit i.e., apparent unawareness or denial of any loss or deficition physical functioning.
    - *Special relationships:* Loss of ability to judge distances or size or localized object of space, impaired right-left discrimination.
    - *Loss of proprioceptive skills:* Lack of awareness or where various body parts are in relationship to each other, and the environment, e.g. telling time, judging distance, right and left discrimination, memory of locationary object.
- *Cognitive emotional:* Emotional liability and unpredictability behaviors may be socially inappropriate (e.g. crying, jags and swearing):
  - Depression.
  - Memory loss.
  - Short attention of span, early distiatibility.
  - Loss of reasoning, judgement and abstract thinking ability.

The clinical manifestation of transient ischemic attacks (TIA) are as follows:

- Symptoms related to carotid involvement:
  - *Visual disturbances*: Temporary blindness in one eye, blurred vision.
  - *Motor disturbances*: Hemiparesis, localized motor deficits in face or extremities.

– *Sensory disturbances*: Hemianesthesia, sensory deficits in face extremities.
- Symptoms related to vertebral involvements:
  – *Motor disturbances*: Ataxia, dysarthria, dysphagia, unilateral or bilateral weakness.
  – *Visual disturbances*: Diplopia and bilateral blindness.
- Other
  – Brief lapses in level of consciousness.
  – Sensory disturbances.
  – Dizziness.
  – Vertigo
  – Tinnitus.

Management

As usual, diagnostic studies are carried out in stroke are:
- Computed tomography scan for size and location of lesion.
- MRI—To differentiate hemorrhagic or nonhemmorhagic.
- EEG—For knowledge suggestive ischemic infarction.
- PET—Shows the chemical activity of brain and extent of tissue damage.
- Radionuclide scan.
- DSA (digital subtraction angiography)—Visualization of blood vessel involved
- CSF analysis.

To know the evaluation of etiology of CVA, the following are necessary.
- Cerebral blood flow-by doppler ultrasonographs, transcranial doppler carohd duplex and carohd angiography.
- Cardiac assessment-by ECG, cardiac enzyme, echocardiography and Holter monitor (evaluation of arrythmias).

Before diagnostic studies, proper history and thorough physical examination are necessary. For locating signs and symptoms listed in clinical manifestations, the nurses and health care team should take primary prevention as a priority for reducing morbidity and mortality associated with CVA. The goals of stroke prevention include health management for the well individual, modifiable risk factors, prevention of stroke for those with history of TIA, and prevention of additional stroke for those who have had a CVA. Health management focuses on (1) healthy diet, (2) weight control, (3) regular exercise (4) no smoking, (5) limiting alcohol consumption and (6) routine health assessments. Patients with known risk factors such as diabetes mellitus, hypertension, obesity, high serum lipids, or cardiac dysfunction require close management of their illness. Postmenopausal women on estrogen therapy are less likely to experience a CVA as compared with women not on estrogen therapy. Measures designed to prevent the development of thrombus or embolus are also used in patient at risk. Low dose aspirin is used as prophylactic dose of platelet inhibitor. Anticoagulation therapy for patient with atrial fibrillation. Treatment of underlying cardiac problem and surgical intervention for patients with aneurysm risk of bleeding, i.e., with TIAs from carotid disease carotid endarectus, transluminal angioplasty and extracranial and intracranial bypass may be done as precaution.

Emergency Management of stroke carried out for patients with etiology of sudden vascular compromise causing disruption of blood flow to the brain (may be thrombosis, trauma, aneurysm, embolism and hemorrhage). Assessment finding will reveal that patients are:
- Altered level of consciousness.
- Weakness, numbness, or paralysis of portion of the body.
- Speech or visual disturbances.
- Severe headache.
- Increased or decreased heart rate.
- Respiratory distress.
- Unequal pupils.
- Hypertension.
- Facial drooping on affected side.
- Difficulty in swallowing.
- Seizures.
- Bladder or bowel incontinence.
- Nausea and vomiting.

The nursing interventions carried on during emergency initially are:
- Ensure patent airway.
- Remove dentures.
- Administer oxygen via nasal cannula or nonrebreather mask.
- Establish IV access with normal saline to maintain BP.
- Remove clothing.
- Obtain CT scan immediately.
- Elevate head of bed 30 degrees of no symptoms of shock or injury.
- Institute seizure precautions.
- Anticipate thrombolytic therapy for ischemic stroke.

Ongoing monitoring includes:
- Monitor vital signs, LOC, oxygen saturation, cardiac rhythm, GC scale pupil size and reactivity.
- Maintain patient warmth.
- Reassure patient and family.

Nursing Management

Nursing assessment includes obtaining subjective and objective data of the person who had a stroke and will include:
- Health history including hypertension, and its management, history of coronary artery disease, diabetes and history of TIA.

- Medication in use, both prescription and over-the-counter drugs (OTC).
- Smoking history.
- Circumstances surrounding the stroke.
- Onset, nature and severity of symptoms.
- Presence of headache-nature and locaton.
- Visual ability-acuity, diplopia, blurred vision.
- Ability to concentrate and follow commands and memory.
- Emotion/affective response.
- Level of consciousness and response to tackle stimuli.
- Family and social support network, financial and insurance status and following to be observed:
- Motor strength—presence of and severeity of paresis or paralysis.
- Coordination—gait and balance.
- Ability to communicate.
- Cranial nerve assessment.
- Bowel and bladder control or incontinency.

Nursing diagnosis are determined from analysis of patient's data. The possible nursing diagnosis may include:
- Altered cerebral tissue perfuse r/t interruption of arterial blood flow.
- Risk for disuse syndrome r/t hemiparesis or hemiplegia.
- Self care deficit: Feeding, bathing, toileting r/t neuromuscular and sensory perceptual impairment.
- Impaired swallowing, r/t oral and neck muscle weakness.
- Impaired verbal communication r/t residual aphasia.
- Sensory—Perceptual alternated r/t altered sensory reception, transmission, integrated.
- Urinary incontinence r/t altered neurological stimulation.
- Impaired adjustment r/t residual disability necessary changes in lifestyle and independence.

Planning: The patient, family and nurse establish the goals of nursing care in a cooperative manner. These goals typically include that the patient will:
- Maintain a stable or improved level of consciousness.
- Attain maximum physical functioning.
- Attain maximum self-care abilities and skills.
- Maintain stable body functions (e.g. bladder control).
- Maximize communication skills and abilities.
- Maintain adequate nutrition.
- Avoid complications of stroke.
- Maintain effective personal and family coping.

Nursing Implementation

Monitoring Cerebral Perfusion

The nurse has to do continuous monitoring of patient's neurological status. Accordingly, the nurse has to maintain patient's patent airway and it is essential to support oxygenation and cerebral perfusion. Nursing intervention includes frequent assessment of airway patency and function, suctioning, patient's mobility, positioning of the patient to prevent aspiration, and encouraging deep-breathing. The environment is kept in quick and restful as possible, and all activities that are known to increase ICP such as coughing, straining, lying prone, isometric muscle contraction, emotional upsets and abrupt head or neck flexion are avoided or minimized. Administer prescribed medication and prevent thrombus formation.

Prevention of the Complications of Immobility and Disuse

Appropriate positioning is a key concern. Positioning is fundamental to preventing complication such as contractures and skin breakdown. Maintain alignment with support of pillows and footboards according to procedures, teach and assist family and patient with positioning techniques to prevent contractures. Administer active or passive range-of-motion exercises to affected extremities.

Promoting Independence in Self-care

Assess document level of self-care to determine extent of problem and plan appropriate intervention. Encourage independence, provide supervision or assistance as needed to avoid development of dependency.

Promoting Safe Swallowing and Adequate Nutrition

The protective swallowing and gag reflexes usually return within a few days after the stroke, but the patient may have ongoing problems managing the complex act of swallowing. The following guidelines can be used for the patient with impaired swallowing.
- Place the patient upright in bed or preferably sitting in a chair for meals.
- Offer mouth care before meals to stimulate saliva flow; Strong-tasting or salty liquids also stimulate saliva flow.
- Position the patient's head and neck slightly forward with the chin tucked in to prevent premature movement of food to the back of the mouth before it is adequately chewed.
- Experiment with food texture. Most patients tolerate a mechanically soft diet better than liquids. Avoid thin liquids. Consider adding thickness to liquid if they are poorly tolerated.
- Encourage the patient to take small bites and chew food thoroughly.
- If hemiplegia is present, food should be placed in the unaffected side of the mouth. If 'pocketing' of food occurs on the affected side, instruct the patient to sweep the affected side with a finger after each bite. Teach the patient to clean the affected side of the

mouth with gauze wipes and perform mouth care after meals. Retained food causes mouth odors, infection and tooth or gum disease.
- Position foods within the patient's visual field if hemianopia is present.
- Keep an accurate intake and output record until the patient is drinking sufficient liquid daily. IV supplementation may initially be needed.
- Monitor the patients weight weekly. Add supplements to diet or liquids to increase calorie and nutrient intake.

Supporting Communication

Communication problem following stroke may include both aphasia and dysarthria. Specific strategies for assisting the patients with aphasia are as follows:
- *Nonfluent expressive aphasia*
  - Allow the patient adequate time to respond. Establish a nonhurried atmosphere.
  - Be supportive and encouraging of the patient's efforts to communicate.
  - Use openended questions at intervals to assess spontaneous communication ability.
  - Involve the family or significant others in exercise to name objects used for routine self-care.
  - Express understanding and support to behavioral responses to frustration such as tears or anger. Remind the patient that speech skills will improve.
  - If the aphasia is severe, a picture board or book may be necessary to communicate by whatever means are successful (e.g. pointing, pantomime). Anticipate the patient's needs when appropriate and verify your interpretation of the patient's meaning.
- *Fluent sensory aphasia*
  - Face the patient and speak slowly and distinctly. Do not increase your volume: hearing is not the problem.
  - Break instructions into component parts and give them one at a time. Repeat as needed.
  - Use gestures appropriately to support your verbal messages.
  - Involve the family in planning and implementing all strategies.
  - Provide support and encouragement when the patient becomes frustrated.
- *General*
  - Provide practice at times when the patient is rested and not fatigued.
  - Offer liberal praise and reinforcement for efforts. Remind patient and family that small gains can still be made months into the rehabilitation process.

Compensatory for Sensory-Perceptual Deficits

A wide variety of sensory-perceptual deficits may be present following stroke; particularly strokes involving the right hemisphere. Specific intervention designed to address the major sensory perceptual deficits in the following guidelines.
- *Hemianopia* (loss of vision in a portion of visual field)
  - Approach the patient from the side of intact vision.
  - Position the patient in the room so that his or her intact visual field faces the door if possible.
  - Teach the patient to move the head from side-to-side (scan) to compensate for diminished visual fields. Scanning is also important with meals.
  - Place objects needed for self-care within the patient's intact visual field.
- *Denial/neglect and body image distortion*
  - Encourage the patient to look at and touch the affected side. Verbally remind the patient to check the position and safety of the affected side during activity.
  - Lightly touch and stimulate the affected side during care.
  - Providing gentle but consistent reminders to include the affected side in care (e.g. bathing, dressing).
  - Monitor the affected side for injuries when the patient is out of bed. A sling may be used to protect the affected side during ambulation.
  - Use a full length mirror to assist the patient to reintegrate an intact body image and to assist with posture and balance.
  - Assist the family to understand the nature of the patient's behavior.
- *Agnosia/apraxia*
  - Encourage the patient to use all senses to compensate for problems in object recognition.
  - Practise the recognition and naming of commonly used objects, and encourage the family to participate in the relearning process.
  - Encourage the patient to participate in self-care.
  - Correct the misuse of any object or task, guiding the patient's hand if necessary.
  - Continue to verbally cue the patient about correct use of any object or self-care tasks.
  - Be aware that memory deficits may make frequent reteaching necessary.
  - Explain the nature of all deficits to the family.

Restoring Continence

Problems with urinary incontinence are common after stroke; but the chances for restoring continence are good because half of the innervation and control pathways to the bladder remain intact. Assess and record patient's continent and incontinent voidings to determine pattern and plan appropriate intervention. Note color and character of urine daily needed to ensure early detection of urinary tract infection and to prevent highly concentrated urine. Provide fluid intake of 2000 ml/day less contraindicated to foster adequate elimination of dilute urine. If indwelling catheter is used, give perineal cleaning and catheter care every shift and as needed to avoid infection and ensure uninterrupted urinary flow. Offer urinal or commode every 2 hours and encourage to empty the bladder and as needed to aid in establishing regular voiding pattern. Assure patient of your willingness to assist with urinary problem to avoid embarrassment and to demonstrate a caring attitude.

Constipation is the most common bowel problem after stroke. Regaining bowel incontinence is reasonable expectation for most patients if a pattern of constipation, impaction, and diarrhea is not permitted to develop. The nurse needs to carefully monitor the patient's bowel elimination pattern and ensure that the patient received adequate daily fluid. A bowel program of stool softner, fiber laxatives and suppositories should be implemented at admission and modify as needed to support bowel regularity.

Promoting Effective Coping

The effects of stroke are usually life altering and can be devastating to the patient and family. Depressions and despair are normal responses to stroke. The patient may experience significant difficulty in responding appropriately to any situation. He may be emotional and cry easily. Here, families need to be helped to understand that these behaviors are outcomes of the stroke and are not viotational acts by the patient. Distraction and shifting the patient's attention can be successful strategies for assisting the patient to regain control.

To evaluate the effectiveness of nursing intervention, compare the patient behavior with those stated in the expected outcome objectives. Successful achievement of patients outcome for the patient with stroke is indicated by:
- Maintain stable vital sign and that he has no signs of increased ICP.
- Is able to move and transfer easily.
- Performs ADL independently.
- Consumes balanced oral diet without any problem.
- Communicate needs effectively.
- Uses technique to compensate for perceptual defects and injury.
- Maintain bladder and bowel continence.
- Participate with family in social interaction.

EPILEPSY/SEIZURE DISORDER

A seizure is a paroxysmal, uncontrolled electrical discharge of neurons in the brain that interrupts normal functions. Seizures are frequently symptoms of an underlying illness. They may accompany a variety of disorders, or they may occur spontaneously without any apparent cause.

Epilepsy is a condition in which a person has spontaneously recurring seizures caused by chronic underlying conditions.

Etiology

The most common causes of epilepsy during the first 6 months of life are severe birth injury, congenital defects involving the CNS infection and inborn errors of metabolism.

In patients between 2 and 20 years of ages, the primary causative factors are birth injury, infection, trauma, and genetic factors. In individuals between 20-30 years of age, epilepsy is a result of structural lesions, such as trauma, brain tumors or vascular diseases. After 50 years of age, the primary cause will be cerebrovascular lesions and metastatic brain tumors. Heredity may lead to epilepsy in a few cases. The common risk factors for epilepsy are as follows:
- Anoxia.
- Cerebral palsy.
- Perinatal problems (toxemia, difficult delivery, low birth weight and hypoxia).
- Congenital central nervous system defects.
- Mental retardation.
- Febrile conditions.
- Family history of epilepsy.
- Head trauma.
- Central nervous system infections.
- Central nervous system tumors.
- Cerebrovascular disease.
- Alcohol or drug abuse.
- Metabolic distubrances.
- Exposure to toxins.
- Degenerative diseases (Alzheimer's disease).

Pathophysiology

A seizure can be caused by any process that disrupts the cell membrane stability of a neuron. The point at which the cell membrane becomes destabilized and an uncontrolled electrical discharge begins is known as seizures threshold. Some people have lower seizures threshold than others and are, therefore, more prone to seizures. In recurring seizures (epilepsy) a group of abnormal neurons (seizures focus) seems to undergo spontaneous firing. This firing spreads by physiologic pathways to involve adjacent or distant areas of the brain. If this activity spreads to involve the whole brain, generalized seizures occurs. The factor that causes this abnormal firing is not clear. Any stimulus that causes the cell membrane of the neuron to depolarize induces a tendency to spontaneous firing. Often the area of the brain from which the epileptic activity arises is found to have scar tissues (gloses). The scarring is thought to interfere with the normal chemical and structural environment of the brain neurons, making them more likely to fire abnormally.

Clinical Manifestations

The specific clinical manifestations of a seizure are determined by the site of electrical disturbance. In 1981, the International League Against Epilepsy (ILAE) proposed a revised classificatioan for epileptic seizures. The major categories are partial (focal) generalized and unclassified. Further, subdivisions within the categories based on the person's clinical behavior during the *ictal* and *interictal* times. Ictal refers to the time during the seizure. *Interictal* refers to the time between seizure activity. Postictal refers to the time immediately after a seizure as the patient recovers.

The types of seizure and their signs and symptoms are as follows:

Partial Seizures

- Simple partial seizures (formerly focal) characterized by no impairment of consciousness, with symptoms of motor, somatosensory or special sensory, autonomic and psychic, which includes focal twitching of extremity, speech arrest, specral visual sensations (e.g. seeing lights), feeling of fear or doom. There is no postictal state.
- Complex partial (formerly psychomotor or temporal lobe seizures) is a simple partial seizure with progression to impairment of consciousness with no other features except features of simple partial seizure and automatism. That is it may begin as simple partial and progress to complex by showing automatic behavior (e.g. lipsmacking, chewing, or picking at clothes). Postictal state as follows.
- *Complex partial generalized to generalized tonic-clonic seizures* begins as complex partial as above, then progresses to tonicclonic as in generalized seizures. Postictal state presents.

Generalized Seizures

Generalized seizures impair consciousness from the start:
- *Absence seizures:* Atypical seizures (formerly petit mal) do not include motor signs and may last less than 1-minute. There will be brief loss of consciousness, staring, unresponsive and no postictal state.
- *Tonic clonic seizures (formerly Grand mal):* Tonic phase involves rhythmic jerking of muscles, possibly tongue biting and urinary and fecal incontinence. May be combination of tonic and clonic movement.
- *Atonic seizures:* In this, there will be impairment consciousness for only few seconds and brief loss of muscle tone, which may cause patient to fall or drop something referred to as drop attacks.
- *Myoclonic seizures:* There will be impaired consciousness for only few seconds or not at all and brief jerking of a muscle group which may cause the patient to fall.

Postictal states represent periods of recovery from the seizures. In this patients may have some degree of confusion, lethargies or inability to follow commands or speak clearly during this period. In some rare cases the patient may experience a prolonged period of weakness involving one or more extremities called Todd Paralysis.

Status epileptical is an episode of seizures activity lasting at least for 30 minutes or repeated seizures without full recovery between seizures. Seizures cause a marked increase in cerebral metabolic activity and demands. These demands may outpace the delivery of oxygen and nutrient from the cerebral blood flow. Prolonged seizures can lead to cellular exhaustion and destruction and lead to death if not effectively treated.

Management

The diagnosis of epilepsy is made from a careful history including the risk factors involved and physical examination supplemented by diagnostic tests (EEG, CT, MRI, PET). Antiepileptic drugs are used to control seizures. The common medications used, their actions and nursing interventions are as given below.

- *Hydantoin (Phenytoin-Dilantin):* These blocks synaptic potentiation and propagation of electrical discharges in the motor cortex and blocks sodium transport and stabilize membrane sensitivity. They are used alone or in combination to manage tonic-clonic, simple partial and complex seizures. Therapeutic range is 10–20 mg/LN. saline takes at least 7–14 days to establish. The nursing intervention during this treatment with hydantoin are:
  - Monitor common side effects including nystagmus, ataxia, fatigue, drowsiness and cognitive impairment.
  - Gastrointestinal systems (nausea, anorexia, vomiting) are common. Drug may be given with meal.
  - Gingival hyperplasia is common side effect. Patients are taught the importance of scrupulous oral hygiene.
  - Regular follow-up for monitoring is encouraged.
- *Barbiturates (phenobarbitol-Luminal):* It depresses post-synaptic excitatory discharge. Used to manage tonic-clonic, simple partial and complex partial seizures and status epilepticus. During these stages, the nurse has to monitor side effects which include sedation, drowsiness and depression.
- *Succinimides (Ethosuximide):* It depresses motor cortex and raises threshold to stimuli used to manage absence seizures. In this, nurse has to monitor side effects (e.g. Anorexia, nausia, vomiting and drowsiness) and caution the patient to never abruptly discontinue the drug as this can precipitate status epilepticus.
- *Others*
  - *Carbamazepine (Tegretol):* Is believed to reduce polysynaptic responses and blocks synaptic potentiation. This is used to manage tonic clonic, simple partial and complex partial seizures. In

this the nurse has to monitor side effects, i.e., drowsiness, dizziness, headache, nausea, anorexia, vomiting. Side effects tend to decrease in severity over time. Regular follow-up encouraged because drug can cause rare but severe bone marrow toxicities.
- *Valproic acid (Depakene):* Increases levels of gamma-aminobutyric acid for membrane stabilization. This is used to manage absence seizures or in combination with other drugs. For tonic-clonic and complex partial seizures. The nursing interventions include—Monitor side effects (anorexia, nausea and vomiting). Teach patient to take drug with meal and watch for CNS side effects such as drowsiness, tremor and ataxia. Regular follow-up is encouraged because drug may cause liver dysfunction and blood dyscrasias.

Antiepileptic Drugs

Several effective antiepileptic drugs are available which have different mechanisms of action. A single drug is effective in most of the cases. Drugs regimen used should be simple and combination of drug therapy should be considered when it is absolutely necessary. The antiepileptic used in various types of epilepsy are presented in the **Table 17.1**.

Table 17.1: Antiepileptic drugs.

Drug	Daily dose	No. of daily doses	Optimal drug level	Selected side effects and idiosyncratic reactions
Generalized tonic-clonic (grand mal) or partial (focal) seizures				
Phenytoin	200–400 mg Adult: 3–5 mg/kg Children: 3–5 mg/kg	1–2	10–20 mcg/ml	Nystagmus, ataxia, dysarthria, sedation, confusion, gingival hyperplasia, hirsutism, megaloblastic, anemia, blood dyscrasias, skin rashes, fever, systemic lupus erythematosus, lymphadenopathy, peripheral neuropathy, dyskinesias
Carbamazepine (extended-release formulation)	600–1200 mg	2–3(2)	4–8 mcg/ml	Nystagmus, dysarthria, diplopia, ataxia, drowsiness, nausea, blood dyscrasias, hepatotoxicity, hyponatremia. May exacerbate myoclonic seizures
Valproic acid (extended release formation)	800–2000 mg	3(2)	50–100 mcg/ml	Nausea, anorexia, diarrhea, drowsiness, alopecia, weight gain, hepatotoxicity, thrombocytopenia, tremors, pancreatitis, headache
Phenobarbital	60–180 mg	1–2	10–40 mcg/ml	Sedation, nystagmus, ataxia, skin rashes, learning difficulties, hyperactivity
Primidone	750–1500 mg	3	5–15 mcg/ml	Sedation, nystagmus, ataxia, vertigo, nausea, skin rashes, megaloblastic anemia, irritability
Lamotrigine	200–500 mg	2	–	Sedation, skin rash, visual disturbances, dyspepsia, ataxia, blood dyscrasias
Topiramate	200–400 mg	2	–	Somnolence, nausea, dyspepsia, irritability, dizziness, ataxia, nystagmus, diplopia, glaucoma, renal calculi, weight loss, hypohidrosis, hyperthermia, fatigue, speech disturbance
Oxcarbazepine	900–1800 mg	2	–	As for carbamazepine
Levetiracetam	1000–3000 mg	2	–	Somnolence, ataxia, headache, behavioral changes
Zonisamide	200–600 mg	1–2	–	Somnolence, ataxia, anorexia, nausea, vomiting, rash, confusion, renal calculi. Do not use in patients with sulfonamide allergy
Tiagabine	32–56 mg	2	–	Somnolence, anxiety, dizziness, poor concentration, tremor, diarrhea
Pregabaline	150–180 mg	2	–	Someolence, dizziness, poor concentration, weight gain, thrombocytopenia, skin rashes, anaphylactoid reactions
Felbamate	1200–3600 mg	3	–	Anorexia, nausea, vomiting, headache, insomnia, weight loss, dizziness, hepatotoxicity, aplastic anemia
Absence (petit mal) seizures				
Ethosuximide	500–1500 mg	2–3	40–100 mcg/ml	Nausea, anorexia, headache, lethargy, unsteadiness, blood dyscrasias, systemic lupus erythematosus, urticaria, pruritus, ataxia
Valproic acid	1500–2000 mg	3	50–100 mcg/ml	See above
Clonazepam	1–6 mg	1–2	20–80 ng/ml	Drowsiness, ataxia, irritability, behavioral changes, exacerbation of tonic-clonic seizures
Myoclonic seizures				
Valproic acid	1500–2000 mg	3	50–100 mcg/ml	See above
Clonazepam	1–6 mg	1–2	20–80 ng/ml	See above

Emergency Management of Tonic-Clonic Seizures

Tonic-clonic seizures may be caused by the following needs emergency management.
- *Head trauma:* Hematuria of epidural, subdural, intracranial, cerebral contusion and traumatic birth injury.
- *Drug-related process:* Overdose, withdrawal of alcohol, opiods antiseizure drugs, ingestion and inhalation.
- *Infectious process:* Meningitis, septicimia.
- *Intercranial event:* Brain tumor, subarachnoid hemorrage and stroke, hypertensive crisis and increased ICP secondary to clogged shunt.
- *Metabolic imbalance:* Fluid and electrolyte imbalance and hypoglycemia.
- *Medical disorders:* Heart, liver or kidney disease-systematic diseases.
- *Others:* Cardiac arrest, ideopathic, psychiatric disorder and high fever.

Assessment finding will reveal the:
- Aura-Peculiar sensation that preceds seizures.
- Loss of consciousness.
- Bowel and bladder incontinence.
- Tachycardia.
- Diaphoresis.
- Warm skin.
- Pallor, flushing or cyanosis.
- Tonic phase-continuous muscle contractions.
- Hypertonic phase-extreme muscular rigidity lasting 5 to 15 seconds.
- Clonic phase—rigidity and relaxation alternate in rapid succession.
- Postictal phase—lethargy, altered level of consciousness.
- Confusion and headache.
- Repeated tonic clonic seizures for several minutes.

Initial nursing interventions will include:
- Ensure patient airway.
- Assist ventilation if patient does not breath spontaneously after seizures. Anticipate need for intubation if gag reflex is present.
- Suction as needed.
- Stay with patient until seizures have passed.
- Protect patient from injury during seizures. Do not restrain. Pad side rails.
- Anticipate administration of phenobarbital, phenytoin or benzodiazephine to control seizures.
- Remove or loosen tight clothing.

And ongoing monitoring instituted as follows:
- Monitor vital signs, LOC, O_2 saturation, GCS, pupil size and reactivity.
- Reassure and orient the patient after seizures.
- Never force an airway between a patient's clenched teeth.
- Give dextrose for hypoglycemia.

The following guidelines will help the nurse while taking care of patient in status epilepticus:
- Protect airway and provide oxygen. Position the patient on side to prevent aspiration. Place on oral airway if the teeth are not clenched. Administer oxygen by mask of respiratory depression occurs from seizures or medication used to control seizures, intubation may be necessary.
- Establish IV access for medication delivery and fluids.
- Draw blood for electrolytes, arterial blood gases and toxicology to rule out metabolic causes for seizures.
- Administer benzoidiazepines usually lorazepam (Ativan) 4 to 8 mg over 2 to 4 minutes or diazepam (valium) 5 to 20 mg over 5 to 10 minutes to stop seizures. These drugs are fast acting and will control seizures until anticonvulsant drugs reach therapeutic levels.
- Administer anticonvulsants usually phenytoin 15 to 20 mg/kg in normal saline at 50 mg/min. maximum rate at the same time as the benzoidiazepines to begin establishing therapeutic levels. Phenytoin can cause significant hypotension and cardiac dysfunction. Place the patient on a monitor during loading doses.
- Continue the search for an underlying cause of seizures.

Patient and Family Education

The patient with seizures disorders should be taught the following:
- Medications must be taken as prescribed. Any and all side effects of medications should be reported to the health care provider. When necessary, blood drawings are done to ensure that therapeutic levels are maintained.
- Use of nondrug technique, such as relaxation therapy and biofeedback training to potentially reduce the number of seizures.
- Availability of resources and the community.
- Need to wear a medicalert bracelet, necklace and identification card.
- Avoidance of excessive alcohol intake, fatigue and loss of sleep.
- Regular meals and snack in between if feeling is shaky, faint or hungry.

Family members should be taught the following:
- First aid treatment of tonic-clonic seizures. It is not necessary to call ambulance or send the patient to the hospital after a single seizure unless the seizure is prolonged, another seizure immediately follows or extensive injury has occurred.
- During an acute seizure, it is important to protect the patient from injury. This may involve supporting and protecting the head, turning the patient to the side, loosening constricting clothing, and easing the patient to the floor if seated.

HEADACHE

Headache is probably the most common type of pain experienced by humans. Headache is a common symptom of many neurologic conditions and is also a separate disease process.

Etiology

Headaches are classified by the international society on primary and secondary. Primary headaches are not associated with any other known pathological cause. Examples are *migraine, tension,* and *cluster* headaches. Secondary headaches are caused by known pathology such as meningitis, tumors or subarachnoid hemorrhage.

- *Tension-type headache:* Occurs at any age and is associated with stress. Onset often in adolescence, related to tension or anxiety. There will be no family history. It is episodic, vary with stress; duration is variable. There is no prodrome (early manifestation) of impending disease. The pain is usually bilateral, occurring most often in the back of the neck. It is usually bilateral, occurring most often in the back of the neck. It usually does not interfere with sleep. The pain is often described as a tight, squeezing, bandline pressure. It is sustained, chronic, dull and persistent. The headache occurs intermittently for weeks, months or even years. Many patients have a combination of migraine and tension-type headache with features of both occurring simultaneously.
- *Migraine headache:* Migraine occurs more often in women than men and most commonly begins between adolescence and at the 40 years. They demonistrate a strong hereditary pattern, but no specific genetic link has been identified. It is episodic, tends to occur with stress or life crisis it lasts. Lasts hours to days. It occurs slowly. Pain becomes severe with one side of head affected more than other. There is prodromal, i.e. vision field defects, confusion, paresthesia, and associated symptoms like nausea, vomiting, chills, fatigue, irritability, sweating and edema. There are two types of migraine headache: migraine without aura (formerly called common migraine) and migraining with aura (formerly called classic migraine, i.e. with prodrome).

    Migraine headaches in many cases have no precipitatory events. However, for other patients, the headache may be precipitated or triggered by stress, excitement, bright light, menstruation, alcohol or certain foods such as chocolate or cheese.
- *Cluster headache* is one of the most severe forms of head pain. No epidemiological pattern has been identified occurs in early adulthood, precipitated by alcohol or nitrate use, more common in older men. Episodes clustered together in quick succession for few days or weaks with remissions that lasts for months. It lasts a minute to a few hours. Pattern of pain is intense, throbbing, often unilateral pain begins in intraorbital region and spread to head and neck. There is no prodrome but associated with flushing, tearing of eyes, nasal stuffiness, sweating, swelling of temporal vessels.

Pathophysiology

The pathophysiology of headache is not full understood. Some structures of the head are incapable of sensing pain. The structures that are capable of feeling pain are, skin, muscles, periosteum of the skull, eyes, ears, nasal cavities and sinuses, meninges, cerebral blood vessels, and cranial nerves with sensory function. Pain is caused by traction, stretching of movement of structures or by vasodilation of blood vessels. Serotonin is the primary neurotransmitter found in the pathways involved in headache, but its role is not fully understood.

Migraine is believed to be caused when cerebral blood vessels narrow and blood flow is reduced to some areas of the brain. The initial vasoconstriction is followed by significant vasodilation and inflammation of the blood vessels which triggers a release of serotinin and causes headache. Migraine vary in duration, frequency and intensity from patient to patient and from episode to episode in the same patients.

Cluster headaches are thought to be similar to migrains but episodes are brief, usually lasting 45 minutes or less. They occur in 'Cluster' periods of weeks or months. Tension headaches are the results of the stress-induced muscle tension over the neck, scalp and face of the patient. These headaches are associated with the stresses of daily life. Some headaches are preceded by prodromal signs and symptoms called 'aurae'—The aura occurs before the acute attack and may include visual field defects such as "flashing lights" Photophobia, confusion or paresthsis. Aurae typically last for an hour or more. Their symptoms are associated with the reduction and cerebral blast flow that precedes the vasodilation of the migraine.

Clinical manifestations are discussed in types (see aetiology) and secondary headache, manifests associate an underlying disease.

Management

The diagnosis of headache is made from the patient's history, complete history, clinical examination (often negative). Inspect for local infections, palpation of tenderness, hardened arteries and bony swellings. Auscultation for bruits over major arteries. Assessment parameters for headache are development by the International Headache Society are as follows:

- *Headache characteristics:* Time of onset, location, frequency, severity, duration, quality (deep, superficial, steady, throbbing, stabbing, burning), situations or activities that make the headache better or worse.

- *Presence of an aura:* Duration, relation to onset of pain.
- *Associated symptoms occuring before, during or after a headache:* Nausea, vomiting, photophobia, visual disturbance, dizziness, incoordination, redness of the eye, facial symptoms (sweating, paleness, flushing), fatigue, or sleepiness, moodswings, weakness and paresthesia.
- *Potential precipitating factors:* Change in eating pattern, dietary substances (e.g. tyramines, nitrates), relationship to menstrual cycle, sexual intercourse, pregnancy, menopause, phychosocial stressors, change in sleep pattern, weather changes, hot or cold wind, attitude, lights and smog.
- *Activities of daily living patterns:* Eating, sleeping, exercise and relaxation.
- *Drug history:* Over-the-counter and prescribed headache medication, other medications (nitroglycerine, hormone replacement) alcohol and drug use and smoking history.
- *Medical history:* Asthma, peptic ulcer, motion sickness, head injury, seizure disorder, sleep walking. Raynaud's disease, irritable bowel syndrome, infertility, skin problems. Pain in neck, head or throat, abdominal distress: anxiety, depressions and insomnia.
- *Family history:* History of headache and other medical problems.

While nursing assessment, nurse should keep in mind the above stated parameters and she/he can suggest the patient keep a diary of headache episodes with specific details including complete description of each headache, precipitating events, associated symptoms, and in women, the relationship with menstrual cycles. This type of record can be of great help in determining the type of headache.

Nursing diagnosis: For the patient with headache may include.
- Pain related to headache as manifested by complaint of steady throbbing or severe crushing pain.
- Anxiety related to lack of knowledge about headache details.
- Hopelessness related to chronic pain, alteration of lifestyles and ineffective treatment.
- Sleep pattern disturbance related to pain.

Planning: The overall goals are that the patient with headache will:
- Have reduced or no pain.
- Experience increased comfort and decreased anxiety.
- Demonstarte understanding of triggering events and treatment strategies.
- Use positive coping strategies to deal with chronic pain.

Nursing Intervention

Headaches may result from an inability to cope with daily stresses. The most effective therapy may be to help patients examine their lifestyle, recognize stressful situations and learn to cope with them appropriately. Precipitating factors can be identified and ways of avoiding them can be developed. Daily exercise, relaxation periods, and socializing can be encouraged, since each can help decreased the recurrene of headache. The nurse can suggest alternative ways of handling the pain of headache through technique such as relaxation, meditation, yoga, and self hypnosis.

Medications for the treatment of headache fall into two broad categories: Symptom relife and prevention.a.
- *Symptomatic treatment:* Following drugs are used:
   a. Non-narcotic analgesics (aspirin, acetaminophen, and ibuprofen).
   b. Analgesic combinations (butalbital).
   c. Muscle relaxants.
   d. Serotonin receptor agonists (Sumatriptan, naratriptan, rizatriptan).
   e. Alpha-adrenergic blockers (ergatramine tartrate, i.e., afergot).
   f. Vasoconstrictors (isometheptone, i.e. midrin).
   g. Corticosteroids (dexamethosone).
   (Note: a, e, f, g are used in migraine and e, f and oxygen used in cluster headache).
   h. Metodopramide (Reglan).
- *Prophylactic:* Treatment includes the following:
   a. Tricyclic antidepressants (dexepin, amitriptyline).
   b. Beta-adrenergic blockers (Propranol-Inderal).
   c. Biofeedback.
   d. Muscle relaxation training.
   e. Psychotherapy (ede are not drugs).
   f. Calcium channel blockers (isoptin).
   g. Divalp..... (b, c, d, e, f, g, h are used in migraine).
   h. Yoga, meditation, electric counter stimulation).
   i. Corticosteroids (Prednisone).
   j. Lithium.
   k. Alpha-adrenaline blockers) (i, j, k, l are used in cluster headache).
   l. Serotonin antagonists.

Nursing intervention during medication are: advise the patients to take prescribed dose and the nurse has to observe the side effects as follows:
- *Ergot alkaloids* may be taken as soon as migraine symptoms begin. In this, nausea is common side effect. Patient may also need to use antiemetics. Ergot has a cumulative effect. Use sparingly and monitor for signs and symptoms of ergotism-numbness, and tingling, weakness, and muscle pain.
- *Metaclopramide* increases gastrointestinal mobility to decrease the evidence of nausea and vomiting. During this medication, patients should avoid driving or other hazardous activity after taking drug.
- *Serotonin* receptor agonist, causes vasoconstriction. This drug contraindicates in pregnancy and coronary

artery disease. Teach the patient to take drug at first sign of a headache.
- *Beta blockers* inhibit vasodilation and serotonen uptake. Propranolol is the first drug of choice for prophylaxis of migraine. This may cause cardiac dysfunction; monitor for bradycardia, orthostatic hypertension lethargy and depression.
- *Tricyclic antidepressants*: Block uptake of serotonen and catecholamines. They are most effective for migraine associated in tension headache. It is alternative if beta-blockers are not tolerated. These may cause dry mouth, drowsiness and urinary retention.

For the patient whose headaches are triggered by food, dietary counseling may be provided. The patient is encouraged to avoid foods that provoke headaches such as vinegar, chocolate, onions, alcohol (red wine) excessive caffeine, cheese, fermented or marinated food, monosodium glutamate and aspartome. Patients should avoid smoking and exposure to triggers such as strong perfumes, volatile solvents, and gasolene fumes. Cluster headaches' attacks may occur at high altitudes with low oxygen levels during air travel. Ergotamine, before the plane takes off, these may be decreased likelihood of these attacks. The following is the teaching guide for the patient with headache, used by the nurse while giving the patient and family education.

- Avoid factors that can trigger a headache.
  - Food containing amines (cheese, chocolate), nitrates (meat), vinegar, onion, fermented or marionated food.
  - Monosodium glutamate.
  - Caffeine.
  - Nicotine.
  - Ice cream.
  - Alcohol (particularly red wine).
  - Emotional stress.
  - Fatigue.
  - Medications such as ergot containing and mono-amineoxidase inhibitors.
- Able to describe the purpose, action, dosage and side effects of medication taken.
- Able to self-administer sumatriptan subcutaneously if prescribed.
- Use stress reduction technique such as relaxation.
- Participate in regular exercise.
- Keep diary or calender of headaches and possible precipitatory event.
- Contact health care provider if the following occur:
  - Symptoms become more severe, last longer than usual or are resistant to medication.
  - Nausea, vomiting, change in vision or fever occur with headache.
  - Problem with medication.

MULTIPLE SCLEROSIS

Multiple sclerosis (MS) is a chronic, progressive, degenerative disorder of the central nervous system (CNS) characterized by inflammation of the white matter of the CNS.

Etiology

The cause of MS is unknown, although an underlying viral infection has been suggested as a cause. It is also related to immunologic and genetic factors and is perpetuated as a result of intrinsic factors (e.g. faulty immunoregulation). The susceptibility to MS appear to be inherited, multiple unlinked genes confer susceptibility to MS.

The role of precipitating factors such as exposure to pathogenic agents in the etiology of MS is controversial. The possible precipitating factors include infections, physical injury, emotional distress, excessive fatigue, pregnancy and a poorer state of health.

Pathophysiology

Multiple sclerosis causes scattered demyelination of the white matter of the CNS. It is characterized by chronic inflammation, demyelination and ghiosis (scarring) in the CNS. The primary neurophthologic condition is an immune mediated inflammatory demyelinating process that some believe, may be triggered by a virus in genetically-susceptible individuals. The acute inflammation reduces the thickness of the myelin sheath that surround the axons and nerve fibers and impulse conduction is slowed and/or blocked. Astrocytes or scavenger cells that remove the damaged myelin and scar tissues form over the damaged areas. Natural healing may restore some of the functions of the myelin or the lesions may continue to interfere with nerve conduction. This partial healing accounts for the transitory nature of early disease symptoms. Eventually nerve fibers may generate so that permanent damage occurs and overt disabilities increase. The blood-brain barrier usually protects the brain from immune cell activity. In MS, however, the barrier is breached and activated T-cells, antibodies and macrophages attack the fatty myelin sheath and the oligodendrocytes that produce it. The CNS damage is thought to be caused by a delayed type of hypersensitivity response, a cell-mediated immune response. The course of MS is highly variable and unpredictable. Site of inflammatory demyelination can occur usually anywhere in the brain and spinal cord and MS produces a greater range of signs and symptoms that any other neurological diseases.

Clinical Manifestations

The onset of MS is often insidious and gradual, with vague symptoms that occur intermittently over months or years. The clinical manifestations vary according to the areas of the CNS invoked. Some patients have severe long-lasting symptoms easily in the course of the disease. Other may experience only occasional and mild symptoms for several years after onset. A classification scheme that identifies the variety causing MS has been developed.

- Relapsing/remitting MS Disease: exacerbations occur over 1 to 2 weeks and then gradually resolve over 4 to 8 weeks, usually returning the patient to baseline or near-baseline functioning. It is characterized by clearly defined relapses with full recovery or with sequelae and residual deficit on recovery.
- Relapsing/progress MS disease exacerbations occur, but the patient does not return to baseline and is left with increasing amounts of residual disability. It is characterized by the disease progression from onsets with occasional plateaus and temporary minor improvement.
- Secondary/chronic progressive MS disease is characterized primarily by spinal cord and cerebellar symptoms which are progresive and rarely remit. It is characterized by relapsing-remittant followed by progression with or without occasional relapses, minor remissions and plateaus.
- Progressive relapsing/stable MS is characterized by progressive disease from onset, with clear acute relapses, with or without full recovery; Periods between relapses are characterized by continuing progressing.

The following are the symptoms of multiple sclerosis.
- *Sensory symptoms*
  - Numbness and tingling on the face or extremities.
  - Decreased proprioception.
  - Paresthesis (burning, prickling).
  - Decreased sense of temperature, vibration and depth.
- *Motor symptoms*
  - Weakness or a feeling of heaviness in the lower extremities.
  - Paralysis.
  - Spasticity and hyper reflexes.
  - Diplopia.
  - Bowel and bladder dysfunction (retention, or urge, incontinence).
- *Cerebellar symptoms*
  - Spasticity and hyper reflexes.
  - Incoordination, ataxia, in lower extremities.
  - Slurred speech dysarthria.
  - Scanning speech (slow with pauses between syllables).
  - Nystagmus.
  - Dysphagia.
- *Neurobehavioral symptoms*
  - Emotional liability, euphoria, depression.
  - Irritability.
  - Apathy.
  - Poor judgement, inability to solve problems effectively.
  - Loss of short-term memory.
- *Others*
  - Opticneuritis (visual clouding and visual field deficits).
  - Impotence, sexual dysfunction.
  - Fatigue (extremely common, ranges from mild to disabling).

Management

Diagnosis is based primarily on history and clinical manifestation. Certain tests currently used are:

CSF analysis, evoked response test (AEP- auditory evoked potential VEP-visual evoked potential, SSEP-Somatosensory evoked potential), CT scan and MRI (ask to see the sclerotic plaques).

Nursing assessment may be made by collecting subjective and objective data based on clinical manifestation. The possible nursing diagnosis will be:
- Impaired physical mobility: r/t muscle weakness.
- Self-care deficits r/t muscle spasticity and neuromuscular deficit.
- Risk of impaired skin integrity r/t immobility.
- Sensory-perceptual alteration r/t visual disturbance.
- Altered urinary eliminate (Retention or incontinence).
- Constipation r/t immobility.
- Sexual dysfunction r/t neuromuscular deficit.
- Self-esteem disturbance r/t prolonged debilitating conditions.
- Altered family processes r/t changing family roles, etc.

Drugs used for managing symptoms of MS are as follows:
- Spasticity:
  - Baclofen (Licresal)
  - Dantrolene (Dantrium)
  - Diazepam (Valium).
- Tremors
  - Hydraxyzine (Vistaril)
  - Isoniazid (INH)
  - Trihexyphenidyl (Artane)
  - Primidone (Mysoline).
- Spastic Pladder and urge, incontinence:
  - Oxybutynin
  - Imipramine (Tofranil)
  - Pro-pantheline (Probanthine)
- *Urinary Retention:* Bethenicoal chloride (urecholine).
- Antidepressants:
  - Amitriptyline (Elavil)
  - Imipramin (Tofranal)
  - Trazodone (Desuyrel)
  - Fluoxetin (Proleu)
  - Paroxetine (Paxil)
  - Sertraline (Zoloft).

- Fatigue:
  - Amantadine hydrochloride (Symmetrel)
  - Pemoline (Cylert).
- Other
  - Stool softner
  - Laxatives.

The drugs used for reducing the frequency of severity of relapses of multiple sclerosis are as follows:
- Acute exacerbations. Short course of high-dose corticosteroids are used, which include:
  - Methylprednisolone (Medrol) IV daily for 3 to 7 days with or without the following taper of oral prednisolone.
  - Oral prednisolone tapered over 2 to 4 weeks.
  - Crticotropoin (ACTH) by IV infusion or IM gradually tapered over 2 to 4 weeks.
- For decreasing relapses: usually used are:
  - Interferon beta-16 (Betaseron) SC.
  - Interferon beta-1a (Vvinex) 1g SC.
  - Copolymer 1 and injectable polymer (effecting if started early).
  - Azathioprine (Imuron)-an anti-inflammatory and immunosuppressive.
- For halting disease progression drug used are:
  - Cyclophosphamide (Cytoxan)
  - Cyclosporin (Sandimmune)
  - Clad sporin (Leustatin), etc.

In addition, various nutritional measures that have been advocated in the management of MS include vitamin B_{12}, vitamin C and diet consisting of low-fat and gluten-free food and raw vegetables. A nutritious well-balanced diet is essential. Surgical measures are followed nursing management of neurosurgical nursing is carried out.

Patient education should be focussed on building general resistance to illness including, avoid fatigue, extremes of heat or cold, and expose to infection. The last measures involve avoiding exposure to cold climate and to people who are sick, as well as vigorous and early treatment of infection when it does occur. It is important to teach the patient to:
- Achieve a good balance of exercise and rest
- Eat nutritious and well-balanced meals
- Avoid the hazards of immobility (contractures and pressure ulcers).

Patient should know that treatment regimens, the side effects of medication and how to watch them, and drug interactions and new over the counter medications. The patient should consult a health care provider before taking any non-prescriptive drugs.

PARKINSON'S DISEASE

Parkinson's disease, a form of Parkinsonism is named after James Parkinson who in 1817 wrote a classic "shaking palsy" a disease for which the reason is still unknown. It is a chronic degenerative disorder that primarily affects the neurons of the basal ganglia. It is a syndrome that consists of slowing down in the initiation and execution of movement (Bradykinesia), increased muscle tone (rigidity), tremor and impaired postural reflexes. The famous internationally known boxer Mr Mohmed Ali suffered from this disease.

Etiology

Parkinson's disease affects men and women about equally and usually occurs after the age of 50 with a median age of onset of about years. Actual etiology of the disease remains unknown. The possible causes of Parkinson's disease may be:
- A genetic component has recently been proposed. (Heredity). The disease usually begins insidiously and then progresses.
- Primary Parkinson's disease is idiopathic, but variety of other categories exist.
- Symptoms of Parkinson's may develop in response to the use of antipsychotic drugs (or neuroleptic agents); following an encephalitis infection in response to brain trauma, tumors, hydrocephalis or ischemia; in association with rare metabolic disorders; and in response to arteriosclerosis.
- Neurotoxin such as cyanide, manganese and carbon monoxide have also been proposed as possible causes of disease.

Drug-induced Parkinson's can follow reserpine (Hydropres)-methyldopa (Aldomet), haloperidol (Haldol) and phenothiazine (Thorazine) therapy.

Pathophysiology

The Pathology of Parkinson's disease is associated with the degeneration of the dopamine-producing neurons in the substantial nigra of neurun an area within the basal ganglia. Destructions of dopaminergic neurons in the substantia nigra significantly reduces the amount of available straital dopamine. Dopamine (DA) and acetylcholine (ACh) are primarily neurotransmitters that are responsible for controlling and refining motor movements and have opposing effects. Dopamine has inhibitory effect and acetylcholine has excitatory effects. When the excitatory activity of ACh is inadequately balanced by DA, and individual has difficulty in controlling and initiating voluntary movements. Cellular degeneration in Parkinson's disease also leads to impairment of the extrapyramidal tracts that control semiautomatic and coordinated movements.

Clinical Manifestations

The onset of Parkinson's disease is gradual and insidious, with a gradual progression and prolonged course. In the beginning stages, a mild tremor, a slight limp or a decreased arm swing may be evident. Later on the disease, the patient may have shuffling, propulsive gait with arms flexed and loss of postural reflexes. In some patients, there may be a slight change in speech pattern. The following are the 'classic' clinical manifestations of Parkinson's disease.

- *Tremor:* (often the first sign affects handwriting).
  - Non-intentional, present at rest but usually not during sleep.
  - Characterized by rhythmic movements of 4 to 5 cycles per second.
    * Movement of the thumb across the palm gives a "Pill rolling" character.
    * Tremor also seen in limbs, jaw, lips, lower facial muscles and head.
- *Rigidity* (often the second sign)
  - Increased resistance to passive motion when the limbs are moved through their range of motion.
  - Muscles feel stiff and required increased effort to move.
  - Discomfort or pain may be perceived in muscle when rigidity is severe.
  - "Cogwheel" rigidity refer to ratchet-like rhythmic contractions of the muscle that occur when the limbs are passively stretched.
- *Bradykinesia (Akinesia)*
  - Slowness of active movement.
  - Difficulty in initiating movement.
  - Often the most disabling symptom: interferes with ADK and predisposes patient to complication related to constipation, circulatory stasis, skin breakdown and other related complications of immobility.
- *Postural instability*
  - Changes in gait
    * Tendency to walk forward on the toes with small shuffling steps.
    * Once initiated, movement may accelerate almost to a trot.
    * Festination may occur, which propels the patient either forward or backward propulsively until falling is almost inevitable.
  - Changes in balance:
    * Stooped over posture when erect.
    * Arms are semiflexed and do not swing with walking.
    * Difficulty in maintaining balance and sitting erect.
    * Cannot 'right' or brace self to prevent falling, when balance is lost.

Complications

Many complications of Parkinson's disease are caused by the deterioration and loss of spontaneity of movements.

- Dysphagia leading to malnutrition or aspiration.
- Venereal debilitation leads to pneumonia, urinary track infection and skin breakdown.
- Decreased mobility affects gait.
- Lack of mobility leads to constipation, ankle edema, and contractures.
- Orthostatic hypotension with loss of postural reflexes lead to fall on injury.
- Bothersome complications include seborrhea, dandruff, excessive sweating, conjunctivitis, difficulty in reading, insomnia, incontinence and depressions.
- Side effects of drugs—dyskinesia, weakness and akinesia.

The complication may be secondary manifestations of Parkinson's disease are as follows:

- Facial appearance.
  - Expressionless.
  - Eyes store straight ahead.
  - Blinking is much less frequent than normal.
- Speech problems.
  - Low volume.
  - Slurred, muffled.
  - Monotone.
  - Difficulty with starting speech and word finding.
- Visual problems
  - Blurred vision.
  - Impaired upward gaze.
  - Blepharospasm - involuntary prolonged closing of the eyelids.
- Fine motor function
  - Microphagia handwriting progressively decreases in size.
  - Decreased manual dexterity.
  - Clumsiness and decreased coordination.
  - Decreased capacity to complete ADL.
  - Freezing—sudden involuntary inability to initiate movement can occur during movement or inactivity.
- Autonomic disturbance.
  - Constipation—hypomotility and prolonged gastric emptying.
  - Urinary frequency or hesitancy.
  - Orthostatic hypertention (dizziness, fainting and syncope).
  - Dysphagia (neuromuscular incoordination).
  - Drooling (results from decreased swallowing).
  - Oily skin.
  - Excessive perspiration.
- Cognitive/behavioral.
  - Depression.
  - Slowed responsiveness.
  - Memory deficits.
  - Visual-spacial deficits.
  - Dementia.

Management

The diagnosis of Parkinson's disease is made directly from the patient's history and symptoms. No definite diagnostic test exists, and the diagnosis may be confirmed primarily from the patient response to medication.

The common medications used for Parkinson's disease and their action and nursing intervention are as follows (**Table 17.2**):

- *Anticholinergics* are used to relieve tremors. They antagonize the transmission of acetylcholine in the CNS; most effective in decreasing rigidity, selective action but still have systematic anticholinergic effects. Example: Trihexyphenidyl, cycrimine, procyclidine, benztropine, biperiden. The side effects of these drugs, usually dry mouth, blurred vision, constipation, delirium, changes in memory, confusion, anxiety, agitation, hallucination. During this treatment, nurse has to monitor the incidence and severity of the side effects; avoidance of drugs with similar actions, (e.g. antihistamine, sominex, antispasmodics like donnadral, bellergal, tricyclic antidepressants like tofoamil, elavil, etc.
- *Antiviral* amantadine (Symmetril)-block the uptake and storage of catecholamines, allowing for the accumulation of dopamine. Positive effects may not be least beyond 3 months. Here, the nurses have to monitor for effectiveness and severity of side effects, e.g. mental confusion, visual disturbances, nervousness, insomnia, dry mouth, nausea, edema orthostatic hypotension.
- *Antihistamine* reduces the tremor and rigidity. The drugs used are: Diphenhydramine (Benedryl), orphenadrine, chlorphenaxamine, Phenindamine. Sedation is the side effect and the nurse has to take same precautions as for anticholenergic drugs.

Table 17.2: Commonly used drugs for treatment of Parkinsonism.

Drug (action)	Daily dose in mg	Side-effects
Levodopa preparations (replaces the lost neurotransmitter dopamine)		
• Levodopa (500 mg)	1500–6000	Nausea, vomiting, agitation, confusion, psychosis, postural hypotension, dyskinesias, arrhythmias. GI and cardiac side-effects are less with preparations containing decarboxylase inhibitor (carbidopa, benserazide) or catechol-o-methyltransferase inhibitor (entacapone)
• Carbidopa plus levodopa (10 + 100, 25 + 100, 25 + 250)	300–1000 of levodopa	
• Levodopa plus entacapone (25/100/200)	-do-	
• Decarboxylase inhibitor (benserazide *plus* levodopa, 25 +100 ; 12.5 + 50)	600–800 of levodopa	
• Controlled release carbidopa plus levodopa (50 + 200)	200–800 of levodopa	
Amantadine	100–200	Anorexia, confusion, psychosis, pedal edema, livedo reticularis, restlessness, disturbance of cardiac rhythm (potentiates the effect of endogenous dopamine)
Anticholinergics		
• Trihexyphenidyl	4–8	Dry mouth, blurred vision, sphincter disturbance, nausea, vomiting, constipation, palpitations
• Procyclidine	7.5–15	
• Benztropine	1.0–1.5	
Antihistaminics		
• Diphenhydramine	50–200	Giddiness, mild sedation
• Orphenadrine	150–200	
Dopamine agonists		
A: Ergot alkaloids		
• Bromocryptine	5–10	Nausea, vomiting, postural hypotension, confusion
• Pergolide	0.1–0.2	Cardiac arrhythmias may occur in addition with pergolide
B: Nonergot alkaloids		
• Ropinirole	12–24	Nausea, somnolence, edema, dyskinesia, confusion and sleep attacks
• Pramipexole	1.5–4.5	
MAO-B-inhibitor (redues the rate of removal of dopamine)		
• Selegiline	5–10	Confusion, hallucinations, postural hypotension
• Rasagiline	1 mg	
Apomorphine		
• Subcutaneous injection	1–6	Nausea, vomiting, confusion, psychosis

- *Dopamine agonists* include drugs such as bromocriptine merylate, pergolide (Permax), pramipexole (Mirapex), used to reduce bradykinesia, and tremor and rigidity. They directly stimulate dopamine receptors and increase the effect of levadopa, minimize the fluctuations in drug responses. Possible side effects are: orthostatic hypotension, nausea, vomiting, toxic psychosis, limb edema, phlebitis, dizziness, headache, insomnia. The nurse has to monitor the side effects and take precautions accordingly.
- Dopaminergic (Ex. Levadopa, Carbidopa-Levadopa) used to relieve bradykinesia, tremor and rigidity. They resotore deficient dopamine to the brain. Carbidopa blocks peripheral conversion of levadopa. Possible side effects are: Nausea, dyskinesia, hypotension. Palpitation, arrythmias, agitation, hallucination, confusion (older patient), drymouth, sleep disturbances. The nurse has to monitor side effects, take measures accordingly by using guidelines for safe use of levellopalisted as given below (after MAO).
- *Monoamine Oxidase inhibitors (MAO)* (E.g. Selegiline-(eldepryl)-MAO-blocks the metabolism of dopamine, may slow the underlying disease process. This is also used for relieving symptoms like bradykinesia; rigidity, tremors. Side effects and precautions are taken similar todopaminergic drugs. Particularly, monitor for incidence of orthostatic hypotension. Do not exceed prescribed dose. The some may be given in combination with levadopa as the disease progresses.

The below given guidelines should be followed for the safe use of levodopa:

- Levodopa is best absorbed in an empty stomach. If nausea occurs, it can be taken with food.
- Dry mouth is common side effect. Chewing gum and hard candy can counter this effect.
- Depression and moodswings may occur. Report the incidence of these or other cognitive-behavioral changes such as insomnia, agitation or confusion to health care provider.
- Avoid the use of alcohol or minimize alcohol intake. It is believed to antagonize the effects of levodopa.
- Avoid protein ingestion near the time for medication administration. Some protein aminoacids are believed to inhibit the absorption of levodopa. A pattern of low-protein breakfast and lunch with a high-protein dinner has improved symptoms in selected patients.
- Be alert to the possibility of orthostatic hypotension. Change positions slowly. Avoid steam baths sauna, and hot tubs. Experiment with the use of support stockings to support venus return.
- Avoid vitamin supplementation with products that contain Vitamin B_6 (Pyridoxine). Pyridoxine increases the conversion of levodopa in the liver, which decreases the amount of available for conversion to dopamine in the brain.
- Consult the primary care provider and pharmacists about the use of all other drugs. Levodopa has multiple adverse drug interactions.

The possible nursing diagnosis are as follow and perform nursing intervention and evaluation accordingly.

- Impaired physical mobility (r/t) rigidity, bradykinesia and akinesia.
- Self-care deficits r/t Parkinson symptoms.
- Impaired verbal communication r/t dysarthias and tremor or bradykinesia.
- Constipation r/t weakness of abdominal and perineal muscle, lack of exercise and side effects.
- Altered nutrition and body requirement r/t dysphagias.
- Diversional activity deficit r/t inability to perform usual recreational activity.
- Sleep pattern disturbance r/t Medication's side effects.

In addition, the following health education is provided to the patient and family member, regarding activity, exercises, safety, nutrition, elimination, etc.

- *Activity and exercise*
  - Perform range of motion exercises to all joints for three times daily.
  - Massage and stretch muscles to reduce stiffness.
  - Use a broad base of support when ambulating, cautiously and consciously lift and down the feet when ambulating.
  - Pay attention to posture. Try walking with the hands clasped behind.
  - Explore the use of assistive devices.
  - Avoid staying in one position for prolonged time and keep altering position regularly.
- *Safety*
  - Examine the home environment for risk of injury.
  - Modify the environment to improve and remove hazards.
  - Consider installing devices such as raised toilet seat, and grab bar.
  - Change positions slowly if orthostatic hypotension develops.
  - Be alert to the side effects of heat, stress and excitement on severity of symptoms.
- *Nutrition*
  - Monitor weight once a week.
  - Evaluate dysphagia and modify diet to increase ease of chewing and swallowing if appropriate.
  - Practice swallowing and take small bites.
  - Provide an unhurried atmosphere and allow additional time for meal.
  - Follow a plan of small, frequent meals, if fatigue is a problem during meals.
  - Avoid eating high-protein meals at times of medication administration.
  - Do not use supplements containing pyridoxine (Vit. B_6).

- Ensure adequate fiber and fluid intake to prevent constipation.
- Manage drooling problems with soft clothes.
- *Elimination*
    - Monitor bowel elimination pattern.
    - Use diet, exercises and fluids to ensure regularity if possible.
    - Use stool softeners if needed.
    - Keep a urinal or commode at the bedside.
    - Respond promptly to urge to urinate, and be sure to empty the bladder, at least every 2 to 4 hours. Bradykinesia may result in episodes of incontinence.
- *Cognitive/behaviors*
    - Monitor for depression. Report its presence to health care provides.
    - Monitor change in sleep pattern, thought disorders, development of any other manifestations, convusion, hallucination—Report to health care provider.
- *Communication*
    - Exercise the voice regularly by singing or reading aloud.
    - Attempt to project the voice and alter volume and pitch.
    - Consult a speech therapist if vocal problems are severe.

MYASTHENIA GRAVIS

Myasthenia Gravis (MG) is a disease of the neuromuscular function characterized by the fluctuating weakness of certain skeletal muscle groups. It is a rare chronic disease that affects the myoneural junctions. The prevalence is estimated to be from 43 to 84 persons per million. (For example, unfortunately our Mega Star of the Millennium Mr Amitabh Bachchan is one among those who suffered from MG during 1980s).

Etiology

Myasthenia Gravis is caused by an autoimmune process that results in production of antibodies directed against the Acetylecholone (ACh). Receptors and a reduction in the number of Ach receptor (AChR) sites at the neuromuscular junctions, i.e. myoneural junctions. This results in the classic disease features of weakness and fatigue of selected voluntary muscles. The exact cause is not known but thymus tumor and viral infection are suspected as precipitating an attack.

Pathophysiology

Effective muscle contraction is contingent on adequate amounts of acetylcholine (ACh), a neuromuscular transmitter, being available at the postsynaptic membrane to generate an action potential that can spread along the length of the muscle and culminate in muscle contraction. Mitochondria in the motor nerve axons synthesize ACh, which is released when the nerve is stimulated. The ACh crosses the myoneural junction and binds with an ACh receptor (AChR) on the postsynaptic membrane to initiate the action potential. Acetylcholinesterase (ACh E) is also released into the synaptic cleft. The AChE breaks down the ACh, which limits the duration of the muscle contraction. The number of AChR sides are significantly reduced in persons with MG as a result of the destructive effects of an antibody mediated autoimmune attack that specifically target the AChR sites. As a result, the stimuli may lack sufficient amplitude to trigger an effective action potential in some muscle fibers. The strength of muscle responses is weakened and with the repeated stimuli to amount of ACh readily decreases resulting in muscle fatigue.

Clinical Manifestations

The classic symptoms of MG are muscle weakness and generalized fatigue. The primary feature of MG is easy fatigability of skeletal muscle during activity. Strength is usually restored after a period of rest. The muscle motor often involved are those used for moving the *eyes and eyelids, chewing, swallowing, speaking, and breathing*. Ptosis and diplopia are common early findings and the disease is occasionally limited to the eye muscles. Muscles innervated by the cranial nerves are often affected and it may be impossible for the patient to keep the mouth closed to chew and swallow for prolonged period. The mobility of the facial muscles also is affected and face may take on an expres-sionless appearance. Attempts to smile, may result in the classic myasthenic 'snarl'. The patient's voice is often weak, and as fatigue sets in, it may become difficult for the patient even to swallow saliva effectively. Weakness of the neck tends to cause the head to bend forward.

Weakness of the arm and hand muscles may first become apparent during self care activities such as shaving or combing the hair. Symptoms develop rapidly but early in the course of the disease, they also are relieved easily with rest. As the disease progresses, fatigue becomes evident with less and less exertion. The muscles of the trunk and lower limbs may also become involved, creating difficulties with walking and even sitting. The distal muscles are rarely affected as severely as proximal muscles.

During a disease, exacerbation of muscle weakness of the intercostal and diaphragm may become so severe that intubation and mechanical ventilation are necessary. Exacerbations of disease can be triggered by upper respiratory infection, emotional stress, secondary illness, trauma, surgery, pregnancy and even menstruation. There is no accompanying sensory loss in the affected area.

The major complication of MG results from weakness in areas that affect swallowing, and breathing. Aspiration, respiratory insufficiency, and respiratory infection are the major complication. An acute exacerbation of this type is termed as "myasthenic crisis".

Management

The simplest diagnostic test for MG is to have the patient to look upward for 2 to 3 minutes. If the problem is MG, there will be an increased drop of the eyelids, so that the person can barely keep the eye open. After a brief rest, the eyes can open again. Complete history and physical examination (following fatigability and weakness). In addition, electromyogram (EMG) Tensilon test (reveals improved muscle contractability after giving AhE intravenously) are used to dignose MG.

Drugs used in MG are usually anticholenergic agents, corticosteroids and immunosuppressive agents. Surgical measure used in MG is thymectomy. Plasma pheresis is also used in the treatment of MG. The common drug used for MG is pyridostigmine (Mestinon).

The nurse can assess the severity of MG by asking the patient about fatigability, which body parts are affected, and how severely they are affected. The patient's coping abilities and understanding of the disorder should also be assessed. The objective rate should include respiratory rate and depth and oxygen saturation. ABG analysis, PFT and evidence of respiratory distress in patient with acute myasthenia crisis. Muscle strength of all face and limb muscles should be assessed on the basis of swallowing, speech (volume and clarity) and cough and gag reflexes. The possible nursing diagnosis will be as follows:

- Ineffective breathing pattern r/t intercostal muscle weakness (IMW).
- Ineffective airway clearance r/t intercostal muscle weakness and impaired cough and gag reflex.
- Impaired verbal communication r/t weakness of larynx, lips, mouth pharynx-jaw.
- Altered nutrition of body requirement r/t impaired swallowing and weakness.
- Sensory perceptional alteration r/t ptosis and gaze.
- Activity intolerance r/t muscle weakness and fatiguability.
- Body image disturbance r/t inability to maintain usual life style and role responsibility.
- The possible goals of nursing care will be to have return of normal muscle endurance.
- Avoid complication and
- Maintain quality of life appropriate to disease cause.

Nursing Intervention

The patients with MG who is admitted to the hospital usually has a respiratory tract infection or in an acute myasthenic crisis. Nursing care is aimed at maintaining adequate ventilation, continuing drug therapy and watching side effects of therapy.

As with chronic illnesses, care focuses on the neurologic deficits and their impact on daily living. A balanced diet with food that can be chewed and swallowed easily should be prescribed. Semi-solid foods may be easier to eat than solid or liquid foods. Scheduling doses of medication, so that peak action is reached at meal time may make eating less difficult. Diversional activities that require little physical effort and interests of patients should be arranged.

Education should focus on the importance of following: medical regimen, potential adverse reactions to specific drugs. Planning activities of daily living to avoid fatigue, the availability of community resources and complication of disease and therapy and what to do about them. Following guidelines may be helpful in taking care of the patient with myasthenia gravis.

- Use of Mestinon (choice of dugs) safely and appropriately:
  - Take the drug with food or fluid.
  - Take the drug before meals to permit maximum effect for chewing and swallowing.
  - Adjust drug dosage and time of administration within set parameters in resposne to individual pattern of weakness.
  - Do not take any other medications, including over the counter products without proper approval of health care provider. Many drugs can compromise neuromuscular transmission and will worsen MG. (e.g. Local anesthetics, aminoglucocides, beta blockers, calcium chanel blockers).
- Modify diet as needed in response to swallowing problems.
  - A soft diet is usually well tolerated.
  - Eat slowly and take small bites.
- Balance rest and activity throughout the day in response to weakness.
  - Plan for additional rest periods.
  - Seek out energy conservation strategies for routine activities.
- Keep medical alert identification with you at all times.
- Know the symptoms of cholenergic and myasthenic crisis and contact physically.
- Be alert to disease response to periods of stress-infection, temperature extremes, and hormonal swings (e.g. menstruation or pregnancy).

ALZHEIMER'S DISEASE

Alzheimer's disease is a type of dimentia that is characterized by progressive deterioration in memory and other aspects of cognition.

Etiology

The etiology of Alzheimer's disease is still unclear. There is possibility of genetic etiologies. At least four chromosomes (1,14,19,21) are involved in some forms of familial Alzheimer's disease. Inheritance of the apo E4 genotype is a major risk factor for developing this disease. Estrogen protects against the development of disease and leads to slow progression of disease has been suggested and role of NSAIDs in reducing the risk of this disease. However, long-term NSAID leads to gastrointestinal and kidney problems.

Pathophysiology

Pathologic changes associated with Alzheimer's disease, include neurofibrillary tangles and beta-amyloid plaques in the cerebral cortex and hippocampus. The neuritic plaque is cluster of degenerating axonal and dendritic nerve terminals that contain an abnormal protein (B-amyloid). Neurofibrillary tangles are seen in the cytoplasm of abnormal neurons. These bundles of protein are in the form of paired helical filaments. There is also excessive loss of cholinergic neurons, particularly in regions essential for memory and cognition.

Clinical Manifestation

An initial sign of Alzheimer's disease is a subtle deterioration in memory. Inevitably this progresses to more profound memory loss that interferes with the patients' ability to function. Recent events and new information cannot be recalled. Some patients develop psychotic symptoms. Personal hygiene deteriorates as does the ability to maintain attention. Later in the disease, long-term memories cannot be recalled, and patient loses the ability to recognize family members. Eventually, ability to communicate and to perform activities of daily living is lost. The progression of the deterioration which eventually leads to death, varies but can last as long as 20 years.

Management

The diagnosis of Alzheimer's disease is a diagnosis exclusive when all other possible conditions that can cause mental impairment have been ruled out and the manifestation of dementia persists the diagnosis of this disease can be made. CT scan and MRI scan may show brain atrophy and enlarged ventricles. Neuropsychologic testing can help document the degree of cognitive dysfunction in early stages.

Nursing assessment will include the following.
- Past health history: Repeated head trauma, exposure to metals (Alluminium Previous CNS infection).
- Medications: Use of any drug to mitigate symptoms, tranquilizers hypnotics, antidepressants and antipsychotics.
- Positive family history and emotional stability.
- Nutritional metabolic: Anorexia, malnutrition and weight loss.
- Elimination-incontinence.
- Activity exercise: Poor personal hygiene, gait instability, weakness, inability to perform ADL.
- Sleep-rest: Frequent night time awakening, day-time napping.
- Cognitive erceptual: Forgetfulness, inability to cope with complex situation, difficulty in problem solving, depression, and suicidal ideation.
- General: Disheveled appearance and agitation.
- Neurologic: Loss of recent memory, disorientation to date and time, flat affect, lack of spontaneity, impaired abstraction, cognition, and memory, loss of remote memory, restlessness and agitation. Inability to recognize family members and friends, nocturnal wanderings, repetitive behavior, loss of social graces, stubborness, paronea, belligerency, later on- Aphasia, agnosia, alexia, apraxia, seizures, limb rigidity and flexor posturing.

The possible nursing diagnosis are:
- Altered thought processes r/t effects of dementia.
- Self care deficits r/t memory deficit.
- Sleep pattern disturbance r/t memory deficit.
- Risk for injury r/t impaired judgement—Possible gait instability.
- Rest for violence: Self or other directed r/t sensory overload, misinterpretation.
- Ineffective individual coping r/t depression.
- Risk for ineffective management of therapeutic management.

AMYOTROPHIC LATERAL SCLEROSIS (ALS)

Amyotrophic Lateral Sclerosis (ALS) is a rare progressive neurologic disorder characterized by loss of motor neurons. It is also referred to as Loubehrig's disease after the, New York Yankee baseball player who died from this disease.

Etiology

ALS occurs in 2 or 3 persons per 100,000 annually. Men have a higher incidence of ALS than women. The onset is between 40 and 70 years of age. The cause is unknown, but theories of causation includes exposure to heavy metals, vital infections, lympoma, gammopathy and hexosaminidase, and HIV infection.

Pathophysiology

The term amyotrophic refers to the weakness and atrophy that occur from the degeneration of alpha or lower motor neurons. For unknown reasons motor neurons in the brainstem and spinal cord gradually degenerate in ALS. The dead motroneuron cannot produce or transport vital signals to muscle. Consequently, electrical and chemical messages originating in the brain do not reach the muscles to activate them. ALS causes progressive degeneration of both the upper and lower motor neurons from demyelination and scar tissue formation. The disease gradually destroys motor pathways but leaves sensations and mental status intact. Lower mentors usually affect first resulting weakness and atrophy. The muscles of the upper body are affected much earlier than legs.

Clinical Manifestation

The primary symptoms are weakness of the upper extremities, dysarthria, and dysphagia. Muscle wasting and fasciculations result from the denervation of the muscles and lack of stimulation and use. The disease is relentlessly progressive and eventually involves the upper motor neurons, which causes increased weakness and spasticity in affected muscles. Hyperactive reflexes, jaw clonus, tongue fasciculations and a positive Babinski's reflex may be present. As the muscle of the neck, pharynx, and larynx becomes increasingly involved, slurring of the voice occurs, which gradually worsens to dysarthria and dysphagia. Paralysis is inevitable, and death usually results from pneumonia and respiratory failure within 5 years of diagnosis.

Management

ALS is diagnosed by a process of elimination because no definitive diagnostic tests exist. Muscle biopsies may be performed to determine the source of muscle weakness and an EMG will show muscle denervation fibrillation and fascioulation. Blood studies typically show elevation in the levels of creatinine phosphokinase.

There is no cure for ALS and treatment is primarily directed towards symptom relief. Rilusole (Rilutek) has recently been approved for use in ALS treatment. It is believed to extend the life of ALS patients. The specific interventions are directed at management of complications.

The focus of nursing care is on supporting self care abilities of the patient and the coping resources of the entire family. General interventions are targeted at maintaining good general health, supporting nutrition, promoting adequated sleep, appropriately-balancing activity and rest, and introducing use of self-help devices as they become appropriate. And take measures according to symptom arising appropriately, and patient and family education also include taking of symptomatic measures accordingly.

GUILLAIN-BARRÉ SYNDROME

Guillain-Barré syndrome (GBS) is an acute inflammatory polyneuropathy characterized by varying degrees of motor weakness of paralysis. It primarily affects the motor components of the cranial and spinal nerves and is known by variety of other names, which include, Landry-Guillain-Barré-Strohl syndrome, Postinfectious polyneuropathy, ascending polyneuropathic paralysis. It affects the peripheral nervous systems and results in loss of myelin (a segmental demyelination) and edema and inflammation of the affected nerves-causing a loss of neurotrans mission to the periphery.

Etiology

GBS is a rare disorder with an incidence of 1.5 to 1.9 per one lakh population. The etiology of this disorder is unknown, but it is believed to be cell-mediated immunologic reaction directed at the peripheral nerves. The syndrome is frequently preceded by immune system stimulation from a viral infection, trauma, surgery, viral immunization, human immunodeficiency virus (HIV) or lympoproliferative neoplasms. These stimuli are thought to cause an alteration in the immune system resulting in sensitization of T-lymphocytes to the patient's myelin causing myelin damage.

Pathophysiology

In GBS an immune-mediated response triggers destruction of the myelin sheath surrounding the peripheral nerves, nerve roots, root ganglia, and spinal cord. Collections of lymphocytes and macrophages are believed to be responsible for the myelin stripping. Demyelination occurs between the nodes of Ranvier, which impair or blocks the transmission of impulse from node to node. The nerve axons are generally spared and recovery takes place, although process of re-myelination occurs slowly. In severe forms of the disease, wallerian degeneration occurs that involves the axons, making recovery slower and more difficult. In a small percentage of patients the disease does not resolve and become chronic and recurrent. In this, lymphocytes are basically normal and return to complete functioning after an illness.

Clinical Manifestation

There are four major forms of GBS. Each reflects a different degree of peripheral nerve involvement.
- Ascending GBS is the most common form. Weakness and numbness begin in the legs and progress upward. Fifty percent of patients experience respiratory insufficiency. Sensory involvement is also usually present.
- Pure or motor GBS similar to the ascending form, but no sensory involvement is present. It is usually milder form of disease.
- Descending GBS begins with weakness in the muscles controlled by the cranial nerves and then progresses downward. The respiratory system is quickly impaired. Sensory involvement is present.
- Miller-Fisher syndrome; a variant of GBS is rare and primarily involves the eyes, loss of reflexes and severe ataxia.

Symptoms of GBS usually develop 1 to 3 weeks after an upper respiratory or gastrointestinal infection. The patients with GBS have symmetrical muscle weakness and flaccid motor paralysis. The paralysis usually starts in the lower extremities and ascends upwards to include the thorax, upper extremities and face. Progression of GBS to include the lower brainstem involves facial, abducens, oculomotor, hypoglossal, trigeminal and vagus nerves. This involvement manifests itself through facial weakness, extraocculomotor, eye movement difficulties, dysphagia and paresthesia of the face and patient may have difficulty in swallowing, speaking and breathing.

Pain and paresthesia are present when sensory nerves are involved. The pain can be categorized as paresthesias, muscular aches, and cramps, and hyperesthesias. Pain appears to be worse at night. Tingling or a pin and needle sensation is common. Pain may lead to a decrease in appetite and may interfere with sleep. Pain requires narcotics or analgesics.

Now autonomic dysfunction is recognized as a common problem with GBS and may include dysrhythmias, blood pressure instability, tachycardia or bradycardia, flushing, sweating, urinary retention, and paralytic ileus. GBS does not affect the patient level of consciousness, alertness and cognitive functioning. GBS generally progresses through three stages. The initial period lasts from 1 to 3 weeks and ends when no further physical deterioration occurs. A plateau period follows, which lasts from a few days to few weeks. The recovery period can last from 6 months to well over 1 year. The remyelination of damaged nerves occurs during the recovery phase. Permanent dificits may remain.

Complications

The most serious complication of GBS is respiratory failure, which occurs on the paralysis progresses to other nerves that innervate thoracic area. Respiratory or urinary tract infections may occur. Fever is generally first sign of infection. Immobility from the paralysis may cause problem such as paralytic ileum, muscle atrophy, deep vein thrombosis, pulmonary emboli, skin breakdown, orthostatic hypotension and nutritional deficiency.

Management

The diagnosis of GBS is made from the clinical presentation supported by a history of recent viral infection, elevation in the levels of protein in the CSF and results of EMG studies.

The management of GBS is largely supportive and aimed at preventing complication until recovery process can begin.
- Respiratory support is always the priority intervention.
- Corticosteroid therapy is often used to attempt to reduce the autoimmune inflammation, but steroid has not been proven to be beneficial.
- Plasmapheresis is used in first 2 weeks of GBS. With plasmapheresis, blood is removed and filtered of antibodies, immunoglobuline fibrinogens and other proteins.
- IV administration of high-dose immunoglobuline has also shown to be as effective as plasmopherons and has the advantages of immediate availability and greater safety.
- Recovery is accelerated by early institution of plasmapheresis and IV therapy.
- Corticosteroids and ACTH are used to suppress the immune response but appear have little effect on the prognosis and duration of disease.

Assessment of the patient is the most important aspect of nursing care during the acute phase. The nurse must monitor the ascending paralysis, assess respiratory function, monitor ABGs, and assess the gag, cornea and swallowing reflexes during the routine assessment. Monitoring blood pressure, cardiac rate and rhythm is also important in acute phase, and report and any autonomic disfunction also be assessed and reported to the concerned.

Nursing diagnosis of patient with GBS may be: Inability to sustain spontaneous ventilation r/t progression of disease process:
- Inability to sustain spontaneous ventilation r/t progression of disease process.
- Risk for aspiration r/t dysphagia.
- Pain r/t paresthesias.
- Impaired verbal communication r/t intubation or paralysis of muscles of speech.
- Fear r/t uncertain outcome.
- Self-care deficit r/t inability to use muscles to accomplish ADL.

Here nurse has to follow the measure to treat respiratory failure which may include endotracheal intubation, meticulous suctioning technique may be used to prevent infection. Through bronchial hygiene and chest physiotherapy, help clear secretions and prevent respiratory deterioration. If fever develops, sputum culture should be obtained and sent to laboratory. Good communication should be maintained with the patients. If urinary retention occurs, intermittent catheterization is preferred. Nutritional needs must be met in spite of possible problems associated with delayed gastric emptying, paralytic ileus and potential for aspirations if the gag reflex is lost. Throughout the course of illness, the nurse needs to provide support and encouragement to the family and patient because residual problem and relapses are common.

TRIGEMINAL NEURALGIA (TIC DOULOUREUX)

Trigeminal neuralgia affects the fifth cranial nerve and causes intense paroxysmal pain in one or more of the branches of trigeminal nerves. Then CN has both motor and sensory branches. The sensory branches are involved in trigeminal neuralgia. Primarily, the maxillary and mandibular branches.

Etiology

No etiology has been found for the disorder although variety of risk factors have been identified. Major initiating pathologic events may include nerve compression by tortuous arteries of the posterior fossa blood vessels, demyelinating plaques, herpes virus infection, infection of teeth and jaw, transmission infarction. The effectiveness of antiseizures drug therapy may be related to the ability of these drugs to stabilize neuron membrane and decrease paroxysmal afferent impulses of the nerve.

Pathophysiology

The trigeminal nerve exists the pons and merges into the gassenar ganglion before it separates into its three major branches. It is the largest of the cranial nerve (CN) and has both motor and sensory fibers. Trigeminal neuralgia primarily affects the maxillary and mandibular branchehs of the nerve. The pain occurs abruptly lasts from few seconds to a few minutes and can recur at any time. Pain typically described as intense, piercing, burning or like a lightening bolt; the pain affects only one side of the face and there are no accompanying motor or sensory deficits in the region served by the nerve.

Clinical Manifestation

The classic feature of trigeminal neuralgia is an abrupt onset of paroxysms of excruciating pain described as a burning knife like or lightening, like shock in the lips, upper or lower gums, cheek, forehead or side of the nose. Intense pain, twitching, grimacing, and frequent blinking and tearing of the eye occur during the acute attack (giving rise to the term "tic"). The attacks are usually brief, lasting only from seconds to 2 or 3 minutes and are generally unilateral. Recurrences are unpredictable, they may occur several times a day or weeks or months apart. After the refractory (Pain free) period, a phenomenon known as clustering can occur. Clustering is characterized by a cycle of pain and refractoriness that continues for hours.

The painful expisodes are usually initiated by a triggering mechanism of light cutaneous stimulation at a specific point along the distribution of the nerve branches. Precipitating stimuli include chewing, teeth-brushing, a hot or cold blast of air on the face, washing the face, yawning or even talking. Touch and tickle seem to predominate as causative triggers rather than pain or changes in temperature. As a result, the patient may eat improperly, neglect hygienic practices, wear a cloth over the face, and withdraw from interaction with other individuals. The patient may sleep excessively as a means of coping with the pain. This pain disrupts the lifestyle, patients may even commit suicide.

Management

History and physical examination help to make diagnosis and brain or CT scan, audiologic evaluation. EMG, CSF analgesics, arteriography, posterior myography and MRI are used as diagnostic measures.

There is no definitive treatment for trigeminal neuralgia. Treatment attempts to prevent or block the pain episodes in the most minimal invasive way. The majority of patients obtain adequate relief through antiseizure drugs such as carbamazepine (Tegretol), phenytoin (Bilantin) and valproate (Depekene). Clonazepam, Baclofen.

Nerve block is another possible treatment of trigeminal neuralgia.

If a conservative approach is not effective, fitting surgical measures are available.
- Glycerol injection into one or more branches of trigeminal nerve.
- Retrogasserian rhizotomy for permanent anesthesia.
- Suboccipital craniotomy.
- Percutaneous radiofrequency rhizotomy for total pain relief.
- Microvascular decompressing for pain relief without loss of sensation.
- Gamma knife radiosurgery.

The nursing intervention include assessment of attacks of pain and its characteristics, management of pain, maintenance of nutritional status of patient, and taking suitable hygienic measure and education. Patient and family regarding disorder and management.

BELL'S PALSY

Bell's palsy refers to a peripheral facial paralysis, acute benign cranial polyneuritis. It is a disorder characterized by a disruption of the motor branches of the facial nerve (CNVII) or one side of the face in the absence of any other diseases such as stroke.

Etiology

The aetiology of disease is unknown; but it is generally believed to be a type of localized inflammatory reaction. There is evidence that reactivated herpes simplex virus (HSV) may be involved in majority of cases. The reactivation of HSV causes inflammation of edema, ischemia and eventually demyelination of the nerve, creating pain and alteration in motor and sensory function.

Pathophysiology

The facial nerve is primarily composed of motor nerve that innervates the muscles of expression on the face.

Sensory branches supply the anterior two-thirds of the tongue. Bell's palsy is characterized by a rapid weakening or paralysis of the facial muscles on one side of the face, which creates a mask-like appearance. The eye on the affected side tears constantly, and the person has difficulty in swelling secretions. The paralysis may develop over a period of 24 to 36 hours or be fully present when a patient wakes from sleep.

Clinical Manifestation

The onsets of Bell's palsy is often accompanied by an outbreak of herpes vesicles in or around the ear. Patient may complain of pain around or behind the ear. In addition, manifestation may include fever, tinnitus, or hearing difficult. The paralysis of the motor branches of the facial nerve typically results in flaccidity of the affected side of the face, with dropping of the mouth accompanied by drooling. An inability to close the eyelid with an upward movement of eyeball when closure is attempted is also evident. A widened palpebral fissure (the opening between the eyelids), flattening of the nasolabial gold, and inability to smile, frown or whistle are also common. Unilateral loss of taste is common. Decreased muscle movement may alter chewing ability and although some patients may experience loss of tearing or excessive tearing, pain may be present behind the ear on affected side especially before the onset of paralysis.

Complication can include psychologic withdrawal because of changes in appearance, malnutrition and dehydration, mucus membrane trauma, corneal abrasions, muscle stretching and facial spasms and contractures.

Management

There is no definitive test for diagnosing Bell's palsy. The diagnosis and prognosis are indicated by observation of the typical pattern of onset and signs and testing of percutaneous nerve excitability of EMG.

There is no definitive treatment for Bell's palsy, treatment for Bell's palsy includes moist heat, gentle massage and electrical stimulation of the nerve. Stimulation may maintain muscle tone and prevent atrophy. Care is primarily focussed on relief of symptoms and prevention of complication. Corticosteroid, especially predisone are started immediately and the best results are obtained if corticosteroids initiated before paralysis completes. When patient improves, they can be tapered off over 2-week period. Analgesics may be administered for pain management. Anti-HSV infection drug acyclovir, valacyclovir and Famiciclon are used if it is present.

The patient with Bell's palsy does not usually require inpatient hospitalization. The following nursing interventions are used throughout the course of disease:
- Mild analgesic can relieve pain.
- Hot wet packs can reduce the discomfort of herpic lesions aid circulation and relieve pain.
- The face should be protected from cold and drafts.
- Maintenance of good nutrition—Patient may be taught to chew food on unaffected side.
- Thorough oral hygiene.
- Teach patient to safely use of heat, massage and TENS at home.
- Instruct about safe use of corticosteroids.
- Teach importance of protecting eyes from infection and other supportive measures.

SPINAL CORD INJURY

The spinal column is a circular bony ring that provides excellent protection for the spinal cord from most low-intensity injury. The vertebrae are dense bony structures with multiple articulations that provide for a wide range of head and neck movements, but these articulations also create points of weakness that are vulnerable to a variety of types of injury. The close anatomical proximity of the spinal cord to the vertebrae, muscles and ligaments increases the chance of injury to any of the supporting structures will also result in injury to the cord itself.

Etiology

Spinal injuries occur most commonly when excessive force is exerted on the spinal column, resulting in excessive flexion, hyperextension, compression or rotation.

The population at risk for spinal cord injury is primarily young adult men between ages of 15 and 30 years and those who are impulsive or risk taken in daily living. Individuals at risk for spinal cord injury include motor cyclists, skydivers, football players, police personnel, divers and military personnel. Coordination exists between alcohol and drug abuse and spinal injuries that substantial abuse is present in the majority of motor vehicle accidents that result in spinal cord injury (SCI) as well as many other accidents' diving incidents, and episodes of violent trauma.

Events that cause abrupt forceful acceleration and deceleration are common initiating factors for SCI. Injuries to the spinal cord can be classified in a variety of ways that take into account damage to both the vertebrae and the underlying spinal cord. Most injuries are the results of sudden and often violent external trauma, but the persons who have chronic conditions affecting the vertebrae such as stenosis, arthritis, or osteoporosis are also at a high risk for injury.

Mechanisms of Injury

- Hyperflexion injuries are frequently the result of sudden deceleration as might be experienced in a head on collision or from a severe blow to the back of the head. The head and neck are forcibly hyperflexed and then may be snapped backward into forced hyperextension. These injuries are typically seen in C-5-6 area of the cervical spine. They may result in

fracture of the vertebrae, dislocation and or tearing of the posterior ligaments.
- Hyperextension injuries are frequently acceleration injuries as are seen in rear end collisions or as the result of falls in which the chin is forcibly struck. These injuries tend to cause significant damage because the downward and backward area of the head's movement is so great. C-4-5 is the area of the spine most commonly affected.
- Compression injuries cause the vertebrae to squash or burst. They usually involve high velocity and affect both the cervical and thoracolumbar regions of the spine. Blows to the top of the head and forceful landing on the feet or buttocks can result in compression injury.
- Rotational injuries are caused by extreme lateral flexion or twisting of the head and neck. The tearing of ligaments can easily result in dislocation as well as fracture, and soft tissue damage frequently complicates the primary injury. The result can be a highly unstable spinal injury. Many SCI involve more than one type of directional force.

Types of Spinal Cord Damage

The injuries that can affect the spinal cord are concussion, contusion, laceration and transection.
- *Cord concussion:* The cord is severely jarred or squeezed as is frequently seen with sports related injuries e.g. football. No identifiable pathological changes are detectable in the cord but a temporary loss of motor or sensory function, or both can occur. The dysfunction resolves spontaneously within 24-48 hours.
- *Cord contusion:* This injury is frequently caused by compression. Bleeding into the cord results in bruising and edema. The extent of damage reflects the adequacy of the overall perfusion to the cord and then severity of the inflammatory response.
- *Cord transection:* A complete or incomplete severing of the spinal cord with loss of neurological function is below the level of the injury. The cord segment in which neurological function is preserved.

Spinal Cord Syndrome

There are many unique and specific syndrome can occur in SCI. They represent types of localized spinal damage although it is unusual to see any of these syndromes in their pure form.
- Central cord syndrome reflects damage primarily to the central gray or white matter of the spinal cord. It is believed to be resulting from edema formation that occurs in response to the primary injury and puts pressure on the anterior horn cells. It usually occurs in older adults who experience a hyper extensive injury, typically in the cervical region. The resulting motor deficit is more severe in the upper extremities than in the lower, particularly in the hand. The amount of sensory impairment is highly variable. Bowel and bladder function may or may not be affected. Improvement over the time is expected.
- Anterior cord syndrome typically results from injury or infarction involving the anterior spinal artery, which perfuses the anterior two-thirds of the spinal cord. It can also result from tumors and acute discherniation. The resultant damage includes motor paralysis with loss of pain and temperature sensation. Position, vibration, and touch sensation remain intact.
- Posterior cord syndrome is an extremely rare syndrome in which proprioceptive sensation is the position and vibration are lost due to damage to the posterior column of the spinal cord.
- Brown-sequard's syndrome results from unilateral injury usually of the penetrating type, that involves just half of the spinal cord. There is a resulting loss of motor ability plus touch, pressure, and vibration sensation on same side as the injury but loss of pain and temperature sensations on the opposite side.
- Conus medullaris syndrome results from damage to the sacral region of the spinal column and the lumbar nerve roots that comprise the cauda equina. It creates a lower motor neuron injury with flaccid paralysis of the bowel and bladder and loss of sexual function. Motor function in the sensory involvement is rarely present.

Pathophysiology

Trauma to the spinal cord produces both primary and secondary injury processes. The primary damage results from the initial mechanical insult and is usually irreversible. Bruising and compression are the most common types of injury. The cord is rarely transected at the time of primary injury, but the initial insult initiates a self-destructive process that frequently results in a worsening of the injury. This is primarily the result of a progressive slowing of blood flow to the cord.

The primary compression, stretching, jarring or tearing of the spinal cord causes small hemorrhages in the gray matter of the cord. Edema causes the blood blow to the cord to slow in a matter of minute. Hypoxia develops rapidly which often leads to tissue necrosis.

Secondary cord injury results from the body's natural responses to injury and inflammation, which can have dramatic negative consequences for the spinal cord. Capillary permeability increases in response to trauma which allows fluid to move into interstitial spaces. Edema impairs the microcirculation and worsens the ischemia. The developing hypoxia stimulates the release of vasoactive substances such as catecholamines, histamin and endorphins from the injured tissue, which further decreases blood flow in the microcirculation and may induce vasospasm. Proteolytic and lypolytic enzymes are also released from the injured cells. Which can clog the microcirculation and worsen the edema, ischemia and necrosis. The enzymes actively work to clear cellular debris, which can include removal of neural tissue that is then incapable of regeneration.

This secondary injury process can destroy the full thickness of the spinal cord at the level of injury and further extends its effects severe and cord segments above and below the original level of injury. The process of secondary injury is initiated immediately after the original insult and progresses rapidly. Blood flow to the injured spinal cord is further compromised by the upset of spinal shock.

Spinal Shock

Spinal shock represents a temporary but profound disruption of spinal cord functions, which occur immediately after injury, typically within 30 to 60 minutes. It is a state of a reflexion characterized by the loss of all neurological function below the level of the injury. Spinal shock causes a complete loss of the motor, sensory, reflexes, and autonomic functioning. The severity of shock varies depending on the extent and level of the primary injury, but injuries at T6 or above usually result in more severe forms. Spinal shock is the direct result of the neuronal injury and is not preventable. The clinical manifestation of spinal shock are as follows:

- Flaccid paralysis: Affects all skeletal muscles below the level of injury.
- Loss of spiral reflex activity: Paralytic ileus, loss of bowel and bladder tone.
- Sensory loss below the level of injury: Pain, temperature, touch, pressure and proprioceptive senses, somatic and visceral sensations. Bradycardia (results from unopposed parasympathetic vagal (slowing of the heart).
- Bradycardia (results from venous pooling in lower extremities and splanchnic circulation, related to loss of vasomotor tone).
- Loss of temperature control.
  - Warm, dry skin
  - Inability to shiver or perspire.
  - Poikilothermia: the body assumes the temperature of the external environment.

Clinical Manifestations

The clinical manifestations of the spinal cord injury are dependent on the level of the injury and whether the injury is complete or incomplete. The terms paraplegia' tetraplegia (previously quadriplegia) are used to describe the functional consequence of spinal cord injury (SCI).

Generally there will be poikilothermia and warm, dry flushed extremities below the level of injury (Spinal shock). Other manifestations related to level and degree of injury are as follows: RS Lesions at C1 to C3 give rise to apnoea, inability to cough.

- Lesion at C4 gives rise to poor cough, diaphragmatic breathing.
- Lesion at C5 to T6 give rise to hypoventilation, decreased respiratory reserve.
- Lesions above T5 leads to bradycardia, hypotension, postural hypotension, and absence of vasomotor tone.
- Lesion above T5 also leads to decreased or absent bowel sounds (paralytic ileum) abdominal distention, constipation, fecal incontinence and fecal impaction.
- Lesions between T1, L2 leads to flaccid bladder (acute stages) spasticity with reflex bladder emptying (later stages).
- Lesion above C8: resulting in flaccid paralysis and anesthesia. Below the level of injury resulting in tetraplegia.
- Lesion below C8 leads to hyperactive deep tendon reflexes, bilaterally positive Babinski's test.

Mixed loss of voluntary motor activity and sensations and muscle atomy (in flaccid state), contractures (in spastic state) will be present. In addition, priapism, loss of sound functions also occur.

Management

The initial goals for the patient with a spinal cord injury are to sustain life and prevent further cord damage. Spinal cord injury is initially diagnosed on the basis of the presenting symptoms. Systemic, neurogenic and spinal cord shock must be treated. For injury at the cervical level, all body systems must be maintained until the full extent of the damage can be evaluated. Treatment of spinal cord injury may be medical or surgical.

Emergency Management

Patient may come to hospital with blunt injury or penetrating injuries. Blunt injuries include, compression, flexion, extension, or rotational injuries to spinal column, due to motor vehicle accidents pedestrian accidents, falls and diving.

Penetrating injuries may be stretched, torn, crushed or lacerated spinal cord due to gunshot wounds and stab wounds.

During this, the nurse has to make the following assessment of findings.

- Pain, tenderness, deformities or muscle spasms adjacent to vertebral column.
- Numbness, paresthesias.
- Alterations in sensation; temperature, light, touch, deep pressure and proprioception.
- Weakness or heaviness in limbs.
- Weakness, paralysis or flaccidity of muscles.
- Spinal shock.
- Cuts, bruises, open wounds overhead, face, neck or back.

- Neurogenic shock, hypotention, bradycardia, dry flushed skin.
- Bowel and bladder incontinence.
- Urinary retention.
- Difficulty in breathing.
- Priapism.
- Diminished rectal sphincter tone.

Nursing Intervention

- Ensure patent airway.
- Stabilize cervical spine.
- Administer oxygen via nasal cannula or nonbreather mask.
- Establish IV with two large-bone catheters and infuse normal saline or lactated Ringer's solution as appropriate.
- Assess for other injuries.
- Control external bleeding.
- Obtain cervical spine radiographs or CT scan.
- Prepare for stabilization with cranial tong and traction.
- Administer high-dose methyl prednisolone, and ongoing monitoring includes:
    - Monitor vital signs, level of consciousness, oxygen saturation, cardiac rhythm, urine output.
    - Keep warm.
    - Monitor for urinary retention and hypertention.
    - Anticipate need for intubation if gag reflex is absent.

Following emergency management, patient should be prepared and assisted to perform the following diagnostic measure:

- Complete neurologic examination.
- ABG analysis.
- Electrolytes, glucose, hemoglobin, and hematocrit levels.
- Urinalysis.
- Anteroposterior, lateral and odontoid spinal X-ray studies.
- CT Scan.
- Myelography.
- MRI.
- EMG to measure evoked potentials.

Following measures should be taken if confronted with cervical cord injury.

- Immobilization of vertebral column by skeletal traction.
- Maintenance of heart rate (Example atropine) and blood pressure (e.g. dopamine).
- Methylprednisolone therapy to reduced edema.
- Insertion of nasogastric tube and attachment to suction.
- Intubation (if indicated by ABGs).
- Administration of oxygen by high humidity mask.
- Introduction of indwelling catheter.
- Administration of IV fluids.

In addition, following ambulatory care should be followed:

- Stress ulcer prophylaxes.
- Physical therapy (range of motion exercises).
- Occupational therapy (splints and ADL training).

CHAPTER 18

Nursing Management of Oncological Conditions

INTRODUCTION

The word 'Onco' originated from Greek word 'Onkos' means 'Mass' relating to tumors. Oncogene, a gene which in certain circumstances can transform a cell into a tumor cell, oncology is the study and treatment of tumors, may be benign or malignant. If it is malignant, people used to call it as cancer. Cancer was recognized in ancient times by skilled observers who gave it the name "Cancer" (Latin word Cancer-crab) because it stretched out in many directions like the legs of a crab. The term cancer is an "umbrella" word used to describe a group of more than 270 diseases in which cells multiply without restraint, destroy healthy tissue endangering life. The psychological and physiological impact on cancer patients and their families results in profound changes in their lifestyles. Cancer may result in death for some and mutilation for others. The legends, surroundings, malignant diseases often focussing on its incurability help foster feelings of hopelessness and dread. Yet, much progress has been made in prevention, early detection and treatment of cancer and research continue in these areas.

Oncology nurses must have a broad base of knowledge in both pathophysiology and psycholosocial arena. They care for patients of all ages, both gender and in a variety of settings. The oncology nurse feels and fills the role of care provider, manager, researcher, teacher and consultant. To provide comprehensive care, the nurse must have accurate knowledge about prevention, control and treatment of cancer. Nurse has to teach about cancer in all settings. In addition to teaching, the nurse has an active role in treatment and control programs of cancer. To be effective as a helping person, the nurse must be aware of the emotional impact that the diagnosis of cancer has on the patient and family, because this emotional response affects every aspect of nursing care. Cancer nursing challenges the creativity, skill and commitment of the nurses.

CANCER

The word Cancer, often abbreviated Ca, is a term that frightens most people. Cancer is synonymous with the term "malignant neoplasma". Other terms suggest malignant neoplasm includes tumor, malignancy, carcinoma and aberrect cell growth. Strictly speaking, these words are not interchangeable.

Cancer is a disease of the cell in which the normal mechanisms of control of growth and proliferation are disturbed. This results in distinctive morphological alteration of the cells and aberration in tissue pattern. Cancer is a collective term describing a large group of diseases characterized by uncontrolled growth and spread of abnormal cells. This group of diseases:

- Arise from any tissue or organ
- Differ greatly from one another in appearance and growth
- May follow very different courses of developments in their host.
- Respond differently to the variety of therapies applied to them.

The word 'neoplasm' is derived from Greek words neos: new, and plasis: molding. Thus, neoplasm is defined as an abnormal new growth or formation of tissue that serves no useful purpose and may harm the host organism.

A neoplasm may be either benign or malignant.

- Benign is defined as a usually harmless growth that does not spread or invade other tissues.
- Malignant is defined as a harmful tumor, capable of spread and invasion of other tissues far removed from the site of origin.

In addition, some other important terms used in cancer are:

- Anaplastic refers to those tumor cells that are completely undifferentiated and bear no resemblance to cells of tissues of their origin.
- Hyperplasia refers to an increase in the number of normal cells in a normal arrangement in a tissue or organ, usually leads to an increase in the size or part and an increase in functional activity.
- Metaplasia refers to the replacement of one type of fully differentiated cell by another fully differentiated cell in another part of the body where the second cell type does not normally occur.
- Dysplasia refers to an alteration in the size, shape, and organization of differentiated cells; cells lose their regularity and show variability in size and shape, usually in response to an irritant; cells may revert to normal when the irritant is removed, but may transform to neoplasia.
- Metastasis refers to the ability of neoplastic cells to spread from the original site of the tumor to distant

organs, spreading as the same cell type as the original neoplastic tissue.
- Carcinoma refers to a form of cancer that is composed of epithelial cells that tend to infiltrate surrounding tissues and may eventually spread to distant sites.
- Oncogenes refer to cancer genes that are altered versions of normal genes.
- Proto-oncogenes refer to repressed oncogenes existing in normal which can be activated by many different factors and cause the host cell to become malignant.
- Tumor refers to usually synonymous with neoplasm.

Pathophysiology of Cancer

The exact cause and method of the development of cancer are unknown. Cancer is a group of many diseases of multiple causes that can arise in any cell of the body capable of evading regulatory control over proliferations and differentiation. The two major dysfunctions present in the process of cancer of "defective cellular proliferation (growth)" and "defective cellular differentiation".

Defective Cellular Proliferation

Cancer cells usually proliferate in the manner and at the same rate of the normal cells of the tissue from which they arise. However, cancer cells respond differently than normal cells to the intracellular signals that regulate the state of dynamic equilibrium. Cancer cells divide indiscriminately and haphazardly. Sometime, they produce more than two cells at the time of mitosis. The loss of intracellular control of proliferations may be result of a mutation of the stem cells. The stem cells are viewed as the target or the origin of cancer developed. The DNA of the stem cell is substituted or permanently rearranged. When this happens the stem cell is mutated and has the potential to become malignant. It will usually proliferate at the rate of the tissue origin, and some subpopulation can promote tumor progression to generate malignant cells. The malignant cells can differentiate to form normal tissue cells **(Table 18.1)**.

Defective Cellular Differentiation

Cellular differentiation is normally and orderly a process that progresses from a state of immaturity to a state of maturity. Because all body cells are derived from the fertilized ova, all cells have the potential to perform all body functions. As cell differentiates, this potential is repressed and the mature cell is capable of performing only specific functions. Genes that are important regulators of these normal cellular processes are the "cellular oncogenes or proto-oncogenes" Mutations that alter the expression of genes or their products can activate proto-oncogenes to function as 'oncogenes' (tumor inducing genes) by inducing mitosis but inhibiting differentiation of the cell.

The proto-oncogene has been described as the genetic lock that keeps the cell in its mature functioning state. When this lock is 'unlocked' it may occur through exposure to carcinogens or oncogenic viruses, genetic alterations and mutations occur. The abilities and properties that the cell had in fetal development are again expressed. Although oncogens and oncogenic products, contribute to normal cell function, oncogens intefere with normal cell expression under some conditions, causing cell to become malignant. The comparison of the characteristics of normal and malignant cells **(Table 18.1)** are as follows:

The cause and development of each type of cancer are likely to be multifactorial. It is not known how many tumors have chemical, environmental, genetic, immunologic, or viral origin. It is common belief that the development of cancer is rapid, haphazard event. Although scientists have learned a great deal about the causes of cancer, the exact mechanism by which these agents transform healthy cells into neoplastic cells remains obscure. One accepted perception is that cancer develops as a result of genetic alteration from one or more causes, resulting in uncontrolled cellular reproduction and growth. When a defective cell divides, the new cells contain defective genetic code within the DNA. Overtime defective cells divide and multiply and the malignancy grows.

Carcinogens are substances that when introduced into the cell cause changes in the structure and function of the cells that lead to cancer. It is not a simple cause and effect mechanism. However, the natural history of cancer is an orderly process causing several stages and occurring over a period of time. There are three identified stages of carcinogenesis, i.e. initiation, promotion and progression.

Initiation

The first stage, initiation, is an irreversible alteration in the cells' genetic structure resulting from the action of a chemical, physical or biologic agent. This altered cell has the potential for developing into a clone of neoplastic cells. Most carcinogens (pl. see etiology) are detoxified by protective a enzymes and are harmlessly excreted. If this protective mechanism fails, carcinogens enter the cells' nucleus and may irreversibly bind to DNA. DNA repair is possible. However, if repair does not occur before all divisions, the cell will replicate into daughter cells, each with the same genetic alterations. After this damage of DNA cells are more susceptible to progression into malignancies. Irreversibly initiated cells do not display their changes and are not detectable until exposed to a promoting agent.

Promotion

Promotion is usually the result of a second factor acting on the initiated cell. A single alteration of the genetic structure of the cell is not sufficient to result in cancer. At least one

Table 18.1: Characteristics of normal and malignant cells.

Normal cells	Malignant cells
Mitotic cell division	
• Mitotic cell division leads to two daughter cells	• Mitosis leads to multiple cell that may or may not resemble the parent, multiple mitotic spindles
Appearance	
• Cells of same type homogeneous in size, shape	• Cells larger and grow more rapidly than normal, pleomor-and growth phic, i.e. heterogeneous in size and shape
• Cells cohesive, form regugular pattern or expansion	• Cells not as cohesive, irregular
• Uniform size to nucleus	• Larger, more prominent nucleus
• Have characteristics pattern of organization	• Lack of characteristic pattern of organization of host cell
• Mixture of stem cells (Precursors) and well-differentiated cells	• Anaplastic, lack of differen tiated cell characteristic, specific functions
Growth pattern	
• Do not invade adjacent tissue	• Invade adjacent tissues
• Proliferate in response to specific stimuli	• Proliferate in response to abnormal stimuli
• Growth in ideal conditions (e.g. nutrients, oxygen, space, correct biochemical environments)	• Growth in adverse conditions such as lack of nutrients
• Exhibit contact inhibition	• Do not exhibit contact inhibition
• Cell birth equals or in less than cell death	• Cell birth exceeds cell death
• Stable cell membrane	• Loss of cell control as a result of cell membrane charges
• Constant and predictable cell growth rate	• Erratic cell growth rate
• Cannot grow outside specific environment, e.g. breast or lymphatics or seed to distant sites and grow in other sites	• Able to break off cells than migrate through blood stream cell growth and only in breast
Functions	
• Have specific and designated purpose	• Serve no useful purpose
• Contribute to the overall being of the host, parasitic	• Do not contribute to the well-being of the host
• Cells function in specific pre-determined manner (e.g. cells in thyroid secrete thyroxine)	• If cells function at all, do not function normally or they may actually cause damage. (e.g. malignant lung cancer cells secrete ACTH, causing excessive stimulated...cortex)
Others	
• Develop specific antigens, characteristic of particular cell formed	• Develop antigens completely different from normal cell
• Chromosomes remain constant throughout cell division	• Chromosomal aberrations occur as cell matures
• Complex metabolic and enzyme pattern	• Have more primitive and simplified metabolic and enzyme pattern
• Cannot invade, erode or spread	• Invade, erode and spread
• Cannot grow in the cells and inflammation	• Grow in presence of necrosis presence of necrosis or inflammation
	• Exhibit periods of latency that vary from tumor to tumor
	• Have own blood supply and supporting stroma

or more mutation must occur in cells in which a mutation already occurred. The chances of this occurring, given the billions of cells in the human body, seem highly unlikely. However the odds of cancer development are increased with the presence of promoting agents.

Promotion—The second stage in the development of cancer is characterized by the reversible proliferation of the altered initiated cells and consequently, with an increase in the initiated cell population likelihood of second cell mutation is increased. Some agents are called complete carcinogens because they produce both initiation and promotion. However, promotion may occur after very long periods of latency, which varies with the type of agent, dose, and characteristics of the target cell. Promoting agents work by changing the expression of genetic information within the cell, increasing DNA synthesis, increasing the number of copies of a particular gene, and altering cellular communication. Often exposure to the promoting agent is under the control of the client as with the tobacco, alcohol and dietary.

An important distinction between initiation and promotion is that the activity of promoters is reversible. This is a key concept in cancer prevention. Promoting factors include such agent as dietary fat, obesity, cigarette smoking, and alcohol consumption. Prolonged stress may also be a promoter. The withdrawal of these factors can reduce the risk of neoplastic formation.

Progression

Progression is the final stage in the nature/history of a cancer; it involves the morphologic and phenotypic changes in cells, which are associated with increasingly malignant behavior leading to invasion of surrounding tissue and metastasis to distant body parts. In other words, this stage is characterized by increased growth rate of the tumor, as well as by increased invasiveness and metastasis.

Metastasis can occur via the vascular system, lymphatic system and the process of implantations. Metastasis via the vascular system occurs in a variety of ways, which includes:

- Proliferating cancer cells in draining lymph nodes may enter a large collecting lymph vessel, such as thoracic duct, that empties into the larger veins leading to the heart.
- Surrounding tissue may be invaded from the primary site of the cancer cells. The cancer cells penetrate the blood vessels and are released into blood stream.
- Cancer cells aggregates are trapped in the small capillaries of the tissues and organs.
- Through the segregation of proteolytic enzymes, cancer cells penetrate the walls of the capillary and enter the adjacent tissue where they begin to proliferate.

The lymphatic spread occurs in a manner similar to vascular spaces in the body, conducting particles and fluid into lymph nodes. Cancer cells that break free from tissue or invade a lymph vessel almost always become trapped in the meshwork in the draining lymph node. If these cancer cells proliferate, the result is lymphadenopathy. Continued proliferation may result in the release of cancer cells into the lymph vessels leading from the lymph node to the next lymph node up the chain.

Implantation may occur when cancer cells become embedded along the serosal surfaces of body organs, such as the peritoneal cavity or the pleural cavity. During the surgical procedure, implantations may also occur in the primary organ or in the regional area if the environment is suitable.

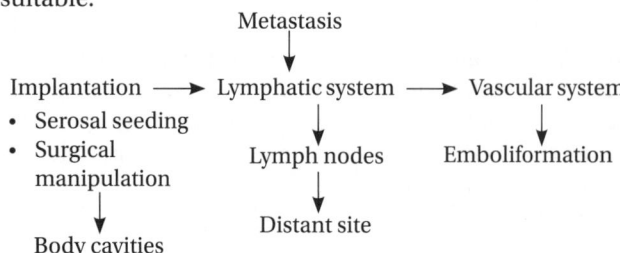

Etiology of Cancer

There are approximately 150 types of cancers found in human beings and there are probably at least 500 different cancer-causing agents. Some of the causes on the basis of several studies are as follows:

Viruses

The study of viruses in tumors has lead investigators to discover oncogenes. Oncogenes are small segments of genetic DNA that can transform normal cells into malignant cells, independently or incorporated into a virus. Viruses probably do not, as a single agent cause cancer. However, viruses may be one of multiple agents acting to initiate carcinogenesis. Certain DNA and RNA viruses termed 'oncogenic' can transform the cells they infect and induce malignant transformations. It has been found that viruses have been associated with hepatocellular carcinoma (hepatitis G. Virus) T-cell lymphoma, T-cell leukaemia, Burkitt's lymphoma (Epstein-Barr virus), nasopharyngeal carcinoma, and cervical cancer.

Chemical Carcinogens

The chemical carcinogens thought to cause cancer in human beings due to close and prolonged contact and persons who are affected usually are workers in industries where these chemicals are used as by-products. The chemical carcinogens and associated neoplasm are as follows **(Table 18.2)**.

Table 18.2: Chemical carcinogens and affecting organ.

Carcinogen	Affecting organ
Cigarette smoking	Lungs, upper respiratory tract, bladder, cervix, etc.
Asbestos	Mesothelioma, lung
Acrylonitrile	Lung, colon, prostate
Arsenic	Skin, lung, liver
Benzene	Leukemia
Cadmium	Prostate, kidney
Chromium compound	Lung
Nickel	Lung, nasal sinuses
Uranium	Lung
Aflatoxin	Liver
Nitrates	Stomach
Chloromethyl ethers	Lung
Isopropyl oil	Nasal sinuses
Benzidene	Bladder
Vinyl chloride	Angiosarcoma of liver
Radiation	Numerous locations
Polycyclic hydrocarbons	Lung, skin
Mustard gas	Lung

Physical Carcinogens

Physical carcinogens cause cellular damage just as chemical carcinogens. The classification of physical carcinogen exists:
- Ionizing radiation
- Ultraviolet radiation, and
- Foreign bodies.

Excessive exposure to ionizing radiation can cause permanent DNA mutation and transformation into a malignant growth. Most radiation from natural resources (radon, cosmic, terrestrial and internal radiation). Certain malignants have been correlated with radiation as carcinogenic agents are leukaemia, lymphonce, thyroid cancer, childhood cancer (if exposed) bone cancer (exposed persons include radiologists, radiation chemises, uranium miners).

Ultraviolet radiation from the sun can cause changes in DNA structure that can lead to malignant transformation if it is not repaired. Basal and squamous cell carcinomas of the skin as well as melanoma are linked to ultraviolet exposure.

Foreign bodies that are not biodegradable, such as asbestos fibers and bekelite disk and cellophane implants can induce the development of cancer by stimulating reactions to constant tissue damage such as scar formations, thus increasing the probability of neoplastic formations.

Drugs and Hormones

Certain drugs and hormones have also been identified as carcinogens **(Table 18.3)**. Drugs that are capable of interacting with DNA (e.g. alkylating agents) as immunosuppressive agents, have the potential cause neoplasm in human beings. And certain hormones administered to women has also been linked to the development of cancer. Certain cancers related to drug and hormone exposure in human beings are as follows:

In addition to the carcinogen described above, there are also certain predisposing factors that influence the host susceptibility to various etiologic agents.

- *Age:* There is an increasing incidence of cancer in the young and in persons more than 55 years of age. Many cancers such as prostate, and colon cancer and some chronic leukemia occur in older people. Testicular cancer is found in men between 20 and 40 years of age. Ovarian cancer is most common in women over 55 years of age. Many cancers occur mainly in childhood, e.g. Ewing's sarcoma, certain acute leukemias, Wilms' tumor and retinoblastoma.
- *Sex:* Women are most susceptible to certain types of cancer than men, i.e. cancer cervix, cancer breast, etc.
- *Occupation:* People in certain occupations are more susceptible to certain cancers because of their greater contact with specific carcinogens. For example, industrial workers, who expose to certain physical and chemical carcinogens.
- *Heredity:* Actually, none of the specific types of cancer are considered heredity. But there are a number of cancers that provide evidence of inheritable predisposed to cancer. Fanconi anemia, atelangiectasia, and xeroderma pigmentosum are examples of autosomal recessive conditions that predisposes persons to a variety of malignancies. Fasmilial polyposis, coli retinoblastoma, Wilms' tumor, and neurofibromatosis are examples of autosomal dominant disorders that follow classic mendelian patterns of inheritance. Breast, overian and colon cancers may also show a familial pattern.
- *Diet and nutrition:* A diet high in fat may be a factor in the development of breast, colon and prostate cancer. Excessive alcohol, especially when accompanied by cigarette smoking, increases the risk of cancers of mouth larynx, throat, esophagus and stomach has been noted as area of world where salt-cured smoked, and nitrate cured goods are eaten frequently. People

Table 18.3: Carcinogen drugs and associated cancer.

Carcinogen	Associated cancer
Radioisotopes	
Phosphorus (32 p)	Acute leukemia
Radium, mesothorium	Osteosarcoma, sinus carcinoma
Thorotrast	Hemangioendothelioma of liver
Immunosuppressive agent	
Antilymphocyte serum	Reticulum-cell sarcoma
Antimetabolites	Epithelial cancer of skin
Alkylating agents	Viscera, acute myelogenous
Corticosteroids	Leukemia
Cytotoxic drugs	
Phenylalanine mustard	Bladder cancer
Cyclophosphomide	Acute melogenous leukemia
Hormones	
Synthetic estrogen prenatal	Vaginal and cervical
Synthetic estrogen-	Endometrial carcinoma postnatal (adenosquamous type)
Androgenic-anabolic steroids	Hepatocellular carcinoma
Diethylstilbestrol (DES)	Vaginal cancer
Others	
Arsenic	Skin, liver cancer
Phenacetin containing drug	Renal pelvis carcinoma
Coal tar ointments	Skin cancer
Diphenyl hydantoin	Skin cancer
Chloramphenicol	Leukemia
Amphetamine	Hodgkin's disease

who have more weight have an increased risk of colon breas prostate, gallbladder, ovary and uterine cancer.

Studies have shown that daily consumptions of vegetables and fresh fruits is associated with decreased risk of lung, prostate bladder, esophagus, colorectal, and stomach cancers. High fiber diet may reduce the risk of colon cancer.

- *Stress:* Studies suggest that stress may increase the risk of cancer. Chronic physical and emotional stress preys on the hypothalamus, the portion of the pituitary gland that regulates hormone and immune systems. Increased stress causes hormonal and immunologic changes or both, which may in turn may spur the growth and proliferation of cancer cells.
- *Precancerous lesions:* Common precancerous lesions include pigmented moles, burn scars, senile keratoses, leukoplakia, and benign adenomas or polyps of the colon or stomach. These lesions need to be periodically assessed for malignant changes.

Classification of Cancer

Neoplastic tumors classified according to behavior of tumor (benign or malignant) anatomic site, histologic analysis (grading) and extent of disease (staging). This classification systems are intended to provide a standardized way:

- To communicate the status of cancer to all members of health team.
- To assist in determining the most effective treatment plan.
- To serve as a factor in determining the prognosis, and
- To compare like groups for statistical purposes.

Benign and Malignant

Tumors can be classified on the basis of behavior as benign or malignant. In general, benign neoplasm, are well differentiated and malignant neoplasms range from well differentiated to undifferentiated. The difference between benign and malignant tumors are as follows; on the basis of their characteristics **(Table.18.4)**.

Anatomic Site Classification

In the anatomic classifications of tumors, the tumor is identified by the tissue origin, the anatomic site and the behavior of the tumor, i.e. benign or malignant. Carcinoma originates from embryonical ectoderm

Table 18.4: Difference between benign and malignant tumor.

Benign tumor	Malignant tumor
Speed of growth	
They grow slowly usually continue to grow throughout life unless surgically removed; may have periods of remission	They usually grow rapidly, tend to grow relentlessly through life, rarely, neoplasm regress spontaneously
Mode of growth	
Growth by enlarging and expanding, always remaining localized, never infiltrates surrounding tissues	Grows by infiltrating surrounding tissues; may remain localized (in situ) but usually infiltrates other tissues
Cell characteristics	
Usually well-differentiated; mitotic figure absent or scanty mature cells; an aplastic cells absent, cell function poorer in comparison with normal cells from which they arise, if neoplasm arises in glandular tissue, cell may secrete hormones	Usually poorly differentiated large number of normal and abnormal mitotic figures present, cells tend to be anaplastic, i.e. young embryonic type; cells too abnormal to perform any physiologic functions; occasionally a malignant tumor arising in glandular tissue secretes hormones
Recurrence	
Recurrence extremely unusual when surgically removed	Recurrence common following surgery because tumor cells spread into surrounding tissues
Metastasis	
Metastasis never occurs	Metastasis very common
Effect of neoplasm	
Not harmful to host unless located in area where it causes compression of tissues or obstruction of vital organs, does not produce cachexia (weight loss, dabilitation, anemia, weakness, wasting)	Always harmful to host. Results in death unless removed surgically or destroyed by radiation or chemotherapy, causes disfigurement, disrupted organ function, nutritional imbalance may result in ulceration, sepsis, perforations, hemorrhage, tissue slough, almost always produces cachexia which leaves person prone
Prognosis	
Prognosis is very good speed of diagnosis, poor indicated when cells still resemble normal cells and there is no evidence of metastasis	Depends on cell type and tumor generally removed surgically

(skin and glands) and endoderm (mucous membrane linings of the respiratory tract, GI tract and genitourinary tract). Sarcoma originates from embryonal mesoderm (connective tissue, muscle, bone and fat). Symphomas and leukemias originate from the hematopoietic system. The classification of tumor by tissue origin is as given **(Table 18.5)**.

Histologic Analytic Classification

The histologic grading of tumors, the appearance of the cells and the degree of differentiation are evaluated. For many tumors, four grades are used.
- *Grade I:* Cells differ slightly from normal cells (mils displasia) and are well differentiated.
- *Grade II:* Cells are more abnormal (moderate displasia) and moderately differentiated.
- *Grade III:* Cells are very abnormal (severe dysplasia) and poorly differentiated.
- *Grade IV:* Cells are immature and primitive (anaplaxia) and undifferentiated, cell of origin difficult to determine.

Extent of Disease Classification

The extent of disease classification is often called 'staging'. The clinical staging classification determines the extent of the disease process of cancer by stages:
- Stage '0': Cancer in situ. It is defined as a neoplasm of epithelial tissue that remains confined to the site of origin.
- Stage I : Tumor linked to the tissue of origin, localized tumor growth.
- Stage II: Limited local spread.
- Stage III : Extensive local and regional spread.
- Stage IV: Metastasis.

This type of classification is used as a basis for staging in cancer of cervix and Hodgkin's disease.

The TNM classificatiaon system represents the standardization of the clinical staging of cancer. It is used to determine the extent of disease process of cancer according to three parameters. Tumor size (T), degree of regional spread to the lymph nodes (N) and presence of metastasis (M). TNM system has been used in cancer of breast **(Table 18.6)**.

Prevention of Cancer

The nurse plays a prominent role in all the levels of prevention of cancer. Cancer nursing is directed towards the prevention and early detection of neoplasm as well as the care of the patient in treatment, recovery or advanced stage of cancer. At present, it is not possible to prevent all types of cancer, but some cancers can be prevented by avoidance of recognized carcinogens and by altering health behaviors.

Table 18.5: Classification of tumor by tissue origin.

Tissue origin	Benign	Malignant
Connective tissue	—	Sarcoma
♦ Embryonic fibrous tissue	Myxoma	Myxosarcoma
♦ Fibrous tissue	Fibroma	Fibrosarcoma
♦ Adipose tissue	Lipoma	Liposarcoma
♦ Cartilage	Chondroma	Chondrosarcoma
♦ Bone	Oesteoma	Osteogenic sarcoma
Epithelium tissue	—	Carcinoma
♦ Skin and mucous membrane	Papilloma	Squamous cell carcinoma
♦ Glands	—	Basal cell carcinoma
	—	Transitional cell carcinoma
	Adenoma	Adenocarcinoma
	Cystadenoma	Cystadenocarcinoma
♦ Pigmented cells malanocytes	Nevus	Malignant melanoma
Endothelium	—	Endothelioma
♦ Blood vessels	Hemangioma	Hemangioendothelioma
		Hemangiosarcoma
		Kaposi's sarcoma
♦ Lymph vessels	Lymphangioma	Lymphangiosarcoma
		Lymphangioendothelioma
♦ Bone marrow	—	Multiple myeloma
		Ewing's sarcoma
		Leukemia
♦ Lymphoid tissue		Malignant lymphoma
		Lymphosarcoma
		Reticulum cell sarcoma
Muscles tissue		
♦ Smooth muscles	Leiomyoma	Leiomyosarcoma
♦ Striated muscle	Rhabdomyoma	Rhabdomyosarcoma
Nerve tissue		
♦ Nerve fibers and sheaths	Neuroma	Neurogenic sarcoma
	Neurinoma	
	Neurofibroma	Neurofibrosarcoma
♦ Ganglion cells	Ganglioneuroma	Neuroblastoma
♦ Glial cells	Glioma	Glioblastoma
♦ Menenges	Meningioma	Malignant meningioma
Gonads	Dermoid cyst	Embryonal carcinoma
		Embryonal sarcoma
		Teratocarcinoma

Table 18.6: TNM staging classification system.

Tumor	
T0	No evidence of primary tumor
TS	Carsinoma in situ
T1, T2, T3, T4	Ascending degrees of tumor size and involvement
Nodes	
N0	No evidence of disease in lymph node
N_{1a}, N_{2a}	Disease found in regional lymph nodes, metastasis not suspected
NX	Regional lymph nodes cannot be assessed clinically
Metastasis	
M0	No evidence of distant metastasis
M_1, M_2, M_3	Assending degrees of metastatic involvement of the host, including distant nodes

Primary Prevention

Primary prevention of cancer is activity taken to prevent the occurrence or reduce the risk of cancer in healthy persons. Activities in this area of health promotion include identifying risk factors, reduction and cancer prevention programmes. For example the dietary changes to reduce cancer which include:

- Increased intake of high-fiber foods such as fruits and vegetables and whole grain cereals. Dark green and deep yellow fruits and vegetable rich in vitamin A and C (cabbage, broccoli, cauliflower, Brussels sprouts, and kohlrabi).
- Reduced intake of salt-cured, smoked and nitrite-cured foods, fats and oils especially from animal sources; alcoholic beverages and excess calories leading to obesity.

So, one important aspect of the nurse and other health care provider is to educate the public to do the following:

- Reduce or avoid exposure to known or suspected carcinogens and cancer-promoting agents.
- Eat balanced diet that includes vegetables (green, yellow and orange), fresh fruits, wholegrains, adequate amount of fiber, and low level of facts and preservatives.
- Participate in regular exercise regimens.
- Obtain adequate, consistent, periods of rest (at least 6 to 8 hours per night).
- Have a health examination on consistent basis that includes health history physical examination and specific diagnostic tests for common cancers, i.e., lung cancer, colon and rectal cancer, prostate cancer, cervical cancer and breast cancer, etc.
- Eliminate, reduce or change the perceptions of stressors and enhance the ability to positively cope with stressors.
- Enjoy consistent periods of relaxation and leisure.
- Know the seven warning signals of cancer- which include "CAUTION" as follows:
  1. Change in bowel or bladder habits.
  2. A sore that does not heal.
  3. Unusual bleeding or discharge.
  4. Thickening or lump in the breast or elsewhere.
  5. Indigestion or difficulty in swallowing.
  6. Obvious change in a wart or more.
  7. Nagging cough or hoarseness.
- Learn and practice self-examination of breast and testicles.
- Seek immediate medical care if cancer is suspected.

In some occupations, the employees may have contact with carcinogenic substances such as asbestos, chromium, ether, vinyl chloride and benzyprene, etc. In such industries, proper regulation and protective measures can be taken accordingly to reduce the risk of cancer.

The nurses can have a definite impact in convincing people that a change in the lifestyle pattern will have a positive influence on health.

Secondary Prevention

Secondary prevention of cancer is focused on the early diagnosis of which early detection and screening are the major components. Screening and detection programmes are concentrated on some of the most common cancers including cancers of the breast, cervix, colon/rectum, prostate, skin and oropharynx.

The screening for specific cancer sites which have high risk profile are as follows:

Lung: The risk of lung cancer can occur with a person of:
- History of 20 pack years of smoking (1 pack a day for 20 years).
- Exposure to air-born carcinogens especially asbestos, uranium, hydrocarbon.
- Age range 40-80 years.
- Chronic lung disease.

The method of screening any such case will be observation by patient for change in respiratory status, increased frequency of infections and change in cough, sputum, breathing, and voice. Some doctors advise annual chest X-rays.

Colon and rectum: The risk of colon and rectal cancer occurs with a person's:
- History of familial polyposis, ulcerative colitis, Crohn's disease.
- Personal or family history of colon or rectal cancer.
- Taking diet high in fat and low in fiber.
- Age range 40–75 years.
  The method of screening will be
- Blood test on stools every year after age of 50 years.
- Digital rectal examination annually after age of 40 years.

- Sigmoidoscopic examination (preferably flexible) every 3-5 years after 50 years.
- Observations by patients for change in bowel pattern, i.e. diarrhea, constipation, pain, flatus, black tarry stools, bleeding.

Prostate: The risk of prostatic cancer occurs with presence of prostatic hyperplasia and presence of prostatic infection. The methods of screening of such case will be;
- Digital rectal examination of age 40 years and annually thereafter.
- Prostate specific antigens blood test every year.
- Observation on men aged 50 and older, for dysuria, blood in urine, difficulty in producing stream of urine.

Cervix: The risk of cervical cancer occurs with a person
- Who has a history of early intercourse (before the age of 20 years) with multiple partners.
- Who maintains poor personal hygiene including poor menstrual hygiene.
- Who has history of herpes virus type II infections and cervical dysplasia.
  For such cases screening measures will include:
- Pap test and pelvic examination every year for those who are or have been sexually active or who have attained the age of 18 years.
- Calposcopy if suspicious area is noted.
- Observation by patient for abnormal vaginal bleeding or discharge, pain, or bleeding with sexual intercourse.

Endometrium: The risk of endometrial cancer occurs with a person's having infertility, ovarian dysfunction, obesity, uterine bleeding, estrogen therapy over long period of time, diabetes and age range 30–80 years.

By such cases, screening measures will include:
- Pap test every year.
- Pelvic examination every year.
- Endometrial biopsy every year for women of menopause.
- Observation by patient for abnormal uterine bleeding, pain, change in menstrual pattern.

Skin: The risk of skin cancer occurs with person, having prolonged exposure to sun, and previous radiation exposure; fair, thin skin, and positive family history of dysplasia nevus syndrome.

For such cases, screening measures include, self examination monthly with suspicious lesions evaluated promptly, physical examination every year, and observation by patient for sore that does not heal, change in wart or mole.

Breast: The risk of breast cancer occurs with persons who are caucasian, who has early menarche, late menopause, fibrocystic disease, and infertility, more than age of 30 years for first pregnancy, and who has a personal history of breast cancer mother or sister with history of breast cancer, obesity, and whose age range is 35–65 years.

The screening measure will be:
- Monthly breast self-examination.
- Breast examination by health professional every 3 years for women aged 20–40 and every year after the age of 40.
- Baseline mammogram of age 40 and every 1–2 years between ages 40–49 and every year after the age of 50.
- Observation by patient for lungs or thickening discharge from nipple, pain in the breast.

In order to assume the expected role in cancer prevention and early detection programmes, the nurse must keep informed about the trends in the incidence of cancer and advances being made. If the nurse is to have a significant impact, the challenge needs to be recognized and strategies must be developed to teach cancer control effectively.

To sum up, the early detection of cancer in asymptomatic population according to American Society Guidelines (1995) are as follows:
- *Chest X-ray:* It is no longer recommended for smokers to screen for lung cancer, but can be done.
- *Sputum cytology:* -do-
- *Physical examination:* For both male and females, after the age of 40 years, yearly including examination of skin, lymph nodes, mouth, thyroid, breast, testes, rectum and prostate.
- *Health teaching:* For both male and females, who attained the age of 20 years. It has to be done every 3 years to teach about proper diet, exercise, healthy habits, breast and testicular self-examinations, avoidance of sunlight, and smoking cessation.
- *Breast self examination:* For females who have attained menarchy or 20 years and above, every month after menses before menopause; after menopause, monthly on any specified day such as the first or last of the month.
- *Mammography:* For women who are between 35 and 40 years of age, baseline mammogram; between 40 and 49 years mammogram should be done every 1–2 years and yearly after 50 years; high risk women should check with their physicians.
- *Pap smear:* For females who are above 18 years of age, and sexually active women should have pap smears regardless of age, should be performed yearly until there are three negative examinations in a row; at this point, they can be performed yearly or as physician advises.
- *Pelvic examination:* For females who are between 20–40 and 40 and above, every 3 years, earlier if sexually active, yearly after 40 years.
- *Endometrial tissue sample:* For female at menopause, high-risk women (obese, abnormal uterine bleeding, estrogen therapy, history of infertility, diabetes, hypertension, failure to ovulate) should have this test performed at menopause.

- *Testicular self-examination:* For males, monthly, on a set date such as the first of the month following a shower.
- *Breast physical examination:* For females every 3 years for those who are between 20 and 39 years and annually for those who are above 40.
- *Digital rectal examination:* For both male and females who are above 40, annually rectal cancer and prostate in men.
- *Fecal occult blood:* For both males and females those who are above 20 years, done on advice of physician.
- *Proctoscopy, flexible sigmoidoscopy:* For both men and women who are above 50 years every 3–5-years.

Diagnosis of Cancer

A diagnostic plan for the person in whom cancer is suspected, includes health history, identification of risk factors, physical examination and specific diagnostic studies.

Health History

The health history includes particular emphasis on risk factors, such as family history of cancer, exposure to or use of known carcinogen (e.g. cigarette smoking and exposure to occupational pollutants or chemicals, disease characterised by chronic inflammation (e.g. ulceration colities) and drug ingestions (e.g. hormone therapy). Other important information related to dietary habits, ingestion of alcohol, lifestyle and patterns and degree of coping with perceived stressors.

Physical Examination

The physical examination should be thorough and particular attention should be given to the respiratory system, the gastrointestinal systems, including colon, rectum, and liver, the lymphatic system (including spleen), the breast, the skin, the reproductive system of the male (testicles, prostate) and of the female (cervix, uterus, ovary and the musculoskeletal and neurologic systems.

When a malignant tumor is in the early stages, there are often few manifestations. Clinical manifestations usually appear once the tumor has grown to a sufficiently large size to cause one or more of the following problems:
- Pressure on surrounding organs or nerves
- Distortion of surrounding tissue
- Obstruction of lumen of tubes
- Interference with the blood supply of surrounding tissues
- Interference with the organ function
- Disturbance of body metabolism
- Parasitic use of the body's nutritional supplies
- Mobilization of the body's defensive responses, resulting in inflammatory changes.

Common clinical manifestations that may arise secondary to cancer include weight loss, weakness or fatigue, CNS alterations, pain and hematologic and metabolic alterations. Close assessment of such manifestations may reveal that they are directly or indirectly related to the tumor growth.

Anorexia, weight loss, weakness and fatigue are related to the body's inability to consume and use nutrients appropriately. Mechanical interference by tumors, malabsorption, paraneoplastic endocrine secretions (such as excessive secretions of thyroid hormone) and tumor, use of nutrient, may all contribute to a cycle that must be interrupted to avoid general physical debilitation.

Pain may occur as a result of obstruction or destruction of a vital organ, pressure on sensitive tissues or bone, or involvement of nerves. If it occurs and is not adequately treated, it may become constraint and progressively severe.

The client who has difficulty with vision, speech, co-ordination or memory may be experiencing primary or metastatic CNS disease. Increased intracranial pressure caused by tumor growth may cause headache, lethargy, nausea, and vomiting.

Unexplained anemia often indicates a malignancy. Hematologic changes also include leukopenia, leukocytosis, and bleeding disorders. Which in some diseases may occur before local manifestations. Metabolic manifestations also signify the possibility of malignant disease.

A localized tumor usually produces manifestations related to increased pressure or obstruction in a single region. Metastatic disease and extensive tumors of major organs may display a variety of local and systemic manifestations.

Diagnostic Studies

Diagnostic studies to be performed will depend on the suspected primary or metastatic site (s) of the cancer. The common diagnostic studies that may be included in the process of diagnosing cancer include the following:
- Cystologic examination, e.g. pap smear
- Basic X-ray studies for identifying the destructive tumors of the GI, respiratory and renal tracts
- Complete blood count
- Proctoscopic examination
- Liver function studies
- Radiographic studies, e.g. mammogram, (in breast cancer)
- Radioisotopic scans (for liver, brain, bone, lung cancer)
- Computed tomography (CT) scan
- Magnetic resonance imaging (MRI)
- Antigen skin testing (to know the presence of oncofetal antigens)
- Bone marrow examination
- Lymphangiography
- Biopsy (surgical excision of a small piece of tissue for microscopic examination, i.e. needle biopsy, incisional biopsy, excisional biopsy).

Treatment of Cancer

When caring for the patient with cancer, the nurse should know the goals of the treatment plan to appropriately communicate with and support the patient. The goal of cancer treatment is 'cure', 'control' or palliation.

The Major objective of cancer therapy is to treat the client effectively with appropriate therapy for sufficient duration so that cure results with minimal functional and structural impairment. When cure is the goal, it is expected that after treatment the patient will be free of disease and will have a normal life. Many kinds of cancer have the potential to go into permanent remission with an initial course of treatment or with treatment extending for several weeks, months or years. (e.g. Basal cell carcinoma of skin is usually cured by surgical removal of lesion or radiation therapy.)

When cure is not possible, important alternative goals are:
- To prevent metastasis
- To relieve manifestations
- To maintain a high quality of life for as long as possible.

Here, the control is the goal of the treatment plan for many cancers considered to be chronic. The patient undergoes the initial course of therapy and is contineud on maintenance therapy for a period of time or is followed closely so that early signs and symptoms of recurrence can be detected. These cancers are usually, not cured., but they are controlled by therapy for long periods of time (e.g. chronic lymphocytic leukemia).

Palliation can also be a goal of the cancer treatment plan. With this treatment, goal, relief of symptoms and the maintenance of a satisfactory quality of life are the primary objective rather than cure or control of the disease process. For example, radiatioan therapy given to relieve the pain of bone metastasis.

The goals of cure, control and palliation are achieved through the use of four treatment modalities for cancer, which includes:
- Surgery
- Radiation therapy
- Chemotherapy
- Biologic response modifiers.

Surgery

Surgery is the oldest form of cancer treatment and for many years it was the only effective method of cancer diagnosis and treatment. It is also an integral part of the rehabilitation and palliation of patients with cancer. The types of surgical procedures used in surgical management of cancer are as follows:

- *Biopsy* is the surgical removal of a piece of tissue from the questionable area, and the tissue sample is sent to the pathology laboratory for diagnostic verification. The sample of tissues can be obtained through the needle biopsy or incisional biopsy or excisional biopsy.
- *Reconstruction/Rehabilitative surgery* Advances in reconstructive surgery offer a different perspective on rehabilitation to the patient who has experienced curative surgery. Here, performing the repair of defects from previous radical surgical resection. It can be performed early (as in head and neck surgery). Restoration of form and function is possible in varying degrees depending on the site and extent of surgery. Reconstructive surgery may be performed concurrently with the radical procedure or delayed for optimal outcome. The major goal of reconstructive surgery is to improve the patient's quality of life by restoring maximal function and appearance.
- *Palliative surgery* refers to a surgery that attempts to relieve the complications of cancer. Because of surgical procedures carry an inherent potential for morbidity, use of surgery in palliative care is carefully considered and used only if the risk-benefit ratio is favorable. Palliative surgery can benefit the clients with cancer and improve quality of life include the procedure than reduce pain; relieve airway obstruction, relieve obstructions in the GI and GU tract; relieve pressures on the brain and spinal cord; prevent hemorrhage remove infected and ulcerating tumors and drain abscess. Example of palliative surgical procedure are cordotomy, colostomy, laminectomy, etc.
- *Adjuvant surgery* refers to the use of various surgical techniques to facilitate the overall management. These procedures are used to provide supportive care throughout the disease process of cancer. These procedures include:
  - Insertion of feeding tubes in the esophagus or stomach.
  - Creation of a colostomy to allow a rectal abscess to heal.
  - Suprapubic cystotomy for the patient with advnced prostatic cancer.
  - Vascular access devices.
  - Radiotherapy implants.
  - Peritoneal access.
  - Ventricular access.
  - Drainage of peritoneal or pleural effusions.
- *Surgery for primary lesions* is the removal of the primary site of malignancy. The goal of therapy is cure. This depends on the biology of that particular cancer. For example basal cell carcinoma of skin, early tumor of the rectum or colon.
- *Surgery for metastatic lesion* or resection of metastatis is used in selected case where a cure can be obtained or reasonable prolongation of survival is possible. The primary cancer must be under control. The decision to proceed is influenced by the type of histology,

number of lesions, their locations and whether they are bilateral, solitary metastatic lesions that appear in the lungs, liver or brain can be removed to effect a surgical cure.

- *Preventive/prophylactic surgery* is the removal of lesion, that if left in the body are apt to develop into cancer. Certain conditions or diseases increase the risk of cancer occurrence so significantly that removal of the target organ is justified to prevent cancer development. For example, polyps in the rectum. Clients with high risk factors may consider prophylactic surgery (e.g. prophylactic mastectomy, or oophorectomy).
- *Curative surgery* is the removal of the primary site of malignancy and any lymph nodes to which the neoplasm has extended. Such surgery may be all that is required. For example, radical neck dissection, lumpectomy, mastectomy, pneumonectomy, orchiectomy, thyroidectomy and bowel resection.
- *Debulking surgery* is the removal of bulk of the tumor; should be performed before the start of chemotherapy whenever possible. This procedure may be used if the tumor cannot be completely removed (e.g. attached to a vital organ). This type of procedure makes the adjuvant therapy more effective.

Radiation Therapy (RT)

Radiation therapy (RT) is a local treatment modality for cancer. RT is the use of high energy ionizing rays to treat a variety of cancer. Ionizing radiation destroys the cell's ability to reproduce by damaging the cells DNA. Rapidly dividing cells, such as some cancer cells are more vulnerable to radiation than more slowly dividing cells. Furthermore, normal cells have greater ability than cancer cells to repair the DNA damage from radiation. In addition to the DNA effects, a complex chain of chemical reactions occurs in the extracellular fluid resulting in the formation of free radicals. Well oxygenated tumor show a much greater reaponse to radiation than poorly oxygenated tumors. Oxygen free radicals formed during ionization interact readily with nearby molecules causing cellular damage including genetic material.

Radiation is the emission and distribution of energy through space or a material medium. The energy produced by radiation, when absorbed into tissue, produces ionization and excitation. This local energy is sufficient to break chemical bonds in DNA, which leads to biologic effect. The major target of radiation effect is DNA. The ionization that occurs eventually causes damage to DNA, which renders cells incapable of surviving mitosis. Loss of proliferative capacity yields cellular death at the time of division. Cellular death is dependent on the cell going through its mitotic cycle. Thus death occurs at different rates for different cell types. This is true for both normal cells and cancer cells. However, cancer cells are more likely to be dividing because of the loss of control of cellular divisions. Furthermore, these cells are unable to repair the radiation damage to DNA. Therefore, cancer cells are more likely to be permanently damaged by the cumulative doses of radiation. Normal tissues are usually able to recover from radiation damage of therapeutic doses are kept within certain ranges.

Goals of radiation therapy: The goals of radiation therapy are cure, control and palliation. To accomplish these treatment goals, radiation therapy can be used alone or as an adjuvant treatment modality in combination with surgery chemotherapy and biologic response modifiers.

- Cure is the goal when radiation therapy is used alone as a curative modality for treating patients with basal cell carcinoma of the skin, tumors confined to the vocal cord, and Stage I or II A Hodgkin's disease. Radiation therapy can be combined with surgery and chemotherapy to cure certain cancers such as Stage II B, III A and III B, Hodgkin's disease, Ewing's sarcoma, head and neck cancer and Stage I and II breast cancer.
- Control of the disease process of cancer for a period of time is considered to be a reasonable goal in some situations. Initial treatment is offered at the time of diagnosis, and additional treatment is given each time symptoms of disease recur. Most of the patients enjoy a satisfactory quality of life during symptom-free period. It can be combined with surgery to further enhance the local control of cancer. It can be given preoperatively, intraoperatively and also postoperatively as assessed accordingly.
- Palliation is often the goal of RT. The patient can be treated to control the distressing symptoms that are occurring as a result of disease process. Tumors can be reduced in size to relieve symptoms more as pain and obstruction. Example of the use of RT for palliatives include the relief of:
  - Pain associated with bone metastasis
  - Pain and neurologic symptoms associated with brain metastasis
  - Spinal cord compression
  - Intestinal obstruction
  - Superior vena cava obstruction
  - Bronchial or tracheal obstruction
  - Bleeding (e.g. bladder and intrabronchial).

Types of radiation therapy: Radiation therapy can be administered from a variety of sources. Sources can be classified into those used outside (i.e. external RT) and those used close to the surface of the body or inside the body (Internal RT).

External radiation: Radiation treatment can be given by external beam radiation delivered from a source placed at some distance from the target site. It is usually administered by high energy X-ray machine (e.g. the betatron and linear accelerator) or machine containing a radioisotope (cobalt 60).

The main advantage of high-energy radiations is its skin-sparing effect. This means that the maximum effect of radiation occurs within the tumor deep in the body and not on the skin surface. Neutron beam therapy is delivered from a cyclotron particle accelerator is currently used to treat many types of cancer (tumor in salivary gland, prostate, lung).

Internal radiation: Internal RT involves the placement of specially prepared radioisotopes directly enter near the tumor itself. This is known as brachy therapy in which the implantation or insertion or radioactive materials directly into the tumor or in close proximity of the tumor. An implant may be temporary with the source placed into a catheter or tube inserted into the tumor area and left in place for several days. This method is commonly used for tumors of the head and neck, and gynecologic malignancies.

There are two types of internal RT:
1. Sealed-source in which the radioactive material is enclosed in a sealed container. Sealed source RT includes intracavity and interstitial therapy. In intracavity therapy, the radio-iostopes, usually cesium 137 or radium 226, is placed into an applicator, then placed in body cavity for a carefully calculated time usually 24 to 72 hours (e.g. used to treat cancer of uterus or cervix).

   In interstitial therapy, the radioisotope of choice (iridium 192, iodine 125, cesium 137, gold 198 or radon 222) is placed in needles, beads, seeds, ribbons or catheters and then implanted directly into the tumors (e.g. as used in prostate cancer).
2. Unsealed-sources RT are used in systemic therapy. Radioisotopes may be administered intravenously into a body cavity or orally. For example, sodium phosphate P32 is administered intravenously to treat polycythemia vera.

   Iodine 131 is given orally in very low doses to treat Graves' disease.

Measurement of radiation: There are different units which are used to measure radiation as follows:
- Curie (ci)—A measure of the number of atoms of a particular radioisotope that disintegrate in one second.
- Rontgen (R)—A measure of the radiation required to produce a standard number of ions in air; a unit of exposure to radiation.
- Rad—Measurement of radiation dosage absorbed by the tissue.
- Rem—Measurement of the biologic effectiveness of various forms of radiation on the human cell (1 rem = 1 rad).
- Gray (Gy)—100 rads - 1 Gy.

The grays and centigrays are the units currently used in clinical practice.

Safety precautions in radiation therapy: There are three key principles to follow to protect nurses and others from excessive radiation exposure, viz. distance, time and shielding.
- *Distance:* The greater distance from the radiation source, the less exposure dose of ionizing rays. The intensity of radiation decreases inversely to the square of the distance from the source. For example, if a person stands 4 ft from a source of radiation, the person is exposed to approximately 1/4 the amount of radiation the person would receive at 2 ft.
- *Time:* Minimal exposure time should be promoted, although patient care needs must still be met. A nurses exposure is generally limited to 30 minutes of direct care per 8 hours shift.
- *Shielding:* The dose of X-rays and gamma rays is reduced as the thickness of the lead shield is increased. In practice, nurses have found that leadshielding can be cumbersome to work with. So it is better to maintain maximum distance from the radioactive source and limiting duration of exposure as safety measure.

The following guidelines will help protecting staff and others from radiation:
- Place the client in a private room—It prevents undue exposure to other clients and to nurses caring for these clients.
- Plan care well so that minimal time is spent in direct contact with the client. Do not spend more than 30 minutes per shift with the client.
- Stand at the client's shoulder (for cervical implants) or at the foot of the bed (for head and neck implants) avoiding close contact with unshielded areas.
- In case, if you must have prolonged contact with the client or if you will be exposed to an unshielded area, use a lead shield.
- Do not care for more than one client with a radiation implant at one time.
- All health care personnel should wear appropriate monitoring devices.
- The room should be marked with appropriate signs stating the presence of radiation, do not allow children under 18 or pregnant women to visit; limit visitors' time to 30 minutes at a distance of at least 6 feet from the radioactive source; do not care for these patients if you (female nurse) are pregnant.
- Carefully check all linens or other materials from the bed for the presence of implants.
- Keep long handled forceps and lead-lined container available on the nursing unit or in the client's room while the implant is in place.

Nursing Management of Client Receiving Radiation Therapy

Nurse plays two roles in the management of patients who have received radiation therapy, such as providing education and minimizing the side-effects.

1. *Providing education:* In addition to emotional impact of cancer diagnosis, the clients may experience fears of being burnt or becoming radioactive. The nurse, through education, can dispel such common fears and misconceptions. Because XRT can neither be seen nor felt during the treatment, hence, the client may become apprehensive that the treatment is not effective. If cancer is not causing any physical manifestations, then the client again would not have any evidence of the effect of treatment. The nurse must tell them the parameters of the efficacy of treatment.
2. *Minimise side-effects*: In general, skin reactions varying from mild erythema to moist desquamation, and fatigue are common side-effects of XRT to any site, therefore, nurse must educate the patients about skin care within the teratment field as follows:
    - Keep your skin dry.
    - Do not clean/wash the treatment area unless permitted. If permitted, gently wash the skin with soap and pat dry. Do not use hot water.
    - Do not remove the lines or ink marks placed on your skin.
    - Avoid the use of powder, lotion, cream, alcohol and deodorant on the treated skin.
    - Wear loose-fitting clothes to avoid friction over the area.
    - Do not put tape to the treatment area if dressings are applied.
    - Shave with an electric razor. Do not use pre-shave or after-shave lotion.
    - Protect your skin from direct exposure to sunlight.
    - Consult your radiation therapist or nurse about specific complaint related to skin reactions.

Chemotherapy

Chemotherapy is the systemic treatment of cancer with chemicals, i.e. drugs. Here the use of antineoplastic drugs to promote tumor cell destructions by interfering with cellular function and reproduction. It includes the use of various therapeutic agents and hormones.

The goal of chemotherapy is to destroy as many tumor cells as possible with minimal effect on healthy cells. It can be used for cure, control, and palliation. The objective of chemotherapy is to reduce the number of cancer cells present in the primary tumor site(s) and metastatic tumor site(s). Several factors will determine the response of cancer cells to chemotherapy as given below:
- *Mitotrio rate of the tissue* from which the tumor arises. The more rapid the mitotic rate, the greater response to chemotherapy. Chemotherapy is the treatment of choice for acute leukemia, choriocarcinoma of the placenta, Wilms' tumor (used in conjunction with surgery) and neuroblastoma. These cancer cells have a rapid rate of cellular proliferation.
- *Size of the tumor:* The smaller the number of cancer cells, the greater the response to chemotherapy.
- *Age of the tumor:* The younger tumor, the greater the response to chemotherapy. Younger tumors have a greater percentage of proliferating cells.
- *Location of the tumor:* Certain anatomic sites provide a protected environments from the effects of chemotherapy. For example, only few drugs cross the blood brain barrier (nitrosoureus and bleomycin).
- *Presence of resistant tumor cells:* Mutation of cancer cells within the tumor mass can result in varient cells that are resistant to chemotherapy. Resistance can also occur because of the biochemical inability of some cancer cells to convert the drug to its active form.
- *Physiologic and psychologic status of the host:* A state of optimum health and positive attitude will allow better withstand aggressive chemotherapy.

Classification of Chemotherapy

Chemotherapeutic agents generally are classified according to their pharmacologic action and effect on the cell generation cycles. However, the method by which cancer cells are inhibited or destroyed is not always unknown.

The two major categories of chemotherapeutic drugs are cell cycle-nonspecific and cell cycle-specifer. The cell cycle non-specifiers have their effect on the cells that are in the process of cellular replication and proliferation, as well as on the cells that are in the resting phase. The cell cycle-specific have their effect on cells that are in the process of cellular replication or proliferation. These drugs are effective at only one specific phase of cell cycle.

The common drugs used as chemotherapeutic agents are as follows **(Table 18.7)**:
- Alklating agent:
    - Nitrogen mustard (Mechlorethamine)
    - Cyclophosphamide (Cytoxan)
    - Chlorambucil (Leukeran)
    - Busulfan (Myleran)
    - Melphalan (Alkeran)
    - Thiotepa (Thiotepa)
    - Ifosfamide (Ifex).
- Antimetabolites:
    - Methotrexate
    - 6 Mercaptopurine (6 MP)
    - 6 Thioguanine (6 TG)
    - 5 Fluorouracil (5 Fu)
    - Cystosine arabinoside ((A-RA-C) Cytosar-4)
    - Fludarabine phosphate
    - Deoxycoformycin (Pentastatin).
- Antitumor antibiotics:
    - Deunorubicin (Cerubidins)
    - Doxorubicin (Adriamycin)
    - Dactinomycin (Cosmegen)

Table 18.7: Antineoplastic drugs: Classification, mode of action, side-effects and management.

Drugs	Action	Side-effects	Nursing interventions
I. Alkylating agents			
• **Nitrogen mustard,** e.g., mechlorethamine, chlorambucil, cyclophosphamide, busulfan, melphalan, ifosfamide	Prevent DNA replication and transcription of RNA	• **Blood toxicity**, e.g., anemia, leukopenia, thrombocytopenia, pancytopenia	• Monitor blood counts biweekly • Look for signs of infection, bleeding and anemia • Provide rest periods intermittently and a good night sleep • Promote good personal hygiene
• **Aziridines,** e.g., thiotepa		• **Gastrointestinal toxicity**, e.g., nausea, vomiting, diarrhoea, tenesmus	• Administer antiemetics, H_2-blockers • Proper hydration. Give IV fluids and maintain intake the output chart • Provide small frequent meals • Record the amount and frequency of vomiting
		• **Reproductive toxicity**, e.g., change in libido, infertility	• Inform the client about the infertility as a temporary or permanent side-effect • Warn danger to the growing foetus, hence avoid pregnancy • Counseling, if needed
		• **Genitourinary toxicity**, e.g., hemorrhagic cystitis, renal impairment	• Encourage hydration. Encourage frequent emptying of bladder • Inform that hemorrhagic cystitis is temporary side-effect • Administer urothelial protective agents
II. Antimetabolites			

• **Folate antagonist,** e.g., methotrexate
• **Purine analogue,** e.g., 6–thioguanine, azathioprine, fludarabine, pentostatin
• **Pyrimidine analogues,** e.g., cytosine arabinoside, 5-flurouracil
	Interfere with DNA synthesis by interfering with synthesis of nucleic acid and block the enzyme necessary for synthesis of essential factors necessary for incorporation to DNA	• **Haemopoietic toxicity,** e.g., anaemia, leucopenia, pancytopenia or bone marrow suppression
		• **GI tract toxicity,** e.g., mucositis, stomatitis, diarrhoea, nausea and vomiting
			The nursing interventions of these toxicities have been discussed above
			
			• **For mucositis/stomatitis**
			  – Inspect the oral cavity for soreness, change in taste
			  – Teach good oral care, i.e., instruct mouthwash after each meal, use soft toothbrush and use soft oral anaesthetic gel
			  – Report if oral infection occurs
			  – Advise soft non-irritating nonspicy food, rich in proteins, calories and fiber
			• **For diarrhoea**
			  – Maintain hydration. Record urine output
			  – Monitor and document the frequency and amout of stools
			  – Administer anti-diarrhoeal agents
			  – Low residue, high protein diet
			  – Promote meticulous skin care of perianal area, and good personal hygiene

III. Antitumour antibiotics			
• **Anthracyclines,** e.g., doxorubicin, daunorubicin, idrarubicin	Interfere with synthesis of nucleic acids and inhibit RNA and DNA synthesis	• **Haemopoietic toxicity,** e.g., anaemia bone marrow suppression	• Read alkylating agent toxicity and nursing interventions
• **Others,** e.g., dactinomycin, bleomycin, mitomycin, picomycin		• **GI tract,** e.g., mucositis/stomatitis, nausea, vomiting	• Read nursing management of antimetabolites above
		• **Skin toxicity,** e.g., alopecia and tissue necrosis due to extravasation	• Warn about the potential loss of hair and ways of minimising it or wear alternative wig • Extravasation of drug has been discussed in route of administration of chemotherapy
		• **Cardiac and pulmonary toxicity**	• Assess cardiac and pulmonary status • Do not exceed the prescribed dose

Contd...

Contd...

Drugs	Action	Side-effects	Nursing interventions
Hormonal agents			

• **Corticosteroids,** e.g., prednisolone, diexamethasone, methylprednisolone
• **Androgens,** e.g., flutamide bicalutamide
• **Antiestrogens,** e.g., tamoxifen, torimefine
	Androgens and antiestrogens	Toxicities include fluid retention and masculinization	• **For fluid retention**
			  – Warn against potential weight gain
			  – Weigh the client biweekly
			  – Maintain intake and output
			  – Diuretics, if advised
			• **Virilisation in female**
			  – Masculine voice, facial hair, clitoris enlargement is expected. Reassure the client and inform these side-effects
			  – Give psychological support

• **Aromatase omjobotprs,** e.g., letrozole, anastrozole
• **Gonadotropin-releasing hormones,** e.g., leuprolide, anastrozole
	Antiandrogens and estrogens	Fluid retention, feminization and uterine bleeding	• **Fluid retention** - Read above
			• **Feminization**
			  – Inform about the chances of gynaecomastia, change in voice, distribution of hair and fat
			  – Psychological support
			• **Uterine bleeding**
			  – Provide support and reassurance

	Steroids		Nursing intervention. Read corticosteroids in endocrinology
Biologic agents			
• **Hematopoietic growth factors,** e.g., G-CSF and GM-CSF	These stimulate bone marrow recovery after chemotherapy. These have anti-proliferative activity in addition to anti-viral and immunomodulatory activity. Augment T-cells activities and enhance functions of natural killer cells	• Mild to moderate flu-like symptoms • Rash • Transient increase in liver enzymes • Thrombocytopenia	• Bone pain is cumbersome side-effect. Use analgesics to relieve pain • Toxicity is transient • Reassurance and support
• **Interferons alpha and beta**	These have anti-proliferative activity in addition to anti-viral and immunomodulatory activity	• A flu-like syndrome • Tachyphylaxis (response decreases after administration of few doses)	• Use analgesic and antipyretic for myalgia and fever • Use the lowest dose prescribed
• **Interleukins (IL-2)**	Augment T-cells activities and enhances function of natural killer cells	• **Increased capillary** permeability producing hypotension, edema, ascites, weight gain • **Skin toxicities,** e.g. rash, pruritis	• Fluid management • Antiallergic medications • Salt restriction • Weigh the client frequently • Look for edema

• **Monoclonal antibodies**
  – Enzymes, e.g., L-Asparaginase
  – Taxanes, e.g., paclitaxel, docetaxel
  – Methylhydrazine derivative, e.g. procarbazine, temozolomide
  – Others, e.g. hydroxyurea, interferon, amasacrine, monoclonal antibodies

Principles of use of chemotherapy
• Combination of chemotherapy is preferred to single drug chemotherapy
• Complete remission is the minimum requisite for cure and increased survival
• The first phase chemotherapy should be aggressive as it offers maximum chance for significant benefit
• Maximum doses of the drugs should be used to attain maximum benefit. Dose reduction just to minimize the toxicity is akin to 'killing patients with kindness'
• Chemoprevention shows promise in prevention of head and neck cancer.

- Bleomycin (Blenoxane)
- Mitomycin (Mutamycin)
- Picamycin (Mittracin, mitramycin)
- Idarubiun (Idamycin)
- Mitoxantrone (Novamtrone).
• Hormonal agents:
  - Androgens
    • Testosterone propionate
    • Fluoxymesterone (Halotestin)
    • Dromostanolone (Drolban)
    • Testosactone (Teslac)
    • Methyltestosterone.
  - Corticosteroids
    • Cortisone acetate
    • Prednisone (Meticorten)
    • Dexamethosone (Dedadron)
    • Methyl prednisolone sodium (Solu-Medrol)
    • Hydrocartison sodium succinate (Solu-cortef).
  - Estrogen
    • Diethylstilbestrol (DES)
    • Ethinyl estradiol (Estriny).
  - Progesterones
    • Hydroxy progesterone caporate (Prodrox)
    • Megestrol (Megace)
    • Metroxyprogesterone (Provera)
    • Estramustine (Emcut).
  - Estrogen antagonists
    • Tamoxifen (Norvadex)
    • Leuprolide (Lupron).
  - Antiadrenal
    • Amino gluthimide.
• Vinca alkaloids
  - Vincristine (Oncovin)
  - Vinblastine (Velban)
  - Vindesine sulfate.
• Epipodophyllotoxins
  Etoposide (VP-16).

Nursing Intervention in Chemotherapy

Alkalating agents are cell cycle non-specific and act against already formed nucleic acid by cross-linking DNA strands, thereby preventing DNA replication and transcription of RNA. The major toxin of alkalatings are dependent upon drugs given which include hematopoietic anemia, leukopenia, thrombocytopenia, GI-nausea and vomiting, diarrhea, reproductive infertility, change in libido, Gucystitis and renal toxicity.

The nursing intervention for these toxicities are:
• Hematopoietic toxicity:
  - Monitor WBC, RBC, platest count biweekly for pancytopenia
  - Observe for signs and symptoms of infections, bleeding, anemia
  - Provide rest periods and 8 hours sleep per night
  - Teach benefits of good personal hygiene
  - Provide comfort and suggestion measures.
• Gastrointestinal toxicity:
  - Document nausea and vomiting times and amount
  - Administer antiemetic drug PRN
  - Hydrate to 2000 ml/24 hour if not contradicted
  - Record intake and output
  - Avoid noxious odors
  - Use relaxation techniques or distractions
  - Provide small frequent meals.
• Reproductive toxicity:
  - Inform of possibility of temporary or permanent infertility and danger to growing fetus.
  - Provide reproductive counseling as needed.
• Genitourinary toxicity:
  - Inform that hemorrhagic cystitis can occur with cytoxan and ifosfamide therapy.
  - Administer mesna (urothelial protection agent) to help to prevent cystitis.
  - Encourage hydration and complete and frequent emptying of bladder.

Antimetabolites act by interfering with synthesis of chromosomal nucleic acid, antimetabolites are analogs of normal metabolites and block the enzyme necessary for synthesis of essential factors or are incorporated into the DNA or RNA and thus prevent replication are cycle-specific.

The major toxicities of antimetabolites are dependant on drugs given which are as follows:
• Hematopoietic
  - Bone marrow suppression
  - Anemia
  - Leukopenia
  - Thrombocytopenia
• Gastrointestinal
  - Mucositis/stomatitis
  - Diarrhea
  - Nausea and vomiting.

The nursing intervention of these toxicities are as stated in alkalating agents and in addition to the above, the following has to be performed.

For Mucositis and Stomatitis

• Inspect oral cavity daily for presence of sores, change in taste and sensation.
• Teach oral care and encourage immediately after meals and at bed time, soft toothbrush and prescribed mouthwash (Peroxide, oral saline, baking soda and water or provide anesthetic agent for mouth sores (e.g. Stomatitic cocktail).
• Report signs and symptoms of oral infection.
• Soft diet with non-irritating foods high in protein, calories, offer high caloric liquid supplements.

For Diarrhea

- Low residue diet, high protein and calories maintain hydration
- Monitor and document number and frequency stools
- Administer antidiarrheal medication as needed
- Provide meticulus skin care in perirectal area
- Promote good hygiene habits.

Antitumor antibiotics interfere with synthesis and function of nucleic acids and inhibit RNA and DNA synthesis. These are cycle specific. The major toxicities of antitumor antibiotics include:

- Hematopoietic: Bone marrow suppression
- GI: Mucositis/Stomatitis, anorexia, nausea and vomiting
- Integumentary—Alopecia, tissue necrosis (if extravasate)
- Cardiac and pulmonary toxicity.

In addition to above stated nursing interventions, for other chemotherapeutics, the added nursing interventions for:

- *Integumentary*: For alopecia, warn of potential for hair loss and ways of minimizing loss.
  For Extravasation
  - Monitor IV infusion to prevent infiltration. When infiltrated stop immediately and institute agency protocol to prevent tissue necrosis notify doctor immediately and keep extravasation kit available at all times.
- Cardiac toxicity may occur with bleomycin (Pneumonitis and progressive pulmonary fibrosis), should not exceed a lifetime dose of 400 iu. Assess respiratory status and document changes.

Hormonal Agents

- Androgens alter pituitary function and directly affects the malignant cell. Toxicities of androgens include fluid retention and masculinization.
- Corticosteroids use in lymphoid malignancies and have indirect effects on malignant cells. The major toxicities include fluid retention, hypertension, diabetes, and increased susceptibility to infection.
- Oestrogen and progesterone suppress testosterone production in males and alter the response of breast cancer to prolectin and promote differentiation of malignant cells. The major toxicities include fluid retention, feminization and uterine bleeding.
- Estrogen anagonists compete with estrogens for binding with oestrogen receptor sites on malignant cells. Toxicities are minimal with occasional headache and hotflash.
- Antiadrenals. Produce the equivalent of a medical adrenalectomy, thereby inhibiting the formations of estrogen and androgenesis and function of nucleic acids and inhibit RNA and DNA synthesis. These agents are cycle non-specific toxicity in adrenal insufficiency.

The nursing interventions during chemotherapy with harmful agent are:

- For fluid retention:
  - Warn of potential weight gain
  - Weight biweekly
  - Maintain intake and output if needed.
- For feminization in males: Inform about chance of gynecomastia—change in voice, distribution of body fat and hair and cardiovascular problem.
- Assess fears and concerns and provide psychological support as needed.
- For *virilization* in females:
  - Discuss the risk for facial hair, lowered voice, clitorial enlargement - fluid retention.
  - Assess fears and concerns and provide psychological support.
- For uterine bleeding:
  - Prepare postmenopausal woman for occurrence
  - Provide support and reassurance.
- For diabetes:
  - Inform patient of potential occurrence
  - Monitor blood sugar changes.
  - Observe signs and symptoms of diabetes.
- For adrenal insufficiency:
  - Instruct on need to comply with replacement therapy while on medication.
  - Reassure that need for therapy will cease when drug is discontinued.

Vinca alkaloid bind to proteins within the cells causing metaphase arrest thus inhibiting RNA and protein synthesis. Major toxicities are bone marrow suppression and alopecia (See nursing intervention as stated above).

Epiplodophyllotoxins cause breaks in DNA and RNA protein cross links. The major toxicities are neurological, i.e. neurotoxicity, muscle weakness, peripheral neurities, paralytic ileus, loss of deep tenden reflexes.

The nursing intervention for neurological toxicities will include:

- GI
  - Check for peristalsis frequently.
  - Determine usual pattern of bowel elimination
  - Facilitate elimination with laxativeregimens.
- Peripheral
  - Observe for numbness, tingling inextremities
  - Institute safety measure (e.g. wearing shoes, using cane or walker for ambulation)
  - Seek assistance for ambulation as needed
  - Teach signs and symptoms to report to concerned doctor
  - Provide supportive care and reassurance.

Guidelines for Care of Client with Chemotherapy

- Teach the patient and significant others:
  - Signs and symptoms of infection, thrombocytopenia.
  - How to read thermometer and when to notify the doctor.

- Good hygienic practices—cleansing the perinium from front to back, change underwear daily and handwashing.
- Information about prescribed drugs—name, dose, side effects, importance of taking as prescribed.
- Use of antiemetics.
- Importance of medical follow-up and blood studies.
- Available support group for chemotherapy patients.
• Prevent infection
  - Good hygiene especially handwashing—patient, family, health personnel.
  - Prevent exposure to people with known infection (other staff, family, etc.).
  - Meticulous Aseptic technique during IV infusion and dressing changes.
  - Avoid use of aspirin or acetaminophen to prevent masking fever.
  - Maintain intact skin and mucous membrane:
    ◆ Avoid bumping and breaking the skin
    ◆ No injections
    ◆ Keep finger nails short, to prevent small skin breaks (nurses, patients other care givers).
    ◆ Avoid anal intercourse
    ◆ Avoid enemas, rectal medications, rectal thermometers
    ◆ Avoid excessive friction and provide vaginal lubrication during sexual intercourse (use water soluble jelly...).
  - Maintain meticulous oral hygiene:
    ◆ Maintain teeth and gums in good condition.
    ◆ Use mouthwash or oral irrigations with normal saline... baking soda or sodium bicarbonate solution.
    ◆ Use mycostatin tablets or suspension as necessary.
    ◆ Relieve dryness, drink water and other fluids.
    ◆ Use artificial saliva as needed in form of spray.
    ◆ Stimulate saliva with gum, candies, buttermilk, yoghurt.
    ◆ Brush teeth with soft toothbrush (small soft bristle) or use foam stick or swab.
    ◆ Brush teeth in short horizontal strokes at least for 3 to 4 minutes, at least 3 times a day.
    ◆ Use fluoridated toothpaste or rinse to prevent caries.
    ◆ Use water pik under low pressure or irrigation, if platelet count is low.
  - Maintain optimal respiratory functions, encourage, turn, cough and deep breathe (if confined to bed).
• Maintain optimal gastrointestinal function:
  - Give antidiarrheal medication as needed.
  - Plan daily bowel regimen for constipation, give stool softener as prescribed.
  - Treat stomatitis coral nystatin, or other prescribes.
  - Oral irrigations every 2 hours.
  - Soft, bland foods, cold liquids, tolerated by some persons.
  - Treat nausea and vomiting.
    ◆ Give antiemetics 30 to 45 minutes before chemotherapy, use large doses.
    ◆ Use auditory or diversional stimulation (music slides, phonograph).
    ◆ Give antiemetics around the clock for severe nausea and vomiting.
    ◆ Use texation techniques were hypnosis, therapeutic touch.
    ◆ Eat foods which can minimise nausea and vomiting.
• Minimising or preventing alopecia:
  - Encourage use of wigs, scarves, eyebrow pencils, false eyelashes.
  - Avoid frequent shampooing, combing, or brushing.
  - Use soft-bristle hair brush.
  - Advise against permanent and hair coloring. (increase rate of hair loss).
• Minimising or preventing urinary effects:
  - Hemorrhage, cystitis, renal toxicity.
  - Force fluids when take cyclophosphamide.
  - Take cyclophosphamide early in the day.
  - Check serum creatinine or 24 hour urine for creatinine clearance before giving cisplatin and streptolorecin.
• Minimising reproductive effects:
  - Provide birth control information and reproductive counseling.
  - Provide informatioan about sperm banking before initiation of therapy for male patients.

Administration of Chemotherapy

Chemotherapy can be administered by several routes.
- Oral : Ex. cyclophosphomide
- Intramuscular : Ex. bleomycin
- Intravenous : Ex. doxorubicin, vincristine
- Intracavitary : Ex. radioisotopes, alkalating (pleural, peritoneal) agents
- Intrathecal : Ex. methotrexate, cytosine, arbinoside
- Intraarterial : Ex. DTIC, 5-Fu, methotrexate, fluxuridine
- Perfusion agents : Ex. alkalysing, alkalating
- Continuous infusion : Ex. 5-Fu, methostreate, cytosine, arbinoside
- Subcutaneous : Ex. cytosine arabinoside
- Topical : Ex. 5-Fu cream
- Intraperitoneal : Ex. methotrexate, 5-Fu

Mostly used common routes are IV and oral. One of the major concerns with the IV administration of antineoplastic drugs is possible irritation of vessel wall by the drugs, or even worse, extravasation (infiltration of drugs into tissues surrounding the infusion site), causing local tissue damage. Many chemotherapeutic drugs are vesicants agents that when accidentally infiltrated into the skin cause severe local tissue breakdown and necrosis. Some guidelines to promote safe use of chemotherapeutic drugs by IV administration follows:

- Know specifics about the safe administration of chemotherapy.
- Start an IV infusion and normal saline solution or 5% dextrose in water or saline solution with a small lumens short needle or catheter. Ensure that recent venipunctures have not been performed to the proximal to the IV. Avoid using on arm that has poor lymphatic drainage or that has previously received radiation therapy.
- Select a vein that is larger enough to promote infusion without irritating the intima of the vein. When a vesicant is administered, avoid the veins in the hand, wrist, and antecubital area.
- Instruct the patient to immediately report any changes in sensation especially burning or stinging pain.
- Check for blood return before infusing the chemotherapeutic drug. However, a blood return does not always indicate an intact vein.
- If more than one drug is to be used, give the vesicant agents. First, when the vein is at its optimum integrity. (note this method is controversial, so confirm with the concerned).
- Slowly push those drugs that are to be given by the push or bolus method. Give in small increments (0.5 to 1.0 ml). Pause 30 to 60 seconds after each increment and allow the IV infusion to flush the vein, check blood returns, and again gently push 0.5 to 1.0 ml of the medication. Repeat until the medication has been given and allow the IV infusion to flush the vein for several minutes.
- Avoid continuous peripheral IV infusion of vesicant agents. If given peripherally, the administration of vesicant agents must be motivated directly at all times.
- Stop the IV infusion immediately if the patient complains of a burning or stinging pain or if an infiltration is suspected. If the drug is an irritant, check for blood return and if present continue to administer the drugs. If it is vesicant, stop the infusion and begin appropriate extravasation procedure.
- If extravasation occurs:
    - Stop the IV infusion immediately; notify the doctor or use the standing written orders for the treatment related to the specific vesicant agent.
    - Remove the IV infusion tubing and aspirate any remaining drug with a new syringe.
    - Inject the prescribed antidote (if one is available) in the infusion needle or in a 'pincushion' fashion in the skin surrounding the needle site.
    - Apply a topical corticosteroid cream, if prescribed.
    - Elevate the site.
    - Apply cold compresses for the first 24 to 48 hours unless a vinca alkaloid has been infiltrated; heat is applied following extravasation of vinca alkaloids.
    - Document the extravasation.
    - Observe site at designated intervals
    - A plastic surgeon may be consulted, depending on the extent of anticipated damage.

Principles of Chemotherapy Administration

- Combination chemotherapy is far superior to single agent chemotherapy.
- Complete remission is the minimum requisite for cure and even increased survival.
- The first round chemotherapy offers the best chance for significant benefit, therefore, the initial therapy should be the type with maximum effectiveness.
- Maximum doses of drugs are used to attain maximum tumor cell kill; Dose reduction to minimised toxicity has been called "killing patients with kindness".
- Neoadjuvant or induction chemotherapy is always recommended for some specific cancer (e.g. breast cancer).
- Chemoprevention shows promise in prevention of some second primary cancers (head and neck).

Side effects of radiation therapy and chemotherapy: The common side effects of radiation therapy and chemotherapy classified according to systemwise are as follows:

Gastrointestinal System

- *Dryness of the mucous membranes of the mouth*: When salivary glands are located in the radiation treatment field, they are frequently damaged. This may be a permanent side effect of the radiation therapy and it can be quite disturbing because it is difficult to eat, swallow, and talk when the mucous membranes are dry. Artificial saliva is available.
- *Stomatitis and mucositis*: This problem occurs when epithelial cells of the oral mucosa and intraoral soft tissue structures are destroyed by chemotherapy or radiation therapy. These cells are extremely sensitive because of their normal high cell turnover rate. Mucositis can precipitate complications of infection and hemorrhage.
- *Esophagitis*: Inflammation and ulceration of mucous membranes or esophagus as a result of rapid cell destructions occur as a side effect of chemotherapy and radioactive therapy to the area of the neck, chest and back.

- *Nausea and vomiting*: The vomiting center in the brain is stimulated by products of cellular breakdown that occurs in response to chemotherapy and radiation therapy. The drugs used in chemotherapy also stimulate the vomiting center. Destruction of the epithelial lining of the GI tracts occurs in response to both these therapies to chest, abdomen and back. A strong psychologic impacts is associated with nausea and vomiting and the high stress level associated with concern cancer and cancer treatment.
- *Anorexia*: It is site specific side effect of radiation therapy dry mouth, mucositis, esophagitis, nausea, vomiting, and diarrhea occur. Side effects of chemotherapy include nausea, vomiting, stomatitis, esophagitis, and diarrhea. Fatigue, pain and infection are present. Alteration in the sensation of taste occurs when tumors release waste products into the blood stream. Psychological and social impact of cancer and cancer therapy result in an increased level of stress and changes in the usual lifestyle pattern.
- *Altered taste sensations*: Due to destruction of the taste buds in the treatment field occurs in radiation therapy. The amount of taste alterations or loss depends on the radiation dosage and the extent field. Complete loss of taste often occurs. Taste changes may be a permanent outcome of therapy. Waste products occur in response to cellular destructions from radiation therapy and chemotherapy. These waste products are thought to be responsible for alteration in task sensations.

  Reduction in the amount of saliva occurs because of the locatioan of the salivary glands in the treatment field. Food must be in solution to be tasted.
- *Diarrhea*: Due to denuding of the epithelial lining of the small intestine occurs as a side effect of both the therapies to the abdomen or the lower back.
- *Constipation*: Due to dysfunction of the antonomic nervous system from neurotoxic effects of plant alkaloids (vincristine, vinblastine) occurs.
- *Hepatotoxicity*: Toxic effects of certain chemotherapy drugs such as methotrexate, mitomycin, 6-MP and cytosine arabinoside are product.

Hematopoietic System

- *Anemia*: These therapies result in depressant effect on bone marrow function. Malignant infiltration of bone marrow by cancer occurs. Ulceration, necrosis and bleeding of neoplastic growth occurs.
- *Leukopenia*: As stated earlier, these therapies result in depressant effect on bone marrow. The effect is especially significant because of the short span of white blood cells. Infection is the most frequent cause of morbidity and death in the patient with cancer. Usual sites of infection are the respiratory and genitourinary system.
- *Thrombocytopenia*: Depressant effect on bone marrow functions may lead to malignant infiltrations of the bone marrow. Abnormal destruction of circulating platelets is present. When platelet count decreases spontaneous bleeding can occur.

Integumentary System

- *Alopecia*: Alopecia occurs as a side effect of some chemotherapy agents and radiation therapy to the skull. Hair loss that occurs in response to radiation therapy is usually permanent. The hair begins to fall out during the first week of therapy, and this may progress to complete hair loss.
- *Skin reaction*: Extravasation of vesicant chemotherapeutic drugs (e.g. doxorubicin) gives intravenously causes severe necrosis of tissues exposed to the drug.

Genitourinary Tract

- *Cystitis*: This problem occurs when the epithelial cells of the lining of the bladder are destroyed as a side effect of chemotherapy (e.g. cyclophosphomide) and as a side effect of radiation therapy when the bladder located in the treatment field. Clinical manifestation of urgency, frequency, and hematuria are present.
- *Reproductive dysfunction*: This problem occurs as a result of the effect of chemotherapy on the cells of the testes or ova or as a result of the effect of radiation therapy when the cells of the testes or ova are located in the treatment field. Symptoms of cancer and cancer therapy include fatigue, diarrhea nausea, vomiting, anxiety, fear and pain.
- *Nephrotoxicity*: Necrosis of proximal renal tubules present as a result of an accumulation of drugs (e.g. cisplatin) in the kidney.

Nervous System

- *Increased intracranial pressure*: This problem may result from radiation edema in the CNS. This phenomenon is not well understood but is easily controlled with steroids and pain medication.
- *Peripheral neuropathy*: Paresthesia, areflexia, skeletal muscle weakness and smooth muscle dysfunction (e.g. paralytic ileus, constipation) can occur as a side effect of plant alkaloids (e.g. vimblastine, vincristine) and cisplatin.

Respiratory System

- *Pneumonitis* When the lungs are located in the treatment field, radiation pneumonitis may develop 2-3 months after start of treatment. It is characterized by a dry, hacking cough, fever and exertional dyspnea.

  After 6-12 months, fibrosis will occur and will be persistently evident on X-ray. The patient with fibrosis is more susceptible to respiratory infection. This problem can also occur as a result of chemotherapy (e.g. bloomycin, busulfin).

Cardiovascular System

Pericarditis and myocarditis: This problem is an infrequent complication when the chest wall is radiated. It may occur up to one year after treatment.

Procedure Guidelines—Administering IV Chemotherapy

- Examine the site for erythema or selling. Over a period of days to weeks, the site can become mottled and lead to necrosis.
- Stop the infusion of the chemotherapeutic agent.
- Aspirate all residual chemotherapeutic agent in the IV needle/catheter.
- Administer antidote inject intradermally in circular motion around the extravasation site to prevent leakage of drug to surrounding tissues (if appropriate or inject via the IV catheter).
- Antidote may prevent tissue necrosis. If unable to aspirate from IV catheter, catheter may be blocked and antidote will not reach extravasation.
  Do not inject an antidote via the IV catheter if unable to aspirate the chemotherapeutic agent
  Remove the needle.
  Apply ice or heat to the site, depending on the chemotherapeutic agent which has extravasated.

Follow-up Phase

1. Document drug dosage, site and any occurrence of extravasation including estimated amount of drug extravasated, management. Photograph if possible.
2. Observe regularly after administration for pain, erythema, induration, and necrosis.
3. If only a small amount of drug extravasated and frank necrosis does not occur, phlebitis may still result, causing pain for several days or induration at the site that may last for weeks or months.
4. Monitor for other side effects of infusion.
   - Patient may describe sensations of pain, stretching, or pressure within the vessel, originating near the venipuncture site or extending 7.5-12.5 cm (3-5 inches) along the vein.
   - Discoloration-red streak following the line of the vein (called a flare reaction) or darkening of the vein.
   - Itching, urticaria, muscle cramps, or pressure in the arm.
5. a. Caused by irritation to the vein.
   b. Flare reaction common with doxorubicin (andriamycin).
      Darkening of vein may occur with 5-fluorouracil (5-FU)
   c. Caused by irritation of surrounding subcutaneous tissue.

In addition please refer chapters, specified against following cancer conditions:
- Lung cancer (Ch. 3, Pg. 57).
- Oral cancer (Ch. 4, Pg. 102).
- Esophageal carcinoma (Ch. 4, Pg. 112).
- Cancer of the stomach (Ch. 4, Pg. 120).
- Colorectal cancer (Ch. 4, Pg. 134).
- Leukemias (Ch. 6, Pg. 234).
- Renal tumor (Ch. 7, Pg. 260).
- Neoplasms of the female reproductive tract (Ch. 8, Pg. 292).
- Breast cancer (Ch. 8, Pg. 304).
- Testicular cancer (Ch. 8, Pg. 312).
- Cancer of the prostate (Ch. 8, Pg. 316).
- Cancer of the thyroid gland (Ch. 9, Pg. 347).
- Malignant lesions of skin (Ch. 10, Pg. 385).
- Musculoskeletal tumors (Ch. 11, Pg. 443).
- Eye tumors (Ch. 15, Pg. 538).
- Acoustic neuroma (Ch. 16, Pg. 548).
- Intracranial tumors (Ch. 17, Pg. 582).
- Spinal cord tumors (Ch. 17, Pg. 583).

CHAPTER 19

Management of Emergency and Disaster Nursing

EMERGENCY NURSING

The emergency nurse has had specialized education, training, experience, and expertise in assessing and identifying patients' health care problems in crisis situations. In addition, the emergency nurse establishes priorities, monitors and continuously assesses acutely ill and injured patients, supports and attends to families, supervises allied health personnel, and teaches patients and families within a time-limited, high-pressured care environment. Nursing interventions are accomplished interdependently, in consultation with or under the direction of a physician or nurse practitioner. The strengths of nursing and medicine are complementary in an emergency health care staff members work as a team in performing the highly technical, hand-on-skills required to care of patients in emergency situations.

The nursing process provides a logical framework for problem solving in this environment. Patients in the ED have a wide variety of actual of potential problems, and their condition may change constantly. Therefore, nursing assessment must be continuous, and nursing diagnoses change with the patient's condition. Although a patient may have several diagnoses at a given time, the focus is on the most life threatening ones; often, both independent and interdependent nursing intervention nursing interventions are required.

Issues in Emergency Nursing Care

Emergency nursing is demanding because of the diversity of conditions and situations that present unique challenges. These challenges include legal issues, occupational health and safety risks for ED staff, and the challenge of providing holistic care in the context of a fast-paced, technology-driven environment in which serious illness and death are confronted on a daily basis. Another dimension of emergency nursing is nursing in disasters. With the increasing use of weapons of terror and mass destruction, the emergency nurse must expand his or her knowledge base to encompass recognizing and treating patients exposed to biologic and other terror weapons and anticipate nursing care in the event of a mass casualty incident.

Documentation of Consent and Privacy

Consent to examine and treat the patient is part of the ED record. The patient must consent to invasive procedures (e.g., angiography, lumbar puncture) unless he or she is unconscious or in critical condition and unable to make decisions. If the patient is unconscious and brought to the ED without family or friends, this fact should be documented. Monitoring of the patient's condition, as well as all instituted treatments and the times at which they were performed, must be documented. After treatment, a notation is made on the record about the patient's condition on discharge or transfer and about instructions given to the patient and family for follow-up care.

At the time of consent, the patient is usually also provided a statement of the privacy policy of the health care agency, according to federal law. Patients involved in violent events are often provided with an alias and access to the medical record, both paper and electronic, is limited to protect the privacy of the patient. A patient may also request extra privacy by limiting access to his or her room and by choosing not to receive phone calls, mail, flowers, other gifts, or certain visitors.

Limiting Exposure to Health Risks

Because of the increasing numbers of people infected with hepatitis B and C and with human immunodeficiency virus (HIV), health care providers are at an increased risk for exposure to communicable diseases through blood or other body fluids. This risks is further compounded in the ED because of the common use of invasive treatments in patients who may have a wide range of conditions and who frequently cannot provide a comprehensive medical history. All emergency health care providers must adhere strictly to Standard Precautions for minimizing exposure.

The reemergence of tuberculosis as a major health problem is complicated by multi-drug-resistant tuberculosis and by tuberculosis concomitant with HIV infection. Early identification and adherence to transmission-based precautions for patients who are potentially infectious are crucial. Nurses in the ED are usually fitted with personal high efficiency particulate air (HEPA) filter masks to use when treating patients with airborne diseases.

The potential for exposure to highly contagious organisms, hazardous chemicals or gases, and radiation related to acts of terrorism of natural or manmade disasters presents additional risks to ED staff.

Violence in the Emergency Department

Not only do Ed staff members encounter patients who are violent from substance abuse, injury, or other emergencies, but they may also encounter violent situations in the rest of the environment. Patients and families waiting for assistance are frequently emotionally volatile. Often, waiting rooms are the sites where feelings of dissatisfaction, fear, and anger are channeled violently. Some EDs assign security officers to the area and have installed metal detectors to identify weapons and protect patients, families, and staff. It is not unusual for a patient or family member to come to the ED armed. Nurses and other personnel must be prepared to deal with such circumstances.

Safety is the first priority. Protecting the ED on a daily basis prevents any untoward events from occurring. Protection of the department provides protection for the patients, families, and staff. It is essential that all nurses be aware of the environment in which they are working.

Metal detectors, silent alarm systems, and secured entry into the department assist in maintaining safety. Members of gangs and feuding families need to be separated in the ED, in the waiting room, and later in the inpatient nursing unit to avoid angry confrontations. Security officers should be ready to assist at all times. The ED should be able to be locked against entry if security is at all in question.

Patients from prison and those who are under guard need to be handcuffed to the bed an appropriately assessed to ensure the safety of hospital staff and other patients. The same assessment and care that are provided to patients with hand or ankle restraints are provided to patients with handcuffs. In addition, the following precautions are taken:
- Never release the hand or ankle restraint (handcuff).
- Always have a guard present in the room.
- Place the patient face down on the stretcher to avoid injury from head-butting, spitting, or biting.
- Use restraints on any violent patient as needed.
- Administer Medication if necessary to control violent behavior until definitive treatment can be obtained.

In the case of gunfire in the ED, self-protection is a priority. There is no advantage to protecting others if the caregivers are also injured. Security officers and police must gain control of the situation first, and then care is provided to the injured.

Providing Holistic Care

Sudden illness or trauma is a stress to physiologic and psychological homeostasis that requires physiologic and psychological healing. Patients and families experiencing sudden injury or illness often are overwhelmed by anxiety because they have not had time to adapt to the crisis. They experience real and terrifying fear of death, mutilation, immobilization, and other assaults on their personal identity and body integrity. When confronted with trauma, severe disfigurement, severe illness, or sudden death, the family experiences several stages of crisis. The stages begin with anxiety and progress through denial, remorse and guilt, anger, grief, and reconciliation. The initial goal for the patient and appropriate coping. During this stressful time, safety is of prime importance. Close observation and preplanning are essential and security personnel are stationed nearby in the event that a patient or family member responds to stress with physical violence.

Assessment of the patient and family's psychological function includes evaluating emotional expression, degree of anxiety, and cognitive functioning. Possible nursing diagnoses include anxiety related to uncertain potential outcomes of the illness or trauma and ineffective individual coping related to acute situational crisis. In addition to anxiety, possible nursing diagnoses for the family include anticipatory grieving, alterations in family processes, and ineffective family coping related to acute situational crisis.

Patient-focuses Interventions

Clinicians caring for the patient should act confidently and competently to relieve anxiety. Responding to the patient in a warm manner promotes a sense of security. Explanations should be given on a level that the patient can understand, because an informed patient is better able to cope positively with stress. Human contact and reassuring words reduce the panic of the severely injured or ill person and aid in dispelling fear of the unknown.

The unconscious patient should be treated as if conscious; that is, the patient should be touched, called byname, and given an explanation of every procedure that is performed. As the patient regains consciousness, the nurse should orient the patient by stating his or her name, the date, and the location. This basic information should be provided repeatedly, as needed, in a reassuring way.

Family-focused Interventions

The family is kept informed about where the patient is, how he or she is doing, and the care that is being given. Allowing the family to stay with the patient, when possible, also helps allay their anxieties. Additional interventions are based on the assessment of the stage of crisis that the family is experiencing. Measures to help family members cope with sudden death are presented:
- Take the family to a private place.
- Talk to the family together, so that they can mourn together.
- Reassure the family that everything possible was done; inform them of the treatment rendered.
- Avoid using euphemisms such as "passed on". Show the family that you care by touching, offering coffee, water, and the services of a chaplain.

- Encourage family members to support each other and to express emotions freely (grief, loss, anger, helplessness, tears, disbelief).
- Avoid giving sedation to family members; this may mask or delay the grieving process, which is necessary to achieve emotional equilibrium and to prevent prolonged depression.
- Encourage the family to view the body if they wish; this action helps to integrate the loss. Cover disfigured and injured areas before the family sees the body. Go with the family to see the body. Show acceptance by touching the body to give the family "permission" to touch.
- Spend time with the family, listening to them and identifying any needs that they may have for which the nursing staff can be helpful.
- Allow family members to talk about the deceased and what he or she meant to them; this permits ventilation of feelings of loss. Encourage the family to talk about the events preceding admission to the emergency department. Do not challenge initial feelings of anger or denial.
- Avoid volunteering unnecessary information (e.g., the patient was drinking).

Anxiety and denial: During these crises, family members are encouraged to recognize and talk about their feelings of anxiety. Asking questions is encouraged. Honest answers given at the level of the family's understanding must be provided. Although denial is an ego-defense mechanism that protects one from recognizing painful and disturbing aspects of reality, prolonged denial is not encouraged or supported. The family must be prepared for the reality of what has happened and what may come.

Remorse and guilt: Expressions of remorse and guilt are common, with family members accusing themselves (or each other) of negligence or minor omissions. Family members are urged to verbalize their feelings until they realize that there was probably little that they could have done to prevent the injury or illness.

Anger: Expressions of anger, common in crisis situations, are a way of handling anxiety and fear. Anger is frequently directed by the family at the patient, but it is also often expressed toward the physician, the nurse, or admitting personnel. The therapeutic approach is to allow the anger to be ventilated, then assist the family members ot identify their feelings of frustration.

Grief: Grief is a complex amotional response to anticipated or actual loss. The key nursing intervention is to help family members work through their grief and to support their coping mechanisms, letting them know that it is normal and acceptable for them to cry, feel pain, and express loss. The hospital chaplain and social services staff both serve as invaluable members of the team when assisting families to work through their grief.

Emergency Nursing and Continuum of Care

As stated previously, one principle underlying emergency care is that the patient is rapidly assessed, treated, and referred to the appropriate setting for ongoing care. This makes the ED a very temporary point on the continuum of care. Most patients who receive emergency care are discharged directly from the ED to their homes, and emergency nurses must plan and facilitate the patient's safe discharge and follow-up care in the home and the community.

Discharge Planning

Before discharge, instructions for continuing care are given to the patient and the family or significant others. All instructions should be given not only verbally but also in writing, so that the patient can refer to them later. Many Eds have preprinted standard instruction sheets for the more common conditions. These instructions are then individualized for each patient. These instructions may be available in a variety of languages. If they are not available in a language that the patient speaks, an interpreter should be used. Instructions should include information about prescribed medications, treatments, diet, activity, and when to contact a health care provider or schedule follow-up appointments. It is imperative that instructions are written legibly, use simple language, and are clear inthier teaching. When providing discharge instructions, the nurse also considers any special needs the patient may have related to hearing or visual impairments. Alternate formats of instruction (e.g., Large print, Braille, audiotape) should be available to meet the needs of patients with hearing or visual impairments.

Community Services

Before discharge, some patients require the services of a social worker to help them meet continuing health care needs. For patients and families who cannot provide care at home, community agencies (e.g., Home care nursing services, Visiting Nurse Association) may be contacted before discharge to arrange services. This is particularly important for elderly patients who need assistance. Identifying continuing health care needs and making arrangements for meeting these needs and making arrangements for meeting these needs can prevent return visits to the ED and readmission to the hospital.

For patients who are returning to extended care facilities and for those who already rely on community agencies for continuing health care, communication about the patient's condition and any changes in health care needs that have occurred must be provided to the appropriate facilities or agencies. This communication is essential to promote continuity of care and to ensure ongoing care to meet the patient's changing health care needs.

PRINCIPLES OF EMERGENCY CARE

By definition, emergency care is care that must be rendered without delay. In an ED, several patients with diverse health problems—some life-threatening, some not—not present to the ED simultaneously. One of the first principles of emergency care is triage.

Triage

The word triage comes from the French word trier, meaning "to sort". In the daily routine of the ED, triage is used to sort patients into groups based on the severity of their health problems and the immediacy with which these problems must be treated.

ED use various triage systems with differing terminology, but all share this characteristic of a hierarchy based on the potential for loss of life. A basic and widely used triage system that has been in use for many years has three categories: emergent, urgent, and nonurgent. Emergent patients have the highest priority- their conditions are life-threatening and they must be seen immediately. Urgent patients have serious health problems but not immediately life-threating ones; they must be seen within 1 hour. Nonurgent patients have episodic illnesses that can be addressed within 24 hours without increased morbidity (Berner, 2005). A fourth class that is increasingly used is "fast-track". These patients require simple first aid or basic primary care and may be treated in the ED or safely referred to a clinic or physician's office.

A more refined comprehensive triage system has been implemented to incorporate the changes in the use of the ED for both emergency and routine health care. This system has five levels: resuscitation, emergent, urgent, non-urgent and minor. The increaed number of triage levels assists the triage nurse to more precisely determine the needs of the patient and the urgency for treatment.

Assess and Intervene

For the patient assigned to a resuscitation, emergent, or urgent triage category, stabilization, provision of critical treatment, and prompt transfer to the appropriate setting (intensive care unit, operating room, general care unit) are the priorities of emergency care. Although treatment is initiated in ED, ongoing definitive treatment of the underlying problem is provided in other settings, and the sooner the patient is stabilized and moved to the area, the better the outcome.

A systematic approach to effectively establishing and treating health priorities is the primary survey/secondary survey approach. The primary survey focuses on stabilizing life-threatening conditions. The ED staff work collaboratively and follow the ABCD (airway, breathing, circulation, disability) method:

- Establish a patent airway.
- Provide adequate ventilation, employing resuscitation measures when necessary. (Trauma patients must have the cervical spine protected and chest, injuries assessed first.)
- Evaluate and restore cardiac output by controlling hemorrhage, preventing and treating shock, and maintaining or restoring effective circulation. This includes the prevention and management of hypothermia.
- Determine neurologic disability by assessing neurologic function using the Glasgow Coma Scale.

After these priorities have been addressed, the ED team proceeds with the secondary survey. This includes the following:

- A complete health history and head-to-toe assessment.
- Diagnostic and laboratory testing.
- Insertion or application of monitoring devices such as electrocardiogram (ECG) electrodes, arterial lines, or urinary catheters.
- Splinting of suspected fractures.
- Cleansing, closure, and dressing of wounds.
- Performance of other necessary interventions based on the patient's condition.

Once the patient has been assessed, stabilized, and tested, appropriate medical and nursing diagnoses are formulated, initial important treatment is started, and plans for the proper disposition of the patient are made. Many emergent and urgent conditions and priority emergency interventions are discussed in detail in the remaining sections of this chapter.

In addition to the management of the illness or injury, the ED nurse must also focus on providing comfort and emotional support to the patient and family. Included in this is pain management. Effective pain management must be instituted early and should include rapid-acting agents that result in minimal sedation so that the patient can continue to interact with the staff for continued assessment. Moderate sedation can help facilitate short procedures in ED; the patient will not remember the procedure later. The patient is closely monitored during the procedure and then rapidly awakens when it is complete.

Family crisis intervention is essential for all ED patients. Even if a patient's condition is not emergent, the situation may be perceived as such by the family. Every family needs attentions and support. The chaplain and social worker may be available to assist with interventions.

DISASTER NURSING

Meaning

Disaster means that any occurrence that cuases damage ecological disruption, loss of human life or deterioration of health and health services on a scale sufficient to warrant and extraordinary response from outside the affected community or area.

Types

Disaster is an occurrence, either natural or man-made that causes human suffering and creates human needs that victims cannot alleviate without assistance.

Disasters can be natural or man-made. *Natural disasters* include droughts, earthquakes, tsunamis, forest fires, landslides and mudslides, blizzards, hurricanes, tornadoes, floods and volcanic disruptions. *Man-made disasters* includes hazardous substance accidents (e.g., chemicals, toxic gases), radiologic accidents, dam failures, resource shortage (e.g., food, electricity and water), structural fire and explosions and domestic disturbances (e.g., terrorism, bombing and riots), bioterrorism **(Table19.1)**.

Epidemiology of Disaster

Epidemiology is the study of pattern of disease occurrence in human populations and the factors that influence these patterns. Disaster may be studied and analysed using the epidemiological framework of agent, host and environment in an attempt to predict, prevent, or control the outcomes of a disaster. As stated earlier there are two types of disasters: natural and man made. Both types will vary in intensity, severity and impact.

Disaster agent: To apply the epidemiological framework in a disaster situation, the *agent* is the physical item that actually causes the injury or destruction. Primary agents include falling buildings, heat, wind, rising water and smoke. Secondary agents include bacteria and viruses that produce contamination or infection after the primary agent has caused injury or destruction.

Host: In the epidemiological framework as applied to disaster, the host is human kind. Host factors are those characteristics of humans that influence the severity of the disaster's effect. Host factors include age, immunization status, pre-existing health status, degree of mobility and emotional stability. Individuals most severely affected by a disaster are elderly person, who may have trouble leaving the area quickly; young children whose immune systems are not fully developed; and persons with respiratory or cardiac problems. For example, a fire in a nursing home is potentially more lethal than a fire in a college dormitory. In a fire situation, elderly individuals in the nursing home are at greater risk because they are less physically fire and more susceptible to smoke and other consequences than are young college students.

Environment: Environmental factors that affect the outcome of a disaster include physical, chemical, biological and social factors. Physical include the time when the disaster occurs, weather conditions, the availability of food and water and the functioning of utilities such as electricity and telephone service. Chemical factors influencing disaster outcome include leakage of stored chemicals into the air, soil, ground water or food supplies. Biological factors are those that occur or increase as a result of contaminated water, improper waste disposal, insect or rodent proliferation, improper food storage, or lack of refrigeration owing to interrupted electrical services. Social factors are those that contribute to the individual's social support systems. Loss of family members, changes in roles, and the questioning of religious beliefs are social factors to be examined after a disaster.

HOSPITAL EMERGENCY PREPAREDNESS PLANS

Health care facilities are required to create a plan for emergency preparedness and to practice this plan twice a year. Generally these plans are developed under the Environment of Care Committee or Safety Committee and are overseen by an administrative liaison.

Before the basic emergency operations plan (EOP) can be developed, the planning committee of the health care facility first evaluates characteristics of the community to identify the likely types of natural and manmade disasters that might occur. This evaluative process is the responsibility of the local health care facility and its safety committee, safety officer, or emergency department (ED) manager. This information can be gathered by questioning local law enforcement, fire departments, and emergency medical systems and assessing the patterns of local train traffic, automobile traffic, and flood, earthquake, tornado, or hurricane activity. Consideration is also given to possible mass casualties that could arise because of the community's proximity to chemical plants, nuclear facilities, or military bases. Federal, judicial, or financial buildings, schools, and any places where large groups of people gather can be considered high-risk areas.

Table 19.1: Types of disaster.

Natural	Man-made
Hurricanes	Conventional warfare
Tornados	Nonconventional warfare (e.g., nuclear, chemical)
Hailstorms	Tansportation accidents
Tsunami	Structural collapse
Cyclone	Explosions
Blizzards	Fires
Drought	Toxic materials
Floods	Pollution
Mudslides	Civil unrest (e.g., riots, demonstrations)
Avalanches	Terrorists attacks
Earthquakes	
Volcanic	
Communicable disease epidemics	

The emergency preparedness planning committee must have a realistic understanding of its resources. It must determine, for example, whether the facility has or needs, a pharmaceutical stockpile available to treat specific chemical or biological agent. Another scenario that might be anticipated may include the dispersal of a pulmonary intoxicant or choking agent, which would require that emergency operations planners find out how many ventilators are available within the facility and throughout the greater community. The committee might also outline how staff would triage and assign priority to patients when the number of ventilators is limited. Multiple factors influence a facility's ability to respond effectively to a sudden influx of injured patients, and the committee must anticipate various scenarios to improve its preparedness.

Components of the Emergency Operations Plan

Once the initial assessment is complete, the health care facility develops the EOP. Essential components of the plan are as follows:

- *An activation response:* The EOP activation response of a health care facility defines where, how and when the response is initiated.
- *An internal/external communication plan:* Communication is critical for all parties involved, including communication to and from the pre-hospital arena.
- *A plan for coordinated patient care:* A response is planned for coordinated patient care into and out of the facility, including transfers to other facilities. The site of the disaster can determine where the greater number of patients may self-refer.
- *Security plans:* A coordinated security plan involving facility and community agencies is key to the control of an otherwise chaotic situation.
- *Identification of external resources:* External resources are identified, including local, state, and federal resources.
- *A plan for people management and traffic flow:* "People management" includes strategies to manage the patients, the public, the media, and personnel. Specific areas are assigned, and designated person is delegated to manage each of these areas.
- *A data management strategy:* A data management plan for every aspect of the disaster will save time at every step. A backup system for charting, tracking, and staffing is developed if the facility has a computer system.
- *Deactivation response:* Deactivation of the response is as important as activation; resources should not be overused. The person who decides when the facility is able to go from the disaster response back to daily activities is clearly identified. Any possible residual effects of a disaster must be considered before this decision is made.
- *A post-incident response:* Often facilities see increased volumes of patients 3 months or more after an incident. Post-incident response must include a critique and a de-briefing for all parties involved, immediately and again at a later date.
- *A plan for practice drills:* Practice drills that include community participation allow for troubleshooting any issues before a real-life incident occurs.
- *Anticipated resources:* Food and water must be available for staff, families, and others who may be at the facility for an extended period.
- *MCI planning:* MCI planning includes such issues as mass fatality and morgue readiness.
- *An educational plan for all of the above:* A strong educational plan for all personnel regarding each step of the plan allows for improved readiness and additional input for fine-tuning of the EOP (Anteau and Williams, 1997; Dara et al., 2005).

The EOP should also include a structure that defines roles for all employees in each emergency situation. The most common structure is the ICS described earlier but applied at the level of the health care facility itself instead of at the site of the disaster. For example, an administrator, possibly the nurse executive, will act as incident commander within the hospital and coordinate all aspects of the implementation of the plan. Other personnel will be designated to perform key roles, such as resource manager or patient disposition coordinator. Such predetermined organization is essential to minimize confusion, ensure that all key operations are directed, and promote a well-coordinated response.

Initiating the Emergency Operations Plan

Notification of a disaster situation to a health care facility varies with each situation. Generally, the notification to the facility comes from outside sources unless the initial incident occurred at the facility. The disaster activation plan should clearly state how the EOP is to be initiated. If communication is functioning, field incident command will give notice of the approximate number of arriving patients, although the number of self-referring patients will not be known.

Identifying Patients and Documenting Patient Information

Patient tracking is a critical component of casualty management. Disaster tags, which are numbered and included triage priority, name, address, age, location and description of injuries, and treatments or medications given, are used to communicate patient information. The tag should be securely placed on the patient and remain with the patient at all times. The tag number and patient's name are recorded in a disaster log. The log is used by the command center to tract patients, assign beds, and provide families with information.

Triage

Triage is the sorting of patients to determine the priority of health care and the proper site for treatment. In mondisaster situations, health care workers assign a high priority and allocate the most resources to those who are the most critically ill. For example, a young adult who has a chest injury and is in full cardiac arrest would receive advanced cardiopulmonary resuscitation, including medications, chest tubes, intravenous (IV) fluids, blood, and possibly even emergency surgery in an effort to restore life. However, in a disaster, when health care providers are faced with a large number of casualties, the fundamental principle guiding resource allocation is to do the greatest good for the greatest number of people. Decisions are based on the likelihood of survival and consumption of available resources. Therefore, this same patient, and others with conditions associated with a high mortality rate, would be assigned a low triage priority in a disaster situation, even if the person is conscious. Although this may sound uncaring, from an ethical standpoint the expenditure of limited resources on people with a low chance of survival, and denial of those resources to others with serious but treatable conditions, cannot be justified.

The triage officer rapidly assesses those injured at the disaster scene. Patients are immediately tagged and transported or given life-saving interventions. One person performs the initial triage while other EMS personnel perform life-saving interventions. One person performs the initial triage while other EMS personnel perform life-saving measures (e.g., intubation) and transport patients. Although EMS personnel carry out initial field triage, secondary and continuous triage at all subsequent levels of Staff should control all entrances to the acute care facility so that incoming patients are directed to the triage area first. The triage area may be outside the entry or just at the door of the ED. This allows all patients, including those arriving by medical transport and those who walk in, to be triaged. Some patients already seen in the field may be reclassified in the triage area, based on their current presentation.

Managing Internal Problems

Each facility must determine its supply lists based on its own needs assessment. The Red Cross has developed a basic survival/shelter resource kit. The EOP committee should determine the top 10 critical medications used during normal day-to-day operations and then anticipate which other medications may be required in a disaster or an MCI. For example, the health care facility might plan to have available a stockpile of antidotes (e.g., cyanide kits) or antibiotics used in treating biologic agents. Information should be available about stocking or restocking any of the basic and special supplies, how those supplies are requested, and the time required to receive those supplies.

Communicating with the Media and Family

Communication is a key component of disaster management. Communication within the vast team of disaster responders is paramount; however, effective, informative communication with the media and worried family members is also crucial.

Managing Media Requests for Information

Although the media have an obligation to report the news and can play a significant positive role in communication, the number of reporters and newscasters and their support teams can be overwhelming, possibly compromising operations and patient confidentiality. A clearly defined process for managing media requests that includes a designated spokesperson, a site for the dissemination of information (away from patient care areas), and a regular schedule for providing updates should be part of the disaster plan.

The disaster plan helps prevent the release of contradictory or inaccurate information. Initial statements should focus on current efforts and what is being done to better understand the scope and impact of the situation. Information about casualties should not be released. Security staff should not allow media personal access to patient care areas.

Caring for Families

Friends and family members converging on the scene must be care for by the facility. They may be feeling intense anxiety, shock, or grief and should be provided with information and updates about their loved ones as soon as possible and regularly thereafter. They should not be in the triage or treatment areas, but in a designated area staffed by available social service workers, counselors, therapists, or clergy. Access to this area should be controlled to prevent families from being disturbed cultural variables to consider when coping with disaster related injuries and death.

Any disaster or mass casualty incident can be expected to involve members of diverse religious, ethnic, and cultural groups or may be targeted at and predominately affect a specific likewise include members of all religious, ethnic, and cultural backgrounds and should bear in mind that victims may have:
- Language difficulties that increase fears and frustrations.
- Specific religious practices related to medical treatment, hygiene, or diet.
- Specific place/times for prayer.
- Rituals about handling the dead.
- Timing of funeral services.

Some religious communities have plans for emergencies and disasters, and local hospitals should integrate these plans to the extent possible into their emergency operations plans.

The Nurse's Role in Disaster Response Plans

The role of the nurse during a disaster varies. The nurse may be asked to perform duties outside his or her area of expertise and may take on responsibilities normally held by physicians or advanced practice nurses. For example, a critical care nurse may intubate a patient or even insert chest tubes. Wound debridement or suturing may be performed by staff registered nurses. A nurse may serve as the triage officer.

Although the exact role of a nurse in disaster management depends on the specific needs of the facility at the time, it should be clear which nurse or physician is in charge of a given patient care area and which procedures each individual nurse may or may not perform. Assistance can be obtained through the incident command center, and nonmedical personnel can provide services where possible. For example, family members can provide nonskilled interventions for their loved ones. Nurses should remember that nursing care in a disaster focuses on essential care from a perspective of what is best for all patients.

New settings and atypical roles for nurse arise during a disaster; for example, the nurse may provide shelter care in a temporary housing area, or bereavement support and assistance with identification of deceased loved ones. People may require crisis intervention, or the nurse may participate in counseling other staff members and in critical incident stress management (CISM). Special care may be warranted for at risk population during a disaster.

When a disaster occurs, the multiple agencies involved attempt to provide food, water, and shelter to all those affected. People with disabilities have specific needs that require attention. It is recommended that people with disabilities have a personal support network to check on them after a disaster and to provide needed assistance. They should also have a back-up system and an evacuation plan. Agencies need to be aware that service animals are also affected during a disaster and may be brought to shelters with their companions.

Evacuation assistance is imperative for people with disabilities. Directions to personal equipment (e.g., communication devices, medications, oxygen) should be available to rescue personnel. In a rapid evacuation, mobility devices, oxygen, suction, and medications will be needed at the shelters. Special efforts to keep those with vision or hearing impairment informed should be implemented. People skilled in sign language are also valuable resources during a disaster.

Considering Ethical Conflicts

Disasters can present a disparity between the resources of the health care agency and the needs of the victims. This generates ethical dilemmas for nurses and other health care providers. Issues include conflicts related to the following:

- Rationing care
- Futile therapy
- Consent
- Duty
- Confidentiality
- Resuscitation
- Assisted suicide.

Nurses may find it difficult to not provide medical care to the dying, or to withhold information to avoid spreading fear and panic. Clinical scenarios that are unimaginable in normal circumstances confront the nurse in extreme instances. Other ethical dilemmas may arise out of health care providers' instinct for self-protect and protection of their families. For example, what should be pregnant nurse do when incoming disaster victims have been exposed to radiation, yet too few nurses are available?

Nurses can plan for the ethical dilemmas they will face during disasters by establishing a framework for evaluating ethical questions before they arise and by identifying and exploring possible responses to difficult clinical situations.

CHAPTER 20

Critical Care Nursing

EVOLUTION OF CRITICAL CARE NURSING

Since the earliest days of nursing, the sickest patients have been placed near the nurse's station, underlining the importance of frequent assessment and rapid intervention. From the development of postoperative wards and polio centers to triage centers during various wars, to the evolution of the coronary care unit, this concentration of highly specialized caregivers with access to unique technology has remained the guiding principle for the evolution of critical care environment.

The delivery of critical care as we know it today originated from the need to centralize specially trained personnel and equipment in a separate area of the hospital to optimize the care of critically ill and injured patients. Nurses began to group their most unstable patients closer to the nurse's station so they provide "watchful vigilance" or intensive observation. The concept of gathering patients together for care can be traced back to Florence Nightingale.

It is common, in small country hospitals, to have a recess or small room leading from the operating theatre in which the patients remain until they have recovered, or at least recovered from the immediate effects of the operation.

Critical care units or intensive care units were designed to meet the special needs of acutely and critically ill patients. The concept of clustering the most acutely ill is not new. Florence Nightingale recommended grouping acutely ill patients together. During poliomyelitis and tuberculosis pandemics earlier in 20th century, special units were established, equipped with technical apparatus to manage the airway and ventilate the patient and staffed by specialized care providers. During World War II and Vietnam War trauma units were developed for battle casualties.

In the 1960s, technical developments allowed for more accessible monitoring of electrocardiogram (ECG), arterial and central venous pressures, and arterial blood gases. Coronary care units were developed for patients with acute myocardial infarction. In these units patients were continually monitored for cardiac dysrhythmias and nurses were trained to identify and aggressively manage dysrhythmias. By the 1970s, the intensive care unit (ICU) was a standard component of most general hospitals. Since that time, technologic advances have continued at a rapid pace, bringing improved monitoring capabilities and new strategies to manage life-threatening problems.

The term critical care nursing is often used interchangeably with the term ICU nursing. The critical care nurse is responsible for diagnosing life-threatening conditions and instituting appropriate treatment. Today the technology and equipment available in the ICU are extensive and continually evolving. In ICUs the capability exists to continuously monitor ECG, blood pressure, oxygenation, and temperature. More advanced monitoring devices allow for the measurement of stroke volume, ejection fraction, end tidal carbon dioxide, and oxygen consumption. Patients may be receiving continual support from the ventilator, cardiac assist devices, or dialysis machines.

Now *critical care unit* continues to be a unique, high-paced environment in which the most sophisticated medical, nursing, and technical interventions are integrated to combat life threatening illness. These units are referred to as intensive care units (ICUs), critical care units, coronary care units, and other names that identify the type and intensity of patient care. The one constant is that the role of nursing is critical to success. Through vigilant observation of a patients ever-changing condition, the critical care nurse monitors the complex treatment regimen, quickly identifies problems and initiates appropriate therapies, and intervenes to prevent or correct life-threatening situations. However, the focus of critical care nursing practice is no longer only on the patients critical illness or injury. Critical care nurses have broadened their focus to include preventive care and risk modification to decrease future patient hospitalizations.

Critical care nurse and critical care nursing offers challenge and excitement to the role of the nurse. Physicians have relied heavily on the skills of critical care nurses and respect them for their expertise. Aside from job satisfaction, salaries are highly rewarding in some parts of the country.

Critical care units should be staffed by highly trained and skilled nurses. Specialized critical care units have been developed to meet the needs of individual patients. The size and number of critical care units vary from one institution to another. Categories of some of these specialized units are listed:

- ICU: Intensive care unit.
- CCU: Coronary care unit.
- MICU: Medical intensive care unit.
- SICU: Surgical intensive care unit.
- PICU: Pediatric intensive care unit.
- NICU: Neonatal intensive care unit.
- PMU: Progressive medical care unit.
- PSU: Progressive surgical care unit.
- BU: Burn unit.

Some of the functions of skilled critical care nurses include:
- Performing basic bedside care meeting biopsychosocial needs.
- Identifiying cardiac arrhythmias.
- Administering and adjusting medications.
- Initiating and maintaining intravenous therapy.
- Performing cardiopulmonary resuscitation.
- Performing defibrillation.
- Completing physical assessment.
- Taking health histories.
- Interpreting 12-lead electrocardiograms.
- Monitoring hemodynamic Swan-Ganz catheter.
- Maintaining arterial lines and pressure interpretation.
- Monitoring intra-aortic balloon pumps.
- Providing patient/family teaching.
- Interpret and order diagnostic lab tests.
- Make nursing diagnoses.
- Identify community resources.
- Collaborate with the physician reagarding treatment.
- Prescribe symptomatic treatment in select situations.

Roles and functions of critical care nurses vary from state to state depending on the nurse practice act. In some states, Licences laws dictate, in part, the level of nurse eligible for employment in critical care units. The nursing administration office of the institution establishes the job description and qualification based on the nurse practice act of the state.

Job opportunities are abundant because there are not enough qualifed nurses to meet the job openings in all parts of the country. Salaries depend on the geographic location but are usually higher than those for RNs on a general medical/surgical unit.

The critical care nurse cares for patients and the families of patients with acute and unstable physiologic problems in an environment equipped for technically advanced methods of assessing and managing patient problems. Critical care nursing as that specialty dealing with human responses to life-threatening problems. The specialty requires knowledge of physiology, pathophysiology, pharmacology, and the ability to use advanced technology to accurately measure physiologic parameters. It is important that the nurse understand the assumptions on which measurements depend and determine if those assumptions are correct for each specific patient. The nurse provides ongoing assessment and early recognition and management of complications while fostering healing and recovery. Appropriate actions by an astute nurse can prevent complications. The nurse must be able to provide psychologic support to the patient and the family. To be effective the critical care nurse must be able to communicate clearly and work as a team member.

Critical care nursing is concerned with human responses to life-threatening problems, such as major surgery, trauma, infection, and shock, as well as prevention of potential life-threatening conditions. The critical care nurse is a patient advocate responsible for ensuring that all critically ill patients and families receive optimal care through a process of establishing goals for patient care and providing mechanisms to assess the patients progress toward the goals. Clinical competencies for critical care nurses include clinical judgment and reasoning skills coupled with the ability to think critically and make decisions. The critical care nurse relies on specialized skills and knowledge to monitor and support the patient's physiologic stability of patients and provides an interface between the patient and technology. The nurse tailors clinical practices to the needs of each individual patient and family through collaboration with the health care team members to meet desired patient outcomes. Today's critical care is provided by a multidisciplinary team of health care professionals, including physicians, respiratory therapists, social workers, and clergy. The critical care nurse is an integral part of this team in coordinating care activities for patients and families.

Nursing practice in the ICU often follows a primary care model with the patient cared for by a limited group of nurses who become intensely familiar with the patient's condition and needs and needs of the patient's family. That primary care nurse spends most working hours near the patients bedside. Specialization in ICU nursing usually requires formal training and mentored clinical practice, followed by an internship. Training takes place in a variety of settings. Only a small percentage of baccalaureate nursing programs include critical care as a separate course, often with a minimal clinical component. The number of associate degree programs offering critical care content is unknown. Many clinical institutions offer ICU preparation, as do continuing education agencies.

Advanced practice critical care nurses generally have a graduate (master's or doctorate) degree. These nurses are employed as patient and staff educators, consultants, administrators, researchers, or practitioners. The critical care clinical nurse specialist role traditionally includes aspects of each of these role components. An important emerging role is the acute care nurse practitioner. These master's prepared nurses provide advanced, comprehensive, risk-appropriate care to selected critically ill patients and their families. The acute care nurse practitioner is prepared to conduct comprehensive health assessments, order and interpret diagnostic tests, diagnose and treat health problems and disease-related symptoms, prescribe and evaluate drugs and treatments, and coordinate care during transitions in settings. They may practice independently (e.g., providing comprehensive care to the chronically critically ill), or collaboratively (e.g., providing symptom management in conjunction with physician specialists).

CRITICAL CARE UNIT/ICU

In earlier days critical care units were small carved out of existing recovery rooms or other areas in the hospital. Soon, however, the ICU emerged as a distinct area for care of complex patients, different from the recovery room in that patients were also admitted from outside the hospital and from other units. The units were staffed 24 hours a day, 7 days a week.

Today's critical care unit is designed, equipped, and staffed to meet the anticipated needs of patients in life-threatening situations. The physical layout is frequently a modified circle that allows for direct visualization of all patients at all times. Patients may be separated into cubicles with glass windows or situated in a large open area with curtains for partitions. The advantage of direct nurse-patient visualization is accompanied by the disadvantages of limited privacy and patient exposure to frequent crisis interventions.

Although direct visualization of patients facilitates patient monitoring, maximizes the use of available staff, and is required by some hospital accrediting organizations, the cost to the patient in terms of sensory overload and loss of control can be significant. Optimal patient care requires maintaining a sensitive balance between the needs of patients and those of caregivers.

The central nurse's station contains sophisticated monitoring and even video equipment that enables nurses to continuously monitor vital data for each patient. Certain technologies are available for constant use at each bedside (e.g., cardiac monitor, oxygen, hemodynamic monitoring equipment, and suction equipment), whereas others must be available within seconds (e.g., defibrillator, ventilator, 12-lead electrocardiogram [ECG] machine, emergency medications). Still other technologies must be available for constant or intermittent use with certain patient populations (e.g., intraaortic balloon pumps, continuous venovenous hemofiltration or hemodialysis, extracorporeal membrane oxygenator, temporary or permanent pacemakers, ventricular assist devices, intermittent conventional hemodialysis, and a variety of pumps for infusion of intravenous fluids or enteral feedings).

The concentration of complex technologic equipment creates a unique hazard in the critical care environment: the risk of electrical microshock. The invasive monitoring and therapeutic interventions used with critically ill patients (e.g., central venous pressure lines, pulmonary artery catheters, and temporary pacemakers) often create a direct pathway to the heart. Direct contact with stray or leaked current could prove fatal, particularly to critically ill patients whose resistance may be further decreased by other breaks in skin integrity or electrolyte imbalances. Critical care nurses are responsible for using electrical equipment properly and safely.

As the need for more specialized and sophisticated critical care equipment grows, the patient often becomes surrounded by a sea of machinery for monitoring and care delivery. A popular feature of newer or remodeled critical care environments is the centralized or headwall power needs for monitoring equipment, oxygen, suction equipment, and electrical outlets; to store equipment; and to provide a workspace at each patient's bedside. With the advent of microprocessing and digital processing, continued research and development of critical care equipment focus on how to provide the most service in the smallest available space.

CRITICAL CARE PATIENT

A patient is generally admitted to the ICU for one of three reasons. First, the patient may be physiologically unstable, requiring advanced and sophisticated clinical judgments by the nurse or physician. Second, the patient may be at risk for serious complications and require frequent and often invasive physical assessment. Third, the patient may be stable but require intensive and complicated nursing support, including ventilation, hemodynamic monitoring, feeding, turning, wound care, and hygiene.

ICUs may serve a variety of patients or specialize in a disease condition (e.g., neurology) or age group (e.g., pediatrics). ICU patients are sometimes clustered by acuity (e.g., acute and unstable versus technology dependent but stable). The patient with myocardial ischemia or infarction or respiratory distress is commonly treated in the ICU, as is the patient with acute neurologic impairment, after cardiac surgery, or after major organ transplantation. Trauma ICUs treat the critically injured. The patient with a medical emergency (e.g., sepsis; diabetic ketoacidosis; drug overdoses; poisonings; thyroid, adrenal, or hematologic crises) is often treated in a medical ICU. The patient with a serious underlying condition may be monitored in the ICU while receiving care for unrelated conditions. The patient who is not expected to recover is not treated in an ICU. The ICU should not be used to treat the patient in a persistent vegetative state, nor should ICU care be used to prolong the natural process of death.

The critical care environment confronts patients with advanced forms of medical and nursing therapies. Although the patient and family are partially aware of the dynamics of critical care, their attention primarily focuses on the confusing and frightening environment: flashing lights, buzzing machines, painful procedures, bright lights, noise, and hyperactivity. The stressors on the patient and family are immense. The recovery period from psychologic stressors experienced in critical care may extend well past discharge from the hospital.

The patient admitted into the ICU is at risk for complications and special problems. Invasive devices carry a risk of infection, particularly in the patient with a compromised immunologic status. Sepsis and multiple organ dysfunction syndrome may follow. Other special problems for ICU patients include anxiety, dependency, impaired communication, sensory-perceptual problems, and sleep difficulties These complications are discussed as follows:

Anxiety: Patients commonly find the ICU frightening. Frequently patients are at risk of dying and fear death. Many patients and families feel uncomfortable in the ICU environment with its equipment, high noise and light levels, and intense pace of activity. The nurse can assist the patient and family with their feelings of anxiety by encouraging them to express concerns, ask questions, and state their needs. The nurse should explain equipment and procedures. The nurse may be able to structure the patients surrounding environment in a way that may decrease anxiety. For example, family members can be encouraged to bring in photographs and personal items.

Dependency: Patients in the ICU commonly are unable to perform self-care activities such as eating, bathing, and oral hygiene. The patient may lack control over bodily functions such as elimination and breathing. The patient is frequently dependent on the nursing staff for access to food, liquids, the bedpan and other needed items. In addition, the ICU patient is frequently connected equipment and placed on bed rest. The degree of dependency experienced by an ICU patient can be distressing. Although the highest priority is the safety of the patient, the nurse should provide as much autonomy as the patients condition allows. Family members can be taught to assist the patient with activities of daily living.

Impaired communication: Inability to communicate can be a distressing problem for the patient who may be unable to speak because of the use of paralyzing drugs or an endotracheal tube. As part of any procedure the nurse should explain what will happen or is happening to the patient. When the patient cannot speak, the nurse should explore alternative methods of communication, including the use of devices such as picture boards, magic slates, or computer keyboards. When speaking with the patient, the nurse should look directly at the patient and use hand gestures when appropriate. Nonverbal communication is important. The ICU is characterized by high levels of procedure-related touch and decreased affection-related or comfort-related touch. Patients have different levels of tolerance for being touched, possibly related to cultural background and personal history. It may be appropriate to provide comforting touch with ongoing evaluation of the patients response.

Sensory-perceptual problems: Transient sensory-perceptual changes are common in ICU patients. Approximately 50% of patients treated in the ICU experience decreased orientation and impaired cognition. The combination of changes in mentation (e.g., hallucinations, delusions) and behavior (e.g., shouting, hitting) has been called ICU psychosis. Patients with ICU psychosis or delirium may demonstrate confusion, irritability, an inappropriate behavior. Factors predisposing the patient to sensory-perceptual changes include sleep deprivation, anxiety, sensory overload, stress and many drugs. Physical conditions such as hypoxemia and electrolyte disturbances can produce similar symptoms, including confusion and irritability. Potassium, calcium, and magnesium imbalances are common in the critically ill patient, and each can result in altered cognition.

The task of the ICU nurse is to identify predisposing factors, whether they be physiologic, psychologic, or environmental, and attempt to improve the patients mental clarity and cooperation with therapy. The use of clocks and calendars may help the patient remain oriented. Although symptoms may be managed pharmacologically with a sedative, hypnotic, or a psychotropic (e.g., haloperidol, [Haldol]) medication, these drugs may decrease the patient's ability to interact with family members. This may deprive patients and families of what may be the short and precious time remaining to discuss intimate and important issues.

Sensory deprivation and overload: To interact optimally with the environment, an individual requires the stimulation of all five senses. The optimal level and variety of this stimulation vary significantly among individuals. Patients in a critical care unit have little or no control over the amount or frequency of stimuli they receive. Too much stimuli can be as undesirable as too little. Critical care environments rarely contain the type of sensory stimuli that are familiar or understandable to patients. Unfamiliar voices, equipment noise, continuous bright lights, and frequent assessment interventions all add to the patients stress level. This level of stimulation does not disappear during the night and is in fact minimally diminished. Years of research indicate that sensory overload and sensory deprivation in the critical care environment frequently result in perceptual distortion, hallucinations, and paranoia.

Staff members may not realize the impact of this level of stimuli and frequently perpetuate it. Staff, of course, is also able to leave the high-energy critical care environment at the end of their shift, whereas the patient is unable to escape it. The nurse needs to be constantly aware of the type and amount of stimuli directed toward the patient and must help maintain the level of stimulation within tolerable limits. Research has found that a concentrated effort by staff to reduce environmental stimuli increases the likelihood of patients being able to sleep. Staff should make every effort to reduce noise and other controllable variables and to help the patient understand this complex environment, thereby reducing the stress of the unknown.

Sensory overload can also result in patient distress and anxiety. Noise levels are particularly high in the ICU. The "meaning" of a noise may determine its stressfulness. For example, meaningful noise is less stressful. The nurse can limit noise and assist the patient in understanding noises that cannot be prevented. Conversation is a particularly stressful noise, especially when the discussion concerns the patient and is conducted in the presence of, but without participation from, the patient. The nurse can restructure the environment to eliminate this source of stress by identifying better places for discussing the patient or by including the patient in the discussion. The nurse can also limit noise levels directly by muting phones, setting alarms appropriate to the patients condition, and eliminating unnecessary alarms. For example, the nurse should silence the blood pressure alarms while balancing, calibrating, and flushing lines and reactivate the alarms when the procedures are complete. Similarly, ventilator alarms should be transiently silenced during endotracheal suctioning procedures. Over-head paging should be limited in patient care areas. Music should be played only if it comforts the patient.

Sleep problems: Nearly all ICU patients experience serious sleep disturbances. Patients may have difficulty falling asleep or have disrupted sleep because of frequent monitoring or treatment procedures. Drugs such as sedatives and hypnotics result in disturbed sleep patterns, including reductions in slow wave and rapid eye movement (REM) sleep. Sleep disturbance is a significant stressor in the ICU, contributing to impaired cognition and possibly affecting recovery. The ICU nurse can structure the environment to promote patient sleep. Strategies include clustering activities, scheduling rest, making physiologic measurements without changing the patients position (when appropriate), limiting noise, and promoting comfort and relaxation.

Sleep deprivation: An essential part of the 24-hour cycle, sleep accounts for approximately one third of a persons life. An adequate amount of uninterrupted sleep is essential to prevent exhaustion or illness and maintain physiologic and psychologic well-being. Rapid eye movement (REM) sleep, important for mental restoration, occurs primarily in the last cycles of uninterrupted sleep and is the likely form of sleep to be affect by sleep deprivation in the ICU.

Hourly intervention is frequently necessary in the critical care unit to maintain physiologic homeostasis. This recurrent disruption in the sleep cycle quickly leads to a lack of REM sleep. Adverse effects of REM sleep deprivation include irritability, anxiety, physical exhaustion, disruption of metabolic functions, and respiratory distress.

The critical care nurse must assess the patient and determine whether adequate periods of uninterrupted time have been provided to promote all stages of sleep. Sleep periods should be included in the care plan and adhered to as such much as possible. Consideration must be given to the importance of interventions versus the necessity of uninterrupted sleep periods. Health care personnel should not subject patients to activity or stressful procedures during the early morning hours unless they are imperative. Visiting times should balance the needs of the patient and family while supporting adequate rest. Recent studies suggest that longer but less frequent visits may be more desirable than the traditional plan of a few minutes each hour.

Acute confusion: The risk of developing acute confusion is high in the critical care setting. The high-technology environment is overwhelming and can be frightening for the patient. The presence of serious or traumatic illness adds additional psychologic and physiologic stress. Confusion is common among all patients in ICUs but especially older patients. It has a rapid onset and is generally reversible but can be distressing for both patient and family. Symptoms of acute confusion include hallucinations (both visual and auditory), restlessness, memory impairment, and fluctuations in the patient's level of awareness.

Initial patient assessment should include information about the patient's mental status before admission. If the patient was able to adequately perform activities of daily living, it is reasonable to expect that he or she can return to that level of function once the acute confusion resolves.

Overwhelming stress is a frequent contributor to acute confusion, and the nurse must try to make the critical care environment therapeutic rather than stressful. In the past patients were physically restrained to protect them from harm. This type of intervention controls the patient's behavior but frequently increases confusion and leads to combativeness, which may necessitate chemical sedation. Interventions ideally focus on removing stressors rather than adding to the problem. Current thinking focuses on alternative to physical restraints. Fostering reality orientation by spending time with the patient and encouraging interaction with family and significant others should be priority with the confused patient. Reality orientation is an ongoing regimen of providing information to the patient at regular intervals as needed.

This intervention is initiated immediately after admission to the ICU and is maintained until the patient can repeat the information on request.

Problem Related to Family Members of ICU Patient

The experience of having a friend or family member in the ICU is physically and emotionally difficult. Families of the critically ill are usually anxious about the patient's condition and prognosis. They have concerns regarding the patient's pain and other discomforts. They may question the quality of care that the patient is receiving. In addition, it is common for families to experience anxiety regarding the financial problems related to planning and providing care in the next phases of the illness. The family will typically be experiencing disruption of their daily routines in order to support the patient. They may be far from their own home, routines, and supportive friends and family members. During these difficult times, they are often asked to make critical decisions.

Lack of information is a source of anxiety for families. The nurse should assess the family's understanding of the patient's status, goals, treatments, and prognosis and provide information as appropriate. The first time the family member visits it is important for the nurse to prepare the visitor for the experience by briefly describing the patients appearance, condition, treatments, tubes, and equipment. Families should be told what to expect regarding the environment (sounds, noise, odors). It is helpful if the nurse can accompany the family members as they enter the room. They should be encouraged to touch, hug, and speak with the patient. Chairs should be provided whenever possible. The nurse should observe the responses of both patient and family to the visit. The patient may be fatigued by the visitors yet unwilling to ask them to leave. The visitors might have a difficult time dealing with a sick loved one and may need help and support. Rather than a rigid open or closed visiting policy, each patient should have a plan tailored to the patients and family's needs.

The family needs information about he way in, which the patient's care is managed and decisions are made. They should have the opportunity to affect decision-making. The family should be invited to meet the health care team members, including physicians, dietian, respiratory therapist, social worker, and physical therapist. The nurse should evaluate the appropriateness of including family members to accept and cope with problems if they observe that providers are caring and competent, that decisions are deliberate, and that they themselves have the opportunity to help shape the course of care.

The nurse should assess the family to determine the appropriate extent of their involvement in care. In some cases this might be limited to sitting with the patient and holding the patients hand during quiet periods. Other family members might welcome the opportunity to participate in physical care such as shaving or oral hygiene. The nurse should encourage such activity. Other contributions include assisting with procedures, ambulation, and feeding. Family involvement should be included in the plan of care.

While working with families, the ICU nurse should assess the response of the family to the stress. Their feelings should be acknowledged and accepted. They should be supported in their decisions. Institutional support systems such as chaplains, social workers, and psychologists may be helpful in assisting the family and patient to adjust. The extent to which the family is involved and supported will in turn affect the patients clinical course in the ICU.

Stressors in ICU

The ICU environment is exceptionally stressful for the nursing staff. The nurses stress stems partially from high expectations: advanced knowledge of physiology related to all body systems, astute observational and physical assessment skills, ability to quickly prioritize and make decisions regarding patient care, and technical proficiency in operating the highly sophisticated equipment. Nurses also increasingly face complex ethical issues that consume their time and emotional energy. In addition, the constant vigilance and emergency ready atmosphere may promote an uneasy sense of impending crisis. Critical care nurses must be able to remain and communicate effectively with the patient and family during crisis situations.

Most critical care nurses select this area of practice at least in part because they feel stimulated by a fast-paced environment that requires them to effectively integrate a detailed knowledge base, excellent assessment skills, and significant technologic proficiency. Manageable stress levels can promote creativity and productivity. However, continuous high-level stress can be as detrimental to the nurse as to the patient in the critical care environment or ICU includes the following:

Patients and Family Stressors

- Unfamiliar environment, new faces.
- Noise, light levels.
- Sensory deprivation or overload.
- Interruption of sleep-wake cycles.
- Inaccessibility of family, friends.
- Lack of privacy.
- Lack of information or understanding of prognosis and care plan.
- Lack of information or understanding of policies and procedures.
- Anticipation of painful interventions.
- Confusion or disorientation related to physiologic factors.
- Impaired communication related to intubation.

- Observation of crisis interventions in other patients.
- Fear related to diagnosis.
- Fear of death.
- Conflict between patient or family goals and staff goals.
- Pain.

Staff Stressors

- Expectations of self.
- Expectations of peers, clinical supervisors, other health care team members, hospital administrators.
- Intricate machinery and techniques.
- Closed, crowded work area.
- Constant contact with seriously ill or dying patients.
- Continual vigilance over multiple patients.
- Constant emergency readiness.
- Sustained high activity level.
- Limited breaks from high-stress unit.
- Limited communication with many patients because of intubation or altered level of consciousness.
- Limited opportunity to communicate with families.
- Isolation from other nurses in hospital.
- Ethical conflicts related to resuscitation and use of life-support equipment.
- Legal issues.
- Exposure to infectious diseases.

In addition to understanding how stressors affect the patient and family, critical care nurses must guard their own physical and psychologic health by recognizing and decreasing their own stress levels. They must develop in ability to understand and respond appropriately to their own needs for support in the daily work environment, as well as the needs of their colleagues. Failure to develop self-care strategies may hamper the nurse's ability to respond appropriately to patient needs and ultimately leads to nurse burnout and exit from the health care field.

Long-term involvement with patients in a critical care environment is a relatively new phenomenon and is accompanied by significant new stressors. Technology currently enables medical science to extend the life of some critically ill patients, such as those awaiting organ transplantation, who may have critical care hospitalizations that extend weeks to months. Consistent nurse caregivers can develop a strong therapeutic relationship with the patient and family and help them cope with the stressors of the critical care environment. Nurses caring for patients on an ongoing basis may even be able to more quickly assess and respond to changes in the patients' condition. However, they may become so close to the circumstances of the patient's illness that their own psychologic health suffers. It is important for clinicians to recognize when ongoing care of a patient results in undue stress and to develop strategies for protecting their mental health. Strategies include:

- Development of support networks among nursing peers.
- Use of employee assistance personnel (counselors, social services personnel, and chaplains: critical stress debriefing) to cope with stressful circumstances.
- Development of interests outside the critical care environment to help keep personal and professional worlds separate.
- Careful self-evaluation of the values, beliefs, and feelings associated with the critical care milieu.
- Use of a multidisciplinary team approach to nursing care, in collaboration with direct caregivers such as physicians; respiratory, speech, and physical therapists; and other care providers such as nutritionists, pharmacists, clergy, social workers, radiology technicians, clerical assistants, and hospital volunteers.
- Acknowledgement of the need to occasionally change assignments to provide respite for the clinician.
- Scheduling of regular clinical care conferences with the patient, significant others, and other multidisciplinary team members to help the patient feel less dependent on the nursing staff. Conferences allow the patient and family to provide important input into the overall care plan and to feel the tangible involvement of various members of the multidisciplinary team. This approach is particularly important for the long-term critical care patient. Care goals can be reevaluated, modifications agreed on, or new goals established.

The death of a critically ill patient can be the source of tremendous emotional stress to the nurse. To help protect against overwhelming stress, when caring for a dying patient the nurse should:

- Examine his or her own feelings about death.
- Listen attentively to the expressed needs of the patient and family.
- Remain available to the patient and family both physically and emotionally.
- Use touch, if culturally acceptable, in caring for the patient and family.
- Reassure the patient and family that the patient will continue to receive skilled and compassionate care even if a do-not-resuscitate decision has been made.
- Attempt to remain nonjudgmental about family or hospital issues.
- Respect the strengths and limitations of the patient-family relationship, which existed long before the patient-hospital relationship.
- Include the family in care.
- Provide for patient and family privacy.
- Provide the opportunity for the family to exercise religious or cultural traditions.

Providing comprehensive care to critically ill patients and their families is a challenging opportunity. The critical care nurse combines the technologic sophistication of this unique setting with a personal, individualized care approach to maximize the positive potential outcomes for the patient.

Ethical Decision Making in Critical Care Nursing

In many ways technologic advances in health care have evolved faster than society's ability to understand the associated ethical dilemmas. Life can be prolonged in ways that were previously impossible, sometimes beyond all known hope of recovery. Tremendous emotional, financial, legal, and social ramifications exist as patients are stabilized in conditions for which long-term health care options are limited. For example, few families and even fewer skilled care facilities have the resources to care for a patient who requires continuous mechanical ventilation.

With the advent of advance directives, nurses frequently assume responsibility for gathering information about the patient's wishes concerning the extent of their care or treatment. Patients frequently have not prepared advance directives or are incompetent to render such a decision, leaving the family and significant others to determine the type and extent of medical care the patient would or would not want in this situation. Critical care nurses frequently assist families with highly emotional decisions such as forgoing resuscitation or withdrawing life support systems. Assisting families with these decisions is painfully complex.

All health care professionals must examine their own beliefs about life and death, termination of life, organ and tissue donation, and use of limited resources. Education and support for the nurse are available from formal classes, support groups, peers and hospital ethics committees. Ethics committees are also available to patients, families, and staff members who wish consultation and support in difficult or divisive situations.

Biomedical advances at times seem to challenge the compassionate aspects of care giving. The critical care nurse is the professional caregiver best qualified to play a pivotal role in identifying and supporting the patient's wishes.

Management of the Patient in Critical Care Unit/ICU

Management of critically ill patients requires establishment of a database, identification of actual and potential nursing diagnoses and collaborative problems, delineation of priorities, definition of outcome criteria, execution of planned interventions, and modification of future interventions and plans on the basis of current outcomes.

The assessment process for the critically ill patient differs from the assessment of other patients only in terms of the technologies used. The cardiac monitor, hemodynamic monitoring lines, and laboratory analyses provide data that the nurse must incorporate into the total patient assessment. Technologies provide adjuncts to the data the nurse gathers through observation, history taking, and physical examination. Monitored data are useless unless correlated with physical findings and integrated into meaningful analysis by the critical care nurse.

The importance of accurate, thorough initial information cannot be overemphasized. However, the multiple sources of data and fluctuating condition of critically ill patients make constant priority reorganization a necessity. The critical care nurse continually updates the database to reformulate short-term goals and interventions.

Patient assessment must be thorough, yet rapid. The nurse must consider the physical and psychologic reactions of an entire organism under stress, while remaining open to the unusual or unexpected. Patient assessment also must be organized and repetitive so that small alterations or deviations from previous findings will be apparent. Finally, the assessment must be individualized, with time and attention given to significant aspects.

The patient may be admitted to critical care as either a direct admission (usually through the emergency department), as a transfer from another patient care division in the same or a different hospital, or as a postoperative admission after certain operations. The critical care nurse integrates data from the patient and family, written history, and the transfer report of other nurses into the patient's initial treatment plan. Consultation between transferring and receiving nursing unit staffs is essential to accomplish this process effectively. These data sources help ensure continuity of care and communication of all issues important to the patient or family. The nurse carefully explores the patient's and family's response to the need for critical care placement. A full patient profile may be deferred until later in the hospitalization, as hemodynamic stabilization is always the first priority of care. The initial contact with the critical care personnel sets the tone for all future interactions and is an invaluable opportunity for the nurse to demonstrate competence and caring and begin to establish a foundation of trust.

The physical assessment of the patient, while augmented by the technology of the intensive care unit, still uses the skills of inspection, palpation, percussion, and auscultation to determine the patients care needs and evaluate responses to interventions. The critical care nurse combines these physical assessment may take place hourly or even more frequently as patient status dictates. All disciplines involved in the patients care participate in the ongoing assessment process. The dynamic and collaborative nature of critical care assessment allows for rapid responses to any changes in patient status, but it may also contribute to the patient's sensory overload. The need to evaluate status changes frequently may leave the patient with little time for rest and privacy. Significant nursing skill is required to balance information gathering and patient rest. It may take years of experience for the nurse to gather and synthesize several pieces of data simultaneously, thoroughly, and rapidly, with the least disruption to the patient.

Monitored data: Nurses in all clinical settings use tools such as stethoscopes, sphygmomanometers, thermometers, and scales to collect patient data. Critical care nurses also have access to tools that are capable of continuous data collection, such as cardiac monitors, hemodynamic pressure lines, intracranial pressure and monitoring devices, and airway pressure monitoring devices. The explosion in critical care technology since the 1970s provides the critical care nurse with amazing quantities of objective data. Digital computerized monitoring systems occupy less space and provide more capabilities than ever before. The most sophisticated patient data management systems take information from all the monitored parameters (ECG, respirations, intraarterial pressure, pulmonary artery pressure, venous oxygen saturation, central venous pressure, intracranial pressure, and body temperature), combine it with manually entered data (such as weight, height, intake and output, and times of drug administration), and produce a wide array of hemodynamic and pulmonary calculations and patient response trends for analysis by critical care practitioners.

Technologic adjuncts to critical care assessment are continuously changing, combining older and well-tested monitoring systems with newer advances. Certain types of monitoring equipment are used in all critical care environments. Waveforms and other data produced by these devices may be viewed continuously on a video screen or be graphed for a permanent record.

Many monitoring systems involve use of fluid, tubing, and transducer equipment, which acts as portals of entry for microorganisms. Strict aseptic technique is essential to prevent complications associated with nosocomial infections

- *Cardiac monitoring:* It is a noninvasive procedure that poses minimal risk to the patient. It consists of placing conductive electrodes on the patient's chest that recognize the electrical activity of the heart and relay it to a video display screen. Depending on the sophistication of the monitoring equipment, the clinician may be able to view the patients ECG and heart rate at the bedside and at remote locations in the critical care unit, monitor changes during activity (with mobile equipment), and set flexible monitoring parameters as changes in cardiac status occur. Parameters may include changes in heart rate and rhythm; in respiratory rate and rhythm; in analysis of dysrhythmias; and in specific ECG segments, such as the ST segment for ischemia recognition. Alarms notify the clinician when preset limits have been reached. Most monitors default to preset limits if the clinician does not set specific alarm parameters and only allow clinicians to silence the alarms for a limited time.
- *Hemodynamic monitoring*: Refers to invasive monitoring of the arterial or venous system. Monitoring is accomplished through catheters that measure changes in air and fluid pressures and can also be used to administer intravenous fluids and obtain arterial or venous blood for laboratory analysis. Transducers connected to the system interpret the air and fluid pressure readings and display the results as waveforms on cardiac monitoring equipment. The two most commonly used hemodynamic monitoring systems are intraarterial monitoring and pulmonary artery monitoring.

  It is important for the nurse to verify the digital display of waveform values with a manual sphygmomanometer, regularly calibrate the transducer equipment with the transducer positioned at specific landmarks on the patients body, and assess the entire system for patency and accuracy. The nurse can obtain measurements with the patient in an up to 30-degree lateral or supine position if the patient is hemodynamically stable. The nurse requires a thorough knowledge of waveform interpretation to appropriately interpret and respond to the values displayed on the screen or on a manual printout. Even minor errors in reading and interpreting values or small problems in the patency of the system, such as a tiny air bubble in the transducer system, can result in inaccurate data and may cause profound complications for the patient.

  Aseptic technique is critical to the maintenance of these systems with the least possible risk to the patient. Ongoing assessment of the patient's response to the equipment is also critical to avoid dangerous complications such as air emboli, bleeding, malposition of catheters, tissue damage, or hemodynamic compromise as a result of foreign body insertion or malposition.
- *Intra-arterial monitoring*: Involves inserting a catheter into an artery, usually the radial or femoral artery, and connecting the catheter to a high-pressure flush system filled with either a heparinized or nonheparinized saline solution. The high-pressure flush counterbalances arterial resistance to maintain patency of the system. Intraarterial systems display a continuous reading of the patient's blood pressure and provide ready access to obtain arterial blood gas or other laboratory specimens.
- *Pulmonary artery monitoring*: Involves inserting a catheter through the subclavian or internal jugular vein and advancing it into the pulmonary artery, usually under fluoroscopic guidance. These catheters have several lumens encased within a larger lumen,

and each opens at a different point along the length of the catheter. Each lumen may be used to attach monitoring and transducer equipment. The large bore of the lumens and placement of the catheter in large arteries permit administration of caustic intravenous solutions that could damage peripheral veins.

A balloon at the distal tip of the catheter if filled with approximately 1 ml of air the natural flow of blood through the patient's heart pulls the balloon into place in the pulmonary artery. When the catheter is correctly placed, the balloon is deflated. Monitoring and transducer equipment is attached to the catheter.

The catheter and monitoring equipment are used to obtain significant data about the patient's hemodynamic and cardiac function. Available data include pulmonary artery and central venous pressure recordings and cardiac output measurements. Combining these values with parameters such as blood pressure and body surface area it possible to calculate additional information that is not directly available from catheter readings. Newer monitoring equipment calculates these values automatically when data are entered into the database, decreasing the chance for error from manual calculation. The pulmonary artery catheter rapidly provides valuable information to evaluate the patients response to vasoactive drugs by providing data about left- and right-sided heart function. It is also significant tool for managing severe cardiac failure and cardiogenic shock.

- *A central venous pressure (CVP)*: Catheter may be used in lieu of a pulmonary artery catheter when evaluation of pulmonary artery pressure and left-sided heart function are not required. CVP catheters may be connected to a transducer and used to measure right-sided heart pressures and deliver intravenous fluids, but they are more limited than pulmonary artery catheters in the scope of data they provide. A newer type of central line is called a peripherally inserted central venous catheter (PICC). The nurse assess and maintains the external portion of the PICC and may instruct patients and families in these techniques for home use. PICC lines are long-dwell catheters that require the same aseptic care as other central lines. They can be used for long-term fluid and medication administration but at present have no monitoring capabilities.
- *Monitoring intracranial pressure (ICP)*: Involves placing a catheter through the skull into either the subarachnoid space or the cerebral ventricle to monitor changes in pressure within the cranial cavity. A transducer and tubing system gather the data, which are displayed on monitoring screens. Newer monitoring systems have the capacity to sense changes in intracranial pressure and display pressure readings on a bedside monitor without the use of fluid-filled pressure tubing and transducer systems. Although insertion through the skull into the cranial cavity is still required, these newer systems reduce the risk of contamination by microorganisms.

  Patients with unstable intracranial pressure may be sensitive to routine nursing interventions such as turning, suctioning, and changing bed position. Continuous display of ICP readings allows the nurse to constantly evaluate the patient's response to all interventions and take prompt action if the patient's pressure reaches unsafe levels. The catheter also can be used to aspirate cerebrospinal fluid fro analysis or culture and to relieve elevated ICP. The nurse is responsible for identifying changes in pressure readings, analyzing trends, evaluating patient responses to interventions or therapies, and preventing complications.

- *Continuous airway pressure monitoring (CAPM)*: Is a simple, noninvasive technique that uses a transducer cable, high-pressure tubing (as used for measuring pulmonary and arterial pressures), and a display monitor. The monitoring equipment is connected to a ventilator circuit at the Y connector near the airway. Standard calibration procedures are used, but the monitoring tubing is filled with air, not fluid, and the transducer can be at any level while calibration is performed. The absence of fluid in the transducer system minimizes the risk of infection. The waveforms produced by CAPM may be continuously displayed, graphed, and compared with hemodynamic waveforms.

  The waveforms produced by the system enable the clinician to continuously monitor the patient's response to various modes of mechanical ventilation and therapeutic interventions. CAPM is also useful in identifying one of the most common complications of mechanical ventilation: patient ventilator asynchrony or intolerance. Asynchrony can result from mechanical malfunction, inappropriate ventilator mode selection and inadequate inspiratory flow rate, airway obstruction from excessive secretions, or patient anxiety or agitation. Asynchrony increases the work of breathing and can result in inadequate gas exchange. When a patient experiences asynchrony, the CAPM waveforms deviate from the expected patterns, altering the nurse to the need for prompt intervention. CAPM can be especially helpful in monitoring sedated, very ill, or chemically relaxed patients who may be unable to communicate patient-ventilator intolerance. CAPM provides the bedside nurse with continuous visual assurance that the patient is receiving adequate ventilation and that chemical relaxation is being delivered at an appropriate dose. Any interruption of ventilation is immediately apparent by waveform absence.

Analysis of the patient's waveforms and comparison with expected waveforms allow the care team to evaluate the patient's response to mechanical ventilation and modify the plan if necessary. Hemodynamic pressure data frequently serve as the foundation of treatment for critically ill patients. However, both real and artificial changes in the hemodynamic waveforms occur in response to pressure in the hemodyanamic waveforms occur in response to pressure gradients produced by the pulmonary and systemic circulation. True pressures can be further obscured by tachypnea and underlying cardiac pathologic conditions. CAPM may be used in these situations to help standardize measurements. Simultaneous graphing of CAPM and pulmonary artery pressures provides a clear visual picture of end expiration. CAPM has thus been shown to be a simple, costefficient and effective adjunct to critical care monitoring.

In using any invasive or noninvasive tools, the nurse must be knowledgeable about the proper use and maintenance of the equipment, including the appearance of the waveform associated with each line, standard interventions used to prevent complications, signs and symptoms of complications, and troubleshooting techniques for when problem develop. The patient risk associated with invasive monitoring lines is significantly reduced when knowledgeable personnel manage the lines. In addition to the various invasive lines used for monitoring, critical care nurses also must be skillful in using central lines for medication, fluid, and nutrition administration.

As monitoring techniques become increasingly sophisticated, the health care provider may be tempted to treat solely based on the numbers and waveforms produced by the equipment. It is essential for the clinician to remember that these data must always be combined with data from routine physical assessment, including the patient's general appearance and subjective response to all therapeutic measures. A flat line on a waveform may be the result of a disconnected wire to tubing rather than a change in the patient's condition. The nurse must remain vigilant and keep one eye on the monitor and one eye on the patient to avoid treating the equipment instead of the patient. The nurse must also tailor the use of each monitoring technique to each unique patient situation.

Nursing Problems and their Interventions

Impaired Gas Exchange

Common nursing objectives for the patient with a diagnosis of impaired gas exchange are:

Patient will:

- Demonstrate satisfactory pulmonary function: Adequate blood oxygenation, hemoglobin saturation, and forced expiratory volume in 1 second.
- Maintain a satisfactory respiratory rate and pattern.

For which nurse in a critical care setting the immediate goal of ensuring a patients survival determines the priorities for intervention; physiologic problems must be addressed first. Once the critical care team has alleviated life-threatening stressors, they can re-evaluate priorities and address other problems. Physiologic priorities are determined by the degree of threat to the person's survival. Certain body systems are more prone to disorders requiring intensive therapeutic interventions that are frequently encountered in the critical care unit. At the most basic level, these priorities can be organized in the same "ABC" framework as basic cardiac life support. Establishment of airway, breathing, and circulation remains the foundation for therapeutic management of the critical care patient. By applying the ABCs of basic life support, the critical care nurse is able to move from the most parsing to least pressing patient problems. When a patients physiologic status begins to deteriorate, clinicians take immediate actions to reverse the problem. Correct positioning of the endotracheal tube with suctioning as needed ensues airway patency. The nurse then assess the patients ability to breathe and the effect of physical restraints or physiologic conditions such as acute respiratory failure. The patients pulse oximetry and blood gases are also monitored for normalcy and early signs of distress.

Decreased Cardiac Output

Common nursing objectives for the patient with a diagnosis of decreased cardiac output are:

Patient will:

- Maintain systolic blood pressure above 100 mm Hg, urine output greater than 30 ml/hr, and cardiac rate and rhythm within acceptable limits.
- Maintain good tissue perfusion.
- Maintain stable vital signs.

For which after initially focusing on airway and breathing management, the nurse addresses circulatory needs, such as the establishment of normal cardiac rhythm, intravenous access for administration of medications, and adequate cardiopulmonary perfusion of vital organs. The critical care clinician may continue to use this basic ABC principle in ongoing assessments to ensure that problems are recognized before complication develop. The nurse improves cardiac output by reducing workload on the heart and increasing venous return. The patient is placed in the semi-Flowler's position. Rest and quiet are important. The nurse continues to assess the blood pressure, capillary refill, urine output, presence of edema, and laboratory values. Maintaining intravenous accesses is important, since most medications and fluids are delivered intravenously.

Anxiety

Common nursing objectives for the patient with a diagnosis of anxiety are:

Patient will:

- Report an increase in psychologic comfort.
- Report a decrease in restless and other behavioral manifestations of anxiety.

For which the initial step in preventing or alleviating psychologic stress is to identify the patients and family's perception of the critical event. Their perceptions will be affected by their individual personalities, current psychologic health, general understanding of the situation and its projected outcome, tolerance for an ambiguity, and normal pattern of coping. Initial perceptions are often significantly affected by previous exposure to similar events, either positive or negative, and general level of familiarity with medical interventions and the hospital environment. The critically ill person, separated from familiar surroundings and dependent on others to meet the most basic needs, becomes partially or totally isolated from usual support systems. Feelings of helplessness, loneliness, and depersonalization, as well as disturbances in body image, are common. Modes of expressing and thereby relieving frustration, anger, hostility, fear or depression are limited by the physical constraints of the critical care environment. Anger and hostility are often indications of fear and anxiety. Depression and withdrawal may be normal signs of hopelessness, loneliness, powerlessness, or loss.

Consistently assigned caregivers can be an effective way to establish a therapeutic relationship with the patient and family. An atmosphere of openness and acceptance that encourages expression of feelings can help patients cope. The nurse talks openly and honestly with the patient to decrease feelings of depersonalization, isolation and alienation. The nurse encourages the patient and family to express their feelings and assists the patient in identifying the fears and concerns that may be causing unusual or inappropriate behavior. The nurse or other health care team members who help patients talk about feelings must be to accept whatever emotionally laden information might be expressed. Nonjudgmental recognition and acceptance of the patient's feelings help reinforce the patients right to the feelings.

Intubated patients are unable to express their feelings freely even when alert and oriented and are therefore particularly vulnerable to psychologic stressors. The nurse must guard against the normal inclination to communicate less with persons who cannot talk easily. Strategies such as keeping a letter board, paper and pencil, or "magic slate" within the patient's reach and providing assistance to the patient help reduces the sense of isolation. However, such methods do not allow the patient to truly express feelings and concerns. The nurse carefully assesses the patient for cues concerning his or her emotional state and anticipates common concerns among critically ill patients. The nurse can verbalize the potential concerns and allow the patient to validate them as appropriate. The direct expression of empathy for the patient and family conveys acceptance and understanding.

Interrupted Family Processes

Common nursing objectives for the patient with a diagnosis of interrupted family processes are:

Patient and family will:
- Identify the stress of having a family member admitted to a critical care unit.
- State community and personal resources available to enhance coping abilities.

The essence of crisis intervention is helping persons cope with a major life crisis that a critical illness may precipitate. Critical care nursing is far broader in scope and more future oriented than crisis intervention alone, but specific situations frequently require the immediacy and limited focus of crisis intervention. At the time of crisis the nurse helps the patient and family establish short-term goals and minimize the number and scope of decisions they must make. As the crisis situation stabilizes, the nurse provides the patient and family with more information and helps them accept additional responsibility for decision-making and goal setting. When the patient and family are knowledgeable about the goals of therapy and understand the patient's diagnosis, current status, and prognosis, they can be involved in many aspects of care planning and can make decisions consistent with the treatment regimen.

Involvement of significant others decreases the patients feelings of powerlessness, frustration, and anxiety. The family is likely to be involved in care giving at some point in the patients recovery, and the maldisciplinary team must begin including them in care planning soon as possible. The patient is reassured by having a loving advocate represent his or her wishes and concerns. Even when a patient is unconscious, visits by key support figures who talk to and touch the patient may have positive, if immeasurable, effects on the patient while ameliorating the family's feelings of helplessness.

The nurse actively involves all alert patients in goal setting and care planning. The nurse seeks to increase the patients feeling of personal control in structuring the daily schedule of activities. The knowledge that nursing staff values the patient's preferences and views the patient as capable of making decisions reinforces the importance of the patient's role in recovery.

The environment of the critical care unit presents multiple stresses to the patient and family. Narcotics and sedatives, anxiety, hypoxia, sleep deprivation, and multiple metabolic derangements all contribute to acute confusion, disturbed thought processes, and perceptual distortions. The nurse uses reality orientation on an ongoing basis to help patients regain their mental stability. Although some environmental factors cannot be altered, the nurse can use a variety of strategies to control the sensory level of the critical care unit.

Critical care units increasingly recognize the importance of visits by the patients significant others in minimizing psychologic stressors. The practice of restrictive and minimal visitation is being policies range from longer and more frequent visitation hours to true open visitation, where the patient and family participate fully in care activities and care team rounds. Although these policies appear to improve the patients and family's trust and therapeutic relationship with the care team, the nurse must be careful to avoid overwhelming the family with the daily stress and sensory overload of the critical care unit. The nurse should encourage significant others to meet their own needs for rest, nutrition, psychosocial support, relaxation, and spiritual renewal. Many significant others need support in their decision to leave the critical care environment at regular intervals, even when visitation policies would allow them to remain.

In the critical care setting the patients psychologic needs often assume priority, and care providers may ignore the patients needs as a social being. Limited visiting hours, the strange technical environment, and the aura of danger in the critical care unit isolate patients from their usual social roles. For the most part, staff members view a person who is critically ill primarily in the patient role. The more significant roles of spouse, parent, child, lover, sibling, friend, or provider may go virtually unrecognized unless staff members initiate interventions to provide continuity in these relationships.

The nurse can foster continuity in social roles through the same types of interventions used to reduce psychologic stress; increasing visits between patient and family; including the family in discussions of disease process, prognosis, and care plans; and encouraging the family to report events and activities occurring in other significant spheres of the patients life. Relaying telephone messages between the patient and distant friends is another way the nurse can help the patient maintain contact with his or her broader external world.

One effective way to prevent disruption in relationship is for the nurse to carefully explain the patients physical appearance and the critical care environment to family or friends before their first visit with the patient in the critical care unit. Visitors need to understand the patient's level of consciousness, ability to communicate, and comprehension. They need to understand the importance of their presence to the patient and the patients need for their support. When visitors approach the bedside, the nurse remains with them if possible to facilitate their initial interaction with the patient. Family frequently needs to be encouraged to touch the patient and offer other physical expressions of their love and support. Fear of hurting the patient or disrupting the multiple monitoring devices can virtually immobilize the family member. The nurse can help family members find safe places to stand and explain the basic purpose of the various lines and tubes. The nurse also encourages the family to speak with the patient, especially unconscious or intubated patients. At each subsequent visit the nurse caring for the patient meets with the family to answer the questions and apprise them of the patients progress.

The critical care nurse also must recognize the inevitability of role changes for some patients and families during a critical illness. Roles of provider, decision maker, employer, and employee may be altered, reversed, or eliminated. Family and friends may need to assume some or all of the patient's responsibilities at this time.

During the critical phase of illness, family members trying to cope with significant role change and additional responsibilities may need help in working through problems. The nurse needs to be sensitive to these problems and provide the family with professional guidance, such as from a social worker, to assist in reorganizing themselves and their resources. The nurse may help the family appoint a temporary family representative, someone who knows and is able to represent the wishes of a family as a whole and who can be contracted in an emergency. The nurse also may help the family plan visiting schedules that meet the patient's needs without preventing family members from fulfilling their own responsibilities. This is a period of great emotional stress for both patient and family.

Patient and family teaching is an integral part of nursing care for the patient in the critical care unit.

Index

Page numbers followed by *f* refer to figure and *t* refer to table.

A

Abacavir 477
Abdomen 95, 214, 334
  acute 127
  percussion of 95
  right upper quadrant of 181
Abdominal aneurysm, ruptured 127
Abdominal bruits 255
Abdominal discomfort 412, 476
Abdominal distension 125, 127, 232, 519
Abdominal paradox 45
Abdominal penetrating trauma 127
Abdominal reflex 568
Abdominal rigidity 127
Abdominal trauma 128, 136
Abducens nerves 566
Ablative therapy 345
Abrasion chondroplasty 422
Abruption placenta 231
Abruptly discontinue medication 417
Abscess 16, 232, 303, 544
  formation 493
  peritonsillar 556
Absorption atelectasis 87
Acapella 90
Acetaminophen 41
Acetazolamide diamox 534
Acetone 506
Acetazolamide 539
Acetylcholine 599, 603
Acetylsalicylic acid 41
Achalasia 111
  management of 112
  treatment of 112
Achilles reflex 568
Achilles tendenitis 428
Aching, chronic 433
Acid causes coagulation 532
Acid suppression, drugs for 118
Acid-base balance 46
Acid-fast
  bacilli 46
  smear culture 46
Acidosis 23, 232, 268
Acne 382
  rosacea 383
  treatment of 382
  vulgaris 382
Acoustic nerve 567
Acoustic neuroma 548, 582, 634
Acquired immunity 451
Acquired immunodeficiency syndrome 327, 457, 459, 469, 473, 475
  dementia complex 331
Acral cyanosis 232
Acrylonitrile 616
Actinic keratosis 384
Acupressure and massage 39
Acupuncture 40
Acute gastritis 114
  etiology of 114
Acute laryngeal edema 558
  treatment of 559
Acyclovir 582
Adalimumab 418
Addison's disease 356
Adenoids, chronic enlargement of 557
Adenovirus 552, 554
Adequate airway, maintenance of 33
Adhesions 133
Adhesive otitis media 546
Adipose tissue 358
Administering analgesics, principles of 41
Administration of analgesics, nurse's role in 41
Adrenal gland, disorders of 352
Adrenal insufficiency 630
Adrenergic agents 534
Adrenergic inhibitors 161
Adrenergic nerve endings 159
Adrenocortical insufficiency 356
Adrenocorticotropic hormone 338, 514
Adrenolytics 159
Aerobic bacteria 15
Aerosol nebulization therapy 90
Agnosia 587, 590
Air pollution 80
Airborne precautions 492
Airway 32, 511
  breathing, circulation, disability (ABCD) method 638
  clearance, ineffective 466
  maintenance of 32
  obstruction 512, 513, 559
  patency 352
Akinesia 600
Albuterol 464
Alcohol 156, 179, 228, 304
  consumption 616
  excessive of 447
  intoxication 28
  withdrawal 516
  recognition of 517
Aldosterone 353
Aldosteronism 355
Alendronates 446
Alkaline phosphatase 96, 142, 401
Alkylating agents 233, 459, 626, 627
Allergen 281, 282, 463
  immune mediator reaction, site of 464
Allergic antibiotic 268
Allergic attack, acute 466
Allergic contact dermatitis 378, 470
Allergic phenomena 378
Allergic reaction 354, 504
Allergic rhinitis 552
Allergic transfusion reactions 467
Allergy 450, 463, 510
  testing 466
Allopurinol 425
Alopecia 370, 398, 418, 633
  preventing 631
Alpha and hemolytic streptococci 195
Alpha blockers 161
  centrally acting 161
Alpha receptors blockers 159
Alpha-fetoprotein 312
Alpha-glucosidase 360
Altered health maintenance 551
Altered mental status 181
Aluminium 125
Alveolar basement membrane 254
Alveolar collapse 512
Alzheimer's disease 604
Ambulatory and home care 484
Ambulatory surgery 500
  discharge criteria 521
Amebiasis 123, 487
Amenorrhea 142, 286
  pathophysiology of 287
  primary 286
  secondary 286
American Rheumatoid Association 417
Amikacin 52, 539
Amiodarone 192
Amitriptyline 41, 433, 598
Amniotic fluid embolus 231
Amoxicillin 250
  trimethoprim sulphate 546
Amphotericin B 268
Ampicillin 581
Amprenavir 477
Amsler grid test 527
Amyloidosis 253
Amyotrophic lateral sclerosis 605
Anabolic steroids 486
Anaerobic bacteria 15
Anakinra 418
Anal fissure 138
Analgesia, patient-controlled 517
Analgesics 228, 250
Anaphylactic shock 32, 172, 463
Anaphylaxis 268, 354, 456, 464
Anareobic organism 554
Anatomic site classification 618
Androgens 352, 353, 628, 629
Anemia 142, 179, 217, 227, 417, 633
Anesthesia
  administration 507
  care provider 506
  general 507
  types of 507
Aneurysm 203
  repair 585
Angina 168, 181
  and myocardial infarction 168*t*
  pectoris 164
Angioma 370
Angiotensin converting enzyme 254
  inhibitors 160, 162
Angiotensin receptor blockers 160
Animal dander 466
Ankle 424
  jerk 568

Ankylosing spondylitis 398, 428, 429
Anomaly, congenital 256
Anorectal abscess 138
Anorectal disorders 137
Anorectal fistula 138
Anorectal surgery 124
Anorexia 125, 142, 181, 428, 622, 633
Anosognosia 587
Anoxia
　acute 231
　severe 575
Anoxic encephalopathies 571
Antacids 109, 125
　plus alginic acid 109
Anterior cord syndrome 610
Anthracycline 627
Anthralgia 431
Anthrax 487
Antiadrenergic drugs 159
Antiarrhythmic drugs 191t
Antibacterial drug 233
Antibiotic 34, 228, 268, 531
Antibiotic therapy 434, 494, 546
　appropriate 196
Antibody 458
　assays 476
　deficiencies 458, 459
　hypersensitivities, tissue-specific 467
　response 451
　role of 453
　types of 461
Anticholinergic nasal spray 553
Anticipated resources 640
Anticoagulants 23
Anticonvulsant drugs 233
Antidepressants 125
Antidiuretic hormone 339, 514
Anti-DNA antibodies 402, 471
Antiemetic drugs 107t
Antiepileptic drugs 593t
Antiestrogens 628
Antifolates 459
Antifungal cream 374
Antigen 451
　administration of 459
Antigen-antibody
　binding 453
　complex 455, 456, 469
　　hypersensitivities 469
　treatment of 469
Antigenic determinant 449, 453
Antihistamines 106, 553
Anti-HSV infection 609
Antihypertensive drugs 159t
Anti-inflammatory drugs 233
Antilymphocytic globulin 459
Antimalarial drugs 430
Antimetabolites 233, 459
Antimicrobial agent 459, 505
Antimicrobial therapy 582
Antineoplastic drugs 627t, 632
Antinuclear antibody 402, 430
Antiplatelet agents 230t
Antipsychotics 125
Antipyretic drugs 196
　administering of 30
Antireflux prosthesis 109
Antiretroviral drugs 483

Antiretroviral therapy 483, 484
Anti-rheumatic drugs 417
　disease modifying 418t
Anti-secretory drugs 109
Antisepsis, methods of 17
Antithymocytic globulin 459
Antithyroids 233
Anti-tubercular drugs 52t
Antitumor antibiotics 233, 626, 627
Antiviral drugs 531
Anulus fibrosus 437
Anuria 245
Anus and prostate 277
Anxiety 37, 83, 182, 262, 285, 352, 646, 653
Aortic aneurysm repair 201
Aortic dissection 204
Aortic regurgitation 199
Aortic stenosis 179, 199
Aortography 204
Aphakia 529, 536
Aphasias, types of 564
Apheresis 468
Aphthous stomatitis 101
Aplastic anemia 221, 227, 233
Appendicitis 127, 128
Apraxia 564, 590
　inability 587
Arginine vasopressin 339
Aromatase omjobotprs 628
Arrhythmias 167, 179, 180
　management of 190
Arsenic 616
Arterial blood gases 46
Arterial disorders 203
Arterial occlusive
　disease, chronic 206
　disorders, acute 205
Arteriovenous malformation 583, 585
Arthalgia 427
Arthodesis 419
Arthritis 421, 424, 430, 450
　drug-induced 447
Arthrocentesis 402
Arthrogram 400, 406
Arthroplasty 419, 422
Arthroscopy 401, 406, 419
Arthrotomy 419
Articular cartilage, loss of 421
Artificial heart chamber 201
Asbestos 616
Ascitis 142, 181
Asepsis 16
　methods of 16
Asherman's syndrome 287
Asparate aminotransferase 142
Aspergillus 544
Aspiration 513
Aspirin 41, 228, 230, 426, 498
Asterixis 142
Asthma 74, 354, 450
Astrocytoma 582
Asymptomatic infection, chronic 475
Asynchrony 652
Asystole 190
Atelectasis 64, 512, 513
Athletes foot 374, 378
Atonic seizures 592
Atopic dermatitis 378

Atrial contraction, premature 186
Atrial fibrillation 187
Atrial flutter 187
Atrial septal defect repair 201
Atrial tachycardia 186
Atrial tumor resection 201
Atrophin 535
Auditory evoked potential 540
Auditory system 539, 540
Augmentin 555
Aura 595
Autoimmune disease 287, 354, 456, 471
Autoimmune disorders 233, 338, 471
　organ specific, classifications of 471
　treatment for 471
Autoimmunity 457, 462
Automatic implantable cardioverter
　defibrillator 201
Autonomic disturbance 600
Autonomic ganglia blocker 159
Autonomic neuropathy 125
Auxiliary nursing 5
Avascular necrosis 485
Azathioprine 228, 417, 418
Aziridines 627
Azotemia 462
Azylfidine 417

B

B cell 458
　immunodeficiency 458
Babinskie's sign 569
Bacillary angiomatosis 330
Bacitracin 375
Back pain, causes of 436
Bacteremia 16, 488, 493
Bacteria 48
　destruction of 17
Bacterial endocarditis 179
Bacterial growth 374
Bacterial infections 328, 374
　treatment of 581
Bacterial sinusitis, symptom of acute 554
Bacterial skin infection 375
Bacterial vaginosis 282, 326
　gardnerella associated 281
Baker's cyst 398
Balanced suspension traction 411
Barbiturates 592
Barium
　enema 97
　sulfate 125
Bartholin's cysts 283
Bartholin's gland 278
Bartholinitis 283
Bartter's syndrome 355
Basal body temperature assessment 280
Basal cell carcinoma 385, 623
Basic aseptic technique 505
Basillar skull fracture 578
Basophils 450
Bell's palsy 608, 609
　treatment for 609
Belsey fundoplication 109, 111
Benzene 616
Benzyamides 106
Benzyl benzoate emulsion 372

Beta adrenergic
   antagonists 534
   blockers 161
Beta blockers 159, 597
Betaxolol 534
Bicarbonate 247
   deficit 27
   excess 27
Biceps reflex 568
Biguanide 360
Bile reflux gastritis 120
Biliary drainage 145
Biopsy 47, 216, 370
Biphosphonates 448
Bipolar modular prosthasis 413
Bismuth 125
Bladder
   cancer 261, 268
   control 589
   neck obstructs 264
   neoplasms 256
Bleeding syndrome 227
Blenoxane 629
Bleomycin 626, 627, 629
Blepharitis 530
Blood
   brain barrier 626
   cells 510
   chemistries 247
   clotting 455
   loss 227
   pool imaging 155
   stagnation of 398
   studies 45, 155, 278
   tests 96
   urea nitrogen 247, 497
Blood components 468
   administrative procedure of 241
   type of 240
Blood pressure 156, 511
   diastolic 156, 181
   systolic 156, 181
Blood transfusion 240, 469, 473, 478
   complication of 243
   safe practice of 469
Blood-borne hepatitis 488
Bloomycin 633
Blunt injury 531
Blur vision 232, 525, 531
B-lymphocytes 449, 453
Body electrolyte component 25
Body fluid, normal control of 25
Body mass index 90
Body size 333
Body's tissue cells 402
Bone 443
   biopsy 403
   cancer 401
   conduction 540
   deformities of 397
   deposition 447
   disease 438, 485, 486
   growth stimulators, use of 409
   mass measurement 401
   mineral deficiency 447
   necrosis 408
   pain 445
   scan 401
   tumor, nursing management of 444

Bone marrow 216, 443, 449
   cancer, type of 461
   infiltration 233
   transplantation 460
Bony enlargement 398
Bordetella pertussis 48
Bordies abscess 434
Borrelia burgdorferi 427
Bouchard's nodes 421
Bowel function, maintain regular 574
Bowel habits, change in 142
Bowel movement, decreased frequency of 125
Bowel obstruction 127
Bowel sounds
   high-pitched 232
   normal 519
Bowen's disease 384, 385
Bowing fracture 407
Brachioradialis reflex 568
Bradycardia 611
Bradykinesia 599, 600
Brain 196, 582
   abscess 582
   fog 433
   infections 575
   inflammation of 580
   injury 586
   neurons 591
   parenchyma 578
   surgery 575
   tissue 575
Brainstem
   auditory evoked potentials 570
   tumors 583
Breast 277, 621
   biopsy 280
   cancer 304, 621, 634
      male 308
   development of 617
   disease, benign 304
   female 277
   fibroadenoma of 302
   infections 303
   male 277
   physical examination 622
   problems of 301
   self examination 302, 621
   size 307
Breath 511
   diaphragmatic 18
   ineffective 551
   retraining 88
Bretylium tosylate 192
Broca's area 564
Bronchiectasis 54, 70
Bronchiolitis obliterans 70
Bronchitis
   acute 47
   chronic 71
Bronchoscopy 47
Bronchospasm 512, 513
Brown-Sequard syndrome 610
Brudzinski's reflex 568
Brudzinski's sign, positive 581
Brufen 41
Bryant's traction 410
Buccal mucosa 403
Buck's extension 410

Buck's traction 410
Buerger's disease 208
Bulge sign 399
Bullous diseases 383
Burkitt's lymphoma 238
Burn 268, 388
   and trauma, extensive 231
   classification of severity of 391
   depth 391
   injury
      electrical 389
      mechanism of 392
   location 392
   management of 393
   nursing of 395
   pain 441
   pathophysiology of 389
   severe 228
   size extent 391
   types of 389
   victim, age of 392
Burr hole 585
Bursal swellings 398
Bursectomy 406
Bursitis 406
Busulfan 626
Busulfin 633
Butarin 41
Butorphanol 41

C

Cadmium 616
Caffeine 41
Calcinosis 431
Calcium 125, 247, 258, 259, 401, 461
   channel blockers 160, 162
   levels 97
   oxalate 259
   phosphate 259
   supplements 125, 448
Calculi 256, 257, 262, 271
Callus 442
   formation 408
Caloric test stimulus 540
Campylobacter 123
Cancer 563, 613
   cells 626
      proliferating 616
   cervix 377
   chemotherapeutic agents 459
   classification of 618
   development of 617
   diagnosis of 622
   etiology of 616
   management of 623
   pathophysiology of 614
   prevention of 619
   primary prevention of 620
   secondary prevention of 620
   therapy 623
   treatment of 613, 623
   type of 614
Candida
   albicans 373, 479, 544
   species 492
Candidiasis 373
   diagnosis of 373

Cannabis derivatives 106
Caplan syndrome 416
Capreomycin 52
Captopril 160
Caput medusae 142
Carbamazepine 592, 593
Carbidopa plus levodopa 601
Carbon dioxide pressure 575
Carbon tetrachloride 268
Carbonic anydrase inhibitors 534
Cardiac and joint replacement surgery 502
Cardiac arrest 586
Cardiac arrhythmias 268
Cardiac catheterization 155
Cardiac contraction, rate of 514
Cardiac dysfunction, primary 514
Cardiac dysrhythmias 183
Cardiac failure 268, 355
Cardiac fluoroscopy 152
Cardiac monitoring 651
Cardiac surgery 201
Cardiac tumor 154
Cardiac valve diseases 179
Cardiogenic shock 167, 172, 178, 268
Cardiomyopathy 179
Cardiopulmonary diseases 354
Cardiovascular disease 485
Cardiovascular disorders, nursing
  management of 149, 515
Cardiovascular system 498, 634
  changes in 390
  nursing assessment of 149
Cardiovascular systolic hypertension 343
Carotenaemia carotenosis 370
Carotid duplex studies 570
Carpal tunnel syndrome 405
Cataract 534
  development 535
  diagnosis of 535
  formation, stages of 535
Cauda equina 437
Caudal anesthesia 507
Causative agent 15
Causative allergic agent 470
Causative organism 489
CD4 cell counts 477
CD4 lymphocytes 474
Cefaclor 555
Cefotaxime 581
Ceftriaxone 581
Cell-mediated cytotoxicity 454
Cells, malignant 615t
Cellular component 241
Cellular edema 268
Cellular immune response 451, 454
Cellular immunity 452
Cellulitis 16
Central cord syndrome 610
Central hearing loss 541
Central nervous system 507, 579
Central respiratory drive, depression of 513
Central venous pressure 651, 652
Cephalosporins 228, 268
Cerebellar symptoms 598
Cerebellar tumors 583
Cerebellopontine tumors 583
Cerebral abscess 581
Cerebral anemia 32

Cerebral angiography 569
Cerebral artery
  anterior 586
  middle 586
  posterior 587
Cerebral blood flow 575, 588
Cerebral disorders 572
Cerebral edema 579, 582
  control of 580
Cerebral hemispheres 583
Cerebral hemorrhage 28, 32
Cerebral ischemia 586
Cerebral palsy 440
Cerebral perfusion
  monitoring 589
  pressure 575
Cerebral tissue perfusion 574
Cerebrospinal fluid 476
  analysis 569
Cerebrovascular accident 125, 585
Cerebrovascular system 586
Cervical
  cancer 292, 621
  polyps 292
  spine 609
    articulations of 415
  surgery 439
Cervicitis 282
Cervix 622
Chalazion 530
Charcot-Marie-Tooth disease 440
Charcots joints 420
Chemical burn 392, 532
  emergency management of 393
  injury 389
Chemical carcinogens 616
Chemokines 456
Chemotaxis 456
Chemotherapy 293, 626
  administration of 631
  classification of 626
  nursing intervention in 629
Chemical injury 531
Chest 214
  pain 44, 149, 167, 232
  physiotherapy 89
  tightness 242
  trauma 60
Chickenpox 381, 487
Chills and fever 475
Chlamydia
  infections 323
  pneumoniae 48
  trachomatis 282, 309, 313, 320, 323, 429, 530
Chlorambucil 626
Chloramphenicol 233
Chloramycin 539
Chlorhexidine gluconate 492
Chloropromazine 41, 233, 380
Chlorpheniramine 547
Cholangiography 98
Cholecalciferol 445
Cholecystitis 127
Cholelithiasis 143
Cholemia 32
Cholera 487
Choline magnesium trisalicylate 41

Cholinesterase inhibition 534
Chromium compound 616
Chronic fatigue syndrome 471, 472
Chvostek's signs 352
Cigarette smoking 616, 622
Ciprofloxacin 250, 434
Cirrhosis of liver 141
Clonazepam 593
Clonidine 159
Clopidogrel 230
Clostridia
  botulinum 15
  tetani 15
  welchii 15
Clostridium
  difficile 123, 492, 518
  perfringens 123
Clozapine 233
Coagulation disorder 142
Coaltar derivatives 380
Cobalamin, deficiencies of 228
Cocaine 179
Coccidioides immitis 330, 479
Cognitive-behavioral interventions 37
Colchicine 425
Cold compress, elevation of 551
Coliform bacteria 426
Collagen diseases 179
Colles' fracture 447
Colon cancer 620
  risk of 618
Colonic disorders 125
Colonoscopy 99
Color vision testing 524
Colorectal cancer 134, 634
Colposcopy 280
Comminuted fracture 407
Common cold 552
Common foot problems, nursing management
  of 442
Compartment syndrome 413
Complement-mediated immune
  responses 456t
Complete blood count 46
Compound fracture 409
Concentration test 246
Condom
  female 481
  male 481
Condylomata acuminata 324
Confidentiality issues 482
Confrontation visual field test 524
Congenital abnormalities 398, 493
Congenital deformities 420
Congestive gastritis 142
Congestive heart failure 167, 268
Conization 280
Conjunctiva 523, 525, 538
Conjunctival hemorrhage 232
Conjunctivitis 525, 530
Connective tissue 619
Consciousness 511
  altered level of 570
  level of 509
  state of 563
Conservative therapy 66
Constipation 29, 125, 517, 591, 633
  management of 125

Constrictive pericarditis 201
Constructional apraxia 564
Constructive surgery 496
Contact dermatitis 354, 377
    causes of 378
    types of 377
Contact injury 532
Contact lens 529
Contact precautions 492
Contusion 532
Conus medullaris syndrome 610
Cor pulmonale 69, 82, 179
Cord concussion 610
Cord contusion 610
Cord injury, secondary 610
Cord transection 610
Cornea 523, 526
    corneal abrasion 526
    corneal opacity 526
    pterygium 526
Corneal ulcer 530
Coronary artery
    bypass graft 201
    disease 163, 179
Coronary care unit 643
Coronoviruses 552
Corticosteroids 23, 107, 228, 417, 537, 544,
    553, 628, 629
Corynebacterium
    diphtheriae 556
    vaginale 281
Coryza 552
Cough 18, 43, 237, 242, 466
    effective 89
    exercises 502
    productive 475
Cranial nerve dysfunction 581
Cranial surgery, types of 585
Craniectomy 585
Craniotomy 585
C-reactive protein 402
Creatine phosphokinase 432
Creatinine clearance 246
Creatinine kinase 155
Creatinine phosphokinase 402
Crepitation 407
Crepitus 421
Crest syndrome 431
Critical care
    nursing 643, 644, 647
    patient 645
    unit 643, 645
Critical incident stress management 642
Critically ill, management of 650
Crohn's disease 127, 132, 354
Cromolyn sodium 464
Cryoprecipitate 241
Cryosurgery 377, 386
Cryotherapy 38
Cryptococcal meningitis 330
Cryptococcosus neoformans 479
Cryptomenorrhea 287
Crypto-orchidism 312
Cryptosporidiosis 487
    cryptosporidium leads to 123
Cryptosporidium muris 330, 479
Culdocentesis 280
Culdoscopy 280

Culdotomy 280
Curative surgery 624
Cushing's disease 352
Cushing's syndrome 352, 354, 358
Cyanide 506
    kits 641
Cyanosis 45, 232, 242, 368, 370
Cyclic neutropenia 233
Cyclobenzaprine 435
Cyclophosphamide 228, 239, 599, 626, 633
    cytotoxin 418
Cyclosporin 418, 599
    nephrotoxicity 271
Cyst 370
Cystic breast disease 301
Cystic fibrosis 70, 76
Cystine 259
Cystitis 251, 633
Cystogram 248
Cystometrogram 248
Cytokines 454, 455
    group of 456
Cytology 46
Cytolysis 456
Cytomegalovirus 70, 320, 328, 475, 479, 487,
    528
Cytoplasm 450
Cytotoxic drugs 424, 617
Cytotoxic hypersensitivity 467
Cytotoxic T-cells 452, 454

D

Dactinomycin 626, 627
Daily living patterns, activities of 596
Dakin's solution 383
Danazol 228
Danger stage experiences 507
Darzolamide 534
Daunorubicin 233
Debulking surgery 624
Decadran 584
Decarboxylase inhibitor 601
Dectomycin 380
Deep breathing exercises 59, 502
Deep coma 31
Deep vein thrombosis 65, 209, 514
Defense 449
Deforman 444
Degenerative arthritis 397, 445
Degenerative disc disease 437
Degenerative diseases 124
Dehydration 268, 493
Delavirdine 477
Delirium 30
Dementia 124
    develops 328
Dental dams 481
Dental problems 100
Deoxypyridinoline, urine for 402
Deoxyribonucleic acids 471, 475
Depression 83, 478
Dermatitis 377
    lesions 378
    medicamentosa 379
        management of 380
    type of 379
Dermatologic disorders 354

Dermatological surgery, nursing management
    of 386
Dermatomyositis 432
Dermatophytosa, types of 373
Destructive lesions 571
Detrusor muscle atrophy 262
Deunorubicin 626
Dexamethasone 107, 584
Diabetes 163, 523, 630
    insipidus 268, 341
Diabetes mellitus 124, 156, 253, 268, 357, 397,
    424, 441, 563
    chronic complications of 362
    classification of 357
    complications of 361
    controlled 375
    diagnosis of 359
    etiology of 357
    hypoglycemia in 363
    management of 359
    treatment of
        type 1 359
        type 2 359
    type 1 357
    type 2 357
Diabetic coma 576
Diabetic foot 364
Diabetic ketoacidosis 361, 645
Diabetic nephropathy 271
Diabetic retinopathy 527
Dialysis therapy 273
Diaphoresis 268
Diarrhea 28, 122, 124, 127, 476, 627, 630, 633
Diarrheal disease 487
Diazepam 41, 107
Diazoxide 160
Dichlorophenamide 534
Diet and body weight 304
Diet and fluids 132
Diet modification 106
Diet therapy 584
Diethylstilbestrol 300
Diffuse axonal injury 579
Digestive disorders, nursing management
    of 93
Digestive system 96
    nursing assessment of 93
    physical examination of 94
Digital rectal examination 622
Dilantin 584
Dilated cardiomyopathy 179
Dioarticular arthritis 427
Diphenhydramine 107
Diplopia 603
Disaster
    agent 639
    epidemiology of 639
    man-made 639
    nursing 638
        types 639
    response plans, nurse's role in 642
    types of 639*t*
Discharge instructions 423, 439
Discharge planning 637
Diskogram 400
Dislocation and subluxation, clinical
    manifestations of 404
Diverticular disease 125

Diverticulitis 130
Dividing cells 624
Dizziness 125, 232, 539, 540, 546, 547
Dobutamine echocardiogram 154
Dolastran 107
Domperidone 107
Dopamine 612
  agonists 601, 602
  receptors inhibitors 107
Double leg lift 436
Dowager's hump 447
Down syndrome 234
Doxorubicin 233, 626, 633
Doxycycline 555
D-penicillamine 418
Drainage accumulation 23
Drainage tube, explanation of 202
Drawer test 399
Dressler's syndrome 167
Drop arm test 400
Droperidol 107
Drug reaction 378
Drug therapy 66, 85, 158, 584
Dry and leathery skin 368
Dual-photon absorptiometry 401
Dumping syndrome 120
Duodenal ulcer 116, 117
Duodenum, peptic ulcer of 117f
Dupuytren's contracture 441
D-xylose absorption test 97
Dynamic splints 419
Dypyridomole thallium scan 154
Dysarthria 564, 606
Dysmenorrhea 285
  primary 286
  secondly 286
Dyspepsia 114, 142
Dyspepsia syndrome 114
Dysphagia 431, 432, 600, 606
Dyspnea 43, 149, 181, 237, 242, 432, 475
Dysrhythmias 431, 514
Dysuria 245, 553

E

Ear
  and mastoid, problems of middle 545
  bleeding, inner 232
  canal 544
  disorders of external 543
  external 540
  infection, external 544
  middle 545
  nose and throat, nursing management of disorders of 539
Earache 539
Ebola 487
Ecchymosis 232, 370, 408, 532
Echoviruses 552
Eclampsia 32
Ectoparasitic disease 320
Ectopic pregnancy, ruptured 127
Edema 150, 182
  and swelling 407
  chronic 406
  progressive generalized 476
Efavirenz 477
Elbow 423
  props 436

Electrical burns, emergency management of 394
Electrolyte 515
  balance 367
Embolism 268
Embryo transfer 301
Embryonic stem cells 457
Emergency and disaster nursing, management of 635
Emergency care, principles of 638
Emergency management 175
Emergency operations plan 639
  components of 640
Emergency surgery 496
Emission tomography, posterior 155
Emmetropia 528
Emotional stress 156
Emphysema 70, 72
Empyema 55
Enalapril 160
Encainide 192
Encephalitis 581, 582
Enchondroma 443
Endocarditis 180, 493
Endocrinal manifestations 335
Endocrine 397
  disorder 340, 447
  system 333, 334, 471
Endocrinopathis 358
Endometrial biopsy 281, 300
Endometrial cancer 295
Endometrial tissue sample 621
Endometriosis 288
Endometrium 621
  postcurrettage loss of 287
Endoscopic examination 47, 99
Endoscopic retrograde cholangiopancreatography 99
Endoscopy 248, 401
Endothelium 619
Endotracheal intubation 559
Endotracheal tube 559
Entamoeba histolytica leads 123
Enteric aerobic gram-negative bacteria 48
Enteric infections 320
Environmental noise control 542
Enzyme deficiency anemia 223
Enzyme-linked immunosorbent assay 329, 476
Eosinophils 450
Ependymoma 582
Epididymitis 309
Epidural analgesia 518
Epidural anesthesia 507
Epigastric pain 181
Epilepsy 591
  causes of 591
  diagnosis of 592
Epinephrine injection 467
Epipodophyllotoxins 629
Episodes, acute 225
Epistaxis 232, 550
Epithelium tissue 619
Epitopes 449
Epstein-Barr virus 237, 475
Erectile dysfunction 319
Ergot alkaloids 596
Eropafenone 192
Erysipelas 16, 375

Erythema 368, 427
  multiforme 380
Erythematous psoriasis 381
Erythmatis 373
Erythrocyte 457
  disorders of 217
  sedimentation rate 401
Erythrocytosis 226
Erythromycin 107
Escherichia coli 48, 123, 195, 249, 313, 544
Esophageal and gastric varices 142
Esophageal carcinoma 112, 634
Esophageal dilation 112
Esophageal hypermotility sclerodactyly 431
Esophageal tumors 113
Esophagitis 632
Esophagogastroduodenoscopy 99, 143
Esophagus, normal 110f
Estotropia 537
Estrogen 629
Etanercept 418
Ethambatol 52
Ethmoid sinus surgery 555
Ethosuximide 592, 593
Ethoxzolamide 534
Eustachian tube 545
Ewing's sarcoma 624
Exacerbations, acute 484
Exercise program 448
Exocrine pancreas, diseases of 358
Exotropia 537
Explorative dermatitis 380
Extracorporeal membrane oxygenation 231, 645
Extra-luminal obstructing lesions 125
Extraocular muscle 523, 526
  testing 524
Extremity exercises 502
Eye 214, 330, 334, 531, 603
  blink 567
  care 34
  crossed 583
  defences, natural 532
  disorders of 523
  drops 502
  examination 417
  infections 530
  inflammation 530
  injuries, first aid of 532
  malignancy, diagnosis of 538
  opening 572
  pink 530
  protection 490
  sclera of 368
  surgery 354
  trauma and injury 531
  tumors 538, 634
Eyelids 525, 603
  allergic reactions 525
  and conjunctiva 523
  blepharitis 525
  blepharospasm 525
  chalazion 525
  dacrocystitis 525
  decreased blink 525
  ectropion 525
  entropion 525
  hordeolum 525

lid lag 525
ptosis 525
stye 525
xanthelasma 525

F

Face 334
   shield 490
Facial and ocular expression 523
Facial bone 445
Facial nerve 567, 608
Factitious hyperthyroidism 342
Family's psychological function 636
Fanconi's syndrome 227
Fat
   and pulmonary emboli 231
   cells 404
   distribution, abnormal 397
Fatigue 37, 150, 181, 222, 427, 428, 476
Febrile nonhemolytic reactions 467
Fecal incontinence 124
Fecal occult blood 622
Felbamate 593
Felty's syndrome 233
Female reproductive
   system, surgeries of 299
   tract, neoplasms of 292, 634
Fertility studies 280
Fetty's syndrome 233
Fever 147, 167, 232, 428
   causes high-spiking 424
   history of 214
   management of 27
Fibroadenoma 303
Fibroids 295
Fibroma 443
Fibromyalgia syndrome 433
Fibrosarcoma 443
Fibrosis 431
Fibrous cartilage 406
Fine-needle aspiration 58
First aid, simple 551
First-generation sulfonylureas 360
Fistulas 291
Fistulectomy 124
Flaccid paralysis 611
Flail chest 61
Flat foot 442
Flecainide 192
Fluent sensory aphasia 590
Fluid
   accumulation of 521
   and electrolyte balance, management
      of 25
   distribution of 25
   electrolyte 353
   intake 25
   loss 25
   replacement 176
   retention 142, 150
Fluid-filled lesions 369
Fluorescein angiography 527
Fluorescent treponemal antibody
      absorption 402
Fluoxetin 598
Flutter mucus clearance device 90
Focal glomerulonephritis 253

Focal impaction 124
Folate antagonist 627
Folic acid 228, 233
   deficiency 220
Follicle-stimulating hormone 336
Follicular pharyngitis 556
Follicular tonsillitis, acute 556
Folliculitis 374
   treatment of superficial 375
Food and fluids 34
Foodborne hepatitis 487
Foot
   amputation of 209
   and ankle, amputation of 209
   disease 487
   drop, prevention of 32
   problem 441
Forefoot 441
Foreign body 23, 281, 531, 544, 617
   perforation 127
Formaldehyde 506
Foscicles 432
Fosinopril 160
Fossa fracture, posterior 578
Foul odor 245
Fracture 406
   cause of 446
   clinical manifestation of 407
   closed 407
   complications of 413
   dislocation 404
   displacement of 408
   fragments 408
   frontal 578
   healing of 401, 408
      complication of 408
   hematoma 408
   immobilization of 411, 413
   impacted 407
   linear 407
   management of 409, 413
   pathological 407, 444
   principles of 408
   reduction 409
   risk for 447
   simple 409
   temporal 578
   type of 408
   unstable 407
Fresh frozen plasma 241
Frontal sinusotomy 555
Frontal sinusitis, acute 555
Fulminant bacterial infections 233
Functional endoscopic sinus surgery 555
Functional incontinence 266
Functional splints 419
Fundus photography 533
Fungal infection 328, 372, 397
Fungal pharyngitis 556
Fungal sinusitis 554, 555
Fungi 48
Fusion inhibitor 477

G

Gaint cell tumour 444
Gait disturbances 397
Gallbladder series 98

Gammopathy 461, 457
Gardnerella vaginalis 281
Gastric contents, aspiration of 512
Gastric suction 268
Gastric ulcer 116, 117
Gastritis 114, 127
Gastroenteritis 127
Gastroesophageal reflux disease 83, 106
Gastrointestinal cells 327, 475
Gastrointestinal function, maintain optimal
   631
Gastrointestinal increased appetite 343
Gastrointestinal malignancy 127
Gastrointestinal motility 390
Gastrointestinal problems 519
Gastrointestinal surgery 502
Gastrointestinal system 93, 272, 498, 622, 632
Gastrointestinal toxicity 629
Gaucher's disease 233
Genetic defects 358
Genetic engineering 457
Genetically transmitted syndromes 529
Genital herpes 320
Genital myeoplasmas 320
Genital warts 324
Genitalia 334
   external 277, 278
   male 276
Genitourinary assessment
   female 275
   male 276
Genitourinary disorders, nursing management
   of 245
Genitourinary system 245, 272
Genitourinary toxicity 629
Genitourinary tract 619, 633
Gentamicin 268, 375, 539
Gestational trophoblastic neoplasia 296
Giant cell tumor, benign 445
Giardia lamblia 123
Giardiasis 123
Gingivitis 100
Glasgow Coma Scale 572
Glaucoma 523, 529, 533
   congenital 533
      primary closure angle 533
      primary open angle 533
      secondary open angle 533
Glenoid fossa 405
Glial cells 327
Glioblastoma multiforme 582
Gliomas 582
Glomerular basement membrane 254
Glomerular capillary permeability,
   decreased 269
Glomerular disease, primary 253
Glomerular dysfunction 271
Glomerular filtrate, leakage of 269
Glomerulonephritis 231, 251, 271
   acute 252, 268
   chronic 253
Glossopharyngeal nerve 567
Glove use 491
Glucagonoma 358
Glucocorticoids 353
Glucocorticosteroids 352
Glucose tolerance, disorders of 358
Glycerine 534

Glycoproteins 312, 453
Gnosia 564
Goiter 345
Gonadotropin-releasing hormone 337, 628
Gonads 619
Gonorrhea 320, 487
    uncomplicated 321
Goodpasture's syndrome 254, 471
Gout 397, 424
    chronic 425
    primary 424, 425
    secondary 425
    treatment of 425t
Gouty arthritis 424
    acute 425
        attacks of 424
Graft disease, post-transfusion 468
Gram's stain 46, 279
Gram-negative bacteria 195
Granulation tissue 408
Granulocytes 241
Granuloma inguinale 324
Granulomatous disease, chronic 458
Graves' disease 342, 470, 527, 625
    ophthalmopathy in 343
Great toe 425
Greenstick fracture 407
Griseofulvin 373
Growth hormone 338
    deficiency, manifestations of 339
    hypersecretion 337
Guanethidine 159
Guillain-Barré syndrome 471, 606
    complication of 607
    diagnosis of 607
Gunshot wound 136
Gynecomastia 142, 308

H

Haemophilus influenzae 48, 426, 530
Haemopoietic toxicity 627
Hair 334
    follicles 367
Hallux valgus 441
Haloperidol 646
Hammer toe 442
Hand
    and foot problems 441
    disease 487
    hygiene 490
    problem 441
    washing 491
Hashimoto's thyroditis 345
Hay fever 552
Head
    and neck surgery 623
    elevation of 551
    trauma 594
Head injury 28, 32, 575, 577, 578
    minor 578
    severe 231
Headache 125, 232, 242, 427, 475, 539, 563, 595, 596
    pathophysiology of 595
Health and burns, general 392
Health and illness, concepts of 8
Health education 112
    with allergies 466

Health history 213, 397
Health illness level 509
Health maintenance 133
Health promotion 484
    practices 276
Health teaching 483, 621
Hearing aids 541
Hearing devices, types of implanted 542
Hearing impairment 540, 542
Hearing loss 540, 541, 545
    conductive 541
    mixed 541
    noise-induced 542
    sudden 541
Hearing problem 542
Heart
    defects, congenital 201
    disease, congenital 154
    sounds, abnormal 242
Heart failure 179
    classification of 180
    clinical manifestations of 181
    left-sided 180
    management of 182
    right-sided 180
    severe congestive 254
Heart rate 511
    increased 517
Heat stroke 231
Heberden's nodes 421
Helicobacter pylori 115, 117
Helper T-cells 454
Hemangioblastoma 583
Hemarthorosis 404
Hematemesis 127, 142, 232
Hematogenous osteomyelitis 434
Hematogenous spread 250
Hematologic malignant disorder 227
Hematological disorders 217, 233, 354, 430
Hematological system, nurses assessment of 213
Hematology 213
Hematoma 370
    formation 579
Hematopoietic growth factors 628
Hematopoietic system 633
Hematopoietic toxicity 629
Hematuria 232, 245
Hemianopia 581, 590
Hemiparesis dysphasia 581
Hemodynamic monitoring 59, 651
Hemolysis, acute 231
Hemolytic anemias 222, 430, 354
Hemolytic disease 467-469
Hemolytic process 231
Hemolytic reaction
    acute 243, 467
    delayed 243, 467
Hemolytic transfusion reaction, acute 467
Hemophilia 229, 397, 420
    A 227, 230
    B 227, 230
Haemophilus 580
    ducreyi 324
    influenzae 48, 80, 458, 554, 580
Hemoptysis 44
Hemorrhage 22, 23, 222, 268
    control of 33
    intraocular 232

Hemorrhagic cystitis 418
Hemorrhagic shock 23
Hemorrhoidal varices 142
Hemorrhoidectomy 124
Hemorrhoids 137
Hemostasis, disorders of 227
Hemothorax 63
Hemotological system 215
Heparin 228
Hepatic disease 23
Hepatic encephalopathy 142
Hepatic system 498
Hepatitis 139, 142, 233, 253, 354
    B 320, 635
        immune globule 326
        vaccine 494
        virus 326, 479
    C 635
        virus 479
    chronic 457
Hepatotoxicity 633
Hereditary spherocytosis 223
Hereditary thrombocytopenia 227
Heredity 617
Hernias 133
Herniated intervertebral disk 438
Herniated vertebral disk 437
Herpangina 488
Herpes genitalis 322
Herpes simplex 376, 479, 488, 581
    stomatitis 101
    virus 328
Herpes zoster 253, 376
    ophthalmicus 528
Hiatal hernia 110
    management of 111
    surgical nursing management of 111
Hiccups 519
Hill gastropexy 109, 111
Hindfoot 442
Hindu surgery 2
Hip 423
    joint 209
        dislocation 404
    spica cast 412
    tilts 436
Hirschsprung's megacolon 125
Histoplasma capsulatum 330, 479
Histoplasmosis 488
Hodgkin's disease 237, 238, 254, 256, 624
Holter monitoring 153
Homeostasis 449
Homosexuality 485
Hookworm disease 488
Hordeolum 530
Hormonal agents 628-630
Hormonal synthesis and action 287
Hormone 304, 617
    testing 278
    therapy 622
Horner's syndrome 526, 587
Hospital emergency preparedness plans 639
Hospital-acquired pneumonia 48
Hospitalization, effects of 13
Host's disease, post-transfusion 468
Host's threshold of reactivity 464
Host's virus-specific immune 475
Hot and cold application 38

House dust 467
  mites 552
Huhner test 280
Human chorionic gonadotropin 278, 296
Human growth hormone 486
Human immune response 492
Human immunodeficiency virus 458, 474, 606, 635
  disease 480
  infection 327, 228, 473, 478
  management of 476
  testing and counseling 482
Human leukocyte antigen 402
Human papilloma virus 293, 318, 320
Humidification and nebulizers 86
Humoral immune 451
Hydralazine 159, 162
Hydrocephalus 584
Hydrochloric acid 114, 116
Hydronephrosis 257
Hydroxyindoleacetic acid 97
Hydroxychloroquine 417, 418
Hydroxyzine 41
Hygiene 32
Hyperbaric oxygen therapy 435
Hypercalcemia 240, 462
Hypercapnia 577
Hyperemia, reactive 387
Hyperextension injuries 610
Hyperflexion injuries 609
Hyperglycemia 485, 497
Hyperglycemic hyperosmalor nonketonic coma 361, 362
Hyperlipidemia 424
Hypernatremia 27, 497
Hyperopia 529
Hyperoxia 509
Hyperparathyroidism 349
Hyperplasia 262, 441
Hyperpyrexia 32
Hypersensitivity diseases 462
Hypersplenism 233
Hypertension 156, 157, 163, 179, 242, 255, 424
  hypoxemia 577
  malignant 268
  secondary 157
  treatment of 515
Hypertensive heart disease 179
Hypertensive nephrosclerosis 271
Hyperthermia 35, 518
Hyperthyroidism 342, 343
Hypertrophy 179
Hypertropia 537
Hyperurecemia 424
Hypoalbuminemia 142
Hypoglossal nerve 567
Hypoglycemia 233
Hypokalemia 27, 514
Hyponatremia 27, 142
Hypoparathyroidism 350
Hypoperfusion 268
Hypopituitarism 32, 338
Hypostatic pneumonia, prevent 20
Hypotension 232, 268, 514
Hypothermia 35, 518
  complication of 518
  risk for 510
Hypotropia 537

Hypouricemia 429
Hypovolemia 23, 180
Hypovolemic shock 172, 413
Hypovolemic states 355
Hypoxemia 512, 513
Hypoxia 23
  stimulates 610
Hypoxic encephalopathies 571
Hystero-salpingectomy 299
Hysterosalpinogram 281

I

Iatrogenic drug intoxication 124
Ibuprofen 41, 228
Idarubicin 629
Idiopathic cyclic edema 355
Idiopathic hypertrophic subaortic stensosis 154
Idiopathic neutropenia 233
Idiopathic pulmonary fibrosis 70
Ifosfamide 626
Illness
  behavior stages 11
  chronic 420, 447
Imipramine 233, 433, 598
Immobility and disuse, complications of 589
Immune aberrations and disease, primary 457
Immune cells 459
  function of 457
Immune complex 469
  disease 462
Immune regulation 450
Immune response 456t
  primary and secondary 459
  type of 456
Immune system 449, 499
Immune thrombocytopenia 240
Immune thrombocytopenic purpura 228
Immunity, types of 450
Immunization programs 492
Immunocompetent cells 459
Immunodeficiency 457
  causes of secondary 459
  diseases 460
  disorder 459
    management of 459
  primary 457, 459
  secondary 458, 459
  severe combined 457
  treatments for 459
Immunogen 451
Immunoglobulin 453
  A deficiency 458
  E 459
  G 459
  reactions to 459
  replacement therapy 459
Immunologic disorders 231
Immunologic transfusion reactions 467
Immunological disorder 430
Immunological problems, nursing management of 449
Immunoserum globulin 241
Immunosuppressant drug, primary 459
Immunosuppression 458
Immunosuppressive agent 617
Immunosuppressive therapies 458

Immunothrombocytopenia purpura 228
Impaired gas exchange 653
Impetigo 16, 374, 488
Impingement syndrome 403
Impotence 142
  management of 319
In vitro fertilization 301
Inadequate dressing technique 23
Indomethacin 41
  naproxen 228
Indwelling catheter, placement of 395
Infection 15, 22, 80, 87, 124, 180, 228, 294, 338, 490, 521, 538, 563, 571, 580
  and inflammation 15
  at fracture side 408
  chain of 489
  control 396
  effects of 15
  recurrent 323
  risk for 459, 460
  sequelae of 487
  signs of 630
  sources of 15
  symptoms of 630
  transmission, preventing 494
Infectious bone diseases 433
Infectious disease 380, 487, 487t, 490, 493, 494, 539
  nursing management of 487
  symptoms of 493
Infectious mononucleosis 239, 452
Infective endocarditis 154, 195
Infertility 300, 493
Inflamed joints 425
Inflammation 16, 262, 415
Inflammatory bowel disease 130
Inflammatory conditions, chronic 457
Inflammatory heart disease 193
Inflammatory strictures 125
Infliximab 418
Influencing pain, factors of 36
Influenza 233, 488, 493, 539, 552
  virus 479
Infusion sets 492
Inguinal region 277
Inhalation injury, emergency management of 393
Inherited nephrotic disease 253
Initiated cell 614
Initiating coughing 59
Injury, type of 406
Inner ear, problems of 548
Insertive sex 480
Insomnia 553
Insulin action 358
Integumentary system 330, 370, 498, 633
Intensive care unit 20, 643
Intercranial bleeding 584
Interferon 450
  alpha and beta 628
  role of 457
Interstitial lung disease 70
Interstitial nephritis, drug-induced 268
Intestinal flora 520
Intestinal obstruction 133
Intra-aortic balloon pumps 645
Intra-arterial
  monitoring 651
  pressure 651

Intra-articular fractions 404
Intracerebral hemorrhage, large 579
Intracranial hematoma 577
Intracranial infections 584
Intracranial pressure 586, 651
    increased 574, 633
    monitoring 652
    normal 574
Intracranial problems 570
Intracranial surgery 584
Intracranial tumor 32, 582, 584, 634
Intraocular melanoma 538
Intratubular obstruction 269
Intravenous immunoglobulin 459
Intravenous pyelography 247
Intussusception 125, 133
Iodine induced hyperthyroid 342
Irbesartan 160
Iris 526
    and pupils 523
    heterochromia 526
    iridokinesis 526
Iritis 428
    chronic 526
Iron
    deficiency anemia 218
    supplements 125
Irritability 232, 352
Irritable bowel syndrome 122, 125
Irritant 281, 282
    contact dermatitis 378
Ischemic bowel, acute 127
Ischemic changes 338
Ischemic heart disease 201
Islet cells 287
Isoniazid 52, 53, 493
Isopropanol 506
Isosorbide dinitrate 166
Isosorbide-5 mononitrate 166
Isospora belli 330
Itching 376

J

Jackhammer operator 435
Jaundice 138, 142, 370, 525
Jock itch 374
Joint
    ankylosis of 426
    capsule articular cartilage 428
    cavity 421
    disease, degenerative 420
    enlargements 421
    erythema 416
    mice 421
    mobility, preserve 419
    pain 416
    replacement 422
    swelling 416
    warmth 416
Jugular venous distention 181, 242
Junctional arrhythmias 187
Juvenile rheumatoid arthritis 424

K

Kanamycin 268, 539
Kaposis sarcoma 330, 386, 528
Kegel exercises 265
Keloid 370
Keratitis 530
Keratoacanthoma 386
Keratometry 524
Kernig's reflex 569
Keroin 373
Khyposis 447
Kidney 196, 257, 259
    dropped 256
    shape, disparity in 255
    size, disparity in 255
Killer T-cells 452, 454
Kinesthetic apraxia 564
Kinesthetic sense 565
Klebsialla 48, 195
    pneumoniae 44, 554
Knee 423
    amputation 209
    involvement 421
    jerk 569
Kussmaul's respiration 45, 269
Kyphotic posture 398

L

Labetalol 159
Labyrinthitis infection 549
Lacrimal system 523
Lactic acidosis 485
Lactic dehydrogenase 155
Lactose tolerance test 97
Lacuna 586
Laminectomies 506
Lamivudine 477
Lamotrigine 593
Landry-Guillain-Barré-Strohl syndrome 606
Language and speech 564
Lansoprazole 118
Laparoscopy 280, 300
Laryngeal edema 513, 558
Laryngeal paralysis 558
Laryngitis
    acute 558
    chronic 558
    management 558
Laryngospasm 513
Latex allergy responses, risk for 465
Laxative abuse 125, 126*t*
Lectin pathways 456
Lederhoses disease 441
Leflunomide 418
Leg exercises 515
Legg-Calve-Perthes disease 420
Legionella pneumophila 48
Leiomyoma 295, 444
Lens 523, 526
    cataract 526
    dislocation 526
    subluxation 526
Lentigo 384
Lentivirus 473
Leomyosarcoma 444
Lesion configuration 370
Lesion distribution 370
Lethargy 427, 475
Leukemia 233, 234, 254, 634
    acute 626
    classification of 234
Leukocytes 450
Leukopenia 142, 633
Leukoplakia 384, 385
Leukotrienes 463
Levetiracetam 593
Levobunolol 534
Levodopa 601, 602
    plus entacapone 601
    preparations 601
Lice manifestation 371
Lichen plasius 381
Lichen simplex chronicus 379
Lichenification 370
Lidocaine 192
Ligament injury 403
Limb
    measurement 399
    removal of 209
Lipase 97
Lipoma 384
Lisnopril 160
Listeriosis 488
Liver 358
    biopsy 100, 143
    disease 231, 355, 369
    function studies 142
    scan 143
Local muscle spasms 406
Loop diuretics 161
Lopinavir 477
Lorazepam 107
Losartan 160
Low back pain 435
    chronic 435, 436
    management of chronic 437
Lower urinary tract 256
Lumbar puncture 635
Lumbosacral strain, acute 435
Lung
    abscess 55
    cancer 57, 634
    risk of 620
    transplant 70
Lupus erythematosus cells 381, 401
Luteinizing hormone secretion 336
Lyme's disease 427, 488
Lymph node 214
    biopsy 216
    enlarged 256
    regional 306
Lymphadenopathy 271, 427, 476
Lymphangiosgraphy 216
Lymphangitis 16
Lymphatic system 616
Lymphedema 236
Lymphocytes recirculate 452
Lymphocytic leukemia
    acute 234
    chronic 234-236
Lymphocytosis 452
Lymphogranuloma venereum 323, 488
Lymphoid tissues 449
Lymphokines 454
Lymphomas 237
    leukemias 354
Lymposarcoma reticuli-cell carcinoma 256

Index

M

Macrocytic anemia 219
Macrophages 327, 458
Malaise 434, 476
  history of 214
Malaria 28, 253, 488
Mammary duct ectasia 303
Mantoux tuberculin skin test 470
Marfan's syndrome 440, 526
Mashimotos thyroiditis 342
Mask 490
Mass 543
  lesions 575
Mast cell
  coated 459
  stabilizer 553
Master's prepared nurses 644
Mastitis, acute 303
Mastoidectomy 547
Mastoiditis 545
Maxillary sinusitis pain 554
McMurray's test 399
Measles 28, 233, 380
Mechanical restriction 513
Mechanical trauma 532
Mechlorethamine 626
Meclizine 107
Mediastinoscopy 47
Medical asepsis 16
Medulloblastoma 582
Megaloblastic anemia 219
Melanocytes, neoplastic growth of 386
Melanoma 386, 538
  large 538
  malignant 384, 385, 538
Melena 127, 232
Melphalan 626
Membranous proliferative
    glomerulonephritis 253
Memory
  cells 454
  problems 433
Menier's disease 548
Menigioma 582
Meningeal tumors 583
Meningitis 360, 580-582
Meningococcal meningitis 488
Meniscal injury 403
Menometrorrhagia 287
Menorrhagia 287
Menstrual and reproductive history 304
Menstrual cycles 284
Menstruation, problems of 284
Mental status 496, 563
Mentholated rubs 39
Meperidine 41
Mesenteric adenitis 127
Metabolic acidosis 27
Metabolic alkalosis 27
Metabolic alteration 586
Metabolic bone diseases 444
Metabolic causes 571
Metabolic disorders 179, 409
Metabolic disturbances 478
Metabolic encephalopathic conditions 575
Metaclopramide 596
Metaplasia 613

Metastasis 620
Metastatic carcinoma 526
Metastatic disease 622
Metastatic lesion, surgery for 623
Metastatic thyroid cancer 342
Metastatic tumors 583
Methazolamide 534
Methotrexate 418
Methoxazole 546
Methyldopa 159
Methylmorphine 41
Methylprednisolone 107
Meticulous oral hygiene, maintain 631
Metoclopramide 107
Metrorrhagia 287
Mexiletine 192
Microaerophilic bacteria 15
Microbial agents, lysis of 449
Microsporum 373
Midfoot 442
Midshaft fracture, uncomplicated 408
Migraine 427, 595
  classic 595
  common 595
  headache 595
Military nursing 4
Military tuberculosis 233
Milwaukee brace 441
Mineral metabolism test 401
Mini Hoffman's system 412
Minoxidil 160, 162
Miosis 534
Miotics 534
Mitomycin 627, 629
Mitotic cell division 615
Mitoxantrone 629
Mitral regurgitation 198
Mitral stenosis 197
Mitral valve
  prolapse 198
  prosthetic dysfunction 154
  regurgitation 154
Mitramycin 629
Modern nursing, beginning of 4
Moist heat 17
Mole melanocytic nevus 370
Monilial vaginitis 281
Monoarticular arthritis 427
Monoclonal antibodies 459, 628
Monoclonal gammopathy 461
Monocytes 327
Mononuclear phagocyte system 213
Mononucleosis 488
Monro-Kellie hypothesis 575
Moraxella catarrhalis 48, 80, 554
Morphine sulfate 41
Mortons neuroma 442
Mortons toe 442
Motility disorders 122
Motor disturbances 587, 588
Motor status 568
Motor symptoms 598
Mouth 214, 334
  attention to 29
  care 34
  disease 487
  problems of 100
Mucositis 627, 632

Mucous membrane 373
  of mouth, dryness of 632
Multicentric neoplasm 386
Multiple endocrine neoplasia 348
Multiple erythematous macule 382
Multiple myeloma 271, 239, 401, 424, 444, 461
  management of 461
  stages of 462
Multiple sclerosis 124, 125, 457, 527, 597
Multisystem disease 253
Muscle
  biopsy 403
  contraction, effective 603
  cramps 397
  fibers 432
  relaxants 433, 435
  spasm 406, 421
    clinical manifestation of 406
  strength 568
  tissue 619
  tumors 444
  weakness 397
Muscular dystrophy 440
Musculoskeletal assessment 397
Musculoskeletal disorders, nursing
    management of 397
Musculoskeletal fatigue 343
Musculoskeletal manifestation 446
Musculoskeletal nursing 397
Musculoskeletal system 399, 400, 415, 433, 498
Musculoskeletal tumors 443, 634
Mutamycin 629
Myalgia 427
Myasthenia gravis 603
Mycobacterial diseases 488
Mycobacterium 488
  avium complex 328, 330
  tuberculosis 48, 51, 328-330, 470
Mycoplasma pneumoniae 48, 488
Myelogenous leukemia, acute 235
Myeloma 444
Myelomenigocele 440
Myeloproliferation disorder 424
Myelosuppressive drugs 227
Myocardial infarction 166, 168, 268, 457
Myocardial ischemia 164
Myocarditis 179, 194
Myoclonic seizures 592, 593
Myofascial pain 433
Myoglobin 155
Myoglobinuria 245
Myomas fibromas 295
Myopathic disease, primary 402
Myopia 529
  high 536
Myringoplasty 547

N

Nails 214
  and hairs 398
Nalidixic acid 380
Naprosyn 41
Naproxen 41
Narcotic analgesics 41, 504
Nasal fracture 551
Nasogastric tube, placement of 395
Natural disaster 639

Natural immune system, dysfunction of 450
Natural immunity 450
Natural killer cells 450, 454
Nausea 125, 142, 181, 232, 434, 517, 539
    and vomiting 104, 127, 167, 633
    postoperative 519
Needlestick prevention 491
Neisseria 580
    gonorrhea 282, 309, 313, 320, 426, 530, 556
    meningitidis 580
Nelfinavir 477
Neomycin 268, 375, 539
Neoplasm 571, 613
Neoplastic disease 231, 407
Nephrolithotomy 259
Nephrological disorders 354
Nephroptosis 256
Nephrosclerosis 256
Nephrosis 355
Nephrotic syndrome 253, 271, 354
    primary 253
    treatment of 254
Nephrotomogram 248
Nephrotoxic injury 268
Nephrotoxicity 633
Nephrotoxin 268
Nerve block 39
Nerve tissue 619
Nervous system 215, 343, 633
    changes in 391
    diagnostic studies of 569
    nursing assessment of 563
Neural hearing loss 541
Neuralgia 376
Neurobehavioral symptoms 598
Neuroblastoma 626
Neurofibroma 582
Neurofibromatosis 125, 440
Neurogenic bladder dysfunction 262
Neurogenic disorders 125
Neurogenic shock 172
Neurologic injury 268
Neurologic system 330, 498
Neurological deficits 447
Neurological diseases 354, 397
Neurological disorder 430
Neurological symptom 427
Neurological system 272
Neurons, abnormal 591
Neuropathic arthropathies 420
Neurosurgery 39
Neurosyphilis 322
Neurovascular impairment
    signs of 411
    symptoms of 411
Neurovascular problems, prevention of 412, 413
Neutropenia 233
Neutrophil 450, 458
    production 459
Neutrophilia 234
Nevirapine 477
Nifedipine procardia 112
Night sweats 434, 475
Nipple discharge test 279
Nissen fundoplication 109, 111
Nitrofurantoin 250

Nitroprusside 160
Nitrosourceus 626
Nocardia 48
Nocturia 245
Noncardiac pulmonary edema 243, 468
Non-diabetes mellitus, hypoglycemia in 363
Nonergot alkaloids 601
Nonfluent aphasia 587
    expressive 590
Non-Hodgkin's lymphoma 238, 330
Nonimmunogenic transfusion reactions 468
Noninvasive interventions 37
Non-narcotic analgesics 41
Nonsteroidal anti-inflammatory drugs 157
Nonstructural scoliosis 440
Nontreponimal serologic tests include 279
Nose 334
    and sinuses, disorders of 550
Nuclear imaging scans 98
Nucleus pulposus 437
Null lymphocytes 454
Numbness 563
Nurse addresses, perioperative 495
Nurse's responsibility 498
Nurse-client relationship, trusting 37
Nursing
    interventions 67
    management 28, 105, 109, 166, 171, 177, 179, 201
    responsibilities 501
Nutrition 33, 371, 602
    and fluids 503
    maintain 574
    promoting 59, 103, 415
Nutritional deficiencies 180, 233
Nutritional deficits 23, 388
Nutritional imbalances 367
Nutritional management 177
Nutritional support 396
Nutritional therapy 90

O

Obesity 163
Oblique fracture 407
Obstructive pulmonary disease, chronic 79
Obstructive uropathy 256
Occipital lobe 583
Occult blood, stool for 143
Occupational lung diseases 56
Ocular malignance 538
Ocular pressure 553
Ocular trauma 529, 536
    types of 531
Oculomotor nerves 566
Ofloxacin 434
Olecranon bursa 425
Oligodendroglioma 582
Oligomenorrhea 287
Oliguria 245, 520
    progressive 232
Olmesartan 160
Omeprazole 118
Oophorectomy 299
Oophoritis 283
Open fracture 407
Open heart surgery 268
Open pneumothorax 62, 63

Operation theatre 22
Ophthalmoscopy 524
Opportunistic infections 476
Opsonization 453, 456
Optic nerve 523, 566
Opticneuritis 598
Oral anaerobes 48, 49
Oral cancer 102, 634
    nursing management of 104
    radiation therapy for 102
Oral candidiasis 101
Oral cavity 94
Oral cholecystogram 98
Oral contraceptives 285, 304
Oral floral 520
Oral hygiene 20, 34
    and comfort, promoting 103
Oral infections 100, 376
Oral inflammation 100
Oral lesions 476
Oral medications 502
Oral rehydration therapy 26
Oral ulcers 430
Orbital fracture 578
Orchitis 310
Orthopnea 181
Orthoses 418
Osetophytes, formation of 437
Osmotic agents 534
Osteitis 444
Osteitis deformans 445
Osteoarthritis 420, 425, 435
Osteochondroma 443
Osteoclastoma 444
Osteoid 408
Osteoma 443
Osteomalacia 397, 444
    development of 444
    rickets 401
Osteomyelitis 397, 401, 433
    acute 434
    chronic 434
    treatment of 434
    type of 433, 434
Osteopenia 485
Osteophytes 421
Osteoporosis 401, 406, 444, 446, 447, 485
    etiology of 446
Osteosarcoma 443
Osteotomy 419
Osteous tissue, interruption of 407
Ostomy surgery 136
Otalgia 544
Otitis 540
    diagnosis of external 544
    external 544
Otitis media 545, 546
    chronic 546
    diagnosis of 546
Otorrhea 539
Otosclerosis 545
    management of 545
Otospongiosis 541
Ovarian cancer 297
Ovarian cyst 296
    ruptured 127
Ovum transfer 301
Oxalate 259

Index

Oxcarbazepine 593
Oxidase inhibitors, monoamine 602
Oxygen
    deficit 23
    free radicals 624
    therapy 59, 466
Oxymetazoline 553

P

Pacemakers, permanent 645
Paget's disease 180, 305, 401, 424, 444-446
Pain 36, 146, 205, 513, 563, 565
    abdominal 125, 142
    and tenderness 407
    control 423, 502
    cranial nerves 565
    management 35, 119, 393, 395
    meaning of 37
    nature of 36
    physiology of 36
    purpose of 36
    relief measures, types of 40
    relief of 202
    superficial 565
    therapy 40
    throbbing 546
    types of 37
Palliative surgery 496, 623
Palmar erythema 142
Palpable fullness 520
Palpable mass 125
Palpation 45, 151, 150
Pamidronate 446
Pancreas, disorders of 357
Pancreatitis 127
    acute 146
    chronic 147
Pancytopenia 227
Panhysterectomy 299
Pantaprazole 118
Papanicolaou smears 279, 288, 621
Papillary muscle
    dysfunction 167
    rupture of 179
Papulosquamous diseases 381
Paraesophageal hernia 110, 110*f*
Parainfluenza 552, 554
Paralysis 205
Paralytic ileus 633
Paraphimosis 317
Parasitic infections 371
Parathyroid gland, disorders of 349
Paraxysmal supraventricular tachycardia 186
Parietal lobe 583
Parkinson's disease 125, 599
    causes of 599
    complications of 600
    diagnosis of 601
    drug-induced 599
    facial appearance 600
    fine motor function 600
    multiple sclerosis 498
    pathology of 599
    secondary manifestations of 600
    speech problems 600
    symptoms of 599
    visual problems 600

Parkinsonism 568
    treatment of 601*t*
Paroxetine 598
Paroxysmal noctural dyspnea 181
Partial seizures 592
Passive acquired immunity 451
Patch test 371
Patellar reflex 569
Pediculosis 371, 488
Pelvic belt 410
Pelvic examination 621
Pelvic exenteration 299
Pelvic floor relaxation 124
Pelvic inflammatory disease 127, 283
Pelvic organ 434
    surgery, types of 506
Pelvic sling traction 410
Pelvic tilt 436
Pemphigus vulgaris 383
Penetrating injury 531
Penicillin 228, 268, 581
Penis 277
    cancer of 318
    congenital problem of 317
    problems of 317
Peptic ulcer 83, 116, 117
    disease 116
    surgical management of 119
    treatment of 118*t*
Perforated tympanic membrane 545
Pericarditis 167, 193, 431
    management of acute 194
Perimenopausal symptoms 276
Perinatal transmission 474
    decreasing risks of 481
Perindopril 160
Perineal descent 124
Perineal muscle exercises 265
Perioesteum 407
Periorbital edema 252
Peripheral edema 142, 242
Peripheral nerve block anesthesia 507
Peripheral neuropathy 142, 476, 633
Peripheral pitting 182
Peripheral pulses 232
Peritoneoscopy 280
Peritonitis 127, 129, 268
Pernicious anemia 563
Persistent hacking cough 181
Persistent meningitis 581
Pes planus 442
Pet allergens, avoid 553
Petechae 142, 232, 370
Petit mal 593
Peyrobie's disease 441
Phagocytes 458
Phagocytic cells 450
Phagocytic defects 458
Phalangeal joints 432
Phalen's sign, positive 405
Phalen's test 400
Pharyngitis, acute 556
Phenothiazine 233
    therapy 599
Phenoxybenzamine 159
Phentolamine 159
Phenylbutazone 233, 380
Phenylephrine 553

Phenytoin 192, 233, 268, 584, 593
Pheochromocytoma 358
Phimosis 317
Phosphorous 247, 401
Photoallergy reactions 380
Photophobia 524, 534, 595
Physical carcinogens 617
Picamycin 627, 629
Pigmented nevi moles 385
Pilonidal sinus 138
Pinguecula 525
Pinworm disease 488
Piroxicam 41
Pituitary adenoma 583
Pituitary gland, hyper function of anterior 334
Pituitary hyperthyroidism 342
Pituitary studies 334
Pityriasis rosea 382
Placenta, choriocarcinoma of 626
Plantar fascia 441
Plantar neuroma 442
Plantar reflex 569
Plantar wart 377, 442
Plantor facitis 428
Plasma
    cell 452, 461
    components 241
    infusion 228
    proteins 453, 461
Plasmacytoma 462
Plaster of Paris 411
Platelet 227, 241
    destruction 228
    production, suppression of 228
    transfusion 228
Pleural effusion 63
    management of 64
Pleurisy 64
Plummer's disease 342
Pneumococcal pneumonia 44, 488
Pneumocystis carinii 476
    pneumonea 329
Pneumocystis jiroveci pneumonia 484, 488
Pneumonia 48, 493
Pneumonitis 633
Pneumothorax 62
Poikilotheremia 205
Poison 32, 530
Poliomyelitis 440
Pollen spores 467
Polyarteritis nodosa 271
Polycethemia 586
Polyclonal gammopathies 461
Polycystic kidney disease 257, 271
Polycystic ovary disease 287
Polycythemia vera 226, 424
Polydipsia 341
Polymenorrhea 287
Polymicrobic endocarditis 195
Polymorphonuclear leukocytes 450
Polymyositis 432
Polymyxin B 268
Polyuria 245, 341
Portal hypertension 233
Posterior cord syndrome 610
Postexertional malaise 472
Postexposure prophylaxis 482
Post-herpetic neuralgia 377

Postprandial hypoglycemia 120
Poststreptococcal glomerulonephritis, acute 252
Potassium 247
   deficiency 142
   sparing diuretics 161
Prazosin 159
Precancerous lesions 618
Precardial temponade 268
Precursor stem cells 459
Prednisone 417
   high dose 228
Pregabaline 593
Pregnancy
   taxemia of 268
   testing 278
Preinvasive disease 298
Premalignant lesions 384
Premenstrual syndrome 284
Presbyastasis 549
Presbycusis 541
Presbyopia 529
Presbyvertigo 549
Pressure ulcer 387, 388
Priapism 320
Primary lesions, surgery for 623
Primary myopathies, treatment of 402
Primidone 593
Procainamide 191
Prochlorperazine 107
Progesterones 629
Prokinetic drugs 109
Prolactin hypersecretion 336
Prolectin deficiency, manifestations of 339
Promethazine 107
Propylthiouracil 345
Prostaglandin 463
   agonists 534
   inhibitors 285
Prostate 622
   cancer of 268, 316, 621, 634
   hyperplasia 264
   problems of 313
Prostatic and bladder tumors 271
Prostatic hyperplasia, benign 268
Prostatic hypertrophy, benign 256
Prostatitis 313
Prosthetic devices 231
Prosthetic eye 538
Protein, type of 461
Proteinuria 232
Proteus 48
   mirabilis 546
   vulgaris 544
Proton pump inhibitors 109, 118
Protozoal 253
   infection 328
Proximal intraphalangeal joints 417
Pruritus 544
Pseudoephedrine 547
Pseudohermaphroditism, male 287
Pseudomonas 195
   aeruginosa 44, 48, 87, 195, 491, 544
   organisms 458
Psoralens 380
Psoriasis 381
   complication 381
   types of 381
   vulgaris 381

Psoriatic arthritis 381, 429
Psychotropics 233
Ptosis 257, 603
Pulmonary angiogram 47
Pulmonary artery
   monitoring 651
   pressure 651
Pulmonary contusion 71
Pulmonary disease 180
Pulmonary disorders 340
Pulmonary edema 44, 512, 513
Pulmonary embolism 64, 167, 179, 180, 212, 513
   management of 66
Pulmonary fibrosis secondary 70
Pulmonary function test 47
Pulmonary hypertension 67, 70, 431
   primary 67
   secondary 69
Pulmonary oedema 390
Pulmonary valve disease 200
Pulmonary ventilation, maintenance of 19
Pulselessness 205
Pulses 334
Punch biopsy 386, 403
Puncture wounds 474
Pupil 526, 534
   anisocoria 526
   dyscoria 526
   function testing 524
   miosis 526
   mydriasis 526
Pupillary reflex 523
Purine analogue 627
Purkinje's fibers 183
Purpura 142, 232, 417
   ecchymosis 380
Pursed-lip breathing 44
Purulent meningitis 32
Pyaemia 16
Pyelolithotomy 259
Pyelonephritis
   acute 268
   chronic 271
Pyrazinamide 52, 53
Pyrexia
   common causes of 27
   signs of 28
   symptoms of 28
Pyridoxine 602
Pyrimidine analogues 627

Q

Quinidine 191

R

Rabies 488
Radiation burn injury 389
Radiation hazard 304
Radiation therapy 40
   and chemotherapy, side effects of 632
   goals of 624
   types of 624
Radical hysterectomy 299
Raloxifene 448
Ramipril 160
Raynaud's disease 208

Raynaud's phenomenon 208f, 416, 431, 432
Reaction, risk of 466
Rebound tenderness 127
Rectal cancer 620
Rectal pressure 125
Rectal prolapse 124
Rectocele 125
Red blood cells 240
Reed-Sternberg cell 237
Reflex incontinence 265
Refractive disorders 528
   aphakia 528
   astigmatism 528
   hyperopia 528
   myopia 528
   presbyopia 528
Refractometry 526
Regional anesthesia 507
Reifer's syndrome 428
Reinsert prosthesis 538
Reiter's syndrome 429
Releasing cell mediators 450
Remberg test 565
Renal allograft rejection 459
Renal angiography 248
Renal artery
   stenosis 255, 355
   thrombosis of 268
Renal calculi 258
Renal compromise 461
Renal disease
   end-stage 271
   intrinsic 424
Renal disorders 430
Renal failure 23, 232, 267, 271
   acute 267, 273
   chronic 271
Renal impairment 271
   drug-induced 424
Renal infarction 271
Renal insufficiency 271
Renal radionuclide imaging 248
Renal reserve 271
Renal trauma 261
Renal tumor 260, 634
Renal vascular obstruction 268
Renal vasoconstriction 268
Renal vein thrombosis 255
Renin-angiotensin-aldosterone system 514
Reno-ureteral surgery 266
Reproductive dysfunction 633
Reproductive problems, male 309
Reproductive system 272, 275
   diagnostic studies of 278
   female 275
   male 275
   nursing management of disorders of 275
Reproductive toxicity 629
Reservoir 489
Resistant tumor cells, presence of 626
Respiratory complications care, postoperative 513t
Respiratory compromise 466
Respiratory distress 478
Respiratory droplets 376
Respiratory failure 78
Respiratory muscle tone 513

Respiratory problems 512
    nursing management of 43
Respiratory rate, respiratory increased 343
Respiratory syncytial disease 488
Respiratory syndrome, severe acute 489
Respiratory system 272, 329, 498, 633
    changes in 390
    diagnostic studies of 45
    nursing assessment of 43
Respiratory tract, foreign body in 32
Respiratory viruses 48
Retina 536
Retinal detachment 536
Retinal lattice degeneration 536
Retinal separations, diagnosis of 536
Retinal vascular system 523
Retinoscopy 526
Retrograde pyelography 248
Retrovirus 473, 474
Rhabdomyolysis 268
Rhabdomyoma 444
Rheumatic heart disease 28, 179, 197
Rheumatoid arthritis 233, 354, 415, 416, 441, 528
    cause of 415
    symptoms of 416
Rheumatoid nodules 416
Rheumatoid synovial disease 405
Rheumatoid arthritis 416
Rhinitis 552
    acute 552
    chronic 553
Rhinophyma 383
Rhinovirus 552, 554
Rhizotomy 496
Rib fractures 61
Rickets 397, 444
Riedel's thyroiditis 345
Rifampicin 52, 53
Ring finger, part of 405
Ringer's lactate 176
Ringer's solution 612
Ringworm 373, 488
Rinne test 545
Risedronate 446
Ritonavir 477
Rocky mountain 488
Rotator cuff
    injuries 405
    tear 403
Rotatory chair testing 540
Rotavirus 123
    gastroenteritis 489
Rubella 489, 539
Russel's traction 410
Rynoductre 142

S

Salmonella 123, 330, 426, 434
    typhosa 381
Salpingectomy 299
Salpingitis 283
Salt depletion, severe 28
Salt diet, high 156
Saquinavir 477
Sarcoidosis 70
Scabies 372, 489
    treatment 372

Scalp 373
    lacerations 577
Scarlatina 381
Scarlet fever 381
Schirmer tear test 527
Schwann cells 582
Schwartz-Bartter syndrome 339
Schwarz's sign 545
Scintigraphic studies 154
Sclera 523
Scleroderma 271, 354, 431
Sclerosing cholangitis, primary 145
Sclerosis 268
Scoliosis 398, 440
    congenital 440
    management of 440
    screening 400
Scopolamine 107
Scrotum, problems of 309
Scurvy 397
Seborrheic dermatitis 379
Seborrheic keratosis 384
Sedantary lifestyles 156, 163
Seizure 232, 563
    disorder 591
    types of 592
Self-antigens, alteration of 471
Sellar tumors 583
Semen analysis 280
Sensation 564
Sensitizing dose 463
Sensorineural hearing loss 541, 549
Sensory
    hearing loss 541
    information 499
    perceptual problems 646
    status 565
    symptoms 598
Sensory-perceptual deficits, compensatory for 590
Sepsis 23, 268, 468, 493, 645
Septic abortion 231
Septic arthritis 426
Septic meningitis 580
Septic shock 172, 268, 493
Septicemia 16, 231, 493
Septum, deviated 550
Seronegative arthropathies 428
Serositis 430
Serotonin 596
    antagonists 106
    reuptake inhibitions 84, 285
Serous otitis media 546
Sertraline 598
Serum
    albumin 143, 241
    aspartate aminotransferase transaminase 402
    complement 402
    creatinine 247
    electrolyte 143
    enzyme levels 432
    estradiol 279
    glutamic pyruvic transaminase 143
    gutamic-oxaloacetic transaminase 402
    lipids, elevated 156
    muscle enzyme test 402
    progesterone 278, 281

sickness 469
    test 401
    uric acid 425
Sexual activity 170
Sexual health 276
Sexual intercourse 480
Sexual related problems 333
Sexual response, stages of 170
Sexual transmission 474
Sexually transmitted disease 320, 473, 474, 478, 493
Sheehan's syndrome 339
Shigella 123
Shock 22, 171, 231, 268
    classification of 172
    distributive 172
    management of 175
    pathophysiology of 173
    prevention of 19
    signs of 408
Shoulder 423
    pain, complain of 405
Shunt procedures 585
Sick children 15
Sick elderly persons 14
Sick role
    assumption of 11
    behavior 12
Sick sinus syndrome 186
Sickle cell
    anemia 224, 271, 424, 586
    disease 224, 253
Siding hiatal hernia 110*f*
Single-lung transplantation 70
Singultus 519
Sinogram 400
Sinus
    arrest 186
    bradycardia 185
    dysrhythmia 186
    exit block 186
    of Valsalva, aneurysm of 201
    rhythm, normal 189*f*
    surgery, types of 555
    tachycardia 185
Sinusitis 554
Sjögren's syndrome 238, 341, 431
Skeletal muscle 358
Skeletal system 272
Skeletal traction 410
Skene's glands 278
Skin 214, 333, 367, 398, 621
    allergic conditions of 377
    and pressure areas 29
    assessment of 367
    biopsy 403
    breakdown, preventing 433
    care 34, 411, 412
        general 383
    cell growth 383
    color, assessment of 515
    disinfecting 492
    flora, normal 491
    infection 374
    integrity, maintaining 415, 575
    lesions 369, 384, 417
    malignant lesions of 385, 634
    manifestation 446

normal 369
patch 166
preparation 503
  bowel of 499
problems 371
rash 476
reaction 379, 380, 633
splints 403
surface, breaks in 369
tags 384
traction 409
tumors of 383
viral infections of 376
Skull
and spine 569
fractures 584
pains 445
Sleep 28
deprivation 647
problems 647
Sliding hiatal hernia 110
Slit-lamp microscopy 524
Smallpox 381, 489, 492
Smoke, avoid 553
Smoking cessation 85
Soft tissue
infection 397
injuries 403, 404
mammographing 279
Solar keratosis 384
Sotalol 192
Speech, promoting 104
Spermatic cord 277
Spermatocele 312
Spider angioma 142
Spinal anesthesia 507
Spinal canal, narrowing of 437
Spinal cord
damage, types of 610
disease 268
injury 124, 440, 609
lesion 125
malformation 262
produces 610
syndrome 610
tumors 583, 634
Spinal injuries 609
Spinal lesions 569
Spinal nerve root 437
Spinal shock 611
Spinal stenosis 437, 438
Spinal surgery, management of 438
Spine, degenerative disorders of 437
Spiral fracture 407
Spiral reflex activity, loss of 611
Splash and spray, avoidance of 491
Spleen 196
disorders of 240
Splenectomy 228
Spondyle arthritis 428
Spondylitis 428
Spondylolisthesis 437
Spondylosis 437
Spongy bone 545
Sprains and strains 403
Sputum
analysis 46
cytology 621
production 44

Squamous cell carcinoma 384, 385
Staphylococcal pneumonia 44
Staphylococcus 375, 530
  aureus 16, 48, 49, 97, 195, 282, 303, 426, 434
  epidermidis 195, 303
Stasis dermatitis 379
Stavudine 477
Stem cell 449, 457, 582
  transplantation 457
Stenosis 268
Stereognosis 564
Stereopsis testing 524
Stereotaxis 585
Sterilisation 17
Steroids 531
Stiff neck 475
Stills disease 424
Stimulating hormone 470
Stimulatory hypersensitivity 470
Stimulatory reactions, causes of 470
Stokes-Adams syndrome 32
Stomach
cancer of 120, 634
gastrin test 96
Stomatitis 627, 632
Stool examination 97
Stool with blood 125
Storage diseases 233
Strabismus 526, 537
Straight leg raising test 400
Streptococcal organism 452
Streptococcal throat infection 452
Streptococcus 546
  bovis 195
  hemolyticus 426
  pneumoniae 48, 49, 80, 195, 554, 580
  pyogenes 453
Streptomycin 52, 53, 539
Stress 618
  echocardiogram 154
  fracture 407
  patients and family 648
  reduction 119
  testing 153
  ulcer prophylaxes 612
Strider 237
Stroke 124, 457, 585
  emergency management of 588
Struma ovarii 342
Subconjunctival hemorrhage 525
Subcutaneous emphysema 59
Subcutaneous nodules 398
Subdural effusion 581
Subdural empheyema 581
Sublingual nitroglycerin 166
Substance abuse 563
Subtentorial masses 571
Subtotal hysterectomy 299
Sucking blood 371
Sulfagalazine 417
Sulfalim 380
Sulfasalazine 418
Sulfonamides 380
Sulfonylurea, second-generation 360
Sulphonamide 268
Sunstroke 28
Suppressor T cells, defective 471
Surgical asepsis 16
  maintenance 508

Surgical procedure, classification of 496
Symptomatic health information 397
Syncope 149, 516
Syndesmophyte 428
Syndrome of inappropriate anti-diuretic hormone 339
Synovectomy 419
Synovial cyst 398
Synovium biopsy 403
Syphilis 321, 489, 539
  serological test for 402
Syringomyelia 440
Systemic acting drugs 124
Systemic antibiotic therapy 547
Systemic disease 271
Systemic disorders 125
Systemic lupus erythematosus 233, 253, 268, 271, 354, 429, 456
  scleroderma 354
  treatment of 401
Systemic metabolic derangements 571
Systemic sclerosis 431
Systemic septicemia 391

T

T cell
  deficiencies 458
  function 460
  mediated hypersensitivity 469
  suppressor 454
  types of 454
Tachycardia 181, 232
Tachypnea 45
Tangential surgery 386
Taste sensations, altered 633
Telangiectasia 370
Telmisartan 160
Temporo-parieto-occipital junction 564
Tendonitis 403
Tendon transplant 419
Tenesmus 125
Tenosynovitis 405
Tension 595
  pneumothorax 62, 63
  type headache 595
Terbutaline 464
Testicles 622
Testicular atrophy 142
Testicular cancer 312, 634
Testicular feminization 287
Testicular self-examination 622
Testicular torsion 311
Testosterone 486
Tetanus 489
  immunization 393
Tetracycline 380
  furosemide 268
Thalassemia 220
Therapeutic management 176
Therapeutic regimen, management of 119
Thermal burn
  emergency management of 394
  injury 389
Thermolabile plastic 412
Thiazide 158, 268
  diuretics 228
    barbiturates 380

Thiazolidinediones 360
Thioamide, antithyroids of 343
Thiotepa 626, 627
Thomas test 400
Thoracentesis 47
Thoracic injuries 60
Thoracic spinal surgery 439
Thoracic surgery, nursing management in 58
Thorax 334
Thorazine therapy 599
Throat, disorders of 556
Thrombocytes 457
Thrombocytopenia 142, 227, 354, 630, 633
Thrombocytopenic purpura 228
Thrombocytosis 227, 229
Thrombophlebitis 209, 294
Thrombopoietin 228
Thrombotic thrombocytopenia purpura 228
Thromboxanes 463
Thyroid 645
  disease 563
  gland 470
    cancer of 347, 634
    disorders of 342
  hormone 622
  lymphoma 348
  tissue, atrophy of 345
Thyroiditis 342, 345
Thyrotoxicosis 179, 180, 470
Tiagabine 593
Tic douloureux 607
Tiludronate 446
Timolol maleate 534
Tinea
  capitis 373
  corporis 373
  cruris 374
  pedis 374
  unguium 374
Tinel's sign 400
  positive 405
Tinnitus 539
  with salicylate 417
Tissue
  damage 450
  handling of 23
  inadequate oxygenation of 367
  oxygenation insufficient 23
  perfusion, altered 580
  swelling of 369
T-lymphocytes 452, 606
  role of 454
Tobramycin 268
Todd paralysis 592
Toe 334
  touches 436
Tolbutamide 233
Tolmetin 41
Toluene 506
Tongue falling back 513
Tonic-clonic seizures 592
Tonometry 524
Tonsillectomy 557
Tonsillitis 557
  complications of 556
Tonsils 557
  and adenoids 557
  chronic enlargement of 557

Tooth and gum disorder 100
Tophaceous deposits 398
Topical agents 507
Topical anesthesia 507
Topiramate 593
Torn meniscus 406
Torsades de pointes 188
Torus fracture 407
Total hip replacement 422
Total hysterectomy 299
Total knee replacement 423
Total parental nutrition 136, 292
Totipotent cells 457
Toxemia 16, 231
Toxic adenoma 342
Toxic diffuse goiter 342
Toxic hepatitis 139
Toxic multinodular goiter 342
Toxicity 571
Toxoplasma gondii 328, 330
Tracheostomy 559
  care 561
  tube 559, 561
Trachoma 530
Transcranial Doppler 570
Transcutaneous electrical nerve stimulation 39, 437
Transdermal nitroglycerin 166
Transfusion reaction 354
Transient ischemic attacks 587
Translucent joint 420
Transochondrial fracture 407
Transverse fracture 407
Trauma 124, 256, 262, 338, 544
Trazodone 433, 598
Trendelenburg's test 400
Treponema pallidum 321
Triceps reflex refers 569
Trichinosis 489
Trichomonas vaginalis 281, 325
Trichomoniasis 282, 325
Trichophyton fungi 373
Tricuspid valve disease 200
Tricyclic antidepressants 597
Trigeminal nerve 567
Trigeminal neuralgia 607, 608
Trimethaphan 159
Trimethoprim 555
Trimetho-prime sulfamethoxazole penicillin 233
Trochlear nerves 566
Trophic stimulation, loss of 345
Troponin 155
Trousseau's signs 352
Tubal embryo transfer 301
Tuberculin skin test 493
Tuberculosis 51, 397, 469, 470, 489
Tubular necrosis, acute 268
Tumor 124, 133, 256, 262, 338, 620
  age of 626
  benign 384, 618, 618*t*
  classification of 619, 619*t*
  inducing genes 614
  location of 307, 626
  malignant 136, 618, 618*t*, 622
  necrosis factor 416, 454
  primary 306
  size of 307, 626
  treatment of 613

Tuning fork tests 545
Tympanoplasty 547
Tympanosclerosis 546
Typhoid fever 233, 381
Tzanck test 383

U

Ulcerative colitis 127, 131, 354, 622
  management of 131
Unconscious patient, nursing management of 32
Unconsciousness 31
  etiology of 32
Undescended testes 312
Upper extremities 606
Upper gastrointestinal
  barium swallow 143
  bleeding 115
Urate crystals 425
Uremia 271
Ureteral obstruction 256, 271
Ureterolithotomy 259
Ureteropelvic junction 258
Ureterovesical junction 258
Ureterovesical reflux 262
Ureters 259
Urethral stricture 256, 262
Urge incontinence 265
Urgent surgery 496
Uric acid 247, 258, 424
  stones 259
Urinalysis 246
Urinary catheter 506
Urinary diversion 266
Urinary effects, preventing 631
Urinary incontinence 263, 590
Urinary problems 520
Urinary retention 125, 262, 598
Urinary stones 258
Urinary system 498
  changes in 390
  inflammatory disorders of 249
Urinary tests 402
Urinary tract
  infection 245, 249
  location of calculi in 258*f*
  malformation 262
  obstruction 271
  trauma of 261
Urinary uric acid 402
Urine
  amylase 97
  bilirubin 97
  collection 246
  culture 246
  cytology 246
  odour 245
  studies 216, 246, 278
  tests 97
Urobilinogen 97
Urology 245
Urticaria 378, 380, 463
Uterine bleeding 630
  dysfunctional 287, 288
Uterine leiomyoma 295
Uterine prolapse 289, 290
Uterine rupture 127
Uterovaginal outflow tract 287

Uterus 622
Uveitis 530

V

Vaginal bleeding 232
Vaginal discharge, care of 35
Vaginal hysterectomy 506
Vaginitis 281, 320
Vague arthralgia 424
Vagus nerve 567
Valproic acid 593
Valsalva's maneuver 23, 158
Valve repair 201
Valvular dysfunction 180
Valvular heart disease 197
Valvular insufficiency 201
Vancomycin 268
Varicella 381
Varicocele 312
Varicose veins 211
Variola 381
Vascular disease 571
Vascular lesions 369
Vascular smooth muscle 159
Vasculitis 271
Vasodilators 159, 161
Vasogenic edema 579
Veins, disorders of 209
Venous stasis ulcer 212
Venous thrombosis 413
    prevention of 30
Ventilation 46, 47
Ventricular aneurysm 167, 201
Ventricular arrhythmias 201
Ventricular assist device 201
Ventricular fibrillation 188
Ventricular sepral defect 179, 201
Ventricular tachycardia 188
Verbal communication problems 509
Verruca vulgaris 377
Vertebrobasilar artery 587
Vertebral fracture 447
Vertigo 232, 539, 563
Vestibular disorders 549
Vestibular neuronitis 549
Vinca alkaloid 629
    bind 630

Vincent's angina 101
Vioform 375
Viral encephalitis 582
    treatment of 582
Viral hepatitis 139, 141
Viral infections 228, 328, 581
Viral load 477, 483
Viral pharyngitis 556
Viral sinusitis 554
Virus 48, 616
Viscera, abdominal 447
Vision
    loss of 590
    peripheral 523
Visual acuity testing 524
Visual assessment, complete 523
Visual changes 563
Visual defects 587
Visual disturbances 587
Visual evoked potentials 570
Visual field
    defect 526, 566
    perimetry 526, 533
Visual impairment 523, 527, 528
    connective disorders 528
    endocrine disorders 527
    etiology 527
    neurological disorders 527
    nurse's role of 529
    pathophysiology 528
    vascular disorders 527
Visual system 523, 524
    diagnostic studies of 526
    nursing assessment of 523
Vital nutrients, tissues of 405
Vitamin 228, 413
    B 413
        deficiency 369
    B6 602
    C 228, 413
    D 413, 417, 445
        deficiency 445
        supplements 448
    E 228
    K 227
        deficiency 231
        supplementation 602

Vitiligo 384
Vitreous traction 536
Vomiting 20, 23, 142, 146, 181, 232, 268, 517
von Willebrand disease 230
Vulvar cancer 298
Vulvar intraepithelial neoplasia 298
Vulvovaginal problems 276

W

Wasting syndrome 328, 478
Watchful vigilance 643
Water intoxication 27
Weight-bearing bones 445
Wernicke's aphasia 564
Wertheim procedure 299
West-Nile virus 489
White blood cell action 450
Wilm's tumor 261, 626
Wolff-Parkinson-White syndrome 187
Wound
    care 20, 393, 395, 422, 423, 438, 439
    drainage 268
    healing of 22
    stressors 23
Wound infection 518
    common organisms of 24
    common sources of 22
    signs of 24
    symptoms of 24

X

Xylocaine 507

Y

Y cell function, decreased 459
Yeast infections 373
Y-glutamyl transferase 143

Z

Zafirlukast 464
Zalcitabine 477
Zidovudine 477
Zonisamide 593
Zygote intrafallopian transfer 301